PHYSICIAN ASSISTANT

A Guide to Clinical Practice

SIXTH
EDITION

Ruth Ballweg, MPA, PA-C Emeritus, DFAAPA

Professor Emeritus
Department of Family Medicine
University of Washington School of Medicine
Seattle, Washington
Director of International Affairs
National Commission on Certification of Physician Assistants
Johns Creek, Georgia

Darwin Brown, MPH, PA-C, DFAAPA

Physician Assistant Educator
Omaha, Nebraska

Daniel T. Vetrosky, PhD, PA-C, DFAAPA

Associate Professor (Ret.) and Part Time Instructor
University of South Alabama
Department of Physician Assistant Studies
Pat Capps Covey College of Allied Health Professions
Mobile, Alabama

Tamara S. Ritsema, MPH, MMSc, PA-C/R

Assistant Professor
Department of Physician Assistant Studies
George Washington University School of Medicine and Health Sciences
Washington, DC
Adjunct Senior Lecturer
Physician Assistant Programme
St. George's, University of London
London, United Kingdom

ELSEVIER

ELSEVIER

1600 John F. Kennedy Blvd.
Ste 1800
Philadelphia, PA 19103-2899

PHYSICIAN ASSISTANT: GUIDE TO CLINICAL PRACTICE,
SIXTH EDITION

ISBN: 978-0-323-40112-8

Notices

Knowledge and best practice in this field are constantly changing. As new research and experience broaden our understanding, changes in research methods, professional practices, or medical treatment may become necessary.

Practitioners and researchers must always rely on their own experience and knowledge in evaluating and using any information, methods, compounds, or experiments described herein. In using such information or methods they should be mindful of their own safety and the safety of others, including parties for whom they have a professional responsibility.

With respect to any drug or pharmaceutical products identified, readers are advised to check the most current information provided (i) on procedures featured or (ii) by the manufacturer of each product to be administered, to verify the recommended dose or formula, the method and duration of administration, and contraindications. It is the responsibility of practitioners, relying on their own experience and knowledge of their patients, to make diagnoses, to determine dosages and the best treatment for each individual patient, and to take all appropriate safety precautions.

To the fullest extent of the law, neither the Publisher nor the authors, contributors, or editors, assume any liability for any injury and/or damage to persons or property as a matter of products liability, negligence or otherwise, or from any use or operation of any methods, products, instructions, or ideas contained in the material herein.

Library of Congress Cataloging-in-Publication Data

Names: Ballweg, Ruth, editor. | Brown, Darwin, editor. | Vetrosky, Daniel T.,
    editor. | Ritsema, Tamara S., editor.
Title: Physician assistant : guide to clinical practice / [edited by] Ruth
    Ballweg, Darwin Brown, Daniel T. Vetrosky, Tamara S. Ritsema.
Other titles: Physician assistant (Ballweg)
Description: Edition: sixth. | Philadelphia, PA : Elsevier, [2017] | Includes
    bibliographical references and index.
Identifiers: LCCN 2016053047 | ISBN 9780323401128 (pbk. : alk. paper)
Subjects: | MESH: Physician Assistants | Clinical Competence | Professional
    Role | Delivery of Health Care--methods | United States
Classification: LCC R697.P45 | NLM W 21.5 | DDC 610.7372069--dc23 LC record available at
https://lccn.loc.gov/2016053047

Content Strategist: Sarah Barth
Content Development Specialist: Joan Ryan
Publishing Services Manager: Patricia Tannian
Project Manager: Ted Rodgers
Design Direction: Patrick Ferguson

Printed in China

Last digit is the print number: 9 8 7 6 5 4 3 2 1

Working together
to grow libraries in
developing countries

www.elsevier.com • www.bookaid.org

CONTRIBUTORS

David P. Asprey, PhD, BA, BS, MA

Professor and Program Director
Physician Assistant Program
College of Medicine, University of Iowa
Iowa City, Iowa

Ruth Ballweg, MPA, PA-C Emeritus, DFAAPA

Professor Emeritus
Department Family Medicine
University of Washington School of Medicine
Seattle, Washington
Director of International Affairs
National Commission on Certification of Physician
    Assistants
Johns Creek, Georgia

Kate Sophia Bascombe, BSc, PGDip

Teaching Fellow
Physician Associate Studies
St. George's University of London
Physician Associate
General Practice
Glebe Road Surgery
London, United Kingdom

Wallace Boeve, EdD, PA-C

Professor
Program Director
Physician Assistant Program
Bethel University
St. Paul, Minnesota

Jonathan M. Bowser, MS, PA-C

Associate Dean of Physician Assistant Studies at the
    School of Medicine
Associate Professor of Pediatrics
Program Director of the Child Health Associate
    Physician Assistant Program
University of Colorado School of Medicine
Denver, Colorado

Anthony Brenneman, MPAS, PA-C

Director and Associate Professor
Department of Physician Assistant Studies and
    Services
Carver College of Medicine
University of Iowa
Iowa City, Iowa

Darwin Brown, MPH, PA-C, DFAAPA

Formerly Assistant Professor
University of Nebraska Medical Center
Physician Assistant Program
Omaha, Nebraska

Michelle Buller, MMS, PA-C

Academic Director/Associate Professor
Physician Assistant Studies Program
Union College
Lincoln, Nebraska

Reamer L. Bushardt, PharmD, PA-C, DFAAPA

Senior Associate Dean for Health Sciences
Professor, Department of Physician Assistant Studies
George Washington University School of Medicine
    and Health Sciences
Washington, DC

Robin N. Hunter Buskey, DHSc, MPAS, PA-C

Senior Physician Assistant
U.S. Department of Justice
Federal Bureau of Prisons Medical Center
Butner, North Carolina

Jill Cavalet, MHS, PA-C

Clinical Associate Professor
Physician Assistant Department
Saint Francis University
Loretto, Pennsylvania

Jeff W. Chambers, PA-C

Physician Assistant
St. Mary's Health Care System
Athens Regional Medical Center
Athens, Georgia

Torry Grantham Cobb, MPH, MHS, DHSc, PA-C

Dartmouth Medical School
Hanover, New Hampshire
Dartmouth-Hitchcock Medical Center
Lebanon, New Hampshire

Roy H. Constantine, PA-C, MPH, PhD

Assistant Director of Mid-Level Practitioners
St. Francis Hospital–The Heart Center
Roslyn, New York
Professor of Health Sciences
Trident University International
Cypress, California

Marci Contreras, MPAS, PA-C

Assistant Professor
Physician Assistant Studies
University of Texas Medical Branch at Galveston
   (UTMB)
Galveston, Texas

Dan Crouse, MPAS, PA-C

Assistant Professor
Department of Family and Preventive Medicine
Director of Clinical Evaluation, Division of
   Physician Assistant Studies
University of Utah
Salt Lake City, Utah

Ann Davis, MS, PA-C

Vice President, Constituent Organization Outreach
   and Advocacy
American Academy of Physician Assistants
Alexandria, Virginia

Justine Strand de Oliveira, DrPH, PA-C, DFAAPA

Professor
Vice Chair for Education
Department of Community and Family Medicine
Professor, Duke School of Nursing
Affiliate Faculty, Duke Global Health Institute
Duke University School of Medicine
Durham, North Carolina

Sondra M. DePalma, MHS, PA-C, CLS, DFAAPA, AACC

Assistant Director of Advanced Practice
Penn State Milton S. Hershey Medical Center
Physician Assistant and Clinical Lipid Specialist
Penn State Hershey Heart and Vascular Institute
Hershey, Pennsylvania

Christine Everett, PhD, MPH, PA-C

Assistant Professor
Duke Physician Assistant Program
Department of Community and Family Medicine
Duke University School of Medicine
Durham, North Carolina

Jennifer Feirstein, MSPAS, PA-C

Clinical Coordinator and Assistant Professor
Department of Physician Assistant Studies
A.T. Still University
Mesa, Arizona

Christopher P. Forest, MSHS, PA-C, DFAAPA

Director of Research
Assistant Professor of Clinical Family Medicine
Keck School of Medicine
University of Southern California
Division of Physician Assistant Studies
Primary Care Physician Assistant Program
Alhambra, California

April Gardner, MSBS, PA-C

Assistant Professor
Program Director and Academic Coordinator
Department of Physician Assistant Studies
University of Toledo
Toledo, Ohio

Constance Goldgar, MS, PA-C

Associate Professor
University of Utah Physician Assistant Program
Salt Lake City, Utah

Earl G. Greene III

Managing Attorney
Law Offices of Idleman and Greene
Omaha, Nebraska

Noelle Hammerbacher, MS

Freelance Examination Editor/Technical Writer
Philadelphia, Pennsylvania

Virginia McCoy Hass, DNP, FNP-C, PA-C

Assistant Clinical Professor
Former Director, Nurse Practitioner Program
Former Interim Director, Physician Assistant Program
Betty Irene Moore School of Nursing
Family Nurse Practitioner and Physician Assistant
   Programs
Sacramento, California

Erin Hoffman, MPAS, PA-C

Assistant Professor
Department of Physician Assistant Education
University of Nebraska Medical Center
Omaha, Nebraska

Trenton Honda, MMS, PA-C

Director and Assistant Clinical Professor
Physician Assistant Program
Northeastern University
Boston, Massachusetts

Theresa Horvath, MPH, PA-C

Associate Professor and Program Director
Department of Physician Assistant Studies
Hofstra University
Hempstead, New York

Hannah Huffstutler, PA-C, MHS

Assistant Professor
Department of Physician Assistant Studies
University of South Alabama
Pat Capps Covey College of Allied Health
    Professions
Mobile, Alabama

Emily Joy Jensen, MMSc, PA-C

Surgical and Inpatient Physician Assistant
Piedmont Transplant Institute
Piedmont Atlanta Hospital
Atlanta, Georgia

James C. Johnson III, MPAS, PA-C

Assistant Professor
Department of Physician Assistant Studies
High Point University
Congdon School of Health Sciences
High Point, North Carolina

Gerald Kayingo, PhD, PA-C

Director for the Master of Health Services-Physician
    Assistant Program
Assistant Clinical Professor
Betty Irene School of Nursing at University of
    California, Davis
Sacramento, California

Kathy A. Kemle, MS, PA-C

Assistant Professor
Family Medicine
Mercer University
Macon, Georgia

Bri Kestler, MMS, PA-C

Assistant Professor
Department of Physician Assistant Studies
University of South Alabama
Mobile, Alabama

William C. Kohlhepp, DHSc, PA-C

Professor of Physician Assistant Studies
Dean, School of Health Sciences
Quinnipiac University
Hamden, Connecticut

David H. Kuhns, MPH, PA-C, CCPA, DFAAPA

Consultant on International Physician Assistant
    Education
Advisor to the University of Aberdeen (Scotland)
    Physician Assistant Program
Advisor to the Royal College of Surgeons in Ireland
Advisor to the European Physician Assistant
    Cooperative (EuroPAC)
Adjunct Faculty, Arcadia University Physician
    Assistant Program
Glenside, Pennsylvania

Luppo Kuilman, MPA

Master Physician Assistant Program
School of Health Care Studies
Hanze University of Applied Sciences
Groningen, The Netherlands

Barbara Coombs Lee, JD, FNP

President
Compassion and Choices
Denver, Colorado

Susan LeLacheur, DrPH, PA-C

Associate Professor of Physician Assistant Studies
School of Medicine and Health Sciences
The George Washington University
Washington, DC

Jason Lesandrini, PhD(c)

Executive Director of Medical and Organizational
    Ethics
WellStar Health System
Adjunct Faculty, Department of Physician Assistant
    Studies
Mercer University
Atlanta, Georgia
Adjunct Faculty, Department of Physician Assistant
    Studies
Philadelphia College of Osteopathic Medicine
Suwanee, Georgia

Erin Nicole Lunn McAdams, PA-C, MHS

Assistant Professor
Department of Physician Assistant Studies
University of South Alabama
Pat Capps Covey College of Allied Health
  Professions
Mobile, Alabama

Nancy E. McLaughlin, MHA, DHSc, PA-C

Assistant Professor
Department of Physician Assistant Studies
Philadelphia College of Osteopathic Medicine
Philadelphia, Pennsylvania

Steven Meltzer, BA, BHSc, PA-C

Director, Outreach and Eastern Washington
Education Programs
MEDEX Northwest Physician Assistant Program
University of Washington
Spokane, Washington

Anthony A. Miller, MEd, PA-C

Professor and Director
Division of Physician Assistant Studies
Shenandoah University
Winchester, Virginia

Margaret Moore-Nadler, DNP, RN

University of South Alabama
College of Nursing
Community Mental Health
Mobile, Alabama

Dawn Morton-Rias, EdD, PA-C

President and CEO
National Commission on Certification of Physician
  Assistants
Johns Creek, Georgia

Karen Mulitalo, MPAS, PA-C

Associate Professor
Program Director
Division of Physician Assistant Studies
Department of Family and Preventive Medicine
University of Utah School of Medicine
Salt Lake City, Utah

Debra S. Munsell, DHSC, PA-C, DFAAPA

Associate Professor
Program Director, Master of Physician Assistant
  Studies Program
Louisiana State University Health Sciences Center
New Orleans, Louisiana

Lillian Navarro-Reynolds, BS, MS

Assistant Professor
Physician Assistant Program
Oregon Health Sciences University
Portland, Oregon

Kevin Michael O'Hara, MMSc, MS, PA-C

Assistant Professor
Physician Associate Program
Yale School of Medicine
New Haven, Connecticut

Courtney J. Perry, PharmD

Assistant Professor
Department of Physician Assistant Studies
Wake Forest School of Medicine
Winston-Salem, North Carolina

Ron W. Perry, MS, MPAS, MEd, DFAAPA, PA-C

Program Director, Interservice Physician Assistant
  Program (IPAP)
Graduate School, Health Readiness Center of
  Excellence
Army Medical Center & School, Joint Base San
  Antonio
San Antonio, Texas

Maura Polansky, MS, MHPE, PA-C

Program Director, Curriculum Development,
  Department of Clinical Education
Program Director, Office of Physician Assistant
  Education
The University of Texas MD Anderson Cancer
  Center
Houston, Texas

Michael L. Powe, BS

Vice President, Reimbursement and Professional
  Advocacy
American Academy of Physician Assistants
Alexandria, Virginia

Brenda Quincy, PhD, MPH, PA-C

Associate Professor
College of Pharmacy and Health Sciences
Butler University
Indianapolis, Indiana

Michael Rackover, MS, PA-C

Theodore C. Search Emeritus Professor
Physician Assistant Program
Philadelphia University
Philadelphia, Pennsylvania

Stephanie M. Radix, JD

Senior Director, Constituent Organization Outreach
    and Advocacy
American Academy of Physician Assistants
Alexandria, Virginia

Scott D. Richards, PhD, PA-C, DFAAPA

Founding Chair and Director
Department of Physician Assistant Studies
School of Health Sciences
Emory & Henry College
Marion, Virginia

Robin Risling-de Jong, PA-C, MHS

Assistant Professor
Department of Physician Assistant Studies
University of South Alabama
Mobile, Alabama

Tamara S. Ritsema, MPH, MMSc, PA-C

Assistant Professor
George Washington University School of Medicine
    and Health Sciences
Washington, DC

Elizabeth Rothschild, MMSc, PA-C

Assistant Professor
Physician Assistant Division
Department of Family and Preventive Medicine
Emory University School of Medicine
Atlanta, Georgia

Barbara Saltzman, PhD, MPH

Assistant Professor
Public Health and Preventive Medicine
University of Toledo College of Medicine and Life
    Sciences
Toledo, Ohio

Patty J. Scholting, MPAS, MPH, PA-C

Assistant Professor
Physician Assistant Program
University of Nebraska Medical Center
Omaha, Nebraska

Craig S. Scott, PhD

Professor of Biomedical Informatics and Medical
    Education
University of Washington School of Medicine
Seattle, Washington

Freddi Segal-Gidan, PhD, PA-C

Assistant Clinical Professor of Neurology and
    Gerontology
University of Southern California (USC) Keck
    School of Medicine
Los Angeles, California
Director of Rancho/USC California Alzheimer's
    Disease Center (CADC)
Rancho Los Amigos National Rehabilitation Center
Downey, California

Edward M. Sullivan, MS, PA-C

Physician Assistant
J. Kirkland Grant Obstetrics and Gynecology Practice
Sunnyvale, Texas

Stephane VanderMeulen, MPAS, PA-C

Associate Professor
Founding Program Director
Physician Assistant Program
Creighton University School of Medicine
Omaha, Nebraska

Daniel T. Vetrosky, PhD, PA-C, DFAAPA

Associate Professor (Ret.) and Part Time Instructor
University of South Alabama
Department of Physician Assistant Studies
Pat Capps Covey College of Allied Health
    Professions
Mobile, Alabama

Lisa K. Walker, MPAS, PA-C

Director, Physician Assistant Studies Program
Massachusetts General Hospital Institute of Health
    Professions
Boston, Massachusetts

Natalie Walkup, MPAS, PA-C

Assistant Professor
Associate Program Director
Department of Physician Assistant Studies
University of Toledo
Toledo, Ohio

Jennifer B. Wall, MSPAS, PA-C

Assistant Professor
Department of Physician Assistant Studies
The George Washington University
Washington, D.C.

Chantelle Wolpert, PhD, MBA, PA-C, GC

Assistant Professor and Research Coordinator
Department of Physician Assistant Studies
School of Health Sciences
Emory & Henry College
Marion, Virginia

Johnna K. Yealy, MSPAS, PA-C
Physician Assistant Program Director
University of Tampa
Tampa, Florida

Gwen Yeo, PhD
Director Emerita, Senior Ethnogeriatric Specialist
Stanford Geriatric Education Center
Stanford University School of Medicine
Stanford, California

Joseph Zaweski, MPAS, PA-C
Assistant Dean and Program Director
Physician Assistant Program
School of Nursing and Health Professions
Valparaiso University
Valparaiso, Indiana

Olivia Ziegler, MS, PA
Assistant Chief, Academic Affairs
Physician Assistant Education Association
Washington, DC

FOREWORD

Thirty-one years ago, doctors were in short supply. Nurses were even scarcer. The old model of the doctor, a receptionist, and a laboratory technician was inadequate to meet the needs of our increasingly complex society. Learning time had disappeared from the schedule of the busy doctor. The only solution that the overworked doctor could envisage was more doctors. Only a doctor could do doctors' work. The lengthy educational pathway (college, medical school, internship, residency, and fellowship) must mean that only persons with a doctor's education could carry out a doctor's functions.

I examined in some detail the actual practice of medicine. After sampling the rich diet of medicine, most doctors settled for a small area. If the office was set up to see patients every 10 to 15 minutes and to charge a certain fee, the practice conformed. If the outcome was poor, or if the doctors recognized that the problem was too complex for this pattern of practice, the patient was referred.

Doctors seeing patients at half-hour or 1-hour intervals also developed practice patterns and set fee schedules to conform. The specialists tended to treat diseases and leave the care of patients to others. Again, they cycled in a narrow path.

The average doctors developed efficient patterns of practice. They operated 95% of the time in a habit mode and rarely applied a thinking cap. Because they did everything that involved contact with the patients, time for family, recreation, reading, and furthering their own education disappeared.

Why this intense personalization of medical practice? All doctors starting practices ran scared. They wanted to make their services essential to the well-being of their patients. They wanted the patient to depend on them alone. After a few years in this mode, they brainwashed themselves and actually believed that only they could obtain information from the patient and perform services that involved physical contact with the patient.

During this time I was building a house with my own hands. I could use a wide variety of materials and techniques in my building. I reflected on how inadequate my house would be if I were restricted to only four materials. The doctor restricted to a slim support system could never build a practice adequate to meet the needs of modern medicine. He or she needed more components in the system. The physician assistant (PA) was born!

Nurses, laboratory technicians, and other health professionals were educated in their own schools, which were mostly hospital related. The new practitioner (the PA) was to be selected, educated, and employed by the doctor. The PA—not being geographically bound to the management system of the hospital, the clinic, or the doctor's office—could oscillate between the office, the hospital, the operating room, and the home.

A 2-year curriculum was organized at Duke Medical School with the able assistance of Dr. Harvey Estes, who eventually took the program under the wing of his department of Family and Community Medicine. The object of the 2-year course was to expose the student to the biology of human beings and to learn how doctors rendered services. On graduation, PAs had learned to perform many tasks previously done by licensed doctors only and could serve a useful role in many types of practices. They performed those tasks that they could do as well as their doctor mentors. If the mentor was wise, the PA mastered new areas each year and increased his or her usefulness to the practice.

Setting no ceilings and allowing the PA to grow have made this profession useful and satisfying. Restricting PAs to medical supervision has given them great freedom. Ideally, they do any part of their mentors' practice that they can do as well as their mentors.

The PA profession has certainly established itself and is recognized as a part of the medical system. PAs will be assuming a larger role in the care of hospital patients as physician residency programs decrease in size. As hospital house staff, PAs can improve the quality of care for patients by providing continuity of care.

Because of the close association with the doctor and patient and the PAs' varied duties, PAs have an intimate knowledge of the way of the medical world. They know patients, they are aware of the triumphs and failures of medicine, and they know how doctors think and what they do with information collected about patients. For these reasons, they are in demand by all businesses that touch the medical profession. One of the first five Duke students recently earned a doctoral degree in medical ethics and is working in education. The world is open, and PAs are grasping their share.

We all owe a debt of gratitude to the first five students who were willing to risk 2 years of their lives to enter a new profession when there was little support from doctors, nurses, or government. From the beginning, patients responded favorably, and each PA gained confidence and satisfaction from these interactions. Patients made and saved the profession. We hope that every new PA will acknowledge this debt and continue the excellent work of the original five.

Eugene A. Stead Jr., MD
The late Dr. Stead was the Florence McAlister Professor Emeritus of Medicine, Duke University Medical Center, Durham, North Carolina. This Foreword was published in the previous edition, and is being reprinted.

PREFACE

Welcome to the sixth edition of *Physician Assistant: A Guide to Clinical Practice!*

The sixth edition recognizes that our students increasingly do not enter PA school with years of experience as health professionals. Ten new chapters have been written to provide guidance to students regarding clinical environments, key pieces of medical knowledge, and preceptor expectations before they start on each core rotation and four common elective rotations. We have also added a new section called "Your Physician Assistant Career" which provides resources for students as they near the end of their training. Chapters include "Leadership Skills for Physician Assistants," "Be a Physician Assistant Educator," "Professional Service" and an overview article on the future of the profession.

The history and utilization of this publication mirror the expansion of the physician assistant (PA) profession. The first edition, published in 1994, was the first PA textbook to be developed by a major publisher and was at first considered to be a potential risk for the company. Ultimately, it came to be seen as a major milestone for our profession. Our first editor, Lisa Biello, attended the national PA conference in New Orleans and immediately saw the potential! She made a strong case to the W.B. Saunders Co. for the development of the book. Quickly, other publishers followed her lead. Now there are multiple PA-specific textbooks and other published resources for use in PA programs by practicing physician assistants.

The first edition was written at a time of rapid growth in the number of PA programs and in the number of enrolled PA students. Intended primarily for PA students, the textbook was also used by administrators, public policy leaders, and employers to better understand the PA role and to create new roles and job opportunities for PAs.

The second edition was expanded and updated to reflect the growth of the PA profession.

The third edition included eight new chapters and a new format. This format included Case Studies, which illustrated the narrative in "real-life" terms; Clinical Applications, which provided questions to stimulate thought, discussion, and further investigation; and a Resources section, which provided an annotated list of books, articles, organizations, and websites for follow-up research. With the third edition, the book became an Elsevier publication with a W.B. Saunders imprint.

The fourth edition had a totally new look and was also the first edition with an electronic platform. Most important, the textbook's content was reorganized to make it more responsive to the new Physician Assistant Competencies, which were approved by all four major PA organizations in 2006. New sections on professionalism, practice-based learning and improvement, and systems-based practice address specific topics delineated in the competencies. Sections covering materials that had become available in other books (e.g., physical examination and detailed history-taking skills) were omitted. Significant new material was added on the international PA movement, professionalism, patient safety, health disparities, PA roles in internal medicine and hospitalist settings, and issues in caring for patients with disabilities.

The new content for the fifth edition included chapters on the electronic health record, population-based practice, the new National Commission on Certification of Physician Assistants specialty recognition process, health care delivery systems, and mass casualty/disaster management.

Many PA programs find the textbook useful for their professional roles course and as a supplement to other core courses. PA students have found the chapters on specific specialties helpful in preparing for clinical rotations. PA graduates thinking about changing jobs and encountering new challenges in credentialing will find a number of relevant examples. All practicing PAs will find the new material useful as they continue their lifelong learning in a rapidly changing health care system. Health care administrators and employers can benefit from an overview of the profession, as well as information specific to PA roles and job descriptions. Policy analysts and health care researchers will find a wealth of information at the micro and macro levels. Developers of the PA concept internationally will find what they need to adapt the PA profession in new settings. Finally, potential PAs can be informed and inspired by the accomplishments of the profession.

Although Dr. Eugene Stead died in 2005, we have decided to continue to use the foreword that he wrote for this book. Encouraged by Dr. Stead and by countless colleagues, students, and patients, we hope that this textbook will continue to serve as a significant resource and inspiration for the PA profession.

Ruth Ballweg, MPA, PA-C Emeritus, DFAAPA
Darwin Brown, MPH, PA-C, DFAAPA
Daniel Vetrosky, PhD, PA-C, DFAAPA
Tamara Ritsema, MPH, MMSc, PA-C

ACKNOWLEDGMENTS

As we reach the sixth edition, we want to thank the many individuals—across time—who have made this book possible. Much of the success of this book has had its roots in physician assistant (PA) educational networks. Not only did we want to create a book that would be a critical resource for PA students and educators, but also we wanted to create new publishing opportunities for many of our colleagues to become contributors. A major strength of the book has always been the inclusion of a wide range of faculty members from PA programs from all regions in the United States. We especially want to acknowledge the contribution and leadership of Sherry Stolberg, who served as our coeditor for the first, second, and third editions, and Ed Sullivan, who was with us through the fifth edition. When Sherry and Ed stepped down, Darwin Brown and Dan Vetrosky were recruited as new coeditors. For this sixth edition, Tamara Ritsema has joined our group. They have brought new energy, new ideas, and new contacts to the subsequent editions of the book, for which we are grateful.

This textbook would not be possible without the support of our colleagues, students, friends, and loved ones who have helped us to continue to move this project ahead. The patience and good humor of our spouses, Jeanne Brown, Penelope Vetrosky, and the late Arnold Rosner, have been critical to this project. Our children, Pirkko Terao, Dayan Ballweg, and Alex, Tim, and Jackson Brown, provided us with their valuable opinions and perspectives.

We gratefully acknowledge our editors over time, including Lisa Biello, Peg Waltner, Shirley Kuhn, Rolla Couchman, John Ingram, Kate Dimock, and Sarah Barth, and content development specialists, Janice Gaillard and Joan Ryan. The input from these individuals has resulted in the substantial improvements in this publication over time. Although new authors have joined us for each edition, contributors to prior editions of this book deserve our appreciation for their participation.

Physician Assistant: A Guide to Clinical Practice has benefited from the feedback of PA educators and students. We hope you will continue to provide us with your opinions and suggestions.

CONTENTS

SECTION I

OVERVIEW

CHAPTER 1

MAXIMIZING YOUR PHYSICIAN ASSISTANT EDUCATION

Ruth Ballweg • Daniel T. Vetrosky

OVERVIEW AND INTRODUCTION

Congratulations on choosing to be a physician assistant (PA) as we celebrate 50 years of the PA profession! As educators who have also enjoyed clinical practice as part of our professional roles, we welcome you to our career and challenge you to explore it fully during your PA education. As many senior PAs say, with great enthusiasm: "I had no idea where the PA career would take me or the many options and opportunities that would come along. Who knew?"

Our goal is for this sixth edition of *Physician Assistant: A Guide to Clinical Practice* is to be both a textbook and your lifelong "go-to" resource on PAs and the profession that remains on your bookshelf throughout your career. In the early days of the PA profession, there were no textbooks or resources specifically for PAs. We relied on resources for physicians and medical students, and faculty members photocopied handouts they had developed individually or that they had borrowed from their colleagues in other programs. Fortunately, the Saunders Publishing Company saw the potential for a PA textbook, and in 1994, the first edition of this book was released. The editors were pleased to receive numerous communications from PA students expressing enthusiasm, pride, and even relief that there was "finally a book for PAs" sitting on the shelves of their college bookstores and libraries.

The early editions of the book were only available in hard copy. We're delighted that it's now available in both a hard copy and a downloadable version. This eliminates the need for you to carry around the heavy printed version of the book and allows you to have just what you need available on your computer screen for use in the classroom, study sessions, and clinical rotations. You'll always have it with you! Be sure to check out the book's additional features in the online version.

This edition includes additional primers on how to best use many of the unique and latest teaching and learning approaches that are features of a constantly evolving PA educational methodology.

In addition to the skilled faculty members in your program, whom you know well, you'll also benefit from experiences from other faculty members and health care leaders beyond your own program. We've purposely recruited a wide range of experts from the United States and several other countries. You can expect to see even more international involvement in future editions as PA utilization, education, and regulation expand beyond the U.S. nexus of our profession.

A lot of the stress of PA education is not knowing what PAs really do. This book will help with that! Our goal as editors is to show you a bigger world of what PAs have been, are currently, and can become. Some of the chapters are about cutting-edge topics you didn't know you'd need. You'll probably have a different view about the relevance of these issues by the time you graduate and start your first job.

You'll find that you need the book's various sections at different times in your education and PA career. Section I features an overview of our career. You may find these topics assigned early in your PA program as your faculty introduce you to PA history. Although we've come a long way in our 50 years, there is still work to do in the further development and regulation of PAs in new roles. Section I will provide you with background about how we got to where we are. We hope it will inspire you to consider PA and community leadership roles throughout your career. You'll learn the principles behind PA education and why it's different from medical school. You'll find out how to be safe in clinical settings. You'll find out the complexities of how PAs are allowed to work because of PA program accreditation, national certification by the National Commission on Certification of Physician Assistants (NCCPA), licensure at the state level, and privileges at the institutional level. You'll develop greater understanding of physician–PA supervisory relationships, and you'll have appreciation for the long-term challenges that we faced and continue to face for appropriate payment for our services. Finally, you'll learn about the importance of being part of an interprofessional team. These first chapters may be especially helpful to share with your family and friends who may not yet understand as much as they would like to about the PA profession.

Section II focuses on medical knowledge. This section is not intended to substitute for the many outstanding medical textbooks available to all types of clinical students. Some chapters in Section II are examples of how this book serves as a resource for topics and skills you didn't know you'd need. As PA educators, we're proud of our responsibility to design the PAs of the future. New health care systems will need PAs who understand evidence-based medicine and research methodology. Keeping people healthy becomes more important as more and more people have access to health care. Common clinical procedures are included to give some examples of the broad procedural skill sets of PAs. The description of PA prescriptive practice has a similar role.

Genetics will play a greater role in medicine and our genetics chapter provides updated information that you can integrate into your practice. Other marketable skill areas this text will enhance include chapters on chronic care, alternative and complimentary medicine, end-of-life issues and the changing health care environment.

PAs are known for their outstanding communication and people skills. Section III is designed to reinforce the communication experiences that PA students receive throughout their education and practice. This section provides important background about the appropriate use and value of electronic medical records. Tools such as patient education, cultural sensitivity, and cultural competence are also available in this section.

Section IV focuses on clinical rotations. These chapters are not intended as a substitute for other textbooks on these medical and surgical specialties nor are they there to supplant your program's rotation manuals. For the sixth edition, we've asked our authors to rewrite these chapters to focus specifically on what a students need to know for each of these rotations. We've included the rotations that are required by the Accreditation Review Commission on Education for the Physician Assistant (ARC-PA) as well as examples of the most common electives. We believe that this section will be especially popular.

Professionalism is the subject of Section V. Professionalism is a hot topic in all clinical education programs and is often a topic that students may not have previously considered.

We've focused on professionalism as it applies to PAs specifically. Similarly, this section considers ethics and malpractice relative to PA practice. The chapter on stress and burnout describes the issues of adopting an extremely responsible clinical role in a relatively short period of time. This section also recommends strategies for recognizing and managing these concerns in yourself as well as friends and colleagues. Finally, this section reviews the issue and range of postgraduate programs.

Section VII on systems-based practice has several functions. The initial chapter on health care delivery systems is designed to provide students with information about changes in the health care delivery system, primarily in response to the regulations concerning the provision and access to health care as defined by the Affordable Care Act. This is a rapidly evolving topic with a range of regional differences. Recognizing the underlying principles of these changes will help students and practicing PAs to make employment decisions about the type of setting in which they'd be the best fit.

Other chapters in this section have been written to allow readers to explore settings and populations where PAs are employed and practice. In addition to providing background for job choices, this section is also written to encourage PAs to understand and appreciate the wide range of employment opportunities and challenges that are available to PAs.

Finally, Section VIII will help new graduates as they move into clinical practice. New PAs describe several years of transition as they move from being students into the world of clinical practice. It's reasonable to expect that this transition will take 2 to 3 years. Even in the early stages of a PA career, there are opportunities to move into leadership and professional service. This is a time to think about the potential of involvement in PA education, as a preceptor, or as a part- or full-time faculty member. The last chapter explores our future. As authors and teachers, we are excited that you will be a part of it.

We would like to offer some general pieces of advice that we hope will further maximize your experience as a PA student and as a PA:

a. In class and in clinic: go early, stay late.
b. Get to know your faculty members—be transparent.
c. Get to know each of your classmates—schedule a time with each of them one on one at least once in the first quarter or semester of school.
d. Stay caught up—pay attention to objectives in your courses. They're designed to guide you in what you need to know and in how to spend your precious time.
e. Meet as many PAs as you can. They will be role models and mentors.
f. Most important, learn from you patients. Again, welcome to this wonderful career!

KEY POINTS

- The principle and culture of medical and clinical roles is about lifelong learning. We've designed this book to promote this concept.
- We encourage you to develop a support system of peers, senior mentors, supervising doctors, and others to serve as a foundation for the long-term decisions that you make about your career.
- Effective leaders are needed to promote access and health care quality.
- The PA profession has moved ahead because PAs have been willing to say "yes!" to leadership opportunities. Please consider leadership as part of your PA career.

CHAPTER 2

HISTORY OF THE PROFESSION AND CURRENT TRENDS

Ruth Ballweg

What was to become the physician assistant (PA) profession has many origins. Although it is often thought of as an "American" concept—recruiting former military corpsmen to respond to the access needs in our health care system—the PA has historical antecedents in other countries. Feldshers in Russia and barefoot doctors in China served as models for the creation of the PA profession.

FELDSHERS IN RUSSIA

The *feldsher* concept originated in the European military in the 17th and 18th centuries and was introduced into the Russian military system by Peter the Great. Armies of other countries were ultimately able to secure adequate physician personnel; however, because of a physician shortage, the large numbers of Russian troops relied on feldshers for major portions of their medical care. Feldshers retiring from the military settled in small rural communities, where they continued their contribution to health care access. Feldshers assigned to Russian communities provided much of the health care in remote areas of Alaska during the 1800s.[1] In the late 19th century, formal schools were created for feldsher training, and by 1913, approximately 30,000 feldshers had been trained to provide medical care.[2]

As the major U.S. researchers reviewing the feldsher concept, Victor Sidel[2] and P.B. Storey[3] described a system in the Soviet Union in which the annual number of new feldshers equaled the annual number of physician graduates. Of those included in the feldsher category, 90% were women, including feldsher midwives.[3] Feldsher training programs, which were located in the same institutions as nursing schools, required 2 years to complete. Outstanding feldsher students were encouraged to take medical school entrance examinations. Roemer[4] found in 1976 that 25% of Soviet physicians were former feldshers.

The use of Soviet feldshers varied from rural to urban settings. Often used as physician substitutes in rural settings, experienced feldshers had full authority to diagnose, prescribe, and institute emergency treatment. A concern that "independent" feldshers might provide "second-class" health care appears to have led to greater supervision of feldshers in rural settings. Storey[3] describes the function of urban feldshers—whose roles were "complementary" rather than "substitutional"—as limited to primary care in ambulances and triage settings and not involving polyclinic or hospital tasks. Perry and Breitner[5] compare the urban feldsher role with that of U.S. physician assistants (PAs): "Working alongside the physician in his daily activities to improve the physician's efficiency and effectiveness (and to relieve him of routine, time-consuming tasks) is not the Russian feldsher's role."

CHINA'S BAREFOOT DOCTORS

In China, the *barefoot doctor* originated in the 1965 Cultural Revolution as a physician substitute. In what became known as the "June 26th Directive," Chairman Mao called for a reorganization of the health care system. In response to Mao's directive, China trained 1.3 million barefoot doctors over the subsequent 10 years.[6]

The barefoot doctors were chosen from rural production brigades and received their initial 2- to 3-month training course in regional hospitals and health centers. Sidel[2] comments that "the barefoot doctor is considered by his community, and apparently thinks of himself, as a peasant who performs some medical duties rather than as a health care worker who performs some agricultural duties." Although they were designed to function independently, barefoot doctors were closely linked to local hospitals for training and medical supervision. Upward mobility was encouraged in that barefoot doctors were given priority for admission to medical school. In 1978, Dimond[7] found that one third of Chinese medical students were former barefoot doctors.

The use of feldshers and barefoot doctors was significantly greater than that of PAs in the United States. Writing in 1982, Perry and Breitner[5] noted:

Although physician assistants have received a great deal of publicity and attention in the United States, they currently perform a very minor role in the provision of health services. In contrast, the Russian feldsher and the Chinese barefoot doctor perform a major role in the provision of basic medical services, particularly in rural areas.

The "discovery" in the United States that appropriately trained nonphysicians are perfectly capable of diagnosing and treating common medical problems had been previously recognized in both Russia and China. We can no longer say that PAs "perform a very minor role in the provision of health services." In contrast, the numbers of both feldshers and barefoot doctors have declined in their respective countries owing to a lack of governmental support and an increase in the numbers of physicians.

DEVELOPMENTS IN THE UNITED STATES

Beginning in the 1930s, former military corpsmen received on-the-job training from the Federal Prison System to extend the services of prison physicians. In a 4-month program during World War II, the U.S. Coast Guard trained 800 purser mates to provide health care on merchant ships. The program was later discontinued, and by 1965, fewer than 100 purser mates continued to provide medical services. Both of these programs served as predecessors to those in the federal PA training programs at the Medical Center for Federal Prisoners, Springfield, Missouri, and Staten Island University Hospital, New York.

In 1961, Charles Hudson, MD, proposed the PA concept at a medical education conference of the American Medical Association (AMA). He recommended that " assistants to doctors" should work as dependent practitioners and should perform such technical tasks as lumbar puncture, suturing, and intubation.

At the same time, a number of physicians in private practice had begun to use informally trained individuals to extend their services. A well-known family physician, Dr. Amos Johnson, publicized the role that he had created for his assistant, Mr. Buddy Treadwell. The website for the Society for the Preservation of Physician Assistant History provides detailed information on Dr. Johnson and tells more about how Mr. Treadwell served as a role model for the design of the PA career.

By 1965, Henry Silver, MD, and Loretta Ford, RN, had created a practitioner-training program for baccalaureate nurses working with impoverished pediatric populations. Although the Colorado program became the foundation for both the nurse practitioner (NP) movement and the Child Health Associate PA Program, it was not transferable to other institutions. According to Gifford, this program depended ". . . on a pattern of close cooperation between doctors and nurses not then often found at other schools."[8] In 1965, therefore, practical definition of the PA concept awaited establishment of a training program that could be applied to other institutions.

DEVELOPMENTS AT DUKE UNIVERSITY

In the late 1950s and early 1960s, Eugene Stead, MD, developed a program to extend the capabilities of nurses at Duke University Hospital.[9] This program, which *could* have initiated the NP movement, was opposed by the National League of Nursing. The League expressed the concern that such a program would move these new providers from the ranks of nursing and into the "medical model." Simultaneously, Duke University had experience with training several firemen, ex-corpsmen, and other non–college graduates to solve personnel shortages in the clinical services at Duke University Hospital.[9]

The Duke program and other new PA programs arose at a time of national awareness of a health care crisis. Carter and Gifford[10] described the conditions that fostered the PA concept as follows:

1. An increased social consciousness among many Americans that called for the elimination of all types of deprivation in society, especially among the poor, members of minority groups, and women
2. An increasingly positive value attached to health and health care, which produced greater demand for health services, criticism of the health care delivery system, and constant complaints about rising health care costs
3. Heightened concern about the supply of physicians, their geographic and specialty maldistribution, and the workloads they carried
4. Awareness of a variety of physician extender models, including the community nurse midwife in America, the "assistant medical officer" in Africa, and the feldsher in the Soviet Union
5. The availability of nurses and ex-corpsmen as potential sources of manpower
6. Local circumstances in numerous hospitals and office-based practice settings that required additional clinical-support professionals

The first four students—all ex-Navy corpsmen—entered the fledgling Duke program in October 1965. The 2-year training program's philosophy was to provide students with an education and orientation similar to those given the physicians with whom they would work. Although original plans called for the training of two categories of PAs—one for general practice and one for specialized inpatient care—the ultimate decision was made to focus on skills required in assisting family practitioners or internists. The program also emphasized the development of lifelong learning skills to facilitate the ongoing professional growth of these new providers.

CONCEPTS OF EDUCATION AND PRACTICE

The introduction of the PA presented philosophical challenges to established concepts of medical education. E. Harvey Estes, MD,[11] of Duke, described the hierarchical approach of medical education as being "based on the assumption that it was necessary to first learn 'basic sciences,' then normal structure and function, and finally pathophysiology . . . ." The PA clearly defied these previous conventions. Some of the early PAs had no formal collegiate education. They had worked as corpsmen and had learned skills, often under battlefield conditions. Clearly, their skills had been developed, often to a remarkable degree, before the acquisition of any basic science knowledge or any knowledge of pathologic physiology.

The developing PA profession was also the first to officially share the knowledge base that was formerly the "exclusive property" of physicians. Before the development of the PA profession, the physician was the sole possessor of information, and neither patient nor other groups could penetrate this wall. The patient generally trusted the medical profession to use the knowledge to his or her benefit, and other groups were forced to use another physician to interpret medical data or medical reasoning. The PA profession was the first to share this knowledge base, but others were to follow—such as the NP.[11]

Fifty years later, it is common to see medical textbooks written for PAs, NPs, and other nonphysician providers. Such publications were relatively new approaches for gaining access to medical knowledge at a time when access to medical textbooks and reference materials was restricted to physicians only. The legal relationship of the PA to the physician was also unique in the health care system. Tied to the license of a specific precepting physician, the PA concept received the strong support of establishment medicine and ultimately achieved significant "independence" through that "dependence." In contrast, NPs, who emphasized their capability for "independent practice," incurred the wrath of some physician groups, who believed that NPs needed supervisory relationships with physicians to validate their role and accountability.

Finally, the "primary care" or "generalist" nature of PA training, which stressed the acquisition of strong skills in data collection, critical thinking, problem solving, and lifelong learning, made PAs extraordinarily adaptable to almost any patient care setting. The supervised status of PA practice provided PAs with ongoing oversight and almost unlimited opportunities to expand skills as needed in specific practice settings. In fact, the adaptability of PAs has had both positive and negative impacts on the PA profession. Although PAs were initially trained to provide health care to medically underserved populations, the potential for the use of PAs in specialty medicine became "the good news and the bad news." Sadler and colleagues[12] recognized this concern early on, when they wrote (in 1972):

> The physician's assistant is in considerable danger of being swallowed whole by the whale that is our present entrepreneurial, subspecialty medical practice system. The likely co-option of the newly minted physician's assistant by subspecialty medicine is one of the most serious issues confronting the PA.

A shortage of PAs in the early 1990s appeared to aggravate this situation and confirmed predictions by Sadler and colleagues[12]:

> Until great numbers of physician's assistants are produced, the first to emerge will be in such demand that relatively few are likely to end up in primary care or rural settings where the need is the greatest. The same is true for inner city or poverty areas.

Although most PAs initially chose primary care, increases in specialty positions raised concern about the future direction of the PA profession. The Federal Bureau of Health Professions was so concerned about this trend that at one point, federal training grants for PA programs required that all students complete clinical training assignments in federally designated medically underserved areas.

MILITARY CORPSMEN

The choice to train experienced military corpsmen as the first PAs was a key factor in the success of the concept. As Sadler and colleagues[12] pointed out, "The political appeal of providing a useful civilian health occupation for the returning Vietnam medical corpsman is enormous."

The press and the American public were attracted to the PA concept because it seemed to be one of the few positive "products" of the Vietnam War. Highly skilled, independent duty corpsmen from all branches of the uniformed services were disenfranchised as they attempted to find their place in the U.S. health care system. These corpsmen, whose competence had truly been tested "under fire," provided a willing, motivated, and proven applicant pool of pioneers for the PA profession. Robert Howard, MD,[13] of Duke University, in an AMA publication describing issues of training PAs, noted that not only were there large numbers of corpsmen available but also using former military personnel prevented transfer of workers from other health care careers that were experiencing shortages:

> ... the existing nursing and allied health professions have manpower shortages parallel to physician shortages and are not the ideal sources from which to select individuals to augment the physician manpower supply. In the face of obvious need, there does exist a relatively large untapped manpower pool, the military corpsmen. Some 32,000 corpsmen are discharged annually who have received valuable training and experience while in the service. If an economically sound, stable, rewarding career were available in the health industry, many of these people would continue to pursue such a course. From this manpower source, it is possible to select mature, career-oriented, experienced people for physician's assistant programs.

The decision to expand these corpsmen's skills as PAs also capitalized on the previous investment of the U.S. military in providing extensive medical training to these men.

Richard Smith, MD,[14] founder of the University of Washington's MEDEX program, described this training:

> The U.S. Department of Defense has developed ways of rapidly training medical personnel to meet its specific needs, which are similar to those of the civilian population. ... Some of these people, such as Special Forces and Navy "B" Corpsmen, receive 1400 hours of formal medical training, which may include nine weeks of a supervised "clerkship." Army corpsmen of the 91C series may have received up to 1900 hours of this formal training.

> Most of these men have had 3 to 20 years of experience, including independent duty on the battlefield, aboard ship, or in other isolated stations. Many have some college background; Special Forces "medics" average a year of college. After at least 2, and up to 20, years in uniform, these men have certain skills and knowledge in the provision of primary care. Once discharged, however, the investment of public funds in medical capabilities and potential care is lost, because they work as detail men, insurance agents, burglar alarm salesmen, or truck drivers. The majority of this vast manpower pool is unavailable to the current medical care delivery system because, up to this point, we have not devised a civilian framework in which their skills can be put to use.[14]

OTHER MODELS

Describing the period of 1965 to 1971 as "Stage One—The Initiation of Physician Assistant Programs," Carter and Gifford[10] have identified 16 programs that pioneered the formal education of PAs and NPs. Programs based in university medical centers similar to Duke emerged at Bowman Gray, Oklahoma, Yale, Alabama, George Washington, Emory, and Johns Hopkins and used the Duke training model.[8] Primarily using academic medical centers as training facilities, "Duke-model" programs designed their clinical training to coincide with medical student clerkships and emphasized inpatient medical and surgical roles for PAs. A dramatically different training model developed at the University of Washington, pioneered by Richard Smith, MD, a U.S. public health service physician and former Medical Director of the Peace Corps. Assigned to the Pacific Northwest by Surgeon General William Stewart, Smith was directed to develop a PA training program to respond uniquely to the health manpower shortages of the rural Northwest. Garnering the support of the Washington State Medical Association, Smith developed the MEDEX model, which took a strong position on the "deployment" of students and graduates to medically underserved areas.[15] This was accomplished by placing clinical phase students in preceptorships with primary care physicians who agreed to employ them after graduation. The program also emphasized the creation of a "receptive framework" for the new profession and established relationships with legislators, regulators, and third-party payers to facilitate the acceptance and utilization of the new profession. Although the program originally exclusively recruited military corpsmen as trainees, the term *MEDEX* was coined by Smith not as a reference to their former military roles but rather as a contraction of "*Medicine Extension*."[16] In his view, using *MEDEX* as a term of address avoided any negative connotations of the word *assistant* and any potential conflict with medicine over the appropriate use of the term *associate*. MEDEX programs were also developed at the University of North Dakota School of Medicine, University of Utah College of Medicine, Dartmouth Medical School, Howard University College of Medicine, Charles Drew Postgraduate Medical School, Pennsylvania State University College of Medicine, and Medical University of South Carolina.[15]

In Colorado, Henry Silver, MD, began the Child Health Associate Program in 1969, providing an opportunity for individuals without previous medical experience but with at least 2 years of college to enter the PA profession. Students received a baccalaureate degree at the end of the second year of the 3-year program and were ultimately awarded a master's degree at the end of training. Thus, it became the first PA program to offer a graduate degree as an outcome of PA training.

Compared with pediatric NPs educated at the same institution, child health associates, both by greater depth of education and by law, could provide more extensive and independent services to pediatric patients.[10]

Also offering nonmilitary candidates access to the PA profession was the Alderson-Broaddus program in Philippi, West Virginia. As the result of discussions that had begun as early as 1963, Hu Myers, MD, developed the program, incorporating a campus hospital to provide clinical training for students with no previous medical experience. In the first program designed to give students both a liberal arts education and professional training as PAs, Alderson-Broaddus became the first 4-year college to offer a baccalaureate degree to its students. Subsequently, other PA programs were developed at colleges that were independent of university medical centers. Early programs of this type included those at Northeastern University in Boston and at Mercy College in Detroit.[16]

Specialty training for PAs was first developed at the University of Alabama. Designed to facilitate access to care for underserved populations, the 2-year program focused its entire clinical training component on surgery and the surgical subspecialties. Even more specialized training in urology, orthopedics, and pathology was briefly provided in programs throughout the United States, although it was soon recognized that entry-level PA training needed to offer a broader base of generalist training.

CONTROVERSY ABOUT A NAME

Amid the discussion about the types of training for the new health care professionals was a controversy about the appropriate name for these new providers. Silver of the University of Colorado suggested syniatrist (from the Greek *syn*, signifying "along with" or "association," and *iatric*, meaning "relating to medicine or a physician") for health care personnel performing "physician-like" tasks. He recommended that the term could be used with a prefix designating a medical specialty and a suffix indicating the level of training (aide, assistant, or associate).[17] Because of his background in international health, Smith believed that "assistant" or even "associate" should be avoided as potentially demeaning. His term *MEDEX* for "physician extension" was designed to be used as a term of address, as well as a credential. He even suggested a series of other companion titles, including "Osler" and "Flexner."[14]

In 1970, the AMA-sponsored Congress on Health Manpower, attempted to end the controversy and endorse appropriate terminology for the emerging profession. The Congress chose *associate* rather than *assistant* because of its belief that *associate* indicated a more collegial relationship between the PA and supervising physicians. *Associate* also eliminated the potential for confusion between PAs and medical assistants. Despite the position of the Congress, the AMA's House of Delegates rejected the term *associate*, holding that it should be applied only to physicians working in collaboration with other physicians. Nevertheless, PA programs, such as those at Yale, Duke, and the University of Oklahoma, began to call their graduates *physician associates*, and the debate about the appropriate title continued. A more subtle concern has been the use of an apostrophe in the PA title. At various times, in various states, PAs have been identified as *physician's assistants*, implying ownership by one physician, and *physicians' assistants*, implying ownership by more than one physician; they are now identified with the current title *physician assistant* without the apostrophe.

The June 1992 edition of the *Journal of the American Academy of Physician Assistants* contains an article by Eugene Stead, MD, reviewing the debate and calling for a reconsideration of the consistent use of the term *physician associate*.[18]

The issue concerning the name resurfaces regularly, usually among students who are less aware of the historical and political context of the title. More recently, however, a name change has the support of more senior PAs who are adamant that the title *assistant* is a grossly incorrect description of their work. Although most PAs would agree that *assistant* is a less than optimum title, the greater concern is that the process to change it would be cumbersome, time consuming, and potentially threatening to the PA profession. Every attempt to "open up" a state PA law with the intent of changing the title would bring with it the risk that outside forces (e.g., other health professions) could modify the practice law and decrease the PA scope of practice. Similarly, the bureaucratic processes that would be required to change the title in *every* rule and regulation in each state and in every federal agency would be incredibly labor intensive. The overarching concern is that state and national PA organizations would be seen by policymakers as both self-serving and self-centered if such a change were attempted. This has become a particularly contentious issue among PAs since NP educators have chosen to move to a "doctorate in nursing practice"

by 2015. In 2011, American Academy of Physician Assistants (AAPA) President Robert Wooten sent a letter to all PAs describing a formal process for collecting data regarding PA "opinions" about the "name issue" on the annual AAPA census for review by the AAPA's House of Delegates.

The "name" is currently back on the list of PA "hot topics" as new PA programs in other countries have adopted the name "physician associate." The United Kingdom PAs were the first to make this change based on advice from medical organizations that "physician assistant" was not a correct description. In addition, the fact that personal secretaries were termed "personal assistants" further muddied the waters. In 2013, the United Kingdom PAs became physician associates, and the New Zealand PAs followed them. Other non-U.S. PA programs and organizations are considering this change, which may make the term "physician associate" easier to support in the United States. Currently, U.S. PA organizations are promoting the use of the term *PA* rather than the spelled out words for *physician assistant* to facilitate the transition if needed.

PROGRAM EXPANSION

From 1971 to 1973, 31 new PA programs were established. These startups were directly related to available federal funding. In 1972, Health Manpower Educational Initiatives (U.S. Public Health Service) provided more than $6 million in funding to 40 programs. By 1975, 10 years after the first students entered the Duke program, there were 1282 graduates of PA programs. From 1974 to 1985, nine additional programs were established. Federal funding was highest in 1978, when $8,686,000 assisted 42 programs. By 1985, the AAPA estimated that 16,000 PAs were practicing in the United States. A total of 76 programs were accredited between 1965 and 1985, but 25 of those programs later closed (Table 2.1). Reasons for closure range from withdrawal of accreditation to competition for funding within the sponsoring institution and adverse pressure on the sponsoring institution from other health care groups.

Physician assistant programs entered an expansion phase beginning in the early 1990s when issues of efficiency in medical education, the necessity of team practice, and the search for cost-effective solutions to health care delivery emerged. The AAPA urged the Association of Physician Assistant Programs (APAP) to actively encourage the development of new programs, particularly in states where programs were not available. Beginning in 1990, the APAP created processes for new program support, including new

TABLE 2.1 Distribution of Closed Physician Assistant Training Programs by State

State	Program
Alabama	University of Alabama, Birmingham
Arizona	Maricopa County Hospital Indian HSMC, Phoenix
California	U.S. Navy, San Diego (now Uniformed Services PA Program in San Antonio), Loma Linda University PA Program
Colorado	University of Colorado OB-GYN Associate Program
Florida	Santa Fe Community College PA Program*
Indiana	Indiana University Fort Wayne PA Program
Maryland	Johns Hopkins University Health Associates
Mississippi	University of Mississippi PA Program
Missouri	Stephens College PA Program
North Carolina	Catawba Valley Technical Institute, University of North Carolina Surgical Assistant Program
North Dakota	University of North Dakota
New Hampshire	Dartmouth Medical School
New Mexico	USPHS Gallup Indian Medic Program
Ohio	Lake Erie College PA Program Cincinnati Technical College PA Program
Pennsylvania	Pennsylvania State College PA Program, Allegheny Community College
South Carolina	Medical University of South Carolina
Texas	U.S. Air Force, Sheppard PA Program
Virginia	Naval School Health Sciences
Wisconsin	Marshfield Clinic PA Program

*Transferred to another sponsoring institution (University of Florida, Gainesville).
From Oliver DR. *Third Annual Report of Physician Assistant Educational Programs in the United States, 1986–1987.* Alexandria, VA: Association of Physician Assistant Programs; 1987.

program workshops, and ultimately a program consultation service (Program Assistance and Technical Help [PATH]) to promote quality in new and established programs. These services were ultimately disbanded as the rate of new program growth declined.

The PA profession has engaged in an ongoing and lively debate about the development of new PA programs. The difficulty lies in the impossibility of making accurate predictions about the future health workforce, a problem that applies to all health professions. By 2011, 159 programs were accredited compared with 56 programs in the early 1980s. Expanded roles of PAs in academic medical centers (as resident replacements), in managed care delivery systems, and in enlarging community health center networks have created unpredicted demand for PAs in both primary and specialty roles. The major variable, aside from the consideration of the ideal "mix" of health care providers in future systems, has to do with the *number* of people who will receive health care and the *amount* of health care that will be provided to each person. When, for example, the Affordable Care Act, signed into law by President Obama in 2010, was fully implemented on schedule in 2014, the demand for all types of clinicians rose dramatically. These projections are driving the expansion of current programs and the development of new ones. By 2015, there were more than 200 PA programs with more than 100,000 PAs having graduated from U.S. PA programs.

Unfortunately, much of the concern about the health care workforce has focused primarily on physician supply (see "Physician Supply Literature" in the Resources section) without including PAs and NPs in economic formulas. As a result, American medical and osteopathic schools have been urged to expand their class size and to create new campuses to serve underserved groups. PA programs are concerned about the impact of medical school growth on access to clinical training sites, as well as on the development of PA jobs. Overall, however, it appears that new models of medical training that include increased emphasis on interdisciplinary teams and greater integration of medical students, residents, and PA students on most patient care services will be beneficial for the PA profession.

FUNDING FOR PROGRAMS

The success of the Duke program, as well as that of all developing PA programs, was initially tied to external funding. At Duke, Stead was successful in convincing the federal government's National Heart Institute that the new program fell within its granting guidelines. Subsequently, Duke received foundation support from the Josiah Macy, Jr. Foundation, the Carnegie and Rockefeller Foundations, and the Commonwealth Fund.[10]

In 1969, federal interest in the developing profession brought with it demonstration funding from the National Center for Health Services Research and

Development. With increasing acceptance of the PA concept and the demonstration that PAs could be trained relatively rapidly and deployed to medically underserved areas, the federal investment increased. In 1972, the Comprehensive Health Manpower Act, under Section 774 of the Public Health Act, authorized support for PA training. The major objectives were education of PAs for the delivery of primary care medical services in ambulatory care settings; deployment of PA graduates to medically underserved areas; and recruitment of larger numbers of residents from medically underserved areas, minority groups, and women to the health professions.

Physician assistant funding under the Health Manpower Education Initiatives Awards and Public Health Services Contracts from 1972 to 1976 totaled $32,669,565 for 43 programs. From 1977 to 1991, PA training was funded through Sections 701, 783, and 788 of the Public Health Service Act. Grants during this period totaled $87,927,728 and included strong incentives for primary care training, recruitment of diverse student bodies, and deployment of students to clinical sites serving the medically underserved. According to Cawley,[19] as of 1992 "This legislation . . . supported the education of at least 17,500, or over 70% of the nation's actively practicing PAs." Unfortunately, this high level of support did not continue and with lesser funding for primary care, programs followed medical schools into specialty practice models. Today the majority of the nation's PAs— and the programs from which they graduated—have unfortunately not been exposed to the primary care values and experiences that characterized and defined the early PA concept.

During the period of program expansion, the focus of federal funding support became much more specific, and fewer programs received funding. Tied to the primary care access goals of the Health Resources and Services Administration (HRSA), PA program grants commonly supported less program infrastructure and more specific primary care initiatives and educational innovations. Examples of activities that were eligible for federal support included clinical site expansion in urban and rural underserved settings, recruitment and retention activities, and curriculum development on topics such as managed care and geriatrics.

An important trend was the diversification of funding sources for PA programs. In addition to federal PA training grants, many programs have benefited from clinical site support provided by other federal programs, such as Area Health Education Centers (AHECs) or the National Health Service Corps (NHSC). Also, many programs now receive expanded state funding on the basis of state workforce projections of an expanded need for primary care providers.

Unfortunately, federal Title VII support for all primary care programs (including family medicine, pediatrics, general internal medicine, and primary care dentistry) began to erode in the late 1990s. Federal budget analysts believed that the shrinking number of graduates choosing primary care employment was a signal that federal support was no longer justified. The federal Title VII Advisory Committee on Primary Care Medicine and Dentistry—which includes PA representatives—was formed to study the problem and recommend strategies. Title VII and Title VIII Reauthorization was delayed until the passage of overarching health reform legislation in 2010.

Physician assistant programs immediately benefited from available funding through traditional 5-year training grants and two one-time only grant programs for (1) educational equipment, including simulation models and teleconferencing hardware, and (2) expansion grants to add more training slots for students who were willing to commit themselves to primary care employment. For the first time, PA training grants were expanded from 3 years to 5 years but were limited to $150,000 per grant.

ACCREDITATION

Accreditation of formal PA programs became imperative because the term *physician assistant* was being used to label a wide variety of formally and informally trained health personnel. Leaders of the Duke program—E. Harvey Estes, MD, and Robert Howard, MD—asked the AMA to determine educational guidelines for PAs. This request was consistent with the AMA's position of leadership in the development of new health careers and its publication of *Guidelines for Development of New Health Occupations.*

The National Academy of Science's Board of Medicine had also become involved in the effort to develop uniform terminology for PAs. It suggested three categories of PAs. Type A was defined as a "generalist" capable of data collection and presentation and having the potential for independent judgment; type B was trained in one clinical specialty; type C was determined to be capable of performing tasks similar to those performed by type A but not capable of independent judgment.

Although these categories have not remained as descriptors of the PA profession, they helped the medical establishment move toward the support of PA program accreditation. Also helpful were surveys conducted by the American Academy of Pediatrics and the

American Society of Internal Medicine determining the acceptability of the PA concept to their respective members. With positive responses, these organizations, along with the American Academy of Family Physicians and the American College of Physicians, joined the AMA's Council on Medical Education in the creation of the "educational essentials" for the accreditation of PA training programs. The AMA's House of Delegates approved these essentials in 1971.

Three PAs—William Stanhope, Steven Turnipseed, and Gail Spears—were involved in the creation of these essentials as representatives of the Duke, MEDEX, and Colorado programs, respectively. The AMA appointed L.M. Detmer Administrator of the accreditation process. In 1972, accreditation applications were processed, and 20 sites were visited in alphabetical order, 17 of which received accreditation. Ultimately, the accreditation activities were carried out by the Joint Review Committee, which was a part of the AMA's Committee on Allied Health Education and Accreditation (CAHEA). John McCarty became the Administrator of the ARC-PA in 1991 and has been the first PA to serve in this role. Later, the Joint Committee was renamed the Accreditation Review Committee (ARC). In 2000, the ARC became an independent entity, apart from the CAHEA, and changed its name to the Accreditation Review Commission. Current members of the ARC include the Physician Assistant Education Association, AAPA, American Academy of Family Physicians, American Academy of Pediatrics, American College of Physicians, American College of Surgeons, and American Medical Association.

CERTIFICATION

Just as an accreditation process served to assess the quality of PA training programs, a certification process was necessary to ensure the quality of individual program graduates and become the "gold standard" for the new profession. In 1970, the American Registry of Physician's Associates was created by programs from Duke University; Bowman Gray School of Medicine; and the University of Texas, Galveston, to construct the first certification process. The first certification examination, for graduates from eight programs, was administered in 1972. It was recognized, however, that the examination would have greater credibility if the National Board of Medical Examiners administered it. During this same period, the AMA's House of Delegates requested the Council of Health Manpower to become involved in the development of a national certification program for PAs. Specifically, the House of Delegates was concerned

that the new professional role should be developed in an orderly fashion, under medical guidance, and should be measured by high standards. The cooperation of the AMA and the National Board of Medical Examiners ultimately resulted in the creation of the National Commission on Certification of Physician Assistants (NCCPA), which brought together representatives of 14 organizations as an independent commission. Federal grants contributed $715,000 toward the construction and validation of the examination.[10]

In 1973, the first NCCPA national board examination was administered at 38 sites to 880 candidates. In 1974, 1303 candidates took the examination; in 1975, there were 1414 candidates. In 1992, 2121 candidates were examined. In 1997, the examination was administered to 3728 candidates. In 2002, 4918 candidates took the Physician Assistant National Certifying Examination (PANCE) (3995 first-time takers). In 2006, 5495 candidates (4522 first-time takers), and, in 2007, an estimated 5836 candidates took the PANCE, of whom 4736 were first-time takers. In January 2014, Dawn Morton Rias, NCCPA CEO, announced the certification of the 100,000th physician assistant (PA-C) in the nation since the organization's inception nearly 40 years ago.[20]

Now administered only to graduates of ARC-PA–accredited PA programs, the NCCPA board examination was originally open to three categories of individuals seeking certification:

- Formally trained PAs, who were eligible by virtue of their graduation from a program approved by the Joint Review Committee on Educational Programs for Physician's Assistants
- NPs, who were eligible provided that they had graduated from a family or pediatric NP/clinician program of at least 4 months' duration, affiliated with an accredited medical or nursing school
- Informally trained PAs, who could sit for the examination provided that they had functioned for 4 of the past 5 years as PAs in a primary care setting. Candidate applications and detailed employment verification by current and former employers provided data for determination of eligibility.[21]

Since 1986, only graduates of formally accredited PA programs have been eligible for the NCCPA examination.

The NCCPA's assignments include not only the annual examination but also technical assistance to state medical boards on issues of certification. The NCCPA's website, NCCPA Connect, includes a listing of all currently certified PAs as a resource for employers and state licensing boards.

The NCCPA also administers a recertification process, which includes requirements to complete and register 100 hours of continuing medical education (CME) every 2 years and to pass for recertification examinations on a specified schedule. Originally every 6 years, since 2014, the NCCPA has begun a transition to a 10-year recertification and exam cycle. Since recertification was mandated in 1981, PAs have been required to retest every 6 years. The 10-year process now includes CME requirements obtained through self-assessment or performance improvement.

A recent development for the NCCPA is the development of voluntary recognition for specialty training and education. Called Certificates of Added Qualification (CAQ), the process is modeled after similar acknowledgments in Family Medicine. The NCCPA's decision to create the CAQ was based on a long process that involved requests from PA specialty groups, a history of inquiries from institutional credentialing and privileging bodies, a series of meetings involving partnerships between specialty PAs and supportive parallel physician organizations, and a long exploration of possible options.[22]

The final decision—to try the CAQ process with five specialties—was sharply criticized by the AAPA, which feared that any specialty process threatens the generalist image. Ultimately, the NCCPA decided that it was better for them to move in this direction rather than have external for-profit organizations create certification processes without PA input. The five specialties chosen were cardiovascular surgery, orthopedics, nephrology, psychiatry, and emergency medicine. Teams composed of representatives of MD and PA specialty organizations worked together to create the CAQ process. Subsequently, CAQs in pediatrics and hospital medicine have been added.

In 2005, the NCCPA created a separate NCCPA Foundation to promote and support the PA profession through research and educational projects. The Foundation supports the work of the NCCPA for the advancement of certified physician assistants and the benefit of the public. PA Foundation activities have included a PA Ethics Project with the Physician Assistant Education Association, a Best Practice Project focusing on the relationships between PAs and their supervising physicians, and a research grants program.

In 2010, the NCCPA welcomed the Society for the Preservation of Physician Assistant History and was moved into its infrastructure. The Society is now headquartered at the NCCPA offices in Johns Creek, Georgia. Originally founded in 2002 as a free-standing organization for educational, research, and literary purposes, the Society's mission is to serve as the preeminent leader in fostering the preservation, study, and presentation of the history of the PA

profession by creating and presenting an online virtual repository of historic and current information on the PA profession. The Society's projects include an archive of PA historical items, the extensive website on PA history designed to serve as a resource for PA students and practicing PAs and researchers, as well as the PA History Center housed in the North Carolina Academy's headquarters in Raleigh-Durham, North Carolina. An 11-member board governs the Society and provides leadership for history activities with support from NCCPA staff.

ORGANIZATIONS

American Academy of Physician Assistants

What was to become the AAPA was initiated by students from Duke's second and third classes as the American Association of Physician Assistants. Incorporated in North Carolina in 1968 with E. Harvey Estes, Jr., MD, as its first advisor and William Stanhope serving two terms as the first president (1968–1969 and 1969–1970), the organization's original purposes were to educate the public about PAs, provide education for PAs, and encourage service to patients and the medical community. With initial annual dues of $20, the Academy created a newsletter as the official publication of the AAPA and contacted fellow students at the MEDEX program and at Alderson-Broaddus.

By the end of the second year, national media coverage of emerging PA programs throughout the United States was increasing (Fig. 2.1), and the AAPA began to plan for state societies and student chapters. Tax-exempt status was obtained, the office of president-elect was established, and staggered terms of office for board members were approved.

Controversy over types of PA training models offered the first major challenge to the AAPA. Believing that students trained in 2-year programs based on the biomedical model (type A) were the only legitimate PAs, the AAPA initially restricted membership to these graduates. The Council of MEDEX Programs strongly opposed this point of view. Ultimately, discussions between Duke University's Robert Howard, MD, and MEDEX Program's Richard Smith, MD, resulted in an inclusion of graduates of all accredited programs in the definition of *physician assistant* and thus in the AAPA.

At least three other organizations also positioned themselves to speak for the new profession. These were a proprietary credentialing association, the American Association of Physician Assistants

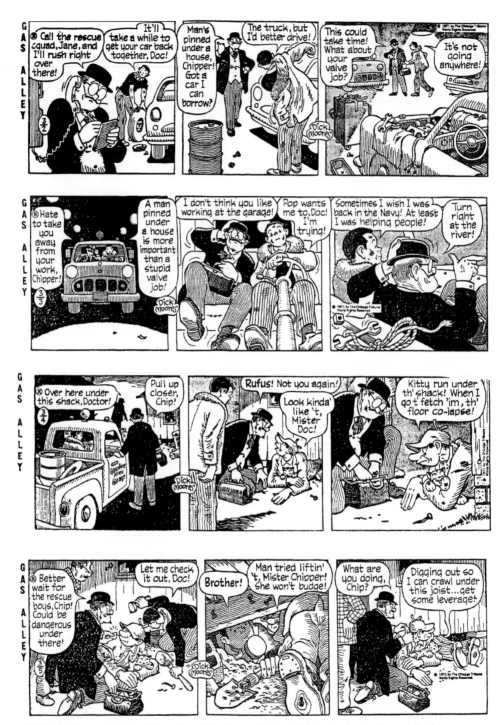

FIG. 2.1 ■ The comic strip "Gasoline Alley" is credited with introducing to the public the concept of the physician assistant in 1971, when leading character Chipper Wallet decided to become one. (Tribune Media Services. All Rights Reserved. Reprinted with permission.)

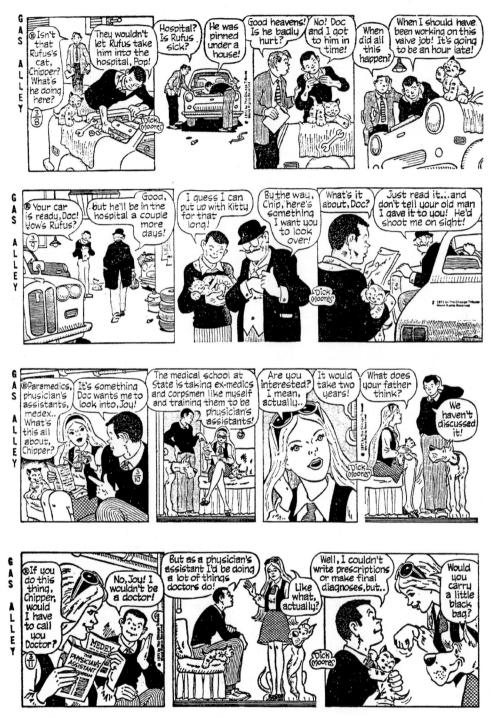

FIG. 2.1, cont'd

(a group representing U.S. Public Health Service PAs at Staten Island); the National Association of Physician Assistants; and the American College of Physician Assistants, from the Cincinnati Technical College PA Program. AAPA President Paul Moson provided the leadership that "would result in the emergence of the AAPA as the single voice of professional PAs" (W.D. Stanhope, C.E. Fasser, unpublished manuscript, 1992).

This unification was critical to the involvement of PAs in the development of educational standards and the accreditation of PA programs. During Carl Fasser's term as AAPA president, the AMA formally recognized the AAPA, and three Academy representatives were formally appointed to the Joint Review Committee.

During the AAPA presidency of Tom Godkins and the APAP presidency of Thomas Piemme, MD, the two organizations sought funding from foundations for the creation of a shared national office. Funding was received from the Robert Wood Johnson Foundation, the van Ameringen Foundation, and the Ittleson Foundation. Because of its 501(c)(3) tax-exempt status, APAP received the funds for the cooperative use of both organizations. "Discussions held at that time between Piemme and Godkins and other organizational representatives agreed that in the future, because of the limited size of APAP . . . funds would later flow back from the AAPA to APAP"[23] (W.D. Stanhope, C.E. Fasser, unpublished manuscript, 1992). Donald Fisher, MD, was hired as executive director of both organizations, and a national office was opened in Washington, DC. According to Stanhope and Fasser, "a considerable debt is owed to the many PA programs and their staff who supported the early years of AAPA."

AAPA constituent chapters were created during President Roger Whittaker's term in 1976. Modeled after the organizational structure of the American Academy of Family Physicians, the AAPA's constituent chapter structure and the apportionment of seats in the House of Delegates were the culmination of initial discussions held in the formative days of the AAPA. The American Academy of Family Physicians hosted the AAPA's first Constituent Chapters Workshop in Kansas City, and the first AAPA House of Delegates was convened in 1977.

Throughout its development, the AAPA has been active in the publication of journals for the profession. As the first official journal of the AAPA, *Physician's Associate*, was originally designed to encourage research and to report on the developing PA movement. With the consolidation of graduates of all programs into the AAPA, the official academy publication became the *PA Journal, A Journal for New Health Practitioners*. In 1977, *Health Practitioner*

became the official magazine of the AAPA followed by *Physician Assistant* in 1983 and the *Journal of the American Academy of Physician Assistants* in 1988. A monthly online publication, *PA Professional*, has more recently been created by the AAPA to feature news, policy issues, and the successes of individual PAs. *Clinician Reviews* and *Physician Assistant*, published by external publishers, also offer medical articles and coverage of professional issues for PAs. In addition to formal publications, the AAPA's website provides the most current information about current practice, policy, and advocacy issues for PAs and their employers.

Governed by a 13-member board of directors, including officers of the House of Delegates and a student representative, the AAPA's structure includes standing committees and councils. Specialty groups and formal caucuses bring together academy members with a common concern or interest.[24]

The AAPA's Student Academy is composed of chartered student societies from each PA educational program. Each society has one seat in the Assembly of Representatives, which meets at the annual conference and elects officers to direct Student Academy (SAAPA) activities.

The Academy also includes a philanthropic arm, the Physician Assistant Foundation, whose mission is to foster knowledge and philanthropy that promotes quality health care.

The annual AAPA conference serves as the major political and continuing medical education activity for PAs, with an average annual attendance of 7000 to 9000 participants. A list of past and present AAPA presidents is provided in Table 2.2. A history of conference locations is given in Table 2.3. Table 2.4 lists presidents of the SAAPA from the AAPA.

Legislative and leadership activities for the AAPA take place at an annual leadership event, which also provides the opportunity for lobbying of state congressional delegations in Washington, DC.

Key to the success of the AAPA is a dedicated staff at the national office in Alexandria, Virginia. Under a chief executive officer who is responsible to the AAPA Board of Directors, senior vice presidents and vice presidents manage Academy activities related to governmental affairs, education, communications, member services, accounting, and administration.

Association of Physician Assistant Programs to Physician Assistant Education Association

The APAP evolved from the original American Registry of Physician's Associates. The Registry was originally created "to determine the competence

TABLE 2.2 **AAPA Presidents**

1968–1969	William D. Stanhope, PA	1993–1994	Ann L. Elderkin, PA
1969–1970	William D. Stanhope, PA	1994–1995	Debi A. Gerbert, PA-C
1970–1971	John J. McQueary, PA	1995–1996	Lynn Caton, PA-C
1971–1972	Thomas R. Godkins, PA	1996–1997	Sherrie L. McNeeley, PA-C
1972–1973	John A. Braun, PA	1997–1998	Libby Coyte, PA-C
1973–1974	Paul F. Moson, PA	1998–1999	Ron L. Nelson, PA-C*
1974–1975	C. Emil Fasser, PA-C	1999–2000	William C. Kohlhepp, MHA, PA-C
1975–1976	Thomas R. Godkins, PA	2000–2001	Glen E. Combs, MA, PA-C
1976–1977	Roger G. Whittaker, PA*	2001–2002	Edward Friedmann, PA-C
1977–1978	Dan P. Fox, PA	2002–2003	Ina S. Cushman, PA-C
1978–1979	James E. Konopa, PA	2003–2004	Pam Moyers Scott, MPAS, PA-C
1979–1980	Ron Rosenberg, PA	2004–2005	Julie Theriault, PA-C
1980–1981	C. Emil Fasser, PA-C	2005–2006	Richard C. Rohrs, PA-C
1981–1982	Jarrett M. Wise, RPA	2006–2007	Mary P. Ettari, MPH, PA-C
1982–1983	Ron I. Fisher, PA	2007–2008	Gregor F. Bennett, MA, PA-C
1983–1984	Charles G. Huntington, RPA	2008–2009	Cynthia Lord
1984–1985	Judith B. Willis, MA, PA	2009–2010	Stephen Hanson, MPA, PA-C
1985–1986	Glen E. Combs, PA-C	2010–2011	Patrick Killeen, MS, PA-C
1986–1987	R. Scott Chavez, PA-C*	2011–2012	Robert Wooten, PA-C
1987–1988	Ron L. Nelson, PA-C	2012–2013	James Delaney, MPA, PA-C
1988–1989	Marshall R. Sinback, Jr., PA-C	2013–2014	Lawrence Herman, PA-C
1989–1990	Paul Lombardo, RPA-C	2014–2015	John McGinnity, MS, PA-C
1990–1991	Bruce C. Fichandler, PA	2015–2016	Jeff Katz, PA-C
1991–1992	Sherri L. Stuart, PA-C	2016–2017	Josann Pagel, MPAS, PA-C
1992–1993	William H. Marquardt, PA-C		

*Deceased. From American Academy of Physician Assistants, Alexandria, VA; 2016.

TABLE 2.3 **American Academy of Physician Assistants National Conference Locations**

1973	Sheppard Air Force Base, Texas	1996	New York, New York
1974	New Orleans, Louisiana	1997	Minneapolis, Minnesota
1975	St. Louis, Missouri	1998	Salt Lake City, Utah
1976	Atlanta, Georgia	1999	Atlanta, Georgia
1977	Houston, Texas	2000	Chicago, Illinois
1978	Las Vegas, Nevada	2001	Anaheim, California
1979	Fort Lauderdale, Florida	2002	Boston, Massachusetts
1980	New Orleans, Louisiana	2003	New Orleans, Louisiana
1981	San Diego, California	2004	Las Vegas, Nevada
1982	Washington, DC	2005	Orlando, Florida
1983	St. Louis, Missouri	2006	San Francisco, California
1984	Denver, Colorado	2007	Philadelphia, Pennsylvania
1985	San Antonio, Texas	2008	San Antonio, Texas
1986	Boston, Massachusetts	2009	San Diego, California
1987	Cincinnati, Ohio	2010	Atlanta, Georgia
1988	Los Angeles, California	2011	Las Vegas, Nevada
1989	Washington, DC	2012	Toronto, Canada
1990	New Orleans, Louisiana	2013	Washington, DC
1991	San Francisco, California	2014	Boston, Massachusetts
1992	Nashville, Tennessee	2015	San Francisco, California
1993	Miami Beach, Florida	2016	San Antonio, Texas
1994	San Antonio, Texas	2017	Las Vegas, Nevada
1995	Las Vegas, Nevada	2018	New Orleans, Louisiana

From American Academy of Physician Assistants, Alexandria, VA; 2016.

TABLE 2.4 Student Academy Presidents

1972–1973	J. Jeffrey Heinrich	1994–1995	Ernest F. Handau
1973–1974	John McElliott	1995–1996	Beth Grivett
1974–1975	Robert P. Branc	1996–1997	James P. McGraw, III
1975–1976	Tom Driber	1997–1998	Stacey L. Wolfe
1976–1977	John Mahan	1998–1999	Marilyn E. Olsen
1977–1978	Stephen Nunn	1999–2000	Jennifer M. Huey-Voorhees
1978–1979	William C. Hultman	2000–2001	Rodney W. Richardson
1979–1980	Arthur H. Leavitt, II	2001–2002	Abby Jacobson
1980–1981	Katherine Carter Stephens	2002–2003	Andrew Booth
1981–1982	William A. Conner	2003–2004	Annmarie McManus
1982–1983	Michael J. Huckabee	2004–2005	Lindsey Gillispie
1983–1984	Emily H. Hill	2005–2006	Trish Harris-Odimgbe
1984–1985	Thomas J. Grothe	2006–2007	Gary Jordan
1985–1986	Gordon L. Day	2007–2008	Gary Jordon
1986–1987	Patrick E. Killeen	2008–2009	Michael T. Simmons
1987–1988	Keevil W. Helmly	2009–2010	Kate Lenore Callaway
1988–1989	Toni L. Deer	2010–2011	Michael Shepherd
1989–1990	Paul S. Robinson	2011–2012	Peggy Diana Walsh
1990–1991	Jeffrey W. Janikowski	2012–2013	Emilie Suzanne Thornhill
1991–1992	Kathryn L. Kuhlman	2013–2014	Nick Rossi
1992–1993	Ty W. Klingensmith Flewelling	2014–2015	Melissa Ricker
1993–1994	Beth A. Griffin	2015–2016	Elizabeth Prevou

From American Academy of Physician Assistants, Alexandria, VA; 2016.

of Physician's Associates" through the development of a national certifying examination. After these functions were subsequently assumed by the National Board of Medical Examiners, and ultimately the NCCPA in 1972, the Registry became the APAP.

Led by Alfred M. Sadler, Jr., MD, as its first president, the APAP evolved as a network within which member programs could work on "curriculum development, program evaluation, [and] the establishment of continuing education programs"; the APAP was also developed to "serve as a clearing house for information and define the role of the physician assistant." Similar to the Association of American Medical Colleges, the APAP (now the Physician Assistant Education Association [PAEA]) represents educational programs; the American Medical Association and the AAPA represent individual practitioners.

For many years, the educational offices were located in the AAPA building in Alexandria, Virginia. A change in both the name and the structure of the organization occurred in 2004. The APAP became the PAEA. Initially, the organization relocated to separate office space in Alexandria. In 2015, the PAEA moved to Washington, DC, to join the American Association of Medical Colleges (AAMC)

in its new building. Governed by an eight-member board of directors, including a student representative, the PAEA holds its major annual meeting in the late fall, as well as meetings in conjunction with the AAPA's May annual meeting. APAP presidents are listed in Table 2.5.

The PAEA offers an online directory of PA programs as a resource for program applicants. In 2001, the organization began a nationwide centralized electronic application process (CASPA) to streamline PA program application. The goal was for CASPA to serve the same function as the American Medical College's Application Service (AMCAS) process used extensively by U.S. medical schools. CASPA now serves as both the medical school admissions gateway and the provider of important data regarding the applicant pool and long-term graduate career trajectories.

A major function of PAEA is also the support of PA program faculty. An online newsletter, *PAEA Networker*, provides information on PAEA activities and educational opportunities. PAEA's formal publication, the *Journal of Physician Assistant Education*, offers articles on a range of PA educational issues. PAEA also promotes professional development and scholarly activity through the Faculty Development and Research Institutes.

TABLE 2.5 Physician Assistant Education Association Presidents			
1972–1973	Alfred M. Sadler, Jr., MD	1995–1996	James Hammond, MA, PA-C
1973–1974	Thomas E. Piemme, MD	1996–1997	J. Dennis Blessing, PhD, PA-C
1974–1975	Robert Jewett, MD	1997–1998	Donald L. Pedersen, PhD, PA-C
1975–1976	C. Hilmon Castle, MD	1998–1999	Walter A. Stein, MHCA-PA-C
1976–1977	C. Hilmon Castle, MD	1999–2000	P. Eugene Jones, PhD, PA-C
1977–1978	Frances L. Horvath, MD	2000–2001	Gloria Stewart, EdD, PA-C
1978–1979	Archie S. Golden, MD	2001–2002	David Asprey, PhD, PA-C
1979–1980	Thomas R. Godkins, PA	2002–2003	James F. Cawley, MPH, PA-C
1980–1981	David E. Lewis, Med	2003–2004	Paul L. Lombardo, MPS, RPA-C
1981–1982	Reginald D. Carter, PhD, PA-C	2004–2005	Patrick T. Knott, PhD, PA-C
1982–1983	Stephen C. Gladhart, EdD	2005–2006	Dawn Morton-Rias, EdD, PA-C
1983–1984	Robert H. Curry, MD	2006–2007	Anita D. Glicken, MSW
1984–1985	Denis R. Oliver, PhD	2007–2008	Dana L. Sayre-Stanhope, EdD, PA-C
1985–1986	C. Emil Fasser, PA-C	2008–2009	Justine Strand de Oliveira, DrPH, PA-C
1986–1987	Jack Liskin, MA, PA-C	2009–2010	Ted Ruback, MS, PA
1987–1988	Jesse C. Edwards, MS	2010–2011	Kevin Lohenry, PhD, PA-C
1988–1989	Suzanne B. Greenberg, MS	2011–2012	Anthony Brenneman, MPAS, PA-C
1989–1990	Steven R. Shelton, MBA, PA-C	2012–2013	Contance Goldgar, MS, PA-C
1990–1991	Ruth Ballweg, PA-C	2013–2014	Karen Hills, MS, PA-C
1991–1992	Albert F. Simon, Med, PA-C	2014–2015	Stephanie VanderMeulen, MPAS, PA-C
1992–1993	Anthony A. Miller, MEd, PA-C	2015–2016	Jennifer Snyder, PhD, PA-C
1993–1994	Richard R. Rahr, EdD, PA-C	2016–2017	William Kohlhepp, DHS, MHA, PA-C
1994–1995	Ronald D. Garcia, PhD		

From Association of Physician Assistant Programs, Alexandria, VA; 2016.

TRENDS

Although the first PA programs were developed with the primary purpose of training male military corpsmen, the demography of the profession soon changed, largely because the PA profession developed in historical context with both the women's and the civil rights movements. Early articles and promotional materials for PAs described the new provider almost universally as "he." In 1966, Eugene Stead, MD, explained:

> *Our intent is to produce career-oriented graduates. Since the long-range goals of most females remove them from continued and full-time employment in the health field, we anticipate that the bulk of the student body will be males. This is not meant to exclude females, for those who can present credentials, which would assure the Admissions Committee of proper intent should be considered in the same light as male applicants.* [25]

In fact, there were many "career-oriented" women seeking exactly this type of training. By the mid-1970s, the PA profession was quickly evolving—fueled not only by the need for changes in the health care system but also by the attraction to the profession of strong, motivated women seeking a new and open-ended health career. PA program brochures included photographs of both male and female students, and marketing for the PA profession began to focus on the diversity of individuals entering the profession. In 1972, 19.9% of PA students were women; in 1976, 32.8% were women; and by 1982, the distribution of graduates was nearly equal.[26,27] The percentages of women entering U.S. medical schools for the same years were 16.8%, 23.8%, and 30.8%, respectively.[28] By the late 1990s, there was some thought that the PA profession might become a female-dominated profession because women filled more than 60% of the training slots. The move to master's degrees seems to have accelerated the increase in the number of women in PA programs. Researchers have yet to fully explore this phenomenon and its potential impact on the PA profession.

Physician associate programs also immediately focused on recruiting minority candidates for PA training. PA programs to train American Indians and Alaskan Natives were established at Indian Health Service hospitals in Phoenix, Arizona, and Gallup, New Mexico. Programs were also established at Drew University, Howard University, and Harlem Hospital with initiatives to train African Americans for inner-city practice. In addition, federal funding guidelines encouraged other PA programs to emphasize the recruitment and training of minority PAs. Since 1987, 20% of all PA students have been minorities. Nevertheless, the recruitment of minorities into the PA profession is an ongoing issue. In 1977, Ruth Webb of the Drew program challenged "each and every PA to accept the responsibility for seeking out five minority applicants during the coming year. Your minimum goal would be to have at least one of them accepted into your parent program."[29] This challenge is equally appropriate today as an ongoing issue.

NATIONAL HEALTH POLICY REPORTS

Two national reports, one by the Institute of Medicine in 1978 and the other by the Graduate Medical Education National Advisory Committee (GMENAC) in 1981, had a major impact on both PAs and NPs.

In 1978, the National Academy of Sciences Institute of Medicine (IOM) issued its "Manpower Policy for Primary Health Care." Strongly supporting PAs and NPs, the IOM statements included the following recommendations[30]:

- For the present time, the numbers of PAs and NPs being trained should remain at the current level.
- Training programs for family physicians, PAs, and NPs should continue to receive direct federal, state, and private support.
- Amendments to state licensing laws should authorize, through regulations, PAs and NPs to provide medical services, including prescribing drugs when appropriate and making medical diagnoses. PAs and NPs should be required to perform the range of services they provide as skillfully as physicians, but they should not provide medical services without physician supervision.

Emphasizing the value of primary care, the IOM report stressed that even with the projected increase in the supply of physicians, PAs and NPs have an important role to play in the delivery of primary care.[30]

Charged by the U.S. Secretary of Health, Education, and Welfare, a national advisory committee began in 1976 to examine the physician supply issue. The report by GMENAC, published in 1981 and seen as a major turning point in the history of American health care, projected an oversupply of physicians by 1990. Strategies for correcting this oversupply included reducing medical school enrollments, limiting the use of foreign-trained physicians, and reviewing the need to train nonphysician providers. According to Cawley,[31] "Many people who supported PAs during the times of physician shortage viewed an excess of physicians as signaling the discontinuation of federal funding for PA programs and the exit of PAs from the medical scene." Although federal funding was not completely eliminated, it was significantly reduced, from $8,262,968 in 1980 to $4,752,000 in 1982. The reduced funds could assist only 34 programs rather than the previous 43, and the amounts per program were significantly cut.

In retrospect, there were significant flaws in the assumptions of the GMENAC process. Among the issues that could not be predicted were the impact of HIV, the greater usage of physician services, the shortening of physician workweeks, and the changing lifestyles of physicians. As a result, questions remain about the existence of a physician shortage, and the general understanding is that the United States has a physician maldistribution. As Cawley states, "Any perceived negative impact of the rising physician numbers on the vitality of the PA profession has failed to occur."[32] According to Schafft and Cawley,[32] "The most significant outcome of the study was a gradual awareness that the profession would have to reevaluate its mission and redirect its efforts to validate its existence."

CURRENT ISSUES AND CONTROVERSIES

The development of any new career brings with it controversies and concerns. The late 1960s heralded the creation of the PA and the successful implementation of the pilot projects that would serve as the foundation for subsequent PA training. In the 1970s, enthusiastic new PAs pioneered the role in a variety of settings, practice acts were put in place in most states, and professional organizations were established at national and state levels. The 1980s saw both the continued training of PAs and questions about where PAs fit in the health care system. Although the GMENAC report resulted in a backlash against PAs and NPs through fewer federal dollars for training, the late 1980s found PAs being used in a wider range of practice settings than had ever been dreamed of by the founders.

During the 1990s, our attention was focused on training and utilization; however, there was a growing appreciation for the political context of health care in a rapidly changing society. Federal health workforce policy documents were paralleled by similar state documents that acknowledged state-specific issues. Most frequently, these documents called for a maintenance or expansion of the primary care workforce and acknowledgment of the valuable roles that PAs played in health care systems based on our generic primary care training, our adaptability, and our willingness to rapidly respond to the needs of specific health care "niches." In the second decade of the 21st century, we continue to market the profession as a major solution to health care access issues. Doctors in all medical specialties—many who have now trained alongside PAs—are seeking PAs as a non-negotiable part of their practice team. The Affordable Care Act and the Triple Aim—emphasizing (1) better care for individuals, (2) better health for populations, and (3) reductions in per capita costs—are creating an unprecedented demand for our services.

CONCLUSION

The social change theory, which holds that "it takes society 30 years, more or less, to absorb a new technology into everyday life,"[32] can be applied to PAs. Created during a time of chaos within the health care system, the PA profession is now, more than ever, a solution to access, efficiency, and economic problems in health care. Although consumers are not yet 100% informed about PAs, more and more have been the recipients of PA care. Evolving health care delivery systems—with emphasis on quality and efficiency—require that PAs be part of the provider mix. The range of opportunities for PA employment is limitless in both primary care and

the specialties. International applications of the PA movement, including demonstration projects and the creation of educational programs, create opportunities to increase global health care access. Maintaining a flexible, responsive stance will continue to be the most important strategy for the PA profession—domestically and internationally.

CLINICAL APPLICATIONS

1. Research the history of the PA profession in your state. What, if any, was the involvement of the state medical association in the creation of the practice "environment"? Who were the key PAs in the formation of the state academy? If one does not exist, prepare a chronological list of state academy presidents and conference locations.
2. Keep a longitudinal diary of the issues that are your personal, local, state, regional, and national concerns regarding the PA profession. These might include specific licensure or reimbursement issues or even your personal reflections on the changes occurring across time. Use this diary as a personal history of your PA career. You might want to include your successful application to PA school as the first item in this diary.

KEY POINTS

- The PA concept has its roots in similar roles first created in Russia by Peter the Great (feldshers) and in China (barefoot doctors). In addition, roles such as the purser's mate in the U.S. Merchant Marine and informal physician extender roles in the offices of individual physicians paved the way for the AMA to consider a new role in American medicine.
- Several models of PA training and practice eventually coalesced into the PAs that we know today. Duke University focused on an academic medical center role, the MEDEX program trained PAs to work in rural and underserved communities with an emphasis on primary care, the University of Colorado created a pediatric role, Alderson Broadus worked to recruit individuals from small Appalachian communities, and the University of Alabama designed a surgical program. The PA movement is supported by four distinct organizations—each with its own well-defined role: the American Academy of Physician Assistants (AAPA); the Physician Assistant Education Association (PAEA), formerly known as the Association of Physician Assistant Programs (APAP); the National Commission on Certification of Physician Assistants (NCCPA); and the Accreditation Review Commission on Education for Physician Assistants (ARC-PA.)
- New models of health care developed in response to the Affordable Care Act have created the need for expanded numbers of PAs in both primary care and specialty settings. New PA leadership roles are emerging in hospitals, large health care systems, corporations, and governmental agencies.
- The PA profession is developing globally to solve country-specific health care issues and concerns. Global connections are rapidly being created among individuals, PA programs, PA organizations, and health care delivery systems to promote this growth through consultations, online communication, site visits, and social media.

References

1. Fortuine R. *Chills and Fevers: Health and Disease in the Early History of Alaska*. Fairbanks: University of Alaska Press; 1992.
2. Sidel VW. Feldshers and feldsherism: the role and training of the feldsher in the USSR. *N Engl J Med*. 1968;278:935.
3. Storey PB. *The Soviet Feldsher as a Physician's Assistant*. Washington, DC: Geographic Health Studies Program, U.S. Department of Health, Education, and Welfare Publication No. (NIH); 1972.
4. Roemer MI. *Health Care Systems in World Perspective*. Ann Arbor, MI: Health Administration Press; 1975.
5. Perry HB, Breitner B. *Physician Assistants: Their Contribution to Health Care*. New York: Human Sciences Press; 1982.
6. Basch PF. *International Health*. New York: Oxford University Press; 1978.
7. Dimond EG. Village health care in China. In: McNeur RW, ed. *Changing Roles and Education of Health Care Personnel Worldwide in View of the Increase in Basic Health Services*. Philadelphia: Society for Health and Human Values; 1978.
8. Gifford JF. The development of the physician assistant concept. In: *Alternatives in Health Care Delivery: Emerging Roles for Physician Assistants*. St. Louis: Warren H. Green; 1984.
9. Fisher DW, Horowitz SM. The physician assistant: profile of a new health profession. In: Bliss AA, Cohen ED, eds. *The New Health Professionals: Nurse Practitioners and Physician's Assistants*. Germantown, MD: Aspen Systems Corp; 1977.
10. Carter RD, Gifford JF. The emergence of the physician assistant profession. In: Perry HB, Breitner B, eds. *Physician Assistants: Their Contribution to Health Care*. New York: Human Sciences Press; 1982.
11. Estes EH. Historical perspectives—how we got here: lessons from the past, applied to the future. *Physician Assistants: Present and Future Models of Utilization*. New York: Praeger; 1986.
12. Sadler AM, Sadler BL, Bliss AA. *The Physician's Assistant Today and Tomorrow*. New Haven, CT: Yale University; 1972.
13. Howard R. *Physician Support Personnel in the 70s: New Concepts*. In: Burzek J, ed. Chicago: American Medical Association; 1971.
14. Smith RA, Vath RE. A strategy for health manpower: reflections on an experience called MEDEX. *JAMA*. 1971;217:1365.
15. Smith RA. MEDEX. *JAMA*. 1970;211:1843.
16. Myers H. *The Physician's Assistant*. Parson, WV: McClain Printing Company; 1978.
17. Silver HK. The syniatrist. *JAMA*. 1971;217:1368.
18. Stead EA. Debate over PA profession's name rages on. *J Am Acad Physician Assist*. 1992;6:459.
19. Cawley JF. Federal health policy and PAs: two decades of government support have contributed to professional growth. *J Am Acad Physician Assist*. 1992;5:682.
20. *NCCPA News Release*, January 14, 2014. http://www.nccpa.net/Upload/PDFs/Press%20Release%20202014%20CAQ%20Recipients.pdf.
21. Glazer DL. National Commission on Certification of Physician's Assistants: a precedent in collaboration. In: Bliss AA, Cohen ED, eds. *The New Health Professionals: Nurse Practitioners and Physician's Assistants*. Germantown, MD: Aspen Systems Corp; 1977.
22. National Commission on Certification of Physician Assistants. Specialty Certificates of Added Qualifications (CAQs). https://www.nccpa.net/Specialty-CAQs.
23. Stanhope WD. The roots of the AAPA: the AAPA's first president remembers the milestones and accomplishments of the academy's first decade. *J Am Acad Physician Assist*. 1993;5:675.
24. American Academy of Physician Assistants. *Constitution and Bylaws. Membership Directory 1997–1998*. Alexandria, VA: American Academy of Physician Assistants; 1997.
25. Stead EA. Conserving costly talents: providing physicians' new assistants. *JAMA*. 1966;19:182.
26. Light JA, Crain MJ, Fisher DW. Physician assistant: a profile of the profession, 1976. *PAJ*. 1977;(7):111.
27. Selected Findings from the Secondary Analysis. *1981 National Survey of Physician Assistants*. Rosslyn, VA: American Academy of Physician Assistants; 1981.
28. American Medical Association. Annual report on medical education in the United States, 1987–88. *JAMA*. 1988;260:8.
29. Webb R. Minorities and the PA movement. *Phys Assist*. 1977;2:14.
30. Stalker TA. IOM report: the recommendations and what they mean. *Health Pract Phys Assist*. 1978;2:25.
31. Schafft GE, Cawley JF. *The Physician Assistant in a Changing Health Care Environment*. Rockville, MD: Aspen Publishers; 1987.
32. Cringely RX. *Accidental Empires*. New York: HarperCollins; 1993.

The resources for this chapter can be found at www.expertconsult.com.

CHAPTER 3

INTERNATIONAL DEVELOPMENT OF THE PHYSICIAN ASSISTANT PROFESSION

David H. Kuhns • Luppo Kuilman

The U.S. physician assistant (PA) profession, created 50 years ago at Duke University, is rooted firmly in the compressed medical curriculum originally developed by the military to quickly train medics and corpsmen. The profession was further influenced by the history of Russian feldschers and the use of Chinese barefoot doctors. The PA movement has since grown globally in response to specific access, quality, and efficiency needs in many countries. Perhaps it is the timing that now, when the need for skilled medical providers continues to grow worldwide, the harsh economic realities reinforce the idea that not everyone can become a doctor, nor can everyone afford to have a doctor treat every ailment. Jane Farmer's evaluation of the Scottish PA pilot considered the international PA movement by saying that "the current wave of international development in deploying and training PAs can . . . be viewed in alternative ways. First, it could be viewed as a 'fashion.' The PA profession is neatly packaged, emanates from the United States (as many health system fashions do), has some assiduous 'product champions,' and is promoted in a panacea-like way. Alternatively, PAs can be viewed as *the* profession, designed as uniquely adaptable (i.e.,

moving from the United States to other parts of the world at this time *expressly because* it can meet the world's current health workforce gaps)."[1]

This chapter reviews international PA models that are close analogs of the American PA and therefore knowingly excludes many other nonphysician clinicians (NPCs) who contribute substantially to health care delivery around the world. It is important to acknowledge that no slight is intended by this distinction. Rather, it is our attempt to say the role of all NPCs, including PAs, is on a continuum. NPCs can be viewed as either complementing existing health services provided or actually substituting services for those usually performed by physicians, especially as is often necessary in many developing countries. This chapter focuses on models that typically provide complementary services with linkages to supervising or collaborating doctors and surgeons.

It is also important to acknowledge that this is intended as an overview of the current state of affairs as of the summer of 2016. It is not intended to be a comprehensive, in-depth report on the PA model worldwide.

The chapter first examines countries where either, after 15 to 20 years of experience, rapid and significant advances are being made or the concept is in developmental stages where there is little to report. We also explore some of the common and diverse issues and challenges faced as the PA model evolves.

CANADA

Canada's PA profession, still in its early stages, has a solid foundation and is expected to continue to grow throughout the Canadian health care system. As of June 2016, there are about 500 Canadian Certified Physician Assistants (CCPAs) who were trained through either Canadian or American programs. (U.S. PAs are eligible to take the Canadian Certification Exam, but unfortunately, Canadian-trained PAs do not yet have access to the National Commission on Certification of Physician Assistants [NCCPA] exam.)

Canadian PAs are health care clinicians academically and nationally qualified to provide medical services to patients in a wide range of settings and in a variety of roles. All PAs work in collaboration with a physician; the scope of practice is determined by observations and comfort levels and in the negotiated role required of the physician practice and PA qualification. The scope of practice is summarized as duties authorized by a physician that the physician is qualified to perform and is comfortable delegating. A PA can collect a history, order appropriate diagnostics, reach a differential diagnosis, and prescribe appropriate treatment.[2]

The Canadian PA model was developed in the military during the Korean War as an advanced medical technician called a *medical assistant*. The training transitioned to the present PA concept in 1984 and was further revised in 2002.[3] The Canadian Forces program is taught at the Canadian Armed Forces Health Services Training Center and is restricted to serving members of the Canadian Forces. Three, soon to be four, civilian university programs are located at the University of Manitoba (2008) and in Ontario (McMaster University, 2008) and the Consortium for PA Education (2010). The Consortium is housed in the Department of Family Medicine at the University of Toronto's School of Medicine and includes partnerships with the Northern Ontario School of Medicine and the Michner Institute for Applied Health Professions. Alberta's University of Calgary has a program in development potentially starting in September 2016. All programs are 24 to 25 months in duration and deliver curricula that support the Canadian Association of Physician Assistants'

(CAPA) scope of practice statement and *Canadian Medical Education Directives for Specialists (CanMEDS)* PA competencies. In 2003, the Canadian Medical Association (CMA) Board of Directors approved an application from the Canadian Association of Physician Assistants (CAPA) to include PAs within the CMA accreditation. The CMA first accredited the PA program delivered by the Canadian Forces Medical Services School in 2004.

The Physician Assistant Certification Council of Canada (PACCC) administers and oversees certification for PAs in Canada and provides quality assurance for the entry-to-practice examination. The CCPA designation is recognized as the national standard process (CMA Accreditation Report). As part of the professional recognition requirements, CAPA structured the PACCC to establish an independent national certification examination and registry. The first national examination was held in 2005. In 2009, CAPA refined its National Competency Profile and PA Scope of Practice. The national competency profile (NCP) defines the core competencies that a generalist PA should possess on graduation and is the accepted standard in Canada.[4]

Each province and territory has its own medical act that further delineates the degree of delegation and supervisory requirements. For example, Manitoba first introduced PAs in 1999 under the title of Clinical Associate. In 2009, those regulations were amended to permit practice under the title of PA. Also in 2009, the College of Physicians and Surgeons of New Brunswick amended the New Brunswick Medical Act (1981) to include PAs. Alberta is the only Canadian province with a voluntary PA (nonregulated) registry that is held by the College of Physicians and Surgeons of Alberta. Efforts are currently under way to regulate PAs in Ontario, where they currently practice under the supervision of a physician and are only able to perform controlled acts under delegation. Other provinces are in various stages of considering the PA career as an appropriate clinician for their governmentally controlled health systems.

The highest concentration of PAs (50%) in Canada is found in Ontario. What started as the first emergency medicine projects in 2007 has since expanded to include various demonstration projects in family medicine and community health teams, medical and surgical specialties, and long-term care facilities.[5] New Brunswick has introduced PAs into emergency departments. Alberta has several pilot projects introducing PAs into occupational industrial medicine.

Canada's certified PAs report working in 32 medical or surgical subspecialties. It is estimated that 38%

are in primary care roles, 13% are in internal medicine specialties, 18% are involved in surgical practice, and 19% are in emergency medicine. Just fewer than 50% of Canada's PAs report serving communities of less than 250,000, with 34.5% in populations under 50,000 (CAPA 2014 National Survey).

A significant advance for Canadian military PAs came in 2016 when PAs transitioned from their status as senior enlisted noncommissioned members and warrant officers to the newly identified officer occupation within the Canadian Armed Forces.[6,7]

UNITED KINGDOM

The first PAs to work in the United Kingdom were two Americans who in 2003 were recruited for primary care posts. They worked in the Black Country, so called from its days as an industrial hub but now an economically distressed and medically underserved area of England's West Midlands; this area encompasses Birmingham, England's second largest metropolitan area. A larger scale demonstration project followed in Scotland from 2006 to 2008, with 20 experienced American PAs deployed across a number of specialties.[8] It was from these projects that the U.K. PAs, UK Association of Physician Assistants (UKAPA), the first professional body, was created by expatriate American PAs to provide necessary continuing medical education and to encourage advancement of the PA profession.

Initial efforts by the British at "growing their own" PAs started in 2002 with pilot training programs for what were then called *health care practitioners* (HCPs), precursors to the PA role, at St. George's University of London and Kingston University. The HCP model then evolved into the medical care practitioner (MCP) and then to the PA, with the University of Wolverhampton as the first to identify its curriculum as a PA program in 2004. The first substantive programs, as defined by class size with cohorts of 10 or more, were launched in 2008 when the University of Birmingham and University of Wolverhampton and then as St. George's in London relaunched with a similar sized cohort in 2009. Notably, the St. George's program was the only one to be led by a U.S.-trained PA. These programs followed a national curriculum and were taught at the postgraduate diploma (PgDip) level.[9]

Despite the emphasis on the creation of PA programs, there was initially significantly less effort devoted to the broad types of advocacy required to create a new health profession. These include (1) role development and gaining the broad support of doctors; (2) the development of a national regulatory

processes and the authorization of clinical privileges such as prescribing; (3) the creation of other forms of professional recognition such as certification, recertification, and credentialing at the health systems level; and (4) the authorization of a reimbursement structure to pay for the services of PAs.

A setback to the British PA movement was the closure of the PA program at the University of Birmingham in 2011, the consequence of loss of the original champions within the university's hierarchy and opposition from certain quarters within the local National Health Service (NHS). The University of Wolverhampton's program was also suspended at the same time. Meanwhile, on a much more positive note, the St. George's program in London had doubled its entry cohort number, and a new program was launched at the University of Aberdeen, Scotland, in October 2011.

The transition of the title of "physician assistant" to "physician associate" came upon the recommendation of the NHS's Health Education England (HEE). Within the NHS structure, the "assistant" role denotes lesser qualified, less trained individuals with lesser academic credentials and reflects lower pay scales. It also was intended to clarify the role from those informally trained "physician assistants" ("medical assistants" in U.S. terminology) who were working in some NHS hospitals.

After a couple of years of the United Kingdom's PA profession languishing in the doldrums of governmental apathy, the winds of change slowly started to build. A renewed interest in PAs came from cities and regions across the whole of the country, especially as hospitals were feeling the strain of the work hour restrictions on their house officers and doctors in training. First to reclaim their status was the program at the University of Birmingham with a relaunch in January 2014. They continued the momentum of making up for lost time by increasing their cohorts to two intakes per year, which they have since continued to this time, the only U.K. program to do so. The University of Wolverhampton restarted in September 2014, and the University of Worcester joined the effort at the same time. Only a few months later, the sixth program was up and running at the University of Plymouth. This dramatic shift in fortunes was helped along with additional support by the first national strategic PA workforce conference, hosted by HEE, on Physician Associates in the Workplace held in Birmingham in October 2014. This was followed in 2015 when growing support for the PA profession came from the United Kingdom's Minister of Health and was manifest in a demand for 1000 PAs for the primary care workforce alone by 2020. To meet this demand, the number of universities offering PA programs tripled from just 5 in 2015 to 15 in 2016 and is expected to double again by 2017. Also of significance is that although the number of English and Scottish programs has since increased exponentially, there are now new programs being established in Wales and Northern Ireland, where previously there were none.[10]

Another milestone was achieved in April 2016 when the First Annual Physician Associate Educators Conference was held at the University of Worcester. With the recent explosion of PA programs across the United Kingdom, it was thought that it was time for a renewed vision of increased cooperation and collaboration on setting academic standards among the current and new program.

U.K.-trained PAs were originally expected to work in primary care, which at the time was anticipating a significant shortage of workers in underserved areas. Accordingly, the Competency and Curriculum Framework developed by the Department of Health was focused on primary care. However, implementation of the European Working Time Directive, which significantly limited work hours for doctors in training to less than 48 hours per week, has increased the demand for PAs to work in hospital and specialty practices; fewer are working in general practice (outpatient medicine). Revisions to the CCF are presently under way to reflect the shift to a broader approach, including hospital-based practice.[11]

Unfortunately, despite more than a decade of scores of PAs working in the NHS, there is still no official recognition by the U.K. government or by the nongovernmental medical licensing bodies such as the General Medical Council. The original professional organization UKAPA has since transformed into the Faculty of Physician Associates (FPA) of the Royal College of Physicians. As such, the FPA holds a "managed voluntary register" as a means of identifying the PA workforce; it provides the necessary continuing education U.K. PAs need to maintain their qualification. Until officially recognized, U.K. PAs face the hardships of not having prescriptive practice or being able to order diagnostic imaging, thus limiting their overall effectiveness. Despite these challenges, demand for PAs continues to increase. As of June 2016, there are about 300 PAs in the United Kingdom, including about 20 Americans.

Newly graduated PAs will have an initial qualifying examination, modeled after the Physician Assistant National Certifying Exam (PANCE) in the United States. The United Kingdom's version is a two-part process, a 200-question multiple-choice examination and a 12-station Objective Structured Clinical Examination (OSCE). Of potential interest to American PAs is that at present, PAs who are already currently NCCPA certified are able to apply to become a member of the Managed Voluntary Register (MVR) without first having to undergo the UK examination process.

A novel idea to further use American PAs in advancing the UK's PA role in the NHS was the creation of the National Physician Associate Expansion Program (NPAEP) (http://npaep.com). This program was intended to recruit more than 200 American PAs to go to the United Kingdom for a period of 2 years, effectively doubling the existing PA workforce. The overall goal of the program was to expand the use of PAs across a number of sites in the NHS. However the projected faced many obstacles including meeting the desired recruitment numbers. The project was implemented in mid-2016.

THE NETHERLANDS

Around the turn of the millennium, the Netherlands government predicted upcoming shortages in the medical workforce. To address the imbalance between the demands and supply of Dutch medical care providers, the PA role was first introduced in 2001.[12] Since then five Master Physician Assistant (MPA) programs have been started at universities of applied sciences. The first MPA program started at the University of Applied Sciences Utrecht in 2001 followed by the HAN University of Applied Sciences located in Nijmegen in 2003. Then in 2005, three more MPA programs opened at the Inholland Graduate School in Amsterdam; the Hanze University of Applied Sciences, Groningen; and the Rotterdam University, University of Applied Sciences. With reference to this last MPA program, it should be mentioned that from 2005 to 2009, the program had a primary focus on clinical midwifery. However, since 2009, Rotterdam University also developed a traditional generic MPA program and maintained the midwifery program.[13] In total, the five Dutch MPA programs have an annual enrollment of approximately 125 students. These enrolling students must meet the admission criteria of (1) being a holder of a bachelor's degree in either nursing or paramedicine and (2) having a minimum of 2 years of relevant professional, clinical experience after their undergraduate training.

In the Netherlands the MPA program is a 30-month curriculum, based on the National Training and Competency Profile MPA. This profile is tailored to the professional roles of the CanMEDS, including (1) medical expert, (2) communicator, (3) manager, (4) collaborator, (5) scholar, (6) health advocate, and the overarching role of (7) professional. These seven professional roles are described by a definition, delineation, and related competencies. Each of these professional roles is linked to the task areas as defined within the Professional Profile Physician Assistant by the Dutch Association of Physician Assistants (NAPA). According to the Framework for Qualifications of the European Higher Education Area, the MPA programs in the Netherlands are designated as second-cycle programs and entail a total study load of 150 European Credits, equal to 4200 clock hours. PA training in the Netherlands differs from other traditional international PA models in the integration of their didactic and clinical education, known as a *dual program*. At the day of enrollment to the MPA programs, the students are also employed as paid PA trainees. While students on campus (1 day per week) are learning the core knowledge and skills required for all PAs, each student simultaneously receives additional clinical expertise in a designated medical specialty by actually learning in that area the rest of the working week. Students are contracted through a "training and employment contract" with a minimum of 32 hours per working week. On top of this, students are expected to engage in self-study. As a result, PA students have both didactic (to acquire generic competencies, modeled to the medical curriculum) and clinical days (to acquire specialty competencies, analogues to that of training medical residents) interspersed throughout the duration of their training. Fully qualified PAs are known as MPAs. Dutch PAs work across all areas of medicine, including general practice, and because of their unique approach to their training, are found in subspecialty areas in greater numbers than PAs elsewhere.[14,15]

In the past 15 years, the Dutch PA profession has grown to more than 1000 clinicians. Under the leadership of the NAPA, the Dutch PA profession has made significant advances. The most substantial professional milestone as reached in 2012: PAs are enabled by law to practice medicine autonomously, albeit at all times in collaboration with a medical doctor. Granting this independent practice is a result of a change in the Individual Health Care Professional Act and involves authorization to perform medical procedures, including prescription of medications, which formerly belonged within the realm of physicians only. This assigned professional autonomy is anchored in a temporary legislative change and will be evaluated in the year 2017.[16]

At the time of graduation, PAs can voluntary enroll in NAPA's Quality Register. The Quality Register contributes to ensuring the quality of professional practice by keeping track of developments in the profession (i.e., by means of continuing medical education [CME]). Being enlisted into the Quality Register indicates the PA to be a graduate of a Dutch Flemish Accreditation Organization–accredited MPA program and is clinically active at time of registration. The registration period covers a term of 5 years after which a re-registration is required. Only those who have been practicing as PAs with a minimum of 16 hours per working week and have followed CME totaling 200 hours (40 hours per year) in the last registration period of 5 years are considered for re-registration.

LIBERIA

First established in 1965, the first and only Liberian PA program at the Tubman National Institute of Medical Arts grew from a collaboration among the national government, World Health Organization, and UNICEF. The political instability, civil wars, and public health crises have resulted in intermittent disruptions to the training program. Nonetheless, the PA model remains integral to health care delivery, especially in rural and remote areas of the country. Of particular note, while the nation's resources were otherwise overwhelmed, Liberian PAs played a major and essential role in the treatment centers for the Ebola outbreak in 2014 to 2015; as a result, many PAs became infected, often because of lack of proper protective equipment, including 14 who died in service to their country.[17]

INDIA

Until the first scholarly article in 2012[18] that reported on the Indian PA educational system and professional workforce, the Indian PA movement remained largely invisible. The first PA training program had actually started in 1992 under the auspices of the Madras Medical Mission, guided by Dr. K.M. Cherian, a renowned cardiac surgeon. Dr. Cherian worked with American PAs during his training in the United States. Almost 25 years later, there are more than 1100 qualified PAs in India nationwide; however, many of them are working with pharmaceutical or medical device companies rather than as clinical PAs. The Indian programs are hosted by training institutes and facilitated by affiliated universities granting the degrees. Similar to the American experience, a range of academic credentials are associated with Indian PA training. Programs range in length from 2 to 4 years. They also vary from baccalaureate to postgraduate diploma (as per the U.K. approach). Master's degree level programs were in existence in the earlier days but were downgraded because there were few applicants.

Because there is not yet a formal accreditation process for PA programs, there is a reported exponential growth of a wide range of programs promoting themselves as educating PAs primarily for economic motives. The first International Conference on Physician Assistants was sponsored by the Indian Association of Physician Assistants (IAPA).

Under the purview of the Indian Ministry of Health and Family Welfare the National Initiative for Allied Health Sciences (NIAHS) task force has been primarily created to bring in regulation in the education and practice of all allied health care programs with a long-term vision of creating a governance council. In addition, a PA task force was initiated in 2015 with the purpose of defining and establishing a national standardized curriculum. The result is the *Model Curriculum Handbook—Physician Associate*, which is currently in the final stage of development and will soon be presented to the government. Alongside standardizing the curriculum and acquiring the PA profession's governmental recognition, it includes the necessary title protection. In line with several other nations, the Indian PA workforce has opted to exchange the indication of *assistant* to *associate*. The current definition of physician associates in India, as is laid down by the IAPA, is as follows: "Physician Associates are health care professionals trained in a medical model who practice medicine as part of the healthcare team. They are qualified and competent to perform preventive, diagnostic, and therapeutic services with physician supervision."

Although the lion's share of the Indian PA workforce has its roots in surgical specialties, with an emphasis on cardiothoracic surgery, nowadays a shift is observed to other disciplines, such as emergency medicine, general medicine, general surgery, obstetrics and gynecology, and orthopedics.[19] Because most PAs are still employed in private practice, they are therefore barely visible to the public, government, and health administrators responsible for planning primary health care.

GHANA

In 2009, the medical assistant (MA) profession in Ghana celebrated the historical landmark of their workforce's presence in the health care system spanning 4 decades. Initially, the program was designed for nurses as an advanced study lasting 18 months. Enrollment was open for nurses who had at least 3 years of work experience. Because of an increasing demand of MAs, the program was redesigned in 2007, also enabling high school graduates and other health workers to enter MA training, parallel to the existing

program. This new "direct admission program" offered via the Kintampo Rural Health Training Center is a 4-year curriculum that includes intensive clinical internships in the last year. After completion of the training, MAs are mainly deployed in primary health care centers in rural areas. The workload of MAs is demanding, with an average of 90 to 150 consultations per working day. Because MAs conduct a supervisory role to nurses, midwives, and community health workers, they are the attainable key figures of a health center 24 hours a day. In 2005, the very first two bachelor PA programs were initiated at the Cape Coast University and Central University College.[20] Now after more than a decade, colleges and universities offer a PA program, often referred to as a *B.Sc. Physician Assistantship*. The PA profession in Ghana is known to have three types of PAs—namely, PA Medical (the earlier known medical assistants as well as graduates of the "new" PA programs), the PA Dental (formerly Community Oral Health Officers), and PA Anesthesia (also known as Nurse Anesthetists). As of 2015 the Ghanaian PA workforce included 2500 clinicians, of whom more than 70% were registered as PA Medical. After graduation, PAs can obtain a license to practice through the Medical and Dental Council, designated by the Ministry of Health as the regulatory body to regulate PA training and practice in Ghana. To get licensed, PAs have to sit for the "Licentiate Examination."[20] The PAs Medical are predominantly stationed in primary care settings, with the majority serving communities in the rural and remote parts of Ghana.[20] Given the content areas assessed in the "Licentiate Examination," the PAs Medical appear to be trained to the medical curriculum and can be considered fellow PAs, as adapted to meet the local needs of the Ghanaian health care system.

SOUTH AFRICA

The PA equivalence in South Africa are called *clinical associates* (CAs), a concept first considered by the National Health Council in 2002.[21] CAs were formally introduced by their Health Ministry in 2008 as a means to address chronic health workforce shortages, especially in rural and otherwise underserved areas of the country. The "brain drain" of the medical workforce of South Africa had resulted in a loss of almost 40% of their doctors through immigration in the past 15 years.

Three South African programs were created simultaneously to bring significant numbers of graduates into the workforce in multiple sites throughout the country. Programs at Johannesburg's University of the Witwatersrand, the University of Pretoria, and Walter Sisulu University in the Eastern Cape Province are all are offered in partnership with national and provincial departments of health, as well as the South Africa Military Health Service (SAMHS). All CA programs follow a 3-year curriculum, which is competency based and delivered in a variety of formats. This leads to a bachelor of clinical medical practice degree. Qualified CAs are registered with the Health Professions Council of South Africa. The first cohorts of CAs graduated in January 2011 and are now working in district hospitals.[22] (Perhaps it is because the South African government is driving the CA project that it has faced fewer challenges than other international PA projects.)

AUSTRALIA

As of 2016, PAs remain a promising addition to the health workforce in Australia, although progress has been slow. Acceptance of the PA role continues to move forward at a restrained pace in a historically conservative health care culture. Even with solid support from influential health workforce leaders, scholars, and many in the medical community, a major question has yet to be completely answered to the satisfaction of governments and various health care organizations: Does this delegated medical practice model fit in the Australian health care context?

The Australian health care system is structured quite differently from that of the United States. Measured by a range of external evaluations and benchmarks, it functions remarkably well. Since 1984, Australia has had a publicly funded universal health care scheme called Medicare. Health care services are provided with a complex mix of government and private financing and service provision. The Commonwealth (federal) government funds the bulk of public hospital services, but the public hospitals are controlled and operated by the six state and two territorial governments. The Medicare Benefits Scheme (MBS) heavily subsidizes out-of-hospital services for primary care and specialty services and pays for free universal access to public hospital care. Primary care services are privatized and provided by general practitioners (GPs) who function as sanctioned gatekeepers. Specialists who work in both public and private health settings may only be accessed with a referral from a GP. The federally funded Prescription Benefits Scheme (PBS) subsidizes the cost of medications. Approximately 55% of the total population of 23.9 million is covered by optional private health insurance that affords beneficiaries access to private hospital care and flexible ancillary services.[1,22]

Australia is consistently noted to be close to the top in studies comparing health outcomes and health system efficiency.[23] Sensible social policy and a fairly resilient economy have had a positive influence, but despite these beneficial circumstances, serious problems do exist within the fragmented health care system:

- Health care costs are on an ever increasing, unsustainable path.
- Public health care is notably deficient in some states and generally strained in all.
- Urban public hospitals tend to be underresourced and overburdened.
- Waiting times for nonemergent care and elective surgeries in public hospitals can be excessive.
- There is a significant shortage of health care providers in rural and remote areas. A policy of imposing forced rural placements with oppressively extended visas durations on international medical graduates has made little overall difference.
- Australia's land mass is almost identical to that of the contiguous United States, and access to health care services for the 13% of the population living in outer regional, rural, and remote areas is consistently challenging.[22,24]
- Indigenous Australians, accounting for 2.5% of the total population, are much less healthy by all indicators and have a significantly lower life expectancy.

Proponents firmly believe that PAs could make significant contributions to a number of different underserved areas suffering from the serious misdistribution of doctors, including rural and remote practice, primary health care services, Aboriginal medical services, and struggling urban public hospitals.

The lack of acceptance of PAs partially stems from circumstances not common to the United States. In contrast to the United States, Australia does not have a shortage of doctors. According to the World Health Organization (WHO) in 2011, Australia had 3.3 doctors per 1000 people compared with 2.5 per 1000 for the United States, but significant problems with underutilization and misdistribution negate the oversupply.[25] Furthermore, the number of medical schools has increased from 10 to 19 since 1999, and class sizes have ballooned over the same period. Reasons for the increase are unclear and controversial, but the situation has led to opposition of PAs from the Australian Medical Association (AMA) and the Australian Medical Students Association (AMSA) over perceived competition for clinical training resources and potential jobs. However, compared with more than 3400 medical school graduates annually, the small number of PA graduates is scarcely noticeable. Despite similar negative treatment of nurse practitioners from the same PA-resistant medical community over the past 2 decades, major nursing organizations also oppose including PAs in the Australian health care scheme. Nurse Practitioners in particular view PAs as redundant and a direct threat to their employment opportunities.

Two Australian states, Queensland and South Australia, completed PA pilots between 2009 and 2010. Four years after the release of independent evaluations containing mostly positive outcomes, the Queensland government became the first to develop significant policy changes enabling physician assistants to practice within the public health system, Queensland Health. The South Australia state government has yet to record any forward momentum.

The first PA program in Australia began at the University of Queensland (UQ) in Brisbane in 2009. The 2-year master's degree program graduated two cohorts totaling 34 students before it closed in 2012. There is now a single educational program at James Cook University (JCU) College of Medicine & Dentistry in Townsville, Queensland. The 3-year bachelor of health science (PA) course has been adapted specifically for mature age students with previous health care and tertiary academic experience living distantly. Similar to UQ, the average age of students to date at JCU is approximately 36. Paramedics account for the largest group of students enrolled followed by nurses. Nine students graduated from the first JCU class. At the time of writing, JCU has two active cohorts totaling 15 students. An additional intake of 18 students started the course in February 2016. The JCU course is a fully integrated component of the College of Medicine & Dentistry. Teaching and administrative resources are shared, including PA academics teaching medical students in the 6-year medical bachelors—bachelor of surgery (MBBS) course. The JCU College of Medicine & Dentistry strongly adheres to a philosophy of social accountability and focuses on supplying medical and PA graduates to underserved populations; in particular, rural, remote, tropical, and indigenous Australia. A 2013 comparative study showed that JCU medical graduates take up training and eventual employment in rural and remote areas in numbers far superior to any other Australian university.[26]

The emerging PA profession is receiving essential but incremental support from certain segments of the medical profession and health care advocates. Always a supporter of PA development, in 2011, the Australian College of Rural and Remote Medicine (ACRRM) became the first major health care professions organization to champion the PA model with a formal policy statement. The Rural Doctors Association of Australia (RDAA) has endorsed the ACRRM policy. The Grattan Institute, an independent think tank dedicated to influencing public policy, has released several reports and opinion papers that outline the utility of PAs and recommend their incorporation in to the health care system.[3]

Sadly, Australia is currently in an economic downturn. Health care reforms are under significant review at both the federal and state government levels, complicating the steps toward formal recognition of PAs but also presenting opportunities for inclusion and innovation. Changes in Medicare reimbursement may eliminate the greatest impediment to PA employment—the lack of remuneration from Australia's single-payer system. The Commonwealth government has proposed a major shift in Medicare reimbursement from fee for service to predominantly performance-based disbursements for primary care services. With this policy change, doctors potentially will be able to use PAs to provide care to subsegments of patient populations such as chronically ill and older individuals.

Initiated by students at UQ, the influence of the Australian Society of Physician Assistants (ASPA) has continued to grow from its inception in 2010 and is now the official representative professional body of Australian PAs. Even though fewer than 10 Australian PAs are working clinically in Queensland, the organization continues to promote and lobby for professional recognition and the development of policy and regulations to support the future PA workforce. Current undertakings include creation of a self-regulatory board, developing a clear path to indemnity coverage, advancing novel employment and funding models and continuing professional development (CPD) opportunities and recognition. Most important, ASPA is applying to the Medical Services Advisory Committee for access to Medicare reimbursement privileges. Strengthening ties with its primary supporting organization, ACRRM, and seeking the backing of other key health care associations is a priority for ASPA. Presently, ASPA is corresponding or actively interacting with the Australian Health Care Reform Alliance (AHCRA), the Royal Australian College of General Practitioners (RACGP), the AMA, and Queensland Health. After the outcome of application for Medicare reimbursement, the ASPA plans to lobby for prescriptive privileges under the Pharmaceutical Benefits Scheme. In alignment with professional organizations in the United Kingdom and New Zealand, the ASPA endorsed a name change to *physician associate* in November 2015.

KINGDOM OF SAUDI ARABIA

The first PA program in the Middle East, offered by the Medical Services Directorate of the Ministry of Defense and Aviation in the Kingdom of Saudi Arabia, was launched in September 2010 at the Prince Sultan Military College of Health Professions in Dharhan, Saudi Arabia. A team of experienced American PA educators follows a traditional American-style PA model curriculum, with a 28-month postgraduate curriculum. The program, a collaborative effort with the Prince Sultan Military College of Health Sciences and the George Washington University Medical Faculty Associates in the Department of Emergency Medicine, trains 40 PAs per year, with their eventual deployment across all divisions of the Saudi military.[25] This is hoped to be the first of several PA programs for the country. The first class graduated in February 2013. Of particular interest is that Saudi PAs will be known as *assistant physicians* (APs) because of an issue with how the original PA title is translated into Arabic.

FEDERAL REPUBLIC OF GERMANY

The first German PA program opened its doors at Steinbeis University Berlin (SUB) in 2005. SUB is a private university, and the PA program established an official relationship with the German Society for Orthopedic and Trauma Surgery. Until recently, there were just three programs in Germany. The total number of graduates from 2005 until 2016 was 269. Whether these graduates have remained active as PAs in clinical practice is unknown. Currently, German PAs have a relatively limited scope of practice, requiring direct supervision by the attending medical doctor. Germany's medical hierarchy has been generally reluctant to entrust any significant aspects of medical practice to nonphysicians. Despite this barrier, the German PA profession is steadily growing because of access and efficiency pressures within the medical system.

Similar to the Netherlands, PA programs in Germany are offered through universities of applied sciences. All PA programs offer bachelor's degrees because the majority of health professionals are trained at a vocational level. By 2015, two of the original PA programs (SUG and the Baden-Wuerttemberg Collaborative State University) in Karlsruhe remained open.[26] The third program, through Mathias Hochschule Rheine University of Applied Sciences, has been restructured through the Praxis Hochschule University of Applied Sciences.

Beyond the original three programs, four other PA programs currently enroll students and expect to graduate their first classes sequentially in 2017, 2018, and 2019. These programs include the University Medical Center Hamburg-Eppendorf, Fresenius University of Applied Sciences in Frankfurt am Main, State Academy Plauen, and Fresenius University of Applied Sciences offered in Munich. It appears that PA training in Germany largely relies on the initiative of private universities. The absence of a national accreditation process means that there is not yet the assurance of a standardized curriculum across schools. Future challenges to PA practice are upcoming because of the governmental structure of Germany. Similar to the United States, Germany has a federal system of government with 16 separate states, each with its own constitution and regulatory processes. Despite a recent resolution by the Germany Medical Association, calling PA "a profession," the nationwide establishment of the PA profession in Germany will not be complete until all 16 states have "signed on" (unpublished data, Samantha Keller, president and CEO, German Association of Physician Assistants).

NEW ZEALAND

Based on Australian developments as well as New Zealand doctors' experiences in working with PAs during U.S. residency training, New Zealand's first moves were to develop two pilot projects. In 2011, the first pilot, a 1-year nongovernmental project at Counties Manakau (Middlemore) Hospital in Auckland, selected two U.S. surgical PAs to provide pre- and postoperative care on a busy surgical teaching service. Supported by the Ministry of Health's Health Workforce New Zealand, the second project recruited seven U.S.-trained PAs for a 2-year commitment from 2013 to 2015. Six PAs worked in primary care in small cities or rural communities on the North Island, and one emergency department PA worked in a rural hospital on the South Island. Funding for each project included an evaluation process and written report summarizing the activities.[27]

The short duration of the Middlemore pilot was a major drawback in that there was insufficient time for the institution and its staff to develop a broad understanding of the role despite the outstanding performance of the two PAs. The in-depth evaluation of the Ministry of Health's second primary care pilot was designed with mixed methodology to evaluate the PA role in multiple settings and to provide guidance to Health Workforce New Zealand on future directions for the PA profession in New Zealand. Although the report was positive, by the summer of 2016, Health Workforce New Zealand had not yet moved ahead authorization for regulation or the creation of PA programs.[28]

In the meantime, a new cadre of U.S. PAs has replaced the PAs in the settings that employed PAs in the Health Workforce Pilot, and these PAs are functioning under the "delegatory practice" rules for doctors. The absence of prescriptive rights is a barrier to full utilization. The New Zealand Medical Association is a strong proponent of PAs, and the Medical Council of New Zealand stands ready to begin a regulatory process upon the receipt of a formal request from the Ministry of Health. The professional body for PAs in New Zealand has endorsed the title "physician associate" and is continuing to work for PAs to formally recognized and related. As a first step, the creation of a registry is in progress.

AFGHANISTAN

Afghanistan, with a history of more than 30 years of armed conflict and the extensive disruption of its national medical infrastructure, is one of the most underresourced health systems in the world. With only 2.1 physicians per 10,000 population, compared with a regional average of 11 physicians per 10,000 population,[28] the need to quickly increase the overall size of the health workforce is essential.

As part of the effort to address some of these inequities, the NATO Training Mission in Afghanistan developed a PA course, which was launched in October 2010. The primary goals of this program are to both increase the overall numbers of clinicians and to improve the skill levels of the clinicians in the Afghan National Army.[29]

The Afghan PA program, located at the National Military Hospital Compound in Kabul, offers a 12-month didactic curriculum, derived from existing U.S. and Canadian military medical courses and then augmented with a month-long pharmacology course. In addition, there is a 16-week clinical phase, offering experience in "sick call" and emergency medicine and trauma. A Tactical Combat Care Course will complete the training, with the expectation that PAs will be ready to face the challenges of providing medical care in a war zone.[25]

It is expected that they will eventually graduate 65 qualified PAs per cohort. Of particular note is that the program has both male and female students. Although female PAs will not be part of active combat units, they will work in district military hospitals.

According to Canadian Forces PA, Master Warrant Officer Kelly Humphreys, who served as PA Adviser to the Armed Forces Academy of Medical Sciences (AFMAS), "The AFMAS PA program could address many of their health care shortfalls in the urban areas, as well as out in the more remote locations" (personal communication, K. Humphreys, November 19, 2011). Plans are under way for the eventual expansion of the PA model into the civilian medical system in Afghanistan as well.

ISRAEL

Jewish American PAs welcomed the news that the Israeli government has been exploring introducing the role of PAs (and NPs) as a means to address current medical workforce shortages, including in emergency medicine, surgery, internal medicine, and pathology. This was especially encouraging given the strong opposition that had initially come from organized medicine, including the Israeli Medical Association. However, given the chronic state of overcrowding of hospitals and the increasing demand for services, the government has since moved forward with efforts to promote the PA role.[30] To this end, Israel's Ministry of Health's training department developed the first PA program in the spring of 2016 at Tel HaShomer's Sheba Medical Center.[31]

The curriculum is intended to upskill a cadre of experienced paramedics through a 6-month training course to have them identified and functioning as PAs. This represents a classic scenario in which the PA model has been *adapted* to meet the local needs rather than adopted straight from the American model.

BULGARIA

With a history of more than 130 years of incorporating feldschers, a secondary education level medical practitioner, into primary care and hospital-based medicine across their national health system, Bulgaria has, since 2014, developed its first two formal university-based, 4-year bachelor's level PA training programs based on the American PA curriculum. Since January 2016, PAs are now included on the register of regulated professions.

REPUBLIC OF IRELAND

The Republic of Ireland is the newest entry into the developing PA role in Europe. Although still at the embryologic stage of the profession, Ireland, as with many other European countries, is dealing with a combination of factors that make it fertile ground for the introduction of the PA role. Ireland faces a recovering economy, an aging population, recently enforced work-hour restrictions on house officers, and the emigration of many of its qualified doctors and surgeons. With the goal of achieving improved service delivery and better continuity of care, the Department of Health approved a 2-year pilot project with four expatriate PAs, three Canadian and one American, employed in surgical subspecialties in Dublin in July 2015. Anticipating a favorable environment, the first Irish PA training program based in Dublin and awarding a 24-month Master of Science in Physician Associate Studies degree was launched in January 2016 at the Royal College of Surgeons in Ireland. By the autumn of 2016, the Irish Society of Physician Associates was established. It remains to be seen how the Irish PA clinical role will develop to meet the ever-increasing needs of both primary and secondary care throughout Ireland.

WHERE NEXT?

Spain, Belgium, and China have recently shown interest in developing the PA role. The coming years will likely see further expansion of the PA role as nations look for ways to address the growing demands on their medical delivery systems and as they continue to explore options to achieve cost-efficient and effective health care systems.

ACKNOWLEDGMENTS

A debt of gratitude is owed to the following contributors to this chapter: Ruth Ballweg, MPA, professor emeritus, Department of Family Medicine, University of Washington, Seattle, Washington; Allen Forde, PA-C, MPAS, senior lecturer, James Cook University School of Medicine & Dentistry, Townesville, Australia; and Ian Jones, MPAS, CCPA, PA-C, program director, University of Manitoba Physician Assistant Program.

KEY POINTS

- The PA profession continues to grow and can now be found in various stages of development in numerous countries in the world.
- Individual countries may need to "adapt, not adopt" the traditional PA role to make it fit with their specific health care needs and challenges.
- The full implementation of the PA role in a "new" country is not complete until it includes
  - The creation of educational programs
  - Development of the new role and the acceptance of doctors
  - The development of regulatory processes, including program accreditation, licensure and registration, and a national or regional certification process separate from educational programs
  - Mechanisms that provide for professional liability coverage for PAs and privileges such as prescriptive authority
  - A plan for reimbursement for the services of PAs
- Experience has proven that such processes always take longer than estimated.
- The potential for unanticipated governmental delays caused by "changes in governments" or transitions in leadership within agencies such as Ministries of Health should be viewed as inevitable in the developmental process.
- Although doctors are likely allies in PA development, other professions may see PA development as threatening and therefore may create turf wars and other obstacles. The most common opposition groups are nursing and "junior doctors."
- It's often easier to develop and implement the PA profession in smaller countries with less complicated governments (e.g., the Netherlands) than it is in countries with complex federal systems (e.g., Canada) allowing regulation at the state, provincial, or territorial level.

References

1. Farmer J, Curry M, West C, et al. *Evaluation of Physician Assistants to NHS Scotland*; 2009. http://www.abdn.ac.uk/crh/upl oads/files/PA%20Final%20report%20Jan%2009%20version %205.pdf. Accessed December 2011.
2. *Canadian Association of Physician Assistants: Scope of Practice and National Competency Profile*. Ottawa: Canadian Association of Physician Assistants; 2009.
3. Hooker R, MacDonald K, Patterson R. Physician Assistants in the Canadian Forces. *Mil Med*. 2003;168(11):948.
4. Jones IW, Hooker RS. Physician assistants in Canada: update on health policy initiatives. *Can Fam Physician*. 2011;57:e83.
5. Mikhael N, Ozon P, Rhule C. *Defining the Physician Assistant Role in Ontario*. HealthForce Ontario; 2007.
6. Physician Assistant Certification Council of Canada. http://www.capa-acam.ca.

7. Government of Canada. Canadian Armed Forces creates new officer occupation for Physician Assistants. http://news.gc.ca/web/article-en.do?nid=1079489.

8. *United Kingdom Association of Physician Assistants: Evaluation of Physician Assistants to NHS Scotland: final report.* UHI Millennium Institute; 2009. https://static1.squarespace.com/static/544f552de4b0645de79fbe01/t/54b544e0e4b0c1225eb116ce/1421165792194/Scotland-PA-Final-report-Jan-09.pdf. Accessed 26 June 2016.

9. UK Association of Physician Assistants website. www.ukapa.co.uk. Accessed October 12, 2012.

10. Aiello M, Roberts K. Development and Progress of the United Kingdom Physician Associate Profession. *JAAPA*. In press.

11. Merkle F, Ritsema T, Bauer S, et al. The physician assistant: shifting the paradigm of European medical practice? *HSR Proceedings in Intensive Care and Cardiovascular Anesthesia*. 2011;3(4):255.

12. van Vught AJ, van den Brink GT, Wobbes T. Implementation of the physician assistant in Dutch health care organizations: primary motives and outcomes. *Health Care Manag (Frederick)*. 2014;33(2):149–153.

13. Hooker RS, Kuilman L. Physician assistant education: five countries. *J Physician Assist Educ*. 2011;22(1):53–58.

14. Timmermans MJ, van Vught AJ, Van den Berg M, et al. Physician assistants in medical ward care: a descriptive study of the situation in the Netherlands. *J Eval Clin Pract*. 2015. http://dx.doi.org/10.1111/jep.12499.

15. Simkens ABM, van Baar ME, van Balen FAM, Verheij RA, van den Hoogen HJM, Schrijvers AJP. The physician assistant in general practice in the Netherlands. *J Physician Assist Educ*. 2009;20:30–38.

16. van den Driesschen Q, de Roo F. Physician assistants in the Netherlands. *JAAPA*. 2014 Sep;27(9):10–11.

17. Oliphant J. "Present": Ebola's impact on PAs in Liberia. *Clinician Reviews*. 2015;25(9):41–42. http://www.clinicianreviews.com/specialty-focus/infectious-disease/article/present-ebolas-impact-on-pas-in-liberia/e5d7d256748acb4bfec72cfa6ef031f4.html.

18. Kuilman L, Sundar G, Cherian KM. Physician assistant education in India. *J Physician Assist Educ*. 2012;23(3):56–59.

19. Sundar G. Physician assistants in India: triumphs and tribulations. *JAAPA*. 2014;27(4):9–11.

20. Adjase ET. Physician assistants in Ghana. *JAAPA*. 2015 Apr;15(4):28. http://journals.lww.com/jaapa/Fulltext/2015/04000/Physician_assistants_in_Ghana.1.aspx.

21. Clinical Associates. A new kind of health professional in South Africa. http://www.kznhealth.gov.za/Clinical_Associate/clinical_associates.pdf.

22. Clinical Associates website. http://www.twinningagainstaids.org/documents/CABoolketFinal_lowres.pdf. Accessed January 4, 2012.

23. Merkle F, Ritsema T, Bauer S, et al. The physician assistant: shifting the paradigm of European medical practice? *HSR Proceedings in Intensive Care and Cardiovascular Anesthesia*. 2011;3(4):255.

24. Kuhns D, Tozier W, Hearn D. *Physician Assistants and Military Medical Services (Poster) for the Annual Conference of the American Academy of Physician Assistants*; June 1-4, 2011. Las Vegas.

25. Nondo H, Jebakumar A, Fernandez J. Physician assistant education in the Kingdom of Saudi Arabia. *Journal of Physician Assistant Education*. 2013;24(4):22–25.

26. Duale Hochschule Baden-Württemberg Karlsruhe/Baden-Württemberg Cooperative State University Karlsruhe. http://www.dhbw-karlsruhe.de/allgemein/newssingle/article/studiengang-physician-assistantarztassistent-organisiert-tagung/64/. Accessed October 12, 2012.

27. New Zealand Ministry of Health. Phase II of the Physician Assistant Demonstrations Evaluation Report. http://www.health.govt.nz/publication/phase-ii-physician-assistant-demonstrations-evaluation-report.

28. World Health Organization. http://www.who.int/gho/countries/afg.pdf. Accessed November 20, 2011.

29. NATO Training Mission—Afghanistan. http://ntm-a.com/wordpress2/archives/2175. Accessed November 20, 2011.

30. Berkowitz O, Jacobson E, Fire G, Afek A. Physician assistants in Israel. *JAAPA*. 2014;27(12):7–8.

31. Coming soon: Physician assistants, T. Dvorin, *Israel National News*. 20 Dec 2015. http://www.israelnationalnews.com/News/News.aspx/205211#.V20KEKb2a-s.

CHAPTER 4

PHYSICIAN ASSISTANT EDUCATION: PAST, PRESENT, AND FUTURE CHALLENGES

Anthony A. Miller • Olivia Ziegler

OVERVIEW OF PHYSICIAN ASSISTANT EDUCATION

Physician assistant (PA) education has matured and grown significantly since its humble beginning in 1967 with the graduation of three ex-Navy corpsman students at Duke University. By the end of 2015, the number of programs grew to nearly 200 with an estimated enrollment of 20,700 students (Physician Assistant Education Association [PAEA] research staff). The typical PA program is 27 months in duration with more than 2000 hours of clinical education and offers a master's degree upon graduation.[1] Resident tuition and fees for PA education are much lower in publicly supported schools than private schools, with average costs for students of $48,831 and $87,357, respectively. Typically, students begin their PA education at the graduate level, but some colleges and universities offer 3 + 2 or 4 + 2 options in which the candidate is accepted to the PA track at the freshman level and subsequently completes both a bachelor's and a master's degree.

Getting into PA school is quite competitive. There are more than six candidates for each seat. The typical PA student is white, female, aged 26 years, and with an undergraduate grade point average of 3.52.[1] Most PA students would qualify for medical school.

The quality of PA education is ensured by rigorous standards required through accreditation by an independent organization, the Accreditation Review Commission on Education for the Physician Assistant (ARC-PA). The ARC-PA has its roots in the Joint

Review Committee on Education for the Physician Assistant (JRC-PA) established in 1971 under the auspices of the American Medical Association's (AMA's) Committee on Allied Health Education and Accreditation (CAHEA). In 1991, the ARC-PA became an independent body. The most recent (fourth) edition of the Standards for PA Education became effective in September 2010. The Standards establish the minimum requirements for PA education in terms of resources, operations, curriculum, and evaluation and assessment. Although accreditation is voluntary, technically all PA programs must achieve and maintain accreditation because only graduates of accredited PA programs may take the national certifying examination, which is required for licensure in all states. The ARC-PA Commission, which sets policy and makes accreditation decisions, is composed of 22 members representing organized medicine, the PA profession, and the public.[2] In addition to oversight of education at the PA program level, colleges and universities are reviewed and accredited by regional accrediting agencies. Regional accreditation ensures standards are met regarding curriculum, faculty qualifications, and general operations of the colleges and universities. If an institution loses accreditation by the regional agency, it would jeopardize eligibility for transfer of credits and participation in the federal student loan programs.

The PAEA serves as the only advocacy organization for PA education at large. It was founded in 1972 as the Association of Physician Assistant Programs (APAP). Governed by a 12-member elected board, the PAEA provides a wide range of products and services for its member programs. Some of the services PAEA provides include faculty development workshops, testing products (e.g., End of Rotation Exams), various research reports to inform members and the public, and an annual education forum conference that provides faculty with an opportunity to learn about the latest teaching and evaluation strategies. PAEA also provides oversight for the Centralized Application Service for Physician Assistants (CASPA), which serves as the portal for admission to most PA programs. PAEA's mission is to pursue excellence, foster faculty development, advance the body of knowledge that defines quality education and patient-centered care, and promote diversity in all aspects of PA education.[3]

BRIEF HISTORY OF PHYSICIAN ASSISTANT EDUCATION

Overview

Significant advancements and innovations are often attributed to thought leaders who responded to a need and filled the gap. In addition to the actions taken by leaders in the PA education movement, one must also consider what other influential events were occurring around the same time that either provided a stimulus for innovation or the right environment for the innovation to take hold. For each decade starting in the 1960s, a summary of the historical context is reviewed followed by key events that occurred in PA education.

1960s

Historical Context

Although many factors may have influenced the development of the PA profession at that time, the 1960s witnessed a time of significant change in the health care arena. Beginning in the 1950s, the U.S. health system began to see growth in the numbers of hospitals as innovations in medicine and treatment shifted the role of hospitals from a caretaking role to a curative role. By the 1950s, hospitals employed more people than the steelmaking, rail, and auto industries combined.[4] In July 1965, President Lyndon Johnson signed the Medicare and Medicaid bills into law, which opened the health care doors for many elderly and poor individuals. The original Medicare program provided for hospital (Part A) and outpatient (Part B) insurance that was expected to provide coverage for more than 19 million individuals aged 65 years and older.[5,6]

The need for more health care providers was recognized as physicians began to be attracted to specialties born out of advances in technology and innovations such as open heart surgery using a heart–lung machine (1953), coronary artery bypass (1967), the beginnings of successful transplant surgeries, and long-term hemodialysis (1960) to name just a few.[7] During the same time, combat medics and corpsmen who served in the Vietnam War were seen as having a strong foundation to fill the gaps in health care.

Physician Assistant Education Events

Although one can find prototypes of the PA profession that were either formally or informally (e.g., apprentice model) prepared, the first formal educational program is generally considered to be the Duke program in North Carolina. Under the leadership of Dr. Eugene Stead, the first class of four PA students began their journey in 1965. Two years later, the first three formally trained PA graduates entered the workforce. Shortly after the first program at Duke launched, Dr. Richard Smith founded the MEDEX model of PA education at the University of Washington in 1969. The MEDEX model combined a short period of classroom study with a longer apprentice-like period with a potential physician employer. Other education models were established at by Dr. Hugh Myers at Alderson-Broaddus (the first baccalaureate program) and by Dr. Henry Silver at the University of Colorado (the first graduate-level program). The University of Colorado was first established as a Child Health Associate program with a 3-year curriculum to prepare individuals to work primarily in pediatrics. Early in the PA profession's history, specialty PA programs were also developed. In 1967, the first entry-level program in surgery was launched at the University of Alabama. Later surgical programs were initiated at Cornell Medical Center in New York and Cuyahoga Community College in Ohio. There were also other entry-level specialty programs in fields such as orthopedics and urology.[8] These subspecialty programs only existed for a short while, and only the three surgery-focused programs survived past 2000.

1970s

Historical Context

During the 1970s, the federal government needed to respond to the increasing demand for health care services spurred on by the enactment of Medicare and Medicaid, as well new health care services available through the advent of technology. In 1970, the National Health Service Corps was established to help address the lack of doctors in rural and inner city areas.[9] In 1971, the Comprehensive Health Manpower Act was passed, creating significant funding for the development of additional PA educational programs. By 1973, the war in Vietnam was coming to a close, which would eventually lead to a decrease in the number of medics and corpsman that would be available to enter the profession. Technological advances in medicine, such as improved antirejection medications for solid organ transplantation, the development of the computed tomography scanner, and the advent of in vitro fertilization, meant that medical care was now available for diseases that previously would have caused death. Increased demand for medical care meant increased demand for medical care providers, such as PAs.

Physician Assistant Education Events

The 1970s could be characterized as the decade for the professionalization of the PA career. During this time, PA advocacy associations were launched, and the foundations were laid for PA education accreditation and the national certification examination. During the same time, the first growth spurt of

educational programs was seen, including the launch of the first postgraduate "residency" program for PAs at Montefiore Hospital in 1971.

Early PA leaders and the AMA's Council on Medical Education recognized the need for some mechanism to evaluate the quality of educational programs. In 1971, the first accrediting body, the JRC-PA, was established under the auspices of the AMA's CAHEA. The *Essentials of Accredited Educational Program for the Assistant to the Primary Care Physician* were adopted and approved by the AMA's House of Delegates to provide a written document, which was used for determining whether or not a program met minimum requirements.

In the early years of the profession, there was also a need to ensure to state regulators, doctors, and patients that PA graduates had the background knowledge and skills to practice in their chosen field. The Registry of Physicians' Associates, formed in 1970, issued certificates of approved programs and administered examinations to ensure competency of informally trained PAs. Later, the Registry was incorporated into the American Academy of Physician Assistants and was dissolved as the National Commission on Certification of Physician Assistants (NCCPA) began to take on the PA certification role in 1975.

In 1972, the first and only organization for representation and advocacy of PA education was formed with 16 charter members. Through funding by the Robert Wood Johnson Foundation, the APAP (later changed to the PAEA) was able to establish a home with the American Academy of Physician Assistants (AAPA) in Arlington, Virginia. The initial role of APAP was to facilitate faculty development and sharing of ideas about curriculum, teaching, and evaluation. However, the APAP at this time was incorporated into the fabric of the AAPA, and as such the AAPA also took an active role in PA initial and continuing education. One example was *The Development of Standards to Ensure the Competency of Physician Assistants*, which was a five-volume report funded by the federal government and included a role delineation for PAs. The role delineation provided a foundation for mapping PA program curricula.[10]

1980s

Historical Context

In 1980, the widely disseminated report of the Graduate Medical Education National Advisory Committee (GMENAC) to the Health and Human Services was issued. The Committee predicted a physician surplus and recommended that medical schools decrease enrollment in the entering class by 10% to 17%. It further recommended that nonphysician health care provider enrollments be capped and called for further research on PAs, nurse practitioners (NPs), and CNMs. The Graduate Medical Education National Advisory Committee (GMENAC) also contained some positive recommendations regarding PAs, including in the report recommendations to the states to broaden the scope of PA practice and authorize limited prescriptive authority. In addition, the report contained a recommendation that "Medicare, Medicaid, and other insurance programs should recognize and provide reimbursement for the services of NPs, PAs and nurse-midwives in those states where they are legally entitled to provide these services" (recommendation 14 of the nonphysician provider panel).[11]

In 1986, through the Omnibus Budget Reconciliation Act, PL 99-210, PAs and NPs were approved to receive reimbursement under Medicare. Reimbursement for Medicare services was made to the practice that hired the PA, not the provider. PAs were reimbursed at 85% of the physicians' rate for hospital and nursing home care and 65% of the physicians' rate for first assistant in surgery services. PAs providing services in certified rural health clinics were reimbursed at 100%. Reimbursement for PA services provided increased job opportunities for PAs. The improved PA job market stimulated interest in the profession by potential PAs and caused universities to develop new PA programs to meet the increasing demand.

Physician Assistant Education Events

During the 1980s, there was a slowing in the growth of PA educational programs in response to GMENAC (Fig. 4.1). PA education at that time was still provided predominantly in academic medical centers. In 1985, 21 of 33 existing PA programs were housed in medical schools (http://www.arc-pa.org/acc_programs). In 1985, under the leadership of Dr. Denis Oliver at the University of Iowa, the first national survey of PA education and PA education programs was conducted and published. It has been published consistently since then. In 2015, the 30th program survey report was released by the PAEA.

1990s

Historical Context

Although health maintenance organizations (HMOs) can trace their roots back to as early as 1910 in Tacoma, Washington, there was a rapid growth of HMOs in the 1990s. The rise of HMOs was spurred in part by the need to bring down health care costs as they reached 13.4% of gross domestic product in 1993 and were predicted to reach 20% by the end of the decade.[12] Because the financial model is supposed to favor prevention, many HMOs began to use PAs.

In addition, policymakers became increasingly aware that the dramatic increase in health care costs was not matched by improved patient outcomes. In September 1993, President Bill Clinton announced his intention to lead a major health care reform initiative to address these concerns. Unfortunately, his reform plan did not gain the support of Congress.[13]

Physician Assistant Education Events

Beginning in the mid-1990s, there was another spurt in the development of new PA programs. During this decade, an additional 65 programs enrolled their first

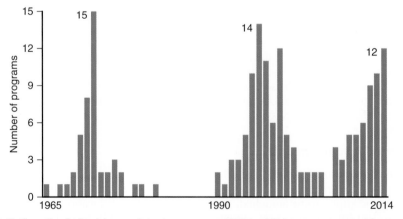

FIG. 4.1 ■ Growth of physician assistant programs, 1965 to 2014, as represented by year first class enrolled). (From Physician Assistant Education Association. *By the Numbers: 30th Report on Physician Assistant Education Programs in the United States, 2015.* Washington, DC: Author; 2015.)

classes. During the 1990s, there was an increasing realization that the tremendous growth in PA programs was resulting in a high number of PA faculty who were qualified by clinical experience but lacking in teaching skills. The APAP was offering workshops and seminars but formalized these activities in 1998 under the APAP Faculty Development. Initial faculty development workshops were designed primarily to assist faculty with basic skills such as writing better examinations, development of syllabi, and working effectively in the academic environment. There were also extended leadership workshops for individuals new to the program director role. Today, there are at least 15 to 20 different "courses" ranging from clinical coordination skills to use of simulation for teaching and evaluation (http://www.paeaonline.org/events/pando-workshops).

In 1998, *US News and World Report* (*USNWR*) released its first ranking of graduate-level PA programs. Although there was (and continues to be) much skepticism surrounding the *USNWR* methodology, inclusion of PA programs in the rankings helped legitimize PA education within academia.

2000s

Historical Context

The 2000s were marked by continued advancements in medicine, many related to discoveries from the Human Genome Project. Personalized medicine became a real possibility for the first time. The terrorism threats after September 11, 2001, and several subsequent cases of anthrax infection resulted in significant federal funding and research into combating threats related to bioterrorism.

This decade is also marked by a national concern for health care quality as evidenced by the release of the seminal report by the Institute of Medicine (IOM), *Crossing the Quality Chasm: A New Health System for the Twenty-first Century*, which pointed out the human and financial cost of medical errors. In 2008, Berwick, Nolan, and Whittington proposed a paradigm for improving the nation's health system. They proposed what is now commonly called the "Triple Aim: improving the experience of care, improving the health of populations, and reducing per capita costs of health care" (IOM, *Crossing the Quality Chasm*).

Prompted by concerns about medical errors and patient safety from overworked physician residents as well as a petition by the American Medical Student Association and others to the U.S. Occupational Safety and Health Administration (OSHA) in 2001, the Accreditation Council on Graduate Medical Education (ACGME) began to look at resident and patient issues relative to workload.[14] It was not until 2003 that the ACGME established tighter restrictions on the hours residents could work and be on call. These restrictions were later tightened further in 2011 and contributed in part to the need for more PAs in academic medical centers and teaching hospitals.

Physician Assistant Education Events

One of the seminal events that occurred early in this decade was the endorsement of the master's degree as the standard entry-level degree to the profession by the PAEA (then the APAP) in October 2000.[15] From 2000, the percentage of graduate-level PA programs increased from 49% to 93%. In March 2000, the ARC-PA left the Commission on Accreditation of Allied Health Educational Programs (CAAHEP) to become an independent organization.

The increased interest in PA education by students helped to spawn the CASPA in 2001. This service allows applicants to PA educational programs to file one application and have it disseminated to as many as programs as they choose. Since the launch of CASPA, the number of applicants to PA schools has increased. In the 2005 to 2006 cycle, there were 7933 applicants, and this rose dramatically to 22,997 by the 2014 to 2015 cycle.

The endorsement of the master's degree as the proper degree for PAs in 2000 did not end the discussion about degrees. The decision of the NP profession to endorse the Doctor of Nurse Practice (DNP) degree as the entry-level degree for NPs spurred further discussion regarding a clinical doctorate for PAs. In March 2009, representatives of the entire PA community and others came together for the Doctoral Summit. The purpose of the summit was "to develop recommendations to the profession on whether the clinical doctorate is appropriate as an entry-level degree, as a postgraduate degree, or not at all." The outcome of the summit was that that PA profession unified around four recommendations: (1) opposition of the entry-level doctorate, (2) re-endorsement of the master's degree as the entry-level and terminal degree for the profession, (3) support of postgraduate clinical doctorates, and (4) recommendation to explore bridge programs to allow PAs advanced standing in medical schools.[16]

2010s

Historical Context

One of the most influential events during this decade was the passage of the Affordable Care Act in 2010. This act fundamentally changed health care with provisions that increased access to health insurance for millions, allowed young adults to stay on their parents' insurance plans until the age of 26 years, outlawed denial of health insurance coverage based on preexisting conditions, and required coverage for preventive health measures. In addition, the law directed the federal agency charged with administering Medicare to find and implement measures to decrease the costs of health care.

Physician Assistant Education Events

The 2010 decade will likely be remembered for the third spike in PA program growth, particularly among private, nonprofit colleges and universities not associated with medical schools. During this decade, there were calls for health care to be increasingly delivered by teams of health professionals. Although physicians and PAs have worked as teams since the inception of the profession, there was a recognition that the team needed to be expanded. Two important reports were released in 2011 by the Interprofessional Education Collaborative: *Core Competencies for Interprofessional Practice*[17] and *Team-Based Competencies: Building a Shared Foundation for Education and Clinical Practice*.[18] Unfortunately, the PA profession was excluded from the initial members of the collaborative formed in 2009 but was invited to participate in events and became a member in early 2016. During this decade, PA partnerships were strengthened with organized medicine as evidenced by the joint position statement of PAEA and the Society for the Teachers of Family Medicine.[19] In April 2014, as further evidence of the strengthening of PA and physician partnerships, the PAEA relocated its headquarters to the same building with the Association of American Medical Colleges (AAMC) and the American Dental Education Association (ADEA).

CHARACTERISTICS OF PHYSICIAN ASSISTANT EDUCATION

Physician assistant education is "minds on" and "hands on" from the first day. In a short and intense period of time, PA educators train students to practice in a complex world; they teach students to analyze data, care for patients, work in teams, and demonstrate their own value. Perhaps most critically, they teach students to develop a learner mindset: how to learn, how to reflect, and how to adapt. The PA education model of the past 50 years has done a laudatory job creating new PA graduates with knowledge of health and disease ready to practice in an ever-changing health care landscape. PA education achieved this by being adaptable, planning for growth in the profession, and watching for changes in clinical practice that could potentially affect the future of health care and the PA profession.[20]

Adaptability is a theme deeply woven into the fabric of the PA profession. One only needs to reflect on the beginning of the PA profession to recognize how quickly change occurs. Early PA graduates could not have foreseen the significant advances that have occurred in both education and clinical practice in the past 50 years. The willingness and ability of PA programs to undergo constant change is unique. The profession, supported by accreditation standards, has always encouraged PA programs in different types of institutions (from public to private and from community colleges to academic medical centers) to evaluate their institutions' missions and the unique needs of their communities and to regularly implement the changes required to respond to the needs of society.

The differences among PA programs are perhaps most notable at the student application and admission phase. There is a significant variation in admission requirements across all PA programs. Each program has set prerequisites that identify applicants who are most likely to succeed at that particular institution and to progress through the program's unique curriculum and help the program meet its mission. Multiple studies have pointed out the diversity of prerequisite course requirements.[21,22] Although some have argued that the lack of prerequisite standardization may decrease the number of applicants to PA programs, data from the Central Application Service for Physician Assistants do not bear this concern out. In fact, the application pool grew nearly 40% in the early part of the century and continues to grow 6% to 9% a year.[23,24]

Physician assistant programs include a number of different admission requirements to help identify ideal applicants for their programs. Historically, the PA profession has been thought of as a "second career," attracting individuals with years to decades of experience in other fields such as nursing, emergency medicine, and rehabilitation. It remains true today that most matriculants have been employed or have volunteered in a health care field. However, as the profession has grown and the number of applicants has increased, we have seen a decrease in both the average age of matriculants and the average health care experience required by programs.[25] Programs have adapted to attract and accept a younger generation of students.

A unique challenge in PA education is the short time during which students move through the curriculum to graduate and become clinicians. The average length of a PA program is just under 29 months, split between didactic and clinical education.[1] This short training period gives programs very little time to deliver a significant amount of education and students very little time to grow into their new professional identities. In addition, unlike doctors, PAs do not typically undergo postgraduate residency training.

Physician assistant education provides students with an ongoing stream of appropriately sequenced active-learning experiences. Just over half of all PA programs integrate clinical training experiences into the didactic year.[1] These introductory clinical experiences put students in the community with a preceptor-mentor to help hone history taking, physical examination, differential diagnosis, presentation, and therapeutic skills before entering their formal clinical rotations. Many programs also provide students with early clinical experiences via service learning activities. Service learning fosters a greater understanding of population health, culturally and socioeconomically appropriate care, and the role that service plays in the practice of medicine.

In today's curriculum, students are part of the patient-centered team in almost every clinical setting. PA programs, their institutions, and community partners have long shared a common culture of teaching and learning. Providing students with clinical practice experiences would not be possible without strong community partnerships; hospitals, clinics, and preceptors all share in the responsibility with PA programs to provide clinical training of PA students. During the formal clinical education phase, students learn clinical skills, leadership, and professionalism. This intersection between education and practice is an important one, if for no other reason than that many PAs obtain their first PA jobs from a doctor or PA with whom they trained in the clinical year.

Historically, PAs have been educated in a one-on-one clinical training model, meaning each individual clinical student is assigned to an individual clinical preceptor. This model has served the profession well for decades. However, it was designed to train a much more limited population of students at a time when there was not as much competition for training sites. Today, opportunities for students to get to know and assume responsibility for the management of patients is becoming more and more limited. In today's competitive clinical training environment, there is an emphasis on developing new and innovative clinical training models that better use current resources and continue to provide students with authentic roles in patient care.

CURRENT ISSUES IN PHYSICIAN ASSISTANT EDUCATION

Clinical Sites

Today there are a number of challenges to effective clinical site and preceptor recruitment and retention. More than half of all PA program directors report that they are very concerned about having sufficient numbers of clinical training sites and preceptors for students.[26] A changing health care environment that emphasizes increased accountability for patient outcomes combined with decreased reimbursement for clinical services has placed limitations on the number of supervised clinical training placements available to PA programs. Additionally, there has been significant growth in the sheer number of learners in the clinical environment, leading to unintended competition within and among health professions for supervised clinical training placements.[27] This challenge pushes PA educators to develop creative ways to best use current resources. Potential solutions include designing interprofessional clinical training experiences that accommodate multiple students in a shared rotation. Collaboration with clinical practices also expands opportunities in clinical training. PA programs must build partnerships with clinical sites whereby it is understood that all parties have a shared stake in training PA students. The goals of educators and employers are mutual and synergistic—both are working together for the preparation of well-qualified future PAs. Practices need to be reminded that precepting students is one excellent way to discover and select the best students for employment after graduation.

Last, PA educators should look to the students in their classrooms as future preceptors. PA educators should foster a culture of teaching and learning in each one of our students. PA students are already taught that this is a career of lifelong learning. If being a PA means being a lifelong learner, then it also means being a lifelong teacher. Teaching makes up an important part of our overall professional identity and should be part of our ongoing professional development after graduation. All PAs don't choose to be full-time educators, but our profession is, by its very nature, one in which we teach. We teach people every day—our colleagues, patients, administrators, and students. A study published by the Robert Graham Center shows that PA students are highly influenced by their clinical preceptors, and PA programs should actively teach their students to embrace clinical teaching as part of their professional identities.[28,29]

Expansion of Physician Assistant Programs

As the student applicant pool and job market have continued to grow, colleges and universities sought ways to meet the demand for PA education. There are three fundamental ways that PA education can expand. First, the capacity of existing programs can be increased to accommodate more students. Over the past 15 years, the average class size of U.S. PA programs has increased nearly 20%, rising from 40 in 2000 to 47.5 in 2014. In 2010, the federal government created a grant program called Expansion of Physician Assistant Training (EPAT) in conjunction with the passage of the Affordable Care Act. With this funding, PA programs that expanded their class sizes were able to offer student stipends up to $40,000. Twenty-seven programs were awarded funds for 5 years.

Another way programs were able to expand was to create satellite or distant campuses. First conceived by the University of Washington MEDEX) program, these campuses allowed schools to expand their enrollment and at the same time meet the need for education in other communities. The MEDEX program first established a satellite program in Sitka, Alaska, in 1993. Other programs soon followed suit by setting up distant campuses generally in more rural communities. Barry University was the first to establish a distant campus outside the continental United States. In 2011, the university established a satellite campus in St. Croix. The accreditation of the distant campus is linked to that of the main campus.

The third mechanism for expansion of PA training is to develop new PA programs. Most new PA programs that were developed during the current decade are at private, not-for-profit universities that are not affiliated with an academic medical center. Since 2000, there has been an increase in 83 accredited PA programs across the United States (http://www.arc-pa.org/acc_programs).

Faculty Development

As the number of PA programs grows, so does the need for PA faculty. Just as there is a science to medicine, there is also a science of teaching. PA faculty need professional development in the areas of teaching, management, and leadership. Faculty should undergo training in how to incorporate interactive teaching strategies and write effective written and practical tests. Faculty must also learn to create balance in their own lives among teaching, clinical practice, community service, and research.[30]

Recruiting young, diverse, clinically active faculty can be challenging. Many PAs are simply unaware of the role, responsibilities, and opportunities associated with faculty positions. New faculty face learning essentially a new profession. Sources of stress for new faculty include teaching a large number of classes, demands to perform research and to publish, their new role as advisor to students, and the mysteries of the academic promotion process. However, many PA faculty enjoy the schedule flexibility; experience teaching students; and the opportunities for community service, research, and leadership.[1]

There is a growing emphasis on preceptor development as a pathway to core faculty positions. PA students, new graduates, and clinically active PAs should seek out training and development opportunities that prepare them to be clinical preceptors. PAs are nimble and well positioned to meet the rapidly evolving preceptor and faculty workforce needs. But we must embrace the teaching as an important part of our overall professional identity.

Diversity

Recruiting and building a diverse workforce is an important priority across all health professions because diversity in the workforce can decrease health disparities in the community.[31]

The PA profession, which grew philosophically out of a desire to improve access and quality of care for underserved patients, has had a commitment to building a diverse workforce from its very first days. Many early programs, in fact, received federal funding with the intent to increase the number, diversity, and geographic distribution of primary care providers, as well as to increase the number of underrepresented minorities in the PA profession. The first African American PA graduated from Duke in 1968, and by the mid-1970s, there were several programs established in both African American and Native American communities.[31]

As a result of this early interest in decreasing health disparities, PA programs had a higher percentage of underrepresented minority students enrolled in their programs during the 1980s and 1990s than other health profession programs.[31] Today, however, although there are still several minority-serving PA programs, PA program admissions have not been able to keep up with the diversification of the United States. According the U.S. Census Bureau, for example, just over 13% of the population in America is black or African American, but only 11.7% of the 2015 incoming PA class reports the same race. Additionally, the profession has slowly become primarily female, with the Census Bureau reporting only

50.8% of the American population as female but 72% of the incoming class reporting as female.[1,32]

Improving diversity in the PA workforce requires ongoing research and implementing changes at the community, institution (colleges and universities), program, and policy levels. PA programs and their parent institutions need to look to their communities to develop objectives that match the needs of the community, working with the community to both recruit new students and train current students. At the institutional level, we need improved strategies to promote diversity. PA program admissions committees must continue to institute policies and practices that specifically target diversity objectives. PA programs should also continue to build curricula that focus on improving PA students' ability to practice in racially and ethnically diverse communities. Additionally, at the policy level, we need to reduce financial barriers to health profession training, looking to Congress and federal funding programs (e.g., the Health Resources and Services Administration Title VII) to provide increased support for underrepresented students and for new graduates working in medically underserved areas. We should also look to enhance diversity-related accreditation standards and apply real sanctions if those standards are not met. Research remains critical; it provides the necessary data to support enhanced diversity efforts, holding us accountable for outcomes and reinforcing support among all stakeholders. Last, we must look not only to increase the diversity of the incoming class but also to seek to recruit diverse faculty and assure that diverse PAs have representation on admission panels and on the Accreditation Review Commission.[33]

Distance Education

Traditional PA education has been place bound, meaning that the entire curriculum was offered on the college or university campus. Even when most of the PA programs were offered at medical schools, most of the clinical training was done close by. In the past 30 years, however, distance education has become an increasingly popular model in higher education. Although PA education has not fully embraced distance education, some schools have established satellite campuses as described later. Delivery of instructional content varies at these campuses, with some hiring an entire team of faculty for the distant site and others using video conferencing technology (VCT). Some schools combine instruction by local faculty with VCT.

Only a few PA programs use distance education as the primary mode of instruction. The University of North Dakota offers a significant portion of it curriculum online, and students are only on campus after a 1-week orientation for four 2- to 5-week intervals during the remainder of the program (http://www.med.und.edu/physician-assistant/design-and-history.cfm). In 2015, Yale's PA program proposed a "blended" curriculum that would be a combination of online courses and clinical training. Along with this new educational model, Yale's proposal would have increased Yale's class size by more than 300 students per class. As of the writing of this chapter, the Yale program has yet to receive approval by the accrediting agency (http://news.yale.edu/2015/03/10/yale-launch-its-first-national-online-pa-program).

Arguments in favor of distance education include that it increases access to educational opportunities for individuals who may be place bound and that the learning outcomes are similar to those delivered via more traditional approaches. Those objecting to distance education as a primary delivery mode for PA curriculum cite potential issues of monitoring professional and interpersonal behaviors desired in a health care provider such as compassion and caring as well as evaluation of clinical skill competencies such as venipuncture, suturing, or physical examination techniques.

Doctoral Degree

Almost before the ink was dry on the resolution passed by the PA educators in October 2000 to designate the master's degree as the terminal degree for the profession, there was the beginning of discussions regarding a clinical doctorate for PAs. In 2000, pharmacy educators had decided to offer the Pharm D as the sole degree for pharmacists. The physical therapy profession had also decided in 2000 that its entry-level degree would be the Doctor of Physical Therapy (DPT) (*Today's Physical Therapist: A Comprehensive Review of a 21st-Century Health Care Profession*). In 2004, the American Association of Colleges of Nursing (AACN) called for the advanced practice nursing educational programs to move to the DNP by 2015 (*Fact Sheet: The Doctor of Nursing Practice*).

Although there were periodic communications in social media and in print, it was not until March 2009 when the PA profession formally examined the desirability of moving to a doctoral degree. A doctoral summit was convened with nearly 50 participants by two of the four PA organizations (AAPA and PAEA) to address the specific goal of "Develop[ing] recommendations to the profession on whether the clinical doctorate is appropriate as an entry-level degree, a postgraduate degree or not at all." One of the four recommendations was to oppose the entry-level doctorate for PAs.[16]

So what is the controversy surrounding the doctoral issue? Certainly, having a doctoral degree credential provides a certain prestige to the holder. Some argue that the number of credit hours and depth of learning experienced by typical PA students entitles them to a degree commensurate with that level of effort. Whereas the average number of semester credits in a PA program is slightly over 104, the minimum credits for a master's degree in public health is 42 semester credits (Accreditation Criteria for Public Health Programs, 2011). Some argue that PAs should have academic credential parity with nurse practitioners and pharmacy and other related professions because it would provide many benefits, including improved scope of practice and reimbursement for services.

Concerns regarding the clinical doctoral degree include the potential awkward clinical moment when a patient is introduced to his or her physician provider—Dr. Smith—and his or her PA provider—Dr. Jones. Another potential concern is that access to PA education may be constrained for certain disadvantaged populations that have experienced hurdles to higher education in the past. To date, there are no educational programs offering an entry-level clinical doctorate. However, one postgraduate emergency medicine program in Texas offers a clinical doctorate, and some institutions offer add-on doctoral degrees such as the Doctor of Health Science (DHS) degree. This issue is expected to remain unsettled over the near future.

LOOKING FORWARD: EMERGING ISSUES

Technology in Medicine and Education

Physician assistant educators are constantly challenged to keep up with not only the latest innovations and technology related to teaching, learning, and evaluation but also the latest clinical developments. In 2015 alone, the Food and Drug Administration (FDA) approved 45 novel drugs and nearly the same number of new medical devices (FDA). Recently, the availability of lower cost handheld ultrasound units is challenging the tried and true stethoscope as a diagnostic tool. Mobile devices such as the iPhone now have applications and attachments to enable electrocardiograms and capturing of retinal images. New research findings regularly result in changes to clinical practice guidelines. The rapid pace of change means that it is possible for some knowledge and clinical techniques taught in PA school to be outdated shortly after the PA graduates.

Mainstream computer technology, such as mobile phones, tablets, and laptops, has greatly influenced education by making information more accessible and providing more platforms for the delivery of instruction. Advances in video technology and Internet speed have allowed PA programs to deliver instructional content to satellite campuses, provide remote visits to clinical training sites, and provide educational content for the students to access at a time convenient for them. Nearly every school now uses some form of a learning management system (LMS) (e.g., Blackboard, Canvas) to deliver instructional content and to provide students with opportunities to interact remotely through discussion boards. Clinical experiences are now tracked via computer applications. Finally, the lower cost and increased availability of high-tech simulation devices and mannequins are providing realistic opportunities to practice clinical skills such as venipuncture and endotracheal intubation as well as training to work in teams in critical care scenarios. Studies have shown that high-fidelity simulation increases team effectiveness and clinical skill proficiency before real patient encounters.[34]

Cost of Education: Student Debt

Although the job market and pay for PAs are good, the cost of education continues to rise, resulting in an increasing debt load for PA graduates. In 2005, the average resident and nonresident tuition costs for the entire program were $34,167 and $41,723, respectively. Ten years later, the tuition had almost doubled to $64,961 and $75,964. Over the same time frame, incidental costs (books, equipment, and so on) had also increased significantly from $5018 to $8872 (PAEA 20th and 30th Annual Reports). Fig. 4.2 shows the historical trends in PA education costs. According to a report of newly certified PAs by the NCCPA, more than 54% had educational debt

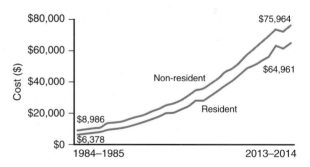

Note: These numbers were not adjusted for inflation.

FIG. 4.2 ■ Cost of physician assistant education, 1984 to 2014. (From Physician Assistant Education Association. *By the Numbers: 30th Report on Physician Assistant Education Programs in the United States, 2015.* Washington, DC: Author; 2015.)

after PA school between $75,000 and $175,000, with 12.5% reporting debt higher than $175,000.

Compounding the challenges to financing PA education is the fact that ceiling for federal loans (e.g., Stafford) is lower for PA students than for several other health professions. The lifetime limit for PA students is $138,500 compared with $224,000 for graduate students in public health. This means that students often need to finance their education through more costly loans such as the Grad-Plus loan program.

It is not clear if salaries will be able to keep pace with rising tuition and debt. In an effort to determine if student debt had an impact on graduate deployment into primary care specialties, the PAEA commissioned a study by the Robert Graham Center (http://www.graham-center.org/rgc/home) in 2014. The results indicated that the amount of debt had some influence but was not the major factor in specialty choice and geographic location decisions.[35]

Role of Simulation

Simulation is also playing, and will continue to play, an important role in providing students with clinical training experiences. The effectiveness of simulation has been well established, but currently the cost is high, and accreditation standards limit the use of simulation to replace clinical training. PA programs are working to integrate simulation as both a supplementation and enhancement to clinical training experiences. PA programs will also need to both develop more varied and validated simulations, as well as provide more formalized training for faculty on the development and use of simulation.

Leadership

The practice of medicine involves good communication, flexibility, hard work, and a passion. These skills are integral parts of the PA's identity and set up PAs to have excellent clinical relationships, both with other providers and with patients. These same skills also transition well into leadership positions. For decades, PAs have been called on to serve in leadership roles such as membership on hospital committees, state professional boards, or licensing boards. In today's rapidly changing health care landscape, PAs are also being called on to take leadership positions in health-focused enterprises (e.g., information technology), care-delivery organizations, the pharmaceutical industry, and the government. PAs are assuming higher level leadership roles and influencing the business of health care more than ever before. At the national organization levels, the AAPA has even

developed a Center for Healthcare Leadership and Management to provide professional development and advisory services to PAs in leadership and management positions.

Although PA education primarily focuses on clinical knowledge and skill development, leadership skills are also routinely taught in PA school. The Competencies for the Physician Assistant Profession, endorsed by all four national PA organizations, define the core knowledge, skills, and behaviors PAs should possess to practice in the health care field.[36] Although the document does not include leadership as a competency, it does emphasize the need for leadership skills. The competencies of "interpersonal and communication skills," "professionalism," and "systems-based practice" all clearly identify leadership skills. The Competencies for the Physician Assistant Profession document state: "[F]oremost, [professionalism] involves prioritizing the interests of those being served above one's own." And "systems-based practice" calls for leadership skills as PAs "work to improve the larger health care system of which their practices are a part." These competencies are an important part of PA education and the lifelong continuing education and professional development of PAs in practice.[36]

Maximizing the effectiveness of PAs in these newer leadership positions, however, will require an increased focus on leadership education. Beyond teaching the core interpersonal, communication, professionalism, and system-based practice skills, PA programs should also consider teaching hard leadership skills such as systems thinking, strategy setting, change management, and financial oversight.[37] Additionally, the Center for Creative Leadership reports that the health care sector's top priority for leadership development is improving the ability to lead employees and work in teams.[38] Team-based leadership requires having a good understanding of the other health professions, participative management, and both building and mending relationships. Continued development of interprofessional education models is therefore critical to developing future leaders.

Physician assistant students can take direct steps to get additional leadership training and experience in PA school. There are many leadership opportunities at the program, state, and national levels. Students should talk to their faculty advisors to help identify student specific leadership roles such as with the Student Academy of AAPA (SAAAPA) or fellowship training such as with the PAEA Student Health Policy Fellowship. Taking proactive steps as students will help move future graduates and the profession toward new and exciting leadership roles in the health care sector. Assuming higher level leadership roles and influencing the business of health care provides an opportunity to impact change at the highest level. As leadership opportunities for PAs grow, it is important that PAs not lose their clinical identities. PAs must hold on to their clinical identity and love for patient care. These attributes, along with executive skills, will produce leaders who can effectively lead and shape their organizations.

CONCLUSION

Physician assistant education has made significant strides since its humble beginning in 1965. Today it is one of the fastest growing professions in the United States. However, it is unclear how long this rapid growth will be sustainable. As of early 2016, there does not seem to be any slowing of growth in PA education, with 55 new programs in development and large numbers of applicant to PA programs. The expansion of access to health care through the Affordable Care Act, the aging of the U.S. population, and the retirement of baby boomer physicians are expected to contribute the continued growth of the PA profession. With this growth, PA programs will continue to be challenged to recruit and retain high-quality faculty and clinical training sites.

Physician assistant education must continue its tradition of high quality and adaptation to the needs of society. Teaching methods must continue to engage students and prepare clinicians for the needs of patients and the health care system, not just for immediately after graduation but also for a lifetime of clinical practice. Students need to embrace the concept of lifelong learning because the practice of medicine is in a constant state of change.

KEY POINTS

- The popularity of the PA profession has and continues to lead to a significant growth of PA programs.
- The growth of PA programs and other health professions has strained the capacity of clinical training sites to provide high-quality education and challenges PA programs to recruit and retain faculty.
- Because medicine and medical education are in a constant state of change, educational programs must continually evolve to meet the needs of students and the patients they will eventually serve.
- Physician assistant education and other health professional education must continue to find ways to prepare students to work in effective teams.

References

1. Physician Assistant Education Association. *By the Numbers: 30th Report on Physician Assistant Educational Programs in the United States, 2015*. Washington, DC: Author; 2015.
2. Accreditation Review Commission on Education for the Physician Assistant. *About ARC-PA*. http://www.arc-pa.org/about.
3. Physician Assistant Education Association. *About PAEA*. http://www.paeaonline.org/about-paea.
4. Stevens RA. Health care in the early 1960s. *Health Care Financing Rev*. 1996;18(2):11–21.
5. United States Department of Health and Human Services. History. https://www.cms.gov/About-CMS/Agency-Information/History/index.html?redirect=/History/.
6. Gluck MG, Reno V, eds. *Reflections on Implementing Medicare*. Washington, DC: National Academy of Social Insurance; January 2001.
7. National Kidney Foundation. https://www.kidney.org/transplantation/transaction/Milestones-Organ-Transplantation.
8. Fasser CE. Historical perspective of PA education. *J Am Acad Phys Assist*. 1992;5(9):663–670.
9. Nach BJ. *The Comprehensive Health Manpower Training Act of 1971: Panacea or Placebo?* 22 Cath. U. L. Rev. 1973;829. http://scholarship.law.edu/lawreview/vol22/iss4/6.
10. American Academy of Physician Assistants. *The Development of Standards to Ensure the Competency of Physician Assistants*. vols. I–V. Arlington, VA: Author; 1979.
11. Graduate Medical Education National Advisory Committee. *Report of the Graduate Medical Education National Advisory Committee to the Secretary*. Hyattsville, MD: U.S. Department of Health and Human Services; 1980.
12. Stanton MW, Rutherford MK. *Reducing costs in the health care system: learning from what has been done. Agency for Healthcare Research and Quality*; 2002. Research in Action Issue 9. AHRQ Pub. No. 020046. http://archive.ahrq.gov/research/findings/factsheets/costs/costria/costsria.pdf.
13. Starr P. What happened to health care reform? *American Prospect*. 1995;20:20–31. https://www.princeton.edu/~starr/20starr.html.
14. Accreditation Council for Graduate Medical Education. *ACGME Highlights Its Standards on Resident Duty Hours*, May 2001. https://www.acgme.org/acgmeweb/tabid/363/Publications/Papers/PositionPapers/HighlightsItsStandardsonResidentDutyHours-.aspx.
15. Miller AA, et al. Association of Physician Assistant Programs Degree Task Force Final Report, September 28, 2000. *Perspective on Physician Assistant Education*. 2000;11(3):169–177.

16. Physician Assistant Education Association. *PA Clinical Doctorate Summit Final Report and Summary*. Alexandria, VA: Author; 2009.

17. Interprofessional Education Collaborative Expert Panel. *Core Competencies for Interprofessional Collaborative Practice: Report of an Expert Panel*. Washington, DC: Author; 2011.

18. Interprofessional Education Collaborative. *Team-Based Competencies: Building a Shared Foundation for Education and Clinical Practice. Conference Proceedings*. Washington, DC: February 16–17, 2011.

19. Keahey D, et al. Educating primary care teams for the future: family medicine and physician assistant education. *J Phys Assist Educ*. 2012;23(3):33–41.

20. Miller AA, Glicken AD. The future of physician assistant education. *J Phys Assist Educ*. 2007;18(3):109–116.

21. Jones PE, Miller AA. Physician assistant education: a call for standardized prerequisites. *Perspective on Physician Assistant Education*. 2002;13(2):114.

22. Dehn RW. Applicants are slip sliding away. *Clin Advis*. 2002;5(5):152.

23. Ruback T, Coombs J, Keck M, et al. Central application service for physician assistants: five-year report. *J Phys Assist Educ*. 2007;18(3):52–59.

24. Physician Assistant Education Association. *CASPA: for Programs*. http://www2.paeaonline.org/index.php?ht=d/sp/i/141724/pid/141724.

25. Hamann R. *Brief Report: Matriculating Student Survey. Work and Health Care Experience*. Washington, DC: Physician Assistant Education Association; 2013. http://paeaonline.org/wp-content/uploads/2015/09/IssueBriefWorkHealthCare.pdf. Assessed February 27, 2016.

26. Physician Assistant Education Association. *Issue Brief: Payment of Clinical Sites and Preceptors in PA Education*. http://www.paeaonline.org/wp-content/uploads/2015/09/PaymentClinicalSites-PreceptorsPAEducation.pdf.

27. Physician Assistant Education Association. *Recruiting and Maintaining U.S. Clinical Training Sites: Joint Report of the 2013 Multi-Discipline Clerkship Training Site Survey*. http://paeaonline.org/wp-content/uploads/2015/10/Recruiting-and-Maintaining-U.S.-Clinical-Training-Sites.pdf.

28. Ziegler OW. Lifelong learners = lifelong teachers: precepting is part of our identify. *PA Professional*. September 2014.

29. Robert Graham Center. *The Impact of Debt Load on Physician Assistants Project Report: Executive Summary*. http://www.graham-center.org/content/dam/rgc/documents/publications-reports/reports/impact-debt-physician-assistants.pdf.

30. Essary AC, Coplan B, Liang M, et al. The professional development needs of faculty of physician assistant programs. *J Phys Assist Educ*. 2009;20(4):40–44.

31. Mulitalo KE, Straker H. Diversity in physician assistant education. *J Phys Assist Educ*. 2007;18(3):46–51.

32. United States Census Bureau. Quick Facts United States. http://quickfacts.census.gov/qfd/states/00000.html.

33. Smedley BD, Butler AS, Bristow LR. *In the Nation's Compelling Interests: Ensuring Diversity in the Health-Care Workforce*. Washington, DC: National Academies Press; 2004.

34. Lateff F. Simulation-based learning: just like the real thing. *J Emerg Trauma Shock*. 2010;3(4):348–352.

35. Robert Graham Center. *The Impact of Debt Load on Physician Assistants*; 2014. http://www.graham-center.org/content/dam/rgc/documents/publications-reports/reports/impact-debt-physician-assistants.pdf.

36. Physician Assistant Education Association. *Competencies for the Physician Assistant Profession*; 2012. http://www2.paeaonline.org/index.php?ht=a/GetDocumentAction/i/161748.

37. Jain SH. The skills doctors and nurses need to be effective executives. *Harvard Business Review*. https://hbr.org/2015/04/the-skills-doctors-need-to-be-effective-executives.

38. Fernandez CSP, Peterson HB, Holmström SW, et al. *Developing Emotional Intelligence for Healthcare Leaders*. Center for Creative Leadership. http://cdn.intechopen.com/pdfs-wm/27249.pdf.

The Faculty Resources can be found online at www.expertconsult.com.

SAFETY IN CLINICAL SETTINGS

Darwin Brown

This chapter provides information to prepare physician assistant (PA) students for safe clinical experiences. Health professional students are typically required to hone many skills by working and practicing on real patients. Students are sometimes placed in "educational" situations with minimal supervision and asked to perform procedures for which they are not adequately trained. Such circumstances place students at risk for injuries ranging from needlestick to more substantial injuries.

All PA programs require students to provide basic health information when they are admitted. The only confidential student health information that can be disclosed to the program involves immunizations and results of tuberculosis (TB) screening. Programs do not have access to other types of health information on students. Students usually complete a health status form describing any medical concerns or significant items in their medical history. In addition, programs require an immunization record, with special emphasis on the currency of rubeola, rubella, and tetanus booster. Most, if not all, programs require students to obtain the hepatitis B vaccine before enrollment. TB testing is also performed on entry into the program and is repeated annually. The Accreditation Review Commission for the Education Physician Assistant directs these basic requirements as part of the PA program's accreditation process and by the educational institution with which the program is affiliated.

Before enrollment or at orientation, many programs require students to undergo background checks, drug screening, or both. These procedures help to ensure a safe environment within the educational institution.

Students may receive required information on sexual harassment, bloodborne pathogens, safety, and the Health Insurance Portability and Accountability Act (HIPAA). PA programs cover these topics to ensure a level of student health and safety. The greatest potential for exposure to risk starts when students begin clinical rotations. The exposures may include infectious agents (hepatitis, human immunodeficiency virus [HIV], TB), physical injury (needlestick, laceration, latex allergy, physical attack by a patient), and emotional abuse (verbal abuse, belittlement, sexual harassment). Programs differ in the ways they educate, prevent exposures, and protect students. In the following sections, safety issues important to the clinical portion of a PA training program are explored.

ROTATION SAFETY

To maintain your safety on clinical rotations, common sense is the rule. Be aware of your surroundings at all times, especially when at a new location. Ask your preceptor to review clerkship safety policies. Ask questions regarding who has access to the clinic space, whether chaperones are required for male and female examinations, what to do in case of an emergency, and what to do if you sustain an injury.

Remember to have your needlestick injury protocol available on rotations.

UNIVERSAL PRECAUTIONS

One area often neglected by students is the consistent use of universal precautions. Universal precautions are infection control guidelines designed to protect health care providers from exposure to diseases spread by blood and certain body fluids.[1] Implemented in the 1980s as HIV infection became more prominent, universal precautions eliminated concerns about which patients might require precautions because of infection and which patients were not infected. Simply put, universal precautions require that you assume everyone may be able to transmit hepatitis B, HIV, or other infectious agents, and therefore, the same precautions are used for all patients. The types of exposures for which universal precautions should be used and for which they are not necessary can be found in Table 5.1.

Universal precautions involve the use of personal protective equipment such as gloves, gowns, masks, and protective eyewear, which can reduce the risk of bloodborne pathogen exposure to the health care student's skin or mucous membranes. As a student and future professional, it is incumbent on you to use universal precautions whenever appropriate. If you are performing phlebotomy, suturing a laceration, or performing a punch biopsy, these precautions are in place to protect you from exposure to infectious agents, but they are effective only if you use them consistently.

TABLE 5.1 **Universal Precaution Requirements**	
Universal Precautions Required	**Universal Precautions Do *Not* Apply**
Semen	Feces
Vaginal secretions	Nasal secretions
Synovial fluid	Sputum
Cerebrospinal fluid	Sweat
Pleural fluid	Tears
Peritoneal fluid	Urine
Pericardial fluid	Vomitus unless contaminated with blood
Amniotic fluid	Saliva unless contaminated with blood

From Centers for Disease Control and Prevention. 2007 guideline for isolation precautions: preventing transmission of infectious agents in healthcare settings. http://www.cdc.gov/hicpac/pdf/isolation/Isolation2007.pdf.

INTERNATIONAL TRAVEL

Increasing numbers of health care students travel outside the United States as part of their clinical experience. International rotations are frequently seen as exciting and exotic adventures. These types of experiences provide students with a unique appreciation of diverse cultures, intensive language development, and opportunities to observe uncommon diseases. Most traveling students have a wonderful experience, bringing back lifetime memories and a desire to return to these areas in the future. However, to enjoy this type of clinical experience, you must consider your safety a priority and devote a portion of your preparation time to this goal.

Many international clinical destinations are in developing countries that may pose safety concerns. Before you leave the United States, participate fully in the planning of your trip. Check with your medical insurance company to determine if you are covered for emergency care while abroad. Evacuation back to the United States can easily cost $10,000 or more, depending on your location and medical condition. If you are not already covered by such insurance, purchase a policy that provides medical coverage and evacuation if necessary. The U.S. Department of State (http://www.state.gov/travel) is an excellent resource for information on traveling to foreign countries, including facts on medical emergencies and evacuation.

NEEDLESTICK AND SHARPS INJURIES

Needlestick and sharps injuries are the most common method of transmitting bloodborne pathogens between patients and health care providers; therefore, they pose a significant risk to health care workers and students. According to the Centers for Disease Control and Prevention (CDC), approximately 385,000 needlestick and other sharps-related injuries occur each year in hospital-based situations.[2] Needlestick and sharps injuries are primarily associated with transmission of hepatitis B, hepatitis C, and HIV, but other types of infections can also result.[3] Health care students are at especially high risk for needlestick injuries because of their relative inexperience; exposure rates have been reported as between 11% and 50% of students.[4] One PA program found that 22% of its students had some type of exposure, 60% of which were percutaneous injuries.[5]

The most important points of this discussion of student safety are prevention of needlestick injuries and reporting of an injury if one occurs. Prevention of needlestick and sharps injuries has improved significantly through the adoption of safer needles, protocols on handling sharps, and improved provider education on safety techniques. It is incumbent on PA educational programs to train their students in safe procedures and to establish a comprehensive response process for handling expected injuries.

Physician assistant students must take advantage of their programs' training opportunities in areas of phlebotomy, initiation of intravenous lines, suturing, and other procedures that involve needles and sharps. Usually, training in these techniques takes place far in advance of actual clinical experience. Students should be closely supervised to ensure that they are performing appropriate procedures for which they have been trained and that they are doing so correctly. It is natural to want to impress the supervisor or preceptor, which can lead students to perform procedures for which they are not yet qualified. To remain safe, students must be aware of these behaviors and understand their roles in caring for patients.

Physician assistant programs are required to provide students with a process for reporting and seeking medical care in the unfortunate event of a needlestick injury. Current recommendations call for the student to be evaluated and given appropriate postexposure prophylaxis within hours after an exposure.[6] PA programs provide this information; however, it is imperative that you keep it readily available so that you can make appropriate contacts when the need arises. Exposures that occur in a training hospital are usually handled quickly, but injuries in a rural site without access to appropriate prophylactic medications can be a challenge. Any student who will be in a rural clinical location needs to be familiar with the program's needlestick reporting process.

A troubling concern identified in the medical literature is the failure of health care workers and students to report needlestick and sharps injuries.[7,8] Reasons for not reporting include fear of losing insurance or employment, concerns about effectiveness of postexposure prophylaxis, and a tendency to deny personal risk.[7,9] Failure to report even what is considered an inconsequential exposure can have a significant impact on future ability to practice. Although it may seem inconvenient, reporting provides several benefits to both the student and the health care entity. Reporting an incident may be useful for future insurance and disability claims. It typically results in the student being evaluated medically and helps the institution assess internal systems that may prevent similar exposures for other health care workers.

CASE STUDY 5.1

During a busy Saturday morning in the emergency department (ED) of a rural community hospital, a senior PA student was busy suturing a laceration on the scalp of a male patient. The patient was being held by local law enforcement for drug dealing. He had been in a fight at the jail, resulting in his laceration. The patient was somewhat uncooperative, and while the PA student was placing a suture, the patient moved suddenly, causing the bloody needle to deeply puncture the student's gloved right middle finger. The student called for a nurse to assist him and to monitor the patient while he spoke with the family physician covering the ED. He asked the physician what he should do and was told to thoroughly clean the puncture site and then contact his program for advice. The student remembered he had been given a needlestick emergency contact card with a toll-free telephone number to call in case of an injury. After cleaning the site, he called the appropriate number and was given information about testing, follow-up, and postexposure prophylaxis, as well as points to discuss with the patient about having his blood tested for infectious diseases. The patient refused to consent to testing for HIV and hepatitis B and C. The student underwent baseline testing and decided to begin HIV prophylaxis medication. He was counseled on the risk for developing HIV, the need for safe sexual practices, and length of time for follow-up. He completed the postexposure prophylaxis without incident, and his HIV test result remained negative 1 year later.

TUBERCULOSIS SCREENING

As part of any type of formal health care training, students are required to be screened for TB annually.[10] For PA students, this is required as part of a PA program's accreditation. TB is still a significant disease process for which health care workers are at increased risk. According to the CDC, in 2014, health care workers accounted for 3.7% of reported TB cases nationwide.[11] The rate of health care student conversion while in training is unknown, but because of increased risk for exposure, all health care workers and students are screened annually.

The CDC recommends that groups considered to be at high risk undergo targeted tuberculin testing using the purified protein derivative (PPD) tuberculin skin test for latent TB infection. Three cut points have been recommended for defining a positive tuberculin reaction: induration of 5 mm or more, 10 mm or more, or 15 mm or more. For individuals at the highest risk for developing active TB,

5 mm or more of induration is considered a positive result. For groups with the lowest risk for contracting TB, a skin reaction is considered positive if it is 15 mm or more of induration (Table 5.2).[12] You will undoubtedly learn more about TB during your training; however, it is important to have an understanding of the rationale for your annual tuberculin skin testing.

LATEX ALLERGY

Latex is ubiquitous in the health care system. It has been used in all facets of medicine for several decades. The use of latex soared during the 1980s and 1990s as latex gloves were recommended as protection against bloodborne pathogens, including HIV.[13] As use of latex products increased, so did the incidence of allergic reactions associated with latex proteins. Commonly, latex gloves are coated with cornstarch powder as a dry lubricant. The latex protein particles easily stick to the powder and aerosolize when the gloves are removed, resulting in latex allergy reactions, which can be local (skin), respiratory, or both.

The actual prevalence of latex allergy is difficult to pinpoint. Data on occupational health care subgroups range from 0.5% to 24%. This wide range can be attributed to several issues related to the quality of the research studies and inconsistencies in the definition of "latex allergy."[14]

CASE STUDY 5.2

During routine annual testing for TB, a senior PA student was noted to have 17 mm of induration on her tuberculin skin test. Records showed that she had tested negative for TB at entry into the PA program and again after completing her first year in the program. She had spent the past 12 months in clinical rotations locally, regionally, and internationally. She denied any known exposure to anyone with active TB, although she had spent 4 weeks in Guatemala within the previous 3 months. She denied any suspicious symptoms, weight loss, night sweats, or cough. Her chest radiograph was interpreted as normal. She was counseled by student health personnel on the need to begin isoniazid and pyridoxine. She agreed to take the state-provided medications for the recommended 9 months. She tolerated the medications well without adverse effects and completed the regimen without incident.

Three types of clinical syndromes are associated with latex exposures. The majority of reactions involve an irritant dermatitis caused by the rubbing of gloves on the skin. This type is not immune mediated and is not associated with allergic symptoms.

A second form is the result of a delayed (type IV) hypersensitivity reaction, causing a contact dermatitis within 24 to 48 hours after exposure. Individuals

---

TABLE 5.2 Targeted Tuberculosis Testing and Interpreting Tuberculin Skin Test Results

Positive IGRA Result or TST Reaction ≥5 mm of Induration	Positive IGRA Result or TST Reaction ≥10 mm of Induration	Reaction ≥15 mm of Induration
HIV-infected persons	Recent immigrants (<5 yr) from high-prevalence countries	Persons with no risk factors for tuberculosis*
Recent contacts of a TB case	Injection drug users	
Persons with fibrotic changes on chest radiograph consistent with old TB	Residents and employees of high-risk congregate settings (e.g., correctional facilities, nursing homes, homeless shelters, hospitals, and other health care facilities)	
Organ transplant recipients	Mycobacteriology laboratory personnel	
Persons who are immunosuppressed for other reasons (e.g., taking the equivalent of >15 mg/day of prednisone for 1 month or longer, taking TNF-α antagonists)	Children younger than 4 years of age or children and adolescents exposed to adults in high-risk categories	

*Although skin testing programs should be considered only among high-risk groups, certain individuals may require tuberculin skin test (TST) for employment or school attendance. An approach independent of risk assessment is not recommended by the Centers for Disease Control and Prevention or the American Thoracic Society.
IGRA, Interferon-gamma release assay; *TB*, tuberculosis; *TNF*, tumor necrosis factor.
From Centers for Disease Control and Prevention. Targeted tuberculosis testing and interpreting tuberculin skin test results. http://www.cdc.gov/tb/publications/factsheets/testing/skintestresults.pdf.

with a history of atopic disease are at greater risk for this type of reaction. The most serious and least common presentation is the immediate (type I) hypersensitivity reaction. This is mediated by immunoglobulin E response specific to latex proteins. As the process escalates, histamine and other systemic mediators are released, possibly resulting in anaphylaxis.

Since awareness of latex allergies has grown, so too has the replacement of latex examination gloves with powder-free, low-protein gloves and latex-free gloves. If you have a latex sensitivity or allergy, you should carry a medical alert bracelet that can identify your allergy for health care providers. Avoid latex gloves and other products, and notify your supervisor or preceptor of your condition. Finally, if your reaction is severe, obtain a prescription for an epinephrine self-injection pen for use in an emergency.

STUDENT MISTREATMENT

Health care students are intelligent, compassionate, excited, and eager to learn. However, as Silver[15] wrote in 1982, medical students become "cynical, dejected, frightened, depressed, or frustrated" over time. He noted these changes were similar to those found in abused children, which may result from enduring unnecessary and harmful abuse. The term "medical student abuse" is now commonly referred to as "student mistreatment."

Knowledge of medical student mistreatment dates back to the 1960s. Several studies have explored the phenomenon and provided a better understanding of what constitutes mistreatment.[16–19] Students who reported mistreatment had more anxiety, depression, difficulty with learning, thoughts of dropping out, and drinking problems.[17–19] These data suggest that mistreatment can have significant negative effects on students.

Since 1991, the Association of American Medical Colleges (AAMC) has included the topic of medical student mistreatment on its annual questionnaire to graduating medical students. The questionnaire covers mistreatment related to the following areas: general, sexual, racial/ethnic, and sexual orientation. In the 2015 AAMC Medical School Graduation Questionnaire, 65.8% of graduates believed they were humiliated or embarrassed at some point during their education.[20] A recent study by Mavis[18] found that over a 10-year period, on average, 17% of medical students reported being personally mistreated during their medical education, and of those, 31% reported the incident.

Only recently have data been gathered about the mistreatment of PA students. Asprey[21] surveyed a group of senior PA students regarding mistreatment in six categories (Box 5.1). Although conclusions were limited by low response rates, a total of 79% of students admitted to having experienced at least one form of mistreatment during their training. Interestingly, Asprey's findings were consistent with those in medical students, in that the PA students reported similar rates of general mistreatment. However, PA students reported sexual mistreatment (50.4%) as the most common form of abuse, closely followed by verbal mistreatment (47.5%). In addition, those responsible for the mistreatment were physicians (33%) followed by PA program faculty (17.7%).[21]

An important distinction concerns the perception of mistreatment. Do students and preceptors agree on what constitutes mistreatment?[18] In a study that used five video vignettes depicting potentially abusive situations, the authors surveyed physicians, resident physicians, nurses, and students to determine their perceptions.[22] They found good agreement regarding abuse in the belittlement, ethnic insensitivity, and sexual harassment scenarios. This study suggests that authority figures and students often agree on what constitutes mistreatment in a clinical situation.

A large proportion of mistreatment appears to go unreported. Studies have identified several reasons for students not reporting: They did not recognize the experience as mistreatment at the time that it happened, did not think reporting would make a difference, feared the reporting could adversely affect their evaluation, and believed that reporting would be more trouble than it was worth.[16,18,19,23]

Reporting an episode of mistreatment is an individual decision. Students often think that their position does not allow them to report behavior by a superior because of possible repercussions. However, in the current health care climate, most organizations have well-defined procedures for handling disruptive providers. These policies are primarily directed at physicians but include anyone within the organization who receives a formal complaint.

SEXUAL HARASSMENT

One form of student mistreatment that deserves special attention is sexual harassment. Federal law protects students from sexual harassment by instructors, staff, and other employees of an educational institution. As with any other form of student

BOX 5.1 PHYSICIAN ASSISTANT SURVEY QUESTIONS BY CATEGORY OF MISTREATMENT

VERBAL MISTREATMENT

- Have you been belittled, humiliated, or denigrated verbally?
- Have you been verbally threatened with harm?

PHYSICAL MISTREATMENT

- Have you been physically abused (e.g., hit, pushed, slapped, kicked)?

SEXUAL MISTREATMENT

- Have you been subjected to unwanted or inappropriate verbal comments, such as slurs, lewd comments, or sexual jokes?
- Have you been subjected to unwanted sexual advances (repeated requests for sexual interactions or activities)?
- Have you been physically touched in an unwanted sexually oriented manner (e.g., groped, fondled, kissed)?
- Have you been sexually assaulted (e.g., raped, forced to perform sexual acts)?
- Have you been asked for sexual favors in return for grades, positive evaluations, recommendations, and so on?
- Have you been subjected to unwanted or inappropriate verbal comments, such as slurs, lewd comments, sexual jokes, and so on on the basis of your sexual orientation?
- Have you been denied educational or training opportunities solely on the basis of your sexual orientation?

- Have you been assigned lower evaluations or grades solely on the basis of your sexual orientation?

GENDER-BASED MISTREATMENT

- Have you been denied educational or training opportunities on the basis of your gender?
- Have you been assigned lower grades or negative evaluations solely on the basis of your gender?

RACE-ORIENTED MISTREATMENT

- Have you been subjected to unwanted or inappropriate verbal comments on the basis of your race or ethnicity?
- Have you been denied educational or training opportunities on the basis of your race or ethnicity?
- Have you been assigned lower grades or negative evaluations solely on the basis of your race or ethnicity?

RELIGION-BASED MISTREATMENT

- Have you been subjected to unwanted or inappropriate verbal comments on the basis of espoused religious beliefs?
- Have you been denied educational or training opportunities solely on the basis of your espoused religious beliefs?
- Have you been assigned lower grades or evaluations solely on the basis of your espoused religious beliefs?

---

mistreatment, consequences of sexual harassment can be far-reaching.

Inappropriate sex-based behaviors in all areas of higher education have been well documented. The types of sexual harassment behaviors reported include offensive body language, flirtation, unwelcome comments on students' dress, outright sexual invitations, propositions, sexual contact, sexual bribery, and sexual assaults.[23] In addition, exclusion from educational opportunities based solely on gender and discriminatory grading has been reported.[24,25]

The U.S. Department of Education's Office of Civil Rights 2001 guidelines define two types of sexual harassment: quid pro quo and hostile environment.[26] Quid pro quo sexual harassment occurs when an employee of the school explicitly or implicitly applies conditions to a student's participation in an educational program or activity on the basis of the student's submission to unwelcome sexual advances; requests for sexual favors; or verbal, nonverbal, or physical contact of a sexual nature.[26] Hostile environment can be further defined to include persistent,

severe, or pervasive unwelcome sexual conduct that limits a student's ability to participate in or benefit from an educational program or activity or that creates a hostile or abusive educational environment.[26] The statistics describing the extent of sexual harassment in medical training are based primarily on experience from medical schools and resident training programs. In 2015, the AAMC's Medical School Graduation Questionnaire found, specific to sexual mistreatment, 6.4% reported having been denied opportunities for training or rewards because of their gender on one or more occasions, 4.7% had been subjected to unwanted sexual advances by school personnel on one or more occasion, 14.1% had been subjected to offensive sexist remarks or names on one or more occasion, and 6.2% believed they had received lower evaluations or grades solely on the basis of their gender rather than performance.[20] The good news is that although the numbers are impressive in total, the overall percentages have declined in general over the past 4 years. Other researchers have found that a larger number of students are sexually

Harassment

On the basis of race, color, gender, age, national origin, disability, gender orientation, genetic information, veteran status and religion is prohibited.

Hostile work environment is created by severe and pervasive conduct, which may include the following:

- Jokes with sexual, racial, or inappropriate content;
- Epithets, slurs, profanity, and name calling;
- Demeaning or sexually suggestive pictures (whether real or virtual), objects, writings, e-mails, or faxes;
- Unwelcome love letters, gifts, or requests for dates;
- Unwelcome behavior that any "reasonable person" would find offensive.

Misuse of power to gain sexual favors is a form of sexual harassment.

How to address harassing behavior ...

- Notify your supervisor
- Contact the Affirmative Action Office in Human Resources—Employee Relations
- Faculty may report complaints directly to the Chair of the Faculty Senate Grievance Committee

Factors to note ...

- A single incident can be enough to be harassment
- Harassers may include supervisors, co-workers, faculty, students, and non-employees
- We expect students and employees to be free from harassment whenever or wherever individuals are engaged in activities on behalf of the university, including off-site events
- We will take immediate action to eliminate harassment
- We will not permit retaliation against any individual who in good faith complains of harassment

If you have questions about harassment, you may contact ...

FIG. 5.1 ■ Sexual harassment bookmark. (Courtesy Carmen Sirizzotti, MBA, at UNMC.)

harassed during their medical education, ranging from 11% to 21% of male students and 35% to 64% of female students.[27,28] In addition, the effects of sexual harassment may be profound for the individual student, affecting performance; inducing feelings of anger, fear, and guilt; and leading to personal and professional dissatisfaction.[28]

Few data exist specific to PA students and sexual harassment experiences. Asprey's survey of 22 PA programs regarding mistreatment among soon-to-be graduates found that 50% of senior PA students experienced some type of sexual mistreatment during their training.[19]

The surprising conclusion to be drawn from these data is that sexual harassment continues to be a problem in professional graduate education. PA students,

male and female, should be aware of their programs' policies on mistreatment and sexual harassment. Legal protections are in place that provide for a nonhostile educational environment where students can feel safe. In addition, students should be aware of what constitutes sexual harassment (Fig. 5.1). If you have concerns about an experience, speak with a PA program faculty member, the school's ombudsman, or the school's human resources department. PA program faculties have a responsibility to develop professional attitudes and behaviors in their students as much as expanding their medical knowledge. Failure to enforce program policy may perpetuate sexism within our profession and result in producing PAs who treat their patients and colleagues with disrespect.

PATIENT SAFETY WHILE ON ROTATIONS

Patient safety concepts have become integrated into the practice of medicine since the Institute of Medicine published two groundbreaking books exploring this issue.[29,30]

The need for these tools and system changes have been well documented. All PA programs provide education on the importance of patient safety awareness and techniques. The role of students, who are transiently involved in patient care during clinical rotations, has only recently been explored. Although educated on the importance of patient safety and specific skill sets, one study found that 56% of medical students would not speak up when witnessing a possible adverse event, and an equally large percentage were afraid to ask questions if things did not seem right.[31] The power dynamics between students and preceptors is a significant barrier for students to challenge and raise concerns about an unsafe practice. However, our ultimate goal as health care professionals is the safety of our patients, and it is incumbent on all students to question anyone if they perceive an unsafe practice. For more information on patient safety and medical errors, see Chapter 39.

KEY POINTS

- Entering the clinical phase of training is an exciting time; however, the practice of medicine and surgery is an inherently dangerous activity.
- Physician assistant students must be properly immunized, educated about safety concerns, and vigilant about their own safety when starting clinical rotations.
- Physician assistant students must be aware of their own limitations and lack of experience, especially when volunteering to learn new skills.
- Locate and review your program's needlestick and blood and body fluid exposure policy. Make sure you have a copy of the emergency contact information with you at all times.
- Students should report any type of injury sustained during clinical training immediately and complete appropriate paperwork in a timely fashion.
- Students are encouraged to report any type of mistreatment that may occur during their training to program faculty or other appropriate resources in their institutions.
- If you question the safety of any procedure or process for a patient, you have an obligation to speak up and question anyone.

References

1. Siegel JD, Rhinehart E, Jackson M, Chiarello L. The Healthcare Infection Control Practices Advisory Committee, Guideline for isolation precautions: preventing transmission of infectious agents in healthcare settings, 2007. http://www.cdc.gov/hicpac/pdf/isolation/Isolation2007.pdf.
2. Panlilio AL, Orelien JG, Srivastava PU, et al. Estimate of the annual number of percutaneous injuries among hospital-based healthcare workers in the United States, 1997–1998. *Infect Control Hosp Epidemiol*. 2004;25(7):556.
3. Collins DH, Kennedy DA. Microbiological hazards of occupational needlestick and other "sharps" injuries. *J Appl Bacteriol*. 1987;62:385.
4. Cervini P, Bell C. Brief report: needlestick injury and inadequate postexposure practice in medical students. *J Gen Intern Med*. 2005;20:419.
5. LaBarbera D. Accidental exposures of physician assistant students. *J Phys Assist Educ*. 2006;17:40.
6. Kuhar DT, Henderson KD, Struble KA, et al. U.S. Public Health Service. Updated US Public Health Service guidelines for the management of occupational exposures to human immunodeficiency virus and recommendations for postexposure prophylaxis. *Infect Control Hosp Epidemiol*. 2013;34(9):875–892.
7. Sharma GK, Gilson MM, Nathan H, Makary MA. Needlestick injuries among medical students: incidence and implications. *Acad Med*. 2009;84(12):1815.
8. Bernard JA, Dattilo JR, LaPorte DM. The incidence and reporting of sharps exposure among medical students, orthopedic residents, and faculty at one institution. *J Surg Ed*. 2013;70(5):660–668.
9. Osborn EHS, Papakakis MA, Gerberding JL. Occupational exposures to body fluids among medical students, a seven-year longitudinal study. *Ann Intern Med*. 1999;130:45.
10. Screening for tuberculosis and tuberculosis infection in high-risk populations: recommendations of the Advisory Council for the Elimination of Tuberculosis. *MMWR Recomm Rep*. 1995;44(No. RR-11):19.
11. Centers for Disease Control and Prevention. *Reported Tuberculosis in the United States, 2014*. Atlanta, GA: U.S. Department of Health and Human Services, Centers for Disease Control and Prevention; 2015.
12. Centers for Disease Control and Prevention. Targeted tuberculosis testing and interpreting tuberculin skin test results. http://www.cdc.gov/tb/publications/factsheets/testing/skintestresults.pdf.
13. Behrman AJ, Howarth M. Latex allergy. eMedicine. http://emedicine.com/emerg/topic814.htm.

14. Statham BN. Epidemiology of latex allergy. In: Chowdhury MMU, Marbach HI, eds. *Latex Intolerance: Basic Science, Epidemiology, and Clinical Management.* New York: CRC Press; 2005.

15. Silver HK. Medical students and medical school. *JAMA.* 1982;247:309.

16. Komaromy M, Bindman AB, Harber RJ, Sande MA. Sexual harassment in medical training. *N Engl J Med.* 1993;328:322.

17. Silver HK, Glicken AD. Medical student abuse. Incidence, severity, and significance. *JAMA.* 1990;263:527.

18. Mavis B, Sousa A, Lipscomb W, Rappley MD. Learning about medical student mistreatment from responses to the medical school graduation questionnaire. *Acad Med.* 2014;89(5):705.

19. Nagata-Kobayashi S, Sekimoto M, Koyama H, et al. Medical student abuse during clinical clerkships in Japan. *J Gen Intern Med.* 2006;21:212.

20. Association of American Medical Colleges. 2015 Medical School Graduation Questionnaire. https://www.aamc.org/download/440552/data/2015gqallschoolssummaryreport.pdf.

21. Asprey DP. Physician assistant students' perceptions of mistreatment during training. *J Phys Assist Ed.* 2006;17:5.

22. Ogden PE, Wu EH, Elnicki MD, et al. Do attending physicians, nurses, residents, and medical students agree on what constitutes medical student abuse? *Acad Med.* 2005;80(suppl):S80.

23. Balwin Jr DC, Daugherty SR, Rowley BD. Residents' and medical students' reports of sexual harassment and discrimination. *Acad Med.* 1996;71(suppl 10):S25.

24. Cook DJ, Liutkus JF, Risdon CL, et al. Residents' experiences of abuse, discrimination and sexual harassment during residency training. *CMAJ.* 1996;154:1657.

25. Rees CE, Monrouxe LV. A morning since eight of just pure grill: a multischool qualitative study of student abuse. *Acad Med.* 2011;86(11):1374.

26. U.S. Department of Education. Revised sexual harassment guidance. Harassment of students by school employees, other students, or third parties, Title IX; 2001. http://www2.ed.gov/about/offices/list/ocr/docs/shguide.html.

27. Lubitz RM, Nguyen DD. Medical student abuse during third-year clerkships. *JAMA.* 1996;275:414.

28. Richman JA, Flaherty JA, Rospenda KM. Perceived workplace harassment experiences and problem drinking among physicians: broadening the stress/alienation paradigm. *Addiction.* 1996;91:391.

29. Institute of Medicine. *To Err Is Human: Building a Safer Health System.* Washington, DC: National Academies Press; 1999.

30. Institute of Medicine. *Crossing the Quality Chasm: A New Health System for the 21st Century.* Washington, DC: National Academies Press; 2001.

31. Bowman C, Neeman N, Sehgal NL. Enculturation of unsafe attitudes and behaviors: student perceptions of safety culture. *Acad Med.* 2013;88(6):802.

CHAPTER 6

ASSURING QUALITY FOR PHYSICIAN ASSISTANTS: ACCREDITATION, CERTIFICATION, LICENSING, AND PRIVILEGING

Constance Goldgar • Dan Crouse • Dawn Morton-Rias

CHAPTER OUTLINE

INTRODUCTION

Health insurance plans are becoming broader in regard to the scope of treatments they cover. These changes include mental health and behavioral health parity; fewer restrictions on preexisting conditions; and the coverage of supplemental services, such as physical therapy, massage therapy, acupuncture, and other holistic health services. Insurers want to be certain that clinicians have the appropriate education and background to qualify them to perform treatments and procedures.

Credentialing is a systematic process of collecting and verifying qualifications for individual professionals, and groups of professionals or organizations, including educational programs. The purpose of credentialing is to assess background and legitimacy for a professional or entity to provide services and grants

the right, through a title or credit, to provide specific services. Credentialing affects physician assistant (PA) students initially while they are enrolled in their programs of education from the standpoint of accreditation of the PA education program. Subsequently, when PA graduates enter the health care marketplace, an individual level of credentialing occurs nationally through passing the Physician Assistant National Certification Examination (PANCE) and the processes whereby graduates gain access to state, insuring, and employing institutions. PA students, PA graduates, and the institutions charged with educating them must understand and accept the significant responsibility of credentialing that allows them the right to perform or provide services. This chapter discusses two separate and distinct credentialing procedures: the credentialing (accreditation) of PA programs by the

Accreditation and Review Commission on Education for the Physician Assistant (ARC-PA) and the credentialing of individual PAs by the National Commission on Certification of Physician Assistants (NCCPA), state licensing boards, and specific institutions.

PHYSICIAN ASSISTANT EDUCATION PROGRAM ACCREDITATION

Accreditation is the process of credentialing PA programs, which is defined as official recognition and approval or vouching that a program maintains standards that qualify the graduates for professional practice and provides them with credentials. PA programs have undergone remarkable professional growth that belies the relatively short history (~50 years) of the profession. In terms of acceptance and privilege to practice clinically, the accreditation process that evaluates PA programs is fundamental to the safety of patients as well as the PA profession's success.[1]

Accreditation Review Commission on Education of the Physician Assistant

Accreditation is a voluntary, formal process of external peer review, encompassing evaluation of an institution or education program to determine whether it meets the standards set up by the accrediting body. If the program or institution meets the standards set, the accrediting body grants recognition that established qualifications and educational standards have been met. The ARC-PA is the recognized accrediting agency that protects the interests of the public and PA profession and the welfare of students by defining the standards for PA education and evaluating PA educational programs within the territorial United States to ensure their compliance with the standards.[2]

Accreditation of PA programs began in 1971 when *Essentials of an Accredited Educational Program for the Assistant to the Primary Care Physician* were developed under the auspices of the American Medical Association's (AMA's) Subcommittee of the Council on Medical Education's Advisory Committee on Education for Allied Health Professions and Services. Many evolutions to PA program accreditation have occurred since that time. On January 1, 2002, the Accreditation Review *Committee* on Education for the Physician Assistant became the Accreditation Review *Commission* on Education for the Physician Assistant. This may have been a minor name change but was a monumental step forward because the ARC-PA became a freestanding accrediting agency for the evaluation and accreditation of PA educational programs in the United States. The ARC-PA is the sole authority for PA program accreditation.

BOX 6.1 THE GOALS OF THE ACCREDITATION REVIEW COMMISSION ON EDUCATION OF THE PHYSICIAN ASSISTANT

- Foster excellence in PA education through the development of uniform national standards for assessing educational effectiveness.
- Foster excellence in PA programs by requiring continuous self-study and review.
- Assure the general public, as well as professional, educational, and licensing agencies and organizations, that accredited programs have met defined educational standards for preparing PAs for practice.
- Provide information and guidance to individuals, groups, and organizations regarding PA program accreditation.

PA, Physician assistant.

The role of the ARC-PA is the following:
1. Establish educational standards using broad-based input.
2. Define and administer the process for comprehensive review of applicant programs.
3. Define and administer the process for accreditation decision making.
4. Determine if PA educational programs are in compliance with the established standards.
5. Work cooperatively with its collaborating organizations.
6. Define and administer a process for appeal of accreditation decisions.[2]

The goals of the ARC-PA (Box 6.1) dovetail with its mission to "protect the interests of the public and PA profession, and the welfare of students by defining the standards for PA education and evaluating PA educational programs . . . to ensure their compliance with those standards."[2]

In its role in accrediting PA programs, the ARC-PA encourages excellence in PA education by establishing and maintaining minimum standards of quality for educational programs. The ARC-PA cooperates and collaborates with several organizations to establish, maintain, and promote appropriate standards of quality for educational programs. Endorsed by a broad consensus within the medical community, the standards represent current, nationally accepted guidelines for all aspects of program operation. Because medical education and the health care system are both in major transformation, the standards continue to evolve to meet the needs of patients and society. The ARC-PA regularly reviews the content of the standards and seeks feedback on their validity and clarity from its sponsor organizations and members of the PA education community. Periodic reviews may result in the creation, elimination, or readaptation of a specific standard.[3]

The standards, initially adopted in 1971, have been revised many times over the years, with its most recent major revision in 2010 and many clarifying changes in the interim. A copy of the most current standards (fourth edition) is available in PDF downloadable format at http://www.arc-pa.org/documen ts/Standards4theditionwithclarifyingchanges9.2014 %20FNL.pdf. The standards are under continuous scrutiny and are amended frequently. Please see the website for the most current edition.

The ARC-PA standards constitute the minimum requirements to which an accredited program is held accountable and provide the basis on which ARC-PA confers or denies program accreditation. The standards are used to develop, evaluate, and require continuous self-analysis of PA programs. To offer curricula of sufficient depth and breadth to prepare all PA graduates to practice in a dynamic health care arena, the standards reflect that a commonality in the core professional curriculum of programs remains desirable and necessary.[1] The standards are designed to allow programs to remain creative and innovative in program design and in the methods used to enable students to achieve student learning outcomes and program expectations and acquire competencies needed for entry into clinical practice.[3]

As delineated in the standards, PAs are academically and clinically prepared to practice medicine with the direction and responsible supervision of a doctor of medicine or osteopathy. The physician–PA team relationship is fundamental to the PA profession and enhances the delivery of high-quality health care. Within the physician–PA team relationship, PAs make clinical decisions and provide a broad range of diagnostic, therapeutic, preventive, and health maintenance services. The clinical role of PAs includes primary and specialty care in medical and surgical practice settings. PA practice is centered on patient care and may include educational, research, and administrative activities.[3]

The professional curriculum for PA education includes basic medical, behavioral, and social sciences; patient assessment and clinical medicine; supervised clinical practice; and health policy and professional practice issues. The standards encompass current, nationally accepted guidelines for all aspects of PA program operation, including institutional responsibilities, admissions processes, faculty qualifications, curricular components and design, expected competencies for students, supervised clinical practice, classroom laboratory and library facilities, clinical affiliations, student issues, fiscal stability, program publications, record-keeping systems, and administration.

The Accreditation Review Commission on Education of the Physician Assistant Standards

The ARC-PA standards are organized into three main sections: (1) administration, (2) curriculum and instruction, and (3) evaluation. Each of these components has sets of pertinent standards denoted with a concise statement of the principles that represent each standard. The administration section primarily consists of institutional responsibilities, resources, and support, including faculty, personnel, and operational aspects of the program within the sponsoring institution. The section on curriculum and instruction outlines commonalities of aspects of the preclinical curriculum, including providing applied course content for core biomedical knowledge, clinical problem solving, patient assessment, and student learning outcomes as expected by the individual program. This section also addresses supervised clinical education with clinical preceptors in the community in designated experiences both across the lifespan and in a variety of specified settings. The evaluation section address the program having an ongoing "robust and systematic process of ongoing self-assessment" to assess how effectively the program performs quality improvement throughout all aspects of the program. The process must include self-identification by the program of its strengths and weaknesses through analysis of collected data. Plans for remediation of weaknesses and continuous improvement are made apparent in this section.

The Accreditation Process

The ARC-PA accreditation process is designed to accomplish the following:
- Encourage educational institutions and programs to continuously evaluate and improve their processes and outcomes.
- Help prospective students identify programs that meet nationally accepted standards.
- Protect programs from internal and external pressures to make changes that are not educationally sound.
- Involve faculty and staff in comprehensive program evaluation and planning and stimulate self-improvement by setting national standards against which programs can be measured.[4]

TABLE 6.1 Collaborating Organizations of the Accreditation Review Commission on Education of the Physician Assistant That Comprise the Commission and Number of Commissioners Allotted

Collaborating Organization	Number of Commissioners Allotted
American Academy of Family Physicians	2
American Academy of Pediatrics	2
American Academy of Physician Assistants	3
American College of Physicians	2
American College of Surgeons	2
American Medical Association	2
Physician Assistant Education Association	3
Public Commissioner	2
Institutional Dean	1
At-large commissioners	4

The accreditation process that evaluates PA programs is fundamental to the profession's success, protects the interests of the public, and fosters excellence in PA programs. This voluntary process is available only to qualified PA programs sponsored by a single institution. The sponsoring institution must be accredited by a recognized regional accrediting agency and be authorized by this agency to confer a graduate degree to graduates of the PA program.[5]

The Commission

The ARC-PA confers or denies program accreditation. ARC-PA commissioners are elected by the ARC-PA from a selection of nominees from ARC-PA collaborating organizations (see Table 6.1 for representative organizations). Each commissioner serves a 3-year term, which is renewable for an additional 3-year term. At-large commissioners are elected for a single 3-year term and are not eligible for reelection. The usual work of the ARC-PA occurs over two meeting periods yearly, in March and in September. The work of the commission is integral to the operation of the ARC-PA; commissioners participate in the decision-making process through many activities including but not limited to review and presentation of program files, site visits of new and continuing programs, evaluation

reports, and reports requested from programs as a result of previous ARC-PA accreditation action or review.[6]

Types of Accreditation Site Visits

There are different categories of accreditation as noted in Table 6.2. Provisional accreditation (for new programs) consists of three sequential steps beginning the accreditation process. The first step, Accreditation–Provisional, is granted with an Initial Provisional Visit when a newly proposed program demonstrates sufficient evidence for program planning and resources to fully meet the ARC-PA standards; this typically occurs 6 to 12 months before the enrollment of students. As the program prepares for the graduation of its first cohort of students and has demonstrated continued progress in complying with the standards, a second review by ARC-PA confirms Accreditation–Provisional status. The Final Provisional Site Visit usually occurs 18–24 months after gaining Accreditation–Provisional status and includes continued compliance with the standards plus a "robust self-assessment process." If the program has fulfilled all ARC requirements the commission may grant Accreditation–Continued status.[7]

Continuing accreditation is for established programs that have been accredited. Revisions to this process have been ongoing since 2012. Beginning in September 2016, all accredited programs will submit a self-study report 2 years in advance of "validation site visits." These site visits will be "customized" for individual programs based on historical accreditation as well as the submitted self-study reports. All accredited programs will have validation visits, but depending on various factors, many programs will have the validation visit every 7 years.[7]

In addition to the Provisional Site Visits, other site visits by the ARC-PA include validation visits and focused visits. Validation visits occur for programs with Accreditation–Continued status and can be called at the discretion of the ARC-PA at any time to review any issues of program compliance with the standards, need for clarification of information submitted by programs via the portal, or demonstration of continuous oversight of processes and outcomes of education. Focused visits may also be done at any time to assess any issues related to specific standard(s) identified through a site visit or in response to any concerns. For programs that may be considering expansion to a distant campus, a site visit would be conducted at the site of the proposed campus and may include or require a concurrent visit to the main program campus.[7]

TABLE 6.2 **Accreditation Review Commission on Education of the Physician Assistant Categories of Accreditation**	
Category of Accreditation	**Description**
Accreditation–Provisional	Granted when the plans and resource allocation, if fully implemented as planned, of a proposed program that has not yet enrolled students appear to demonstrate the program's ability to meet the ARC-PA standards or when a program holding Accreditation–Provisional status appears to demonstrate continued progress in complying with the standards as it prepares for the graduation of the first class (cohort) of students.
Accreditation–Continued	Granted when: 1. A currently accredited program is in compliance with the standards, 2. A program holding Accreditation–Probation status has demonstrated that it is again in compliance with the standards, or 3. A program holding Accreditation–Provisional demonstrates compliance with the standards after completion of the provisional review process.
Accreditation–Clinical Postgraduate Program	Granted when a new or currently accredited clinical postgraduate program is in compliance with the *Standards for Clinical Postgraduate Programs*.
Accreditation–Probation	Granted with a temporary limit of 2 years when a program holding accreditation status of Accreditation–Provisional or Accreditation–Continued does not meet the standards and when the capability of the program to provide an acceptable educational experience for its students is threatened.
Accreditation–Administrative Probation	Granted temporarily when a program has not complied with an administrative requirement, such as failure to pay fees or submit required reports. A program with this status must comply with administrative requirements in a timely manner, as specified by the ARC-PA, or it may be scheduled for a focused site visit or risk having its accreditation withdrawn.
Accreditation–Withheld	Granted when an entry-level program, seeking Accreditation–Provisional or a clinical postgraduate PA program seeking Accreditation–Clinical Postgraduate Program is not in compliance with the standards.*
Accreditation–Withdrawn	Granted when an established program is determined no longer to be in compliance with the standards and is no longer capable of providing an acceptable educational experience for its students or when the program has failed to comply with ARC-PA accreditation requirements, actions, or procedures.*
Voluntary Inactive Status	Granted to programs that temporarily suspend instruction and cease to matriculate students. The conditions of this status are determined by program circumstances necessitating this status.

ARC-PA, Accreditation Review Commission on Education of the Physician Assistant.
*The program may choose to voluntarily withdraw from the accreditation process within the 30-day appeal time frame.

Accreditation–Probation is a temporary status that lasts 2 years and is granted to a program that has either Accreditation–Continued or Accreditation–Provisional status but the program has failed to meet the standards. Accreditation–Administrative Probation is likewise granted temporarily when a program is out of compliance more specifically with an administrative requirement (e.g., did not pay fees, did not submit required information). When on probation, any failure to comply with accreditation requirements in a timely manner may have a focused site visit or have its accreditation status withdrawn.[7]

The last two types of accreditation are Accreditation–Withheld and Accreditation–Withdrawn. Accreditation–Withheld may occur when a program seeking Accreditation–Provisional is not able to comply with the standards. Accreditation–Withdrawn denotes that an established program is not in compliance with the standards and cannot provide an "acceptable educational experience for its students" or cannot comply with accreditation requirements. In either of these instances, a program may voluntarily withdraw from the accreditation process within the 30-day appeal timeframe.[7]

Accreditation decisions are based on the ARC-PA's review of information contained in the accreditation application, the program's self-study report, the report of site visit evaluation teams, any additional requested reports or documents submitted to the ARC-PA by the PA program, and the program's past accreditation history.[3] After review by the commission, a formal notice of accreditation status and the time frame for accreditation are sent to the chief executive officer of the institution and the program director.[3]

After ARC-PA accreditation is granted, periodic reviews and onsite evaluations by an accreditation team are required for maintenance of accreditation. The educational process is improved frequently as programs make modifications to maintain or exceed the accreditation standards or to build on insights gained from an onsite evaluation.[7]

Graduation from an ARC-PA–accredited program benefits students by providing the following:
1. Assurance that the program meets nationally accepted standards
2. Recognition of their education by their professional peers
3. Eligibility for professional certification, registration, and state licensure

Clinical Postgraduate Accreditation

Over decades, the issue of accreditation of postgraduate PA programs has been debated by various stakeholders. In 2007, after much thoughtful deliberation and work studying this issue, the ARC-PA approved accreditation standards for clinical postgraduate PA programs, with the first two programs becoming accredited in 2008.

Accreditation of clinical postgraduate programs is voluntary and represents one method of external validation and assessment of quality. Additional specialty education and training that occur in formal postgraduate PA programs or residencies is not required for successful physician–PA teams to provide specialty medical or surgical care. As it currently exists, the ARC-PA accreditation process is labor and resource intensive for postgraduate programs and may not be the first priority for a program's sponsoring institution.[8] Therefore, in 2014, the ARC-PA decided to hold the current clinical postgraduate PA program accreditation in abeyance, which applies only to programs with the status of Accreditation–Clinical Postgraduate Program and those that received correspondence from ARC-PA with a formal timeline to attain accreditation by the commission. The ARC-PA is not accepting any new programs into the accreditation process. All determinations of clinical postgraduate PA program eligibility, curriculum reviews, and administrative reviews are suspended pending the results of a designated work group's report.[8]

Further information on PA program accreditation can be found at http://www.arc-pa.org or by directly contacting the ARC-PA, 12000 Findley Road, Suite 150, Johns Creek, GA 30097.

NATIONAL CERTIFICATION

Since 1974, NCCPA has served as the profession's certification body, work underpinned by a passionate belief that certified PAs are essential members of the health care delivery team, providing millions of patients' access to more affordable, high-quality health care. As a certification organization, the NCCPA exists to serve the interest of those patients and the public by providing a reliable indicator that those certified by the NCCPA have demonstrated that they possess and continue to maintain the knowledge and cognitive skills to practice safely and effectively.

At the inception of the PA profession, pioneers charting the course for the developing profession affirmed their commitment to clinical excellence; professional regulation; national, state, and local recognition; and patient acceptance. Toward that end, in 1972, the National Board of Medical Examiners (NBME) and the AMA convened representatives from fourteen organizations, including the American Academy of Physician Assistants (AAPA), the Association of Physician Assistant Programs (APAP), and several physician and health industry organizations, to discuss the need for an independent certifying authority for the PA profession. They discussed the development of a representative-based, independent "commission" in the certification process that would:
- Develop a certification examination.
- Determine eligibility to sit for the examination.
- Establish a standard for successful completion of the examination.
- Publicize the availability of the examination.
- Issue certificates to successful candidates.
- Maintain a registry of certified PAs.
- Develop mechanisms to attest to certification to employers and state licensing boards.
- Develop processes for assuring maintenance of knowledge and skills.
- Develop mechanisms for periodic recertification.
- Develop examinations in specialty areas when justified.
- Assist state licensing boards to facilitate interstate mobility.

Following the discussion, the participants concurred, without dissent, that such a commission needed to be free standing and not a part of any existing organization. Three years later, the NCCPA was formed to fulfill that role.[9]

Established as a not-for-profit organization in 1974, the NCCPA is dedicated to assuring the public that certified PAs meet professional standards of knowledge and clinical skills. All U.S. states, the District of Columbia, and the U.S. territories rely on NCCPA certification criteria for licensure or regulation of PAs.

To attain certification, PAs must pass the PANCE. Administered year round at testing centers across the United States, PANCE is a multiple-choice test that comprises 360 questions that assess medical and surgical knowledge. After passing PANCE, PAs are issued an NCCPA certificate, entitling them to use the Physician Assistant-Certified (PA-C) designation until the end of the second year after its issuance. To maintain NCCPA certification and retain the right to use the PA-C designation beyond the date of the initial certificate's expiration, they must follow a multifaceted process, involving documentation of continuing medical education (CME) hours and, after 6 to 10 years, successful completion of a recertification exam.

As the PA profession evolved and grew, so did the NCCPA and the certification process. Over time, the NCCPA took several steps to shore up the integrity of the certification process, including the institution of random CME audits, assumption of all CME logging duties for PAs maintaining certification, requiring new graduates to become certified within 6 years or six attempts (in a move away from lifetime eligibility), and enacting a more comprehensive disciplinary policies. Simultaneously, the NCCPA has become a more service-driven organization that now boasts a fully interactive website, high satisfaction ratings among PAs, and quick response times for those using NCCPA services.

Imbued with a strong sense of responsibility to ensure that PAs meet professional standards of knowledge and skills, the NCCPA will continue to strive to meet the needs of its stakeholders efficiently, effectively, and honorably.

History of the National Commission on Certification of Physician Assistants[9]

1971: Upon recommendation of its Goals and Priorities Committee, the NBME approves development of a certifying examination for the assistant to the primary care physician. Barbara J. Andrew, PhD, is chosen to direct the project. Edmund D. Pellegrino, MD, is appointed by John P. Hubbard, MD, president of the NBME, to chair a Special Advisory Committee that includes representatives of the AMA.

1973: The NBME administers the first certifying examination for assistants to the primary care physician to 880 candidates, 10% of whom are graduates of nurse practitioner programs. The exam consists of multiple-choice questions and patient management problems using invisible ink technology to expose pertinent information.

1974: Fourteen national health organizations come together to form the NCCPA to provide oversight regarding eligibility and standards for the NBME examination and to assure state medical boards, employers, and the public of the competency of PAs. Thomas E. Piemme, MD, is elected the first president. David L. Glazer is selected as the first executive director.

1975: A national office is opened in Atlanta, Georgia, and sponsorship of the PANCE is transferred to the NCCPA. The NCCPA and NBME introduce reliable observational checklists into the PA certification examination to assess candidates' ability to perform a physical examination. It is the first medical professional examination to do so, and the first PA-C certificates are issued.

1981: The NCCPA introduces the Physician Assistant National Recertifying Examination (PANRE), which certified PAs are required to take every 6 years. PAs who fail the exam are recertified for 2 years but are required to retake the examination within that time period, a strategy that helped establish the profession's credibility with regulatory boards and others.

1983: The PANCE is redesigned to include three components: a general knowledge core, an extended core in either surgery or primary care, and observational checklist clinical skills problems (CSPs).

1990: The NCCPA and AAPA assign a joint task force to develop "Pathway II," a take-home version of the recertification examination.

1997: The NCCPA redesigns the PANCE, eliminating CSPs because of the complexity and cost of administration at the designated test centers. At the same time, it eliminates the extended core components in primary care and surgery. Instead it introduces a new "stand-alone" voluntary Surgery Examination, allowing PAs to earn "special recognition." For the first time, the examination is offered twice each year—once in the spring and once in the fall.

1998: Pathway II pilot testing is completed, and the alternative examination is administered by the NCCPA as an alternative to the PANRE. The NCCPA begins requiring PAs to pass the recertifying examination within two attempts.

1999: The PANCE is administered for the first time by computer at multiple sites across the country through a process developed by the NBME and already in place for the licensing of physicians. The computer-based examination soon becomes universal for certification and licensure of all health professionals throughout the country.

2000: The PANRE and the Surgery Examination are administered for the first time by computer. The NCCPA launches a new web-based CME logging system and provides secure online access for PA-C designees to their certification maintenance record.

2001: The NCCPA offers a second administration of PANRE and Pathway II each year and implements new certification maintenance requirements to end the practice of renewing certificates for PAs who fail the examination; the NCCPA announces that it will now assume responsibility for recording all CME hours for purposes of certification maintenance, ending 25 years of service by AAPA as an intermediary. The AAPA will continue to approve continuing educational activities for credit.

2002 to 2005: During this period, NCCPA begins to explore process improvement and quality programs, integrating new ways of framing challenges and seeking solutions using data and experience. Consistent application of process improvement principles yields remarkable results for the organization, from dramatic cost savings to leaps in service delivery and reductions in vulnerability to human error through optimization of technology—processes that continue to be assessed and enhanced as needs and innovations emerge. The NCCPA also leads work to identify the competencies required for successful PA practice, inviting participation of the AAPA, Physician Assistant Education Association, and ARC-PA in the endeavor. The resultant document, "Competencies for the PA Profession," influences curricula, CME programs, certification requirements, and accreditation standards.

2006: The NCCPA creates a supporting foundation to contribute to the development and advancement of the PA profession in new ways for the ultimate benefit of patients. In its first year, the NCCPA Foundation produces an award-winning video-based educational program provided to all PA programs on the subject of ethics. Its content is based on real-world issues that require disciplinary action by NCCPA.

2007: The NCCPA makes the decision to bring exam development—a critical cornerstone of the certification process—in house for the first time in the organization's history. Doing so enables improvements to the quality and validity of key components of the process while lowering the cost of test item development.

2009 to 2010: The NCCPA becomes more active internationally, engaging Ruth Ballweg, MPH, PA-C, to liaise with those working throughout the world on the development of the PA profession and assessment programs to support it. The NCCPA hosts its first international meeting at its headquarters near Atlanta to discuss certification, test item banking, and other regulatory issues with international PA program representatives. NCCPA also continues to lead efforts to address PAs practicing in specialties. Expansion of the growth of PA practice in specialty areas challenges the NCCPA to assemble physician and PA leaders to participate in a discussion on PA specialty practice. This endeavor evolves to include the design of a strategy to address this call.

2011: The NCCPA launches a new Certificate of Added Qualifications (CAQ) program through which PAs in five specialties—cardiovascular and thoracic surgery, emergency medicine, nephrology, orthopedic surgery, and psychiatry—can achieve a new form of recognition by documenting their specialty experience, skills, and knowledge. The first CAQ examinations are held nationally on September 12, 2011. Also in 2011, the Society for the Preservation of Physician Assistant History (PA History Society) becomes a supporting organization to the NCCPA. The Society transfers its archive, library, and museum collection from the Duke University Medical Center and the Eugene A. Stead, Jr. Center for Physician Assistants, located in Durham, North Carolina, to the Society's new headquarters at Johns Creek, Georgia, adjacent to the NCCPA and ARC-PA national offices. The archival function of the PA History Center is assumed by the Society.

2012: The NCCPA reaches a major milestone and certifies its 100,000th PA. The NCCPA collaborates with the newly renamed NCCPA Health Foundation to enhance the NCCPA's data collection and management process beyond the collection of demographic and limited practice data on all PAs. In May 2012, the NCCPA launches the PA Professional Profile through which PAs provided a much broader range of professional and practice data, quickly creating the world's the most robust data source on PAs and PA practice.

As a result of this groundbreaking work for the PA profession, the NCCPA is able to produce the following reports:
- 2013, 2014, and 2015 Statistical Report on Recently Certified PAs
- 2013, 2014, and 2015 Statistical Profile on Certified PAs
- 2014 State Report and 2015 due for release at the end of 2016
- 2015 Specialty Report

2014: PAs begin transitioning to a new 10-year certification maintenance process, including new requirements for self-assessment and performance improvement (PI) CME, additions intended to expand the breadth of PA competencies encompassed by the certification maintenance process. Dawn Morton-Rias, EdD, PA-C, joins the NCCPA as president and CEO, becoming the first PA to serve as the NCCPA's chief staff officer.

2015: The NCCPA launches its first mobile app (Apple and later Android) so that PAs may log CMEs and access certification maintenance details anywhere, any time. The NCCPA also dramatically expands PA involvement of all aspects of the NCCPA's work. Throughout 2015, the NCCPA continues to enhance its technological and psychometrics infrastructure and begins exploration of the use of technology-enhanced test items. The NCCPA launches a new effort to answer: How can we maintain the generalist nature of the PA-C credential through a recertification model that serves the public interest and better reflects the current state of PA practice in which more than 70% of PAs are practicing outside of primary care? The board of directors begins a comprehensive analysis of this question, conducting the most detailed analysis of PA practice in the profession's history. In November 2015, the NCCPA publishes a possible new approach to the PA recertification exam process for public comment.

2016: While gathering PA feedback on potential changes to the PANRE, the NCCPA hears concerns from PAs about the burdens of the certification maintenance process. The NCCPA conducts an in-depth review of existing SA and PI activities, with particular emphasis on the gaps in availability of practice-relevant options for many PAs. Finding inadequate coverage of self-assessment in 31 specialty areas and of PI-CME in 13 specialty areas, the NCCPA recognizes that this adds a fiscal and time burden to PAs pursuing CME activities within their practice area—an unintended complication of the SA and PI CME requirement. Based on these findings, the NCCPA board votes to make SA and PI-CME now optional and to award additional credit—weighting Self Assessment (SA) and Professional Improvement (PI)-CME more heavily than regular Category 1 CME—in recognition of the value of these more interactive types of CME. The NCCPA's board approves the development of a new PA-C Emeritus credential to be launched by year's end to honor qualified PAs who have retired from clinical practice. The NCCPA launches an effort to define "core medical knowledge" to increase the PANRE's focus on assessing core knowledge that is foundational to all PA practice. Over time, that means the content covered by PANRE will narrow to the essential foundational knowledge and cognitive skills all PAs should maintain regardless of the area in which they practice. This work, which will take several years to fully implement, begins in June 2016. The NCCPA announces that changes to PANRE content and the PANRE exam blueprint will be gradual but steady.

Past and Future

Many operational aspects of the NCCPA certification and recertification processes have changed over the past 40 years. The structure and content of exams have changed over time. Exams once offered only once a year are now available year round. The process of maintaining certification (logging CME hours, making payments, checking on the status of certification requirements) has gotten exponentially easier over time. Data collection and management have been enhanced, and vital information about PA practice is now readily available. Codes of conduct and enforcement through a disciplinary policy have been introduced. PA competencies have been defined and are used as a basis for reevaluation of the certification and certification maintenance processes. Process management and customer service continue to be enhanced. The composition and representation of the board of directors has changed as the profession has matured, reflecting greater input from PAs. Specialty CAQs, mobile apps, and responsive website pages have been developed. A PA-C Emeritus status has been developed. These are just a few of the innovations and improvements that have been possible over the past decades.

Some things haven't changed. The primary focus of the NCCPA is and always will be the public's interest. This understanding guides the NCCPA board of directors as it determines how to most effectively define and deliver certification and recertification exam processes and maintenance of certification programs that reflect practice and support delivery of high-quality, affordable, accessible health care. The NCCPA maintains its commitment to supporting the flexibility PAs have to change specialties during their career spans and to work in multiple specialties concurrently. The NCCPA knows it is vitally important to maintain the generalist nature of the PA-C credential.

Although individuals often view issues from their personal perspective, organizations such as NCCPA have the responsibility to view issues from a more global perspective, with input from PAs and other stakeholders. The NCCPA continually reexamines the content and format of its exams and processes while recognizing that change takes several years. The NCCPA staff, led by a certified PA, knows that

PAs value certification as a demonstration of their continued knowledge and skills and is dedicated to service to the NCCPA and the public it serves.

STATE REGULATION: LICENSURE AND REGISTRATION

Greater recognition of PAs as health care providers has led to the development of state laws and regulations governing their practice. Recognition of PAs in state law and delegation of authority to a state regulatory body that oversees their practice serve two main purposes: to protect the public from substandard practice by PAs and to promote appropriate expanded delegation within the scope of PA practice by assuring consumers, physicians, and others that PAs are competent.[10] In the late 1960s and early 1970s, while the PA concept was beginning to blossom, there was pervasive dissatisfaction with the prevailing method of credentialing health professionals. Sadler and colleagues[11] summed up the mood of the time:

> *At a time when the entire licensure scheme for regulating health personnel is under widespread attack as being archaic, inefficient, and destructive of change, a variety of delegation amendments to state medical practice acts have been enacted as a direct result of the physician assistant movement.[11]*

Through their willingness to remain legally dependent, to accept delegation from physicians, and to work under the supervision and control of the physician, PAs are able to function under broad and flexible legal umbrellas that allow them to perform to their capacity.[10]

During the early 1970s, a patchwork of approaches was initiated, and many states put forth amendments to state medical practice acts that allowed for the delegation of tasks by physicians to assistants. Such initial amendments typically consisted of a brief paragraph allowing PAs to function. Most states also identified an agency that would assume the responsibility for regulation of this profession.

Despite the flexibility of the delegation amendments, it became increasingly clear to many state regulatory agencies that they were inadequate to deal with the tremendous growth in responsibility of the PA profession. Today most states realize the need to reexamine the definition of the scope of PA practice, and most recognize that PAs must engage in clinical decision making to practice effectively. As they rework legislation relative to PA practice, a few states continue to register PAs, thus giving rise to the designation "RPA-C" (the "R" indicating registration

in the particular state), but most states have adopted licensure laws to govern PAs.

Statutory authority to promulgate rules and regulations to accompany such laws is typically given to an agency, such as a state medical board. Through the Administrative Rule Making Act, the rules and regulations that are developed, although easier to change than statutes, carry the same weight as laws. State statutes, rules, and regulations are as varied as the states they represent. Whatever the arrangement, the two most consistent criteria for practice in a particular state remain successful completion of the NCCPA national certifying examination and graduation from an ARC-PA–accredited PA educational program.

Physician assistants are playing an ever-increasing role in the regulation of their own profession. Nine states (Arizona, California, Iowa, Massachusetts, Michigan, Rhode Island, Tennessee, Texas, and Utah) have regulatory bodies strictly for PAs.[10] Nearly all state medical boards have PA committees. Some of the committees are advisory, but others have significant responsibilities in rule making, review of applications, and discipline. There are seats for PAs on 18 other medical, osteopathic, or disciplinary boards.[10] The AAPA strongly endorses the authority of designated state regulatory agencies, in accordance with due process, to discipline PAs who have committed acts in violation of state law. Disciplinary actions include, but are not limited to, suspension and revocation of an individual's license or certificate of registration. The AAPA also endorses the sharing of information among the state regulatory agencies regarding the disposition of adjudicated actions against PAs.[10]

Registration

In the few states where PAs are still registered, issues related to PA practice are addressed either by a subcommittee of a state medical board that has been formed to deal with PA practice or by a state medical board that includes a seat (or seats) for PA representation. The medical board most often functions in an advisory capacity to a state governmental agency, such as a department of commerce or department of business regulation. In rare instances, physicians are regulated by a nongovernmental agency; in such cases, PAs are generally covered by the same arrangement.

Licensure

An increasing number of states are creating separate PA licensing boards as a result of new PA practice acts that replace the initial delegation amendments to medical practice acts. Such boards are usually composed of practicing PAs and practicing physicians who employ or work with PAs. The boards are typically advisory to a governmental agency, which has ultimate authority in the regulation of PAs. PAs are licensed in 48 states, the District of Columbia, and most U.S. territories.[10] They are certified in only one state (Ohio) and registered in one state (Massachusetts).[10] Only five states (Montana, New Hampshire, North Carolina, North Dakota, Ohio) do not have statutes or rules regulating temporary licensure.[10] Temporary licensure for most states allows for new graduates to start work as a PA prior to taking their PANCE exams. This may be a holdover from the earlier days when PANCE was only offered a few times a year. The temporary license typically expires after receiving the results of the test. A few states do allow continuation of a temporary license under certain circumstances. PAs should always review the individual state's statutes and rules before applying for a license.

INSTITUTIONAL CREDENTIALING AND PRIVILEGING

Unless a PA is practicing exclusively in a private medical practice with no regulation, he or she will also be subject to credentialing by the institution in which he or she practices. The Joint Commission on Accreditation of Hospitals and the National Commission on Quality Assurance mandate a credentialing process for licensed providers working within an institution. Typically, a committee of the medical staff administers this process with the technical support of credentialing professionals. The institutional credentialing process, which is also carried out by some third-party payers, verifies the training and experience of providers who see patients in the institution's delivery system. Hospital practice requires a further step: privileging. This second step, administered by the medical staff, requires that providers document their training and experience with specific procedures before being granted the privilege of performing these activities within the system. This often entails providing proof of competency for certain procedures. Providers typically are given expanded privileges over time as they gain additional training and experience with new procedures.

CONCLUSION

Currently, all states have enacted laws or regulations recognizing PAs. The AAPA provides up-to-date summary information on state requirements for PA practice. For further information on a specific state's statutes and regulations, readers are advised to contact the appropriate state agency.

CLINICAL APPLICATIONS

1. Interview the director of your PA program to review the program's accreditation history.
   - When was it first accredited? When is its next accreditation?
   - What are the current evaluation and growth issues for the program?
   - What roles do students play in the accreditation of a program?
   - What changes does your program director foresee in the future accreditation of your program specifically?
2. Bookmark the NCCPA's website on your computer to have easy access to the "blueprint" for the NCCPA PANCE exam. Review the most updated requirements for NCCPA "maintenance of certification," including the time frame and the requirements for CME and other activities.
3. Discuss the process of licensure and registration with a
   - PA in your community who practices in an institutional setting
   - PA practicing in a private ambulatory setting
   Compare and contrast the processes for the two settings, and discuss how periodic review occurs.

KEY POINTS

- While enrolled in PA educational programs, students are primarily focused on learning and examination and less focused on the many levels of credentialing that will impact them as they enter practice, including the accreditation status of "their" PA program, details of the entry-level certification exam (PANCE), state licensure processes and timelines, and requirements for "privileging" by the health systems or hospitals where they will work. This chapter provides the "go-to" information that all PAs need in learning about—and understanding—these processes and the organizations that administer them.

References

1. McCarty JE, Stuetzer LJ, Somers JE. Physician assistant program accreditation - history in the making. *Persp. Physi Assist Educ.* 2001;12(1):24–38.
2. Accreditation Review Commission on Education of the Physician Assistant. Mission, philosophy, goals. http://www.arc-pa.org/about/mission-philosophy-goals/.
3. Standards Accreditation Standards for Physician Assistant Education. 4th ed. March 2010 (effective September 1, 2010). http://www.arc-pa.com/acc_standards/.
4. Accreditation Review Commission on Education of the Physician Assistant. http://www.arc-pa.org/about/about/pas/.
5. Accreditation Review Commission on Education of the Physician Assistant. About PAs. http://www.arc-pa.org/about/pas/.
6. Accreditation Review Commission on Education of the Physician Assistant. ARC-PA commissioners. http://www.arc-pa.org/about/arc-pa-commissioners/.
7. Accreditation Review Commission on Education of the Physician Assistant. http://www.arc-pa.org/accreditation/accreditation_types_review_cycle/.
8. Accreditation Review Commission on Education of the Physician Assistant. http://www.arc-pa.org/accreditation/postgraduate-programs/process/.
9. Historical Information Courtesy of Physician Assistant History Society Archives. 2016. Johns Creek, GA.
10. Physician Assistant State Laws and Regulations. 11th ed. Alexandria, VA: American Academy of Physician Assistants; 2010.
11. Sadler AM, Sadler BL, Bliss AA. *The Physician Assistant Today and Tomorrow: Issues Confronting New Health Practitioners.* 2nd ed. New Haven, CT: Yale University Press; 1972.

CHAPTER 7

PHYSICIAN ASSISTANT RELATIONSHIP TO PHYSICIANS

William C. Kohlhepp • Anthony Brenneman • Stephane VanderMeulen

CHAPTER OUTLINE

One of the defining features of the physician assistant (PA) profession is the relationship between PAs and physicians. When physicians created the PA profession, they envisioned PAs practicing medicine with physician delegation and supervision. Throughout the profession's 50-year history, PAs have consistently embraced the concept of team-based health care. PAs believe that the physician–PA team relationship is fundamental because the framework of practice is designed to assure the delivery of high-quality health care.

The key features of this unique relationship were recognized by the PEW Health Professions Commission in its 1998 report on the PA profession when it pointed to the use of consultation, referral, and review of PA practice by the physician. The report concluded, "The characteristics of this relationship are also considered to be the elements of professional relationships in any well designed health system."[1]

The dimensions of the clinical relationship between PAs and physicians are multifaceted and variable given the setting (solo practice vs. hospital, group vs. solo practice, rural vs. urban, teaching hospital vs. nursing home), the practice (family practice vs. specialty, subspecialty vs. internal medicine, hospitalist vs. emergency medicine), and employer (solo practitioner vs. health maintenance organization [HMO], free clinic vs. boutique clinic, preferred provider organization [PPO] vs. Medicaid). Each setting provides its own unique sets of challenges and opportunities. When practitioners, health care systems, and employers are aware of the unique state rules and regulations governing PAs and communication is open on both sides (employer–employee, partner–supervisor, and so on), then the physician–PA relationship can flourish, leading to high levels of autonomy, satisfaction, high-quality health care, and excellent patient outcomes. In addition to the clinical relationship that exists between PAs and physicians, it is important to realize that their association also exists on other levels, particularly the employment relationship and their relationship as colleagues. Successful team practice depends on all of those involved having a clear understanding of what their responsibilities will include. For a physician, it is an understanding that he or she is to maintain an active license to practice medicine, accept responsibility for the care delivered by the PA, and maintain a delegation agreement with the PA that is fluid and should be modified as changes occur. For a PA, it is working within the scope of practice delegated by the physician, establishing and maintaining clear lines of accountability, and seeking guidance when needed. Physician–PA team practice can most effectively operate if team members appropriately allocate their time and talents. "The most effective clinical teams are those that utilize the skills and abilities of each team member most efficiently."[2]

HISTORICAL PERSPECTIVE

The physician–PA relationship has evolved since the inception of the PA profession. The team-based model of care that exists today differs from the original concept envisioned by Dr. Eugene Stead of Duke University, who is generally credited with founding the PA profession. In an early monograph describing his vision for the PA's role, Dr. Stead intended for PAs to be trained in laboratories and clinics to perform an array of procedures, diagnostic tests, and medical therapies. Noting that the physician would direct the activities and would be legally responsible for all acts of the PA, it was thought that PAs would provide medical care in clinics, hospital settings, patient homes, and outlying communities. Dr. Stead also discussed administrative duties for which PAs would be responsible, including the organization of "medical care units," managing all aspects and elements of patient care, ranging from technicians and nursing staff to housekeeping and custodial personnel.[3] Although PAs would be trained to recognize certain medical conditions such as heart failure and shock, Stead posed that PAs would not be involved in the clinical diagnosis, decision making, and treatment of medical problems.[3]

The scope of PA practice has evolved since Stead's early vision to include a holistic approach to medical care, spanning all aspects of patient management. The importance of the physician–PA relationship, however, has remained integral to the PA profession. Although he may not have anticipated these changes, Stead made this prescient prediction of the value of PAs to physician practice: "They will be capable of extending the arms and the brains of the physician so that he can care for more people."[4] This statement remains true today.

SHARED KNOWLEDGE BASE

The relationship between physicians and PAs begins at the educational level. Although there is wide variability in the methods of curriculum delivery among PA education programs, the content delivered is based on the medical model. Because there is little discernable difference in the content delivered in both PA and medical education, PAs and physicians possess a shared knowledge base. The basic elements of medical education include knowledge of the basic sciences and evidence-based medicine, patient interviewing and interpersonal communication skills, physical examination skills, medical ethics, critical thinking, and clinical problem-solving abilities. These elements represent the core knowledge base of physicians and PAs alike.

Many PA programs are administratively located within medical schools or academic health centers, and others are associated with hospitals, large health systems, or military medical facilities. It is common for PA students to share classes, faculty, and experiential education sites with medical students. Some programs housed within medical schools have fully integrated the PA curriculum into the medical school's curriculum. Having both been trained in the medical model, physicians and PAs develop a similarity in medical reasoning that eventually leads them to use a consistent approach to patient care in the clinical workplace: "PAs think like doctors."[5-7]

Training side by side builds camaraderie and allows PAs and physicians to understand one another's competence, knowledge, and skill levels. This leads to mutual trust and respect and creates the foundation of the physician–PA relationship.

DEPENDENT PRACTICE VERSUS INTERDEPENDENT PRACTICE

As the profession has matured and health care needs have evolved, so too has the way in which physicians and PAs have formulated practice styles and plans. What once was clearly a dependent practice, relying on one practitioner to supervise a single PA, thereby limiting scope of practice, has evolved to an interdependent practice, in which the PA and physician rely on each other to provide high-quality health care to a wide range of patients in all settings.

The interdependent practice of physicians and PAs over time has shown itself to be a cost-effective, dynamic, and medically sound approach to health care.[7] This interdependent practice assures the patient of a high-level, quality health care experience in the style of the physician while helping to maintain continuity in the system. The physician benefits by being in the best position to determine that care is provided at the standard the physician seeks to provide as well as freeing up the physician to see to the most complex and critical problems.[8] As Kimball and Rothwell have noted, regardless of the structure of their practice, if a PA determines that a patient's condition is beyond his or her expertise, the PA will expedite referral to the physician or another specialist.[9] In its landmark report "Crossing the Quality Chasm," the Institute of Medicine discussed the importance of "communication among members of a team, using all the expertise and knowledge of team members, and where appropriate, sensibly extending roles to meet patient needs." This approach clearly reflects the physician–PA team and all its attributes.[10] This reflects all the interdependent and interconnected roles that the physician–PA team strives to achieve. Through this interdependent role, there is assurance that the PA will receive the appropriate backup when needed; this interdependence reassures the patient that his or her care is continuous, monitored, and of high quality and reassures the physician that care will be provided at the physician's standard of care.

COMMUNICATION, COORDINATION, AND CONTINUITY OF CARE

Communication is vital to a successful interdependent practice. It also requires advanced interpersonal skills and the ability to coordinate care among multiple providers and systems. Interdependent practice can improve patient care, outcomes, and satisfaction for patients and providers. Interpersonal skills, which include all of the hallmarks of professionalism (see Chapter 33), form the foundation of a developing working relationship with the physician and lead to a fully developed, integrated, and interdependent practice.

Without clear lines of communication, the system quickly falls apart, leading toward mistakes; misunderstandings; and at its worst, harm to the patient. Initially, it is important to develop lines of communication that will benefit the physician, the PA, and the patient. This can be done through the development of practice plans, physician delegation of workloads as defined, and regular meetings to discuss current working arrangements. This fluid and ever evolving approach allows for expansion of duties, reassignment of resources, and more clearly defined working roles and relationships leading toward expanded patient services.

In the joint policy statement from the American Academy of Family Physicians (AAFP) and the American Academy of Physician Assistants (AAPA), the associations recognize the need for a shared commitment to achieving positive working relationships. This occurs by first understanding each member's roles and then maintains and enhances the relationship by effective communication.[11] Nowhere is this more obvious than when the physician and PA are located at different sites. Particularly in this situation, the use of technology becomes extremely helpful to support and facilitate communication and the practice of medicine.[11] With the movement toward electronic medical records, communication and delegation of practice will expand with easier access to patient records, as well as improvement in the continuity of care within the practice and throughout the health care system.

Continuity of care has been defined as the "process by which the patient and the physician are cooperatively involved in ongoing health care management toward the goal of high quality, cost-effective medical care."[12] In its joint policy statement, the AAFP says that this continuity is facilitated by the physician-led team.[11]

With its focus on communication, coordination of medical care, and the provision of that care in a continuous model, the physician–PA relationship not only benefits the patient but also helps expand health care and its limited resources.

DELEGATED SCOPE OF PRACTICE

As medical practice has evolved over the years, tremendous change has occurred in the specific tasks to be accomplished by medical professionals, including PAs. Although scope of practice is a key section of the law and regulations in each state, generally the state delegates to physicians the authority to determine the scope of practice for PAs.[13] This approach was reaffirmed by the Federation of State Medical Boards (FSMB), which stated: "Supervising physician should be legally responsible for the delegation of medical tasks, the performance and the acts of omissions of the physician assistant."[14] Although physician delegation is a "major defining characteristic of PA scope of practice," Davis et al note, "PA scope of practice is generally defined by four determinants: PA education, experience, and preference; physician delegation; facility credentialing and privileging; and state law and regulations." Having pointed to the role of the latter, the authors conclude: "Ultimately, the PA-physician team best determines PA scope of practice."[15]

Because the role of the PA in a practice is highly individualized, physicians and PAs who are working together are in the best position to define the PA's scope of practice. They can evaluate the many factors that go into that PA's role, including the type of practice, the setting, the acuity of the patients, the physician's needs and preferences, and the PA's training and experience.[9]

Evaluating the knowledge, skills, and abilities of the PA is a key step in scope of practice delegation. The physician can observe the PA's performance and can make sure the PA possesses the requisite clinical knowledge and accomplishes tasks and procedures in a highly competent manner. This was reaffirmed in the policy statement jointly written by the AAFP and the AAPA, which stated: "The physician evaluates the PA's competency and performance, and together they develop a team approach based on both the PA's and physician's clinical skills and patient needs."[11] In its monograph on the physician–PA relationship written with the AAPA, the American College of Physicians (ACP) stated, "The physician has the ability to observe the PA's competency and performance and plan for PA utilization based on the PA's abilities, the physician's delegatory style, and the needs of the patients seen in the practice."[16]

It must also be recognized that the scope of practice of the PA is not static but evolves over time. Physicians play a key role in the development of PAs by mentoring them in the clinical setting. This effort combined with that learned from formal continuing medical education programs allows PAs to gain the advanced or specialized knowledge needed for their scope of practice to grow and change and to keep up with advances in the medical profession.[17]

Although the attention is often focused on its legal aspects, scope of practice is also a key expression of the physician–PA relationship. How much and what is delegated in the scope of practice is a measure of the level of trust and confidence placed in the PA by the physician.[7] Scope of practice decisions also impact the effectiveness of the physician–PA team. The AAFP–AAPA joint policy statement notes: "The most effective physician-PA team practices provide optimal patient care by designing practice models where the skills and abilities of each team member are used most efficiently."[11]

Scope of practice is also central to optimal patient care. PAs believe that patients are best served when the physician–PA team treats patients in a consistent practice style and the socialization of PAs facilitates their adoption of the individual practice patterns of the physician.[7] It is most important when discussing scope of practice to realize that patients seen by a PA are evaluated and cared for with a level of skill and competency similar to the manner in which a physician would treat a similarly situated patient.[17]

AUTONOMOUS MEDICAL DECISION MAKING

Autonomous decision making has always been an issue for clinical providers other than physicians. In strict definition, autonomy is having the right or power to self-govern or to carry on without outside control.[18] Although this strictly defines autonomy, it fails to recognize the unique team-based approach that the physician and PA maintain. In this model, autonomy is delegated by the physician, allowing the PA to practice medicine as trained, able to make health care decisions within the scope of practice delegated by the physician, without the need for input on these decisions unless the PA determines that the patient will be best served by physician input.

In the AAFP–AAPA joint policy statement, they use the concept of "delegated autonomy" and compare the relationship of the physician–PA practice to that of attending and resident physicians. They outline the key components of this delegated autonomy that should include clear lines of accountability as well as reciprocal responsibilities of seeking and providing supervision and consultation.[11] This term is reflective of an earlier term used by Eugene Schneller, a medical sociologist, who observed PA practice in the early years of the profession. Schneller coined the term "negotiated performance autonomy" for this evolutionary process that leads to increased delegation of scope of practice.[19]

Chumbler and colleagues defined "autonomy of practice" for PAs as "the extent to which PAs can determine independently the range of tasks they will perform."[20] The authors further defined the concept of autonomy of practice as having two components: clinical decision making and prescriptive authority. As the profession has matured, so too has the level of autonomy within delegated roles of the PA. As White and Davis noted, there has been a trend toward more physician-determined scope of practice as delegated activities have increased instead of trying to list in state and federal law all activities performed by a PA. This allows for the original premise of the physician–PA team-based practice to function as originally designed, with "delegated autonomy" determined by the physician's comfort and the PA's demonstrated competence.[7] This trend may be due to physicians being trained alongside of PAs, understanding the PA role better, or the expansion of state and federal laws, as well as the movement of PAs into areas of medicine outside of the traditional primary care scope of training. It is anticipated that these roles will continue to evolve over time as practice plans and laws evolve and the profession continues to mature. This has been noted and borne out in monograph statements from the AAFP[11] and ACP[16] and in works by White and Davis[7] and Chumbler et al.[20]

AGENCY RELATIONSHIP

A recent article on scope of practice includes reference to another key descriptor for the legal relationship between the physician and the PA, noting: "In the eyes of the law, the PA serves as the agent of the physician."[15] Agency is a fundamental legal concept that is relevant to situations when the PA acts on behalf of the physician. Agency has been described as the "fiduciary relation which manifests from the consent by one person to another that the other shall act on his behalf and subject to his control, and consent by the other so to act."[21]

Three factors must be present for an agency relationship to exist between two parties, such as between the physician and the PA. The physician consents to the relationship; the physician accrues some degree of benefits from the acts of the PA; and the physician has some degree of control of, or right to control, the PA.[22] The "assent, benefit, and control test" can be applied even in situations when assent can be implied in the absence of express consent by the physician (e.g., when the physician is hired by the hospital or practice and supervising the PA is one of the assigned duties).[21]

Because they have no independent authority to act but rather gain the basis for action from the physician's authority, PAs must be considered as "agents of the physicians rather than independent practitioners."[23] The question of to whom the liability runs is central to agency analysis. Thus, after an agency relationship is established, both the physician and PA are liable for the acts of the PA.

Establishing the responsibility of the physician for the actions of the PA was a key factor in recognizing that the PA possessed the authority to establish valid patient care orders in the hospital setting. In a key article on the topic, Bissonette recounted several key attorney general opinions that pointed to the agency relationship in regard to patient orders. "The Attorney General in Maryland concluded, 'it must be presumed that a properly credentialed and supervised PA issues orders with the authority delegated to him/her by a licensed physician.' The Michigan Attorney General noted that physician delegation to the PA confers authority to the agent (PA) to do things that otherwise the physician would have to do."[24] A key court decision also relied on this concept to establish PA authority for order writing. The Supreme Court State of Washington held that it was the intent of the legislature to establish PAs as agents of the physician; therefore, every order given by a PA is considered as coming from the physician.[13,23]

PHYSICIAN SUPERVISION: LEGAL BASIS FOR PHYSICIAN ASSISTANT PRACTICE

The physician–PA relationship is a fundamental principle that guides the model of team-based patient care and PA practice. According to the AAPA's Guidelines for State Regulations of PAs, "the guiding principles of supervision must be that it a) protects the public health and safety, and b) preserves the PA's access to physician consultation when indicated."[25] A central theme of the relationship between a physician and a PA is the recognition that the physician is the more comprehensively trained member of the team and therefore holds terminal responsibility for assuring that all members of the team adhere to accepted standards of care. He or she assumes legal liability and professional responsibility for all medical actions of the PA. The legal recognition of the physician–PA relationship is seen in state laws in all 50 states.

Although the physician is ultimately responsible for the acts of the PA, the responsibility to ensure that PAs practice in accordance with ethical, legal, and medical standards is shared and reciprocal. It is the responsibility of the PA to seek advice and consultation when indicated. PAs are often credited with the strength of "knowing their limits" and understanding when physician input should be solicited. It is incumbent upon physician–PA teams to clearly delineate the role and tasks for which the PA is authorized to perform. These are the key factors in delegated autonomy, discussed earlier in this chapter.

The synergic nature of this compact is beneficial for physicians, PAs, and patients. It allows physicians to expand the capacity of their practice, assured that patients will be cared for in accordance with their own style and preferences. It frees the physician to focus on patients with more complex medical problems. For PAs, this arrangement ensures that a constant resource exists to provide guidance and input when difficult or complicated medical problems arise. The physician is always available to assume care of the patient if necessary. Patients can be assured that the style of practice and standard of care they receive are comparable, whether they are being cared for by the physician or the PA, and that physician involvement in their care is available at all times.[8]

Physician assistants are authorized to practice medicine in all 50 states, the District of Columbia, and the majority of U.S. territories. Virtually all state laws mandate physician supervision as a part of PA practice. However, the definition and degree of these relationships vary widely.

CHANGE IN TERMINOLOGY: COLLABORATION

The term "supervision" itself is a barrier to the public's accurate understanding of the profession and the achievement of legal authority for full scope of practice. Pointing to the evolution of the role of the PA over time to reflect a more collaborative relationship between the professions, the AAPA now recommends replacing the term "supervision" with "collaboration." Maintaining the relationship between physicians and PAs, however, remains critically important to the profession.

In an effort to provide states with guidance on revising and updating state laws to allow PAs to effectively function in this changing health care environment, the AAPA has drafted model legislative language. The AAPA's desire to move toward the term "collaboration" rather than "supervision" surfaced in a recent update to that model language that addresses the need for written agreements between physicians and PAs.

> *Collaboration shall be continuous, but shall not be construed to require the physical presence of the physician at the time and place that services are rendered. It is the obligation of each team of physician(s) and PA(s) to ensure that the PA's scope of practice is identified and appropriate to the PA's skill, education and training, and that the relationship with, and access to, the collaborating physician(s) is defined.*[26]

Widespread implementation and utilization of the term "collaboration" will likely take time. The word "supervision" is used in the regulatory and legal language at the federal and state levels of all states.

TYPES OF SUPERVISION AND COLLABORATIVE RELATIONSHIPS

The practice acts of PAs in all states require either a collaborative relationship with a physician or some level of physician supervision. Alaska and the District of Columbia were early adopters of the collaboration language, and additional states are pursuing updates to their statutes to reflect this more contemporary language. Of the states that still use supervisory language,

wide variability exists in the type of physician–PA relationship mandated by law. Supervision can be divided into three general categories: prospective, concurrent, and retrospective. Although perhaps not using these specific terms, each state's laws contain elements of one or more of the following categories that describe the working relationship between physicians and PAs.

Prospective

Agreements, both formal and informal, made between the physician and PA at the time of employment that delineate the duties and responsibilities of both parties constitute the prospective element of collaboration. These agreements are based on the anticipated scope of PA practice and assume the likely or expected scenarios and patient population that will be managed by the PA. Formal agreements are required in many states; however, in all situations, an informal discussion about both parties' expectations should occur early in the PA's employment.

Many states require written agreements, known as delegation agreements or practice agreements. In general, these guidelines delineate the types of patient visits and procedures the PA is authorized by the physician to perform. The duties should generally fall within the physician's own scope of practice and be appropriate to the PA's level of training and competence. The agreement provides for a clear understanding by all parties about what the physician's role and the duties of the PA will entail. Some states require formal approval of the agreement by the state medical board or licensing agency. All parties sign these agreements, and regular maintenance and updating of the documents are required. States usually require that formal agreements be kept on file at the state licensing agency, the practice, or any remote sites where the PA practices. Ideally, the practice agreement should be specific enough to eliminate any ambiguity about each party's responsibilities but flexible enough to allow the physician and PA to design a plan that maximizes the effectiveness of the team and allows both members to practice to the fullest extent of their qualifications.

Another form of prospective relationship involves protocols. The term "protocol" can be confusing because it is sometimes used to refer to delegation or practice agreements. True protocols are detailed clinical protocols that prescribe specific clinical courses of action in the treatment of disease. Some states require the use of protocols to guide PA practice. The use of protocols to guide PA practice is unwarranted and is discouraged by the AAPA.[27] Protocols, by their nature, are rigid and rapidly outdated. Extensive clinical protocols neither enhance the clinical judgment exercised by PAs nor improve the diagnosis and treatment of disease. Requirement of protocols may actually hinder care because it decreases the ability to use clinical judgment and individualize treatment for a specific patient.[27] The use of protocols is too prescriptive and does not allow for the dynamic, patient-specific clinical decision making that is often necessary in today's challenging and constantly changing health care environment.

Concurrent

The oversight and availability of the physician that occurs on an ongoing, daily basis forms the bulk of the element of concurrent collaboration. Medicare's description of the three levels of physician supervision for diagnostic tests provides a reasonable framework for considering the availability of the physician to the PA envisioned.[28]

General supervision means that the physician must be available to the PA at all times. This does not necessarily suggest that he or she must be physically present but should be available by either electronic or telephonic means. All states require general supervision, but wide variability exists regarding the geographic or time limits and the means by which the physician is available. For example, one state may require that the physician stay within 10 miles of the practice site, and another might require that the physician be able to reach the clinic within 15 minutes. Some states require telephone contact, and others may allow text messaging or email contact.

Direct supervision means that the physician must be physically present in the building. Requirements for direct supervision also vary widely. Some states require the physician to be present at all times, and others require direct oversight for either a percentage of the time that the PA practices or a specific amount of time, such as one day per week. Direct supervision requirements may differ if the PA practices at a geographically remote or satellite clinic rather than the "home" clinic and can vary depending on the PA's level of experience, skill, or competence. Occasionally, a limited probationary period of stricter oversight is required.

Personal supervision is the most restrictive form of concurrent supervision, requiring the physician to be present in the room while the PA provides care. Because of the delegatory nature of the physician–PA team, this type of supervision is rarely necessary or required. Occasionally, new graduates are required to be personally supervised for a finite period of time upon hiring. Some states require physician presence in the room when PAs perform surgical or other procedures and during major surgical procedures.

Retrospective

The process of evaluating the performance, clinical activities, and quality of care provided by the PA makes up the final aspect of collaboration, the retrospective element. The evaluation may take place in person, electronically, or telephonically. It involves the periodic review of patient charts, prescriptions, and orders written by the PA and often includes case discussions. The timing, frequency, and magnitude of review are dictated by the state. It can include all charts, a percentage of charts, a representative sample, or certain predetermined types of patient visits. Some states require physicians to co-sign charts, orders, and prescriptions, and others require that the physician sees the patient periodically (e.g., every third visit). This retrospective focus is an integral part of the physician–PA relationship because it provides a mechanism for feedback and quality assurance and ensures that standards of care are being met.

IMPACT OF CHANGING HEALTH CARE SYSTEMS

With the implementation of the Affordable Care Act (ACA), the nation has been moving to provide services to the millions of uninsured Americans who now have health care coverage. Key to expansion of services, the health care system will need to rely more heavily on primary care clinicians, such as PAs. One model for reforming primary care can be seen in the patient-centered medical home (PCMH). Such a model depends on primary care providers who function with great skill and at high levels of efficiency to ensure the needed continuity, comprehensiveness, and coordination of care. In its monograph, the AAFP argued that PAs are well suited to the PCMH.[11] The ability of PAs to succeed in the PCMH setting is grounded in patient-centric focus of the profession, its medical model of education, and its commitment to team practice.[29]

As the PCMH model has evolved, two challenges have surfaced for PAs: full utilization of skills and leadership of patient care teams. To meet the need for increased access to effective primary care clinicians, it is essential for an expansion of the scope of practice for PAs to be able to allow them to fully use their knowledge and skills. In a number of states, outdated supervision requirements hinder such scope of practice changes. As for qualifications to lead PCMH teams, many discussions have occurred, but PCMH policy language clearly permits this approach.[29]

EVOLUTION OF THE PHYSICIAN–PHYSICIAN ASSISTANT RELATIONSHIP

Although the PA profession's commitment to working in team practice with physicians is unwavering,[25] there is an increasing recognition that the manner in which supervision occurs needs to keep up with the changing practice of medicine. Today health care delivery requires a level of efficiency and effectiveness not seen previously. When considering these changes, the AAFP in its statement on the physician–PA team noted: "The most effective teams are defined by physicians at the practice level to maximize the skills of the providers and meet patient needs."[11] In its monograph, the ACP expanded on that theme, stating: "Flexibility in federal and state regulation [is encouraged] so that each medical practice determines appropriate clinical roles within the medical team, physician-to-PA ratios, and supervision processes, enabling each clinician to work to the fullest extent of his or her license and expertise."[16]

It is thus not surprising that achieving adaptability in the physician–PA relationship is the focus of four of the AAPA's six key elements that should be part of every state practice act. Specific changes in two key areas are offered: removing restriction on the ratios of PAs to physicians and ending blanket requirements for chart co-signature.[30] When states use an approach that allows for customization of the health care team, the physician(s)–PA(s) teams can match collaboration to the specific needs of the practice.

As far back as the late 1990s, the American Medical Association Council on Medical Services pointed to the adverse impact on patient care that occurs when ratios are implemented. The council stated: "Supervising physicians are the most knowledgeable of their own supervisory abilities and practice style, as well as the training and experience of [PAs] in their practice.... Specified ratios of supervisory physicians to [PAs] might restrict appropriate provision of care and could reduce access to care."[31] Unique factors to consider in determining the appropriate number of PAs to work in collaboration with one physician include the training and experience of the PA(s), the nature of the practice, the complexity of the patient population, and the physician's supervisory approach.

Although preserving collaboration and oversight is critical, requiring physicians to co-sign every PA-written order or chart removes the doctors' discretion to exercise supervision in the way that works best for their practices. Such co-signature requirements can place unnecessary burden on the physician, which makes less efficient the care delivered by the team. Thus, physician co-signature should only be required when it is deemed to be necessary by the physician, the PA, or the facility. The AAPA believes that establishing supervision requirements such as ratios and co-signature "should be based on the experience of the PA, the complexity of the patient populations, and additional methods of oversight that are already taking place in the practice."[31]

The FSMB agrees that customization of the physician–PA relationship is key to the ability of the team to meet changing needs. The FSMB states in its document "Essentials of the Modern Medical and Osteopathic Practice Act": "A physician assistant should be permitted to provide those medical services delegated to them by the supervising physician that are within their training and experience, form a usual component of the supervising physician's scope of practice, and are provided pursuant to the supervising physician's instruction."[14]

PRACTICE OWNERSHIP

The patient-centered medical home is but one of many changes in health care delivery that has occurred since the founding of the PA profession. Initially, it was assumed that the physician–PA model would involve a designated PA working beside a single physician in a primary care setting. As the use of PAs as members of the health care team has expanded over the past 40 plus years, the model for PA utilization has changed. Today many PAs work for hospitals, group practices, or other business entities. Often, physicians have separate business relationships with the employers of PAs rather than serving themselves as direct employers of PAs.

In an effort to meet patient needs in certain situations, PAs have assumed full or part ownership or become shareholders of a professional corporation. A key requirement to become a shareholder in a professional corporation is for one to be licensed or otherwise legally authorized to provide the services the corporation offers. Thus, when physicians are not willing or able to step forward to maintain the professional corporations under which the practice is established, the PA can step in because he or she possesses the legal authorization. PA involvement in the business of practice ownership has occurred through outright PA ownership of practices through purchase, establishing corporations to own practices, and creating practice arrangements.[32] Even Medicare policies and most state laws now recognize that employment and supervision are separate and unrelated aspects of medical practice. In April 2002, the Medicare program adopted rules that allow PAs to have an ownership interest in an approved Medicare corporation that is eligible to bill the Medicare program.[33]

SUMMARY

Although PA practice has evolved over time, the tenet of PAs practicing in collaboration with physicians remains steady. This interdependent practice assures the patient of a high-level quality health care experience while helping to maintain continuity in the system. Variables affecting this relationship include type of practice, practice setting, individual state laws, and clearly delineated roles and expectations. Many of these variables are easily dealt with through maintaining open lines of communication, good interpersonal skills, and the ability to coordinate care among multiple providers and systems.

An ideal physician–PA relationship uses team-based concepts to maximize the efficiency and effectiveness of the team as a whole, with the ultimate goal of excellent patient outcomes. The role of PAs within the team should optimize the use of their training and skills and allow for appropriate autonomy to practice medicine to the highest extent of their abilities. Future legislation should preserve the physician–PA relationship while providing for the flexibility to create a team to provide excellence in promoting patient health and providing patient care based on the needs of the population and the environment where they practice.

KEY POINTS

- PAs consistently embrace the concept of the collaboration with physicians and believe it is fundamental to high-quality patient care.
- Having both been trained in the medical model, PAs and physicians share a similarity of medical reasoning.
- Scope of practice for the PA is best determined by the physician and PA together with the focus on evaluating both the PA's clinical skills and patient needs.
- PAs exercise "delegated autonomy," making medical decisions within the delegated scope of practice.
- PAs act as the "agents" of the physician, allowing them to act on behalf of the physician, particularly when generating orders for the delivery of care to hospitalized patients.
- To keep up with the changing practice of medicine, the manner in which physician oversight is provided for PAs must evolve, as does the terminology for that effort.

References

1. The PEW Health Care Commission. *Charting a Course for the Twenty-First Century: Physician Assistants and Managed Care.* San Francisco: University of California San Francisco Center for the Health Professions; 1998.
2. American Academy of Physician Assistants. PAs and team practice. https://www.aapa.org/WorkArea/DownloadAsset.aspx?id=2497.
3. Stead E. Physician Assistant History Center. *Exhibits: Development of PA Program at Duke University Medical Center*; July 1964. http://www.pahx.org/pdf/Item145.pdf.
4. Stead E. Physician Assistant History Center. *Exhibits: Development of PA Program at Duke University Medical Center*; September 1964. http://www.pahx.org/pdf/Item143.pdf.
5. White GL, Egerton CP, Myers R, Holbert RD. Physician assistants and Mississippi. *J Miss State Med Assoc.* 1994;35(12):353–357.
6. White GL. Physicians, PAs, and the facts. *J Miss State Med Assoc.* 1997;38(12):460.
7. White GL, Davis AM. Physician assistants as partners in physician-directed care. *South Med J.* 1999;92(10):956–960.
8. Kohlhepp W. Contemporary concepts of physician supervision. *JAAPA.* 2003;16:48–51.
9. Kimball BA, Rothwell WS. Physician assistant practice in Minnesota providing care as part of a physician-directed team. *Minn Med.* 2008;91(5):45–48.
10. Committee on Quality of Health Care in America, Institute of Medicine. *Crossing the Quality Chasm: a New Health System for the 21st Century.* Washington, DC: National Academies Press; 2001.
11. Rathfon E, Jones G, et al. Family physicians and physician assistants: team-based family medicine. *A joint policy statement of the American Academy of Family Physicians and American Academy of Physician Assistants.* February 2011.
12. American Academy of Family Physicians. Continuity of Care, Definition of, AAFP Policies, 2010. http://www.aafp.org/online/en/home/policy/policies/c/continuityofcaredefinition.html.
13. Younger PA. *Physician Assistant Legal Handbook.* Burlington, MA: Jones & Bartlett Learning; 1997.
14. Federation of State Medical Boards. Essentials of a modern medical and osteopathic practice act. https://www.fsmb.org/Media/Default/PDF/FSMB/Advocacy/GRPOL_essentials.pdf.
15. Davis A, Radix SM, Cawley JF, et al. Access and innovation in a time of rapid change. *Ann Health Law.* 2015;24:286–336.
16. American College of Physicians. Internists and physician assistants: team-based primary care. http://www.acponline.org/advocacy/where_we_stand/policy/internists_asst.pdf.
17. American Academy of Physician Assistants. PA scope of practice. https://www.aapa.org/WorkArea/DownloadAsset.aspx?id=583.
18. *Merriam-Webster Dictionary.* Autonomous. http://www.merriam-webster.com/dictionary/autonomous.

19. Schneller, Eugene S. *Physician's Assistant: Innovation in the Medical Division of Labour*. Lexington Books; 1978.
20. Chumbler NR, Weier AW, Geller JM. Practice autonomy among primary care physician assistants: the predictive abilities of selected practice attributes. *J Allied Health*. 2001;30(1):2–10.
21. Wyse RC. A framework of analysis for the law of agency. *Montana Law Rev*. 1979;40:31–58.
22. Harbert KR. Inpatient systems. In: Ballweg R, Sullivan EM, Brown D, Vetrosky D, eds. *Physician Assistant: A Guide to Clinical Practice*. 4th ed. Philadelphia: Saunders Elsevier; 2008.
23. Delman JL. The use and misuse of physician extenders. *J Leg Med*. 2003;24:249–280.
24. Bissonette DJ. The derivation of authority for medical order writing by PAs. *JAAPA*. 1991;4:358–361.
25. American Academy of Physician Assistants. Guidelines for state regulation of physician assistants. https://www.aapa.org/Workarea/DownloadAsset.aspx?id=795.
26. American Academy of Physician Assistants. Model state legislation for physician assistants. https://www.aapa.org/WorkArea/DownloadAsset.aspx?id=548.
27. American Academy of Physician Assistants. Physician assistants and protocols. https://www.aapa.org/WorkArea/downloadAsset.aspx?id=630.
28. Physician Supervision of Diagnostic Tests. Novitas. http://www.novitas-solutions.com/webcenter/content/conn/UCM_Repository/uuid/dDocName:00008247.
29. American Academy of Physician Assistants. Physician assistants and the patient centered medical home. https://www.aapa.org/WorkArea/DownloadAsset.aspx?id=581.
30. American Academy of Physician Assistants. Six key elements. https://www.aapa.org/threecolumnlanding.aspx?id=30.
31. American Academy of Physician Assistants. Ratio of physician assistants to supervising physicians. https://www.aapa.org/WorkArea/DownloadAsset.aspx?id=632.
32. American Academy of Physician Assistants. Physician assistants and practice ownership. https://www.aapa.org/WorkArea/DownloadAsset.aspx?id=631.
33. Powe ML. Financing and reimbursement. In: Ballweg R, Sullivan EM, Brown D, Vetrosky D, eds. *Physician Assistant: A Guide to Clinical Practice*. 5th ed. Philadelphia: Saunders Elsevier; 2013.

The Faculty Resources can be found online at www.expertconsult.com.

CHAPTER 8

HEALTH CARE FINANCING AND REIMBURSEMENT

Michael L. Powe

Over the past 3 decades, numerous legislative, public policy, and insurance company–driven initiatives have been aimed at fundamentally altering the manner in which our nation's health care is financed and delivered. But even though they appeared to be dramatic changes at the time—think back to managed care—those initiatives turned out to be more comparable to marginal modifications to a health care system that seemed to be nearly unmanageable in terms of stemming the rapid increase in costs and an inability to deliver a uniformly high level of quality.

Comprehensive health care reform was enacted in March of 2010 when the Patient Protection and Affordable Care Act (PPACA) was signed into law. Depending on one's point of view, passage of the ACA placed the U.S. health care system on a different trajectory. One's political views may well decide on whether that trajectory is positive or not. Either way, we appear to be entering an era of health system reform that attempts to usher in a structural change to health care financing unlike anything we've seen before.

The way in which physician assistants (PAs), physicians, and other health professionals will be reimbursed for the professional services they deliver is in the midst of unprecedented change. As practices, hospitals, and health systems begin to reinvent themselves and establish new practice and payment models, PAs must understand how they will adapt to a "new normal" in health care.

One of the essential concepts in health care today is value—value-based reimbursement, value-based purchasing, and a shift from fee for service to fee for value. Value in health care can have many different meanings depending on who and where you are in the health care system. In the reimbursement arena, value can be described as the health outcome achieved per the dollars allocated.[1,2]

What is the concept behind value-based reimbursement or value-based payments? It deals with the providing of preventive care and intervention earlier in the disease process, delivering that care in lower cost settings (the office or in the patient's home vs. an acute care setting), and having health professionals focus on improving both individual and population health. All this has to occur while at the same time reducing the number of avoidable emergency department visits and hospitalizations and reducing hospital readmissions.

The appropriate and efficient use of information technology and analytics will have to be in the forefront of a practice's or hospital's reimbursement or revenue cycle management activities in order to achieve success in a value-based payment environment. Increasingly, health professionals and health systems will need the ability to track quality performance metrics, patient outcomes, patient satisfaction, hospital readmissions, and so on.

Financing often refers to the global manner in which we pay for health care. That includes entities, such as employers in the private sector or Medicare and Medicaid in the public sector, and individual consumers who pay for care either through subscribing to health insurance plans or by paying for care through out-of-pocket expenditures. Reimbursement represents the coverage policy and payments made to PAs and health care professionals to deliver care to patients. In this chapter, we focus primarily on reimbursement.

FULL UTILIZATION OF PHYSICIAN ASSISTANTS WILL ENSURE PATIENT ACCESS TO CARE

Physician assistants deliver quality medical and surgical services that would otherwise be provided by a physician. Numerous government and private sector research reports and studies have verified that the quality of care delivered by PAs is equal to that of physicians. In addition, patient satisfaction with care provided by PAs is equal to that of physicians. A survey conducted by Harris Poll in 2014 found that 93% of individuals surveyed who had seen a PA agreed that PAs are trusted health care providers.[3,4] (The online survey was conducted September 15 to 22, 2014, among 1544 adults age 18 years and older living in the United States, including an oversample of 680 adults who have seen a PA or have accompanied a loved one to see a PA in the past 12 months. For a complete methodology, including weighting variables, please contact the American Academy of Physician Assistants [AAPA].)

As policymakers, regulators, and private payers move forward with a number of programs and initiatives designed to improve quality, increase practice efficiencies, and produce better patient outcomes, it is essential that the concept of interdisciplinary, team-based care be at the forefront of the policies and programs. A high-performing, coordinated health care system recognizes the competency, skill set, and capacity of each health professional in order to enhance patient care quality and increase the likelihood of positive clinical outcomes while being cost-effective with resource allocation.

Policies, rules, and regulations that artificially limit the participation and leadership of PAs in these teams only serve to reduce access and create unnecessary and harmful barriers to timely patient care. Quite simply, PAs should be authorized and incentivized to practice to the full extent of their education and expertise in all existing and future care models. Language that is physician centric as opposed to provider neutral and policies that fail to acknowledge the capacity of PAs to practice medicine are counterproductive and will prevent the United States' health care system from achieving the goals of improving quality, lowering costs, and increasing patient access to care.

GOVERNMENT-SPONSORED PROGRAMS

Medicare

Medicare, which provides coverage to more than 55 million people, is a health care program available for older individuals (older than 65 years), people with disabilities who have received cash benefits under Social Security for at least 24 months, and those with permanent kidney failure (e.g., end-stage renal disease). The Medicare program is administered by the federal government and is funded through a combination of Medicare premiums, general fund revenues, and patient deductibles and copayments.

Medicare's coverage is divided into four parts—A, B, C, and D. Medicare Part A pays for hospital facility, equipment, and supply costs; some inpatient care in a skilled nursing facility (SNF); home health care; and hospice care. Medicare Part B pays for professional services delivered by physicians, PAs, and other health care professionals; durable medical equipment; and other medical services and supplies not covered by Part A.

Medicare Part C is a coverage option available to Medicare-eligible beneficiaries that allows private health insurance companies to provide Medicare benefits. These Medicare private health plans, such as health maintenance organizations (HMOs) and preferred provider organizations (PPOs), are known as Medicare Advantage Plans. Also known as Medicare+Choice plans, these plans often offer an enhanced benefit package such as eyeglasses coverage that are not available with traditional fee-for-service Medicare. The trade-off is that whereas Medicare

Part C enrollees have certain plan restrictions and are required to receive their care from health care professionals who are in a particular health plan or network, those who choose the Medicare Part B fee-for-service option can receive care from any health care provider who accepts Medicare.

Medicare Part D is a prescription drug plan created by the Medicare Prescription Drug Improvement and Modernization Act of 2003 that covers certain costs related to prescription drugs. The program provides prescription drug coverage for both brand-name and generic drugs.

Our primary focus is on Medicare Parts A and B because those programs have the most direct impact on reimbursement for medical and surgical services provided by PAs and physicians.

Medicare Part A

Generally, Medicare Part A pays for costs associated with patient expenses incurred at hospitals such as room and board, meals, and the care provided by licensed practical nurses and registered nurses. Part A can also help defray costs related to stays in hospice and nursing facilities and for home health care.

Administratively, payments to hospitals are made by *intermediaries,* who are under contract to the federal government to administer the Part A program in a particular state. These intermediaries are typically private insurance companies that have won competitive bids to administer the Part A program.

Medicare Part B

Medicare Part B pays for professional services delivered by PAs, physicians, and other professionals in hospitals, nursing homes, private offices, or a patient's home. Part B also covers services provided "incident to" the physician's care. Medicare also allows for services provided in the office setting by registered nurses and medical assistants, for example, to be billed "incident to" the PA. Services provided "incident to" the PA are billed under the PA's name with payment at 85%. A more complete explanation of "incident to" billing can be found in the section titled "Incident to" Services in this chapter. As with Part A, Medicare contracts with private insurance companies to administer the Part B program on behalf of the federal government. The insurance companies that process claims and administer the Part B program are called *Medicare administrative contractors (MACs)*.

Most Medicare beneficiaries receive services on what is commonly referred to as a *fee-for-service* basis. The value of the service is determined by the Medicare fee schedule.

Fee for service gives beneficiaries maximum flexibility in selecting physicians and other practitioners of choice. However, the patient's out-of-pocket expenses can be higher under the fee-for-service arrangement.

Medicare beneficiaries must satisfy an annual deductible before Medicare pays for any services they receive. (Some Medicare HMOs and managed care plans may waive the deductible payment.) After the deductible has been met, Medicare covers 80% of the fee schedule amount, and the patient is responsible for the remaining 20%, after meeting the deductible. Medicare's fee schedule amount is generally less than the medical practice's usual charge for the service. This can be illustrated by a list of the typical fees assessed for the patient who fell off a ladder and needed medical care, as described in Case Study 8.1.

CASE STUDY 8.1

Patient: Paul Peterson, Anytown, USA
Practitioner: James Jones, MD, Anytown, USA
Medical problem: Patient was on a ladder changing a lightbulb. Patient fell and hurt his arm.

Services Provided	Office Charge	Medicare Fee Schedule
Office visit	$105	$75

Although the fees the physician normally charges amounted to $105, Medicare's approved fee schedule amounts allowed the physician to charge only $75 for the care received. The actual Medicare payment to the practice would be $60 ($75 × 80%), with the patient being responsible for the 20% (or $15) difference, assuming that the patient has paid his deductible and the physician participates with Medicare (Table 8.1).

For some time, PAs were covered for services delivered in offices or clinics, hospitals, and SNFs and for first assisting at surgery. Rates of reimbursement ranged from 65% to 85%. However, in years past, services provided by PAs in nonrural health professional shortage area offices and clinics were covered only when billed under the "incident to" billing method, which required the constant onsite presence of the physician. In 1997, the Balanced Budget Act extended coverage to all practice settings at one uniform rate.[3] As of January 1, 1998, Medicare pays the PA's employer for medical and surgical services provided by the PA at 85% of the physician's fee schedule in all practice settings. PAs may treat

TABLE 8.1 Medicare Policy for Physician Assistants

Setting	Supervision	Reimbursement Rate	Services
Office or clinic when physician is not onsite	State law	85% of physician's fee schedule	All services PA is legally authorized to provide that would have been covered if provided personally by a physician
Office or clinic when physician is onsite	Physician must be in the suite of offices	100% of physician's fee schedule*	Same as above. PAs may personally perform but are not authorized to supervise other personnel who perform diagnostic tests.
Home visit or house call	State law	85% of physician's fee schedule	Same as above
SNF	State law	85% of physician's fee schedule	Same as above except that only physicians may perform the comprehensive SNF visit
Hospital	State law	85% of physician's fee schedule	Same as above. Medicare's Conditions of Participation limit certain services as physician only such as supervising a cardiac rehabilitation unit.
First-assisting at surgery in all settings	State law	85% of physician's first-assist fee schedule[†]	Same as above
Federal rural health clinic	State law	Cost-based reimbursement	Same as above
HMO or managed care contract (e.g., Medicare Advantage)	State law	Reimbursement is on capitation basis	All services contracted for as part of an HMO contract

*Using carrier guidelines for "incident to" services.
[†]85% of 16% = 13.6% of primary surgeon's fee.
HMO, Health maintenance organization; *PA*, physician assistant; *SNF*, skilled nursing facility.

new Medicare beneficiaries or established patients with new medical problems when billing the service under their name and Medicare national provider identifier (NPI) number. The office bills at the full physician rate and Medicare will pay for the service at 85% based on use of the PA's NPI number.

For the same office visit described in Case Study 8.1, here is how the reimbursement would look if the service were performed by a PA with billing under the PA's name and provider number.

Services Provided	Office Charge	Medicare Fee Schedule
Office visit	$105	$75

The actual Medicare payment to the practice would be $51 ($75 × 85% × 80%), with the patient being responsible for the 20% (or $12.75) difference, assuming that the patient has paid his deductible and the PA participates with Medicare

Medicare payment is made only to the employer of the PA. PAs participating in Medicare are required to accept assignment for their services. Similar to physicians, PAs have the option to opt out of Medicare. When PAs deliver care to Medicare beneficiaries, the PA must have a relationship with a collaborating physician and practice in accordance with state law. When billing is submitted under the PA's name and Medicare provider number at 85%, only general supervision is required. General supervision requires that the physician and the PA have access to electronic (e.g., telephone) communication. The PA's employer can be a physician, physician group, hospital, nursing home, group practice, professional medical corporation, limited liability partnership, or limited liability company. In 2002, the Medicare program expanded the ability of PAs to have an ownership interest in a practice. Rules that became effective in April 2002 allow PAs to own up to 99% of a Medicare-approved corporation that is eligible to bill the Medicare program, if allowed by state law.

"Incident to" Services

Medicare has a long-standing policy of covering medical services provided by PAs in offices and clinics under what is called the "incident to" provision, at 100% of the physician's fee schedule. Even with the expansion of PA coverage at the 85% reimbursement rate in all settings through the Balanced Budget Act of 1997, "incident to" remains an appropriate billing mechanism for PAs as long as Medicare's more restrictive billing requirements are followed. "Incident to" billing allows a PA to treat a patient, bill the service to Medicare under the physician's name, and be reimbursed at 100% of the fee schedule even though the physician never provided hands-on care to the patient during the encounter in which the PA delivered care.

If a medical service provided by PAs is to be billed under the "incident to" provision, the following criterion must be met:
• "Incident to" billing applies in private offices or clinics and not in a hospital or SNF setting.

The physician must personally obtain the history of the present illness, examine the patient, establish a diagnosis, and develop a plan of care during the patient's first visit for a particular medical problem; any established patient who presents with a new medical condition must also be treated and diagnosed by the physician to qualify for "incident to" billing. PAs may provide the follow-up care for the diagnosed medical problem.[5] The physician must be in the suite of offices (direct supervision) when the PA renders follow-up care. *Direct supervision* does not require that the supervising physician be in the same room with the PA or have any interaction with the patient when the PA delivers care, but he or she must be in the office suite and immediately available.

The physician is responsible for the overall care of the patient and should maintain involvement in the patient's care at a frequency that reflects his or her active involvement and participation in the ongoing management of the patient's treatment. The involvement could be reviewing the patient's medical record or having the PA and physician discuss the patient's progress.

Shared Services

When both a physician and a PA deliver an evaluation and management (E/M) service to a hospital inpatient or outpatient or emergency department patient, the physician may bill for the entire service as long as he or she provides a face-to-face portion of the E/M encounter. Payment for the combined service is at 100% of the physician fee schedule. The rules governing the ability to bill a shared visit include the following:
• Only E/M services qualify for shared service billing; procedures or critical care services cannot be billed as a shared service.
• The physician must personally provide some portion of the E/M service in a face-to-face encounter with the patient. The physician's professional service rendered to the patient must be clearly documented in the patient's medical record. Simply having the physician co-sign or review the patient's chart would not be sufficient to support billing under the shared visit billing guidelines. Medicare's national policy requires that the physician "provides any face-to-face portion of the E/M encounter with the patient." Most Medicare MACs ask that both the PA and the physician perform a substantive portion of an E/M visit; however, a "substantive portion" of the care is not defined. One MAC, Wisconsin Physician Services, asks that the physician perform a complete component of care (the history, examination, or medical decision making or plan of care) to qualify for shared visit billing.
• Care delivered by the physician and the PA must occur on the same calendar day, not simply within a 24-hour period of time. (The physician is not required to be in the hospital at the time the PA delivers his or her portion of care.)
• Both the physician and PA must have a common employer or work for the same entity (e.g., same hospital, same group, or solo physician employing a PA).

Certified Rural Health Clinics

In the mid-1960s, both the shortage and maldistribution of physicians had reached a crisis. The supply of physicians had become insufficient to meet the demands of smaller, rural communities. Although PAs were well accepted by residents in these rural communities, Medicare and Medicaid coverage for their services was not available in most cases.

In 1977, Congress passed the Rural Health Clinic Services Act (Public Law 95-210) in an effort to increase the availability of primary health care services to rural areas of the country. Federal certification as a certified Rural Health Clinic (RHC) allows the clinic to be reimbursed by means of a cost-based, all-inclusive methodology, as opposed to the fee-for-service payment system. Under this process, all of the legitimate expenses for the clinic (salaries and personnel expenses, rent, supplies, and so on) are totaled and divided by the number of patients treated in a year. That figure becomes the per-encounter rate that the clinic receives per visit. Medical care provided by a PA in a certified RHC is covered at the same basic rate as that provided by a physician. Physicians who provide care in designated underserved areas receive a 10% bonus payment. At present, that bonus payment is available only to physicians.

Two types of RHCs exist: independent and provider based. An independent RHC is generally a stand-alone clinic that could be owned by a PA. Provider-based RHCs are typically an integral part of a hospital, nursing home, or home health agency that is already a Medicare-certified provider. Each rural health clinic has a per-patient reimbursement rate generally based on the clinic's overall reasonable costs divided by the number of yearly patient encounters. For independent RHCs, there is a maximum per-patient encounter amount that will be paid, which is referred to as a "payment limit," or "cap."

To be eligible for federal RHC status, the clinic must be located in nonurban rural areas with current health care shortage designations. In addition, the clinic must have a PA, a nurse practitioner, or a certified nurse midwife onsite and available to patients at least 51% of the time the clinic is open to treat patients.

Medicaid

Medicaid, authorized by Title XIX of the Social Security Act, is a program jointly funded by federal and state governments that provides medical assistance for low-income individuals, families with dependent children, older individuals, and people with disabilities. Although the federal government sets basic guidelines, establishes a basic set of core benefits, and generally pays 50% to 80% of the cost of Medicaid (depending on the state's per capita income), individual states actually administer the program. The Medicaid program, which began on January 1, 1966, covers nearly 70 million people. Medicaid is the nation's primary public health insurance program for people with low incomes.

In their Medicaid programs, states may cover medical and surgical services provided by PAs. The decision as to whether to cover PAs generally rests with the state, except with respect to federally certified rural health clinics. If a clinic is designated by the federal government as a certified RHC, the state's Medicaid program must cover PA-provided services in the clinic. Presently, all states cover PAs under their fee-for-service or managed care Medicaid plans.

As Medicaid costs rose in the late 1980s and early 1990s, states began to experiment with more cost-effective methods of providing care to beneficiaries; fee-for-service programs were shifted to managed care delivery systems. To make many of these changes, states were required to get permission from the federal government in the form of waivers, which provided states with exemptions from the traditional guidelines of the Medicaid program.

One of the popular concepts that states have used to lower costs, and ideally to improve the quality of care, is to assign Medicaid beneficiaries to a specific health care provider, known as a primary care provider (PCP). The rationale is that beneficiaries will have better continuity of care and will be more likely to access the health care system at the appropriate time and place if one specific provider is responsible for directing their overall care. The PCP can refer the beneficiary to specialist and hospital inpatient care services as required. The federal government allows PAs to serve as PCPs, and some states allow PAs to assume that role within their Medicaid programs.

States have the authority to name PAs as primary care case managers (PCCMs) under the Medicaid program. A PCCM is typically paid a small monthly fee to act as a coordinator of care for beneficiaries.

States may cover PAs at the physician's rate of reimbursement or on a slightly discounted fee basis. Coverage may apply in all practice settings and for all medical services, or there may be limitations (e.g., no coverage for first assisting at surgery or for certain hospital inpatient care).

PRIVATE INSURANCE

Almost all private insurance companies cover medical and surgical services provided by PAs. However, with different payers and plans, including PPOs, HMOs, and fee-for-service programs operating in the United States, there may be differences in both how services delivered by PAs are covered and how claim forms should be submitted. Even within the same insurance company, PA coverage policies can change on the basis of the particular plan type, the specific type of service being provided, and the state or region of the country where the service is delivered. That being said, in fact there are only two basic variations in PA coverage by private payers. The service is either billed under the name of the supervising physician or under the name of the PA. The key is to determine the particular policy for each insurance company. Although some private payers do not individually credential PAs, that does not negatively affect coverage of services delivered. When plans do not credential PAs, they typically want the service billed under the name of the supervising physician, occasionally with a modifier code attached. As mergers and acquisitions continue to consolidate the health care marketplace, coverage policies for PAs are becoming much more consistent throughout the country. It is essential that PAs and their billing personnel obtain the written reimbursement and coverage policy for each payer before submitting claims for service.

Because of the potential variation, it is virtually impossible to present a complete picture of specific private insurance plan coverage policies, as has been done with respect to Medicare. Instead, this section attempts to outline basic concepts that can help in the determination of how medical and surgical services provided by PAs are covered.

Physician Assistant Recognition

The AAPA occasionally receives calls from PAs who have contacted a particular insurance company and been told that PAs are not covered or that a particular PA-provided service won't be reimbursed. Upon closer examination, the medical services provided by the PA were covered, but the insurance company did not pay directly to the PA. Instead, payment for the PA's services was made to the employing physician or employer. The following case study may better explain the potential problem.

CASE STUDY 8.2

A PA once called the AAPA to say that she was told by a major insurance company that the company would not reimburse for a service provided by a PA. The insurance company was immediately contacted by AAPA staff, and the following question was asked: "Are medical services covered when performed by PAs when billed under the physician's name and provider number?" The answer was that yes, of course, those services would be covered. The AAPA staff person indicated that a PA had just called the company and received a response indicating that the service would not be covered. The insurance company representative said that she remembered the call and said that "the person who called had asked if the company paid the PA for providing a medical service. We don't pay the PA; we pay the PA's employer." Was this a simple misunderstanding or an attempt to use semantics to avoid paying a claim? The lesson to be learned is that how you ask the question will often determine the kind of answer you get.

Credentialing, Enrollment, and Recognition

Some confusion may exist regarding terms that describe the relationship between PAs and third-party payers. The issue is how payers recognize PAs and the PAs' ability to deliver and report the care provided to the payers' subscribers. Whereas some payers enroll PAs in their plans, others ask that PAs be credentialed. Not to be confused with the concepts of being credentialed or privileged to provide services in a hospital setting, credentialing with payers refers to the collection of basic information such as educational history, licensing information, and malpractice details.

In general, there is no direct correlation between enrollment or credentialing of PAs and payment for their services; however, the AAPA strongly believes that all PAs should be enrolled and authorized to submit claims under their own names and provider numbers by all payers. In a health care system in which PAs deliver the same services as physicians, PA-provided services should be visible and tracked throughout the system so that the volume, type, and quality of care PAs deliver can be recognized and acknowledged. Billing mechanisms such as "incident to" or shared visit billing with Medicare or private payer policies that require PA-provided services to be billed under the physician lead to a lack of accountability and hide the true impact of PAs on the health care system.

HEALTH CARE REFORM—NEW MODELS OF CARE DELIVERY

There is a recognition that the prevalent reimbursement model currently in use, fee-for-service reimbursement, is largely responsible for the inefficient system of care delivery. Simply put, fee-for-service reimbursement often rewards uncoordinated, high-volume care with little emphasis on quality or outcomes.

Some of the recent health care delivery models have the potential to achieve improved care delivery while also reducing costs. One of the tenets of these new care models includes correlating reimbursement to patient health care outcomes through entities such as accountable care organizations (ACOs) and patient-centered medical homes.

Accountable Care Organizations

An ACO, in general terms, is a local or regional health organization consisting of health care professionals, typically one or more hospitals and related health care entities that have a formal or informal relationship and are jointly responsible for achieving measurable improvements in the quality and cost of health care delivered within a given community. ACOs will have a strong base of primary care professionals but may also provide a wide range of specialty care. ACOs, perhaps with the assistance of public and/or private third-party payers, should have the ability to establish achievable, evidence-based benchmarks for quality and cost for a defined patient population; a formal legal structure allowing them to administer payments; and a system to distribute shared savings, or levy penalties, depending on whether targets are met. In short, an ACO will likely have the capability to impose practice, reporting, and compensation standards on all participating professionals and health care organizations. If the

ACO concept becomes widely accepted, it will fundamentally change PAs, physicians, and other health care professionals in terms of employment relationships—more PAs and physicians will be employed by the hospital or ACO, and the manner in which practices are clinically organized and paid for delivering medical and surgical services.

Patient-Centered Medical Home

The goal of an effective patient-centered medical home (PCMH) is to establish a primary care model of care that improves the value and quality of health care for patients. Conceptually, a PCMH transforms the manner in which health care in general, and primary care in particular, is delivered. The PCMH is responsible for providing and coordinating a patient's total health care needs and, as needed, arranging care with other qualified professionals and health care organizations. A medical home provides comprehensive and integrated care that is patient and family centered, culturally appropriate, committed to quality and safety, cost-effective, affordable, and provided by a health care team led by a PA, physician, or other qualified health care professional.

The PCMH seeks to alter the paradigm of the fractionalized, episodic health care approach that is so prevalent in this country. The belief is that coordinated care leads to better outcomes for patients at a lower cost.

Insurance Exchanges

One of the central components of the PPACA is the creation of health insurance exchanges. These primarily state-regulated programs provide an assortment of health insurance plans to uninsured individuals, those who purchase individual health policies, and small group employers. The exchanges provide an opportunity for consumers to review and compare health coverage options on the basis of the plan's benefit structure, as well as on pricing information such as premiums, deductibles, and coinsurance.

Simply put, an insurance exchange is the formation of a competitive state or regionally based marketplace offering certain consumers an opportunity to purchase health insurance policies, presumably at a more competitive price than that which is available in the current marketplace. In theory, the exchanges will have bargaining power with hospitals and health care systems that rival some of the largest employer group plans. How states choose to implement exchanges and whether the overall concept will work falls back on that well-worn idiom—the devil is in the details.

The PPACA required that each state establish an American Health Benefit Exchange by January 1, 2014. States are expected to establish exchanges, with the federal government maintaining the authority to establish an exchange if a state fails to do so. States can create multiple exchanges, as long as only one exchange serves a specific geographic area. States can also work together to form regional exchanges.

The plans offered by the exchange have to meet minimum essential benefit standards developed by the federal government.

Some of the expected benefits of an insurance exchange include the following:

- Increased selection: Consumers will have access to a choice of health plans.
- Portability: Health insurance coverage will not be linked to employment, making it easier for individuals to maintain coverage even when they change employers.
- Information: Consumers will be able to more directly compare plans and potential government subsidies, making it simpler for them to determine if they qualify for financial assistance.
- Nondiscrimination: Insurers will not be able to discriminate or deny coverage on the basis of health history.
- Competitive pricing: Health plans within the exchange will disperse risk in a manner similar to large group plans, causing premiums to be more competitive.

Pay for Performance and Pay for Reporting

Pay for performance (commonly known as P4P) is a set of Medicare initiatives to encourage quality of care improvements by extending financial incentives to eligible professionals (EPs) and organizations for more effective patient care delivery. Health care service sites, including physicians' offices, ambulatory care facilities, hospitals, nursing homes, home health care agencies, and dialysis facilities may participate in one or more of the P4P demonstration programs. For information about specific P4P programs, including current and upcoming demonstrations, visit http://www.cms.gov/Medicare/Demonstration-Projects/DemoProjectsEvalRpts/.

One major pay-for-reporting program is the Physician Quality Reporting System (PQRS). Authorized by §101 of the Tax Relief and Healthcare Act of 2006, the voluntary initiative allows Medicare-enrolled EPs to participate in the program by using CPT Category II codes, temporary G codes or quality codes on claims forms.

Beginning in 2015, EPs and group practices that do not satisfactorily report PQRS quality measures will be subject to a negative payment adjustment.

Program participation, or lack of participation, affects payments 2 years later. For example, if a group did not satisfactorily report in 2014, it will be subject to a 2% negative adjustment in 2016.

Alternative Payment Models

Alternative payment models (APMs) are payment and care delivery models that seek to change payment systems from volume-based to value-based care models in which quality, efficient resource allocation, and outcomes become the measures of successful care. Reimbursement is geared to financially incentivize high-value care and reduce payments to health professionals, practices, and health systems that fall below established standards. APMs include Medicare Shared Savings Program ACOs, all Centers for Medicare & Medicaid Services (CMS) Innovation Center initiatives except Health Care Innovation awards, certain demonstration programs, advanced primary care medical homes, and certain bundled payment programs. CMS provides an overview of alternative payment models, which can be found at https://www.cms.gov/Newsroom/MediaReleaseDatabase/Fact-sheets/2015-Fact-sheets-items/2015-01-26-3.html. It should be noted that many private payers have developed their own APM models and in some cases are more ahead of Medicare in the implementation of these models.

Merit-Based Incentive Payment System

The Merit-Based Incentive Payment System (MIPS) is a Medicare pay-for-performance program that "measures" Medicare Part B health professionals in four different categories. Each category has a numerical ranking or score; the four scores added together total to a MIPS composite performance score. The total composite performance scores can range from 0 to 100. MIPS essentially combines the various independent CMS incentive programs that currently exist—the PQRS, meaningful use (MU), and Value-based Payment Modifier (VBM)—and adds one other category, clinical improvement. As of January 1, 2019, included professionals will not report PQRS quality measures, attest to electronic health records MU, or deal with the negative payment adjustment associated with the VBM.

Under the MIPS program, each year a PA's composite score would be compared with a performance threshold consisting of the mean or median of the performance rating for all professionals participating in MIPS. Each PA would have to meet or exceed that established threshold to be eligible to receive an incentive payment or higher payment rate. Those

who fall below the threshold would likely see reduced payment rates. Those with composite scores exactly at the threshold would see no payment adjustments.

Payment adjustments can be as high as 4% in 2019 and increase to a maximum of 9% in 2020 and for subsequent years. In 2022, the positive incentive for the highest performers can be as high as 27%, and the payment decrease for low performers can be a negative 9%, which equates to a potential Medicare payment spread of 36 percentage points.

Here is a look at how each of the four measures will be weighted:
- Quality (30 points): PQRS
- Resource use (30 points): Value-based Modifier Program
- Meaningful use (25 points): appropriate use of certified electronic health records technology
- Clinical practice improvement (15 points): demonstrated improvements in care coordination, patient safety, or population management

A Unique Concern for Physician Assistants

Many medical services that are personally provided by PAs are not billed for under the PA's name or NPI number. These services are often legitimately billed for under the name of the physician with whom the PA works, under Medicare's "incident to" provision, for example. That lack of transparency in the billing process could have negative consequences for PAs in programs such as MIPS. It means that the medical care that PAs provide, and their productivity, is essentially "hidden" or not reported within the Medicare claim systems and databases. A PA cannot be adequately evaluated on care quality metrics when the care he or she delivers is attributed to another professional.

The MIPS program will develop a cut-off point based on the number of Medicare services a health professional delivers to beneficiaries, called a "low-volume threshold" (which is different from the performance threshold), to determine which health professionals will not have to participate in MIPS because they serve a relatively small number of Medicare beneficiaries. While this is still under discussion, a figure of 10% has been suggested. That is, if fewer than 10 percent of a PA's patient encounters occur with Medicare Part B beneficiaries, he or she would not be subject to MIPS and therefore not be eligible to receive incentive payments for delivering high-quality care.

However, if a PA treated a high volume of Medicare beneficiaries and most of the services were billed under the physician, it would appear that the PA did not exceed the 10% threshold and, subsequently, is not entitled to a MIPS incentive payment even though the PA's patient mix included a high percentage of

Medicare beneficiaries. The AAPA has repeatedly voiced this concern to CMS officials in both personal meetings and in formal comments, indicating that a remedy for this problem must be found if the MIPS program is to be an accurate reflection of who provides high-quality care. The AAPA believes that the complete recognition of PAs in the delivery and payment process is the appropriate solution.

CONCLUSION

Several terms have been used to describe the significant changes that are occurring and predicted to ensue over the next 5 to 10 years regarding the U.S. health care delivery system. Some call it transformational. Others refer to it as a seismic shift. Irrespective of the terminology used to describe the change, the fact is that we are in the midst of fundamentally altering the manner in which health care is delivered and reimbursed in this country.

The PA profession has proven its ability to deliver quality medical and surgical care to patients. As this country continues to search for solutions to controlling health care costs, the growing availability of expensive technologies, pharmaceuticals, and treatment options, even more payers and health care–related organizations should realize the important role that PAs play in the health care system. One must not forget, however, that to a large extent, health care is a business. Although delivering excellent quality care with positive patient outcomes continues to be the most important aspect of PA practice, it would be short-sighted to overlook the need to implement serious cost and resource controls as part of delivering care. In addition to delivering quality medical care, PAs must be aware of their responsibility to understand their value to their employers specifically and more broadly to the health care system. A better understanding of both the financing and payment mechanisms of the health care system are important steps in achieving that goal. Although acknowledging that an understanding of the financial aspects of health care is important, the most important quality that PAs bring to the health care system has, and will continue to be, a focus on what is best for patients.

In many ways, a health care system that seeks to increase access to cost-effective, high-quality care is tailor made for the enhanced utilization of PAs. It should also be recognized that logic has not always been the driving force in health care policy decisions. Often politics and culture stand in the way of rational behavior. All PAs and PA students must understand the importance of being advocates for the profession as the health care system continues to transform and reinvent itself at both the state and national levels.

CLINICAL APPLICATIONS

1. What are the potential problems with a fee-for-service reimbursement system?
2. What is the difference between Medicare Part A and Medicare Part B?
3. Define Medicare's "incident to" and shared billing concepts, and list the criteria that must be met for reimbursement for services provided by PAs under these two reimbursement methodologies.
4. What are the potential benefits of a value-based payment system to patients and to the health care system globally?
5. Define the major components of the MIPS.

KEY POINTS

- Although clinicians do not like to think of themselves as "business experts," today's health care environment requires that physicians and PAs be well informed about patients' health care coverage to ensure that they receive optimum and affordable care.
- Although Medicare provides for reimbursement for services provided by PAs, there are stringent rules to avoid submission of duplicate bills by the PA and his or her supervising physicians. This can be particularly confusing in academic health centers where there are separate rules for residents.
- Medicaid coverage policies vary from state to state, both for types of health professionals who are reimbursed and for covered services.
- Each third-party payer may have different requirements for different health plans. Knowledge of these differences helps ensure appropriate payment and coverage to the PA's employer.
- New systems of care created by the Accountable Care Act are intended to create clearer reimbursement policies that are designed to increase efficiency, improve quality, and decrease costs while improving health outcomes for patients.

References

1. Wilper AP, Woolhandler S, Lasser KE, et al. Health insurance and mortality in US adults. *Am J Pub Health*. 2009;99:2289–2295.
2. Porter ME, Teisberg EO. *Redefining Health Care: Creating Value-Based Competition on Results*. Boston: Harvard Business School Press; 2006.
3. Medicare Transmittal 1764, August 28, 2002.
4. American Academy of Physician Assistants. New AAPA Survey Conducted by Harris Poll Shows PAs Are Trusted Healthcare Providers Who Improve Access. https://www.aapa.org/twocolumn.aspx?id=3358#sthash.CvDzL7HU.dpuf.
5. Medicare Program Memorandum, Transmittal No. AB-98–15, April 1998

The resources for this chapter can be found at www.expertconsult.com.

CHAPTER 9

THE POLITICAL PROCESS

Ann Davis • Stephanie M. Radix

Please do not skip this chapter just because you never intend to become involved in politics. You have entered medicine during a period of rapid and profound changes in health care delivery. Where there is change, there is politics. Although sometimes politics is described in disparaging tones, being involved in politics is nothing to be ashamed of because, in its truest sense, politics is the art of getting things done. Physician assistants (PAs) are masters at getting things done!

This chapter is not written for elected officials, professional lobbyists, policy wonks, or pundits. It is written for the rest of us. Because it deals with the political process of making laws and regulations, you will find frequent use of words such as *most* and *usually*. Just as there can be a good deal of ambiguity in law, there can be a good deal of it in the making of laws. This lack of predictability can be difficult for PAs because it may seem unscientific. After you work with the process for a while, however, you will be able to predict some outcomes that initially seemed unpredictable, and, as in medicine, you will become comfortable with some level of uncertainty. The chapter is divided into five parts:

• Individual responsibilities
• The role and importance of professional organizations
• The legislative process
• The regulatory process
• Case studies

Because state processes are generally structured along the lines of federal processes, the description of the federal system precedes the description of state mechanisms. In the discussion of state activities, where and how you can exert influence is integrated into the text.

The word *you* is used frequently. Please do not interpret this to mean that anyone expects or wants you to take on the entire government singlehandedly. Although individualism is highly valued in our society, the fact is that government responds best to group influence. You can and should be an important part of the PA group.

This chapter aims to engage you in advocacy as a PA and presents this activity as a two-step process: become informed and become involved.

INDIVIDUAL RESPONSIBILITIES

As a PA, you have a personal responsibility to understand the political process and to use that knowledge to advance the interests of patients. There are many levels of involvement. At a minimum, you should stay abreast of current issues and trends in health care by reading journals, newspapers, and professional publications, and you should vote. You can also provide moral or financial support for the efforts of others who work on your behalf by becoming a member of a

PA organization or advocacy group. You can become one of those workers yourself, participating in the government-related activities of PA and other health care organizations. You can seek appointment to a licensing board or run for public office at the local, state, or national level.

If running for public office is not for you, consider supporting a candidate whose positions on health care and other issues are compatible with your own. There are dozens of ways to support a candidate: becoming a campaign manager or an issues coordinator, hosting a fundraiser, canvassing for votes, working on a phone bank to solicit supporters, organizing a committee of "Physician Assistants for Candidate N," speaking at community functions in support of the candidate, distributing campaign materials, working to "get out the vote" on election day, and, of course, voting.

If campaign work is not attractive or feasible, consider volunteering your services to individuals already elected to federal or state office. One valuable function you can perform is to advise elected officials about health care issues affecting your community. All legislators are called on to make decisions on a wide variety of topics. Having a constituent health care expert as a resource is a great asset.

It is hard to overstate the value of having ongoing contact with elected and appointed officials. If legislators and others in government know you and understand the valuable role that PAs play in health care delivery, they will be more likely to come to your assistance when you need help. Your credibility will have been enhanced if, in the past, you were involved with issues that were not self-serving, such as bicycle safety measures, support for prevention programs, or health care for the homeless. If you know someone has introduced legislation in these or similar areas, offer your personal support. Historically, PAs have been interested in the broader health care issues because resolving these issues has benefited patients. If you maintain a genuine interest in patient welfare, rather than speaking up only when someone threatens your professional "turf," you will earn genuine respect.

You can do several things to influence the legislative and regulatory processes, even when no issues in which you are interested are awaiting legislation. In fact, if you do these things routinely, you will enhance your visibility and credibility.

The first is to maintain contact with your elected representatives. You want them to know who you are and to smile when they see you coming. When you meet with an elected official, it is best to make an appointment and be prepared to discuss a specific issue. Of course, you will not wait until the busiest days of the legislative session, when everything is in turmoil, to make your visit. Personal contact with legislators when they are at home in the district or between sessions is most productive.

A personal visit is not the only option. You may read something about your representative's pet project and contact him or her to voice your support (if, in fact, you are in support). Such support is often remembered. If you receive an interesting piece of information on health care that you think might be useful, pass it along.

You may also do this with regulators. Remember, regulators are all people who are trying to develop or maintain a level of expertise. They need information, so provide it. A good relationship with a legislator, a legislator's staff person, or a regulator is invaluable.

Finally, support your state and national PA organizations. This suggestion is not just another pitch for membership; it is a tactical imperative. When any organization testifies before a governmental body, one of the first questions asked is, "How many people does your society represent?" The larger the number, the more credibility the organization is given. It is also important to know where your professional organizations stand on an issue before you go to your representative's office to voice your opinion. If you are an active member, you may have already influenced the organization's policy-making process. Even if you disagree with the group's final determination, at least you will understand how and why it reached its decision, and you may choose to remain silent rather than undercut its efforts.

There is value in belonging to a professional organization. Organizations and their members have a symbiotic relationship. Organizations need you, and you need them. They know the legislative and regulatory processes, as well as what issues are under consideration, and they most likely have a professional staff. You know the issues from a personal perspective because you confront them daily. Your personal professional perspective as a PA is essential and should be conveyed to lawmakers or regulators, particularly when your association says it is time to call, write, or visit them.

One of the first things you must know about government is that it regulates almost every aspect of your professional life. The most important law affecting you as an individual PA is one passed by the state and implemented by a state licensing board or agency—the PA practice act.

PRACTICE LAWS

Occupational regulation is the prerogative of the state rather than the federal government. Each state licenses, certifies, or registers a number of different professions and occupations, everyone from physicians and architects to barbers and plumbers. The goal of occupational regulation is to protect public health and safety. This is done by granting licenses only to individuals who meet minimum standards of education and skill, by defining a scope of practice, and by disciplining those who break the law or fail to uphold certain professional standards. A licensing or regulatory agency can seek an injunction and ultimately revoke a license to prevent the public from being harmed by a negligent or incompetent practitioner. Lawbreakers may also face civil or criminal penalties.

Physician assistants belong to a regulated profession. In broad terms, this means that an individual seeking to work as a PA must first obtain permission from the state (for the purposes this chapter, the term *state* shall mean all 50 states, the District of Columbia, and the U.S. territories with the exception of Puerto Rico, which does not yet license PAs) and then abide by any conditions of practice that the state has established. For a time, as with other professions and occupations, the term that described the process by which states authorized PA practice varied across the country and included designations such as *licensure*, *certification*, or *registration*. (On October 15, 2015, Senate Bill 110 became effective in Ohio, thus making *licensure* the official regulatory term for PAs in all states.) However, all states now appropriately use the term *licensure* for PAs—the highest form of state professional regulation—thereby eliminating patient confusion and assuring the inclusion of PAs in important state laws that are applicable to licensed health professionals such as participation in loan repayment programs, the provision of care during natural disasters, and the reporting of specified patient injuries to law enforcement, among numerous others. The requirements for securing this permission vary from state to state. However, as a result of efforts by American Academy of Physician Assistants (AAPA) and state PA associations, there is growing uniformity in the laws that govern PAs. Total uniformity is an unrealistic goal because each state writes its laws slightly differently and cherishes its prerogative to do so. The differences in style and content are problems with which every regulated occupation and profession must cope.

The basis for regulation of PAs is found in the language of the PA practice act. The law may be included in the medical practice act, which governs doctors, or it may be a separate section of the state statutes. The law is further amplified by regulations issued by the licensing board. Every PA should have a copy of the current state law and regulations governing his or her practice, which may be obtained from the licensing board or found on the licensing board's website. Ignorance is no excuse if you are ever accused of breaking the law.

Who is responsible for licensing and regulating PAs? In most cases, the regulatory agency is the Board of Medical Examiners, the same entity that licenses physicians. Fewer states have separate PA boards. A handful of states have departments of education or professional regulation that regulate all health practitioners. A list of PA state regulatory agencies is available on the AAPA's website.

In the law and regulations, you will find details about qualifications, applications and fees for licensure, scope of practice, requirements for PA–physician team practice, prescribing and dispensing privileges, criteria for license renewals, protection of the title "physician assistant," and what constitutes a violation of the law and the disciplinary measures that can be invoked, as well as information about administrative procedures and due process. You may also find information on the composition, terms of appointment, and other powers of the regulatory board, allowing you to determine what role PAs play in the state's regulatory system. Most medical boards have PA advisory committees that provide PAs with a way to participate in and contribute to the regulatory process, and a growing number of states include PAs as medical board members.

The two universal requirements for obtaining licensure as a PA are

1. Graduation from an accredited PA educational program
2. Passage of the Physician Assistant National Certifying Examination (PANCE), administered by the National Commission on Certification of Physician Assistants (NCCPA)

The NCCPA examination, although part of a voluntary, private sector certification process, functions as the national licensing examination for PAs. Every state requires that potential licensees have passed it. Although a few states may test PAs on their familiarity with state law, no state administers its own examination to test clinical knowledge.

Your state license must be renewed on a regular cycle, every 1, 2, or 3 years. Some jurisdictions require that you provide evidence that you have maintained your NCCPA certification or that you have completed a minimum number of continuing medical education (CME) credits, and you will need to pay a renewal fee. Keep in mind that the NCCPA certification system must be dealt with separately; do not confuse it with your state license. To maintain certification by the NCCPA, you must pay NCCPA a fee and register 100 hours of CME every 2 years.

It is also necessary to recertify every 10 years by taking an examination. You may use the letters "PA-C" after your name only if you are currently certified by the NCCPA.

The PA law and regulations also include criteria for the formulation and function of the PA–physician patient care team. All state laws require the ready availability of the physician for consultation and, with rare exception, authorize availability via telecommunication. Although no state allows a PA to work without a physician, no state requires that a physician must always be on site while a PA is providing care. Some states do, however, have on-site physician requirements when the PA is performing certain procedures. More details may also be specified if the PA will be practicing in an office or clinic separate from the physician. Ideally, the most effective state laws neither restrict patient access to care nor the PA's access to the physician. This is best achieved when the laws and regulations authorize collaborative relationships, PA scope of practice and prescriptive authority, the ratio of PAs to physicians, and the necessity (if any) for the review of PA-generated charts, orders, or prescriptions to be determined at the practice level.

All U.S. states permit those PAs who have prescriptive authority to sign prescriptions. The law or regulations may place restrictions on the kinds of medications a PA may prescribe. The authority to dispense medications is also regulated by the state. Pharmacists vigorously protect this privilege and make good arguments for a separation of the prescribing and dispensing functions. Therefore, a physician's or PA's ability to provide patients with medications from a supply maintained in the office or clinic is often more easily justified in rural areas or other locations without pharmacy services. Some states do not permit anyone other than a pharmacist to dispense drugs. In nearly all jurisdictions, giving patients drug samples that have been supplied by a pharmaceutical company is not the same as dispensing and is not subject to the same restrictions.

Regulation of the PA profession has been evolving since the first practice act was passed in the late 1960s. The founders of the profession made a conscious political decision to establish a system in which PAs were recognized under the licenses of their supervising physicians. Changes in health care delivery and greater numbers of PAs, as well as the need for administrative efficiency, have persuaded most states to modify this approach. The more modern system, advocated by the AAPA, is one in which licensure is granted to a PA on the basis of his or her credentials (i.e., on proof of meeting the educational and examination requirements of the law). A licensed PA can

practice after he or she has established a collaborative relationship with one or more licensed physicians. Such systems greatly facilitate the rapid deployment of the PA workforce and diminish administrative burdens for licensees and for the state.

Regulation of the profession continues to evolve based in part on the availability of data and studies that confirm PA quality, changes in medical education that place greater emphasis on interprofessional training among medicine, nursing, pharmacy, and so on; the transition of health care systems to "team" practice; and adjustments in the expectations of both physicians and PAs with regard to liability and the belief that PAs should no longer be considered the "agent" of the physician. These developments (and many more) have ultimately resulted in a more modernized approach to the regulation of the profession as evidenced by (1) the largest employer of PAs in the country, the Veterans Health Administration (VHA), enacting new utilization guidelines for PAs practicing in Veterans Affairs (VA) medical facilities; (2) adoption of new policy of the AAPA House of Delegates (HOD) on the role of PAs within the health care team; and (3) revision of the Academy's Model State Legislation for PAs, which describes best practices in the regulation of the profession.

On December 24, 2013, the VHA enacted a directive updating its policy on PA utilization, which included a new definition for PA practice. Among other things, VHA Directive 1063 defines a PA as a credentialed health care professional who provides patient-centered medical care to assigned patients as a member of a health care team. It also states that PAs practice with clinical oversight, consultation, and input by a designated collaborating physician. Last, it also recognizes that although PAs are not licensed independent providers, they are authorized to practice with defined levels of autonomy and exercise independent medical decision making within their scope of practice. Thus, the VA acknowledged that "supervision" does not define the role of the PA accurately. In a historical shift, the relationship as between PAs and physicians is one of "collaboration" in which each member of the medical team works together jointly.

The AAPA HOD has sole authority on behalf of AAPA to enact policies establishing the collective values, philosophies, and principles of the PA profession. It consists of voting delegates from 56 chapters representing 50 states, the District of Columbia and five federal services, 25 officially recognized specialty organizations, eight caucuses composed of individuals sharing a common goal or interest related to health care access or delivery, and the Student Academy. In addition, the current and immediate past House officers are delegates at large and also vote. Elected delegates have an effective voice in AAPA activities by making recommendations to the AAPA Board of Directors, submitting formal resolutions through the procedures outlined by the House officers, participating in open reference committee hearings conducted at the HOD meeting held during AAPA's Annual Conference and volunteering as a member of a reference committee, and researching and reporting on the resolutions and testimony received. In the year following the enactment of the VHA Directive, the AAPA HOD amended its policy on the role of PAs to reflect that PAs are health professionals licensed or, in the case of those employed by the federal government, credentialed to practice medicine in collaboration with physicians.[1] This significant policy change was made partly to guide PAs, AAPA leaders, and professional staff in their navigation of the rapidly evolving team-focused, value-based health care landscape but also to more precisely define the way in which modern PA–physician teams practice medicine. It thus illustrates the progression of PAs' abilities as medical providers, which was previously believed to be absent within the realm of the "supervision" structure. The change was also embraced in order to overcome the misconception held by some legislators, health policymakers, physicians, and patients that given their need for supervision PAs were less safe or provided inferior care in contrast to their physician counterparts despite numerous studies to the contrary.

When the AAPA HOD adopted its new policy on the PA role in 2014, the Academy's Commission on Advocacy was also charged with the important task of updating the AAPA's Model State Legislation for PAs (Model Law). First drafted in 1991, the Model Law was adopted by the AAPA to describe best practices in regulation of the profession, achieve regulatory efficiency, and promote consistency across states. Although it had undergone several revisions over time in order to incorporate changes in program accrediting agencies and to reflect the evolution of PAs practice, it has always reflected two hallmark concepts: that PAs should be licensed to practice medicine and that PA scope of practice should be based on the PA's skills, education, and experience. As of 2015, the updated model state legislation recommends an administrative process in which a PA presents his or her credentials to a state regulatory agency and receives a license in return. The license is renewable, based on meeting state requirements. The model legislation does not propose that the regulatory authority approve or register collaborating physicians. Any licensed physician or group of physicians

(MD or DO) may collaborate with a PA unless the physician's ability to collaborate has been limited by disciplinary action. Under the updated Model Law, a PA's scope of practice is established by what is within the PA's skills, education, and experience. Language describing the PA scope of practice being determined by physician delegation has been deleted. Since its first draft more than 20 years ago, the model legislation authorizes PA prescriptive authority, including controlled substances in Schedules II through V, as well as limited dispensing authority. This authority has been retained. However, language requiring the collaborating physician to assume responsibility for care provided by PAs has been removed. Instead, PAs are responsible for their professional actions. The new model also deletes the concept that a PA should be considered the "agent" of a physician. In the past, rather than amending health law outside the PA practice act, PAs sought to be able to perform specific regulated medical and surgical tasks as the "agent" of a physician. Current advocacy efforts seek to have PAs specifically named in all relevant health law, removing the need for "agency" language. It is stated quite clearly in the model legislation that a physician need not be physically present as long as the PA and physician can contact one another easily. The details of collaboration are left to the PA–physician team.

Augmenting the current language that removes the requirement that PAs practice with physician collaboration when responding to a disaster situation, the new model state legislation extends the same authorization to PAs who are participating in volunteer activities. The new model legislation presents a list of options for regulatory models, with the preferred option being a separate and independent PA Board. The improved Model Law will serve as a guide for states looking to update PA laws and regulations.

Thus, a good state law is one that allows a PA's scope of practice to be determined by what is within his or her skills, education, and experience. It should neither limit a PA's scope via a law, a regulation, or a licensure application that contains a list of permissible tasks that physicians may delegate nor narrow it by a system in which licensing board members are allowed, when reviewing PA practice descriptions, to arbitrarily delete certain procedures on the basis of their personal biases. Last, it should not be restricted by legislators who do not understand the depth and breadth of PA education and training. The AAPA has distilled the aspects of ideal PA legislation into an easy to understand and describe version in its Six Key Elements of a Modern PA Practice Act (Box 9.1.)

BOX 9.1 SIX KEY ELEMENTS OF A MODERN PHYSICIAN ASSISTANT PRACTICE ACT

- Licensure as the regulatory term
- Adaptable collaboration requirements
- Full prescriptive authority
- Chart co-signature requirements determined at the practice level
- Scope of practice determined by the PA's skills, education, and experience
- No restriction on the number of PAs who collaborate with a physician

STAKEHOLDERS TO WORK WITH BEFORE DRAFTING LEGISLATION

- State medical society
- State association of family physicians
- State association of emergency physicians
- Rural health association
- Primary care association
- Hospital association
- AARP
- Large hospitals and health systems
- Advocacy groups
- Other organizations with a particular interest in the topic of your legislation

PA, Physician assistant.
From AAPA, 2015.

INDIVIDUALS: PART OF THE WHOLE

This section provides information on the structure and mission of your professional organizations: the AAPA and the state PA academies. Many PAs also find great value in belonging to an AAPA specialty organization, caucus, or special interest group.

The AAPA, established in 1968, is the national professional society for PAs. At the headquarters in Alexandria, Virginia, a full-time staff carries out the organization's major activities: advocacy and government relations, research and data collection, public education, publications, continuing medical education and professional development, employment, and other member services. One of the Academy's most important functions is to speak for the profession before the U.S. Congress and federal agencies. Even in a representative democracy such as the United States, it is difficult for one person to single-handedly affect the shape of laws and regulations. It is generally true that legislators and bureaucrats are more responsive to organizations that convey the interests of a large group than they are to individuals. Efficiency, accountability, and credibility come into play here. Therefore, the Academy performs an important role when it voices the PA profession's views on federal legislation and regulations.

Lobbying is done daily by the professional staff of the AAPA. At congressional hearings, during individual meetings with lawmakers and their aides, and at meetings with leaders in federal agencies, AAPA staff may be accompanied by PAs who are elected officers of the Academy or who have special expertise or established relationships with legislators or regulators. Coordinating grassroots advocacy is an important part of AAPA's legislative strategy and success on Capitol Hill. Legislative alerts, AAPA social media channels, and Academy publications are used to inform AAPA members about important issues or to request that they contact their congressional representatives or a federal agency about a particular subject. Annually, the AAPA invites members to attend a government affairs and leadership conference in Washington, DC, that includes a day on Capitol Hill. The AAPA welcomes and relies on PAs from across the country to speak for the profession and the patients PAs serve and helps to make this effective by coordinating the profession's federal advocacy and providing training, support, and direction for its members as advocates.

On the state level, PAs' interests are represented by state PA associations. These associations are chartered constituent chapters of AAPA. Among its other projects, each state academy must advance the interests of the profession before the legislature, the licensing board, and other state agencies. A majority of PA state societies employ professional association management staff, lobbyists, and legal counsel. However, even in the chapters with a significant number of paid employees, much of the substantive work is done by the members themselves. The AAPA's advocacy and government affairs staff helps chapter leaders with these projects by providing information, technical resources, and consultation services. For example, the AAPA supplies summaries of state laws, model language, fact sheets, and demographic data, as well as analyses of proposed rules and legislation. The Academy can also assist state chapters by sending statewide email "legislative action alerts" on behalf of the chapter. The Academy's goal is to maximize the ability of PAs to provide care through appropriate state laws and regulations.

FEDERAL LEGISLATIVE PROCESS: HOW A BILL BECOMES LAW

The legislative processes in the U.S. Senate and the House of Representatives are similar, although each chamber has its own rules and traditions. With only

100 members, the Senate seems flexible and informal compared with the 435-member House, in which a strict hierarchy and rigid system of rules are necessary to expedite business.[2]

Legislative proposals may be introduced by senators or representatives when Congress is in session. The bill—prefixed with *HR* when introduced in the House of Representatives and *S* when introduced in the Senate—is given a number that is based on the order of introduction. It is then referred to a committee that has jurisdiction over the bill's subject matter.

The committee is the heart of the legislative process because it is here that a bill receives its sharpest scrutiny. Professional staff expedites the committee's business by researching issues, identifying supporters and opponents, and designing politically acceptable options and compromises. When a committee decides to act on a legislative proposal, it generally conducts hearings to provide the executive branch, interested groups, and individuals with opportunities to formally present their views on the issue. After hearings have ended, the committee meets to "mark up" the bill (i.e., decide on the language of amendments). When a committee votes to approve a measure and send it to the floor, it justifies its actions in a written statement called a *report*, which accompanies the bill. The committee report is useful because it describes the purpose and scope of the bill, explains the committee amendments, indicates proposed changes in existing law, and frequently includes instructions to government agencies on how the language of the new law should be interpreted and implemented.[2]

Most bills never make it out of committee. The enormous volume of legislation (≈25,000 measures in each 2-year Congress) makes it impossible for every bill to be considered. In addition, many are duplicative, lack sufficient support, or are purposefully ignored in an effort to "kill" them. Only a small percentage of all bills introduced are enacted into law.

The route to a vote by the full House of Representatives usually lies through the Rules Committee, which sets guidelines for the length and form of the debate. The Senate, on the other hand, calls up a bill by voting on a motion to consider it or by "unanimous consent," in which the bill comes up for a vote if no one objects. In both houses, bills may be further amended on the floor before the vote on passage. However, because lawmakers rely heavily on the committee system to ensure that issues are carefully and expertly assessed, amendments on the floor need considerable support in order to be approved.

When a bill has been passed, it is sent to the other chamber for action, where the entire legislative process starts over. Often, the House and Senate consider similar bills. If the measures passed by the two bodies are identical, the resultant bill is sent to the White House for the president's signature. Usually, the measures are not identical, and unless the chamber that first passed the bill agrees to the changes made by the second, a House–Senate conference is arranged to resolve the differences.

Conference committees comprise members of the committees that originally considered the bills. Theoretically, the conferees are not authorized to delete provisions or language that both the House and the Senate have agreed to, nor are they supposed to draft or insert entirely new provisions. In practice, however, they have wide latitude. When agreement is reached, a conference report is written that includes a final version of the bill with the conferees' recommendations. Each chamber must then vote on the report. If no agreement is reached by the conferees or if either chamber does not accept the conference report, the bill dies.

A bill that has been approved by both chambers of Congress is sent to the White House. If Congress is in session and the president does not sign the bill within 10 days, it becomes law automatically. If the president favors the bill, he may sign it into law. If he does not like it, he may veto it by returning it to Congress without signature. To override the president's veto, a two-thirds vote in both the House and the Senate is required.[2]

Interested individuals can monitor congressional activity by watching televised floor proceedings or by reading various government documents. Copies of bills, as introduced, reported, and passed, are available from the House and Senate document rooms and may be accessed electronically. The document rooms also have the committee reports that accompany the bills and copies of "slip laws," the first official publication of newly enacted statutes. Hearing transcripts are frequently published by committees. Proceedings on the floor of both chambers are reported daily in the *Congressional Record*, which is available electronically.

STATE LEGISLATIVE PROCESS

Similar to the federal legislative process, the state process is set into motion when a condition is perceived to require change. For example, if a state does not include PAs in the definition of mental health provider, the need for change would be great. As the solution to the problem or to a situation requiring change begins to crystallize, it is put down in writing and becomes a bill or, in some states, a resolution (Fig. 9.1). Although writing a bill is usually considered the

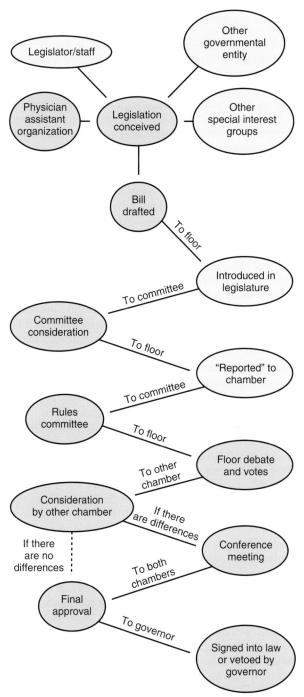

FIG. 9.1 ■ The legislative process, or "how a bill becomes law," designates points in the process at which your involvement is necessary.

The next step is sponsorship. If a representative has written the bill, he or she will usually sponsor it. If your state chapter has written the bill, a sponsor will have to be found. You may select your personal representative, one who is known to be sympathetic to your cause, or a member or chairperson of the committee to which the bill is expected to be referred. Bipartisan sponsorship is a good idea, particularly if different political parties control the state house, the state senate, or the governorship.

After the bill is printed, it has a "bill number" and is placed on the legislative calendar and "introduced." The introduction is a reading of the bill before all the members of the chamber in which it is introduced (all states except Nebraska have bicameral legislatures, i.e., two chambers). In most states, there is a gatekeeper committee, usually the rules or finance committee. If you want to influence when (or whether) a bill is introduced, you need to know which committee performs this function, and, ideally, you must know someone who is assigned to the committee. Alternatively, having a good relationship with the clerk or staff of the committee is invaluable if you want to know when a particular bill is to be introduced. After introduction, the bill's progress can be monitored online at the state legislature's website, and in most states you can sign up to receive email alerts when the bill's status changes.

After it has been introduced, the bill is referred to committee for study. It is here that you and your state chapter become a crucial part of the process. Given the diversity of issues with which legislators are faced, it is impossible for them to know everything about every subject. In the area of medicine, you know much more about PAs than your legislator. Therefore, when your bill is referred to committee, personal contact with the members of the committee to which it has been referred and the chair of that committee is crucial. Do not wait for the actual committee meeting or "hearing" at which your bill will be considered. Legislators need to be well informed about your issue before they are called on to vote.

There are many ways to be in touch with state legislators, but a personal meeting is generally the most effective. If you go to the Capitol, you may not meet with the actual representative but with one of the staff instead. Do not feel slighted. Staff members usually concentrate their activities in particular subject areas to develop considerable specific expertise. The staff member will have some knowledge about the issue and will welcome an opportunity to learn more.

You should remember a few things about making legislative visits. First, they are only the first step. Rarely does one isolated visit send a bill sailing through the legislature. Do not feel compelled

legislator's job, sometimes the best way to get what you need is for a state chapter to work closely with the legislative staff and with AAPA staff in this initial phase. Most legislatures employ professional staff to draft bills requested by senators and representatives.

to "win the battle" during an initial appointment. Keep your visit short and to the point. Be respectful and keep it pleasant. This does not necessarily mean you will agree on everything. That is all right. Offer to send additional information to clarify your position. You may want to leave a one-page statement or briefing on the issue behind. Also, leave your name, address, email, and phone number. Finally, remember to follow up. Always send a prompt note thanking the legislator or staff person for his or her time. Emphasize your areas of agreement and send along any material you promised. If you met with a staff person whom you found particularly pleasant or well informed, a note to the legislator is always appropriate.

Going to visit a legislator requires preparation. Even the best professional lobbyists rarely walk into an office and start talking "off the cuff." Do your homework. What are the pros and cons of the bill? Too many people go into a legislative visit without considering both sides of an issue. That is fine if the legislator agrees with you, but it leaves you unprepared if he or she does not. Think of the questions the opposition might raise and have nonconfrontational answers ready. Consider how this bill is going to affect the legislator's constituents. Does the legislator represent a medically underserved area in which modernizing collaboration requirements, for example, would improve the quality of health care that the constituents are receiving? How does the bill fit into the legislator's health care agenda?

Make sure that you also research information on the legislator. State legislature websites have bios on each member, and you can find additional information online. Go into your meeting with a good understanding of the background, interests, and priorities of the legislator.

Attending a committee meeting can be a revealing experience. Find out in advance whether you and other PA association representatives will be allowed to speak while the meeting is in session. Often you will not, but by watching the give and take during the meeting, you can decide who needs to be targeted for a special visit. In some committees, there is no give and take. The clerk reads off the bill numbers and the committee members vote. All discussions have been held and all decisions have been made before the meeting, which is why it is so important to visit all the committee members as soon as you found out which committee was going to handle your bill.

States are increasingly implementing online systems for submitting opinions or testimony. If this is a communication tool available in your state, make sure to coordinate your message with your state PA organization. "Form letters" or repetitive testimony are not generally compelling. However, emphasizing key points, with examples from your personal practice situation, can make your message more effective.

After a committee approves a bill, it goes to the full chamber. Another series of visits or email or phone contact may be necessary before that vote. You recall that when the bill was introduced, that was its first "reading." Although most states require three separate readings on three separate days, some do not. In some states, the only requirement is that the legislators have possession of the bill for a given number of days, commonly as few as three. This is particularly important to remember at the end of the legislative session, when everything is chaotic and a bill that legislators have had in hand for months may advance from the first to the third reading and a final vote in 30 seconds. In states where many bills are introduced each session, it is important to remember that the legislative calendar is dynamic. It is often perfectly acceptable to do tomorrow's bills in addition to today's.

Legislative calendars and bill scheduling information are located on the state legislature's website. The bill's specific history and text, including amendments to the introduced version, can be found there, too.

For the most part, the full House follows a committee's recommendation on a particular bill. If you do not consider that recommendation wise, then you can contact everyone again and express your concerns. You may be able to get two or three sympathetic legislators to orchestrate the floor debate so that those concerns are brought to the attention of the full chamber.

A bill that passes the first chamber must then be introduced in the second. Everything you did in the first chamber must be repeated: visits, thank you notes, committee meetings, online testimony, more visits. The process may be conducted slightly differently in the two chambers, so be sure you learn the rules.

After a bill has passed both chambers, it must be signed by the governor before it becomes effective. It is perfectly legitimate to attempt to influence the executive chamber. Action here must be planned in advance because the governor may sign the bill the moment it crosses his or her desk. In some states, agencies that will be implementing the bill (e.g., the Health Department) may write memoranda to the governor recommending signature or veto of a particular bill. If you can talk to the person who will be writing the memorandum, you may be able to influence its content. Know what the "vest-pocket veto" provisions are in your state. In some states, if the governor does not sign the bill within a fixed period, it is automatically vetoed.

If your bill is vetoed, there is always the outside chance that two thirds of the members of each house can be persuaded to override the veto. It is a long shot, but veto overrides sometimes happen. See Fig. 9.1 for a condensed depiction of the state legislative process.

This process is described as if it is your organization alone that will have an impact on your bill. Of course, that is not the case. Legislators cannot possibly be experts in all of the areas in which they are asked to cast a vote, so in general, they look to stakeholder groups to help them develop their response to legislation. State PA organizations that have repeated success at the legislature generally report that having the support of critical stakeholder groups before the introduction of legislation is key to positive results. Refer to Box 9.1 for important stakeholders to consider.

FEDERAL REGULATORY PROCESS

The legislative branch of government makes laws that typically contain policy statements and directives. It then delegates to the executive branch—the agencies of the federal government—the authority to implement them. This has been a normal feature of American government since 1790, when the first Congress declared that traders with the Indians should observe "such rules and regulations as the President shall prescribe."[3] Federal regulations generally describe how a program is to be administered. The federal Administrative Procedures Act (APA) guides agencies in their rule making. The APA procedure has four fundamental elements. First, it guarantees that notice of proposed rulemaking is published in the *Federal Register*. Second, it gives "interested persons," which really means everyone, the opportunity to comment on the proposal through at least written submissions. Third, it requires the agency to create a "statement of basis and purpose," justifying and explaining the final rule. Last, it requires publication of the final rule and creates a 30-day gap between publication and the effective date.[3]

Therefore, when a new law is passed, an existing law is amended, or a policy requires clarification, the affected federal agency publishes a notice of proposed rulemaking in the *Federal Register*. The notice includes the proposed rules and their statutory basis; provides background on their content; invites participation from the public through the submission of written comments, data, or arguments; and sets a deadline for the receipt of such comments. Comments must generally be submitted within 30, 60, or 90 days. On the federal level, hearings are seldom held.

Federal agency staff members analyze the comments and may make revisions in the rules on the basis of the information received. When final rules are published in the *Federal Register*, they are prefaced by a discussion of the comments, accompanied by the agency's response to them. For example, in 1989, the Health Care Financing Administration published final rules that changed the Medicare system for certification of nursing homes.[4] The preamble to the rules contained the following discussion:

> *Paragraph (e): Physician Delegation of Tasks*
> Comment: *In proposed section 483.40(e), we would permit physician delegation to physician extenders, that is, physician assistants and nurse practitioners, of tasks that the regulations do not otherwise require to be performed by the physician personally. An overwhelming majority of commenters expressed general support for permitting the delegation of tasks to physician extenders.*
> Response: *We believe that, to the extent feasible, the regulations should be written in a manner that allows for the effective utilization of physician extenders in the nursing home setting. For this reason, we are withdrawing our proposed requirement in section 483.40(b) that all orders be signed by the physician personally. This means that under sec. 483.40(e)(2), requirements concerning physician signature or countersignature of orders are determined by individual State law and facility policy. . . .*

There are exceptions to this procedure (some based in law, others in politics), but it represents the most common method of federal rule making.

General and permanent rules published in the *Federal Register* by the executive departments and agencies of the federal government are codified in the *Code of Federal Regulations*. The *Code* is divided into 50 titles that represent broad areas subject to federal regulation, such as "public health." Each title is further divided into chapters and the chapters into parts covering specific agencies and regulatory areas.[5] The *Code* is always changing in response to either acts of Congress or agency revisions of regulations. The *Federal Register*, published daily, is available in most public libraries, by subscription, and on the Internet. The *Code of Federal Regulations* is sold by the Superintendent of Documents and may also be viewed online.

STATE REGULATORY PROCESS

Agencies, boards, and departments are the regulators at the state level, and they touch what every citizen does every day. They are responsible for inspecting food; keeping the costs of utilities at a given rate;

and of course, governing the practice of medicine.[6] Although almost everyone knows when it is time to contact elected representatives, few know when, let alone how, to interact with agencies. This is crucial because "the rise of administrative bodies has probably been the most significant legal trend of the last century and perhaps more values are affected by their decisions than by those of all the courts. . . . They have become a veritable fourth branch of the Government, which has deranged our three-branch legal theories as much as the concept of a fourth dimension unsettles our three-dimensional thinking."[7] Agencies are here to stay, and it behooves us to learn how to deal with them.

Agencies (the inclusive term used in this chapter for regulatory bodies) are set forth in the Constitution, are created by legislatures, or are created by executive order and sanctioned by the legislature. The powers of the agency come from the body that creates it.[6] The work of agencies and legislatures is intertwined, but the players and processes are different.

First, consider the players. Legislators are elected by the people of the state and stay in office only as long as their work satisfies the voters unless the length of time they may serve is limited by law. Top-level agency personnel are usually appointed by the governor (with confirmation by one or both houses of the legislature) and serve at the pleasure of the governor. Midlevel agency staff members are generally civil service employees, although some political appointments exist at this level as well. Many of these people are career civil servants; they intend to make the government their life's work. Contrast this time frame with that of a legislator, who must think in terms of 2 or 4 years, depending on when he or she is up for reelection. Commissioners or department secretaries, the top-level personnel, may be career civil servants, or they may have aspirations for elected office. As such, their thinking is hybrid: They need to think of the long-term policy implications of their actions, as well as how such actions may influence the governor's reelection in a few years. So legislators and agency personnel think in different time frames and at different paces.

Legislators and bureaucrats also think differently in terms of content. A legislator is elected to represent all the interests of his or her district—the schools, the environment, the businesses. Legislators must also keep overall interests of the state in mind when involved in policy matters or budget negotiations. It is somewhat unrealistic to expect any one person to become expert in all these areas, particularly within 2 or 4 years. Add to that the need to balance the competing interests, and you have an almost impossible task. Contrast this situation with agencies. The subject matter is limited and specific—education, environment, *or* business, not all three. Agency personnel who work with an agency over a long period become quite expert in their specific subject areas. Because of their expertise and the fact that they do not depend on the good will of voters to keep their jobs, agency personnel may be the people who can answer your questions accurately and in great detail—even if they do not give you the answers you want to hear.

But what do agencies do? For this discussion, the focus is on the agency's function in creating rules and regulations. Similar to Congress, state legislatures pass laws (also known as statutes) whose language provides only a skeleton for a given policy. It is the agency's job to flesh out this skeleton by promulgating detailed rules and regulations.[8] The legislature may pass legislation for PAs that says, "A physician assistant is anyone who is licensed by the State Board of Medicine as a PA." But how does one get licensed? This is the sort of thing that will be detailed in state regulations. For example, to be licensed as a PA, one must submit an application documenting that he or she is a graduate of a PA program, has passed an examination, and is of good moral character. Regulations, in most cases, have the force of law.

Just as you can influence the legislative process, you can affect the regulatory process. The process is quite well defined in most states. With a few exceptions, states follow the 1981 modifications of the Model State Administrative Procedures Act (MSAPA), which sets forth a specific rule-making process that includes public notification and public comment. Your elected representative should be able to refer you to the agency in your state that is charged with enforcing your state Administrative Procedures Act. If you anticipate a protracted exchange on a regulatory level, it is wise to review the provisions of this act with the help of an attorney who knows administrative law.

After a law has been passed, an agency (or agencies) is charged with developing the regulations necessary for its implementation (Fig. 9.2). Usually, the staff of a bill's sponsor can tell you who is going to be writing the regulations. This is the time to get involved; it is much easier to influence what gets written than it is to change what has been written. Your initial contact with the regulator should focus on gathering and giving information. Are there any special concerns the agency needs to address in writing these regulations? What outside pressures (e.g., budgetary implications) might be brought to bear on the drafting? When does the agency intend to promulgate the regulations?

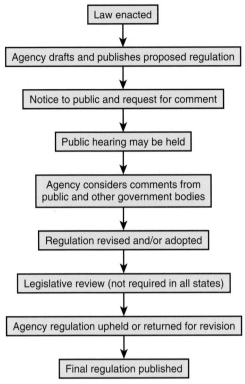

```
          Law enacted
               │
               ▼
Agency drafts and publishes proposed regulation
               │
               ▼
   Notice to public and request for comment
               │
               ▼
       Public hearing may be held
               │
               ▼
   Agency considers comments from
   public and other government bodies
               │
               ▼
    Regulation revised and/or adopted
               │
               ▼
Legislative review (not required in all states)
               │
               ▼
Agency regulation upheld or returned for revision
               │
               ▼
     Final regulation published
```

FIG. 9.2 ■ Procedures for state rule making.

Unless you know the political atmosphere in which the regulator is operating, you cannot supply really useful information. You know the language of PA practice, and the regulator knows the language of regulation. You need to work together. If you disagree with the regulator, fine; there are ways to deal with that. Over time, you will find that being helpful and reasonable with regulators will help to create an atmosphere in which public protection and reasonable regulation of the profession find common ground.

After the initial regulations are written, the MSAPA requires that interested parties be notified. Notification can take many forms. In larger states, the proposed regulations can be published in a register or some other regular publication that includes nothing but proposed regulations. In smaller states, they might be published in a newspaper that has statewide circulation. Agencies also generally post proposed regulations on their websites. In states that have adopted MSAPA, if you have notified the agency in advance that you want to know about any rules it promulgates, your name is added to its mailing list. If you have not made such a request, do not assume that just because the agency personnel know that you are interested in PA issues that they will notify you.

Although it is the agency's responsibility to notify the public, that responsibility does not extend to personal notification. It is also unwise to rely on your agency "contacts" to inform you of a proposed rule. Their primary responsibility is to the agency. If they know your organization is going to make the rule-making process more complicated, they might not notify you in advance.

A comment period follows notification, during which anyone may submit written feedback to the agency. Similar to all other written communication with government, comments should be succinct and unemotional. Your state PA organization may also be submitting comments, so you should try to express your ideas in concert with theirs. "In concert" does not mean using a form letter or parroting what the organization says. Your own thoughts and insights will be more persuasive.

Depending on the statute that was passed and on the particular state administrative procedures act, public hearings may be required. During the public hearing, interested individuals may comment on the proposed regulations. Individual testimony is usually limited to 5 or 10 minutes, including questions and answers. The agency will ask you to submit a written copy of your testimony. When you testify, it is best not to read from your written copy. Paraphrase what you have written and answer any questions the regulators may have. Some people find public testimony intimidating. You might find it useful to watch testimony before state or federal agencies before presenting testimony yourself. It is much easier if you are well prepared and remember that the regulators work for you. In some cases, you may wish to bring in experts from the AAPA or another organization that has had experience with the issue.

After the comment period and hearings, the regulation as initially drafted, or a modification of the proposed regulation is published and subsequently adopted. Some states have a time frame within which a regulation must be adopted or the process terminated.

In many states, the legislatures have not welcomed the rise of the administrative agencies just described. In an effort to curb what they saw as usurping of legislative mandates, they have adopted sunset laws and legislative oversight procedures. In a sunset law, the statute authorizing the existence of a regulatory agency expires in a fixed number of years unless it is reviewed and reauthorized by the legislature. In states with legislative oversight provisions, a committee of the legislature reviews all proposed regulations. State PA organizations have used these opportunities successfully to achieve needed change.

As you might expect, the regulatory process just described is somewhat neater than the reality. Some variations on the theme follow. All of the steps in the process have time limits. Perhaps the proposed rule needs to be published in only two consecutive weekly issues of the newspaper. Any PA group should make sure that one of its members is reading proposed rules on a regular basis. Most states have emergency adoption provisions that allow an agency to circumvent the time limits.[6] It only makes sense that if the state health department detects an increase in tuberculosis cases in August, it is not going to want to wade through the entire process, which may take 90 days, before requiring tuberculosis skin testing for students entering preschool. Usually, emergency rules are effective for only 120 days, with the option of one extension, after which time the agency must go through the notification and comment process. The state regulatory process is depicted in Fig. 9.2.

As has been said, regulatory policy is developed by a diverse array of participants, including agencies, state legislatures, courts and regulatory boards. Although nearly all regulatory actions taken by state actors have no antitrust ramifications, as with anything, there are always some exceptions.

The mission of the Federal Trade Commission (FTC) is to prevent business practices that are anticompetitive or deceptive or unfair to consumers and to enhance informed consumer choice and public understanding of the competitive process without unduly burdening legitimate business activity.[9] The FTC also encourages competition in the health care arena to increase access to health care, improve the quality of patient care, foster innovation in product development and service delivery, and help control costs. The FTC achieves these goals through analysis, advocacy, and enforcement. For example, in 2010, the Alabama Board of Medical Examiners (ALBME) proposed a rule to establish standards for the practice of interventional chronic pain management to require that interventional pain management services be provided exclusively by physicians. Asserting that "it is not the procedures, but the purpose and manner in which the procedures are utilized that demand the ongoing application of direct and immediate medical judgment, which constitutes the practice of medicine," the proposal sought to restrict the interventional treatment of pain to licensed medical doctors and doctors of osteopathy and prohibited them from delegating the authority to utilize such procedures (i.e., injection of local anesthetics, peripheral nerve blocks, and spinal facet joint injections) to diagnose, manage, or treat chronic pain patients to nonphysician personnel. The FTC opposed the proposal and submitted comments urging the state medical board to reject the proposed

rule. "Unnecessary restrictions on the ability of physicians to provide pain management . . . are likely to reduce the availability, and raise the prices, of pain management services in Alabama," potentially burdening patients with cancer and chronic pain, patients in rural areas, hospice patients and others with restricted healthcare access," the agency wrote. Given the strong weigh-in by the FTC, the ALBME ultimately decided to table the proposal.

The composition of regulatory boards can also have antitrust consequences. Boards that are composed of individuals who have no monetary interest in the profession that is being regulated or boards that merely act in an advisory capacity typically allow states to circumvent any conflict with federal antitrust laws. However, the overwhelming majority of licensing boards are predominantly composed of active members of their respective professions. For this reason, the implication of federal antitrust laws on regulatory actions taken by state actors has received a great deal of attention in recent years, as evidenced by the latest decision of the U.S. Supreme Court (SCOTUS) in *N.C. State Board of Dental Examiners v. Federal Trade Commission* (FTC), 135 S. Ct. 1101 (2015).

Established by state law to regulate the practice of dentistry, the majority of the North Carolina Board of Dental Examiners (board) are practicing dentists who therefore have a potential inducement to restrict competition from nondentist providers of teeth-whitening services. In the 1990s, dentists in the state began offering teeth-whitening services, which were quite profitable. Although the state's Dental Practice Act does not specify that teeth whitening is the practice of dentistry, when nondentists began to offer the services at significantly lower prices, dentists complained. The board subsequently issued cease-and-desist letters to the nondentist teeth-whitening service providers, suggesting that their provision of teeth-whitening services constituted the unlicensed practice of dentistry, which was a crime. The FTC brought an administrative complaint alleging that the board's actions to prevent nondentists from the teeth-whitening services market constituted antitrust violations, but the board argued that as a state agency it had antitrust immunity. The Supreme Court rejected the board's argument and affirmed the FTC's findings.[10] According to the Supreme Court's decision, state boards consisting of a controlling number of active market participants in the profession the board regulates are only exempt from the application of federal antitrust liability when two criteria are met. There must be (1) clear articulation and affirmative expression of the challenged restraint as state policy and (2) active supervision of the policy by a state agency or state official that is not an active market participant in the market that is being regulated. A state regulatory board is not in and of itself sovereign. Therefore, boards that are managed by active market participants must closely evaluate any anticompetitive activities and ensure adequate supervision by the state before taking action.

Before the Supreme Court Decision in the *North Carolina Dental Board v. FTC* case, the ALBME had enacted telehealth rules, which were considered to be some of the strictest in the country. Some of the restrictions included:

- A requirement that first-time visits between a patient and physician be in person
- A mandate for physicians to obtain a special-purpose license in order to practice medicine across state lines, thus treating its practice as a specialty versus a tool
- A prohibition against physicians having special-purpose licenses from supervising PAs or collaborating with certified registered nurse practitioners (NPs) or certified nurse midwives
- A prohibition against physicians with special-purpose licenses from using PAs or certified registered NPs or certified nurse midwives as patient site presenters (the individual at the patient site location who introduces the patient to the distant site provider for examination and to whom the distant site provider may delegate tasks and activities)

After the SCOTUS decision, the ALBME immediately suspended enforcement of its telehealth rules, stating that it planned to seek legislation to address telemedicine in the upcoming legislative session.

Hopefully, the SCOTUS decision will inspire other states with unnecessary and anticompetitive barriers to PA practice to follow suit and therefore expand patients' access to care. The AAPA will continue to monitor the effects of the SCOTUS decision and work with its constituent organizations to utilize this Supreme Court action to remove practice barriers.

CASE STUDIES

Examples of the political process, advocacy, and the "get informed, get involved" strategy are presented in the following case studies of actual events.

CASE STUDY 9.1 OBTAINING FULL PRESCRIBING AUTHORITY IN HAWAII

On August 22, 2014, the U.S. Drug Enforcement Administration (DEA) announced its decision to reclassify hydrocodone combination products from Schedule III to Schedule II in a rule that was slated to become effective on Oct. 6, 2014. At that time, the state of Hawaii was only one of 10 U.S. jurisdictions that did not allow PAs to prescribe Schedule II controlled medications. In addition, although the Hawaii Medical Board (HMB) had previously agreed to amend the state's regulations to allow PAs to prescribe Schedule II medications, the regulatory proposal was merely in its drafting stages and had yet to be implemented. As a result of the effective date of the DEA's rule, PAs in Hawaii would no longer be able to prescribe vital pain medications for their patients. This inability also had the potential to impact the state's already overcrowded emergency departments, surgical practices, urgent care clinics, and other health care practices, particularly in rural areas where the effect would be most severe. Thus rule implementation became an urgent matter, and the Hawaii Academy of PAs (HAPA) met with its then Governor Neil Abercrombie's staff to ask them to encourage the HMB to expedite the changes to the regulations. HAPA also generated grassroots support by using the AAPA's Legislative Action Center to request all PAs in the state to write a letter to the governor that included personal examples of how the rule change would impact their patients.

HAPA leadership also met with the governor's office and the Chair of the state's Senate Health Committee to urge rapid implementation of regulations authorizing PAs to prescribe Schedule II medication and to discuss ways to prevent or minimize the impact of the federal rule change.

The meeting also included critical stakeholders from

- The Health Committee Task Force on Narcotics
- The Hawaii Department of Commerce and Consumer Affairs
- The Hawaii County Medical Society
- The Hawaii Medical Association
- The HMB

At this meeting, the HAPA suggested two solutions. In the first instance, the governor could issue an executive directive giving PAs emergency Schedule II prescriptive authority because emergency powers in the state grant the governor broad discretion to waive laws in emergency situations to protect the public's health, safety, and welfare. The governor's office agreed to present the issue to the Hawaii attorney general's office for an opinion to determine if such an emergency situation existed. The chair of the senate health committee was also of the opinion that the issue constituted a federal emergency that had been imposed on the patients of Hawaii given the rapid implementation of the federal rule. As a result, he also agreed to discuss the situation in great detail with the attorney general.

The second possible solution was to quickly implement the rule change previously approved by the HMB authorizing PAs to prescribe Schedule II controlled medications because all of the meeting participants agreed that rapid implementation was vital for patients. The governor's office agreed to work with the HMB and the state agencies involved to expedite the implementation of the HMB rule change, which required a 30-day public notice. The AAPA also submitted a letter to the governor supporting urgent action to authorize PAs to prescribe Schedule II medications.

In the end, the attorney general's office did not advise that an Executive Directive was indicated; however, the rulemaking process was expedited, and by April 2015 Governor David Ige signed the regulatory proposal authorizing PAs to prescribe Schedule II controlled medications, thus giving PAs in Hawaii full prescriptive authority. The rule revisions became effective on April 16. HAPA's persistence, comprehensive and inclusive strategy, and effective relationship with the HMB were critical to the achievement of their goal on behalf of the profession and patients.

CASE STUDY 9.2 HARMONIZING LAWS THAT IMPACT PA PRACTICE IN OREGON

The Oregon Society of PAs (OSPA) found that they were fielding many questions about PA scope of practice. This was increasing as the number of PAs in the state and the range of specialties in which PAs practice grew. Time and again, OSPA was asked, "Can PAs do this?" Just as frequently, OSPA was contacted by a PA who had been told that PAs could not perform a specified service or sign a state-required form.

The problem was not the PA practice act or rules. The PA chapter of Oregon law allows PAs to perform a medical service if their supervising physician approves it unless PAs are specifically prohibited. However, in many sections of law outside of the PA practice act, the language was vague about which providers may perform certain medical functions, often referring only to "physicians" or "physicians and nurse practitioners." Without explicit mention of PAs or direct cross-reference to the PA practice act, these individual statutes gave the impression that PAs were not allowed to perform normal functions related to the profession.

The OSPA advocacy leadership team agreed that they needed to amend laws outside of the PA law to specifically name PAs, and the OSPA board of directors agreed. The Oregon Revised Statutes includes 838 chapters in 17 volumes. However, electronic searching made the process possible. A group of 12 PAs and the OSPA lobbyist searched the statutes to find places where specifically adding PAs would improve PA practice and patient care. Fifty chapters were determined to be relevant.

The OSPA drafting group wanted the bill to be noncontroversial and budget neutral, so they focused on areas of law where adding PAs would be logical and not represent an increase in scope of practice. The changes fell into five categories:
- Professional responsibilities, that is, changing "physician–patient relationship" to "provider–patient relationship"
- Treatment of special populations
- Insurance law for common treatment referrals and rural payment models
- Ordering provisions for home health and staffing of hospice
- Certifying health and disease status, family leave applications, and signing forms

The OSPA drafting group determined that 75 separate provisions met the criteria, and a 40-page bill was prepared. In general, the bill added "and physician assistant" to a list of authorized providers or changed "physician" to "licensed healthcare provider."

The Oregon state legislature has a regular session in odd-numbered years and a shorter budget-focused session in even-numbered years. Although short sessions, which are limited to 35 days, are more challenging, the OSPA team decided that the problem was urgent and growing. Also, they wanted to build on a 4-year successful presence at the legislature. OSPA had supported bills that had passed in the three previous sessions and built effective relationships with legislators. They also relied on a lobbyist who had good insights on current and future priorities and personalities at the capitol. After evaluating all variables, OSPA decided to seek introduction of the bill in the 2014 legislative session.

The advocacy group agreed on some basic principles. They focused on a clear and streamlined description of the bill and articulated how it would improve care and access for patients. A cohesive team led the effort and found a core group of supporting organizations, which included the Oregon State Medical Association.

The strategy worked. The legislation, which improved 75 key provisions of Oregon statute, was introduced on February 3, 2014, and was signed into law by Governor Kitzhaber on March 6. The bill became effective on July 1, 2014.

CONCLUSION

Contrary to what we hear every day about the failure of government, the system does work. It works because individuals and organizations keep doing their part to make it work. We hope this chapter will make it easier for you to be effective and even excited about your part in advocacy. The goal of this chapter was to help you "get informed." Take the next step—get involved!

KEY POINTS

- Understanding the political process is the responsibility of health care providers. Many aspects of health care are governed by laws and regulations, and it is your responsibility to understand the process and know how to impact it.
- Groups of like-minded individuals are more effective than individuals themselves, and coalitions of groups are more effective still.
- The communication and advocacy skills that PAs use to help patients understand diagnoses and treatments can be used to help change laws and regulations. If you see a law or regulation that gets in the way of PA practice and patient care, point it out and help change it.
- Being involved in the political process can be rewarding and fun! Consider being part of your state chapter government affairs committee or running for office. Many PAs have served on school boards and city councils and as mayors. There have been PA state legislators, speakers of the state house of representatives, and a PA in Congress. You could aspire to be the first PA President of the United States!
- As with everything, keep patients first. When you focus your advocacy on improving health and health care, you will keep a firm foundation.

References

1. American Academy of Physician Assistants. https://www.aapa.org/WorkArea/DownloadAsset.aspx?id=2147486552. Accessed November 18, 2015.
2. Congressional Quarterly's Guide to Congress. 6th ed. Washington, DC: Congressional Quarterly; 2007.
3. Koch Jr CH. *Administrative Law and Practice*. St. Paul, MN: West; 1997.
4. 54 Federal Register 5342. Washington, DC: U.S. Government Printing Office.
5. 42 CFR § 61.1. Washington, DC: U.S. Government Printing Office.
6. Breyer S, Stewart R, Sunstein C, Vermeule A. *Administrative Law and Regulatory Policy: Problems, Text, and Cases*. New York, NY: Aspen; 2006.
7. Jackson JR (dissenting). Federal Trade Commission v Rubberoid. 343 US 470 487 (1952).
8. Christoffel T. *Health and the Law: A Handbook for Health Professionals*. New York: Macmillan; 1982.
9. Federal Trade Commission. https://www.ftc.gov/about-ftc. Accessed November 20, 2015.
10. Radix S. *Antitrust Immunity Not a Given for State Licensing Boards*. PA Professional; May 2015.

The resources for this chapter can be found at www.expertconsult.com.

CHAPTER 10

INTERPROFESSIONAL PRACTICE AND EDUCATION

Christopher P. Forest

Physician assistant (PA) students who train in the early 21st century are being prepared as never before for interprofessional practice (IPP) via interprofessional education (IPE) (Box 10.1). IPE is a newer concept in medical education; therefore, PAs who graduated only a few years ago will not have had the same experience in IPE as current students and doctors. Working as a part of a team with other professions is so important that the Accreditation Review Commission on Education for the Physician Assistant states that the PA curriculum must include "instruction to prepare students to work collaboratively in interprofessional patient centered teams ... [and] include opportunities for students to apply these principles."[1] Other health profession education accrediting bodies have similar requirements (Box 10.2).

Why does working collaboratively require new advances in medical education? Don't all medical professionals work in teams already? Unfortunately, the concept of teams in the United States has traditionally been limited to the group of providers at a specific location or within a specific specialty practice. The team has not been defined as a group of people who work together across professional boundaries to care for one patient. Although specialists, for example, may send a letter of recommendations for the patient back to a primary care doctor, the concept of truly integrated care for the patient is rarely implemented. This fragmentation of care is potentially dangerous for the patient. As a result, policies have recently been implemented to provide incentives for better integration of patient care throughout the system.

This chapter is designed to introduce PA students to IPP and IPE. Because instruction in IPP and IPE is a newer approach, do not be surprised if you bring something new to settings that don't currently use interprofessional teams. Feel free to discuss these concepts with preceptors and employers, but avoid being judgmental with them. This chapter will provide you with the basic principles of IPE as well as practical ways to implement the competencies in the clinical environment as a student and as a PA.

BACKGROUND AND RATIONALE FOR INTERPROFESSIONAL PRACTICE AND INTERPROFESSIONAL EDUCATION

The population of adults older than the age 65 the United States is estimated at more than 40 million, and this is expected to double to 83.7 million

BOX 10.1 TERMINOLOGY

Interprofessional education (IPE) "occurs when two or more professions learn with, about, and from each other to enable effective collaboration and improve health outcomes."[19] IPE is intended to prepare students for interprofessional collaborative practice in the workforce.

Interprofessional practice (IPP) is often referred to as interprofessional collaborative practice. This occurs "when multiple health workers from different professional backgrounds work together with patients, families, care givers and communities to deliver the highest quality care." Elements of effective IPP include respect, trust, shared decision making, and partnerships.[21]

- **Triple Aim:** A three-pronged approach to optimizing health system performance created by the Institute for Healthcare Improvement. This involves simultaneous efforts to (1) improve the patient experience of care (including quality and satisfaction), (2) improve the health of populations, and (3) reduce the per capita cost of health care.[22] The Triple Aim is a goal for new collaborative health care systems and serves as the filter or lens through which new health care models will be evaluated. (Video Resource: http://www.ihi.org/engage/initiatives/tripleaim.)
- **Client vs. patient:** Health care professionals who don't prescribe medications, such as social workers and occupational therapists, will refer to the patient as their "client." This may seem rather impersonal, but it is more accurate from their perspective.

Interdisciplinary vs. interprofessional: Some professions may use the word "interdisciplinary" instead of "interprofessional." There are subtle differences between these words, but they are often used interchangeably.

by the year 2050.[2] Although the rates of alcohol consumption and cigarette smoking are lower in this generation of elders, overweight and obesity rates have increased.[2] This means that PAs will be treating more chronic diseases in this group, such as diabetes, hypertension, arthritis, and impaired mobility. According to the NIA Health and Retirement Study, in 2008, 41% of the older population had three or more chronic conditions, and 51% had at least one or two chronic conditions.[3]

The traditional model of fee-for service, referral-based care in the United States has been associated with fragmented care; dangerous outcomes; inefficient use of highly trained health professionals; and frustration for patients, particularly for elderly adults. The nation cannot sustain the inefficiency and cost of the traditional fee-for-service system. These realizations spurred the development of the "patient-centered medical home" (PCMH) and other collaborative health care models.[2]

In response to the limitations of the traditional system, the Patient Protection and Affordable Care Act (PPACA), commonly called the Affordable Care Act (ACA), was signed into law by President Obama on March 23, 2010. The ACA provides health care coverage for the poorest Americans by creating a minimum Medicaid income eligibility level across the country and improving the affordability of private insurance with federal subsidies for other uninsured Americans. With more people now insured, there is an increased need for additional primary care providers. Given the shortage of primary care physicians, pressure is being placed on the system to produce sufficient PAs and nurse practitioners to absorb the newly insured patients under the ACA. The U.S. Department of Health and Human Services reported in 2012 that "the number of PAs in the medical workforce (72,000) will be insufficient to meet the future primary care needs." Even with the anticipated 72% growth by 2025, they will only be able to provide 16% of the providers needed to address the projected physician shortage in primary care. Similar increases in the number of physicians who are being trained will also not fully meet the need for new primary care providers.[2]

In addition to providing insurance for previously uninsured patients, the ACA also enacted provisions to encourage collaborative care models. The government has provided financial support to PCMHs to allow them to accommodate the staff expansion required to improve health care coordination.[3] Additional funds were provided to expand training for medical providers (e.g., PAs) and to increase financial reimbursement to PCMHs that provide high-quality comprehensive medical care in collaborative models.[4] As Medicare transitioned away from the inefficient fee-for-service model, it encouraged the formation of accountable care organizations (ACOs) and has experimented with paying them a set amount per patient in order to encourage them to develop a collaborative model that would reduce costs. Under the old fee-for-service approach, doctors and hospitals would be paid extra to care for patients with preventable complications of a surgery, for example. Under the ACA, health systems are no longer rewarded financially for preventable complications. Instead, doctors and health systems are rewarded for providing high-quality preventive care and for good patient outcomes.[5] Studies show that IPP can address the Triple Aim by increasing the quality of care while reducing costs and increasing patient satisfaction.

BOX 10.2 STANDARDS FOR INTERPROFESSIONAL EDUCATION BY HEALTH PROFESSIONS

Physician Assistant: ARC-PA Accreditation Standard B 1.08. The curriculum must include instruction to prepare students to work collaboratively in interprofessional patient-centered teams. Such instruction includes content on the roles and responsibilities of various health care professionals, emphasizing the team approach to patient-centered care beyond the traditional physician–PA team approach. It assists students in learning the principles of interprofessional practice and includes opportunities for students to apply these principles in interprofessional teams within the curriculum.

Medicine: LCME Accreditation Standard 7.9, Interprofessional Collaborative Skills. The faculty of a medical school ensures that the core curriculum of the medical education program prepares medical students to function collaboratively on health care teams that include health professionals from other disciplines as they provide coordinated services to patients. These curricular experiences include practitioners and/or students from the other health professions.

Dentistry: CODA (Commission on Dental Accreditation) Standard 2-19. Graduates must be competent in communicating and collaborating with other members of the health care team to facilitate the provision of health care. Students should understand the roles of members of the health care team and have educational experiences, particularly clinical experiences that involve working with other healthcare professional students and practitioners. 2-19.1 Describe how students interact and collaborate with other health care providers, including but not limited to: a. primary care physicians, nurses, and medical students; b. public health care providers; c. nursing home care providers; d. pharmacists and other allied health personnel; e. social workers.

Social Work: Council on Social Work Education (CSWE) 2015 Educational Policy and Accreditation Standards Competency 1 – Demonstrate Ethical and Professional Behavior. Social Workers also understand the role of other professions when engaged in inter-professional teams ... Social workers value principles of relationship-building and inter-professional collaboration to facilitate engagement with clients, constituencies, and other professionals as appropriate ... Social workers value the importance of interprofessional teamwork and communication in interventions, recognizing that beneficial outcomes may require interdisciplinary, inter professional, and inter-organizational collaboration. Social workers.

Occupational Therapy: Accreditation Council for Occupational Therapy Education (ACOTE®) Standard B.5.21. A graduate from an ACOTE-accredited doctoral-degree-level occupational therapy program must effectively communicate, coordinate, and work interprofessionally with those who provide services to individuals, organizations, and/or populations in order to clarify each member's responsibility in executing components of an intervention plan.

Physical Therapy: Commission on Accreditation in Physical Therapy Education (CAPTE) Standard 6F. The didactic and clinical curriculum includes interprofessional education; learning activities are directed toward the development of interprofessional competencies including, but not limited to, values/ethics, communication, professional roles and responsibilities, and teamwork. This element will become effective January 1, 2018. *Standard 6L3.* The curriculum plan includes clinical education experiences for each student that encompass, but are not limited to, involvement in interprofessional practice. According to these standards, the programs should provide opportunities for involvement in interprofessional practice during clinical experiences and evidence that students have opportunities for interprofessional practice.

Nursing: The Commission on Collegiate Nursing Education (CCNE) Standards for Accreditation of Baccalaureate and Graduate Nursing Programs and the American Association of Colleges of Nursing (ACCN) publish *The Essentials of Baccalaureate Education for Professional Nursing Practice - Essential VI: Interprofessional Communication and Collaboration for Improving Patient Health Outcomes.* The nursing baccalaureate program prepares the graduate to: 1) Compare/contrast the roles and perspectives of the nursing profession with other care professionals on the healthcare team (i.e., scope of discipline, education and licensure requirements); 2) use inter - and intra-professional communication and collaborative skills to deliver evidence-based, patient-centered care. Sample content includes: interprofessional and intra-professional communication, collaboration, and socialization, with consideration of principles related to communication with diverse cultures; teamwork/ concepts of teambuilding/cooperative learning; professional roles, knowledge translation, role boundaries, and diverse disciplinary perspectives.

In contrast to the referral based system of the past 60 years, in the team-based IPP model, the primary care provider functions as part of a multidisciplinary team. After each member of the team evaluates the patient, the team members collaborate on developing a patient care plan. When one team member discusses the plan with the patient, it becomes clear that everyone is working together in the patient's best interest. The patient is clearly at the center of this model and viewed as an integral part of the team. Although long-term health outcomes for interprofessional teams have not been established, studies demonstrate that interprofessional care improves short-term patient outcomes,[6-8] cost efficiency,[9] and health professional satisfaction.[10] Quality of care is improved by reducing redundancies of medical care services, duplication of medications, medication errors, and gaps in services.

To be prepared to function as part of interprofessional teams, students need to *learn with and about other health professions during their training* instead of waiting until they enter the workforce. Early exposure to IPP enables them to develop this team mentality and the relationships needed to enact change. Universities that train health professionals use a variety of strategies and instructional methods to begin to introduce their students to IPP.

Many universities teach interprofessional skills through student-run clinics. Student-run free clinics have proliferated in the United States, with more than 75% of accredited medical schools having at least one student-run free clinic.[11] Many of these are run as interdisciplinary clinics for the health profession students at these universities. In some clinics, a representative of each profession sees the patient in turn; then the students huddle to share notes and develop a treatment plan, which is presented to the attending. In other clinics, students from each profession see the patient together at the same time in the same room and decide on a care plan together. Student-run clinics offer unparalleled opportunities for preclinical students to experience working in interprofessional teams with the safety of preceptor supervision.

Physician assistant students who are able to work in these clinics should take advantage of the opportunity to speak with students from other professions. Students should ask them about their training, what they are currently able to do, and what their scope of practice will ultimately be when they become licensed. Recognizing the roles of each type of health professional is an important competency to master in school, before going out into practice.

BARRIERS TO INTERPROFESSIONAL EDUCATION

For the IPP model to succeed, exposure to IPP must begin when practitioners are still students. Each profession must provide opportunities for students to receive joint training. Unfortunately, health profession educators have found it more difficult than expected to provide IPE. Attempting to blend among different professions reveals practical and philosophical barriers that can make IPE challenging to implement. Some of the barriers include:

- **Structure of traditional education:** Students from each profession are taught in "silos," unaware

of the content of the education and the role of each health profession. These silos promote isolation and inhibit collaboration among the professions. As the health care needs of the community change, each profession adapts to meet those needs. This results in evolving roles and often an overlap of skills among professions. In many cases, health care professionals are unaware of this "role blurring" until they have the opportunity to work side by side with each other. For example, many clinical pharmacists are able to perform a basic physical examination and prescribe under protocol, and many occupational therapists are trained in assessing childhood development, anxiety, and depression.

The first step to overcoming this barrier is to make the effort to learn about the roles and responsibilities of each profession on the student team. You may learn this as part of your curriculum, but you should take advantage of opportunities to volunteer in interprofessional activities to learn directly from other health professionals about their training and scope of practice.

- **Interprofessional accreditation standards:** Although the inclusion of IPE standards in accreditation procedures ought to promote the development of IPE, the variety of standards and the lack of guidance from accrediting agencies about which activities may fulfill this requirement can inhibit the implementation of IPE. For example, some standards may permit a school to simply provide one lecture on roles and responsibilities of different professions or provide a clinical opportunity for students to interact with another health professional. Other standards may require actual clinical training to be conducted interprofessionally. With each profession trying to meet the standards set for them in the context of already overcrowded curricula, it can be difficult for different professions to agree on the IPE activities for the institution.

- **Complexity of academic scheduling:** Arranging time for IPE is an extremely difficult task because of the differences in content, complexity of schedules, and logistics of transportation to a common location. Most students are already in classes 35 to 40 hours per week. Adding a common course is a hardship. For this reason, programs have to be creative, typically incorporating short IPE activities within existing courses. Some common IPE activities include a panel of speakers from different professions, an IPE day where students from different professions participate in workshops and simulated clinical activities, and student-run clinics, which are often scheduled in the evening hours.

- **Attitudes of faculty and administration:** Merging IPE content into existing courses requires time, effort, and changing the way things have always been done. These changes sometimes meet with resistance from faculty or administrators who do not believe in the viability of IPE or who are simply overwhelmed with the demands of running their existing programs. As IPE becomes an accreditation requirement for each profession, faculty will adjust to the new expectations, and IPE will become an accepted part of the curriculum.

BARRIERS TO INTERPROFESSIONAL PRACTICE

Even as the barriers to IPE seem difficult to overcome, the barriers to true IPP are likely even more substantial:

- **Traditional silo structure of health professionals:** The silos that exist in education result in silos in practice. In any given health care environment, doctors talk to doctors, nurses talk to nurses, social workers talk to social workers, and so on. Through experience, they become self-reliant and tend to refer out any questions that they perceive to be beyond their scope of practice. The reality is that even the conditions that they believe are within their scope can be better cared for by an interprofessional team.
- **Fee-for-service reimbursement structure:** Fee for service refers to the system whereby a health care provider, after seeing a patient, bills either an insurance carrier or the patient for services rendered. The traditional system is not set up to receive invoices for consultations from multiple providers or a team. The ACA has resulted in the movement toward a novel reimbursement system that not only reimburses a medical group based on the number of individuals assigned to its site but also will provide bonuses based on performance, improving health outcomes. In other words, there will be financial rewards for offering high-quality health care and preventing disease. Team-based care will be one of the keys to success for this new system.
- **Physical space in health care facilities:** Medical facilities in the traditional system are designed for optimal patient flow for one type of health care professional (e.g., family medicine practice, physical therapy clinic, social work offices). This physical setup works well in the "referral system" model but is not conducive to IPP. New provider offices are being constructed with a more inclusive design that may include onsite facilities for dentistry, physical therapy, occupational therapy, and social work in addition to primary care. How much better might the care that the patient receives be when a health care team is in close proximity of each other, actively informing each other of the patient's progress and revising patient care plans together?
- **Lack of training and experience in IPP:** To a health care provider who is accustomed to working autonomously and directing care for his or her patients, it can be a large adjustment to work on a team, especially when others now have input into your decisions. Functioning as part of a team does not come naturally for many providers. It requires training and experience. In the IPP model, the team leader role may be given to the one with the most team experience rather than always being assigned to the doctor, as has been the tradition. PAs should be prepared to both lead these teams and know how to be a responsible supporting member of the team.

INTERPROFESSIONAL EDUCATION COMPETENCIES

Creating health care reform begins at the root, educating students from multiple professions to learn the IPE competencies and graduate with experience in interprofessional care. The World Health Organization recommends that health care students and medical providers become proficient at the following skills or competencies:[12]

1. **Teamwork:** Acquisition of the knowledge and skills linked to interprofessional collaboration and networking; building trust
2. **Role recognition:** Understanding one's own roles, responsibilities, and boundaries as well as those of other health and social care professionals
3. **Communication:** Effective communication, listening, negotiation, and conflict resolution; facilitation
4. **Learning and reflection:** Transferring interprofessional learning to the clinical setting; learning about team development; and reflecting critically on one's relationship in the team
5. **The patient:** Central role of the patient in interprofessional care; cooperating in best interests of the patient; treating the patient as a partner within the team
6. **Ethics and attitudes:** Ethical issues relating to teamwork; respect; awareness of stereotyping; tolerating differences and misunderstandings

Teamwork

Team Characteristics

Health professionals may work on teams, but that does not necessarily mean that they are engaging in teamwork. The traditional patient referral system is often mistaken with interprofessional collaboration. Referring to specialists and other health care workers doesn't require teamwork and involves gaps in communication. In many cases, it could take weeks or months before receiving a report about how a patient or client is progressing. In a true IPP, each discipline collaborates in the evaluation and management of the patient's condition in real time.

It took the 15 years of National Institutes of Health–funded studies to identify the following seven team characteristics required for primary care practice improvement:
1. Trust: being vulnerable and collaborative
2. Mindfulness: being highly aware of details and openness to new ideas
3. Heedfulness: attention to tasks belonging to one's self and others
4. Respectful interaction: honesty, self-confidence, and appreciation of others
5. Diversity: differences in perspectives and world views of individuals
6. Social and task relatedness: balance of social and work issues)
7. Rich and lean communication: communicating ambiguous information face to face and less ambiguous information using lean channels such as emails or memos[13,14]

Research shows that IPP involves more than just teamwork. It requires interprofessional collaboration, communication, coordination, and networking in order to improve outcomes, increase patient satisfaction, and reduce medical errors.[8,15-19]

Putting Team Theory Into Practice

Many students will have the opportunity to work on interprofessional teams during the course of their studies, possibly at a health fair or student-run clinic. When assigned to work with a new group of students, there are a few issues that the newly formed team should manage together:
- **Leadership:** The physician or medical student assumes leadership in the traditional model. However, for an interprofessional team, leadership is shared, and the team leader takes on the role of a facilitator. It is a good idea for the individual with the strongest facilitation skills to be selected the leader of the group. The leader is responsible for keeping the discussion on track, allowing everyone's voice to be heard, and for follow-up.
- **Hierarchy:** Team members should decide on the following team roles based on interests and abilities: facilitator, scribe, and timekeeper. This may sound very basic, but a team functions more efficiently when one person is responsible for taking minutes and another for keeping track of the time. Clarity of responsibilities is vital to the success of a team.
- **Ground rules:** To be an effective team, the group should agree on ground rules. For example, the team may decide that all members will be given the opportunity to express their opinions on every issue. They may also decide that cell phones should not be answered while in discussion or that no one is allowed to interrupt the person who is speaking, except for the timekeeper.
- **Diversity:** Is diversity a strength or hindrance for this group? For example, differences in scopes of practice and overlapping roles can enhance or complicate the patient encounters. When two members of the team have differing approaches to a health care problem (e.g., complementary and alternative medicine vs. medication), how will the team resolve these issues? When multiple members of the team are capable of taking a social history or performing a depression screen, who will the team elect to perform those functions? Answering these questions prospectively minimizes frustration for both the students and the patients.
- **Assumptions:** What are underlying assumptions about other team members regarding gender, status, seniority, age, and education? Is it safe to assume that the ideal person to lead the team is the eldest, the physician, or the one with the most seniority? The team must take some time early in its formation to identify members with strong facilitation skills and to learn about each other's education and professional abilities.
- **Jargon:** Avoid using profession-specific jargon that other team members may not recognize, such as PERRLA, EOM, and ADLs. Don't make anyone feel ignorant or as if they are an outsider to the group. Jargon causes rifts in communication and relationships. Remain aware of how members of the team are responding to your language, and if they appear confused, take time to explain any terms that may not be commonly used in their profession.

Requirements for a Good Team Leader or Facilitator

Being a good team leader requires that you have the appropriate knowledge base, skills, and attitudes. The team leader has to have a clear understanding of the roles of other health professionals. Although this can be learned from class, it is ideal if the team leader has had experiential knowledge about the roles by actually working with other professions. The primary skill needed is that of being able to communicate with others but also the ability to reflect and facilitate group reflection. The attitudes required of this position include fostering mutual respect, willingness to collaborate, and openness to others' views.[20]

Role Recognition

Being aware of each other's roles, responsibilities, and limitations sets the climate for effective teamwork. One of the first steps in forming a team is to discuss roles and allow each member to have an equal opportunity to educate teammates about their role. During this process, misperceptions are typically clarified, and assumptions are corrected. It helps the team to develop a common vocabulary and helps avert potential conflicts.

Physician assistants often discover that other health professionals are surprised to learn that PAs can perform surgical procedures and prescribe controlled substances. At the same time, PAs may not realize that many pharmacists can examine patients or that occupational therapists can perform cognitive assessments and depression screening. Learning from each other can is enlightening. Sharing about our roles is an essential part of interprofessional learning and helps solidify the team.

Conflict Management

Conflict should be expected when a new team is forming. It is not a stage to be avoided but rather welcomed and addressed. Conflict offers a team the opportunity to overcome a challenge and grow stronger in the process. It's a stage that brings out new ideas and creativity within the group. Knowing to expect conflict gives the team the opportunity to take a proactive approach, creating a plan of action rather than a reactive approach that generates additional stress.

Psychologist Bruce Tuckman proposed the **forming–storming–norming–performing** model for team development in 1965 that identified the stages of development necessary for team growth and ultimately for the team to produce positive results. If you want to be a strong team leader, you should be aware of the following stages of team development and what your role is at each stage.

In the **forming** stage, team members learn about each other and try to find safe patterns for interacting.

The team leader's role is to set a climate in which each member fully participates, roles and tasks are clarified, and communication is encouraged. This stage builds the group identity.

The **storming** stage is characterized by a storm or conflict among team members as they test their roles as part of the group. If the storm is too violent, some teams will never get past this stage. During this time, it is vitally important for the team to keep the goals the team is trying to achieve in mind. This is a time when the team needs to come together to decide how to move forward. It is important to remember that conflict is an opportunity for growth. The team leader's roles at this stage are to focus the team, encourage respect for each other's viewpoints, and facilitate a plan to resolve the conflict.

Norming refers to the stage during which the team collaborates well and becomes a cohesive unit. Everyone understands the mission of the team, and respect grows. The team leader facilitates good communication by being open about issues, encouraging feedback, building consensus, and delegating new tasks.

In the **performing** stage, the team is fully functioning, with each member aware of his or her specific tasks and producing results. The team leader may assess the team, recognize each member's contributions, and assist each member in reaching his or her full potential on the team.

The **transforming** stage is the point at which the team achieves its goal. It's a time for the team leader to honor the team's accomplishments, celebrate personal growth, and determine future directions for the team.

To optimize team performance, these are the recommended steps that a team leader should take:
1. **Build trust.** Take time to hear each other's personal stories and develop an understanding of their personal motivation.
2. **Establish a "conflict culture."** Profile the team and its members, anticipating conflict and preparing for conflict norming.
3. **Manage meetings.** Protect your team from too many meetings. When you must meet, address the issues quickly while encouraging everyone's voice to be heard.
4. **Get commitment.** Don't assume that everyone thinks the way you do. Speak with the team and make issues and tasks very clear. Use cascading communication to ensure that everyone is aware of messages and decisions.
5. **Establish accountability.** Both the team leader and peers are responsible for holding each other accountable for tasks. An effective leader keeps track of team accomplishments and milestones.

Reflection and Team Assessment

Reflection is an essential part of developing an effective team. It gives meaning and focus to the team, fosters a habit of appreciating each other, creates a sense of closure after an emotional or stressful encounter, develops the ability to learn from both positive and negative experiences, creates shared understanding and improved communication, and provides a broader perspective on the experience.

The ideal time to reflect is at the end of the session or end of the day to discuss how everything went. During this time, team members should be encouraged to share about team strengths and weaknesses they observed that day, whether ground rules were observed, situations that enabled effective collaboration, and potential areas of improvement.

When giving feedback to the team, it is recommended that the team leader begin with team self-assessment based on direct observation. The team leader should encourage all to be clear, specific, and balanced with feedback and to use "teach-back" to ensure that the feedback was received as intended.

Centrality of the Patient

The interprofessional model places the patient at the center and considers the patient a part of the team, to be included in the decision-making process. The patient's improved health is the goal of the team, and every action should be performed in the patient's best interest.

Ethics and Attitudes

Ethics is at the core of the practice of medicine. It includes the principle of *primum non nocere*—above all, do no harm. The fee-for-service model was easily susceptible to abuse and breaches of ethics because providers were financially rewarded for providing potentially unnecessary care. Paying teams for delivering high-quality care and better outcomes aligns the financial interests of the providers with the good of the patient. Ethics in this new delivery system will involve respecting the other team members, being cautious not to stereotype them or the patients, and exhibiting tolerance toward the team members with different opinions. It is important to understand that misunderstandings may occur, and in these situations, communication is key to resolving differences among team members.

SUMMARY

Interprofessional education occurs "when two or more professions learn with, about, and from each other to enable effective collaboration and improve health outcomes." As the result of inefficiencies in the traditional fee-for-service or referral system model, the government has restructured health care reimbursement, allowing for more a comprehensive team-based approach conducive to interprofessional care. Health care professions have traditionally been educated in silos; however, with increased accreditation standards requiring IPE, further integration of education and learning activities will be seen.

Interprofessional competencies must be learned during health care education to adequately prepare students for IPP. These competencies include teamwork, role recognition, communication, learning and reflection, centrality of the patient, and ethics and attitudes. PA students should make every effort to develop these competencies and to prepare themselves for potential leadership of interprofessional teams.

KEY POINTS

- IPP is based on students learning to work with other health professionals while still in their training, often via formal IPE activities or by working together in student clinics.
- National-level policy changes are creating new incentives for providers to practice interprofessionally. The goals of these policy changes are to improve quality of patient care, decrease medical errors, invest in preventive care, and improve the patient experience of receiving care.
- Research has shown specific steps that are essential to developing and sustaining effective IPP.

References

1. Accreditation Review Commission on Education for the Physician Assistant. Accreditation Standards for Physician Assistant Education. 4th ed. http://www.arc-pa.org/acc_standards. Accessed February 14, 2016.
2. National Institute on Aging. NIH-commissioned Census Report highlights effect of aging boomers. Available at https://www.nia.nih.gov/print/newsroom/2014/06/nih-commissioned-census-bureau-report-highlights-effect-aging-boomers. Accessed December 16, 2016.
3. West LA, Cole S, Goodkind D, He W. 65+ in the United States: 2010. U.S. Census Bureau, US Government Printing Office, Washington, DC, 2014:23–212. https://www.census/gov/content/dam/Census/library/publications/2014/demo/p23-212.pdf. Accessed January 3, 2017.
4. U.S. Department of Health & Human Services. The Affordable Care Act supports patient-centered medical homes in health centers. Available at http://www.hhs.gov/about/news/2014/08/26/the-affordable-care-act-supports-patient-centered-medical-homes-in-health-centers.html. Accessed March 25, 2016.
5. Davis K, Abrams M, Stremikis K. How the Affordable Care Act will strengthen the nation's primary care foundation. *J Gen Intern Med.* 2011;26(10):1201–1203.
6. Zwarenstein M, Reeves S, Perrier L. Effectiveness of pre-licensure interdisciplinary education and post-licensure collaborative interventions. *J Interprof Care.* 2005;19(suppl 1):148–165.
7. Reeves S, Zwarenstein M, Goldman J, et al. Interprofessional education: effects on professional practice and health care outcomes. *Cochrane Database Syst Rev.* 2008;(1). CD002213.
8. Zwarenstein M, Goldman J, Reeves S. Interprofessional collaboration: effects of practice-based interventions on professional practice and healthcare outcomes. *Cochrane Database Syst Rev.* 2009;3. CD000072.
9. D'Amour D, Oandasan I. Interprofessionality as the field of interprofessional practice and interprofessional education: an emerging concept. *J Interprof Care.* 2005;19(suppl 1):8–20.
10. Cohen SG, Bailey DE. What makes teams work: group effectiveness research from the shop floor to the executive suite. *J Management.* 1997;23(3):239–290.
11. Smith S, Thomas III R, Cruz M, Griggs R, Moscato B, Ferrara A. Presence and characteristics of student-run free clinics in medical schools. *JAMA.* 2014;312(22):2407–2410.
12. Thistlethwaite J, Moran M, World Health Organization Study Group on Interprofessional Education and Collaborative Practice. Learning outcomes for interprofessional education (IPE): Literature review and synthesis. *J Interprof Care.* 2010;24(5):503–513.
13. Lanham HJ, McDaniel Jr RR, Crabtree BF, et al. How improving practice relationships among clinicians and non clinicians can improve quality in primary care. *Jt Comm J Qual Patient Saf.* 2009;35(9):457–466.
14. Safran DG, Miller W, Beckman H. Organizational dimensions of relationship-centered care. Theory, evidence, and practice. *J Gen Intern Med.* 2006;21(S1):S9–S15.
15. Hallin K, Henriksson P, Dalen N, Kiessling A. Effects of interprofessional education on patient perceived quality of care. *Med Teach.* 2011;33(1):e22–e26.
16. Olson R, Bialocerkowski A. Interprofessional education in allied health: a systematic review. *Med Educ.* 2014;48(3):236–246.
17. Reeves S, Perrier L, Goldman J, Freeth D, Zwarenstein M. *Interprofessional Education: Effects on Professional Practice and Health Care Outcomes (update) (Review).* The Cochrane Collaboration. New York: John Wiley & Sons, Ltd.; 2013.
18. Rodger S, Webb G, Devitt L, Gilbert J, Wrightson P, McMeeken J. A clinical education and practice placements in the allied health professions: an international perspective. *J Allied Health.* 2008;37(1):53–62.
19. Steinert Y. Learning together to teach together: interprofessional education and faculty development. *J Interprof Care.* 2005;19(suppl 1):60–75.
20. Oandasan I, Reeves S. Key elements for interprofessional education. Part 1: the learner, the educator and the learning context. *J Interprof Care.* 2005;19 Suppl 1:21–38.
21. World Health Organization. *Framework for Action on Interprofessional Education & Collaborative Practice*; 2010. Available at http://www.who.int/hrh/resources/framework_action/en. Accessed February 14, 2016.
22. Berwick DM, Nolan TW, Whittington J. The triple aim: care, health, and cost. *Health Aff (Millwood).* 2008;27(3):759–769.

The resources for this chapter can be found at www.expertconsult.com.

SECTION II

MEDICAL KNOWLEDGE

EVIDENCE-BASED MEDICINE

Brenda Quincy

At this point in history, when so much information is available with the click of a mouse or with a sweep of a finger, it is important for medical providers to continue to strengthen their capacity for incorporating evidence into their clinical decision making. Although providers have easier access to current information than ever before, the sheer volume of health-related data can quickly become overwhelming for providers who must efficiently care for patients. For this reason, it is important for busy clinicians to have a grasp of the process and principles of evidence-based practice from asking the question, to finding the evidence, to evaluating the quality of the evidence, and finally to incorporating the evidence into clinical decision making.

HISTORY OF EVIDENCE-BASED MEDICINE

The challenges of implementing the best quality evidence into medical decision-making predates the modern medical era. The well-known "scurvy" experiment dates back to the British Navy of the 1740s. A naval surgeon, James Lind, conducted an experiment in search of a cause and a treatment for sick sailors. Although he had a small sample size, he did use important experimental principles, including the establishment of control groups, a clear endpoint, and the inclusion of similar cases, in an attempt to control for potential confounding variables. In his experiment, Lind clearly demonstrated

the importance of citrus in the diet, but it took 7 years for his findings to be published and 40 years before the British Navy included citrus on every voyage. This delay in the implementation of best evidence into clinical practice has been a recurring theme historically.

Another example of early experimental evidence ultimately informing medical practice includes examination of maternal mortality rates by Semmelweis in the middle 1800s. Through a comparison of deliveries performed by physicians and those by nurse midwives, Semmelweis noted that mortality rates from postpartum infection were much higher for pregnant women attended by physicians. He ultimately attributed the increase to the fact that doctors routinely performed postmortem examinations early in the morning before attending their obstetric patients. The introduction of good handwashing practices significantly lowered the mortality rates for mothers whose babies were delivered by the physicians. However, mortality rates increased again when the new practice of consistent handwashing slackened. The historical challenges of implementing practices based on best evidence and sustaining those practices mirrors challenges encountered today.[1]

Historically, collection of high-quality evidence was limited by bias and lack of blinding as individual physicians made observations about interventions and outcomes in their own patients. The earliest reported randomized controlled trials (RCTs) only occurred in the mid to late 1940s and included a streptomycin trial and a whooping cough vaccine trial. The whooping cough trial actually included elements of the placebo control and informed consent, strengthening the rigor of the trial and the validity of the evidence.[1]

It has been a challenge, however, to summarize and communicate research-based evidence to make it usable by practicing clinicians. In 1967, David Sackett, MD, started the first Department of Clinical Epidemiology at McMaster University in Ontario, Canada. Before Sackett's work, epidemiology and biostatistics and their implications in public health were not readily digestible for practicing clinicians. Sackett was among the first to develop practical tools for physicians to apply research evidence to the care of individual patients. Dr. Sackett continued at McMaster University until 1994 when he became the foundation director of the Center for Evidence-based Medicine at Oxford University. After his retirement from Oxford, he returned to Canada and continued to teach clinical epidemiology to students until his death in May 2015.[2]

Another important figure in the history of evidence-based medicine (EBM) is Dr. Gordon Guyatt. Dr. Guyatt was the director of the internal medicine residency program at McMaster University for many years and was the first to coin the term "evidence-based medicine." Throughout the 1990s, an ongoing series of articles was published in the *Journal of the American Medical Association (JAMA)* titled "User's Guides to the Medical Literature." These later led to the development of a textbook summarizing the principles of evidence-based clinical practice. In his work, Dr. Guyatt presented a methodical, easy-to-remember approach to the practice of EBM that many clinicians use today.[3]

Guyatt and others credit three additional researcher-clinicians from an earlier generation who influenced their work in EBM. Dr. Tom Chalmers recognized the value of rigorous study design and randomized trials as early as 1955 in his paper on bed rest and diet for hepatitis. That paper heavily influenced Guyatt's understanding of what he later called clinical epidemiology. Alvan Feinstein from Yale was both a clinician and a researcher who was a key player in the development of an approach to studying the ways medicine is practiced on a daily basis. The third individual was Archie Cochrane. His work as a clinician, an epidemiologist, and a medical school faculty member inspired the later development of the Cochrane Collaboration, which has become a recognized leader in the development of EBM and EBM resources.[4]

EVIDENCE-BASED MEDICINE PROCESS

Effective evidence based medicine incorporates five primary tasks. These are (1) *asking* a clinical question, (2) *searching for* evidence that addresses the question, (3) *assessing* the quality of the evidence, (4) *incorporating* the evidence into a clinical decision, and (5) *evaluating* the process.

Task 1: Asking a Clinical Question

Typically, clinical questions are categorized as background questions or foreground questions. Background questions are very general questions most often asked by new learners or by practitioners encountering an unfamiliar diagnosis or clinical presentation. Background questions commonly begin with who, what, when, where, how, or why. Examples of background questions may include, "Where is the incidence of Lyme disease highest?" or "What are the risk factors for osteoporosis?" The answers to these questions provide background information on a particular topic.

Foreground questions are very specific questions designed to provide guidance for the clinical care of a particular patient or group of patients. A foreground question about Lyme disease, for example, may compare two antibiotic dosing regimens for speed of recovery. A useful acronym for developing foreground questions is "PICO." PICO stands for:

P: Population or patient—How would you describe a patient or population like yours?

I: Intervention—Which intervention are you considering?

C: Comparison—What alternative approaches are you considering for your patient?

O: Outcome—What am I hoping to measure, achieve or affect?

PICO questions can be developed to address a variety of clinical question types, including diagnosis, etiology or harm, prognosis, and treatment. For example, consider a commonly diagnosed disorder such as diabetes mellitus. A physician assistant may have many questions about diabetes. See Table 11.1 for sample PICO questions of each clinical type regarding diabetes. Properly structuring the question at the outset is the key step to obtaining a meaningful evidence-based answer.

Task 2: Searching for Evidence

The search for evidence begins with identifying the type of evidence of interest. Evidence can be broadly divided into two categories, filtered and unfiltered. Filtered evidence is that which has already been

TABLE 11.1 Example PICO Questions of Each Clinical Type Regarding Diabetes

Type of Question	PICO Question
Diagnosis	In patients with type 2 diabetes, is a 24-hour urine collection for creatinine clearance more sensitive than a serum creatinine for detecting early-onset kidney disease?
Etiology or harm	In middle-aged adults, is family history of diabetes a greater risk factor than obesity for the development of type II diabetes?
Treatment	In patients with new-onset type II diabetes, are saxagliptin and metformin more effective than glipizide and metformin at decreasing the risk of renal failure?
Prognosis	In patients with type I diabetes, is a hemoglobin A1c goal of 6.0% more effective than hemoglobin A1c of 7.0% at increasing survival?

TABLE 11.2 Filtered and Unfiltered Sources of Evidence

Filtered (Secondary) Evidence	Unfiltered (Primary) Evidence
Clinical guidelines: National Guidelines Clearinghouse *CATs*: BestBETs *Evidence-based summaries*: UpToDate, Clinical Evidence, Bandolier *Structured Abstracts*: EBM Online, ACP Journal Club *Systematic reviews*: Cochrane Library *Databases*: Trip Database, Essential Evidence Plus	PubMed EBSCO Ovid

gathered and synthesized by experts into a format that is readily usable by clinicians. Clinical guidelines developed by professional bodies are an example of filtered evidence. Other examples include critically appraised topics (CATs), evidence-based summaries, structured abstracts, and systematic reviews. For a list of evidence-based filtered resources, see Table 11.2.

Unfiltered or primary evidence includes original research articles published in peer-reviewed journals. There are variety of databases through which a search for primary literature may be conducted. Table 11.2 contains a list of examples of databases of primary literature. Individual practitioners will need to determine which databases are available through their employing institutions. The focus of the rest of this chapter will be accessing and assessing primary literature.

A systematic approach to searching medical databases is critical to uncovering the evidence. Table 11.3 provides a format for tracking progress through a systematic literature search. The search begins with identifying an available database and then choosing search terms. Start by entering the key words of the PICO question. For example, in the prognosis question, "For patients with stage IV colon cancer, is chemotherapy plus radiation more effective than chemotherapy alone at prolonging survival?" a search of the PubMed database may begin with the search

terms, "stage IV colon cancer" and "survival." Subsequent searches will include these first two terms and add "chemotherapy" and "radiation." For the opening search, record the number of articles identified in the search table as demonstrated in Table 11.3. If after the second search the number of articles identified remains unwieldy, limiters may be added to the search. Limiters may include acceptable dates of publication, desired publication language, human participants, or the study design. Table 11.3 contains an example of the recording of a step-by-step search for the colon cancer prognosis question.

Continue to narrow the search, step by step, until a manageable number of relevant articles is obtained. At that point, the titles and abstracts can be reviewed, allowing the practitioner to eliminate articles that are clearly irrelevant to the clinical question. Full-text articles are then collected for review and appraisal. If the article is not available to you in full text, consult a medical librarian for interlibrary loan options. In this way, it will not be necessary to limit a search to "full-text" articles only and potentially miss some important evidence. Additional primary evidence may also be uncovered through a hand search of reference lists at the end of some of your key articles. More detailed tutorials on searching databases are available on the website for individual databases or through consultation with a medical librarian.

Evidence Essentials

Research Study Design. After the primary literature has been searched and sources of evidence identified, it is important to assess each article for usefulness and validity. Ultimately, the evidence-based practitioner aims to uncover the most valid evidence available to inform clinical decision making. An important

TABLE 11.3 Search Table Example

Database	Search Terms	Limiters	Articles
PubMed	"stage IV colon cancer" and "survival"	None	577
PubMed	"stage IV colon cancer" and "survival"	2010–2015; English language	234
PubMed	"stage IV colon cancer" and "survival" and "chemotherapy"	2010–2015; English language	92
PubMed	"stage IV colon cancer" and "survival" and "chemotherapy" and "radiation"	2010–2015; English language	6

feature of research studies that affects their validity is the study design. Generally, research study designs that address the types of clinical questions in Table 11.1 can be divided into two categories, experimental and observational. Experimental studies are those in which the investigator assigns (preferably randomly) study participants into their respective groups. The classic example of an experimental design is the RCT. RCTs are frequently used to assess the efficacy of new treatments or interventions. In an RCT, study participants are randomly assigned to either the new treatment or one or more comparison groups and then followed over time for the development of the outcome of interest. The rate of occurrence of the outcome is compared in the two groups to determine which treatment is more effective.

Observational study designs are those in which the investigator observes existing groups of patients. The three most common observational designs are cohort, case-control, and cross-sectional. In a cohort study, a group of people with a common characteristic (cohort) is assembled, and the participants are divided into two or more groups based on their level of exposure to the independent variable of interest. These groups are then followed over time to see develops the outcome of interest. *Cohort* studies can be used to address any of the question types in Table 11.1. The independent variable could represent a therapeutic option, in which case one of the study groups would have undergone the therapy of interest, and the other would have experienced an alternative treatment or perhaps none at all. Alternatively, in an etiology question, the groups within the cohort are categorized as exposed or unexposed to some risk factor. Similar to the RCT, the participants in a cohort study are then followed forward in time to determine the rate of development of the outcome of interest. The outcome may be cure or improvement of symptoms in a treatment study, development of disease in an etiology or harm study, or survival or mortality in a prognosis study.

The *case-control* study design is very different from the cohort in that the groups of participants are defined by disease state (the outcome) rather than by exposure. Case-control studies are particularly useful in the examination of rare diseases for possible risk factors. For this type of question, a group of people with a disease (cases) are identified and then matched to a group of control patients. Ideally, the control participants will be like the cases in every respect except that they do not have the disease of interest. Then the cases and control participants are queried for their level of exposure to a possible risk factor. For example, to explore the possible association of maternal exposure to secondhand smoke with the development of congenital anomalies, investigators would assemble a group of women who have birthed babies with congenital anomalies and a group of women who have delivered healthy babies and query both groups of mothers about their exposure to secondhand smoke during their pregnancies.

Cross-sectional studies are the third common type of observational design. A cross-sectional study is sometimes referred to as a "snapshot" or "slice in time" because the exposure and outcome variables are measured at the same point in time for the study participants. Cross-sectional studies can be used to assess disease prevalence but not incidence. The cross-sectional study can be conducted more quickly and cheaply than other study types, but it is often difficult to ascertain the temporal relation between the exposure and outcome because they are measured at the same time. Causality can never be established by a cross-sectional study.

Two additional study designs that are important for evidence-based practitioners to understand are the systematic review article and meta-analysis. These both represent filtered evidence in that the authors have searched out the original research and synthesized the information to address a clinical question. In a systematic review article, the investigators perform a systematic search of *all* of the primary literature on a topic, locate these articles, critically review the articles, and develop a response to their clinical question based on the evidence. In a meta-analysis, this process is taken one step further. The

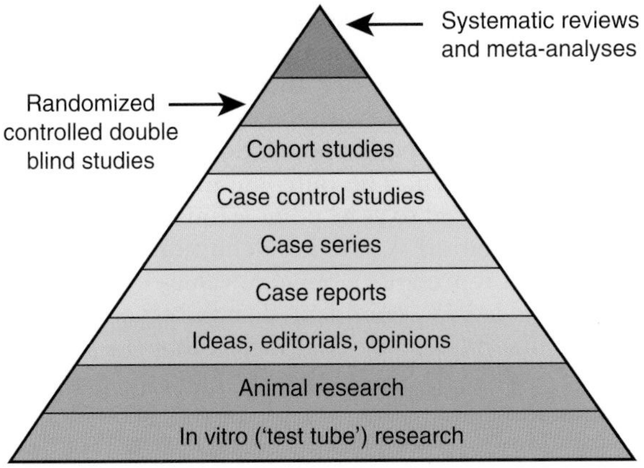
Systematic reviews
and meta-analyses
Randomized
controlled double
blind studies
Cohort studies
Case control studies
Case series
Case reports
Ideas, editorials, opinions
Animal research
In vitro ('test tube') research

FIG. 11.1 ■ Evidence pyramid. (Courtesy SUNY Downstate Medical Center)

investigators not only seek out primary research, but they also seek to gather the original data from the investigators and determine whether it is legitimate to pool those data, repeat the statistical analysis, and come to a new conclusion based on the larger sample size. The strengths and limitations to these approaches are addressed later in this chapter. However, perhaps their greatest strengths are the increased sample size and broader perspective on a clinical question.

Evidence Pyramid. Proponents of EBM have developed an evidence pyramid to help users understand the relative rigor of the various study designs. Of the epidemiologic study designs discussed, the systematic review article and meta-analysis provide the greatest rigor in terms of evidence because of their increased sample size and more representative populations. Among the individual study designs, the RCT is the most rigorous followed by the cohort study, the case-control study, and the cross-sectional study (Fig. 11.1).

Important Concepts in Outcome Measurement

Although evidence-based practitioners need not be a trained statistician to be effective in critical appraisal of the literature, a working knowledge of basic statistical principles empowers them to evaluate the evidence with greater confidence. A few important statistical concepts regard types of data, types of variables and level of measurement. Generally, data can be characterized as qualitative or quantitative. Whereas qualitative data are often represented by words, quantitative data involve numerical expressions. Variables are defined as either independent or dependent. Independent variables are set by the researcher. These often include an intervention in an RCT or an exposure in an observational study. The dependent variable represents the outcome of interest. In the sample PICO questions in Table 11.1, the dependent variables included early-onset kidney disease, type II diabetes, renal failure, and survival.

In addition to being characterized as independent or dependent, variables represent different levels of measurement. A nominal level of measurement involves only one property, and that is classification. When variables are measured at the nominal level, their values are classified into categories. Examples include eye color, vital status (alive or dead), and so on. At the ordinal level of measurement, the additional property of order is present. Variables measured at the ordinal level are classified into categories that have an inherent order. For example, cancer is recorded as stages I to IV. Interval or ratio levels of measurement are marked by their characteristics of equal intervals and a true zero. Variables measured at an interval or ratio level are often further divided into continuous or discrete. Continuous variables represent "amounts," and discrete variables represent "counts." Continuous variables are measured with units; discrete variables have no units. Examples of continuous data include height, weight, and systolic blood pressure. Examples of discrete data include number of pregnancies, number of hospitalizations, and number of surgeries. The level of measurement for the variables included in a research study dictates the type of statistical analysis that is indicated. Consumers of the medical literature are better positioned to confidently appraise research articles when they have a basic understanding of the connection between levels of measurement and statistical analysis. For example, in a study of a new weight loss drug, the outcome of interest may be average weight loss in the group that took the new drug compared with the group that took the standard of care treatment. The dependent variable, weight loss, is a continuous variable, and the outcome would be expressed as the mean number of pounds. The independent variable is the type of treatment, a nominal variable that splits the participants into two groups. The appropriate statistical test is an independent *t*-test, which evaluates the difference between means in two groups. A more detailed explanation of the appropriate statistical test for various levels of measurement may be found elsewhere.

Evidence: Translating the Greek

Most readers of the medical literature are generally familiar with the concepts of *P* value and confidence interval (CI). However, type I (α) and type II (β) errors

Decision	Truth	
	H₀ true	**H₀ false**
Reject the null	Type I error (α)	Correct decision
Fail to reject the null	Correct decision	Type II error (β)

FIG. 11.2 ■ Four possible outcomes for a hypothesis test.

are an important underpinning to the interpretation of study results and are often less well understood. Clinical trials and observational studies are usually founded on some type of a research hypothesis. The research hypothesis may be that New Drug A is more effective than Standard of Care B at preventing a particular outcome. In conducting the study, however, a more specific hypothesis is required. As a result, the researcher tests a null hypothesis (H₀). In this case, the null hypothesis is that there is no difference between New Drug A and Standard of Care B. Before beginning the study, the investigators must decide how great a chance they are willing to take of making a type I error. A type I error occurs when the researchers fail to reject a false null hypothesis. By comparison, a type II error occurs when the researchers reject a true null hypothesis. The degree of risk they are willing to take of making a type I error is generally referred to as "level of significance" or "α." By convention, α is set at 0.05. This means that the investigators are willing to accept a 5% probability that the results occurred by chance alone. Fig. 11.2 depicts the possible outcomes of a research study.

After data collection, the statistical analysis is completed. In the hypothetical study of New Drug A and Standard of Care B, if the outcome of interest is captured by a continuous variable, the t test is the appropriate statistical test. Along with the t statistic, the analysis will generate a P value. If the value of P is less than the α level that was established a priori, the null hypothesis (that there is no difference in efficacy between New Drug A and Standard of Care B) is rejected, and the difference in results between New Drug A and Standard of Care B is deemed statistically significant. In this case, the P value represents the probability that the difference in outcome detected between Drug A and Standard of Care B occurred by chance alone.

As demonstrated in this example, P values are useful for determining whether an effect is present. However, CIs include an additional level of information. When thinking about CIs and hypothesis testing, it is important to remember that research studies are performed on a *sample* of the population about which the research question was asked. Often the entire population is not accessible or the cost

and time required to study the entire population are prohibitive. For this reason, a sample is drawn from the population. Data are then collected and analyzed from the sample with the intent of generalizing the results to the entire population from which the sample was drawn. The outcome measure from the sample is referred to as a "point estimate" of its value for the population. A practical definition for the 95% CI is that it represents a range of values in which the researcher is 95% confident that the true value for the population occurs. That means that the CI provides a sense of the size of the effect and the precision of the estimate.

In addition, a conclusion can be drawn about the statistical significance of the results by considering the CI. If the null value of the point estimate is within the range of values indicated in the CI, the result is not statistically significant. For example, if New Drug A and Standard of Care B represent blood pressure–lowering agents and the results of the study are expressed as a difference in blood pressure lowering between the two drugs, then the null value (the value that indicates there is no difference between the two therapies) is equal to zero. If the study found that New Drug A lowered blood pressure by an average of 8 mm Hg and Standard of Care B lowered blood pressure by an average of 2 mm Hg, then the point estimate for the mean difference in blood pressure lowering between New Drug A and Standard of Care B is 6 mm Hg. If the 95% CI for the point estimate is 3 to 9 mmHg, then the result is statistically significant. However, if the 95% CI is -2 to 14 mm Hg, then the result is not statistically significant because the CI contains the null value of zero. Consider the meaning of the CI—the researcher is 95% certain that the true value for the mean difference in blood pressure lowering between New Drug A and Standard of Care B lies between -2 mm Hg and 14 mm Hg. That means that the true difference may be zero, or in other words, that there is no difference between blood pressure lowering abilities of New Drug A and Standard of Care B. Readers of the medical literature will find that original research articles may include P values, CIs, or both. Although the CI provides additional information regarding the size of the effect, it is important to note that with regard to hypothesis testing the conclusion provided by the CI and the P value will always agree.

Task 3: Evaluating the Evidence

Evaluating the evidence is one of the most critical steps in the practice of EBM. For a busy clinician, the first step when reading a research article is to consider the relevance of the evidence to the clinical question for which you are seeking evidence. A quick look at the abstract will reveal whether the study participants, intervention, comparison, and outcome match those elements of the clinician's current clinical question. If these are not relevant, move on to the next article. If the population, disease, and outcome of interest do not match those elements of the current clinical question but are relevant to other aspects of your practice, you may opt to set the article aside for later review. After you identify a relevant study, you should evaluate the validity of the evidence. In the context of research, validity takes two forms, internal and external. Internal validity addresses whether the results of the research study are accurate for the participants who participated in the study. External validity refers to how confidently the results of the study can be applied to the population from which the study sample was drawn.

In the following section, evaluation of the evidence is discussed for each of the types of research articles mentioned earlier. Each section includes a description of the usual choice of study design for the particular type of article, an explanation of the commonly used outcome measures for the type of study, and a discussion of potential threats to internal and external validity.

Etiology or Harm Article

Etiology or harm articles examine possible risk factors for disease or for complications of an illness. Because in most cases, it is unethical to randomize participants to various levels of exposure to risk factors, observational study designs are usually used to evaluate the etiology of illness. In cohort studies of etiology, participants already have an established exposure level for a potential risk factor. The investigator observes their exposure group membership and follows them forward in time for an outcome. In the case-control design, investigators begin with a group of patients with a particular disease, identify control participants who do not have the disease, and evaluate both groups for exposure to a risk factor.

Commonly Used Outcome Measures. In a cohort study, relative risk is often used to describe the outcome of the study. Relative risk (or risk ratio) is a ratio of the risk of the outcome in the exposed group divided by the risk of the outcome in the unexposed group. For example, in a study of the risk of developing cancer in smokers, the investigators group the participants of the cohort according to their smoking status. They follow the cohort forward in time and count the number of cancer diagnoses in both groups. The risk of cancer in the smoking group is the number of smokers who develop cancer divided by the total number of smokers.

The risk of cancer in the nonsmoking group is the number of nonsmokers who develop cancer divided by the total number of nonsmokers. The relative risk is simply the risk of cancer in the smokers divided by the risk of cancer in the nonsmokers. The relative risk is a user-friendly outcome measure because it is simple and sensible to readers.

Case-control studies cannot employ relative risk because relative risk may only be used with incident (new) cases of disease. In a case-control study, the disease is already present at the beginning of the study. For this reason, the most common outcome measure in a case-control study is the odds ratio. The concept of odds is a bit less intuitive than risk. To help understand the concept of odds, consider an ordinary deck of playing cards. The *risk* of drawing a red ace from the deck is 2 (the number of red aces in the deck) divided by 52 (the total number of cards in the deck). The *odds* of drawing a red ace from the deck are 2 (the number of red aces in the deck) divided by 50 (the number of cards in the deck that are not red aces). In epidemiologic terms, risk is the number of times the disease occurs divided by the number of times the disease could occur. Odds are the number of times the exposure (or disease) occurs divided by the number of times the exposure (or disease) does not occur. Risk is more intuitively sensible (and thereby preferred as an outcome measure), and odds should only be used to describe the level of risk when the disease prevalence is low. To illustrate this further, compare the risk of drawing a club from a deck of cards with the odds of drawing a club. The risk of drawing the club is 13 divided by 52, but the odds of drawing a club are 13 divided by 39. The "prevalence" of a red ace is much lower than the "prevalence" of a club. As a result, the odds of drawing a red ace is a much closer approximation of the risk of drawing a red ace than is the case with the odds and risk of drawing the club. This is an important concept to keep in mind when interpreting the results of a case-control study.

Potential Threats to Validity. Potential threats to both external and internal validity must be considered when evaluating these observational study designs. Because external validity involves generalizing the study results to the population from which the sample is drawn, it is important that the sample be a good representation of the population. Generally, the best way to obtain a representative sample is to randomly select a sample of sufficient size. Unfortunately, in research, obtaining a sample randomly is often not practical. Information about how the sample was obtained may be found in the method section of the paper. To evaluate the representativeness of the sample, readers may refer to the table in the paper where the baseline characteristics of the study sample are often delineated. Because the health care provider is usually interested in applying the results of a research article to a specific patient, the provider can review the information in this table to determine if the study participants are similar to that specific patient. For example, if a specific patient for which evidence is sought by the provider is a young adult but the research article of interest included only participants older than 50 years of age, the external validity or generalizability of the results to the specific patient may be limited.

Threats to internal validity are those that compromise the accuracy of the results for those who are in the study sample. Bias is *systematic* error in research. Some of the more common types of bias include:

1. **Measurement bias:** In both the cohort and case-control designs, it is important to examine how the outcome variables are measured. If a biological measurement is used, the type of laboratory instrument or clinical tool that was used to make the measurement is listed. It is also important to ask whether the study personnel who measured the outcome variables were aware of the group assignment of the participant at the time of measurement. Another potential source of error occurs when the exposure or the outcome variable is determined by review of medical records. Incomplete data or inconsistent expressions of measurement may introduce error into the study.

2. **Confounding:** Confounding variables can also compromise the validity of an observational study. Because group membership in the cohort and case-control study is observed, rather than assigned, the benefits of randomization are lost. As a result, there may be other variables that are differently distributed in the groups that can have an effect on outcome. For example, if the outcome measure is mortality and one group is composed of older participants than the other, the risk of mortality in that group may be influenced by age as much as it is by the exposure of interest in the study.

3. **Loss to follow-up:** Another important consideration in the evaluation of a cohort study is the length and completeness of follow-up. It is essential that the study continue long enough for the potential outcome to occur. It is also important that the follow-up evaluations are complete (the correct measures are used with appropriate timing) and that the timing and types of follow-up measures used are the same in all study groups.

4. **Recall bias:** Recall bias a specific concern for case-control studies. Recall bias occurs when participants who are cases remember their exposures differently from control participants. Patients with disease are more likely to remember their

TABLE 11.4 2 × 2 Table for Calculating Test Characteristics

New Test Result	Truth	
	Disease	No Disease
Positive	True positive	False positive
Negative	False negative	True negative

potentially dangerous exposures than those without disease, falsely increasing the strength of the relationship between the exposure and disease. A classic example of recall bias is that of mothers of babies with congenital abnormalities. They are more likely to accurately recall prenatal exposures than mothers who birth healthy babies.

Diagnosis Articles

Usual Study Design. Studies that examine the diagnostic accuracy of new tests tend to use a design similar to the cohort design. Typically, they enroll a cohort of people who are at risk for the disease of interest. All participants in the study are administered both the new diagnostic or screening test *and* the gold standard test. Then the performance of the new test is compared with the gold standard test.

Commonly Used Outcome Measures. In a study evaluating a new screening or diagnostic test the commonly used measures include sensitivity, specificity, positive and negative predictive value, and likelihood ratio. These measures are best understood in the context of a contingency or 2 × 2 table (Table 11.4). Ideally, in a study of a new diagnostic or screening test, every participant will undergo both the new test and the gold standard test. When the test results are available, each participant is represented in one of the four outcome cells in the 2 × 2 table. If the results of the new test are positive in a patient who really has disease according to the gold standard, that patient is represented in the true positive box. If the new test result is negative in a patient who truly does not have disease according to the gold standard, that patient is represented in the true negative box. Those who have a positive result on the new test but do not have disease according to the gold standard are reflected in the false-positive box. Likewise, those with a negative test result who really do have disease according to the gold standard are recorded in the false negative box. When the data have been collected and recorded in the 2 × 2 table, the test characteristic calculations can be completed according to the formulas in Table 11.5.

TABLE 11.5 Definitions and Formulas for Common Test Characteristics

Test Characteristic	Definition	Formula
Sensitivity	The proportion of people with the disease who have a positive test result	TP/(TP + FN)
Specificity	The proportion of people without the disease who have a negative test result	TN/(TN+FP)
Positive predictive value	The probability of disease in those with a positive test result	TP/(TP + FP)
Negative predictive value	The probability of no disease in those of the negative test result	TN/(TN + FN)

FN, False negative; *FP*, false positive; *TN*, true negative; *TP*, true positive.

Consider the following example. One hundred children with a sore throat are enrolled in a study to evaluate the diagnostic accuracy of a new rapid strep screen. All 100 children undergo both the rapid strep test and the gold standard, throat culture. The throat culture is positive for streptococcal infection in 60 children. Among those with a positive throat culture, 50 have a positive rapid strep test result. The rapid strep test result is also positive in 5 of those with a negative throat culture. To determine the characteristics of this new screening test, complete the 2 × 2 table as follows: The 50 children with both tests positive are the true positives. Because the gold standard was positive in 60 of 100 children, the number of false negatives is 10. If 60 children had a positive throat culture, the remaining 40 children had a negative gold standard result. Five of the 40 children had positive rapid strep results, making those the false positives. That leaves 35 children as the true negatives. Table 11.6 shows how the test characteristics are calculated from this 2 × 2 table.

Interpretation of these results is fairly straightforward if the numerator and denominator are carefully considered. A sensitivity of 83.3% means that out of all of those who truly have strep throat, 83.3% of them will be correctly identified as positive by the new test. Of the children who do not have strep throat, 75% of them will correctly be identified as negative with the new test. Note that predictive values have the test results in the denominator so a positive predictive value of 90.9% means that among children with a positive rapid strep screen 90.9% of them really have strep infection. Likewise, among those with a negative rapid strep screen, 77.8% of them really did not have strep throat. In general, sensitivity and specificity are useful test characteristics when selecting a test to perform, but predictive values are more practical when discussing test results of the patient. The one important caveat to predictive value is that because the denominator of

TABLE 11.6 Test Characteristic Calculations

Rapid Strep	Throat Culture	
	Disease	**No Disease**
Positive	50	5
Negative	10	35
Totals	60	40

Sensitivity = TP/(TP + FN) = 50/60 = 83.3%
Specificity = TN/(TN + FP) = 35/40 = 75.0%
PPV = TP/(TP + FP) = 50/55 = 90.9%
NPV = TN/(TN + FN) = 35/45 = 77.8%
FN, False negative; *FP*, false positive; *NPV*, predictive value; *PPV*, positive predictive value; *TN*, true negative; *TP*, true positive.

TABLE 11.7 Likelihood Ratios

Likelihood Ratio Formula	Example
LR+ = Sensitivity/(1 – Specificity)	**LR+** = 0.833/(1 – 0.75) = 1.11
LR– = (1 – Sensitivity)/Specificity	**LR–** = (1– – 0.833)/0.75 = 0.22

LR, Likelihood ratio.

the calculation includes both people with disease and without disease, the predictive value fluctuates with the prevalence of disease. That important limitation led to a quest for a measure of a test's diagnostic accuracy that is not affected by prevalence and is useful for helping patients understand their probability of disease. The likelihood ratio is the solution. The likelihood ratio positive reflects the probability of disease in someone with a positive test result. The likelihood ratio negative reflects the probability of disease in someone with a negative test result. The formulas for likelihood ratio positive and negative may be seen in Table 11.7.

The likelihood ratios can be used to determine the posttest probability of disease. To do so, begin with

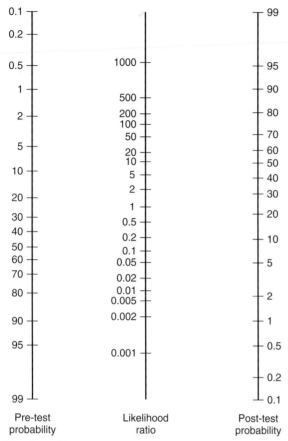

FIG. 11.3 ■ Fagan's nomogram. (Adapted from Fagan TJ. Nomogram for Bayes theorem [letter]. *N Engl J Med* 1975; 293:275.)

the pretest probability of disease. If it is unknown, the prevalence of disease may be used. Using the principles of Bayesian mathematics, the pretest probability of disease (prevalence) is mathematically transformed to pretest odds, multiplied by the appropriate likelihood ratio to obtain the posttest odds, and then converted mathematically to the posttest probability of disease. A much simpler method for using the likelihood ratio to obtain the posttest probability of disease is to used Fagan's nomogram (Fig. 11.3). On the leftmost axis of the nomogram, plot the pretest probability. If the test result is positive, plot the likelihood ratio positive on the middle vertical axis and then draw a line connecting the dots. Extend the straight line across the right vertical axis to determine the posttest probability of disease.

Potential Threats to Validity. When evaluating a study of a new diagnostic or screening test, begin with assessing whether the new test is available and acceptable to patients. In assessing the validity of

the results, consider whether the new test and the gold standard test were applied in a uniformly blind manner to all participants. The "uniformly blind manner" is important because an investigator's foreknowledge of the results of the gold standard may inadvertently influence the performance or interpretation of the results of the new test, potentially compromising the accuracy of the measurement. To accurately populate all four cells in a 2 × 2 table, it is important for every participant to undergo both the gold standard and the new test. Occasionally, the gold standard test is not administered to the participants who have a negative result on the screening test. This usually occurs when the gold standard test is expensive, risky, or less acceptable to patients. When those with a negative screening test result do not undergo the gold standard test, the number of false negatives is unknown, limiting the calculation of the test characteristics. In this situation, readers must carefully review the methods and discussion sections of the paper to determine how the authors address this potential limitation and judge whether the decision was reasonable.

Prognosis Articles

Usual Study Design. Studies of prognosis examine the effects of interventions on the overall prognosis of disease. Mortality is the most common outcome measure. A prognosis study is usually conducted in a prospective manner, using either a randomized controlled or cohort design. A key design feature for prognosis study involves the use of an inception cohort. An inception cohort is a group of patients who are at the same point in the natural history of the disease, preferably right at the onset of disease.

Commonly Used Outcome Measures. Prognosis studies may employ a number of outcome measures, including measures of mortality as well as measures of morbidity or quality of life. When mortality is the outcome, relative risk is a possible measure, but, increasingly, the hazard ratio is used in its place. The hazard ratio is similar to the relative risk in that it examines the risk of death in a group exposed to a particular factor or intervention divided by the risk of death in an unexposed group. The hazard ratio, however, also includes an element of time. The calculation is more complex and is usually performed by a computer program because for each person who experiences the outcome of interest, a measure of his or her time until the event (e.g., person-months) is included in the calculation. Despite this difference, hazard ratios are interpreted similarly to relative risks. A hazard ratio of 1 means that the risk of mortality is the same in the exposed and unexposed groups, a hazard ratio less than 1 means that the exposure was protective, and a hazard ratio greater than 1 indicates that the exposure of interest increases the risk of death.

Potential Threats to Validity. A number of potential biases are important specifically to studies of prognosis. The potential threats to external validity are similar to those already discussed. When assembling a cohort for a prognosis study, it is important that the cohort members are representative of the greater population of people with the given disease. Although random sampling is often not possible, it is important that the researchers consider the potential for a volunteer bias or selection bias in the design of the study and the discussion of the results. Internal validity in a prognosis study can specifically be affected by survivor bias, lead-time bias, and length-time bias. Survivor bias may occur when the cohort included in the study is not an inception cohort. In this case, those who experienced a more serious natural history of the disease are likely to have died before the cohort was assembled. Lead-time bias occurs when patients who were screened for disease before the onset of clinical symptoms appear to have a longer survival time than those who are not diagnosed until clinical symptoms appear when in fact they simply lived longer with the knowledge of disease than their counterparts who were diagnosed at the onset of the clinical manifestation. Length-time bias may occur when patients with more severe disease or a more aggressive type of cancer are likely to die before they can get included in the cohort. This results in a seemingly better prognosis because only those with less severe disease are included in the study. In the design of the study, investigators can make a concerted effort to obtain an inception cohort with every participant screened in the same way and at the same point in the natural history of their disease to minimize these potential biases.

Treatment Articles

Usual Study Design. The RCT is the design of choice for the treatment study. In some situations, randomization of a participant to the treatment or to a comparison group that involves either a placebo or no treatment may be unethical. In this case, an observational cohort design may be used. Key features of RCTs include the random assignment of participants to the treatment group or one or more comparison groups. Random assignment is the gold standard for an experimental study because it provides the greatest probability that the participants in the study groups will be similar in all characteristics other than

the treatment of interest. Effective random assignment helps protect the internal validity of the study.

Commonly Used Outcome Measures. Outcome measures in RCTs depend largely on the type of dependent or outcome variable. If the outcome variable involves a nominal level of measurement of risk (e.g., alive or dead), a relative risk may be the outcome measure of choice. Another option for comparing risks in a treatment and control group is the risk difference. For the risk difference, the risk of the outcome in the control group is subtracted from the risk of the outcome in the treatment group. When the outcome variable is continuous, the outcome measure may be reported as a mean value for that continuous variable. The difference in means in the treatment and comparison groups is evaluated with a t test in the case of two total groups or the analysis of variance (ANOVA) if there are more than two groups.

Number needed to treat (NNT) is an additional measure that is commonly used in RCT to evaluate the efficacy of a new treatment compared with the standard of care. NNT has been developed as perhaps a more user-friendly expression of risk. NNT is easily calculated as 1/ARR, where ARR is the absolute risk reduction. ARR is a term that can be used interchangeably with the risk difference described earlier. As a result, the NNT is simply the inverse of the difference in risk between the treatment and control groups. As an example, if 30 of 100 people in the control group had a myocardial infarction (MI) and 20 of 100 people in the treatment group had an MI, the absolute risk reduction is 30/100 – 20/100 which equals 10/100 or 0.1. That makes the NNT equal 1/0.1 or equals 10. The interpretation of the NNT is relatively straightforward. In this example, for every 10 people treated with the new therapy, one less person will experience an MI.

Number needed to harm (NNH) is similar to the NNT but regards adverse effects to a new therapy. In the previous example, if five of 100 people in the control group experienced bleeding during the trial and 10 of 100 people in the treatment group experience the bleeding, then the risk of bleeding in the control group is 0.05, and in the treatment group, the risk of bleeding is 0.10. That means the NNH = 1/(0.1 – 0.05) = 1/.05 = 20. This means that for every 20 people treated with the new therapy, one additional person will experience bleeding as an adverse effect. Based on their definitions, the best treatments have a high NNH and a low NNT.

Potential Threats to Validity. There are a number of important characteristics of RCTs that need to be evaluated when assessing the quality of the evidence.

As with the previously described study designs, the sampling method must be evaluated. Random sampling is the best way to obtain a sample that is representative of the population. However, this is not always practical or even possible. Concealment of allocation occurs when the treatment group to which a participant will be assigned is unknown at the time of recruitment of participants. This prevents the potential for bias in the selection of participants invited to participate in the study.

Blinding and masking are two other methods to help prevent bias. Blinding occurs when the study participants and the investigator measuring the outcome variable are unaware of whether a particular participant is a member of the treatment or control group. This minimizes the risk of a measurement bias that could occur if knowledge of the participant's treatment group influenced the perceived outcome for either the participant or the member of the research team responsible for measuring the outcome. Masking occurs when the treatment and the alternative are made to look alike so as not to identify the group to which the participant is assigned. In a study comparing two pharmacologic therapies, this may be accomplished by formulating the treatment and the alternative medications to look, smell, and taste alike. Matching the dosing regimen and the monitoring schedule can also help protect the masking. Similar to blinding, masking helps minimize measurement bias.

Random assignment is the key feature of RCTs that minimizes threats to internal validity. Because random assignment ensures that the treatment and control groups will be similar with regard to baseline characteristics, the potential for confounding variables influencing the results of the study is minimized. Other features of RCTs designed to minimize measurement bias include having the same member of the research team measure outcomes in both groups. Thorough follow-up for an appropriate length of time is as important in RCTs as it is in cohort studies. For example, if patients with type II diabetes are treated with two different classes of medications to determine which is more effective at preventing the development of renal failure, they need to be followed long enough for renal failure to occur.

Loss to follow-up is another potential threat to validity of treatment studies. In most articles, readers will be able to locate a flowchart documenting the progression of the sample through the study. A careful review of the flow diagram will show how many participants started the study in each treatment group and how many completed the study. In addition, authors often indicate the number of participants lost at each step in the process and perhaps their reasons for leaving the study. The effect of attrition on the validity of the study depends on proportion of participants lost in each group and their reasons for leaving the study. For example, if several patients in the treatment group dropped out because they did not experience improvement in their symptoms, the beneficial effect of the treatment may be exaggerated without their data included. Commonly, authors will document in the results section or describe in the discussion section what they know about why participants dropped out of the study and anything they know about their outcomes.

Review Articles

Review articles may involve a review of any of the types of studies discussed earlier. The purpose of a review article is to gather the evidence that is already established in the medical literature, synthesize it, and arrive at a more substantiated conclusion.

Usual Study Design. Review articles are either systematic review articles or meta-analyses. The initial steps for these reviews are similar. The review begins with a systematic, comprehensive search of the published literature as described earlier in the chapter. The search is systematic in that is conducted in a step-by-step manner designed to minimize the possibility of overlooking important evidence. It is comprehensive in that the search should involve multiple databases for the purpose of identifying all pertinent evidence. The next step in both types of reviews involves assessing the quality of the studies to determine which should be included in the review article. At this point, the authors of the systematic review article synthesize the evidence to draw a conclusion about what the preponderance of the evidence says regarding the clinical research question. In a meta-analysis, this process is taken one step further in that the researchers contact the authors of the original research articles to request their data. At that point, they determine whether the data are similar enough to be legitimately combined. The next step is to combine the data and repeat the statistical analysis with a substantially larger sample size.

Commonly Used Outcome Measures. The outcome measures in a review article are usually reflective of those in the individual articles that are included in the review. If, for example, the study is a meta-analysis of systematic review articles for which relative risk is the outcome measure, the meta-analysis will report a pooled estimate of the relative risk for the combined data. The systematic review article does not report any new outcomes but rather discusses what the results of the individual original research

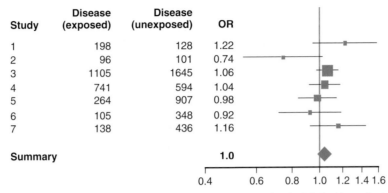

FIG. 11.4 ■ Example of a Forest plot. (Source: Coghlan A. A little book of R for biomedical statistics. Release 0.2. https://media.readthedocs.org/pdf/a-little-book-of-r-for-biomedical-statistics/latest/a-little-book-of-r-for-biomedical-statistics.pdf. 2016. Accessed January 25, 2017.)

articles say together. A few important statistical tests are unique to the meta-analysis and are therefore important in its critical appraisal. These tests include an assessment of the potential for publication bias and an evaluation of the heterogeneity of the data.

Publication bias occurs when studies with negative results or small sample sizes do not get published. One method for minimizing the risk of publication bias is to contact well-known researchers in the field of interest to inquire about unpublished data that are relevant to the clinical question being addressed in the present meta-analysis. The potential for publication bias can be assessed using a funnel plot. A funnel plot is a type of scatter plot in which sample size (or a surrogate for sample size, such as standard error) is plotted on the x-axis and an estimate of effect size is plotted on the y-axis. The scatter of points in the graph usually resembles a funnel. A gap in the funnel shape may indicate a publication bias. Publication bias can also be assessed using a statistical test such as Begg's. The result is interpreted like other hypothesis tests in that if the associated P value is greater than the predetermined level of significance (usually 0.05), there is no evidence of statistically significant publication bias.

Heterogeneity occurs when the results of the individual studies are more different than would be expected from random variation alone. The variation in outcomes may stem from methodological differences or from variation in the sample characteristics among the studies.[5] Two tests commonly used to assess the possibility of heterogeneity include Cochran's Q (indicates whether heterogeneity is present or not) and I^2 (quantifies the degree of heterogeneity). The null hypothesis associated with the Q statistic is that there is no heterogeneity between studies. If the P value associated with the Q statistic is lower than the level of significance chosen before data collection, the null is rejected, and the data are pooled using a random

effects model that takes heterogeneity of data into account. If the P value is higher than the a priori level of significance, the data are presumed homogeneous and combined using a fixed effect model.[6] The value of the I^2 statistic represents the amount of variability that can be explained by heterogeneity. As a result, if I^2 equals zero, the variability present in the estimate can be explained by random differences alone. If I^2 equals 25, then 25% of the variability is due to heterogeneity. Generally speaking, 25% is considered a small degree of heterogeneity, 50% a moderate degree in 75% a high degree of heterogeneity.[6]

An understanding of measures of heterogeneity is important to the critical appraisal of meta-analyses, as is confidence in the interpretation of forest plots. Forest plots are commonly used to depict the results of a meta-analysis. Forest plots can be assembled a number of different ways, but the common elements include a box and whisker-type graphical depiction of the estimate of effect for each of the individual studies and a pooled estimate. See Fig. 11.4 for an example of a forest plot. The forest plot generally includes the outcome measure (OR in Fig. 11.4) for each of the individual studies and the pooled estimate. The whiskers represent the CI for each of the point estimates. The plot generally contains a vertical solid line at the null value (OR = 1) to give readers a quick impression of the overall direction and magnitude of the outcome.

Potential Threats to Validity. Publication bias in a systematic review article or meta-analysis affects the validity of the study in a similar manner to selection bias. Missing data from a study that did not get published because it had a small sample size or negative results may limit the internal and external validity of the review article. As mentioned, publication bias may be minimized by seeking out unpublished data from well-known researchers in the field. However, the downside of including unpublished data is that these findings have not been subjected to the peer review that is an integral part of the publication process. For this reason, the influence of publication bias needs to be weighed carefully.

Another key feature in the critical appraisal of a review article is consideration of the methods used by the authors to search out and critique the original research articles included in the review. Systematic review article and meta-analysis authors should clearly articulate their search strategy in the methods section of the article, including search terms and a list of the databases searched. Ideally, their search strategy will be reproducible for readers. In addition, the authors of the review article should clearly describe their process for appraising the validity of the individual articles included in their analysis. Generally, the review article includes a table (sometimes lengthy) that lists the key features and findings of all the articles included in the review. This is particularly important in the meta-analysis so that readers have the option to review the findings of the individual articles and compare them with the pooled estimate provided by the meta-analysis. Equally important is a discussion of the articles that were excluded from the systematic review or meta-analysis.

Heterogeneity of the data is another important potential threat to the validity of a meta-analysis. As described earlier, there are statistical methods for assessing the influence of heterogeneity. Occasionally, when heterogeneity is too great, the analysts will opt to combine a subset of the individual articles and report the findings of the other studies individually or choose not to report a pooled estimate at all. Critical readers, even without a background in statistics, are able to review the meta-analysis looking for an explanation by the authors of their evaluation of heterogeneity. There should be evidence of some sort of statistical analysis, frequently a Q test or an I^2 statistic. In the event that the data from the individual studies were determined to be heterogeneous, the appropriate way to combine the data is with a random effects model. In addition, the process for developing a pooled estimate of the study outcome should include some sort of weighting to account for variations in sample size or within-study variability. Finally, it is important for the authors of the meta-analysis to be transparent about the way in which they have combined studies with conflicting outcomes. All of these measures help strengthen the internal validity of the meta-analysis.

Task 4: Applying the Evidence

The task of evidence-based medical practice involves identifying the best evidence, combining it with the clinical judgment of the provider, and applying it to an individual patient while considering that patient's unique values and preferences. At this point in the process, when the practitioner has identified high-quality evidence with strong internal and external validity and relevance to his or her particular patient, it is time to use the evidence to inform a specific clinical question. The provider considers the evidence in the light of his or her own clinical experience and then communicates with the particular patient to determine how the proposed treatment fits the patient's unique circumstances. The application of evidence is not intended to occur independent of the provider's best judgment and experience; rather, they are to complement one another. In addition, for the treatment plan to be the most effective, the provider must consider the personal values and preferences of the involved patient. For example, if an elderly patient with cancer has concluded that he has lived a long, fruitful life; that he is ready to die; and that he is uninterested in cancer treatment, it may not matter what the evidence says. In this case, the provider is able to use her assessment of the quality of the evidence to transparently describe to the patient his treatment options and then listen carefully to gain an understanding of the patient's preferences and how his personal values ultimately inform his decision. All of the components of the evidence-based equation (best evidence, clinical judgment, patient's values and preferences) are important.

Task 5: Evaluating the Process

The final important step in the practice of EBM is evaluating the process. To do so, the provider considers the outcomes experienced by his or her patients. It is important to consider whether the individual patient experiences results consistent with those in the evidence that informed the decision or a better or worse outcome. In the event that the outcome for the particular patient is worse than expected based on the evidence, it is important that the provider again uses critical thinking skills in search of an explanation. Perhaps the given patient is less similar than originally believed to those in the studies from which the evidence that supported the decision was drawn or maybe the evidence was not as strong as it appeared to be. Retracing the steps of the critical appraisal will be important to affirm the assessment of the evidence to plan next steps for the patient of interest as well as to inform treatment decisions for future patients. Ultimately, EBM is a continuous cycle of developing new questions, acquiring and appraising evidence, and then again evaluating the process.

KEY POINTS

- The principles and process of EBM emerged from a need to more accurately and efficiently apply best research evidence to the care of individual patients.
- In addition to "best evidence," the clinical expertise of the provider and the values and preferences of the individual patient are critical components of evidence-based practice.
- The five steps of EBM include *asking* a clinical question, *searching for* evidence, *assessing* the quality of the evidence, *incorporating* the evidence into a clinical decision, and *evaluating* the process.
- An understanding of the inherent strengths and limitations of the common research study designs facilitates the critical appraisal of evidence.
- Well-conducted RCTs provide the highest level of evidence for individual studies.

References

1. Doherty S. History of evidence-based medicine. Oranges, chloride of lime and leeches: barriers to teaching old dogs new tricks. *Emerg Med Australas*. 2005;17:314–321. http://dx.doi.org/10.1111/j.1742-6723.2005.00752.x.
2. Thoma A, Eaves FF. A brief history of evidence-based medicine (EBM) and the contributions of Dr. David Sackett. *Aesthetic Surg J*. 2015:1–3. http://dx.doi.org/10.1093/asj/sjv130.
3. Voelker R. Everything you ever wanted to know about evidence-based medicine. *JAMA*. 2015:1783–1785.
4. Smith R, Rennie D. Evidence-based medicine- An oral history. *JAMA*. 311(4):365–367.
5. Higgins JPT, Green S, eds. *Cochrane Handbook for Systematic Reviews of Interventions*. Version 5.1.0 [updated March 2011]. The Cochrane Collaboration, 2011. Available from www.cochrane-handbook.org.
6. Huedo-Medina Tania, Sanchez-Meca Julio, Marin-Martinez Fulgencio, Botella Juan. Assessing heterogeneity in meta-analysis: Q statistic or I2 index? (2006). CHIP Documents. Paper 19. http://digitalcommons.uconn.edu/chip_docs/19.

CHAPTER 12

RESEARCH AND THE PHYSICIAN ASSISTANT

Tamara S. Ritsema

Most physician assistant (PA) students choose to study to become PAs because they want to care for patients. If they had wanted to study for a research-oriented degree, they would have applied for MS or PhD programs in biochemistry, biology, public health, or experimental psychology. Yet even though PA students have enrolled in a clinical training program, they cannot avoid the importance of research to their careers. To engage in high-quality, evidence-based patient care, PAs need to consult research daily. PAs who are interested in improving the quality of care given to patients may become part of a team that conducts new clinical research. PAs who become educators will engage in research on how to better educate students or deploy PA graduates. In short, no PA can escape research.

WHAT IS RESEARCH?

Webster's New World Collegiate Dictionary defines research as "careful, systematic, patient study and investigation of some field of knowledge, undertaken to discover or establish facts or principles."[1] Research can take many forms: basic science research in the laboratory setting, survey research, clinical research, policy research, public health or epidemiological research, anthropological research, educational research, sociological or psychological research, and workforce research. Most PAs will use or perform only a few of these subtypes of research. The research PAs most commonly use and conduct are outlined in the next section.

TYPES OF RESEARCH

Basic Science Biomedical Research

Basic science research performed at many medical schools and research universities and by pharmaceutical companies is the first building block of understanding the pathogenesis of disease, diagnostic strategies, and treatments. These studies are performed at the atomic, molecular, genetic, or cellular levels. They may also involve animal models of anatomy, physiology, genetics, pathophysiology, and treatment. Biomedical research has produced many of the tools we use in the practice of clinical medicine. However, much of what has turned out to be useful for clinicians has actually come from fields other than direct biomedical research. X-rays and magnetic resonance imaging both came from physics. Genetics originated in botany. Discovery of the Ebola virus came from a combination of epidemiology and virology. There is a growing emphasis placed on connecting basic science researchers with clinicians to move basic science discoveries "from bench to bedside" more quickly, and many funding agencies such as the National Institutes of Health are requiring investigators to collaborate more effectively to make this happen. This new approach to biomedical science is called "translational research."

Unlike many physicians at academic medical centers, PAs traditionally have not been very involved in basic science research. Some PAs have worked in a basic science laboratory while studying at a university, but few PAs have the advanced training needed for basic science research. PAs generally choose to become PAs because they are interested in caring for people and are less interested in bench work. A few PAs have basic science PhDs and combine clinical practice and basic science research at academic medical centers, but this arrangement is fairly uncommon. More common are PAs at academic medical centers who are part of teams that engage in translational research. PAs may be involved in advising basic science teams on the clinical implications of a new basic science finding and are often involved in the clinical trials used to assess the innovation.

Clinical Research

Research performed on human subjects with the goal of developing more effective therapies, better diagnostic tests, or better understanding of the pathophysiology of disease is called clinical research. These are the kind of studies that are often highlighted in the health section of newspapers or in online reports of "breaking health news." Clinical trials, cohort studies, and case-control studies are just some of the types of studies included under the banner of clinical research. It is typically not difficult to convince PA students that clinical research is relevant to their practice. Every PA would like to know which chemotherapy regimen is best for stage III breast cancer. All PAs would be thrilled to see an effective vaccine for an illness that has thus far not been preventable. Practicing PAs consume clinical research each day if they are seeking to provide evidence-based care to their patients.

Although all PAs are consumers of clinical research, some PAs are also producers of clinical research. PAs who work at medical schools are often involved in the research mission of the university. Many clinical trials, cohort studies, and case-control studies employ PAs to conduct physical examinations, psychiatric interviews, neuropsychological testing, medication monitoring, observation of participants for adverse events, and performance of many other types of data collection. Doctors often appreciate the generalist background of PAs for these tasks. For example, an orthopedist conducting a clinical trial of a new type of prosthetic hip joint typically does not have much experience in managing diabetes. Yet glucose control can substantially affect wound healing rates. Having a PA on the team who can not only assess the effectiveness of the hip prosthesis but who can also monitor the patient's glucose control expands the range of clinical skills on the research team and provides better quality care for the study patient.

Although PAs often start out in clinical research as simply the person who performs physicals, monitors laboratory results, or collects other data, some of these PAs move up to become investigators themselves. Although federal funders and pharmaceutical companies do not typically allow PAs to be principal investigators, a PA can be one of a group of investigators on the team. To be an investigator, the PA needs to make substantial contributions to the development of the research question as well as the design and evaluation of the research project. Simply collecting a large amount of data according to someone else's protocol does not confer investigator status. PAs who become investigators often have the opportunity to collaborate with investigators from other institutions, to present their work at scientific meetings, and to publish their findings in peer-reviewed journals. Getting involved in clinical research gives PAs a chance to develop new skills, share their knowledge with others, and bring cutting-edge treatments back to their clinics to share with patients (Case Study 12.1).

CASE STUDY 12.1 BRYAN WALKER MHS, PA-C, CLINICAL RESEARCH PHYSICIAN ASSISTANT, DUKE UNIVERSITY HEALTH SYSTEM, DEPARTMENT OF NEUROLOGY

Bryan Walker has served as a clinical research PA in two very different environments. Early in his career, he accepted a job as a clinical PA at a general neurology practice in Maryland. When he started at the practice, the practice did not participate in any clinical trials. Through Bryan's initiative, his practice began to serve as a site for multiple sclerosis (MS) clinical trials. The doctors with whom Bryan worked were pleasantly surprised at the benefits this participation brought to their practice. The sponsors of the trials paid the practice for recruiting patients and enrolling them in the trial. Patients at the practice were delighted by the opportunity to be included in cutting-edge research without having to travel to the large academic medical center in the next city. Because most MS clinical trials compare new medications with existing medications that are known to be effective, no patients get placebo. Patients who have financial limitations were appreciative of the opportunity to receive medications at no cost even if only for the duration of the trial.

Participating with clinical trials also brought benefits to Bryan. To accurately collect data, the studies required that all investigators and subinvestigators become certified in administration of common outcome measures such as the Expanded Disability Status Scale. Obtaining these certifications has increased Bryan's marketability as a research-oriented PA and allowed his practice to be eligible to become a clinical site for even more clinical trials.

Currently, Bryan practices neurology and conducts clinical research at Duke University Hospital in Durham, North Carolina. There he practices clinically about for approximately 70% of his time and works on administrative and research tasks for about 30% of his time. One of his current studies is a multidisciplinary translational research project evaluating the relationship between cerebral volume loss in MS patients and cognitive loss measured at the clinical level. This trial involves radiologists, neurologists, physical therapists, and biostatisticians. The goal is to better correlate magnetic resonance imaging findings with clinical findings to assist clinicians in accurately assessing treatment effects and developing prognoses for patients. Bryan identifies patients for potential involvement in the trial, consents them for inclusion in the study, performs detailed history, conducts standardized physical examinations, and works with the other investigators on protocol development and data analysis.

Bryan enjoys several aspects of his role as a clinical research PA. He loves the prospect of helping to generate new therapeutic options for patients with MS. Although vast improvements have been made in MS care in the past 15 years, there are still patients for whom the existing medications are less than optimal. Enrolling patients in clinical trials sometimes enables him to get care for patients that they would not otherwise receive because of insurance or financial limitations. Investigators have an ethical responsibility to provide the very best care for patients in studies. Sometimes this means that study patients are eligible to receive other services, such as lower cost care by other specialties within the Duke system.

Participating in research has also given Bryan more insight into the skills and interests of other types of health professionals. He has learned more about what a pharmacist, a physical therapist, a social worker, or an occupational therapist can bring to the team. He has learned that he does not have to do everything for the patient himself and that patients are often better served by referral to another type of health professional. Finally, Bryan reports that he enjoys being a researcher because it keeps him intellectually engaged. The research work refreshes his passion for clinical work, and his clinical work refreshes his passion for research.

Bryan says the main drawback to his role as a research PA is "paperwork, paperwork, paperwork." The forms that need to be completed for research patients are far more detailed than those required for clinical care, and completing them can be mind numbing sometimes. Performing research is very time consuming, and as with patient care, he is not always assured of getting out of work right on time.

Bryan's words of wisdom for those considering initiating involvement in research are "Just do it. You will never regret it." He points out that there are many PAs, doctors, and PhDs who are willing to mentor those who are interested in research. Bryan does not hold an MPH or a PhD; he has been trained for his work on the job. He is quick to point out that he, not the doctor, started his practice's involvement in clinical research at his private practice in Maryland and that PAs are ideally suited for being both clinicians and clinical researchers because of the combination of their medical training and their training in team-based care of the patient.

Quality improvement or implementation science research: *Implementation science is the study of methods to promote the integration of research findings and evidence into health care policy and practice.* Implementation science attempts to understand the behavior of health care professionals in the application, adoption, and implementation of evidence-based clinical interventions.[2] Implementation science seeks to help get clinicians to actually do what they know they should do. Many times, no new knowledge is needed to improve outcomes. Instead, developing new approaches that make it easier for clinicians to adhere to best practices is the key to improved patient care. For example, one of the most effective implementation science studies ever performed essentially eliminated the incidence of bloodstream infections in intensive care unit (ICU) patients by instituting standardized practices for central line insertion. Before the intervention, providers in ICUs may have believed they knew how to prevent central line infections, but the study demonstrated that knowledge was insufficient without supporting standard operating procedures designed to reinforce best practices.[3]

Because implementation science is a relatively new discipline, the number of PAs working on these projects is still relatively small. However, PA involvement is likely to increase because PAs are ideally suited for this work. As frontline health care providers, PAs often can identify the simple changes that can have a profound effect on the delivery of clinical care. PAs have the medical training to understand the science behind the changes in implementation and are often involved in development of standard operating procedures for their units or clinics. In teaching hospitals, PAs are sometimes the only medical staff who do not rotate on and off service. Therefore, PAs can help provide and maintain the cultural and procedural changes needed to sustain the intervention for months and years. PAs can develop new procedures, train others in the new approach, and collect data on effectiveness (Case Study 12.2).

CASE STUDY 12.2 STEPHANIE FIGUEROA, MPAS, PA-C, QUALITY IMPROVEMENT AND IMPLEMENTATION SCIENCE RESEARCHER, JOHNS HOPKINS UNIVERSITY SCHOOL OF MEDICINE, DEPARTMENT OF EMERGENCY MEDICINE

Stephanie Figueroa has practiced emergency medicine at the Johns Hopkins Hospital, a large inner-city hospital in Baltimore, Maryland, for nearly 15 years. She serves as the lead PA and assistant director of the observation unit within the emergency department (ED). Stephanie recently had the opportunity to complete a fellowship within the Leadership Academy of the Johns Hopkins Armstrong Institute for Patient Safety and Quality. While working with the Armstrong Institute, she developed and implemented a project to improve the way care is delivered to patients with sickle cell disease who come to the ED for their care. Her project was a classic implementation science project in that she was given no extra financial or clinical resources with which to work. She had to develop a new approach to delivering better quality care more efficiently without extra nursing or provider resources.

Previously, patients who came to the ED at Hopkins may have been seen by a number of different providers who, in the chaos of the ED, would provide inconsistent care. Some doctors and PAs would give the patients large doses of parenteral opiates, and others would simply give one does of oral opiates and discharge the patient. Nurses varied in their willingness to provide opiate pain control to patients who did not yet have a bed assignment in the ED because of assessment requirements regarding narcotic administration that were challenging to meet while patients were in the waiting room. This inconsistency of treatment led to frustration among the patients and the clinical staff alike because neither group knew what to expect from the other at each visit.

Stephanie's project aimed to limit the number of doctors, PAs, and nurses who would care for patients with sickle cell disease by assigning these patients routinely to the observation unit portion of the ED unless the patients were in need of critical care services. This first step was the cornerstone in providing more consistent care to this patient population. In addition, care plans were developed in conjunction with the hematology sickle cell team for patients who came to the ED more often than others with the disease, allowing patients and providers alike to know what the treatment delivered for a typical pain crisis would be. Alternative assessment and treatment space was designated in the observation unit where patients with sickle cell could receive a prioritized medical screening by PAs familiar with sickle cell disease. In addition, PAs would initiate appropriate pain management, allowing patients to receive opiate treatment even if there were no open beds in the main ED or the observation unit. There, nurses could begin to provide narcotic pain medication in a supervised setting while the patient was waiting for a bed to become available. The goal was for patients to receive their first dose of pain medication, after assessment by a PA or doctor, within 90 minutes of arrival to the ED. For patients who were having a particularly bad crisis, they were placed in observation in the unit, and patient-controlled analgesia (PCA) pumps were used for the first time in the ED. PCAs not only remove the burden of the nurses to continually administer pain medications but they give patients the ability to receive timely doses of pain medication in a manner that is safer than bolus after bolus of intravenous narcotics. Standardization of the overall treatment approach to patients with sickle cell disease presenting to the ED in crisis led to consistency in care, thus decreasing the need to negotiate how pain medication would be administered across ED visits.

Removing barriers to aggressively managing patients' pain early in their presentation to the ED has paid substantial benefits for Hopkins patients and staff. Whereas the average time from arrival to first dose of pain medication before the intervention was 2 hours and 45 minutes, now 65% of patients receive pain control within 90 minutes of arrival to the ED. Patient admissions to the hospital have also dropped from 22% of patients presenting with sickle cell pain to around 15% of presentations. These results were accomplished by analyzing the data about sickle cell patients, working with all the stakeholders to identify barriers to providing more timely care, developing new protocols and work flow plans to remove these barriers, collaborating with the hematology service to develop individualized patient care plans, and getting both nurses and providers to take ownership of the project. No one—not patients, not nurses, and not providers—wants to go back to the days before this project was implemented. Patients are getting improved care, and providers and nurses are spending much less time negotiating with patients about their care. Instead they are engaging patients in their care and help to align patients with resources provided by the hematology sickle cell care team to reduce the need for ED visits.

Stephanie has found several sources of satisfaction with becoming a quality improvement researcher. Most of all, she is thrilled with the chance to provide higher quality care for patients along with a better experience for nurses and providers. She loves the opportunity to demonstrate how PAs can be the bridge between the clinical team and the research team. She has told many high-level leaders at the Johns Hopkins medical institutions (including five hospitals) that "PAs are an untapped resource for quality improvement work" and has encouraged them to look within the group of 300+ Hopkins PAs for others who may be able to conduct projects similar to the one Stephanie headed. Stephanie has also enjoyed collaborating with other PAs, nurses, doctors, social workers, case managers, and researchers within emergency medicine and hematology to refine her project to the benefit of patients. She points to the team-based approach in which PAs are trained as key to her ability to negotiate the sometimes complex interdepartmental politics of a major U.S. medical school. Stephanie believes that getting PAs involved in quality improvement work can contribute to professional satisfaction and longevity and that PAs who do this work can really raise the profile of PAs within their institutions.

The difficulties Stephanie finds with this type of work stem predominantly from the lack of visibility of PAs within the health system and the lack of PA role models. PAs who get involved in leadership usually have to blaze their own trail. Leaders generally include doctors and nurses on committees but rarely consider including PAs. When PAs are included in committees or are recruited to be part of a quality improvement team, they are often required to do this on top of their other duties and are often not paid for the time they put into this work. Stephanie says that she "often felt like an eager little dog, nipping at their heels and trying to squeeze my way into the committee room." Her persistence and that of other PAs at Hopkins have paid off because PAs are beginning to be included to a greater degree on health system committees and in quality improvement teams at Hopkins. Stephanie advises PAs to just keep knocking on the doors in their environments to be included in leadership opportunities and quality improvement work. She has been energized by her new roles and believes other PAs would have the same positive experience by contributing to health care quality improvement using innovation steeped in knowledge gained from the clinical practice of medicine.

Health Services Research

Health services research seeks to discover how organizational structures, payment systems, health care processes, information technologies, health reimbursement policies, health care accessibility, and human factors affect the way health care is delivered.

Health services researchers seek to explain the effects of the health care system on the quality, costs, and effectiveness of the care delivered within a population. Health services researchers answer questions such as, "Do copayments for diabetes medications inhibit patients from effectively controlling their diabetes?" "Does the implementation of electronic medical records decrease the number of erroneous prescriptions filled?" or "Are Medicaid patients less likely to receive psychiatric care than patients with private insurance?" Health services research is often multidisciplinary, including health policy specialists, health economists, medical sociologists, health behavior specialists, and clinicians. Health services researchers may collect original data, but increasingly, they are harnessing the power of very fast computers to analyze large federal datasets or mine electronic medical records for extremely detailed data.

Physician assistants who work in health services research nearly all have further training in epidemiology, biostatistics, economics, or statistical programming. Although they may conduct health services research with an MPH or an MBA degree, typically these researchers have obtained a PhD in economics, business, sociology, statistics, political science, or one of the disciplines of public health. PAs' input into health services research is extremely important for enabling these teams to ask the right questions. PA practice is often poorly understood by nonclinicians, and the PA contribution to the health system can be misrepresented by well-meaning but ill-informed scientists.

Workforce Research

Health workforce research is the study of the education, use, and distribution of health care professionals in society. It is a subset of health services research. It seeks to understand the needs for different types of health professionals across the country, the roles each health profession can play within the health system, the most effective approaches for training health professionals, and mechanisms for deploying and retaining health professionals in the area of greatest need. Workforce research seeks to answer questions such as: "What would be the impact of allowing pharmacists to prescribe?" "Can PAs provide preventive care for patients with diabetes as well as doctors?" or "How can we retain primary care PAs in rural areas?" Many PA faculty are engaged in workforce research as our profession is new, and we are still exploring the possibilities and limits of the PA profession within the U.S. health care system, as well as health systems around the world.

Physician assistant workforce research has been the primary research field in which PAs have made a mark. From the earliest days of the profession, PAs and their allies have been performing research to answer questions such as, "Is PA practice safe?" "Are patients reluctant to see a PA?" "Are doctors willing to work with PAs?" and "How can PAs be used effectively in trauma surgery?" The oft-cited statistic that "PAs can perform 85% of a doctor's tasks" comes from a study performed in 1986 by the U.S. government with input from PAs.[4] Unlike in many other types of research, PAs often serve as principal investigators in workforce research. They develop the study question, design the methods that will be used to collect and analyze the data, obtain human subject approval from an institutional review board (IRB), perform the analysis, and publish the data. PAs are eligible to apply for and receive grant funds for workforce research without necessarily working with an MD or PhD.

Physician assistants in workforce research sometimes collect and analyze their own data, but they often use large datasets generated by others to analyze patterns across clinical settings and geographic regions. Federal and state governments, large health insurance groups, and large health systems such as Kaiser Permanente or the Veterans Administration often collect data on patient outcomes and provider characteristics, which can be mined for information about the practices of different health professions. However, it has been a challenge to use many of these datasets to their full potential to assess PAs' contribution to the health system because PAs and doctors work closely together and often see the same patients. This practice style, although beneficial for patients, has made it challenging for researchers to be able to attribute changes in quality of care, length of stay, or cost specifically to the use of PAs on the clinical team. Therefore, although we believe PAs to be cost effective and the dramatic increase in the number of PA positions available within the health system suggests that doctors and health systems find PAs to be cost effective, there are no large national studies that conclusively demonstrate the cost effectiveness of the PA role (Case Study 12.3).

CASE STUDY 12.3 KRISTINE HIMMERICK, PhD, PA-C, HEALTH WORKFORCE RESEARCH PA, UNIVERSITY OF CALIFORNIA SAN FRANCISCO, HEALTHFORCE CENTER

Kristine Himmerick's PA career began in primary care clinical practice followed by a move to PA education and most recently to research about PAs in primary care practice. She was the first PA to be appointed as a postdoctoral research scholar at the University of California San Francisco's (UCSF's) Healthforce Center, a highly regarded health workforce research institute. In her role as a research scholar, she is responsible for collaborating with health economists, health policy experts, statisticians, physicians, nurses, and other health services researchers on developing research studies to evaluate different aspects of the health workforce. Her research examines the role of PAs, nurse practitioners, and physicians in expanding access to primary care for medically underserved patients. At UCSF, she is expanding the reach of her work and collaborating with others to answer broader questions about the role of many types of health professionals, both within California and across the country.

A typical week for Kristine involves meeting with colleagues to design upcoming research projects, writing grant applications to fund investigations, designing survey and other data collections tools, analyzing data, and writing manuscripts and presentations to present findings. The work produced by Kristine and her colleagues at UCSF is targeted for policymakers, health administrators, and insurers to make decisions about funding for patient care and the training and deployment of health professionals. This work is also useful for professional organizations, such as the California Academy of Physician Assistants, to advocate for policy changes affecting PA practice.

Kristine says she enjoys the intellectual freedom that comes with being a workforce researcher and working in an environment where ideas matter. She finds career satisfaction knowing that her work can make a difference in the lives of patient and health care providers. Kristine enjoys working with people who have different types of training to develop high-quality research studies and believes that she often has the opportunity to inform people from other professions about PAs and their role in the health care system. She is surprised to encounter some seasoned health services researchers who are unfamiliar with the PA profession and may still overlook inclusion of PAs in workforce research. She takes delight at broadening their perspectives on what PAs can do for patients. Frequently, she encounters opportunities to encourage colleagues to include PAs and nurse practitioners in studies originally designed to capture only the contributions of physicians. Kris enjoys developing empirical data so that policy recommendations are based on fact and not on supposition.

Similar to all work, there are some challenges to being a health workforce researcher. Negotiating with external funders about the way that the research will be conducted and the fact that specific results cannot be guaranteed a priori can be difficult. Kristine also finds it challenging to merge her career as a high-level researcher with ongoing clinical care as a family medicine PA. Primary care patients have ongoing needs that are not amenable to part-time practice. She is still working to discover the best strategy to combine her clinical practice and research work.

Kristine would like to encourage PAs to get involved in research and other academic pursuits. She believes that despite the relative lack of research training in the PA curriculum that the clinical PAs receive actually lays an excellent foundation for a research career. She says, "PAs have more transferrable skills for research than they may realize. PAs are trained in critical thinking, deductive reasoning, and problem solving. PAs are proficient at thinking on their feet and negotiating complex work environments. These skills are very applicable in the research realm." She encourages PAs to start small by joining a professional committee or participating in local quality improvement efforts in their work environment. For those who wish to go further in a research career, Kris notes the value of building relationships with seasoned research mentors that can provide collaboration opportunities and career guidance.

Educational Research

Educational research is the study of the most effective methods for teaching and learning. It seeks to understand the challenges of communicating new material to students, developing students professionally and personally, assessing student and teacher performance, and improving the educational process. Educational research seeks to answer questions such as: "Is a multiple choice test, a short answer test, or an observed structured clinical examination (OSCE) best for assessing students' knowledge of essential emergency medicine topics?" or "Is in-class or online module instruction more effective for teaching students how to read electrocardiograms?" PA faculty often engage in this type of research as well. Several innovations in medical education, such as competency-based curricula, have actually been developed by PA educators and are now used in the education other health professionals.

Educational research is the second most common type of research performed by PAs. As with workforce research, PAs do not necessarily need to collaborate with a physician or PhD-trained researcher to get approval or funding for this type of research. Many PA educators devote their research efforts toward better understanding the effectiveness of specific instructional or assessment approaches. Although educational approaches taken in medicine, nursing, or pharmacy potentially have relevance to PA education, PA education faces some unique challenges that require us to perform our own research. The brief and intense nature of PA education poses particular challenges not faced by other professions. For example, many educators have struggled to know how best to develop professionalism in PA students. The literature for physician education is only of limited applicability to PA education because of the enormous differences in the time in training for PAs versus MDs (2–3 years from entry to full practice for PAs vs. 7–10 years for MDs). Therefore, several PA educators are performing research around this question. In addition to conducting research on how best to educate students, educational research often focuses on how to best educate faculty to be effective in the classroom. Other areas of study that fall under educational research are questions surrounding retention of faculty, relationships of the PA program to the larger educational institution, and relationships between the PA program and clinical preceptors.

WHY SHOULD PHYSICIAN ASSISTANTS BE INVOLVED IN RESEARCH?

1. **Many key questions about PA practice are unanswered, and PAs should play a role in answering these questions.** Even though PAs have been part of the U.S. health system for 50 years, some basic questions about PA practice still have not been answered in a scientific way. Very little is known about the content of care PAs provide, how PA–MD teams work, how PAs grow in their individual scope of practice, how physicians train newly graduated PAs, how cost effective PA practice is for the health system at large, and the impact of PA practice on public health. We *believe* that the success of the profession (>100,000 PAs trained and practicing) shows that doctors, health administrators, patients, and insurance companies all value PAs as an important part of the health system, but when policymakers or academics ask to see the studies that support this assertion, there is little high-quality evidence to share with them. Neither PA professional organizations nor outside foundations have been able to support the expensive and time-consuming high-quality research that would allow us to answer some fundamental questions about PA practice.

As health services researchers have increasingly become interested in costs of care, they have naturally turned toward attempting to assess the contribution of PAs and nurse practitioners to the health system. Unfortunately, PAs are often not included on the research teams, which can result in the development and publication of seriously flawed research.

Non-PA investigators often don't understand the way PAs are trained (as generalists), how PA services are billed to insurance companies (often under the doctor's name), or that "physician assistant" is not itself a medical specialty. More PAs are needed to be part of multidisciplinary health services research teams to provide guidance to non-PA colleagues about how research questions need to be structured and how data should be analyzed to make valid inferences. Poorly designed studies still have the potential to be used in policy decisions, so this research cannot be safely left to others, no matter how well-intentioned they may be.

2. **Research participation raises the credibility of the profession.** Within medical, academic, and policy circles, the production of original research is a marker of the status and success of a profession. Nearly all health professions have a body of literature that guides practice and policy. The published literature is the place where professions hold their internal discussions about both clinical and professional topics. The quality and seriousness of the profession is judged partly on each profession's contribution. Participating in the execution and publication of research studies contributes not only to the credibility of the profession but can also enhance the personal credibility of a PA with colleagues within and outside the PA profession.

3. **PAs should be involved in research to help patients.** PAs are experts at caring for patients and are experts in team-based medical care. These are the essential ingredients for a successful clinical research enterprise. Every PA has known the sorrow of not being able to offer a better treatment option for a patient who is suffering or dying. All PAs have looked into the eyes of a patient and wished more could be done to help. Getting involved in clinical research allows PAs to advance the science of medicine and potentially benefit patients along the way. PAs are very well suited to being members of the clinical research team and can even be the impetus for a practice to start involvement in clinical trials (see Case Study 12.1). Telling patients that you are working to find answers to their problems is immensely satisfying.

4. **PAs should be involved in research to improve service delivery at their institutions.** Providing medical care in a complex health system can be challenging and frustrating. As health care providers who by definition work in teams, PAs often have ideas for improving integration of health services and delivery of clinical care to patients. PAs should use this detailed system knowledge to get involved in implementing quality improvement techniques in their clinical environments. Improving service delivery and quality of care will not only benefit patients but also all the health professionals who have daily frustrations about working in a poorly functioning environment.

5. **Getting involved in research challenges PAs to continue to grow.** As challenging as the first few years of clinical practice can be, after many years of practice, it can be easy for clinical PAs to wonder "is this all there is for me in medicine?" Getting involved in research or quality improvement projects can be a way to add variety to the day and to stimulate PAs to develop new skills. PAs who work in research often are sent to learn new diagnostic or evaluation skills for particular trials. PAs who do quality improvement projects learn the principles of implementation science. Everyone who does research learns more about data collection, data structures, data cleaning, biostatistics, and epidemiology. PAs who expand their skill sets in these ways are more marketable and are more likely to be engaged in the work they do.

PHYSICIAN ASSISTANT STUDENTS AND RESEARCH

For most PA students, personal participation original research is not a substantial part of their PA education experience. However, there are several ways in which PA students may get involved in research during their time in PA school.

1. **PA students may see clinical research while on clinical rotations.** Clinical research is primarily conducted at academic medical centers, but many private practices serve as clinical sites for research studies. Including private practice sites in the clinical trial allows the clinical trial to draw from a more diverse pool of patients than if the study is only conducted at academic medical centers. Inclusion of a wider variety of patients in the study increases the applicability of the study results to the general population. In addition, participating in clinical trials provides revenue for doctors in private practice and the opportunity to offer new treatments to their patients.

Students who have the opportunity to rotate at either an academic site or a community site that has patients enrolled in clinical studies should ask if they can observe a study visit. Observing how data are collected in a standardized way, how medications are dispensed, and how side effects are dealt with by the study clinician will increase the student's understanding of the clinical trials process. It will also help students explain study participation to patients they may see in their PA careers. Doctors and PAs who practice oncology, infectious diseases, cardiology, and any other subspecialty that cares for patients with life-limiting diseases often speak with their patients about participation in clinical trials because the existing therapies for the illness are not optimal. PA students who are interested in these specialties should make a particular attempt to observe a clinical trial visit during their time as a student.

2. **PA students may be asked to be research subjects.** PA students are often included as subjects in research being performed by their PA program, a group of PA programs, the Physician Assistant Education Association, the American Academy of Physician Assistants, and others. They may be asked to take a survey, participate in an extra OSCE, conduct a role-play exercise, or participate in other assessments. Although this participation may feel burdensome, please seriously consider getting involved. PA student participation can support faculty members to get grant funding, a promotion, a paper published, or a presentation at a national meeting. In addition, supporting PA-related research benefits the profession as a whole, which ultimately will benefit each PA and PA student. Participating as a research subject also gives PA students further insight into the research process itself.

3. **PA students may have the opportunity to turn their capstone projects into publishable papers.** PA programs have different requirements for completion of the master's degree. Some programs require students to develop a clinical review article. Others require students to either propose or actually perform small original research projects. A few students take the next step with their projects and attempt to publish them. Quality clinical review articles can potentially be published in the *Journal of the American Academy of Physician Assistants* (*JAAPA*), *Clinician Reviews*, or *Clinical Advisor*. Research manuscripts can be published in *JAAPA* or other journals that publish original studies.

To get a clinical review article published, the article has to have a "spin"—something novel to entice PAs to read your article. The author needs to provide the reader with new information, not simply the basics of a disease or a treatment that PAs already know. For example, no journal would publish a paper called "Diagnosis and Treatment of Lung Cancer," but a journal editor is more likely to accept a paper called "New Medical Therapies for the Treatment of Metastatic Lung Cancer." PA students need to submit their papers with a faculty member from their institution as a coauthor because journals do not accept solo-author papers from students.

Physician assistant students who wish to publish original research need to know that it will be held to the normal standard for peer-reviewed publications. *Before* conducting research, PA students need to ensure that they have approval from their school's IRB. The IRB is responsible for ensuring that all research conducted by faculty or students meets the standards for ethical and safe research. The IRB may require students to complete some online modules before beginning their research to prepare them to conduct safe and ethical research. Journals will not publish the results of studies that have not received IRB approval.

Physician assistant students should work with a faculty member to write the research design, protocol, and any surveys they wish to administer. Perform the research and then clean the data. Editing the data ensures that there are no duplicate data, biologically impossible measures (the research subject is unlikely to be 68 feet tall, but he or she may be 68 inches tall), or contradictory survey responses. Faculty members can help the student develop the paper into proper research manuscript format and submit it to the journal. After it has been submitted, if the article is deemed of sufficient interest to the journal, it will be sent on to peer reviewers. These reviewers can decide whether to accept the article as is, whether to ask the authors for major or minor changes, or whether to reject the article altogether. The authors will be required to respond to the comments made by the reviewers, revise the manuscript, and resubmit it to the editor. After all concerns have been addressed, the editor makes the final decision about when the paper will be published.

CONCLUSION

All PAs, regardless of their background and their interest level in research, will use research regularly to help their patients, guide their practice, and improve their knowledge base. Most PAs are likely to also have the opportunity to participate in research themselves as either a subject or investigator. Investing some time in better understanding the research process allows PAs to appreciate and enjoy using the literature all the more.

> ## KEY POINTS
>
> - Research affects all aspects of physician assistant practice, including clinical care, health education, health care delivery, and quality improvement. Being able to effectively interpret scientific literature is a key to being able to continue to deliver high-quality care in the course of the PA's career.
> - PAs are increasingly involved in generating their own original research. Several PAs are national leaders in their research fields.
> - PAs who are interested in conducting biomedical, public health, health workforce, health services, or implementation science research should consider obtaining further training in these disciplines to make maximum impact.

References

1. Neufelt V, Guralnik D, eds. *Webster's New World Collegiate Dictionary*. New York: Macmillan: 1997.
2. Fogarty International Center. Frequently Asked Questions about Implementation Science. http://www.fic.nih.gov/News/Events/implementation-science/Pages/faqs.aspx. Published May 2013. Accessed December 9, 2015.
3. Pronovost P, et al. An intervention to decrease catheter-related bloodstream infections in the ICU. *N Engl J Med.* 2006;355:2725–2732.
4. U.S. Congress, Office of Technology Assessment. *Nurse Practitioners, Physician Assistants, and Certified Nurse-Midwives: A Policy Analysis*, OTA-HCS-37; 1986.

The resources for this chapter can be found at www.expertconsult.com.

The Faculty Resources can be found online at www.expertconsult.com.

CHAPTER 13

KEEPING PEOPLE HEALTHY

Natalie Walkup • April Gardner • Barbara Saltzman

In 2013, the Unites States spent $2.9 trillion on health care, or $9255 per person. The amount spent on health care is expected to increase at an average rate of 5.8% per year.[1] The United States spends almost one and a half times as much on health care as any other country. Yet the United States has the highest infant mortality rate of industrialized countries, highest prevalence of overweight children, and highest admission rate for asthma and ranks 43rd for life expectancy. This shows that the United States has one of the most inefficient health care systems worldwide (Fig. 13.1).

The high cost of health care is in part due to the traditional needs-based, medical intervention system in our country. That is, when someone becomes ill, she or he accesses health services, which often cannot treat the issue but only delays further morbidity or mortality. Much of the treatment that is provided could be avoided if preventive medicine was performed with a population or public health approach. Intervening at the population level early on results in less individual morbidity and mortality, also resulting in lower health care expenditures and a healthier population.[2]

The concept of population health has gained attention over the years. The overall purpose of population health is to maintain and improve the health of an entire population by reducing disparities and impacting the determinants of health (Fig. 13.2). This includes focusing on health indicators such as social, economic, and physical environments that influence individuals, communities, and populations of people.[3] The health factors that affect population health include physical environment (air and water quality, housing, transit), social and economic (employment status, education status, income), clinical care (access to care, quality of care, genetics (predispositions), and health behaviors (tobacco use, diet and exercise, and alcohol and drug use).[4] From a population health perspective, each of these determinants needs to be considered in order to have a significant impact on health outcomes.

The Prevention Institute, the California Endowment, and the Urban Institute[5] reviewed the role prevention plays in health care costs and were able to identify key issues associated with health and cost. Most of the illnesses that are associated with the highest health care expenditures are in part preventable (Fig. 13.3 and Table 13.1). The key issues include resources that are being used to influence health are not used efficiently or effectively, a small reduction in disease incidence can lead to substantial savings overall (e.g., a 5% reduction in heart disease can lead to an estimated $974,078,000 savings), effective prevention strategies have already led to a reduction in overall costs, and a reduction in end-of-life care can reduce morbidities.

With the ever expanding opportunities for physician assistants (PA), it is important that PAs recognize their role in population health. PAs need to help transition the focus of medicine to a public health or population health perspective that emphasizes preventive medicine, identifies and corrects disparities, integrates behavior and social sciences, and aims to increase the health of the population as a whole. PAs have the opportunity to engage their communities in

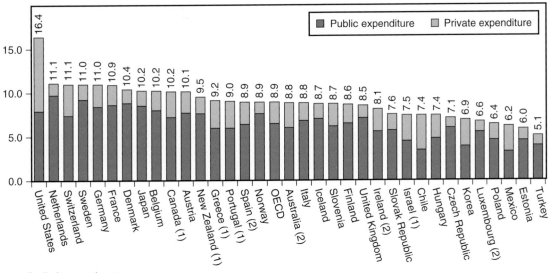

1 Preliminary estimate.
2 Data refer to 2012.

FIG. 13.1 ■ Health spending (excluding investment) as a share of gross domestic product, Organisation for Economic Co-operation and Development countries, 2013. (Focus on Health Spending, Health Statistics 2015, Paris, France: Organisation for Economic Co-operation and Development (OECD). http://www.oecd.org/health/health-systems/Focus-Health-Spending-2015.pdf. Accessed December 5, 2016)

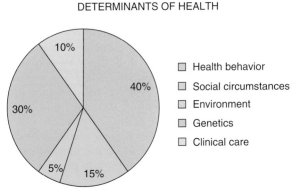

FIG. 13.2 ■ Determinants of health. (Adapted from McGinnis JM, Williams-Russo P, Knickman JR. The case for more active policy attention to health promotion. *Health Aff (Millwood)* 2002;21(2):78–93.)

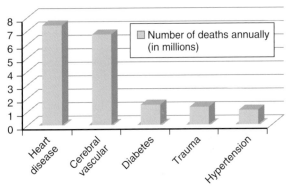

FIG. 13.3 ■ Top causes of death worldwide (2012) associated with the highest preventable health care expenditures. (Reducing healthcare costs through prevention. Los Angeles: Prevention Institute and The California Endowment with The Urban Institute. https://www.preventioninstitute.org/sites/default/files/publications/HE_Health%20Care%20Reform%20Policy%20Draft_040511.pdf. Accessed on Dec. 4, 2016.)

identifying disparities that are affecting their health and address these through community involvement with an emphasis on primary prevention.

PRIMARY, SECONDARY, AND TERTIARY PREVENTION

There are three approaches to prevention: primary, secondary, and tertiary. The primary approach focuses on preventing disease before it develops; tertiary prevention is directed at managing established disease in someone and avoiding further complications (much of how we currently manage patients). To decrease health care expense and increase population and individual health, all three of these prevention methods should be used. However, the emphasis needs to shift from tertiary to primary prevention.

The goal of primary prevention is to impact health outcomes before the onset of disease or injury. This

TABLE 13.1 Top Causes of Death Worldwide (2012) Associated With the Highest Preventable Health Care Expenditures

Disease	Number of Deaths Annually
Heart disease	7.4 million
Cerebrovascular accidents	6.7 million
Diabetes	1.5 million
Trauma	1.3 million
Hypertension	1.1 million

Reducing healthcare costs through prevention. Los Angeles: Prevention Institute and The California Endowment with The Urban Institute. https://www.preventioninstitute.org/sites/default/files/publications/HE_Health%20Care%20Reform%20Policy%20Draft_040511.pdf. Accessed on Dec. 4, 2016.

TABLE 13.2 Prevention Measures

Type of Prevention	Examples of Prevention
Primary	Daily recommended diet and exercise Wearing a helmet when bike riding Vaccines Teeth brushing and flossing Hand washing Smoking or alcohol cessation Prenatal vitamins Condom use
Secondary	Recommended screenings: Pap, mammography, prostate specific antigen, colonoscopy, DEXA scan, blood pressure, glucose, cholesterol Prenatal screenings HIV screening
Tertiary	Improving glucose control in patients with diabetes Rehabilitation after myocardial infarction or injury Providing counseling to victims of rape or PTSD

DEXA, dual-energy x-ray absorptiometry; *PTSD*, posttraumatic stress disorder.

approach classically addresses populations, such as a nationwide campaign to address obesity or targeted at-risk populations, for instance, providing flu vaccines. Because of reaching a large number of individuals, primary prevention can have a substantial impact on economic benefits and is extremely cost effective.[2] Primary prevention can require changes on individual levels as well as policy levels. For example, whereas tooth brushing and flossing are individual prevention measures, adding fluoride to water is a policy prevention change.

Secondary prevention implies that for the specific disease, primary prevention has not been sufficient. The goal of secondary prevention is to identify a disease early in its process in order to maximize the success of treatment and decrease the incidence of morbidity or mortality related to that disease (in other words, identifying a disease while it is still asymptomatic). This includes the routine, recommended screening for cancer, diabetes, and hypertension. In these cases, patients are often without symptoms, and the diagnosis is made through screening methods.

Tertiary prevention is what has traditionally been seen in medicine when a patient presents with symptoms and a disease process is identified, but it is too advanced and a definitive cure is no longer an option. For these patients, the goal of tertiary prevention is to maximize the outcomes and prevent further morbidity from the disease process. An example of this is a patient who presents to the emergency department with chest pain. After a thorough workup, it is determined that the patient is having a myocardial infarction. The damage that has been done to the heart cannot be reversed; however, with appropriate cardiac therapy and rehabilitation, the patient would be able to maximize his or her cardiac output

and prevent further morbidity and mortality associated with the myocardial infarction.

Most patients require a combination of prevention approaches; however, it is the PA's responsibility to recognize common secondary and tertiary issues within his or her practice and consider primary community intervention strategies to address these issues and maximize community health. Often the intervention includes increasing access to health care, community education, and community empowerment to shift the focus from tertiary prevention to primary prevention (Table 13.2).

CASE STUDY 13.1

Lydia, an obstetric/gynecologic PA, is concerned with the prevalence of cervical abnormalities present in her practice. This prevalence has led to many costly and uncomfortable procedures for her patients to better monitor cervical changes. Lydia knows that currently there is no cure for human papillomavirus (HPV), which is strongly correlated with cervical cancer. She decides that her efforts are not enough. Lydia's practice is located next to a major university campus. Although she sees a diverse population of patients, she has a significant portion of university students. Lydia decided to survey the university students to assess what percentage of students have received the HPV vaccine, the only known way to prevent cervical cancer. She found that the majority of the students had not received the three-dose series of the vaccine. In response to her assessment, Lydia established an HPV vaccination clinic on the university campus. Through this clinic, she was able to provide on-campus education about HPV and cervical cancer and offer the vaccine at no cost to all university students and employees who were eligible for the vaccine. Her vaccination clinic was able to increase the vaccination rate of university students by 60%.

Identify the levels of prevention:

Primary: HPV vaccination clinic

Secondary: routine Pap smears

Tertiary: treating and monitoring those already diagnosed with cervical abnormalities

Identify the impact this will have on the community:

Decreasing the prevalence of HPV in an at-risk university population decreases health care expenditures and morbidity on future cervical abnormalities. Lydia addressed the lack of education about HPV, increased access to university students and faculty by putting the clinic on campus, and eliminated the cost barrier. By addressing these determinants, she was able to impact her community's health.

IMMUNIZATION STRATEGIES

Immunization plays a pivotal role in public health, helping to control and eliminate once prevalent communicable diseases that cause illness, hospitalization, morbidity, and mortality for infants, children, and adults. A vaccine works by mimicking a natural disease without acquiring the actual disease in order to stimulate the immune system to combat the natural disease in the case of exposure.[6] Fig. 13.4 illustrates that as the use of vaccination increases, the number of cases of the disease decreases in the population, and oppositely, when vaccinations decrease, there is a rise in the incidence of disease in the population.

Fig. 13.5 illustrates the importance of vaccinating the majority of people in the population and worldwide. Lower numbers of vaccinated individuals lead to continued spread of a disease; however, if most people in the population are vaccinated against a disease, fewer individuals will contract the disease and spread the disease to others. Similarly, unless a disease is completely eliminated, as in the case of smallpox, immunization of the majority of the population must continue, or the disease will reappear with its health-related consequences.

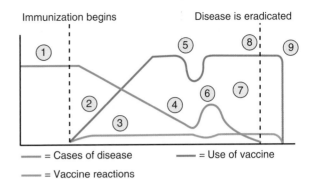

FIG. 13.4 ■ As the use of vaccination increases, the number of cases of the disease decreases in the population. (Chen RT, Rastogi SC, Mullen JR, Hayes S, Cochi SL, Donlon JA, Wassilak SG. The Vaccine adverse event reporting ststem (VAERS). Vaccine1994;12:542-50.)

The Advisory Committee on Immunization Practices (ACIP) is responsible for developing recommendations for childhood and adult vaccinations, which includes the vaccination schedule, dosing and timing of specific vaccinations by age group, and indications and contraindications for receiving vaccinations. The 2016 birth through age 6 years immunization schedule can be accessed at http://www.cdc.gov/vaccines/parents/downloads/parent-ver-sch-0-6yrs.pdf.[7] Guidelines for vaccination of 7- to 18-year-old children can be accessed at http://www.cdc.gov/vaccines/who/teens/downloads/parent-version-schedule-7-18yrs.pdf.[8]

Childhood immunizations prevent communicable diseases. Parents may have many questions about vaccines such as the number of vaccines, risks and benefits of vaccines, side effects of an injection, and if there is a true need for immunizations. Myths and controversies surrounding childhood vaccinations, such as links to autism, lead parents to use caution when considering vaccination for their children. The Centers for Disease Control and Prevention (CDC) provides an educational flyer to help answer the common questions about vaccines. It can be accessed at http://www.cdc.gov/vaccines/events/niiw/ed-resources/downloads/f_provider-qa-color.pdf.[9]

It is important to educate parents on the safety and efficacy of vaccinations; however, parents may continue to have questions about the safety of vaccines or refuse to vaccinate their children. It is important to keep the lines of communication open with parents during office visits. The CDC released a handout for health care professionals to effectively communicate with parents about challenging questions parents may ask about infant vaccinations, which can be found at http://www.cdc.gov/vaccines/hcp/conversations/downloads/talk-infants-color-office.pdf.[10] Parents can also

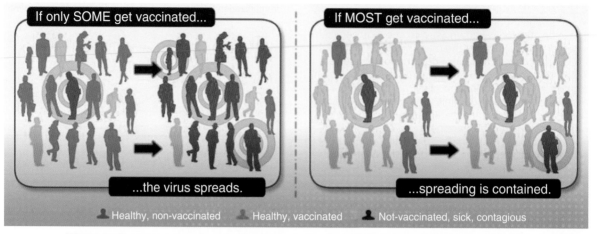

FIG. 13.5 ■ The importance of vaccinating the majority of people in the population and worldwide. ("What would happen if we stopped vaccinations?" Atlanta, Georgia: Centers for Disease Control and Prevention. http://www.cdc.gov/vaccines/vac-gen/whatifstop.htm. Accessed on December 3, 2016.)

be directed to a 6-minute video highlighting parents asking tough questions answered by pediatricians at the following link: http://www.cdc.gov/cdctv/diseaseandconditions/vaccination/get-picture-childhood-immunization.html.[11] Additionally, any vaccine-preventable disease can occur as an isolated incident or in clusters in a community, across the United States, or in any part of the world. It is PAs' responsibility to educate parents who choose not to vaccinate their infants and children about the risks of nonvaccination and the parents' responsibilities for ensuring the best possible health strategies with unvaccinated children. The CDC distributes an excellent educational brochure to inform parents of unvaccinated children of risks and responsibilities of nonvaccination and can be accessed at http://www.cdc.gov/vaccines/hcp/conversations/downloads/not-vacc-risks-color-office.pdf.[12]

Adults are often unaware of their need for vaccinations, and therefore the immunization rates in adults remains low. Patients tend to follow vaccination advice from health care professionals, so it is important to assess vaccination status during every office visit. The adult vaccination schedule for healthy adults and adults with specific diseases is updated and approved annually and can be accessed at http://www.cdc.gov/vaccines/schedules/downloads/adult/adult-combined-schedule.pdf.[13] Additionally, the National Vaccine Advisory Committee issued practice standards regarding vaccinations for all health care professionals to follow to increase adult vaccination rates and decrease serious illness, hospitalization, and death from vaccine-preventable diseases (Table 13.3).

TABLE 13.3 Practice Standards for All Health Care Professionals

1. **Assess** immunization status of all your patients at every clinical encounter.
   - Stay informed. Get the latest CDC recommendations for immunization of adults.
   - Implement protocols and policies. Ensure that patients' vaccine needs are routinely reviewed and patients get reminders about vaccines they need.
2. Strongly **recommend** vaccines that patients need.
   - Share tailored reasons why vaccination is right for the patient.
   - Highlight positive experiences with vaccination.
   - Address patient questions and concerns.
   - Remind patients that vaccines protect them and their loved ones against a number of common and serious diseases.
   - Explain the potential costs of getting sick.
3. **Administer** needed vaccines or **refer** your patients to a vaccination provider.
   - Offer the vaccines you stock.
   - Refer patients to providers in the area who offer vaccines that you don't stock.
4. **Document** vaccines received by your patients.
   - Participate in your state's immunization registry. Help your office, your patients, and your patients' other providers know which vaccines your patients have had.
   - Follow up. Confirm that patients received recommended vaccines that you referred them to get from other immunization providers.

From Centers for Disease Control and Prevention. *Standards for Adult Immunization Practice.* http://www.cdc.gov/vaccines/hcp/adults/for-practice/standards/index.html.

HEALTH DETERMINANTS

Chronic diseases are the leading cause of death and disability in the United States. In 2010, 7 of the top 10 causes of death were chronic, including heart diseases, cancer, chronic lower respiratory diseases, cerebrovascular diseases (stroke), Alzheimer disease, and diabetes mellitus (diabetes), with cancer and heart diseases causing almost 50% of all deaths in this country.[14]

Chronic diseases are those typically lasting longer than 3 months and by and large are not vaccine preventable. These diseases can be managed by medication but usually cannot be cured. Symptoms can often be alleviated or controlled by changes in behavior, including, but not limited to, level of physical activity, smoking cessation, and dietary choices.[15] Genetic susceptibility is an underlying cause of many chronic diseases. Chronic diseases often occur because of a conglomeration of genetic susceptibility in combination with environmental and behavioral factors. Social determinants of health are the nonmedical conditions that have been shown to directly affect health, including residential neighborhoods, school and work environments, and community and religious settings.[15,16] For example, neighborhoods are associated with water quality, lead paint exposure, access to nutritious food choices, and green spaces, all factors that have been identified as affecting health in the literature.[15]

HEALTHY PEOPLE 2020

To formally address all types of determinants of health in the United States, the Healthy People program was initiated in 1979 as a result of Surgeon General Julius B. Richmond's report *Healthy People: The Surgeon General's Report on Health Promotion and Disease Prevention*, emphasizing the role of nutrition, exercise, environmental factors, and occupational safety in advancing health. The Healthy People program has now been in place for more than 30 years and provides 10-year evidence-based health targets for the American population. It emphasizes the overlap between the physical and social environment, behavioral, health services infrastructure, and biology and genetics and their collective impact on health. Healthy People is managed by the Office of Disease Prevention and Health Promotion at the U.S. Department of Health and Human Services. A Secretary's Advisory Board includes 12 members, including nationally known public health experts from across

the country. Objectives of the Healthy People program are developed in conjunction with stakeholders in the greater medical and social community with periods of open comment on objectives as they are developed for the next 10-year program cycle.

In 1990, there were 15 topic areas and 226 measurable objectives. This has expanded to 39 measurable topic areas with nearly 600 measurable objectives in the 2020 program. Objectives cover topics of prevention from all health determinants and levels of prevention. For example, in the diabetes arena, there are measurable objectives, including D-1, reducing the number of new cases (primary prevention), to D-11, increasing the number of patients with diabetes getting HbA1c screenings at least twice a year and increasing the number of patients with diabetes getting annual foot examinations (examples of secondary prevention), and D-2.1, reducing the rate of all-cause mortality among patients with diabetes (tertiary prevention).[17] Healthy People 2020 gives detailed reduction rates providing a baseline rate at the beginning of the period. For example, objective D-1 reports the baseline rate of 8.0 new cases of diabetes per 1000 population ages 18 to 84 years occurring in the past 12 months, as reported in 2006 to 2008 (age adjusted to the year 2000 standard population), with a target for 2020 of 7.2 new cases being diagnosed per 1000 population ages 18 to 84 years, which is a 10% improvement over the 10-year period. These goals are evidence-based, citing sources such as the United States Preventive Services Task Force (USPSTF), CDC, and National Center for Health Statistics in conjunction with the wider body of published evidence of important screening tools and risk reduction activities. Each objective provides links directly to the source used in determining the 10-year goals. Additionally, updates are reported as data are collected to identify the success in reaching the goals. This data are then used to develop the next 10-year cycle objectives.

UNITED STATES PREVENTIVE SERVICES TASK FORCE

The USPSTF is an "independent, volunteer panel of national experts in prevention and evidence-based medicine. The Task Force works to improve the health of all Americans by making evidence-based recommendations about clinical preventive services."[18] The scope of USPSTF includes screening, preventive medicine, and counseling used and offered in the primary care setting. That is, its recommendations are focused on care of healthy adults and children with no signs and symptoms of existing disease. The task force itself does not carry out research but merely uses the available body of evidence to make clinical recommendations based on various demographic and other patient characteristics such as age and sex. The task force evaluates both benefits and harms associated with each clinical test and practice reported on.

Topics can be identified by public nomination and include the identification of new topics, a request to review a topic that has been previously analyzed because of the availability of new evidence or screening tools, or a change in the state of burden on public health by a particular topic.[19] Although topics are accepted throughout the year, there are three meetings per annum at which topics are considered.

After a topic is selected, a rigorous process is undertaken by the task force to develop a recommendation. A research plan is drafted followed by a period of open public comment on the topic, and development of a finalized research plan is achieved. When the plan is finalized, the task force undertakes the review of the available evidence and gives a final recommendation grade. Grades range from A through D, with A indicating the greatest level of certainty for implementation into practice and D discouraging the use. An I statement is issued if the current evidence is insufficient to make a recommendation either for or against a preventive service.[20] After a recommendation is made, it is published and disseminated by the task force.

An example of a task force recommendation includes screening for abnormal blood glucose levels as part of cardiovascular risk assessment in adults aged 40 to 70 years who are overweight or obese. This recommendation only received a grade of B, indicating that "there is high certainty that the net benefit is moderate or there is moderate certainty that the net benefit is moderate to substantial," and clinicians should offer this service. Although the task force identified evidence to support blood glucose screening in overweight and obese adults with diabetes as a tool to prevent the secondary effects of cardiovascular disease, there was a gap in the evidence with only two studies directly measuring the mortality reduction based on screening in asymptomatic individuals.[21]

The task force evaluates the available evidence and summarizes it in a simple form for clinicians to use in their practice to enhance disease prevention and management.

INFLUENCING HEALTH BEHAVIOR CHANGES

Public health and health education specialist professionals use many theories to guide individuals, groups, and communities in changing health behaviors. More than 20 theories are currently in use today to help influence behavior change. Many of these theories use similar concepts to increase knowledge and awareness about diseases and unhealthy behaviors, impact attitudes about health beliefs, teach skills, and ultimately lead to changes in health behaviors. Changing health behavior is a complicated process, and individuals are motivated by different means; therefore, one theory or one type of health promotion program will not work for all. The most popular health behavior models currently in use today include the health belief model, theory of planned behavior, social cognitive theory, and the transtheoretical model.

The popular transtheoretical model is frequently used by clinicians to impact health behavior changes in clinical practice. This model describes the process, or stages, that individuals progress through as they decide to change and adopt a health behavior. The model has been used to change many types of health behaviors including alcohol abuse; substance abuse; smoking; exercise; sedentary lifestyles, obesity, high-fat diets, and weight control; mammography screening; and pregnancy prevention.[4]

The hallmark of the transtheoretical model is the stages of change, which includes the following five stages: precontemplation, contemplation, preparation, action, and maintenance. An individual considering changing a behavior, such as smoking, will move through these five stages with the goal of becoming a nonsmoking person. A person who smokes may understand the risks of smoking and may even understand that she is at risk for smoking-related diseases such as lung cancer or cardiovascular disease, but she still has no intention of taking action within the next 6 months. This first stage is known as precontemplation. Some people in this category may have no information or may be poorly informed about the outcomes of a health behavior, or in the case of our example, a person may be unsuccessful in many attempts to quit smoking. Regardless, people in this stage tend to avoid considering or communicating about the behavior risks.[4] Contemplation is the stage when a person decides to take action and change a behavior in the next 6 months. This person is open to communication about the topic and risks of the behavior but has not committed to change. A person who smokes in this stage would be likely to discuss the risks of smoking and the benefits of quitting with a provider. She would accept informational brochures and suggestions on smoking cessation programs. The third stage, preparation, is when a person decides to take action within the next 30 days. She may have already taken some actions toward this commitment, such as reducing the number of ashtrays and packs of cigarettes in the home or reducing the number of cigarettes smoked daily. Clinically, it is important to identify patients in this stage because they are motivated to make a significant behavior change and will be amenable to suggestions to be successful with that change, such as joining a smoking cessation group and choosing a quit date. Action, the fourth stage of change, is marked by an overt behavior change in the previous 6 months. Our patient has successfully quit smoking; however, she is at significant risk for relapse during this phase. It will be important to address relapse with the patient and provide the needed support to avoid it. The maintenance stage is marked by overt behavior change for longer than 6 months. Relapse is still a concern during this stage and must be addressed; however, the change is more of a habit at this time, confidence to remain tobacco free increases, and relapse is less of a concern than the previous stage. Many health behaviors, including our example of smoking cessation, can apply a sixth stage, termination. This stage is characterized by a complete lack of temptation to return to the previous behavior, and the person has complete confidence in maintaining the new behavior. The patient is known to be in a permanent stage of maintenance.

The transtheoretical model stages of change also include the concepts of decisional balance and self-efficacy. Decisional balance relates to the pros and cons of a behavior change when considering a major change, such as smoking cessation. A person will perform the mental math and weigh the benefits of changing with the costs of changing as she progresses through the stages. If the costs of changing (e.g., losing friends who smoke and concern about withdrawal symptoms) outweigh the perceived benefits of changing (e.g., monetary savings and increased health), the person is unlikely to make the change. Self-efficacy, defined as a person's confidence to successfully perform a health behavior, is a major factor in making a permanent change. High self-efficacy to quit smoking will help our patient toward the goal of becoming a nonsmoker. Additionally, temptation to return to former behaviors can be strong and is seen across all stages. Temptation, especially in the presence of low self-efficacy, can cause a patient to revert to a former stage. Craving cigarettes or going to party where friends are smoking may be a strong temptation for our patient in the action or maintenance phases. Addressing these types of temptations is an important part of relapse education.

CASE STUDY 13.2

Sarah is a senior in college applying to PA programs. She has been so busy maintaining a high grade point average that she has become completely sedentary. She comes to see you, her primary care PA, to discuss her situation. She recognized a couple of years ago that she really needed to start exercising, but she was too busy with homework and did not have the desire to start something new. She also lives in the Midwest and avoids going outdoors over the long winters. About 3 months ago, she realized she needs to make a change and began looking into recreational programs on campus. She picked up some brochures that showed various intramural sports such as basketball, volleyball, and softball. She talked with her friend who participates on a basketball team and thought it sounded like fun; however, she did not join because she was "just too busy." Sarah now understands that she needs to make a significant change in her lifestyle, and she is committed to doing something in the next few weeks.

After a sports physical examination and her discussion with you today, she decides to join an intramural team. Sarah returns to the clinic 7 months later to get her annual flu shot. You ask her about her previous concerns about a sedentary lifestyle. She excitedly explains that she joined the intramural softball team the day after her last appointment. Initially, she found it difficult to go to practice because she was out of shape, but as her skills improved and she made friends, she found the confidence to continue. Additionally, she quit going for a while because she did not want to go to the recreation center in the cold winter, but her friend picked her up for practice. She has been participating in a team sport since her last visit and has recruited three other friends to participate, too!

Identify the stages of change:

Precontemplation: Sarah recognized she needed to start exercising 2 years ago, but she was too busy to make a change.

Contemplation: Three months ago, Sarah became more serious about a behavior change and went to the student recreation center and picked up brochures on intramural activities. She also talked with a friend who participates on a team.

Preparation: Sarah came to you as her PA for a physical examination and to discuss making a change in the next few weeks.

Action: Sarah joined an intramural team, but she had some initial difficulty being fully committed, especially because she was out of shape and did not want to brave the winter weather.

Maintenance: Sarah has maintained consistent participation on a team for the past 7 months and is enthusiastic about maintaining this lifestyle and has recruited others to participate as well.

Identify the following:

Self-efficacy: As Sarah's skills improved and a friend picked her up for practice in the winter months, her confidence to continue participating increased, escalating to the point that she recruited others to join an intramural team.

Temptation: Being out of shape and the winter weather were temptations to discontinue the new health behavior, especially during the action stage.

CONCLUSION

Health education and promotion are essential elements in the practice of medicine for primary care PAs. Focusing on population health can have a significant impact on decreasing health care expenditures in the United States and preventing illness and chronic disease. An essential part of health education and promotion is shifting the focus of medicine to primary and secondary prevention instead of tertiary medicine. A significant part of primary population prevention is incorporating the Healthy People objectives and addressing health determinants as the focus of a PA's practice and providing an emphasis on immunizations and other primary preventive measures.

For a primary care PA, the USPSTF recommendations serve as a clinical guide for preventive medicine and should be referred to for clinical practice. Following these recommendations, PAs should use the transtheoretical model to effectively meet patients at their stage of change. By taking the time to encourage patients to advance through the stages of change and following the Healthy People 2020 objectives and USPSTF recommendations, PAs have the ability to significantly impact the health of individuals and the community they serve.

KEY POINTS

- Public Health focuses on the health of the population rather than the individual patient and yet can have a profound impact on individuals within the population.
- PAs can be the force that helps transition the focus of medicine to a population health perspective that emphasizes preventive medicine, identifies and corrects disparities, integrates behavior and social sciences and aims to improve the health of the population.
- Primary prevention measures impact health outcomes before the onset of disease or injury.
- Immunizations are an essential component to the health of the population. In the age of social media and misinformation, PAs must be armed with the science and facts regarding vaccines. They need to be well equipped to speak with confidence about the life saving benefits as well as the true risks of vaccines. PAs must be equally prepared to have candid conversations regarding the risks to the individual and the community from vaccine refusal. Due to the impact on public health, these are conversations that must not be forgotten, avoided, or skipped due to discomfort or time limitations. They deserve priority. Resources, such as scripts and videos, are available to providers to aid in having these important conversations on CDC.gov and AAP.org.
- PAs should utilize the information and assistance provided by appropriate online resources, such as Healthy People 2020, United States Preventive Services Task Force, and the Centers for Disease Control and Prevention.

References

1. Centers for Medicaid and Medicare Services. *National Health Expenditures 2013 Highlights*; 2015. https://www.cms.gov/Research-Statistics-Data-and-Systems/Statistics-Trends-and-Reports/NationalHealthExpendData/index.html. Accessed on April 14, 2016.
2. DiClemente RJ, Salazar LF, Crosby RA. Health behavior theory for public health. Principles, foundations, and applications. Burlington, MA: Jones & Bartlett Learning, LLC; 2013:3–26.
3. Kindig D, Stoddart G. What is population health? *American Journal of Public Health*. 2003;93(3):380–383.
4. McKenzie JF, Neiger BL, Thackeray R. *Planning, Implementing & Evaluating Health Promotion Programs*; 2013:162–204.
5. Prevention Institute and the California Endowment with the Urban Institute. Reducing healthcare costs through prevention. http://www.preventioninstitute.org/component/jlibrary/article/id-79/127.html. Accessed on April 14, 2016.
6. Centers for Disease Control and Prevention. How vaccines prevent diseases. http://www.cdc.gov/vaccines/parents/vaccine-decision/prevent-diseases.html. Accessed on April 14, 2016.
7. Centers for Disease Control and Prevention. Recommended immunizations for children from birth through 6 years old. http://www.cdc.gov/vaccines/parents/downloads/parent-ver-sch-0-6yrs.pdf. Accessed on April 12, 2016.

8. Centers for Disease Control and Prevention. Recommended immunizations for children from 7 through 18 years old. http://www.cdc.gov/vaccines/who/teens/downloads/parent-version-schedule-7-18yrs.pdf. Accessed on April 12, 2016.

9. Centers for Disease Control and Prevention. Infant immunizations FAQ. http://www.cdc.gov/vaccines/events/niiw/ed-resources/downloads/f_provider-qa-color.pdf. Accessed April 14, 2016.

10. Centers for Disease Control and Prevention. Talking with Parents about Vaccines for Infants Strategies for Health Care Professionals. http://www.cdc.gov/vaccines/hcp/conversations/downloads/talk-infants-color-office.pdf. Accessed on April 14, 2016.

11. Centers for Disease Control and Prevention. Getting the picture: childhood immunizations. http://www.cdc.gov/cdctv/diseaseandconditions/vaccination/get-picture-childhood-immunization.html. Accessed on April 14, 2016.

12. Centers for Disease Control and Prevention. If you choose not to vaccinate your child, understand the risks and responsibilities. http://www.cdc.gov/vaccines/hcp/conversations/downloads/not-vacc-risks-color-office.pdf. Accessed on April 12, 2016.

13. Centers for Disease Control and Prevention. Recommended Adult Immunization Schedule United States. http://www.cdc.gov/vaccines/schedules/downloads/adult/adult-combined-schedule.pdf. Accessed on April 14, 2016.

14. Centers for Disease Control and Prevention. Chronic disease prevention and health promotion. http://www.cdc.gov/chronicdisease/overview/index.htm. Accessed on April 18, 2016.

15. Notterman DA, Mitchel C. Epigenetic and understanding the impact of social determinants of health. *Pediatric Clinics of North America*. 2015;62(5):1227–1240.

16. Healthy People 2020. Washington, DC: U.S. Department of Health and Human Services, Office of Disease Prevention and Health Promotion. https://www.healthypeople.gov/. Accessed on April 12, 2016.

17. Healthy People 2020 [Internet]. Washington, DC: U.S. Department of Health and Human Services, Office of Disease Prevention and Health Promotion. http://www.healthypeople.gov/2020/topics-objectives/topic/diabetes/objectives. Accessed on April 12, 2016.

18. *About the USPSTF*. U.S. Preventive Services Task Force. January 2016. http://www.uspreventiveservicestaskforce.org/Page/Name/about-the-uspstf. Accessed on April 12, 2016.

19. *Nominate a Recommendation Statement Topic*. U.S. Preventive Services Task Force. February 2014. http://www.uspreventiveservicestaskforce.org/Page/Name/nominating-recommendation-statement-topics. Accessed on April 12, 2016.

20. *Grade Definitions*. U.S. Preventive Services Task Force. October 2014. http://www.uspreventiveservicestaskforce.org/Page/Name/grade-definitions. Accessed on April 12, 2016.

21. *Final Recommendation Statement: Abnormal blood glucose and type 2 diabetes mellitus: screening*. U.S. Preventive Services Task Force. December 2015. http://www.uspreventiveservicestaskforce.org/Page/Document/RecommendationStatementFinal/screening-for-abnormal-blood-glucose-and-type-2-diabetes. Accessed on April 14, 2016.

CHAPTER 14

CLINICAL PROCEDURES

Daniel T. Vetrosky • Edward M. Sullivan

This chapter illustrates some of the common procedures performed by physician assistant (PA) students and practicing PAs. It is not designed to be all-inclusive because there are many medical and surgical procedures not covered in this chapter. It is rather a primer for PA students and a refresher for practicing PAs for the procedures commonly performed throughout medical and surgical practices. Wound care, sutures, wound closures (including anesthetics used), wound dressing, universal precautions, and commonly performed procedures are covered. Words of advice for PA students include a willingness to learn any procedure presented during your education and volunteer to assist if you are not asked to perform the procedure. The old adage "see one, do one, teach one" holds quite true during your education and subsequent practice. The information within this chapter is designed to help you understand the aspects of performing these procedures.

The ability to perform clinical procedures is a necessary skill for PA students and practicing PAs alike. Procedures often provide valuable information that may aid in the diagnosis and treatment of a patient's disease. No matter how routine and uncomplicated a clinical procedure may seem to a health care provider, it must always be regarded as a unique and personal experience for the patient.

Preparing the patient for the procedure both mentally and physically presents a challenge to all health care providers. Preparation skills must be developed and applied often. The PA must have a complete understanding of the procedure to be performed, including the indications and contraindications, a command of the anatomy involved, an attention to detail, and an awareness of the goal that is to be accomplished by each procedure.

A majority of all clinical procedures are painful in some way to the patient. Many times, the patient's ability to cope with a procedure lies in the sure hands of the clinician. A positive, gentle manner combined with thoroughness in the explanation will instill confidence in the patient, as well as in the other health care providers assisting with the procedure. A patient who has a complete understanding of what is to be accomplished is much more likely to cooperate with specific requests and is better prepared to handle any difficulties that may be encountered. Finally, no matter how many times a PA student or PA may have performed a clinical procedure, he or she must keep in mind that it may be the first time for the patient and that the better prepared the patient is, the more satisfying the outcome will be.

WOUNDS AND THEIR TREATMENT

Any consideration of an invasive clinical procedure must begin with an understanding of wounds and their healing process. This chapter provides only a brief overview of wounds because a detailed explanation of the pathophysiology is beyond the scope of this discussion. The resource list at the end of the chapter provides sources for more comprehensive study and an in-depth discussion of specific types of wounds.

Definitions

A *wound* can be defined as any break in the normal anatomical relationship of tissues. Wounds can be classified as *internal* (those inside the skin) and *external* (those involving the skin). This chapter concentrates on external wounds because of their relationship to the performance of clinical procedures.

Wounds caused by any clinical or surgical procedure are classified, according to degree of contamination and risk for infection, as clean, clean-contaminated, contaminated, or dirty, as follows:

- *Clean:* A clean wound is typically a surgical incision made under sterile conditions. Clean wounds are generally considered to be relatively new wounds, meaning that they are less than 12 hours old. For the most part, wounds caused by clinical procedures are performed under sterile conditions and therefore can be considered clean.
- *Clean-contaminated:* A wound that begins as a clean wound but has experienced a potential source of contamination is clean-contaminated. One example is the opening of the colon during a bowel anastomosis. In this case, special precautions should be initiated to prevent spillage.
- *Contaminated:* A contaminated wound may have begun as a clean wound or may have been made under nonsterile conditions and has a greater incidence of infection. Some examples are a knife or glass laceration; the bowel opened during an operation with spillage of the contents into the surrounding sterile tissue; and the opening of an abscess, whether accidentally or by design, without containment of the enclosed infected material.
- *Dirty:* A dirty wound presents with an established infection—for example, a soft tissue abscess.

Wound Healing

Wounds heal by forming scars. The process of forming scars is traditionally divided into three main phases:
1. Inflammatory phase, including hemostatic factors

2. Proliferative phase
3. Maturation phase

Inflammatory Phase

Wound healing begins immediately after an injury has occurred to otherwise normal tissue. The inflammatory phase, which usually lasts for 2 to 4 days, serves to cleanse the wound of dead tissue and foreign objects by a sequence of physiologic and biochemical events, beginning with an immediate vasoconstriction to minimize blood loss. This vasoconstriction is brief and is followed by a histamine-induced vasodilatation and a migrating of leukocytes into the wound. The polymorphonuclear neutrophils (PMNs) and mononuclear leukocytes are the source for many of these mediators of the inflammatory response. The primary role of the PMNs and monocytes is to debride the wound of any foreign material. Serum enters the wound from gaps between endothelial cells, aiding the activation of platelets, kinin, complement, and prostaglandin components of the clotting cascade.

Hemostatic Factors

The hemostatic factors of wound healing are all activated immediately after the injury. One of the first is the *activation of platelets*, which adhere to one another and to the edges of the wound, forming a plug that attempts to cover the wound. This plug or clot soon retracts and stops the loss of blood. The kinins are a group of polypeptides that influence smooth muscle contraction, which may induce hypotension. Additionally, they increase the permeability of small blood capillaries, serving to increase the amount of blood flow, which in turn increases the amounts of other hemostatic factors previously mentioned.

Complements are other hemostatic factors whose main job is to produce bacteriolysis and hemolysis by accumulating fluid within the cells, causing them to eventually rupture. *Prostaglandin* acts to increase vasomotor tone, capillary permeability, smooth muscle tone, and the aggregation of platelets. *Fibronectin* aids in the migration of neutrophils, monocytes, fibroblasts, and endothelial cells into the wound and promotes the ability of these cells to adhere to one another, creating a framework of fibrin fibers. Fibronectin is found in abundance within the first 48 hours, gradually decreasing as protein synthesis begins to produce the collagen fibers that will eventually be the scar. The wound appears red and swollen and is painful and warm to the touch during the inflammatory phase, which typically lasts about 4 days. Accordingly, it is difficult to distinguish from an early wound infection at this time.

Fibroblastic or Proliferative Phase

The second phase of wound healing can begin only when the wound is covered by epithelium. This phase begins on or about the fourth day after an injury and continues alongside the maturation phase. An injured patient must have a normal amount of circulating calcium (Ca), platelets, and tissue factor before the second phase can begin. If these three substances are present as blood is exposed to air, prothrombin will be converted to thrombin. Thrombin acts as a catalyst in the conversion of fibrinogen to fibrin fibers, which stabilize the clot.

Fibroblasts are normally located in the perivascular tissue, and when they get into the wound, they produce several substances essential to wound repair, ending with the formation of collagen fibers. *Collagen* is the principal structural protein found in tendons, ligaments, and fasciae. Arranged in bundles, it strengthens and supports these tissues. Collagen levels rise continuously for approximately 3 weeks and have a negative feedback mechanism related to the number of fibroblasts found in the wound. As collagen increases, the number of fibroblasts decreases, eventually causing a decrease in the production of collagen. The rapid gain in tensile strength during this phase is directly related to the remodeling of collagen from a randomly arranged fiber mesh to a more organized formation of fibers that respond to the local stress found at the wound site.

At this stage, although it is less swollen, inflamed, and painful, the wound may look its worst. The scar may appear beefy red and may feel hard and raised. This is normal and should be expected. If the wound remains painful and inflamed at this stage of the healing process, however, some foreign material may have been retained, and reexploration may be warranted.

Maturation Phase

During this third phase of wound healing, metabolic activity remains high, but there is no increase in collagen production. This phase is sometimes referred to as the "remodeling phase" because of the rearrangement of the collagen fibers from their initial haphazard appearance after production to one of more organization. This pattern is determined by the anatomical location of the wound and the amount of stress placed on the skin and the scar at that location.

This phase usually begins at 3 weeks and can be active for 9 to 12 months, depending on the health status of the person. The appearance of the scar becomes less conspicuous as it begins to flatten out and fade and gradually begins to resemble normal skin tissue. The scar becomes more supple and more permanent as the cross-links of collagen are reorganized.

Factors That Affect Wound Healing

The health of an individual can greatly affect the time involved in the healing of a wound. Proper wound closure is paramount to the successful healing of an injury, but many other factors influence this process. The surgical technique, the type of injury, the degree of contamination, and the health status and biochemical makeup of the patient all play important roles in the final outcome of an injury. Suturing and other techniques of wound closure are discussed later in the chapter, but first, some consideration of the biochemical factors and the health status of an individual with a wound are warranted. Some of the factors that directly relate to the healing process are as follows:

- *Oxygen:* Fibroblasts are closely related to the partial pressure of oxygen (PO_2) in the circulating blood. A PO_2 of less than 30 mm Hg severely retards the healing process by lowering the production of collagen in the cytoplasm of the fibroblast. Disease processes such as small vessel atherosclerosis, chronic infection, and diabetes mellitus can be greatly affected by the oxygen delivery system.
- *Hematocrit:* There must be an adequate supply of hemoglobin in the blood to carry oxygen to the tissues.
- *Steroids (antiinflammatory):* Steroids slow the inflammatory phase of the healing process by inhibiting macrophages and fibrogenesis.
- *Vitamin C:* Vitamin C is important to the maturation process of fibroblasts.
- *Vitamin E:* In large doses, vitamin E can decrease the tensile strength of a wound by lowering the accumulation of collagen.
- *Zinc:* Epithelial and fibroblastic proliferation is slowed in patients exhibiting a low serum zinc level.
- *Antiinflammatory agents:* Aspirin and ibuprofen decrease collagen synthesis in a dose-related fashion.
- *Age:* Both tensile strength and wound closure rates decrease as a person ages.
- *Mechanical stress:* Wounds involving the skin over joints, where the stresses are greatly increased by

normal usage, take longer to heal. The delay is caused by the constant stretching and tearing of the collagen mesh, which results in reinitiating the entire wound-healing process.
- *Nutrition:* Poor nutrition results in absence of the essential building blocks of protein for collagen production, prolonging the inflammatory phase and inhibiting fibroblasia. Glucose supplies energy for leukocytes to function. Fats are necessary for synthesis of new cells.
- *Hydration:* A well-hydrated wound, not a wet wound, epithelializes faster than a dry wound. Keeping a wound covered by a dressing enhances the humidity of the wound and speeds the healing process.
- *Environmental temperature:* Wound healing time is shortened by environmental temperatures greater than 30°C. Wound healing time can decrease as much as 20% in temperatures of 12°C or less, owing to vasoconstriction and lowering of the capillary blood supply.
- *Denervation:* Denervated skin is less susceptible to local temperatures and more prone to ulceration. Patients with paraplegia develop massive, rapidly destructive ulcers that can be five times worse than those in patients with intact nervous systems.
- *Infection:* The ability of local tissue defenses to cleanse the wound is greatly diminished by a larger number of pathogenic organisms. Infection prolongs the inflammatory phase of the healing process.
- *Idiopathic manipulation:* Overhandling and rough handling of tissue by health care providers along with tight sutures can result in tissue ischemia and poor healing.
- *Chemotherapy:* Anticancer drugs decrease the fibroblast proliferation.
- *Radiation therapy:* Acute radiation injury is manifested by stasis and occlusion of small vessels, resulting in the formation of ulcers at the point of ischemia.
- *Diabetes mellitus:* Defective leukocyte function and microvascular occlusion may occur secondary to hyperglycemia in diabetes mellitus. High glucose levels interfere with the ability of cells to transport ascorbic acid, resulting in a decrease in the production of collagen.

Wound Anesthesia

Anesthesia is used in a number of different ways. The most common is *local*, whereby just the area around the wound is anesthetized. A *hematoma block* is local anesthetic injected directly into a hematoma. This is primarily used in fractures in which there is some internal bleeding around the fracture site. The anesthetic is allowed to filter throughout the surrounding tissue and fracture site. When an adequate amount of anesthesia has been achieved, the fracture can be set. A *field block* is the injection of an anesthetic around a given surgical operative site. A *nerve block* targets a specific nerve at a distant site from the area of the proposed surgery. A *digital block* administered at the base of the involved finger or toe is used to numb an entire digit. This is especially useful when a laceration of a finger or toe is massive and a local infiltration would result in increased swelling and a more difficult closure. Injection of the anesthetic on both sides of the affected digit will provide effective anesthesia to the area. Last, a *regional block* is used to anesthetize a large specific area; for instance, an epidural block (regional) allows the parturient patient to remain awake during the delivery of her child. A digital block may be referred to as a regional block in some instances. Regional blocks may affect the motor activity of the affected area.

The properties of the ideal local anesthetic are few and simple. It must be easy to administer and have a rapid onset. Its effect must last as long as needed for a given procedure, and it must dissolve completely, with no adverse effects or toxic effects either locally or systemically. Local anesthetics work by blocking depolarization of a nerve impulse. Of the numerous anesthetic agents available on the market today, lidocaine is probably the most widely used for local anesthesia. It is manufactured in a variety of solutions, but the two most commonly used for local anesthesia are 1% and 2%. One percent lidocaine works well in blocking pain stimuli while leaving the sensations of touch and pressure relatively intact. Two percent lidocaine usually blocks all stimuli from a wound area.

Two other agents, procaine hydrochloride (Novocain) and bupivacaine hydrochloride (Marcaine), are well known and warrant some discussion. Novocain has a rapid onset, usually about 4 to 7 minutes, and lasts approximately 1 hour. Lidocaine has an equally rapid onset but may last approximately 3 hours. Marcaine takes longer to reach its anesthetic level but lasts up to 10 hours. Choosing the right anesthetic for the wound takes a significant amount of skill that is developed with years of wound evaluation and experience. The clinician must also be aware of the possible complications involved in the use of these agents. Some general rules to avoid any complications are of value, and the safety of the patient should always be of primary concern, as with the use of any medication.

Use the least amount of local anesthetic to gain the maximum amount of anesthesia for a given wound.

Almost all the local anesthetic agents give the patient a sensation of burning on injection. Before injecting, explain to the patient that this is a normal response. When injecting, go slow and wait for some of the anesthetic effects of the agent to begin working before continuing.

Always aspirate when attempting to inject an agent into the body. If there is a blood return, remove the needle and apply local pressure to ensure hemostasis.

Be aware of the signs of an allergic reaction, such as wheezing, hives, and hypotension. Always be prepared to support the airway with ventilations if necessary. Although a true allergic reaction to lidocaine is rare, extra precautions should be taken if the patient reports any history of this type of allergy.

Be aware of the maximum dosages allowable for local anesthetic medications. The toxic dose of plain lidocaine is 7 mg/kg when it is administered over 1 hour. The common side effects that are associated with lidocaine toxicity include blurred vision, tinnitus, and tremors. Cardiac side effects can also occur, including heart block and a decrease in cardiac output.

The last area for potential complications concerns local anesthetics that contain a vasoconstrictive agent. Epinephrine, in concentrations of 1:100,000 or 1:200,000, is most commonly used to prolong the effects of the local anesthetic. Because of its vasoconstrictive action, it may also be used to control or decrease bleeding. It is this use for which the potential for complications arises. The local anesthetics that contain epinephrine should *never* be used in areas of the body that have terminal vasculature, such as the ears, tip of the nose, fingers, penis, and toes. The vasoconstricting action can lead to tissue death and gangrene in such areas. There is also a higher potential for wound infection because prolonged vasoconstriction delays the highly effective cleansing agents from entering the wound. Adherence to meticulous hemostasis is also important under these conditions to control the potential for increased bleeding after the effects of epinephrine wear off.

The anesthetics mentioned in this discussion are easy to use and readily available. The resource list at the end of this chapter provides in-depth studies of these agents.

Sutures

Numerous types and sizes of suture materials are available. A variety of different sutures may be used to adequately repair any given wound. The selection of suture material depends on the type of wound (clean vs. contaminated), the location of the wound (face vs. arm or leg), and the personal preference of the clinician. The following discussion provides some general principles to help in the selection of a dependable suture for a specific area of the body and a specific type of wound.

Suture Types

Sutures can be divided into two categories, absorbable and nonabsorbable. Absorbable sutures may be either *natural* (e.g., plain catgut, chromic catgut) or *synthetic* (e.g., polyglycolic acid [Vicryl or Dexon], polydioxanone [PDS]). Nonabsorbable sutures may be either *multifilament* (e.g., silk, cotton) or *monofilament* (e.g., nylon, polypropylene [Prolene], stainless steel wire).

When evaluating a wound for primary closure, the clinician must keep in mind the ideal qualities of a suture and must choose the most appropriate suture for each particular wound. The ideal suture:
- Maintains adequate tensile strength until its purpose is served
- Causes minimal tissue reaction
- Does not serve as a nidus for infection
- Is nonallergenic
- Is easy to handle and tie
- Holds knots well
- Is inexpensive
- Is easily sterilized

Absorbable sutures should be used when the suture needs to function for a short time and cannot be recovered when its use is completed, as for the inner layer of a bowel anastomosis. The suture serves only to approximate the mucosa and to assist in temporary hemostasis until the body's hemostatic mechanism can secure permanent hemostasis and wound closure. The suture used most often for this type of anastomosis is catgut. Absorbable catgut sutures, which are obtained from the small intestine of cattle or sheep, generate an inflammatory response within the wound that eventually leads to their absorption. Plain catgut sutures lose approximately 50% of their initial tensile strength in just 7 days. Chromic tanning of plain catgut (chromic catgut), on the other hand, prolongs the absorptive time and the life of this suture to about 3 weeks. The synthetic absorbable sutures (Vicryl, Dexon) do not generate as extensive an inflammatory response as catgut suture material. Their chief advantage is their uniform loss of tensile strength. Research has shown that these sutures lose their strength at a steady rate for about 21 days, at which time they have no residual benefit.

Silk, throughout the years, has been the most commonly used nonabsorbable suture. It is easily

obtained at a lower cost than the monofilaments and is comfortable to work with. Additionally, it holds knots securely. The major disadvantages of using silk include the following:
1. The tissue reaction it stimulates, which, although less than that produced by catgut sutures, is more than that of the synthetic monofilaments
2. It is a multifilament suture that may be associated with an increased risk for inflammation.[1]

A multifilament suture is made of many filaments or fibers intertwined, producing numerous interstices (spaces between the fibers) that, when contaminated with bacteria, serve as a continuous nidus for infection. The interstices are small enough to deter body host defenses but large enough for bacteria to multiply. Cotton suture has the same advantages and disadvantages as silk; however, cotton is slightly weaker than silk initially but maintains its tensile strength in the tissue for a longer period.

Monofilament sutures (nylon, polypropylene [Prolene], poliglecaprone [Monocryl] stainless steel wire) share the advantages of prolonged high tensile strength, low tissue reaction, and lack of interstices. Their chief disadvantages are difficulties for the clinician in handling and tying knots. More throws (seven or eight) are required in a single knot to maintain its security. The monofilaments are also more expensive and are less readily available than silk and cotton.

Suture Sizes

Suture sizes are graded by a number or a zero (e.g., 2, 1, 0, 00 [2-0], 000 [3-0], 0000 [4-0], 00000 [5-0], and so forth); the more zeros, the smaller the diameter of the suture material. Whereas the larger sizes (2, 1) are used for heavier work (i.e., closing fascia layers or placing retention sutures in the abdomen), the smallest sutures (9-0 or 10-0 and smaller) are used exclusively in microvascular surgery.

Choice of Suture

The question remains: What type of suture should be used? Because of the numerous types and sizes of sutures available to the clinician, the choice of sutures for each specific purpose reverts to personal preference and wound closure experience. Because many possible different sutures can be used to close a wound, Table 14.1 is supplied as a general guide for novices in choosing the type of suture according to the anatomical location of the wound.

TABLE 14.1 Suture Size and Type According to Wound Location

Location of Wound	Suture Size	Suture Type
Skin		
Face	5-0, 6-0	Nylon
Hands	4-0, 5-0	Nylon
Scalp	3-0, 4-0	Nylon
Extremities, abdomen	3-0, 4-0	Nylon
Subcutaneous tissue	3-0, 4-0	Vicryl, Dexon
Fascia	0	Prolene
	2-0	Stainless steel wire
	0	Surgilon
Peritoneum*	2-0, 3-0	Vicryl, Dexon
Bowel anastomosis		
Inner layer	3-0, 4-0	Catgut
Outer layer	3-0, 4-0	Silk, propylene

*The peritoneum is usually included with fascia.

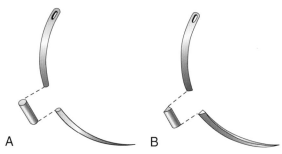

FIG. 14.1 ■ **A,** Tapered needle. **B,** Cutting needle.

Suture Needles

Two basic types of needles are used with suture material in surgery, tapered and cutting (Fig. 14.1). A *tapered needle* has a sharp point and a round body. Tapered needles are less traumatic to the tissues than cutting needles. *Cutting needles* are beveled and have sharp, knifelike edges that make them well suited for skin sutures. A general rule is that cutting needles are used for skin suturing, and tapered needles are used for most other tissues.

Sutures come prepackaged with a label indicating the size, type, and length of the suture and the type and size of the suture needle. Labels are usually color coded according to the type of suture material contained.

Skin sutures should be removed when they have fulfilled their purpose. The longer sutures remain, the more inflammatory the response they generate, which ultimately results in a larger, more noticeable scar. The clinician must weigh the odds of creating an unsightly scar against the chance of a wound dehiscence if the sutures are removed prematurely. The following is a guideline for when to remove sutures according to location:

Face: 3 to 4 days
Scalp: 5 to 7 days
Trunk: 6 to 8 days
Extremities: 7 to 14 days; longer for areas under maximal tension

Wound Closure

Wounds, however they are created, require proper and timely attention to facilitate the best possible outcome. A few general principles can aid in deciding on the best approach for wound closure. Determining the cause of the wound and the possibility of contamination is important. Surgical wounds are almost always closed primarily because of the controlled atmosphere in which they are created. Acute, accidental wounds need much more evaluation before treatment. Often the decision focuses on the size and shape of a wound and the degree of contamination suspected.

Historically, there are three methods of treating wounds, and timing is the most critical aspect to consider when choosing among them.

Primary Closure

The immediate suturing, stapling, or taping of a wound yields the best possible outcome with minimal scarring (Fig. 14.2). Two factors to consider in deciding whether a wound can be closed primarily are the amount of tissue loss and the degree of contamination. Clean surgical wounds fall into this category, as well as lacerations from sharp objects, such as a glass, knife, or sharp piece of metal, in which there is almost no tissue loss and contamination is minimal. Generally, an accidental wound is not closed primarily if it is more than 8 hours old. In instances in which the wounds are in areas with a good vascular supply (i.e., the face and scalp), wounds can still be closed if more than 8 hours old, although each patient needs to be evaluated on an individual basis to determine whether it is appropriate to close primarily.

Delayed Primary Closure

The wound is left open, usually because of a significant amount of bacterial contamination. Through

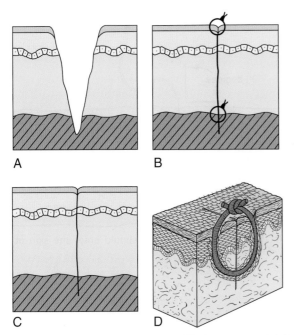

FIG. 14.2 ■ Primary wound closure. Closing a wound primarily—within the first 8 hours—will yield the least possible scarring. **A,** Simple laceration. **B** and **D,** Correct placement of a simple interrupted stitch. **C,** The best possible result of a laceration closed primarily. (**A** and **C** from Westaby S. *Wound Care.* St. Louis: CV Mosby; 1986; **D** from Schultz BC, McKinney P. *Office Practice of Skin Surgery.* Philadelphia: WB Saunders; 1985.)

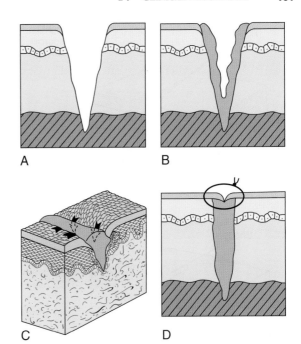

FIG. 14.3 ■ Delayed primary closure results in a larger and more noticeable scar. **A,** Simple laceration. **B** and **D,** The laceration is allowed to granulate. **C,** Correct placement of a simple interrupted stitch on the fourth or fifth day with the absence of any sign of infection. (**A, B,** and **D** from Westaby S. *Wound Care.* St. Louis: CV Mosby; 1986; **C** from Schultz BC, McKinney P. *Office Practice of Skin Surgery.* Philadelphia: WB Saunders; 1985.)

a process that is not fully understood, the wound develops a resistance to infection over the next 4 to 5 days (Fig. 14.3). This development occurs only if the wound is cleansed of all foreign material and is loosely packed with a sterile dressing. The wound is then closed by approximation of the two sides using as little suture as possible.

Healing by Secondary Intention

A wound treated by secondary intention typically involves a large amount of tissue loss or heavy contamination by bacteria. In this case, the wound closes by the process of epithelialization and contraction rather than any type of suturing (Fig. 14.4). The wound is carefully observed throughout the healing process, which may take weeks or months. To promote healing, the wounds are packed with sterile dressings that are changed daily to promote debridement of the wound. All wounds heal in this manner if they can remain free of bacteria and no fistula or sinus tract develops. The cosmetic result of this type of closure is extremely poor, however, and may require consultation with a plastic surgeon to improve the cosmetic result.

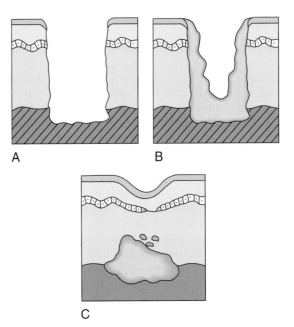

FIG. 14.4 ■ Allowing a wound to heal secondarily is usually done if there is a large amount of tissue loss or an overabundance of bacterial contamination. **A,** Wound with a large amount of tissue loss. **B,** The wound is allowed to granulate completely until epithelialization **(C)** covers the entire area, which may take weeks or months. (From Westaby S. *Wound Care.* St. Louis: CV Mosby; 1986.

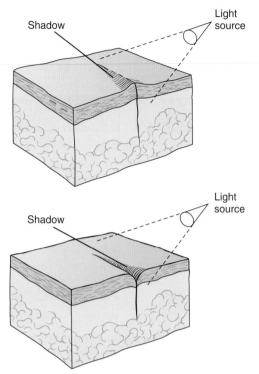

FIG. 14.5 ■ A single centralized lighting source creates a visible shadow. The least amount of scar elevation or indentation can cause a shadow.

Wound Suture

The principles of wound suturing are few and simple. Ideally, when the clinician is evaluating a wound for primary closure, he or she wants to produce the best possible result with the least amount of pain by using the most appropriate material with the least financial cost to the patient. A person's skin is his or her showcase to the world, and wounds and scars create physical changes that often affect self-image. The psychological aftermath of scars can be deeper than the wound itself. Every health care provider must be aware of how an injury has affected the patient. Clinicians can maximize cosmetic results by perfecting their techniques as much as possible. A referral to a plastic surgeon is appropriate for more complicated wounds, especially those involving the face and hands.

Two things make scars visible, color and shadows. The clinician has little control over the color of the patient's skin, but the smaller the scar, the less likely it is that a color change will occur. Shadows, however, are created by a centralized light source catching a subject at an angle. Even the smallest elevation or indentation of a scar makes it visible (Fig. 14.5). The only way for the clinician to address this concern is to make the scar as flat as possible because a flat scar leaves no shadow.

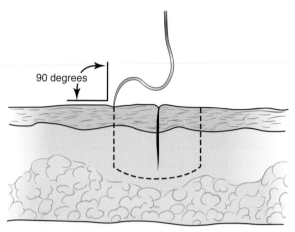

FIG. 14.6 ■ The suture needle should enter the skin at a 90-degree angle to the surface.

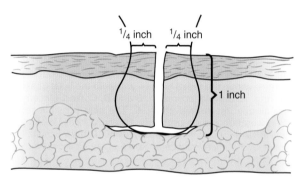

FIG. 14.7 ■ The depth of the stitch should be greater than the width. This principle will help evert the wound edges. In this example, the suture enters and leaves ¼ inch from the wound, for a total width of ½ inch; the depth is 1 inch.

First Principle

The first principle of wound repair is to close the wound in layers, making sure that each layer of skin, from the deep fascia to the epidermis, butts up against its counterpart on the other side. Perfect epithelium-to-epithelium matching and a technique called "everting of the skin edges" give the best possible result (Fig. 14.6). The key is to remove tension from the outer wound edges by placing absorbable sutures inside deep lacerations and matching them layer to layer. This arrangement supports the skin and removes any underlying abnormal pull on the skin. Correctly placed layered stitches can result in a closure that may not even need skin sutures. The skin edges are everted by making sure that (1) the depth of the stitch is greater than the width and (2) the stitch reaches the bottom of the wound.

Adherence to this principle automatically everts the skin edges (Fig. 14.7). As the suture needle is placed in the skin, it should follow a direction that is

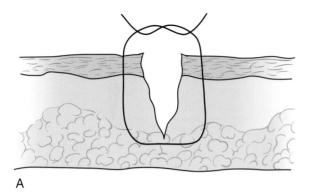

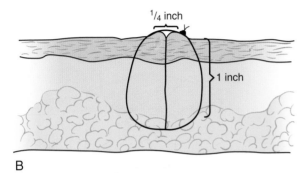

FIG. 14.8 ■ Gathering more tissue within the stitch at the base of the wound **(A)** will create the desired bottleneck effect **(B)** and aid in everting the wound edges.

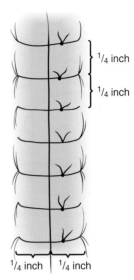

FIG. 14.9 ■ The "quarter-inch rule." Consistency in the spacing between sutures (¼ inch) and the distance of the suture from the wound edge (¼ inch) greatly enhances healing of the wound.

oblique, back, and away from the wound edge. This creates the desired bottleneck effect of the stitch in the wound (Fig. 14.8). In a wound that has been closed with this technique, the tissue will fall back into place when the sutures are removed, and the scar will eventually flatten.

Second Principle

The second principle of wound repair is to match any landmarks that are readily identifiable. Before the first stitch is placed, the wound should be inspected for the location and identification of landmarks (e.g., creases or wrinkles, birthmarks, old age spots, tan lines, hairlines, the vermilion of the lip, eyebrows, eyelids, tattoos). The first stitch should be placed in the landmark or as close to it as possible to match it precisely. Stair-step effects in linear lines, especially on the face, are visible, and extreme caution should be taken to avoid this result.

Third Principle

The third principle is the need for proper placement of the sutures. In the majority of the lacerations seen

in emergency departments (EDs), one side of the wound is longer than the other. Care must be taken in attempting to correct this imbalance. Taking more tissue between stitches on one side than on the other will create what is known as a "dog ear." To avoid a dog-ear effect, it is essential to place the sutures at the same distance along each side of the wound. In the absence of landmarks, measuring may be necessary. A good rule to follow is to measure ¼ inch down one side of the laceration from the apex, place the stitch in the skin about ¼ inch from the wound edge (Fig. 14.9), and then repeat the procedure on the other side. This method gives the most accurate closure possible.

Wound Tension

Wound tension is another aspect of suturing that must always be considered. The amount of tissue captured within a suture loop, no matter how little, creates a potential for ischemia by the overzealous use of force when the knot is tightened. The reduced capillary blood flow within the suture loop can result in tissue necrosis, prolonging the inflammatory response and potentially leading to a breakdown in healing that can result in a dehiscence of the wound. The wound edges should be brought together so that they merely touch because edema created by the inflammatory response increases the amount of tension in the suture loop. Approximating the edges so that dead space is eliminated and tension is minimal should be the goal in each wound closure.

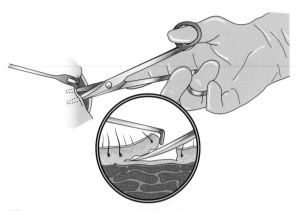

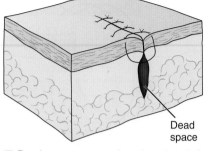

FIG. 14.10 ■ Undermining the skin at different levels releases tension on the entire wound and can give a better result.

FIG. 14.11 ■ Dead space occurs when the stitch fails to reach the base of the wound. The shallowness of the stitch leaves an open area that is an ideal nidus for bacterial growth, leading to infection. Absorbable synthetic sutures are ideal for placement in the base of the wound to eliminate any dead space.

Debridement

Occasionally, a wound may need debridement before primary closure. *Debridement* is the careful removal of dead or damaged tissue in addition to any unwarranted foreign material from the wound. This procedure should be considered when wounds, such as crush injuries, create jagged edges that have obliterated any previously existing landmarks. The goal of the clinician at this point is to create a more manageable wound that will produce a better cosmetic result and minimize the opportunity for any bacterial growth. Occasionally, the margins of a wound will be ragged and contused. The wound can be converted into a nicely incised surgical wound by excision of a 2- to 3-mm wound margin. This can be most easily accomplished by using a #15 surgical blade on a scalpel to cut into the dermis along a predetermined line that is safe to excise. Cut along the line created by the scalpel with a pair of surgical cutting scissors, excising the margins of the wound in a perpendicular fashion. After debridement of the wound, especially if the skin edges are involved, the wound may require undermining of the skin to bring the skin edges together without tension on the wound (Fig. 14.10). Do not excise tissue on the scalp or the eyebrows. This will create a prominent hairless scar.

Dead Space

Dead space occurs when a suture placed in the skin does not encompass the entire wound (Fig. 14.11). Hematomas often develop in the dead space. Hematoma is historically a great culture medium for bacteria. This happens in deep wounds in which the skin suture has not reached the full depth of the wound. In this case, deep sutures using absorbable suture material should be used to eliminate the dead space (Fig. 14.12).

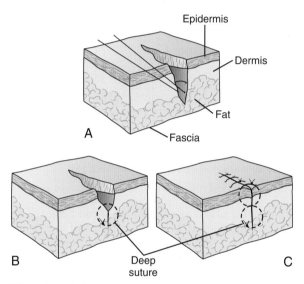

FIG. 14.12 ■ A–C, Proper placement of a deep, internal absorbable suture. Absorbable synthetic sutures are ideal for placement in the base of the wound to eliminate any dead space **(B)**. The wound is then closed primarily **(C)**.

However, caution should be taken to avoid the overuse of deep absorbable sutures because these sutures act as foreign objects, and the inflammatory response around them may result in prolonged healing or wound dehiscence. A few well-spaced deep sutures can remove the dead space and lessen the tension on the outermost layers of the wound, resulting in a minimal "good" scar that will not require revision. Additionally, use of deep sutures should be avoided in grossly contaminated wounds.

Poor Technique

What causes "bad" scars? Understanding how poor technique may cause bad scarring gives the clinician

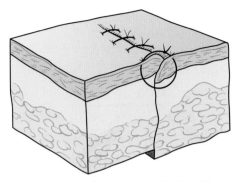

FIG. 14.13 ■ Poor technique can result in rolling of one wound edge over the other. Care must be taken to ensure that equal amounts of tissue on either side of the wound are enclosed within the stitch. The scar resulting from wound edge rolling is readily avoidable if care is taken to match the internal levels of tissue.

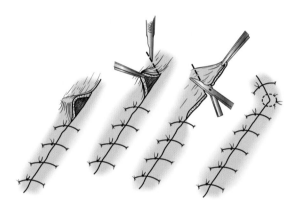

FIG. 14.14 ■ Procedure for eliminating a dog ear. See text for explanation.

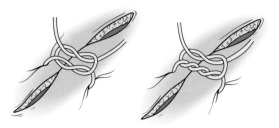

FIG. 14.15 ■ *Left,* Square knot. *Right,* Surgeon's knot.

insight as to what to avoid when closing a wound. Speed is one of the most notorious culprits in the poor results of a wound. The clinician must never sacrifice a good cosmetic result for speed. Rolling one of the wound edges is also a result of poor technique (Fig. 14.13). When one edge of epithelium is rolled under the other, the raw wound edge lying on top of the normal epithelial skin surface will not heal. When the sutures are removed, that portion of the wound will open, resulting in a much bigger scar. With proper eversion of both skin edges, scarring can be minimized. Occasionally, although diligent and adhering to these principles, the clinician will find the remains of a dog ear at the end of a procedure. Plastic surgeons use a procedure to remove the excess tissue, called a "dog-ear maneuver" (Fig. 14.14) as follows:

1. Undermine the area involving the dog ear using blunt dissection (see Fig. 14.10) between the dermal layer and the fascial layer of the skin.

2. Cut a straight line away from the apex of the dog ear, at an angle of 45 to 55 degrees, just the length of the dog ear.
3. Measure the resulting triangular piece of excess skin on that side.
4. Redrape the excess skin to determine just how much of the dog ear should be removed.
5. Cut and remove the excess tissue, and close the new wound primarily.

The basic technique of instrument-assisted wound closure is shown in Figs. 14.15 and 14.16. The key here is to be certain that the first knot laid down on the wound is a square knot. A minimum of six throws or three knots (two throws equaling one knot) should be used with each suture placed in the wound. These principles are crucial to all wound closures. They can be improved and altered as a student becomes more sophisticated in suturing. When wounds are large or have a great amount of tissue loss; however, even the most respected plastic surgeons return to these basics for initial wound closure with difficult wounds.

Special Considerations and Problems in Wound Closure

Triangular Flaps

A commonly encountered problem is a triangular flap with a sharp point. With a triangular flap, care must be taken to protect the distalmost portion of the flap, which has the most compromised blood supply. Accordingly, sutures should not be placed through the skin at the distalmost point. Rather, a stitch is placed transversely under the dermis at the tip of the flap to avoid ischemia, which could develop if sutures are placed over the skin surface. This technique is demonstrated in Figs. 14.17 to 14.20.

Poor Skin Quality

The elderly and those who have been long-term steroid users create a special situation that does not occur in the general population. Their skin is thin and fragile, and it is common to see large, avulsed

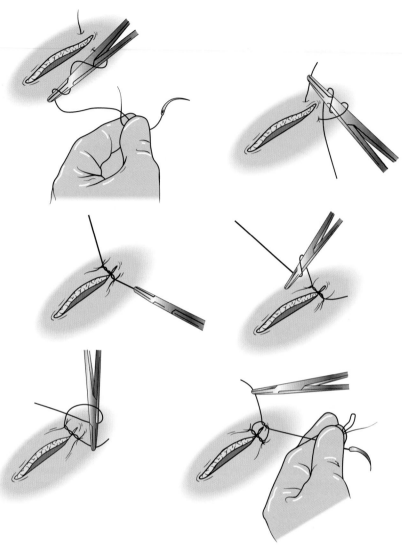

FIG. 14.16 ■ The technique of surgical instrument wound closure.

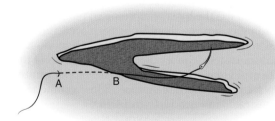

FIG. 14.17 ■ For closure of a triangular flap wound with a sharp point, pass the needle through the skin at point *A* and exit through the dermis at point *B*, which is inside the wound.

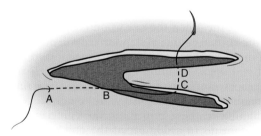

FIG. 14.18 ■ After following the procedure shown in Fig. 14.17, pass the needle transversely through the dermis at the tip of the wound flap from point *C* to point *D*, being careful to maintain the same depth of the suture on both sides of the wound.

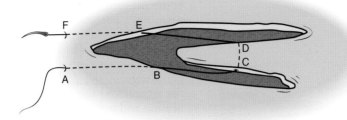

FIG. 14.19 ■ After following the steps in Figs. 14.17 and 14.18, reenter the dermis at point *E* and pass the needle out through the skin at point *F,* approximately the same distance from the wound edge as point *A*. Tie the suture in a normal fashion.

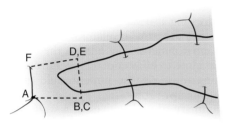

FIG. 14.20 ■ After the steps shown in Figs. 14.17 to 14.19 are completed, the entire wound is sutured closed.

flaps of this type of skin from relatively minor trauma. It is difficult to close these flaps normally because the sutures will tear through the skin, which is friable. Steri-Strips and tincture of benzoin work well. Paint the flap and surrounding skin with benzoin and allow it to dry, being careful not to get any benzoin in the wound itself. Then place the Steri-Strips on the wound, drawing the wound edges close together, and allow them to remain in position for about 3 weeks.

Contaminated Wounds

Some wounds should not be closed primarily. Lacerations of the lower leg caused by objects thrown by a *lawn mower* nearly always get infected. *Human bites* are heavily contaminated with bacteria. *Dog bites* usually involve crush injury and bacterial contamination. A dog's tooth is a blunt instrument, and the biting mechanism is such that the bite does not create a sharp incision. The first effect is to crush the tissue and then puncture it. Because of the angle of closure of the dog's jaw, a bottle-shaped defect in the tissue is created, and there is usually a tearing of the tissue as the bite is completed. Calcareous plaques from the dog's teeth may be deposited deep in the wound and act as foreign bodies. *Wounds more than 12 hours old* are frequently heavily contaminated with bacteria and should not be closed primarily. The

"golden period" for all wounds to be closed primarily is within the first 6 hours of injury.

There are two ways to deal with contaminated wounds. The first is to let the wound heal by secondary intention. This is satisfactory if the wound is small. The second option is to perform a delayed primary closure, as described previously in this chapter. These types of wounds should be anesthetized, irrigated and cleansed profusely, and then dressed. The dressing should be changed every day, and antibiotic treatment should be initiated. After 4 to 5 days, the wound should be reassessed; if there is no evidence of an infection, the wound may be reanesthetized and closed primarily. Avoid the use of absorbable sutures in a wound that is at high risk for infection because they will act like foreign bodies and decrease the resistance of the wound to infection.

The preceding guidelines can be adjusted for facial injuries because the face, with its rich vascular supply, has a high resistance to infection. The major concern here is getting the best cosmetic result. For this reason, most dog bites and wounds more than 12 hours old on the face are closed primarily. Always use antibiotic coverage in these cases.

Skin Glue

There are many skin glue products used today. All of the skin glues are a topical skin adhesive and can be thought of as superglue for the skin. It is easy to use and will leave an airtight, hard coating over the wound when applied correctly.

Skin glue is intended for topical application only to hold closed easily approximated skin edges from surgical incisions, including punctures from minimally invasive surgery, and simple, thoroughly cleansed, trauma-induced lacerations. They can be used in conjunction with, but not in place of, subcuticular sutures. Skin glue should not be used on any wound with evidence of active infection or gangrene

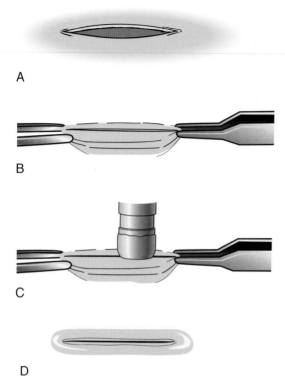

A

B

C

D

FIG. 14.21 ■ Skin glue wound closure technique. **A,** Clean open wound. **B,** Wound edge approximated by retraction with Adson forceps. **C,** Skin glue is applied to the closed wound surface. **D,** The wound is closed, and skin glue is in place.

or on wounds of decubitus etiology. It should not be used on any mucosal surfaces or across mucocutaneous junctions (e.g., oral cavity, lips) or on skin that may be regularly exposed to body fluids or with dense natural hair (e.g., scalp). Other areas to avoid with this material are high–skin tension areas such as the knuckles, elbows, and knees unless the joint will be temporarily immobilized during the healing period (see Fig. 14.21, *A* to *D*).

Dressings

A basic wound dressing consists of four parts. The first part is a nonadherent base that allows the wound to breathe while maintaining a high level of humidity over the wound. The second part is an absorbent gauze sponge that allows the wound to drain and does not obstruct the gaseous exchange that aids in wound healing. An obstructive sponge may result in the drying of the exudate, creating a new wound each time the dressing is changed. The third part is gauze wrapping that allows free movement of gases through the dressing and holds the first two parts in place.

The last part is some sort of adhesive to hold the entire dressing in place. There are several new semipermeable, occlusive, nonadherent dressings on the market. Some are more expensive than others, and the decision as to which dressing to use for a specific wound remains with the clinician's experience and knowledge of the patient. High humidity between the wound and the dressing causes rapid epidermal healing and helps prevent drying of the wound surface, thereby avoiding a "scab," which prolongs the healing process by creating a gas-impermeable state. Repeated removal and re-creation of the "scab" also slows the healing process by creating a new wound each time the scab is removed, thereby reinitiating the inflammatory phase of healing and resulting in a bigger and less cosmetic scar.

The dressing also maintains the heat of the wound by providing a thermal insulator between the wound and the environment. The heat of the wound must remain as close to body core temperature as possible. A dressing must also be impermeable to airborne microorganisms.

In summary, the objectives of a wound dressing are simple and, when they are met, the healing process can be shortened by days. These objectives are as follows:

- To maintain a high humidity between the wound and the dressing
- To remove excess exudate and toxic compounds
- To allow gaseous exchange
- To provide thermal insulation to the wound surface
- To be impermeable to bacteria
- To be free from particles and toxic wound contaminants
- To allow removal without causing trauma during dressing change

Universal Precautions

In 1987, the Centers for Disease Control and Prevention (CDC) published guidelines outlining the steps to take to guard against blood and other body fluid from patients. These guidelines, which were created to decrease infection, are known as *universal precautions.* Universal precaution guidelines address hand washing and the use of gloves, eyewear, and gowns when caring for patients. When performing clinical procedures, it is especially important to keep these guidelines in mind to protect the patient, as well as the clinician. Gloves are required whenever there will be direct contact with blood or other bodily fluids. Similarly, masks and protective eyewear (i.e., goggles or face shields) should also be used whenever there is a risk for exposure to blood or other fluids during a procedure. If a clinician anticipates an even greater exposure, wearing a gown is recommended in addition to the gloves and protective eyewear.[2]

COMMONLY PERFORMED CLINICAL PROCEDURES

This section describes some of the clinical procedures most commonly conducted in the delivery of health care. As the clinician becomes more confident and sophisticated in the ability to perform these tasks, he or she may refine or streamline individual procedures and develop preferences. Each description is simply one proven way to complete a given procedure and obtain the desired results.

Injections

Injections are used to deliver a variety of substances, including drugs, vaccinations, and skin test antigens, through the skin by means of a needle. The types of injections most commonly used are intramuscular (IM), subcutaneous (SC), and intradermal.

Intramuscular Injections

PROCEDURE FOR INTRAMUSCULAR INJECTION

1. Verify the patient and the medication.
2. Fully expose and palpate the anatomic landmarks. The muscle being injected should be at rest and should be non–weight bearing.
3. Prepare the skin with an alcohol wipe, starting at the injection site and extending outward in a circular motion, using the bull's-eye method, for about 5 cm. Allow the skin to dry completely before injection to avoid burning.[2]
4. Fill the syringe with the desired amount of fluid to be injected. (Recommended use of 3- to 5-mL syringe with an 18- to 22-gauge, 1-inch needle.)
   a. Wipe the rubber stopper of the vial of medication with an alcohol wipe.
   b. Pull the plunger of the syringe back to the mark signifying the amount of medication to be withdrawn from the vial, filling the syringe with air.
   c. Insert the needle through the center of the rubber stopper of the vial.
   d. Invert the vial.
   e. Inject air into the vial.
   f. Withdraw the desired amount of medication into the syringe, making it as free of air bubbles as possible.

   g. If medication to be administered is in an ampule: Tap the neck of the ampule to ensure that all of the medication is in the bottom of the ampule. Wrap the neck of the ampule with gauze and carefully break the neck of the ampule. Aspirate the medication from the bottom of the ampule and then remove any air from the syringe. Dispose of the ampule in the appropriate container.[2]
5. Pull the SC tissue slightly to one side.
6. Rapidly plunge the needle perpendicular (a 90-degree angle) into the surface of the skin.
7. Insert the needle to a depth of 1 inch.
8. Aspirate to ensure that the needle is not in a blood vessel. If blood returns, do not inject at this site, but withdraw the needle and apply pressure to encourage hemostasis. Repeat steps 5 and 6.
9. Inject the medication slowly.
10. Withdraw the needle and dispose of in an appropriate chamber.
11. Massage the area briefly with a gauze sponge to promote absorption.
12. Apply a self-adhesive bandage, if necessary.

Indications. Intramuscular injections are used for drugs that are not easily absorbed orally, when an intermediate rate of onset and duration of action are preferred, and when parenteral delivery is necessary.

Contraindications. Intramuscular injections should not be given at any site where a dermatitis or cellulitis exists.

Equipment. The following equipment should be assembled:
• Alcohol wipes
• Syringe of appropriate size depending on the volume to be injected.
• Needle: Selection of needle depends on the depth of insertion and the viscosity of the drug. In general, adults require a 19- to 22-gauge, 1½-inch needle. An obese patient may require a longer needle.
• Medication to be injected
• Sterile gauze sponge
• Self-adhesive bandage
• Needle disposal container

Injection Sites
Deltoid Muscle. Use the main body of the deltoid muscle, which lies lateral and a few centimeters below the acromion. Large volumes (>2 mL) and irritating solutions should not be given at this site.

Gluteal Muscle. The gluteal muscle is the most common and preferred site of injection in adults and in children older than 2 years. A large volume of solution can be injected into the muscle, and the skin over the area is thin and easily pierced. The site for injection into the gluteal muscle should always be in the upper outer quadrant of the buttock to avoid injury to the sciatic nerve and superior gluteal muscles.

Vastus Lateralis Muscle (Lateral Thigh). The vastus lateralis is the preferred injection site in infants. Although it may be used in adults, it is painful because of the firmness of the underlying fascia lata. The injection should be given into the bulk of the muscle.

Possible Complications. The following complications may occur with IM injections:
- Injection into blood vessels may cause a toxic reaction, injury to the vessel, or a hematoma.
- Injection into a deep nerve may cause pain, paresthesias, and possible permanent damage to the nerve.
- The needle may break off and become embedded in the muscle.
- Sterile and septic abscesses at the injection site may occur if equipment is not sterile, the injection site is not properly cleansed, or a site is overused.

Follow-up. No special follow-up is required.

Subcutaneous Injections

PROCEDURE FOR SUBCUTANEOUS INJECTION

1. Verify the patient and medication.
2. Fully expose the area.
3. Prepare the skin with an alcohol wipe, starting at the injection site and extending outward in a circular motion, using the bull's-eye method, for about 5 cm. Allow the skin to dry completely before injection to avoid burning.[2]
4. Fill the syringe with the desired amount of medication to be injected, usually 2 to 3 mL (see instructions for preparing medication under "Intramuscular Injections"). (Recommended use of 3-mL syringe with 24- to 26-gauge, 1-inch needle.)
5. Pinch up the SC tissue into a roll between the thumb and the forefinger to pull SC tissue away from the muscle.
6. Insert the needle with one quick motion at a 45-degree angle to the skin at the midpoint of the roll.

---

7. Advance the needle about three fourths of its length.
8. Release the roll of skin.
9. Aspirate to ensure that the needle is not in a blood vessel. If blood returns, do not inject at this site; withdraw the needle and repeat steps 4 through 7.
10. Inject the medication slowly.
11. Withdraw the needle and dispose of in an appropriate chamber.
12. Apply gentle pressure with a gauze sponge over the site.
13. Apply a self-adhesive bandage, if necessary.

Indications. Subcutaneous injections are to be used for small volumes of drugs that require slow absorption and long duration of action, such as heparin or insulin.

Contraindications. Subcutaneous injections should not be given at any site where a severe dermatitis or cellulitis exists.

Equipment. The following equipment should be assembled:
- Alcohol wipes
- Syringe of appropriate size, depending on the volume to be injected
- Needle: 25 to 27 gauge, ¾ to 1 inch
- Medication to be injected
- Sterile gauze sponge
- Self-adhesive bandage
- Needle disposal container

Possible Complications. Local reactions can occur with repeated injections over the same site.

Follow-up. No specific follow-up is required.

Intradermal Injections

PROCEDURE FOR INTRADERMAL INJECTION

1. Verify the patient and medication.
2. Fill the syringe with the desired amount of solution, usually 0.1 to 0.2 mL (recommended use of 1-mL tuberculin syringe with 27-gauge, ½-inch needle).
3. Clean the ventral surface of the forearm with an alcohol pad using the bull's-eye method. Allow the skin to dry completely before injection to avoid burning.[2]
4. Hold the skin taut between the thumb and the index finger.

---

5. Hold the needle bevel up and angle it about 10 to 15 degrees (almost parallel) to the skin.
6. Insert the needle into the dermis for about two thirds of its length.
7. Inject the solution. A wheal should form immediately.
8. Withdraw the needle. Discard the needle and gauze in an appropriate container.
9. Do not rub the injection site.[2]
10. Record the following information on the patient's chart: type of test, date and time done, and exact location of each test injection mode.

Indications. Intradermal injections are used to test for hypersensitivity to extrinsic allergens and for infection by tuberculosis, nontuberculous mycobacteria, and certain fungal infections.

Contraindications. Intradermal injection should not be given at any site where dermatitis or infection exists. Patients with a previous positive tuberculin skin reaction should not be retested.

Equipment. The following equipment should be assembled:
- Alcohol wipes
- Tuberculin syringe
- Needle: 27 gauge, ½ inch
- Medication to be injected
- Sterile gauze sponge
- Needle disposal container

Injection Sites. The ventral forearm is the most common site used. The back may be used for extensive allergen testing.

Possible Complications. Severe local skin reactions may develop in hypersensitive patients.

Follow-up. Patients should be instructed about when to return to have the skin reaction read, usually in 48 to 72 hours. If the skin reaction is positive, the diameter of the cutaneous induration should be measured and recorded.

Venipuncture

Venipuncture is one of the most frequently performed clinical procedures. It is a skill that can be learned and perfected through frequent practice to minimize patient discomfort. Venipuncture, or phlebotomy, is used to obtain blood samples for diagnostic analysis.

Phlebotomy

PROCEDURE FOR PHLEBOTOMY

1. Wash hands. Verify the patient and labs to be drawn.
2. Position the patient in a sitting or supine position to ensure comfort.
3. Inspect the patient's arms for the optimal venipuncture.[2]
4. Apply the tourniquet 2 to 3 inches above the antecubital fossa (or other venipuncture site) so that it may be removed quickly with one hand. Do not apply the tourniquet too tightly, to avoid causing patient discomfort and blood stasis. The tourniquet should be removed if cyanosis is observed in the arm. In general, it should not remain on for longer than 1 minute.
5. Select the vein site. Palpate and trace the path of the vein with the index finger or use one of the methods previously described.
6. Cleanse the skin with the alcohol pads and allow the area to dry.
7. Put on gloves.
8. Grasp the patient's arm firmly with the nondominant hand, and stabilize the vein using the thumb to anchor the vein by drawing the skin taut.
9. Insert the needle, bevel up, under the skin at an angle of 15 to 30 degrees with a quick motion. A sensation of resistance will be felt followed by ease of penetration as the vein is entered.
10. Transfer the blood as required by equipment chosen.
    a. If using a syringe, withdraw the desired amount of blood into the syringe.
    b. If using a Vacutainer system, hold the Vacutainer needle and unit steady with the hand used to do the venipuncture. Push the vacuum tube forward onto the needle, and look for the inflow of blood into the Vacutainer. Allow the tube to fill until the blood flow ceases. Remove the tube from the holder. If multiple tubes are needed, insert the next tube into the holder, and repeat the procedure. The shutoff valve automatically covers the butt end of the needle, stopping blood flow until the next tube is inserted.
    c. If using a butterfly catheter, remove the cap at the end of the tubing, and attach a syringe. Withdraw the required amount of blood into the syringe.
11. Release the tourniquet.
12. Place a sterile gauze pad just above the venipuncture site.
13. Remove the needle quickly and smoothly, and slide the gauze down to the site with a moderate amount of pressure. Maintain pressure until bleeding has ceased.

14. Apply a self-adhesive bandage.
15. If a syringe was used, fill the appropriate tubes by puncturing the rubber stopper of the tube with the needle and allowing vacuum to fill the tubes.
16. If using tubes containing an additive, mix them immediately by gently inverting them 10 to 12 times each.
17. Make sure all tubes are properly labeled.
18. Used needles should not be recapped but should be disposed of directly into an appropriate needle disposal container, which should be readily available.

Indications. Phlebotomy is used to obtain blood samples for laboratory analysis and to remove blood in the treatment of polycythemia.

Contraindications. Phlebotomy should not be performed if there is evidence of phlebitis, cellulitis, lymphangitis, scarring, recent venipuncture, or venous obstruction at the proposed site of venipuncture. Phlebotomy should not be performed in the same arm in which an intravenous (IV) line is positioned because the IV fluids may dilute the specimen and interfere with the laboratory results.

Equipment. The following equipment should be assembled:
- Tourniquet
- Alcohol pads
- Disposable latex gloves
- Vacutainer needle holder or syringe (5, 10, or 20 mL)
- Vacutainer needle or a 20-gauge needle for the syringe. If a large amount of blood is to be drawn, it is best to use an 18-gauge needle. Needles smaller than 22 gauge should be avoided because the blood sample tends to hemolyze in the small bore. A butterfly needle may be necessary for small veins.
- Properly labeled Vacutainer tubes
- Sterile gauze pads
- Self-adhesive bandage
- Needle disposal container
Important: Know which specific tests are to be collected so that the proper tubes are available.

Site Selection. The arm is the best site for phlebotomy, especially in the antecubital fossa (Fig. 14.22). The superficial veins of the arm are more easily observable and accessible, distinct, and palpable. Size, elasticity, and distance below the skin determine vein selection. In general, the most easily palpable vein, even though it may not be the most visible, should

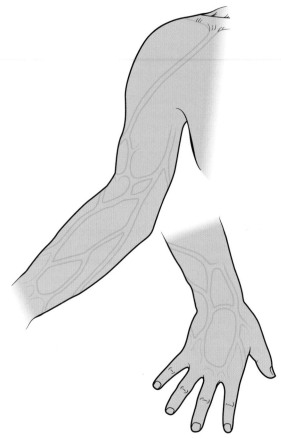

FIG. 14.22 ■ Arm and hand anatomy most commonly used for venipuncture.

be selected for phlebotomy. To aid in selection of a vein, the clinician can:
- Apply the tourniquet first to observe for a suitable vein.
- Have the patient open and close the fist to help pump blood from muscles into the superficial veins.
- Lower the extremity to a dependent position.
- Apply warm, wet towels over the area to encourage venous dilation.
- Gently tap repeatedly over the vein with the tips of the fingers to cause reflex dilation of the veins.
- When a suitable vein cannot be found in the forearm, one of the superficial veins on the dorsal surface of the hand may have to be used. These veins are small and collapse easily, so they should not be used to draw large amounts of blood.

Patient Preparation. The procedure should be explained to the patient to help reduce anxiety and elicit cooperation. The patient should be positioned comfortably with the arm resting on an even, solid surface.

Peripheral Intravenous Catheterization

PROCEDURE FOR PERIPHERAL INTRAVENOUS CATHETERIZATION

1. Verify the patient and the need for IV fluid.
2. Assemble and prepare the IV fluid and tubing. Run the fluid through the tubing to flush all air from the system and recap the end of the tubing.
3. Apply a tourniquet 4 to 6 inches above the proposed site in a way that allows quick removal. The tourniquet should be tight enough to stop venous flow but not arterial flow.
4. Select the vein to be used. The techniques used for phlebotomy can be used to help palpate and visualize a suitable vein for catheterization.
5. Palpate the course of the vein. Make sure it is long enough to accept the catheter to be used.
6. Put on gloves.
7. Cleanse the skin around the insertion site with the antiseptic sponges (i.e., alcohol or povidone-iodine).
8. Inspect the catheter-over-needle unit to ensure that the beveled tip of the metal needle is well beyond the tip of the catheter and that the catheter slides easily.
9. Anchor the vein by gently applying pressure and pulling distally with the thumb of the nondominant hand.
10. Insert the needle, bevel up, through the skin at an angle of 15 to 30 degrees, either on top or to the side of the vein. Insert the needle and the catheter into the vein. A "pop" will be felt, and blood will flow back into the hub of the needle or the "flash" chamber.
11. Advance the needle and the catheter a few millimeters until both have entered the lumen of the vein.
12. Gently and gradually advance the catheter into the vein while withdrawing the needle. Palpate the catheter through the skin as it is advanced inside the vein. Applying gentle pressure just proximal to the end of the catheter prevents blood from leaking back through or around the catheter.
13. Never reinsert the needle into the catheter because this can cause shearing of the catheter.[3]
14. Make sure the entire length of the catheter is inside the lumen of the vein.
15. Release the tourniquet and remove the needle.
16. Attach the IV tubing and check for leakage along the entire system.
17. Secure the catheter in place with tape, and apply an antiseptic or antibiotic ointment to the puncture site. Apply the transparent sterile dressing. Loop and tape the IV tubing onto the forearm to prevent accidental dislodgment of the IV catheter.
18. Label the insertion site with the catheter gauge, date and time of insertion, and initials of the person performing the procedure.

Indications. Peripheral IV catheterization is used to administer fluids, medications, blood, and blood products. In most cases, catheter placement into the vein is preferred over needle placement because a catheter lasts longer and is better tolerated by the patient. The catheter-over-needle unit (Angiocath) is the most common type used. A butterfly IV line may be preferred for patients requiring brief venous access and immediate removal of the line.

Contraindications. Catheters should never be placed where there is cellulitis, phlebitis, lymphedema, or pitting edema of the extremity. Previous mastectomy or other axillary surgery by which ipsilateral venous drainage may have been impaired is another contraindication. Hyperosmolar fluids and agents known to cause chemical phlebitis should not be administered through peripheral veins. Arteriovenous shunts should never be used for placement of routine IV lines.

Equipment. The following equipment should be assembled:
- Tourniquet
- Povidone-iodine (Betadine) antiseptic skin preparation sponges
- Tape to secure the IV line. Prepare two 4-inch lengths of ½-inch-wide tape.
- Catheter-over-needle (Angiocath) unit or butterfly needle of appropriate diameter for the rate and type of fluid to be infused (see "Catheter Selection")
- Bag of IV fluid or blood products with appropriate connecting tubing
- Disposable latex gloves
- Transparent sterile dressing, antiseptic or antibiotic ointment, and labels

Catheter Selection. Considerations in selecting the correct catheter include the size and condition of the vein and the viscosity of the fluid to be infused. The following guideline can be used:
14 to 16 gauge: Trauma or major surgery
16 to 18 gauge: Blood and blood products, administration of viscous medications

20 to 22 gauge: Most patient applications
24 gauge: Pediatric patients and neonates

Site Selection. The veins most suitable for IV therapy are found at the dorsum of the hand, the volar aspect of the proximal ulnar forearm, and the radial aspect of the forearm just proximal to the wrist (see Fig. 14.22 for venous anatomy). In general, the principles below should be followed:
- Use distal veins first.
- Use patient's nondominant arm when possible.
- Avoid veins at areas of flexion, such as the antecubital fossa.
- Select a vein that will not interfere with the patient's daily living activities.
- Select a vein that has not been used previously and is relatively straight.
- Avoid veins in the legs because there is an increased risk for complications, such as thrombophlebitis.

Patient Preparation. Explain the procedure fully to the patient to minimize anxiety and elicit cooperation. The patient should be in a comfortable position with the extremity to be used resting on a solid surface.

Possible Complications. Hematoma formation, extravasation, phlebitis, cellulitis, bacteremia, and sepsis may occur. Daily inspection of the site and aseptic technique are essential to minimize the chances of complications. IV sites should be changed every 3 to 4 days to reduce the probability of phlebitis, or they should be changed at the first signs of phlebitis or infection.

Arterial Blood Gas Sampling

Radial Artery Puncture

PROCEDURE FOR RADIAL ARTERY PUNCTURE

1. Palpate the radial artery, and perform the Allen test to assess the adequacy of the ulnar artery collateral flow to the hand (Fig. 14.23).
   a. Occlude both the radial and ulnar arteries while the patient makes a tight fist and elevates the arm.
   b. Allow the hand to blanch and lower the arm to waist level.
   c. Have the patient open the hand. Release the pressure over the ulnar artery while maintaining pressure over the radial artery.
   d. Normal skin color should return to the ulnar side of the palm within 6 seconds, with color returning to the whole palm quickly. Failure of the hand to regain color within 6 seconds signifies inadequate ulnar collateral circulation, and radial artery puncture is contraindicated.
2. Extend the patient's supinated wrist to about 30 degrees by placing a rolled towel under the wrist to bring the radial artery closer to the surface.[3]
3. Palpate the artery to determine where the pulsation is most prominent.
4. Cleanse the skin over the puncture site with the antiseptic sponges (i.e., alcohol or povidone-iodine).
5. Put on sterile gloves.
6. Anesthetize the skin over the puncture site with the 1% lidocaine. Care should be taken not to inject into the circulation.
7. Relocate the point of maximal impulse with the nondominant hand. Facing the patient, hold the syringe with the dominant hand like a pencil, bevel up.
8. Gently insert the needle through the skin at an angle of 45 to 60 degrees (Fig. 14.24). Advance the needle toward the point of maximal impulse until arterial blood returns into the syringe. The needle and syringe may be advanced until the periosteum of the radius is encountered. If blood returns, allow the syringe to fill itself.
9. If no blood is obtained, slowly withdraw the needle and syringe, and continue to observe for blood return. If this is still unsuccessful, withdraw the needle to a position just under the skin and repeat the attempt, redirecting the needle toward the point of maximal impulse.
10. Collect the desired amount of blood, and remove the needle quickly. Immediately apply direct pressure with a gauze sponge over the puncture site for 10 minutes.
11. Expel all air bubbles from the syringe. Gently roll the syringe between the fingers to mix the blood with the anticoagulant, remove the needle, and dispose of in the appropriate container. Embed the needle in a rubber stopper or place a cap on the end of the syringe, and place the syringe on ice.[3] Make sure the syringe is properly labeled and transported to the laboratory immediately.

Indications. Arterial blood gas (ABG) levels, used in a variety of clinical problems, such as an acute exacerbation of asthma or a suspected pulmonary embolus, may be determined using samples of arterial blood. ABG sampling has become an important and commonly used procedure. The most common site is the radial artery; alternative sites are the brachial and femoral arteries.

Contraindications. Poor collateral circulation in the hand, as determined by the Allen test, or no

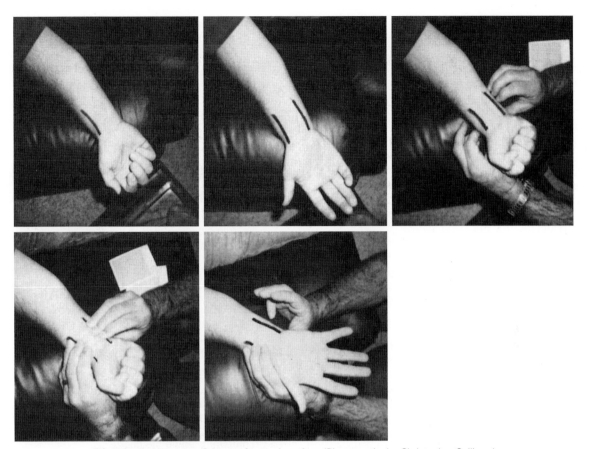

FIG. 14.23 ■ Allen test. See text for explanation. (Photographs by Christopher Sullivan.)

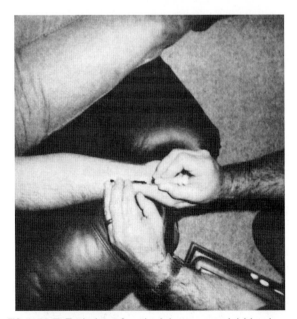

FIG. 14.24 ■ Technique for obtaining an arterial blood gas sample from the radial artery. The needle should enter the skin, bevel up, at an angle of 45 to 50 degrees. (Photograph by Christopher Sullivan.)

palpable pulse in the radial artery, is an absolute contraindication. The Allen test should always be done before a radial arterial puncture (see procedure for the Allen test in box) (see Fig. 14.23). Arterial puncture should not be done over areas of cellulitis or local infection. It is relatively contraindicated in patients with bleeding disorders and patients on anticoagulant and thrombolytic therapy. When essential to management, arterial puncture should be done into the radial artery, with careful monitoring and prolonged postpuncture compression.

Equipment. A prepackaged blood gas sampling kit may be used, or assemble the following:
• Glass or plastic syringe, 3 to 5 mL
• Plastic syringe, 3 to 5 mL, containing 1% lidocaine without epinephrine
• Two needles, 25 gauge, ½ inch
• Heparin, 10,000 U/mL solution, 1 mL
• Povidone-iodine (Betadine) skin preparation spon-ges
• Rubber stopper or a cap for the syringe
• Rolled towel
• Crushed ice

- Sterile gauze sponges
- Sterile gloves

If not using a prepackaged blood gas sampling kit, the syringe to collect the specimen should be heparinized first.[3]

Preparation of the Syringe. To heparinize one 5-mL glass (or plastic) syringe and 25-gauge needle, withdraw 0.5 mL of heparin into the syringe. Hold the syringe with the needle up, pull the plunger to the end of the syringe, and expel all the heparin through the needle. This procedure leaves an adequate amount of heparin in the syringe and needle. Too much heparin left in the syringe gives an artificially low pH.

Patient Preparation. Explain the procedure to the patient to facilitate patient cooperation and reduce anxiety. Tell the patient to expect some discomfort and pain. It is important that the patient keep as still as possible.

Possible Complications. Hemorrhage or hematoma may occur at the puncture site, causing vascular compromise. Hematoma formation can be avoided by providing pressure on the puncture site for 10 minutes after the procedure. Transient spasm may also occur. Thrombosis at the puncture site can lead to ischemia or gangrene of the hand or fingers. Accordingly, the patient should be instructed to notify the physician or PA if the hand becomes numb, painful, cold, or blue. A consultation with a vascular surgeon should be arranged immediately if arterial flow is compromised in any way.

PROCEDURE FOR FEMORAL ARTERY PUNCTURE

Although many believe that femoral artery puncture is the easiest to obtain, it should still be used only when radial arterial blood cannot be obtained. The close proximity of the femoral vein makes inadvertent venous sampling common. There is also a risk for embolization to the distal extremity. Postpuncture bleeding that is undetected can occur. The technique used for femoral artery puncture is similar to that for radial and brachial artery puncture, except for anatomical considerations. The differences in procedure are as follows:

- The patient should be in a supine position with the hip extended and slightly externally rotated. The femoral artery can be palpated just distal to the inguinal ligament in the groin.
- The needle should be inserted perpendicular to the skin surface.

Possible Complications. The possible complications in femoral artery puncture are essentially the same as for radial artery puncture. Any signs of vascular compromise seen in the leg, foot, or toes should prompt an immediate consultation with a vascular surgeon.

Lumbar Puncture

PROCEDURE FOR LUMBAR PUNCTURE

1. Put on the mask, protective eyewear, and sterile gloves, and prepare all equipment. Assemble the manometer and stopcock, and have the specimen tubes ready for use.
2. Position the patient on his or her side with the knees flexed upward and the neck flexed forward toward the chest. Palpate both superior iliac crests; draw an imaginary line between the two to identify the L4 to L5 interspace. Mark the spot with your fingernail or by holding pressure over the site with a pen to mark the spot.
3. Draw up the 1% lidocaine into the 5-mL syringe with the 25-gauge, ½-inch needle.
4. Cleanse and prepare the skin with the iodine solution, starting at the needle site and working outward until a wide sterile field has been prepared. Drape the back.
5. Locate the needle site, and administer the 1% lidocaine. First raise a skin wheal and then infiltrate into the deeper tissues between the spinous processes anticipating the intended track for the spinal needle.[4] Aspirate for blood return before injecting the lidocaine.
6. Hold the spinal needle between the index and middle fingers with one thumb over the stylet and the other thumb stabilizing the needle. Avoid touching the tip and shaft of the needle.
7. Introduce the needle perpendicular to the skin, and advance the needle at an angle of 15 to 20 degrees, directing the needle toward the umbilicus. The bevel of the needle should be up if the patient is in the lateral decubitus position or to the side if the patient is in the sitting position.
8. As the needle is slowly advanced, a distinct "pop" is felt as the needle penetrates through the ligamentum flavum and the arachnoid membrane. If no pop is felt, the stylet should be removed after frequent small advancements to look for CSF return. Advancement too far through the subarachnoid space will result in piercing of the ventral epidural venous plexus, with a subsequent traumatic tap.

9. If bony resistance is encountered, withdraw the needle to the SC tissue, redirect the needle more caudally, and try again.
10. When cerebrospinal fluid (CSF) begins to flow, observe the first few drops of fluid. If the CSF is bloody but it clears after a few drops, the tap was most likely traumatic. If the CSF does not clear the blood clots, replace the stylet, withdraw the needle, and reattempt at a different level. If the CSF does not clear or clot, the patient may have had a subarachnoid hemorrhage, and the CSF needs to be checked for cell counts and the presence of xanthochromia.[4] Do not aspirate because a nerve root might become trapped against the needle and cause injury.
11. Measure the opening pressure.
    a. Have the patient carefully straighten the legs to decrease intraabdominal pressure.
    b. Attach the three-way stopcock to the manometer, remove the stylet, and attach the stopcock and manometer to the hub of the needle. The lever of the stopcock should be toward the patient.
    c. Rotate the lever back toward the clinician. The CSF will fill the manometer, and the opening pressure can be measured. Normal pressure is 65 to 195 mm H_2O. If the pressure is elevated, check the patient's position to make sure it is not causing jugular or abdominal compression. CSF pressure should decrease with inspiration and increase with expiration.
12. Fill the specimen tubes with 0.5 to 2 mL per tube. Drain the CSF from the manometer into the first tube. Remove the manometer, and collect the remaining samples.
13. The first tube should be labeled for cell count and differential, the second tube for Gram staining and bacterial culture, the third for glucose and protein tests, and the fourth tube for a repeat cell count and differential or special studies. If further information is necessary, more samples should be obtained.
14. If therapeutic injection is necessary, inject the solution slowly over 30 seconds after removing at least an equivalent volume of CSF.
15. Replace the manometer and measure the closing pressure.
16. Replace the stylet and remove the needle.
17. Remove residual iodine from the skin and cover the puncture site with a self-adhesive bandage.

Lumbar puncture is an important diagnostic procedure that provides CSF from the lumbar subarachnoid space. It is used diagnostically in both emergency and nonemergency situations and is used therapeutically to give medication intrathecally.

Indications

Lumbar puncture is indicated for the following situations:
- Suspected meningitis
- Follow-up of meningitis therapy
- Suspected subarachnoid hemorrhage
- Aid to diagnosis of neurologic diseases (e.g., multiple sclerosis)
- Diagnosis and staging of neoplastic disease
- Intrathecal administration of antimicrobial or antineoplastic agents
- Administration of spinal anesthesia
- Therapeutic reduction of CSF pressure (i.e., pseudotumor cerebri)

Contraindications

Lumbar puncture is contraindicated by the presence of the following:
- Unexplained increased intracranial pressure (papilledema)
- Suspected intracranial mass lesion (e.g., tumor, abscess, hematoma)
- Suspected spinal cord mass lesion
- Local skin infection over the lumbar area
- Bleeding coagulopathy, thrombocytopenia (platelet count <50,000/cm^3) or anticoagulation therapy (relative contraindication)

Equipment

Prepackaged lumbar puncture kits contain all the equipment needed to perform the procedure. The kits should include the following essential items:
- Spinal needles, 22 and 25 gauge, with stylet
- 25-gauge, ½-inch needle
- 22-gauge, 1½-inch needle
- 5-mL syringe
- 1% lidocaine with epinephrine
- Three-way stopcock and manometer
- Sterile collection tubes (minimum of four)
- Sterile towel and barrier
- Sterile gauze sponges
- Mask, protective eyewear, and sterile gloves
- Povidone-iodine solution and materials for skin cleansing
- Self-adhesive bandage

Patient Preparation

Informed written consent is usually required unless the procedure is an emergency and the patient is confused or lethargic. To reduce anxiety and elicit cooperation, the procedure should be explained fully to the patient before it is begun.

Patient Positioning

Patient positioning is the most important step in performing a successful lumbar puncture. In most cases, the lateral decubitus position should be used. In patients with scoliosis, marked obesity, or ankylosing spondylitis, the sitting position may be more beneficial.

Lateral Decubitus Position
1. Place the patient on his or her side as close to the edge of the bed as possible.
2. The patient should lie in a fetal position with the knees pulled up toward the abdomen and the head flexed forward toward the chest. Forward flexion allows greater access to the interspaces between the spinal processes. An assistant can help support the patient in this position.
3. Put a pillow under the patient's head to keep the spinal axis parallel to the bed.
4. The patient's spine should lie along the edge of the bed, with the bed raised until the spine is at midchest level for the seated clinician.

Sitting Position
1. Have the patient sit on the edge of the bed facing away from the clinician.
2. Have the patient bend over a bedside table with the arms resting on the table and the head, knees, and hips flexed.
3. Raise the bed until the lower lumbar spine is at midchest level for the seated clinician.
4. The sitting position is preferable for obese patients.

Site Selection

The safest site to perform a lumbar puncture is at the L4 to L5 interspace because the spinal cord terminates between L1 to L2 for most adults. The L4 to L5 interspace is also the easiest to identify by drawing an imaginary line between the iliac crest. Although the L4 to L5 interspace is used most commonly, the L3 to L4 and L5 to S1 interspaces can also be used.

To facilitate locating the landmarks before prepping the skin, mark the skin with a ballpoint pen or an impression from a fingernail. The location of needle entry should be the exact midpoint of the interspace between the spinous processes.

Possible Complications

Several complications of lumbar puncture may occur, such as cerebral herniation, bloody CSF, and spinal headache.

Cerebral Herniation. A mass lesion, cerebral abscess, or increased intracranial pressure could result in cerebellar herniation through the foramen magnum upon removal of CSF. An increase in the intracranial pressure is associated with a change in the patient's mental status and evidence of focal neurological findings (i.e., a cranial nerve III palsy). When these conditions are suspected, lumbar puncture should be deferred until a more definitive evaluation can be undertaken with a neuroimaging study to avoid precipitating cerebral herniation.

Bloody Cerebrospinal Fluid. Bloody CSF may occur from a traumatic tap or a subarachnoid hemorrhage. A traumatic tap occurs when the spinal needle passes through the subarachnoid space into the ventral epidural plexus. Features that may signify a traumatic tap rather than a previous intracranial bleed are as follows:
- Normal cerebrospinal pressure
- Decline in amount of blood after several tubes have been obtained
- Decline in the red blood cell count in successive tubes
- Absence of xanthochromia
- Subsequent lumbar puncture at higher interspace, showing clear CSF

Spinal Headache. Spinal headaches are the most common complication associated with lumbar punctures and can be seen in approximately 20% of patients. The headache usually develops in the first 24 hours after the procedure. This usually occurs as a result of persistent CSF leakage through the dura or after the removal of large amounts of CSF. Using the smallest spinal needle possible and prescribing bed rest for 6 to 12 hours after the procedure usually can minimize the risk for headache. Analgesics, bed rest, and oral hydration usually relieve the symptoms.

Follow-up

The patient should be instructed to remain prone for 1 to 3 hours after lumbar puncture to minimize the risk for postpuncture headache. If headache develops, bed rest, oral analgesics, and adequate hydration are indicated. The patient should be instructed to contact a physician if the headache persists. If the headache persists beyond 24 hours despite conservative measures, a blood patch can be performed by an anesthesiologist. A blood patch is performed by slowly injecting 10 to 20 mL of the patient's blood into the epidural space at the original puncture site, effectively sealing any CSF leak. If a therapeutic agent was injected, the patient should be placed in the Trendelenburg position for 30 to 60 minutes after the procedure.

Urethral Catheterization

PROCEDURE FOR URINARY CATHETERIZATION IN MALE PATIENTS

1. Place the patient in a supine position.
2. Put on the mask, protective eyewear, and sterile gloves, and drape the genital area with the sterile towels.
3. Use the antiseptic solution to moisten the cotton swabs with povidone-iodine. Grasp the shaft of the penis with the gloved, nondominant hand; hold it at a 90-degree angle; and retract the foreskin if the patient is uncircumcised. Cleanse the glans from the meatus to the corona of the glans with downward strokes, using a new cotton swab with each stroke.
4. Lubricate the end of the catheter tip with the sterile lubricating jelly. Holding the penis at a 90-degree angle to the body, advance the catheter into the meatus; using gentle pressure, pass the catheter through the urethra and into the bladder until urine returns.
5. If the bladder is markedly distended, it should be drained gradually; generally, no more than 1000 mL of urine should be drained at a time.
6. Inflate the balloon with the sterile water. Pull on the catheter gently to ensure that the balloon is in place.
7. For uncircumcised male patients, be sure to replace the foreskin after the catheter is inserted to avoid constriction.[3]
8. Connect the catheter to the drainage bag. Tape the distal catheter to the inner aspect of the patient's thigh.
9. For patients with an enlarged prostate secondary to benign prostatic hypertrophy, direct instillation of lubricant into the urethra can facilitate passage of the catheter. Additionally, viscous lidocaine may be used to minimize discomfort. Be sure to allow a minimum of 5 minutes after injecting the lidocaine into the urethra for the benefit of the anesthetic.[3]

PROCEDURE FOR URINARY CATHETERIZATION IN FEMALE PATIENTS

1. Place the patient in a supine position with the soles of the feet together.
2. Put on the mask, protective eyewear, and sterile gloves, and drape the genital area with sterile towels.
3. Use the antiseptic packet to moisten the cotton swabs with povidone-iodine. Separate the labia with the gloved, nondominant hand. Cleanse the outside of the labia and the urethral meatus with the swabs. Stroke from anterior to posterior in a downward stroke, using a new cotton swab each time.
4. Lubricate the tip of the catheter with the sterile lubricating jelly. Insert the catheter into the urethral meatus until urine returns, and then advance the catheter another 4 to 5 cm.
5. Collect a urine specimen in the sterile cup, and let the rest of the urine drain into the basin.
6. If the bladder is markedly distended, it should be drained gradually; in general, no more than 1000 mL of urine should be drained at a time.
7. Inflate the balloon with the sterile water. Pull on the catheter gently to ensure that the balloon is in place.
8. Connect the catheter to the drainage bag. Tape the distal catheter to the inner aspect of the patient's thigh.

Indications

The insertion of a Foley catheter through the urethra to the bladder for urinary drainage is a common bedside procedure indicated for treating urinary retention, monitoring urinary output, and performing diagnostic studies.

Contraindications

Urethral disruption secondary to trauma and inability to pass the catheter through the urethra into the urinary bladder are contraindications to the procedure. Suspect a disruption to the urethra with a history of pelvic trauma and evidence of blood at the urethral meatus, the presence of perineal ecchymosis, or if the prostate is nonpalpable on examination.

Equipment

Disposable Foley catheter trays are generally available for use. The essential items are as follows:
- Foley catheter of proper size. Most adults tolerate a 16- or 18-Fr rubber catheter with a 5-mL balloon. (The larger the French number, the larger the diameter.)
- Drainage bag and connecting tube
- Sterile specimen cup
- Sterile syringe containing 5 mL of sterile water
- Sterile lubricating jelly
- Antiseptic cleansing solution (povidone-iodine) and cotton swabs
- Emesis basin or small tray to catch urine
- Sterile towels to drape the area
- Sterile gloves, mask, and protective eyewear

Types of Catheters

Robinson Catheter. Also known as a straight catheter, these catheters are designed to be used once for an "in and out" catheterization.

Coudé Catheters. This type of catheter is bent at the distalmost end to allow smoother insertion in patients who have false passages in the urethra.

Foley Catheters. This type of catheter has an inflatable balloon at the end to keep the catheter in place in the bladder.

Patient Preparation

The necessity for catheterization and the procedure itself should be explained to the patient. Female patients should be supine with both legs raised (lithotomy position). Male patients should be supine with legs flat.

Possible Complications

Infections such as cystitis, pyelonephritis, and bacteremia from long-term indwelling catheters can occur. Traumatic catheterization may cause hematuria, as can occur upon creation of a false urethral passage.

Follow-up

Routine Foley catheter care is important. Keep the urethral meatus area clean, and keep the bag below the level of the bladder to prevent gravity drainage of contaminated urine from the tube into the bladder. Removing the catheter as soon as possible will reduce the risk for infection. Make sure to deflate the balloon before removing the catheter.

Nasogastric Intubation

PROCEDURE FOR NASOGASTRIC INTUBATION

1. Put on the gloves, protective eyewear, and a gown.
2. Determine the tube length needed by measuring from the patient's ear to the umbilicus, and mark the length on the tube.
3. Lubricate the distal end of the tube with the water-soluble lubricant.
4. With the patient's neck slightly flexed, insert the tube into one of the nostrils along the nasal floor and toward the posterior pharynx. When the tip of the tube reaches the back of the throat, resistance is met, and the patient may gag.
5. Have the patient drink small sips of water through a straw, and every time the patient swallows, advance the tube. If the tube slips into the trachea, violent coughing and gagging will occur. Pull the tube back to the level of the pharynx and repeat the attempt. Do not pull the tube entirely out of the nose. The most important step is timing the advancement of the tube with swallowing.
6. Advance the tube into the stomach. Entry into the stomach can be determined when the measured mark on the tube reaches the opening of the patient's nasal passage.
7. Check for the tube's placement in the stomach by aspirating for stomach contents. Inject air down the tube while listening over the epigastrium for the sound of air bubbling into the stomach. If no sound is heard, reposition the tube and inject more air. Obtain a chest radiograph to confirm correct tube placement.
8. Secure the tube to the nose with tape and benzoin. Avoid pressure to the ala of the nose to prevent skin irritation.[3] The tube should not exert pressure or traction on the nostril when the patient moves.

The insertion of a nasogastric (NG) tube is common in both hospital and ED settings. It is an uncomfortable procedure for most patients.

Indications

Nasogastric tubes are inserted to facilitate gastric lavage, for gastrointestinal bleeding, or for treatment of drug overdose, as well as for gastric decompression in association with an ileus or an obstruction.

Contraindications

In semiconscious or fully unconscious patients, NG tube insertion should not be attempted without inserting an endotracheal tube first to prevent aspiration. Massive facial trauma or head trauma with the potential for a basilar skull fracture contraindicates NG intubation. When there is evidence of head or neck injury, obstruction of the nose, throat, or esophagus should be ruled out first. Esophageal burn, such as from the ingestion of corrosive acids or alkali and esophageal atresia or stricture, will also contraindicate insertion of an NG tube.

Equipment

The following equipment should be assembled:
• NG tube of proper diameter. Two types of NG tubes are in common use, the single-lumen tubes (Levin) and the double-lumen sump (Salem's sump) tubes. The single-lumen tubes are best for

decompression, and the double-lumen sump tube is best for continuous lavage or irrigation of the stomach. Both may be used for either purpose. Although sizes of catheters range from 10 to 18 Fr, most adults require a 16- to 18-Fr tube. The limiting factor is the size of the nostril or any deviation of the nasal septa.

- Suction syringe (30 mL) with a catheter tip
- Suction tube and suction device (wall or portable suction)
- Sterile lubricating jelly
- Glass of water and a straw
- Emesis basin
- Disposable latex gloves, goggles, and gown
- Hypoallergenic tape and benzoin

Patient Preparation

The procedure should be explained to the patient, especially the fact that introduction of the tube will produce gagging. Ask patients if they have any symptoms of nasal obstruction, and check for nasal patency to determine which side is the most open. The patient should be in a comfortable sitting position and leaning on a backrest. If the patient is unconscious, position the patient supine with the head slightly elevated. It is important that the patient maintain cervical flexion to enable the entrance to the trachea to be closed when the patient swallows and to allow the tube to enter only the esophagus.

Possible Complications

Accidental placement of the tube into the tracheal airway, aspiration pneumonia, gastric erosion with hemorrhage, and nasal mucosa erosion or alar necrosis may occur with NG intubation. Sinusitis may develop secondary to obstruction of the sinus ostia from the NG tube, which is not typically seen unless the NG tube has been in place for a prolonged time.

Follow-up

The tube should be checked to ensure proper functioning and should be removed as soon as possible. The tube should be kept lower than the nose. Avoid taping the tube to the forehead because this will cause pressure against the ala of the nose, potentially leading to skin breakdown. Proper taping of the tube and frequent monitoring of the tube placement can prevent this complication. If the tube is left in for an extended period, the nostril should be monitored periodically for signs of necrosis.

KEY POINTS

- A clear management plan for treating wounds must be in place.
- Wounds, whether intentional (as in a surgical procedure) or accidental, have common attributes and in most cases can be treated the same way.
- Knowing the anatomy, potential complications, and contraindications before performing any invasive clinical procedure is paramount for the provider and can directly affect the outcome.

References

1. Chen H, Sonnenday CJ. *Manual of Common Bedside Surgical Procedures*. 2nd ed. Philadelphia: Lippincott Williams & Wilkins; 2000.
2. Dehn RW, Asprey DP. *Clinical Procedures for Physician Assistants*. Philadelphia: WB Saunders; 2002.
3. Gomella LG, Haist SA. *Clinician's Pocket Reference*. 11th ed. New York: McGraw Hill; 2007.
4. Lawrence PF. *Essentials of General Surgery*. 4th ed. Philadelphia: Lippincott Williams & Wilkins; 2006.

The resources for this chapter can be found at www.expertconsult.com.

CHAPTER 15

GENETIC AND GENOMIC APPLICATIONS IN CLINICAL PRACTICE

Chantelle Wolpert • Constance Goldgar • Michael Rackover

FROM THE GENETIC AGE INTO THE GENOMIC AGE

Continuing research advances in molecular biology, including genomic sequencing, increases in computing power, and decreases in technology, have propelled what was the genetic age into the genomic age.[1-4] These research advances will fundamentally transform the practice of clinical medicine. This chapter provides an overview of some of these advances and explains their relevance for physician assistants (PAs) practicing in primary care or specialty settings. Relevant subtopics are reviewed, including the language of genetics and genomics, the molecular genetic basis of human disease, the utility of family history data in diagnosis, and a summary and description of various types of genetic and genomic testing currently in use. Finally, a clinical decision-making framework is presented to help PAs determine which clinical situations may benefit from testing; this clinical decision-making framework includes the basic tenets and ethical considerations frequently encountered in such testing situations. Mastery of the information in this chapter enables PAs to (1) use genetic and genomic terms with precision, (2) understand the clinical relevance of the molecular genetic characterization of human diseases, (3) use the diagnostic power of the family pedigree, (4) distinguish between the different types of genetic and genomic testing and when to use them, and (5) appreciate the value of establishing professional relationships with genetic health professionals.

Genetics and Genomics: The Language of Modern Medicine

Genetic and genomic advances have changed the language of medicine. The daily discourse of medicine is dotted with terms such as *sequencing*, *polymerase chain reaction*, and *mutations*. Therefore, understanding genetics and genomics is as important as understanding anatomy and physiology.[5] An understanding of genetic and genomics allows an ever greater level of precision when communicating with patients, colleagues, and other professionals. For instance, the words *allele* and *gene* have been used interchangeably, but they do not represent the same concept. Although humans have approximately 22,000 genes, we also have variations of these genes.[6] Variations or alternate forms of genes are called *alleles*; thus, when referring to a variant of a *gene*, the word to use is *allele*. Similarly, the word *genomic* is now routinely used. What is the difference between *genetic* and *genomic*? In general, *genetic* refers to a single allele or a mutation within an allele. In contrast, the term *genome* refers to the entirety of an organism's genetic information.[1-3] This includes the coding sequences (alleles) and the noncoding sequences—all of the nuclear DNA, mitochondrial DNA (mtDNA), and RNA. The aim of genomics is to understand the structure and function of different genomes (e.g., humans, primates, bacterial) as well as to study the interplay of different genomics in a variety of environments (see Box 15.1).

BOX 15.1 GLOSSARY: GENETIC AND GENOMIC TERMINOLOGY

Allele: Different forms of a gene are called *alleles*. Alleles are variations in the DNA sequence of a gene. For example, A and B are specific alleles for the ABO blood group gene. Allelic variants can be conceptualized similarly to a type of biological maker, such as alpha-fetoprotein or prostate-specific antigen.

Familial clustering: When two or more biological family members have the same or a similar disorder but there is no obvious mendelian pattern of inheritance.

Genes: The fundamental unit of heredity, responsible for transmitting information from one generation to the next in gametes. The coding sequences of DNA are called *genes*. Genes are referred to as *alleles* (see Allele).

Genome: The entirety of an organism's genetic information. This means the coding sequences (i.e., genes) and the noncoding sequences—all the nuclear DNA, mtDNA, and RNA.

Genomics: Aims to understand the structure and functioning of different genomes (e.g., human primates, invertebrates) as well as the interplay of different genomes with different environments.

Heterozygous: The alleles at a genetic locus are different from one another. An individual with blood type AB is heterozygous at the ABO blood group locus.

Homozygous: The alleles at a genetic locus are identical. For instance, an individual with blood type O (i.e., genotype OO) is homozygous for the O allele.

Locus: Genes and their alleles are located on all chromosomes, and the position each one occupies is called a *locus* (plural, loci). For instance, the locus for the allele for β-hemoglobin (HBB) is on chromosome 11p15.5. HBB is a component (subunit) of a larger protein called hemoglobin, which is located on the inside of red blood cells.

Mitochondrial DNA (mtDNA): Mitochondria contain an independent circular genome with 37 alleles. Mitochondria are passed from mothers to both female and male children, and this is referred to as *maternal inheritance.*

Multifactorial inheritance: Any type of non-mendelian inheritance including familial clustering; also referred to as *complex inheritance.*

Mutation: Accidental alterations or changes in our genetic material, DNA. There are three varieties of mutations: no effect, beneficial, or harmful. Most mutations are thought to have no effect on human health. These mutations generally occur in the noncoding region of our genome and are not believed to affect human health. These *no effect* mutations are sometimes called *silent* or *neutral* mutations. Mutations that occur in the coding region of our genome can be *beneficial* or *harmful*. Beneficial mutations confer health benefits; harmful mutations are usually associated with disease.

Polymorphism: A piece of DNA that has more than one form (allele), each of which occurs with at least 1% frequency, is said to be polymorphic (*poly*, many; *morph*, forms). Polymorphisms are a normal part of genetic variability. Polymorphisms of the same gene may or may not have different functions.

Single nucleotide polymorphism (SNP; pronounced "snip"): A polymorphism that involves a change at a base pair of DNA (e.g., from a C to a G or an A to a T). SNPs are the most common type of genetic variation in humans. Some SNPs involve changes in the function of a protein that is made from a gene, but others are silent. Coding SNP (cSNP) is a SNP that occurs in a coding region.

A Genetic and Genomic View of Human Disease

Almost every human disease has a genetic component.[7] Most diseases have a weak genetic component, meaning an individual may be vulnerable (susceptible) to developing a disease. Other diseases have a strong genetic component, meaning an individual has a higher likelihood of developing a disease. The relative strength or magnitude of a genetic effect for a disease can be categorized along a continuum ranging from susceptibility (multifactorial) to causative (mendelian) alleles.[8] Although we typically consider two broad genetic classes of human disease, multifactorial and mendelian,[8,9] it is more appropriate to consider the spectrum of the genetic component of human disease (Fig. 15.1).

Multifactorial genetic diseases account for the majority of health problems in the population.[9] Some examples include hypertension, asthma, coronary artery disease, osteoarthritis, and Parkinson disease. These diseases are associated with *susceptibility alleles*. Susceptibility means an individual is vulnerable (susceptible) to developing a disease. A susceptibility allele confers an increased risk that an individual may develop it, but the susceptibility allele is not sufficient to cause the disorder. Multifactorial genetic diseases usually do not show a recognizable mendelian inheritance pattern (i.e., autosomal recessive, autosomal dominant, or X-linked) on a family pedigree.[9,10] However, sometimes two or more family members may have the same multifactorial genetic disease, which is termed *familial aggregation*.

Mendelian diseases are not rare, but they occur less frequently than multifactorial genetic diseases. Examples include hypercholesterolemia, cystic fibrosis (CF), and sickle cell disease (SCD).[8,11,12] In these diseases, a mutation in one or more alleles is directly associated with the disease, so the term *causative allele* is used. Mendelian diseases typically exhibit a distinct pattern of inheritance (e.g., autosomal dominant, autosomal recessive, X-linked).

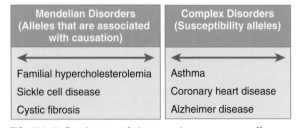

FIG. 15.1 ■ Continuum of the genetic component effect on human disease.

Molecular Genetic Characterization of Human Disease

Human diseases are now being classified according to their molecular genetic characteristics.[13] We are learning more about mechanisms of health and disease from the study of genes that are protective and deleterious. New categories of diseases have emerged, revealing that some diseases once thought to be a single entity are actually multiple distinct diseases that share similar or identical phenotypes.[14] For instance, there are different mendelian or complex subtypes of breast cancer, Alzheimer disease, and Parkinson disease.[14-16] These genetically distinct subtypes of the diseases may necessitate different treatments and have different prognoses.[17]

THE DIAGNOSTIC UTILITY OF FAMILY HISTORY DATA

Taking a family history in pedigree form and learning how to interpret it is the single most useful action PAs can take to use the diagnostic power of genetics.[18-20] The aim of collecting and analyzing family pedigree data is to identify individuals who are at risk for developing or having a multifactorial or mendelian disease. Such identification allows for screening or monitoring and possibly genetic testing, as well as patient education about lifestyle and medical prevention and surveillance practices, with the goal of reducing disease morbidity and mortality. Specifically, family pedigrees allow for the identification of patterns of inheritance, including identifying individuals at increased risk for developing different disorders.[21] When a comprehensive family pedigree is collected, about 30% to 40% will show a significant medical disorder such as coronary heart disease (CHD) or cancer.[22] For this and other reasons, the American Heart Association, for example, recommends regular patient questioning about family history of CHD and stroke.[23] With the growing recognition of the value of family history data, several organizations now recommend that health care providers collect and analyze these data routinely. It is clear from several studies of clinician behavior that the use of family history data is widely underused because of several barriers inherent in our current system, with time, billing, and limitations of the electronic health record seen as the most recognized.[24] Use of a web-based risk appraisal tool for assessing family history and lifestyle factors in primary care is being explored in those clinical settings.[25] The U.S. Surgeon General has led a national educational effort to educate the public about the increasing importance of knowing one's family health history and provides a free web-based, patient-completed questionnaire titled "My Family Health Portrait," which considers six medical disorders—diabetes, colon cancer, breast and ovarian cancer, coronary artery disease, and stroke.[26] The website (https://familyhistory.hhs.gov/FHH/html/index.html) provides patients with a pedigree constructed from the information input, which can be shared with other family members as well as their health care providers. Other methods used by providers to gather family history data include the use of templates in electronic medical records and structured written or electronic questionnaires given to patients. Unfortunately, these methods still require input of data and possible pedigree construction and interpretation, which take time and expertise from health care personnel.

Collecting Family History Data and Creating a Pedigree

Among the ways to collect a family history, the most efficient is a pedigree. This graphic representation of the family history can be a time-saving, inexpensive diagnostic and screening tool. When a clinician is used to taking a pedigree, it usually requires less time than writing out text, is easier to review later, and is often more concise and specific.[27,28] The pedigree allows patterns of disease, if they exist, to be identified more readily. It is a record that can be easily updated or built on over several visits. Pedigrees have internationally standardized symbols that have been in use since 1995. Fig. 15.2 displays an example of a pedigree with common pedigree symbols and nomenclature.

A comprehensive family history includes at least three generations. One usually begins the family history with the patient's health history and then extends to questions about siblings, parents, and children. If the patient is young, grandparents should be included. Questions about relatives should include information found in Tables 15.1 and 15.2. Pertinent health information should be listed for each biological relative.[29] This includes (1) diagnosis, (2) age at onset (AAO) or age at diagnosis (AADx) of the health condition, and (3) age and cause of death.[29] The provider should record all the information the patient

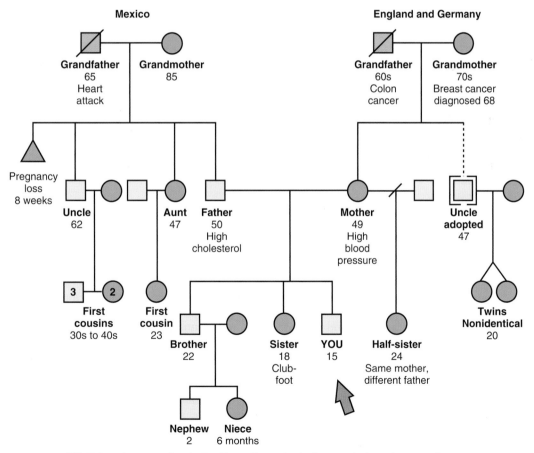

FIG. 15.2 ■ An example of a family pedigree, including symbols and nomenclature.

TABLE 15.1	Typical Information Obtained in Three-Generation Pedigree

Name

Age or year of birth (date of birth is preferable, if known)

Age at death and cause of death

Ethnic background of each grandparent

Relevant health information (see Table 15.2)

Relevant symptoms or diagnoses and age at diagnosis (if known)

Information regarding pregnancies, including infertility, spontaneous abortions, stillbirths, and pregnancy complications

Developmental delay and learning disabilities

Dysmorphic features or congenital anomalies

Consanguinity issues

Date and write your name legibly on the pedigree together with an explanation of any abbreviations

From Rich EC, Burke W, Heaton CJ, et al. Reconsidering the family history in primary care. *J Gen Intern Med* 2004;19:273.

TABLE 15.2	Relevant Health Information to Inquire About When Collecting Family History Data

Alcohol abuse	Drug abuse
Allergies	Emphysema
Alzheimer disease or dementia	Epilepsy or seizures
Anemia	Glaucoma
Asthma	Hearing loss
Arthritis	Heart trouble
Birth defects or malformations	Hemochromatosis or "iron overload"
Any cancer	High blood pressure
Breast cancer	Infertility
Ovarian cancer	Kidney trouble (renal disease)
Uterine cancer	Memory loss or Alzheimer disease
Lung cancer	Mental illness
Colon or rectal cancer	Mental retardation
Prostate cancer	Multiple miscarriages
Thyroid cancer	Neurofibromatosis
Brain cancer	Obesity
Melanoma	Osteoporosis or "hip fracture"
Other cancer	Phenylketonuria or "metabolic" disease at birth
High cholesterol	Sickle cell anemia
Chronic infections	Smoking
Clotting or bleeding problems	Stillborn or infant death
Depression	Stroke
Diabetes mellitus	Violence or domestic abuse
Down syndrome	Other: _____

From March of Dimes. Genetics and Your Practice. Family History. http://www.marchofdimes.com/gyponline.

provides even if it does not seem relevant or may be incomplete at the time. Clarifications and updates can and should be made at a later time.

Pedigree Analysis

Family pedigree data should be evaluated for the following: (1) the presence of significant medical conditions and (2) multiple family members with similar or the same disease. When two or more family members have the same or similar disease, consider the followings questions.

- How closely related are the family members—are they first-degree, second-degree, or third-degree relatives? (See Table 15.3.)
- Is there a clear pattern of inheritance (e.g., mendelian inheritance), or are the family history data suggestive of a *multifactorial disorder* (degree of relatedness of the family members factors in here as well)?
- Is there an earlier AAO than expected for the condition?
- Is there a constellation of related conditions or diseases in relatives (e.g., depression, substance abuse, suicide)?

Table 15.4 refers to genetic "red flags" that aid the clinician in detecting whether an individual may be at-risk for a mendelian or multifactorial disease. When a pedigree shows one or more of these types of findings, the patient's family history can be considered to be a positive family history. The findings may immediately inform clinical decision making or necessitate further investigation or referral. For instance, for a patient with a family history of two or more family members with breast cancer, screening tests such as mammography, magnetic resonance imaging, or ultrasonography can be pursued immediately. Another patient may have a pedigree showing two or more family members with an uncommon neurodegenerative disease. More information about this disease should be sought to determine what, if any, clinical decisions need to be made with the patient. It is important for the PA to review what is known about the genetics for the disorder or disease.

TABLE 15.3 Degree of Genetic Relatedness for Different Relatives	
Degree of Relatedness	**Definition and Relatives**
First-degree relative	• Parent, full sibling, or children (offspring) • A biological relative with whom the patient shares about 50% of his or her DNA
Second-degree relative	• Uncle, aunt, nephew, niece, grandparent, grandchild, or half sibling • A biological relative with whom the patient shares about one quarter of his or her DNA
Third-degree relative	• First cousin, great grandparent, or great grandchild • A biological relative with whom the patient shares about one eighth of his or her DNA

(Wolpert CM, & Speer MC. (2005). Harnessing the power of the pedigree. Journal of Midwifery & Women's Health, 50, 189-196.)

For many diseases, the genetic information may be found in the pathology section of disease reviews; however, a number of reliable resources can help clinicians prepare themselves and their patient for the genetic referral, possible testing, anticipatory management, and longitudinal care (Table 15.5).

The Value of a "Negative" Family History

Sometimes the three-generation pedigree does not reveal any significant medical problems. These "negative" family history pedigree data are still valuable because they provide information that impacts clinical decision making.[19] These negative data suggest that the patient has baseline population risks for developing different diseases, depending on the age of the patient. The data also provide justification for following the standard population screening guidelines and initiating screening tests such as mammography or colonoscopy tests at the recommended ages. All pedigrees need to be updated regularly to make sure that changes have not occurred in the family in the interim and whether updated options may need to be discussed with the patient.

GENETIC AND GENOMIC TESTING

With more than 5000 genetic and genomic tests commercially available today, this specialized testing is now part of clinical practice in primary care settings

TABLE 15.4 "Red Flags" Suggestive of Genetic Disease From Family History Data	
Red Flag	**Clinical Examples**
Family history of known or suspected genetic condition	Neurofibromatosis (NF1) Huntington disease
Multiple affected family members with same or related disorders	Diabetes mellitus type 2 in a father and son Cardiovascular disease in first-degree relatives
Earlier age at onset of disease than expected	Cancers: breast, ovarian, colorectal in 30s Cardiovascular disease: MI in 40s, cerebrovascular accident in 50s
Developmental delays or mental retardation	Fragile X syndrome Rett syndrome
Diagnosis in less-often-affected sex	Breast cancer in men (e.g., BRCA2) Cardiovascular disease (e.g., early-onset MI in women)
Multifocal or bilateral occurrence in paired organs	Breast or ovarian cancer Familial autosomal dominant polycystic kidney disease
One or more major malformations	Trisomy 13 or 21
Disease in the absence of risk factors or after preventive measures	Long QT syndrome Familial hypercholesterolemia
Abnormalities in growth (growth retardation, asymmetric growth, excessive growth)	Turner syndrome Sotos syndrome
Recurrent pregnancy losses (2+)	Inherited thrombophilias Chromosomal abnormalities
Consanguinity (blood relationship of parents)	Hemophilia A Cystic fibrosis
Ethnic predisposition to certain genetic disorders	Tay-Sachs disease Thalassemias

MI, Myocardial infarction.

and across almost all specialties.[30] A working knowledge of the basic tenets of genetic testing is essential for PAs.[21,29,31] This section defines genetic testing; reviews some fundamental background information, including a description of various types of testing; and discusses some ethical considerations associated with genetic testing. This section is not intended to be a comprehensive review of this topic. Genetic testing in

TABLE 15.5 **Genetic and Genomic Web Resources for Clinicians and Patients**		
Resource	**Source**	**Service or Information Provided**
GeneTests: https://www.genetests.org/	GeneTests functions independently of the parent organization, BioReference Laboratories.	• Provides a laboratory directory of >600 international laboratories offering molecular genetic testing, biochemical genetic testing, and cytogenetic testing for >3000 inherited disorders. A clinic directory of >1000 genetics clinics providing diagnosis and genetic counseling services to patients and their families with known or suspected inherited disorders • Links to GeneReviews chapters and other external links such as Online Mendelian Inheritance in Man and the Genetics Home Reference
Gene Reviews: http://www.ncbi.nlm.nih.gov/books/NBK1116/advanced/	Funded and developed by the National Institutes of Health; maintained by the University of Washington, Seattle	• Provides expert-authored organized synopses of known genetic disorders, including descriptions, differential diagnoses, and diagnoses of the condition reviews. Peer reviewed and updated regularly • Provides current information on genetic test use in diagnosis, management, and genetic counseling • Links to genomic databases, patient resources, PubMed citations, policy statements and guidelines, and state laboratory testing centers
Genetics Home Reference: http://ghr.nlm.nih.gov	National Institutes of Health and National Library of Medicine	• Provides consumer-friendly information about the effects of genetic variations on human health • Contains descriptions of >1000 health conditions, diseases, and syndromes • Provides a handbook to help the public learn about mutations, inheritance, genetic counseling, genetic testing, and genomic research • Presents a medical and genetic glossary • Links to reputable genetic resources and organizations
Genetic Alliance: http://www.geneticalliance.org	Not-for-profit network organization with national sponsorships	• The voice of advocacy in genetics for patients and communities • Provides disease information and support database for >13,000 conditions • Contains the ATLAS toolkit to help individuals advocate on behalf of themselves or others to communicate needs, share experiences, and take steps to get what they want and need in areas such as resources, insurance, policies, and so on • Links to publications to help the public, including clinicians, understand and advocate for those affected with genetic conditions
Genetics in the Physician Assistant's Practice: http://www.nchpeg.org/pa/index.php	NCHPEG/Jackson Laboratories	Interactive website written by PAs for PAs with: • Example cases to help apply genetic family history information through reasoning genetic differential diagnoses • Exercises with family history examples

NCHPEG, National Coalition for Health Professional Education in Genetics; *PA,* physician assistant.

children, for instance, necessitates special ethical considerations beyond the scope of this section.

Definition of a Genetic or Genomic Test

Although many different kinds of medical tests may indicate or even provide diagnostic information for a genetic disorder (e.g., kidney ultrasonography can reveal polycystic kidney disease, a peripheral smear can show spherocytosis), for the purposes of this chapter, genetic testing is defined as the analysis of human DNA, RNA, chromosomes, and specific proteins or metabolites to detect a change or changes known to be associated with a genetic disorder.[32]

Technological advances in sequencing the human genome have enabled the emergence of *genomic testing,* which is rapidly replacing *genetic testing.* Genomic testing enables the testing or study of an entire human genome rather than just analyzing single alleles.[30] Hereafter, the term *genetic* will stand for both *genetic* and *genomic testing.* Technological advances have driven down the cost of genetic testing, and the lower cost of genetic testing means it is more likely to be used with increasing frequency as long as the clinical validity and clinical utility of the test are appropriate.[4]

Many argue that genetic testing differs fundamentally from other types of medical testing; this view is referred to as *genetic exceptionalism.*[33] Proponents of genetic exceptionalism put forth the following arguments. First, the impact of genetic testing results extends beyond the index patient to include biological family members. For example, a diagnosis of an autosomal recessive disorder such as SCD, hemochromatosis, or CF also identifies a patient's biological parents as carriers and siblings as potential carriers.[11] Second, certain types of genetic testing can predict the likelihood that an individual will develop a specific disorder (e.g., Alzheimer disease, Parkinson disease).[14,16] This revelation of potential future health could be argued to be somewhat unique to DNA-based testing and, therefore, makes it exceptional from other types of medical testing. These concepts are helpful as we briefly discuss ethical issues in genetic testing.

Ethical Considerations of Genetic Testing

Several special ethical considerations are associated with genetic testing. First and foremost, genetic testing must be voluntary, given the eugenic abuses and atrocities of the past.[34] Individuals have the right *not* to know whether they carry alleles that predispose or affect their current or future health.[35] Genetic testing is never to be associated with eliminating alleles associated with human disease. The genetic mutation rate is constant in humans; therefore, new mutations will always occur, making it impossible to eliminate human genetic disease; identification and management should be the aim of genetic testing.[36] Furthermore, no matter what type of genetic testing is considered or undertaken, individuals must be informed about the benefits, risks, and limitations associated with that particular type of testing.[31] Last, genetic and genomic testing is not routinely done with children in order to protect their rights to make informed and independent decisions when they are adults.[37] As the number of available genetic tests increases and technology advances, these broad ethical considerations will still be applicable.

TYPES OF GENETIC AND GENOMIC TESTS

Carrier Screening

Carrier screening refers to genetic testing used to identify individuals who have an allele associated with an autosomal recessive disease; these individuals are usually referred to as *carriers*. Carrier screening is typically offered to specific populations known to be at higher risk for having particular autosomal recessive disorders (e.g., Tay-Sachs disease, SCD, and CF).[11,38,39] For instance, it is recommended that

individuals with a known Ashkenazi Jewish ancestry be offered carrier screening for a several Jewish genetic diseases.[40] Although targeting different "ethnic groups" or populations is still practiced, the emphasis is now shifting toward universal carrier screening, meaning all individuals, regardless of ethnicity or population, are offered carrier screening.[11,12,41,42] This change occurred, in part, with the recognition that different human migrations have resulted in matings between different populations, and it is therefore impossible for an individual to know his or her entire genetic ancestry without having genetic ancestry testing. In light of several deaths among college athletes who had undiagnosed SCD trait, the National Collegiate Athletic Association (NCAA) recently mandated that all college athletes at Division I and II colleges must have carrier screening for SCD trait or sign a waiver declining testing before they can participate.[12] SCD refers to a group of genetic hematologic disorders characterized by the predominance of sickle hemoglobin (HbS) and is the most common inherited blood disorder in the United States.[12] The clinical manifestations of SCD or even sickle cell trait can cause increased red blood cell hemolysis and acute and chronic vasoocclusive complications.[43] Recommended universal screening underscores the fact that individuals may be carriers or even have this disorder regardless of a perception based on skin color.

Carrier Screening May Reveal Asymptomatic and Symptomatic Individuals

Carrier screening and associated programs have been used for more than 3 decades. Over time, two phenomena have been revealed: (1) carriers can be symptomatic, and (2) carrier screening may identify individuals who have the disorder for which the carrier screening is being done. The intention of carrier screening is to identify individuals who possess alleles associated with autosomal recessive genetic disease. Historically, carriers were not believed to be at risk for medical complications associated with the genetic disease for which they were being screened; the identification of carrier status was primarily to inform personal reproductive decision making.[44] Over time, it is clear that some individuals identified as carriers had symptoms and signs (phenotype) of the genetic disease. For example, individuals with SCD *trait* experience painful vasoocclusive crises, and in some instances, sudden death.[38] Similarly, individuals who were carriers of CF or other disorders such as hereditary hemochromatosis also experience symptoms and or showed signs associated with these disorders.[11,43] Interestingly, individuals identified as having a disorder identified through carrier screening can be asymptomatic or have mild symptoms.

Newborn Screening

Newborn screening done with a heel stick is a specific subtype of carrier screening performed shortly after birth and has become the "poster child" for the benefits of carrier screening, which include early diagnosis in order to offer medical treatment to decrease morbidity and mortality.[45] Newborn screening is done in all 50 states, but each state determines which specific genetic tests are mandated and the types of diseases screened for varies by state. Some diseases screened for includes phenylketonuria (PKU), maple syrup urine disease, and SCD. Both sickle cell trait and SCD are now screened for in all 50 states.[45] Tandem mass spectrometry technology has greatly expanded the number of diseases for which screening can be done.[46,47] As a result, in addition to the state-mandated newborn screening, parents may be offered optional additional newborn screening tests.[46,47] Parents may not understand that this is additional genetic testing and should be educated about this in their informed consent.

Susceptibility and Presymptomatic Testing

It is possible to determine whether individuals, with or without a family history of a specific genetic disorder, are likely to develop it through *susceptibility* or *presymptomatic* testing. A few examples of disorders for which this testing is available include some forms of breast cancer or colon cancer, Alzheimer disease, Parkinson disease, and ataxia.[14-16] Knowing which individuals have a "positive" susceptibility or presymptomatic genetic test and therefore an increased probability of developing a specific disorder allows for ongoing monitoring or surveillance to be done and preventive measures to be undertaken. Depending on the nature of the disorder, this could translate into delaying or even preventing its onset. Previously, it was hypothesized that individuals having this type of predictive testing might experience undue psychological distress from knowing that they had a risk, especially if it was a high risk of developing a specific disorder. Some recent research has indicated that many individuals who have had presymptomatic genetic testing have reported experiencing some heightened anxiety, but this is usually limited in duration, and no long-term negative psychological effects have been noted.[48] Appropriate education and counseling may help mitigate these issues.

Diagnostic Genetic Testing

When an individual is symptomatic or shows signs of a specific disorder, genetic testing can be done to confirm or "rule out" a presumptive diagnosis. A clinical example of such diagnostic genetic testing includes an individual with a history of venous thromboembolism (VTE). A medical evaluation for this patient may include genetic testing for both antithrombin III and factor V Leiden.[49,50] Diagnostic genetic testing may also be used to help "subtype" a disease. In the case of VTE, a set of thrombophilia panels or combinations of the five most common familial thrombophilia mutations is used to determine sometimes-linked inherited thrombophilias. Another example includes forms of ataxia that can be difficult to distinguish clinically from one other; a diagnostic genetic testing panel can be used to identify the specific form of ataxia. Panel testing is also done in oncology for breast cancer. The use of subtyping for diagnostic testing is not inconsequential because a different diagnosis may have a different prognosis or different treatment options.

Prenatal Genetic Testing

Prenatal genetic testing is offered to prospective parents so they can make personal decisions about their pregnancies. Currently, prenatal genetic testing offers the following: (1) fetal testing for hundreds of different genetic diseases; (2) targeted prenatal testing with the fetus if a positive carrier screening test result from one or both biological parents exists; and (3) noninvasive prenatal testing, meaning a DNA sample (e.g., saliva or blood sample) is taken from the mother and not the fetus, eliminating an invasive and risky procedure such as amniocentesis.[46,47] Prenatal genetic testing is primarily confined to an obstetrics clinical setting, is often performed using a variety of testing protocols and algorithms, and has an accompanying myriad of ethical issues to consider.

Regardless of the clinical practice setting, it is essential to be able to refer patients appropriately and understand the different modes of prenatal genetic testing and how rapidly this specialized genetic testing is evolving. PAs are strongly encouraged to contact and collaborate with a prenatal genetic counselor or other genetic health care professional.

Although preimplantation genetic testing is beyond the scope of this chapter, in brief, this type of genetic testing is performed on embryos created in vitro to diagnose particularly serious genetic disorders (e.g., Tay-Sachs disease).[46, 47] Embryos without evidence for the genetic disorder may then be available for implantation. This procedure provides parents an alternative to waiting for prenatal diagnosis and potential termination of fetuses with serious genetic disorders.

Pharmacogenetic and Pharmacogenomic Testing

Just as the term *genetic* refers to a single allele or a mutation within an allele, *pharmacogenetics* and *pharmacogenetic testing* is the analysis of a specific gene or genes, which may predict an individual's response to a specific drug.[51,52] Likewise, *pharmacogenomics* refers to all the genes (or genetic variations) that influence drug responses. Often you will see the terms *pharmacogenomics* and *pharmacogenetics* used interchangeably.

Pharmacogenetic and pharmacogenomic tests are used to predict an individual's response to specific medications and classes of medications to reduce the number of adverse reactions. Knowing whether a patient carries any of these genetic variations can help PAs and other prescribers individualize drug therapy, decrease the chance for adverse drug events, and increase the effectiveness of drugs. Testing is done to identify the presence or absence of allelic variants that code for known drug-metabolizing enzymes. For example, the gene *CYP2C19* codes for the metabolic enzyme cytochrome p450. Different allelic variants of this gene are associated with different medication metabolizer rates. This test determines into which of four different metabolizer profile groups (i.e., poor, intermediate, normal, or ultrarapid metabolizers) an individual fits. Depending on his or her metabolizer rate, an individual may be at increased risk for experiencing side effects with certain medications.

The aim of pharmaco*genomic* testing is to look at allelic variants associated with drug metabolism, not disease; there is no testing for susceptibility or causative genes. Although pharmacogenomic testing makes good sense theoretically, most studies conducted to date have been retrospective, and the level of evidence is not strong enough to determine whether pharmacogenomic testing merits use and is cost effective for use in regular clinical practice. Prospective studies continue to be performed to determine the clinical utility of pharmacogenomic testing.

Direct-to-Consumer Testing

Commercial companies now offer genetic testing for some medical disorders directly to individuals and families. Currently, most of this direct-to-consumer (DTC) genetic testing involves carrier screening (e.g., CF, SCD, hereditary hearing loss) and susceptibility testing (e.g., some types of breast cancers such as *BRCA1* and *BRCA2*). However, to date, limited data are available regarding the psychological impact of this type of DTC genetic testing on individuals,[53] especially without the benefit of genetic counseling and interpretation. In one study, individuals (*n* = 63) were interviewed about their response to *BRCA1* or *BRCA2* genetic testing results.[54] Those who had a positive genetic test (*n* = 32) reported experiencing moderate anxiety, and most reported seeking medical advice and having confirmatory genetic testing done. Most of the individuals (*n* = 25) whose genetic test was mutation positive did not have a personal family history of breast cancer. Notably, these same individuals told family members, and, collectively, 30 relatives underwent medical genetic testing for *BRCA1* and *BRCiA2*; 13 of those 30 relatives were found to have a *BRCA1* or *BRCA2* mutation. Hence, this DTC genetic testing led to the identification of family members who were carriers and at risk for developing one of the cancers associated with *BRCA1* or *BRCA2*.

Direct-to-consumer genetic testing is likely to come into more widespread usage.[1] PAs work with individuals and families who have had DTC genetic testing and want to better understand their test results. Being able to facilitate understanding of risk reports and helping to negotiate how the family member can approach his or her relatives are additional needed clinical skills. Identification of an individual as a carrier through DTC genetic testing necessitates confirmatory genetic testing, likely referral to a genetic specialist, and clarity on how to communicate to potential at-risk relatives.

CLINICAL DECISION-MAKING FRAMEWORK FOR GENETIC TESTING

Thousands of genetic tests for carrier screening, susceptibility, and diagnostic testing are now available. The large number of genetic and genomic tests is overwhelming. How does one determine when and which type of genetic testing to offer? One needs to consider the practical points and let certain facts help guide decision making.

What is the clinical practice setting? In a primary care setting, only a few genetic tests are currently recommended for disorders such as hereditary hemochromatosis, CF, and factor V Leiden thrombophilia.[49,50] PAs in this setting need to be aware of these recommendations and guidelines. The PA must be familiar with and use clinical practice recommendations to determine when specific types of genetic testing should be considered and to whom to offer the genetic testing. Genetic testing guidelines and recommendations are provided through different medical specialty organizations such as the American College of Obstetrics and Gynecology and the American Society of Human Genetics and disease advocacy organizations. It is critical to note that clinical guidelines and recommendations are not meant to be directives or clinical practice standards. They should be viewed as a resource and provide information with which to educate the patient in shared clinical decision making.

Next, direct attention to the individual and his or her family history. The following questions will be useful to use as you contemplate the patient's individual risk:

- Is the individual family history suggestive of a genetic disorder?
- Will the information from a genetic test change medical management or give the patient different options?
- Does the individual want genetic testing, is the patient an adult, and is the voluntary nature of the testing clear to the patient?
- Is there a genetic test available commercially for the disorder? If so, what types of genetic tests are available (e.g., carrier screening, presymptomatic, or diagnostic genetic testing)?
- Is there another nongenetic test that might be more or equally appropriate in terms of clinical validity, utility, and cost?

As noted earlier, genetic testing must be voluntary. It is common, however, for sometimes well-meaning family members to strongly encourage or coerce an individual to have genetic testing. Asking the individual why he or she wants to have genetic testing may help him or her reveal this.

Another important scenario to consider is when genetic testing is requested for a child. As noted, genetic testing is not routinely done on children in order to protect their rights to make informed and independent decisions about genetic testing when they reach adulthood.[38] However, when the medical management of a child would be affected, genetic testing is usually done. When a child may be considered for genetic testing, it is prudent to consult a genetic health professional.

Beyond the issues of deciding whether to test, technical knowledge about the genetic test is needed. As a practical matter, PAs should learn about prevalent genetic disorders and genetic testing that might be done in their clinical setting with their patient population. This can be done by using genetic testing recommendations, valid web-based resources (see Table 15.5), and through consultation and collaboration with local genetic health professionals. Table 15.6 denotes medical specialty areas with examples of common familial and genetic disorders that may be seen in these settings. As in other medical

decision-making instances, if the PA is concerned about whether to proceed with genetic testing, he or she should consult the local genetic health care provider or refer the individual for such testing.

COLLABORATING WITH GENETIC HEALTH PROFESSIONALS AND LIFELONG LEARNING IN GENETICS AND GENOMICS

For all PAs, keeping current with clinically applicable genetic and genomic advances will be a lifelong responsibility and should be part of the clinical management armamentarium. It is imperative to become facile with and use recommended web-based genetic resources to access current, peer-reviewed information about the genetics of different diseases and conditions, available genetic testing, and valid information to support shared clinical decision making with individuals and families (see Table 15.5).

As part of quality care for patients, PAs need to develop a working relationship with local genetic health professionals, including geneticists and genetic counselors. These professionals are a valuable referral resource and provide salient information regarding genetic testing, diagnosis, and longitudinal medical management. To locate a genetic counselor, contact the National Society of Genetic Counselors online at www.nsgc.org.

THE PHYSICIAN ASSISTANT'S ROLE IN THE GENOMIC AGE: PUTTING IT ALL TOGETHER

The ever-evolving tools of genomics can help PAs move into a world where disease susceptibility and risk are identified early, supporting preventive action for patients. Optimal testing, helping determine the course of the disease, and management strategies will be implemented with more precision for the individual patient. The PA role will continue to be on the front line of care, gathering the family history data and interpreting risk for our patients. It will also include genetic screening and the need to educate patients and coordinate care with genetic health professionals. With the shortage of genetic health professionals, we must augment our fundamental knowledge in genetics and genomics to provide genetic care relevant to patients in our practice setting. As health care transforms we will need a health care workforce with the skills and knowledge to make effective use of genomic advances, and PAs must be at the forefront of this vision.

TABLE 15.6 Medical Specialty Areas With Prevalent or Do-Not-Miss Genetic or Familial Diagnoses

Clinical Specialty	Relevant Genetic or Genomic Diagnoses	Clinical Specialty	Relevant Genetic or Genomic Diagnoses
Cardiology	*Arrhythmia syndromes*: atrial fibrillation, Brugada syndrome, long QT syndrome, short QT syndrome, CPVT *Cardiomyopathies*: arrhythmogenic right ventricular dysplasia, dilated cardiomyopathy, hypertrophic cardiomyopathy, left ventricular noncompaction cardiomyopathy, restrictive cardiomyopathy *Coronary artery disease* (and familial hypercholesterolemia) *Familial aneurysms (thoracic) and aortopathies*: syndromic and nonsyndromic—e.g., Marfan syndrome *Congenital heart disease*: isolated and syndromic *Muscular dystrophies and heart disease*	Hematology	*Thalassemias*: α and β *Thrombophilias*: factor V Leiden mutation, prothrombin mutation, MTHFR mutation, protein C or S deficiency, antithrombin III deficiency, dysfibrinogenemia *Hemophilias*: hemophilia A (classic hemophilia, factor VIII deficiency), hemophilia B (Christmas disease, factor IX deficiency) Sickle cell anemia Von Willebrand disease
Dermatology	Neurofibromatosis (type I) Tuberous sclerosis Familial melanoma Ehlers-Danlos syndrome Psoriasis Atopic dermatitis Albinism Vitiligo Alopecia areata	Musculoskeletal and rheumatology	Achondroplasia Spondylolarthropathies: ankylosing spondylitis Osteogenesis imperfecta Muscular dystrophies Ehlers-Danlos syndrome Marfan syndrome Spina bifida Congenital scoliosis Congenital hip dysplasia Clubfoot Osteoarthritis* Scoliosis* Osteoporosis* Rheumatoid arthritis* Systemic lupus erythematosus
Endocrine	Multiple endocrine neoplasia (MEN2 syndrome) Diabetes mellitus, type I Diabetes mellitus, type II	Nephrology and urology	Autosomal dominant polycystic kidney disease Wilms tumor IgA nephropathy End-stage renal disease* Hypertension* Prostate cancer* Bladder cancer*
ENT	*Congenital hearing loss syndromes:* Waardenburg, Ushers, and Alport syndromes *Head and neck cancer* (HPV, p53, nasopharyngeal carcinoma) Acoustic neuroma (NF II) Cleft lip and palate malformations Otosclerosis	Neurology	Huntington disease Neurofibromatosis (type 2) Autism spectrum disorders (ASD) Alzheimer disease* Parkinson's disease* Multiple sclerosis Essential tremor* Epilepsy* Dementia*
Gastroenterology	*Inflammatory bowel disease*: Crohn disease, ulcerative colitis *Familial colorectal cancer syndromes*: familial colorectal cancer,* FAP, Lynch syndrome Hereditary hemochromatosis Cystic fibrosis Wilson disease α_1-Antitrypsin deficiency Celiac disease	Obstetrics	*Prenatal genetic diagnosis*: first- and second-trimester maternal serum screening, prenatal diagnosis of mendelian disorders and neural tube defects, population carrier screening, recurrent pregnancy loss
Gynecology	*Familial breast and ovarian cancer syndromes: BRCA1, BRCA2*, Lynch syndrome		

TABLE 15.6 **Medical Specialty Areas With Prevalent or Do-Not-Miss Genetic or Familial Diagnoses—cont'd**

Clinical Specialty	Relevant Genetic or Genomic Diagnoses	Clinical Specialty	Relevant Genetic or Genomic Diagnoses
Oncology	Refer to cancers related to specific organ system	Psychiatry	Schizophrenia*
			Bipolar disorder*
Ophthalmology	Retinoblastoma		Unipolar major depression*
	Congenital cataracts		Alcohol and substance abuse disorder*
	Congenital glaucoma		Anxiety disorder*
	Retinitis pigmentosa		Autism spectrum disorders*
	Age-related macular degeneration*	Pulmonology	α_1-Antitrypsin deficiency
	Myopia (high myopia)		Cystic fibrosis
	Cataracts*		Asthma*
	Glaucoma*		Sarcoidosis*
			Lung cancer*

*Denotes common disorders that often have a familial component and may be identified with collection and analysis of family history data.

CPVT, Catecholaminergic Polymorphic Ventricular Tachycardia; *FAP,* familial adenomatous polyposis; *HPV,* human papillomavirus; *MEN2,* multiple endocrine neoplasia 2; *MTHFR,* methylenetetrahydrofolate reductase.

CASE STUDY 15.1

Ms. Rodriguez is an incoming freshman student who will be playing Division I volleyball at college. Recently, the NCAA mandated that all college athletes at Division I and II schools must have carrier screening for undiagnosed SCD trait or sign a release before they can play. Ms. Rodriguez states she does not understand why she has to have testing for this SCD trait because she is Hispanic, not black. Also, if she skips the testing, what is the chance that she will have medical problems when she plays volleyball? What do you tell her?

CASE STUDY 15.2

Mr. Smith is 33 years old and recently presented with new-onset seizures. A neurologic workup did not determine an identifiable cause; therefore, the seizures have been labeled idiopathic. Mr. Smith has been prescribed antiseizure medication, which he must take daily to prevent recurrence of the seizures. A first-line medication used to treat idiopathic seizures is carbamazepine. Mr. Smith self-identifies as half-Asian and half-European. This information is clinically relevant because individuals with Asian ancestry who start carbamazepine have an increased risk of developing Stevens-Johnson syndrome compared with individuals without Asian ancestry. Pharmacogenomic testing is available to determine if Mr. Smith is at increased risk of developing Stevens-Johnson syndrome. Should pharmacogenomic testing be used, or might it be better to treat him as if he is at an increased risk based on his self-reported ancestry?

CASE STUDY 15.3

Mr. Schwartz is 58 years old and recently had OTC (over-the-counter) genetic testing for several disorders. He said he did this because he was adopted and curious about knowing his risk for different diseases. His test results showed that he carries a mutation for breast cancer (i.e., *BRCA1*). Now he is nervous and unsure of what this means for him and his two daughters. What do you do? What do you tell him? What do you tell his daughters?

KEY POINTS

Physician assistants can more fully deliver comprehensive and personalized care to patients in the age of genomic medicine by:

- Using the language of genetics and genomics to better interpret and discuss this specialized information with patients and colleagues
- Gathering appropriate family history data in pedigree format to identify and facilitate shared clinical decision making for individuals who may be at risk for developing, having, or transmitting a mendelian or multifactorial disorder
- Upholding the ethical tenets regarding genetic information and testing
- Accessing valid, peer-reviewed genomic resources to inform clinical decision making and maintaining currency with recommendations and guidelines based on important developments in genetic research
- Collaborating with genetic health professionals as part of the team that can facilitate quality care to patients and their family members who may be at risk for genetic or genomic conditions

The resources for this chapter can be found at www.expertconsult.com.

References

1. Genetics Home Reference. http://ghr.nlm.nih.gov/handbook/basics/dna. Accessed March 8, 2016.
2. Genetics Home Reference. http://ghr.nlm.nih.gov/handbook/basics/gene. Accessed March 8, 2016.
3. *What is a cell?* National Library of Medicine (U.S.). http://ghr.nlm.nih.gov/handbook/basics/cell. Accessed December 30, 2015.
4. Lohr S. Google and Microsoft look to change health care. *The New York Times*; 2007. Section C, 2, 179–189.
5. Wolpert CM, Singer ML, Speer MC. Speaking the language of genetics: a primer. *J Midwifery Womens Health*. 2005; 50(3):184–188.
6. Wolpert CM. Genetic nomenclature. In: *Macmillan Reference USA's Science Library: genetics*; 2003.
7. Collins FS. Shattuck lecture: medicine and societal consequences of the human genome project. *The New England Journal of Medicine*. 1999;341:28–37.
8. Online Mendelian Inheritance in Man (OMIM). http://www.omim.org/search?index=entry&sort=score+de%2C+prefix_sort+desc&start=1&limit=10&search=hypercholesterolaemia. Accessed December 30, 2015.
9. Wolpert CM, Melvin E, Speer MC. Complex genetic disorders: evaluating when genetic research findings are applicable for genetic counseling practice. *Journal of Genetic Counseling*. 1999;8:73–84.
10. Taubes G. Epidemiology faces its limits. *Science*. 1995;269:164–169.
11. *Cystic fibrosis*. National Library of Medicine (U.S.). http://ghr.nlm.nih.gov/condition/cystic-fibrosis. Accessed December 30, 2015.
12. *NCAA. 2008–2009 NCAA Sports Medicine Handbook*. Indianapolis: NCAA; 2008a.
13. McClellan J, King MC. Genetic heterogeneity in human disease. *Cell*. 2010;141:210.
14. *Alzheimer Disease search*. Online Mendelian Inheritance in Man (OMIM). http://www.omim.org/search?index=entry&sort=score+desc%2C+prefix_sort+desc&start=1&limit=10&search=Alzheimer+disease. Accessed December 30, 2015.
15. *Breast Cancer search*. Online Mendelian Inheritance in Man (OMIM). Types http://www.omim.org/search?index=entry&sort=score+desc%2C+prefix_sort+desc&start=1&limit=10&search=Breast+cancer. Accessed December 30, 2015.
16. *Parkinson Disease seach*. Online Mendelian Inheritance in Man (OMIM). Types http://www.omim.org/search?index=entry&sort=score+desc%2C+prefix_sort+desc&start=1&limit=10&search=Parkinson+disease. Accessed December 30, 2015.
17. Serrano-Pozo A, Qian J, Monsell SE, Betensky RA, Bradley T. APO E2 is associated with milder clinical and pathological Alzheimer disease. *Journal of the Annals of Neurology*. 2015;24(369):917–929.
18. Guttmacher A, Collins F, Carmona RH. The family history – more important than ever. *The New England Journal of Medicine*. 2004;25(351):2333–2336.
19. Wolpert CM, Speer MC. Harnessing the power of the pedigree. *Journal of Midwifery & Women's Health*. 2005;50(3):189–196.
20. Walter FM, Emery J. Coming down the line – patients' understanding of their family history of common chronic disease. *Annals of Family Medicine*. 2005;3:405–414.
21. Whelan AJ, Ball S, Best L, et al. Genetic red flags: clues to thinking genetically in primary care practice. *Primary Care*. 2004;31:497–508.
22. Hunt SC, Gwinn M, Adams T. Family history assessment: strategies for prevention of cardiovascular disease. *American Journal of Preventive Medicine*. 2003;24:136–142.
23. Pearson TA, Blair SN, Daniels SR, et al. AHA guidelines for primary prevention of cardiovascular disease and stroke: 2002 Update consensus panel guide to comprehensive risk reduction for adult patients without coronary or other atherosclerotic vascular diseases. *Circulation*. 2002;106(3):388–391.
24. Zazove OP, Plegue MA, Uhlmann WR, Muffin MT. Prompting primary care providers about increased patient risk as a results of family history: does it work? *Journal of American Board of Family Medicine*. 2015;28(3):334–342.
25. Baer HJ, Schneider LI, Colditz GA, et al. *Journal of General Internal Medicine*. 2013;28(6):817–824.
26. *My family health portrait*. U.S. Department of Health and Human Services. Accessed December 2, 2016.
27. Facio FM, Feero WG, Linn A, Oden N, Manickam K, Biesecker LG. Validation of My Family Health Portrait for six common heritable conditions. *Genetics in Medicine*. 2010;12(6):370–375.

28. Rackover M, Goldgar C, Wolpert CM, Healy K, Feiger J, Jenkins J. Establishing essential physician assistant clinical competencies guidelines for genetics and genomics. *The Journal of Physician Assistant Education*. 2007;18:47–48.

29. Goldgar C, Clarke K, Wolpert C, Healy K, Malouf E, Harvey E. Web-based module: genetics for the physician assistants' practice. *National Coalition for Health Care Providers for Education in Genetics (NCHPEG) website*. 2009. http://goo.gl/XUkQ VL. Accessed December 7, 2015.

30. GeneTestsTM [Internet]. Available from: https://www.genet ets.org/. Accessed December 30, 2015.

31. Wolpert CM, Schmidt MC. Genomic medicine: understanding the basics of genetic testing. *Journal of the American Academy of Physician Assistants*. 2005;18:42–52.

32. National Library of Medicine (U.S.). Genetics Home Reference [Internet]. Bethesda (MD): the Library; What is genetic testing? Available from: https://ghr.nlm.nih.gov/handbook/te sting/genetictesting. Accessed December 30, 2015.

33. Green MJ, Booth JR. "Genetic exceptionalism" in medicine: clarifying the differences between genetic and nongenetic test. *Annals of Internal Medicine*. 2003;138(7):571–575.

34. Cold Spring Harbor Laboratory. Cold Spring Harbor Laboratory's Image Archive on the American Eugenics Movement. http://www.eugenicsarchive.org. Accessed December 30, 2015.

35. National Human Genome Research Institute (NHGRI). Ethical, Legal, and Societal Implications (ELSI) Research Program. http://www.genome.gov/ELSI/. Accessed December 30, 2015.

36. Cameron LD, Muller C. Psychosocial aspects of genetic testing. *Current Opinion in Psychiatry*. 2009;22:218–233.

37. Wilfond B, Ross LF. From genetics to genomics: ethics, policy, and parental decision-making. *Journal of Pediatric Psychology*. 2009;34(6):639–647.

38. *Sickle cell disease*. Online Mendelian Inheritance in Man (OMIM). http://omim.org/search?index=entry&sort=score+desc%2C+prefix_sort+desc&start=1&limit=10&search=Sickl e+cell+disease. Accessed December 30, 2015.

39. *Tay Sachs disease*. Online Mendelian Inheritance in Man (OMIM). http://omim.org/search?index=entry&start=1&lim it=10&search=tay+sachs+disease&sort=score+desc%2C+prefi x_sort+desc. Accessed December 30, 2015.

40. Jewish Genetic Disease Consortium. http://www.jewishgene ticdiseases.org/jewish-genetic-diseases/. Accessed January 2, 2016.

41. Watson MS, Cutting GR, Desnick RJ, et al. Cystic fibrosis population carrier screening: 2004 revision of American College of Medical Genetics mutation panel. *Genetics in Medicine*. 2004;6(5):387–391.

42. Srinivasan BS, Evans EA, Flannick J, et al. A universal carrier test for the long tail of Mendelian disease. *Reprod Biomed Online*. 2010;21(4):537–551.

43. *Hereditary hemochromatosis*. National Library of Medicine (U.S.). http://omim.org/searchindex=entry&start=1&limit=1 0&search=hereditary+hemochromatosis&sort=score+desc%2 C+prefix_sort+desc. Accessed December 30, 2015.

44. American College of Obstetricians and Gynecologists (ACOG). http://acog.org/About/News=Room/News-Releases/ 2011/All-Women-Should-Be-Offered-Cystic-Fibrosis-Screening-Regardless of Ethnicity. Accessed December 30, 2015.

45. *Newborn screening*. Centers for Disease Control (CDC). http: //www.cdc.gov/newbornscreening/. Accessed December 30, 2015.

46. Dondorp W, de Wert G, Bombard Y, et al. European Society of Human Genetics; American Society of Human Genetics. Non-invasive prenatal testing for aneuploidy and beyond: challenges of responsible innovation in prenatal screening. *European Journal of Human Genetics*. 2015;23:1438–1450.

47. Rochman B. New genetic tests for women who are expecting. *The Wall Street Journal*. October 29, 2015.

48. Green RC, Roberts JS, Cupples LA, REVEAL Study Group, et al. "Disclosure of APOE genotype for risk of Alzheimer's disease." *New England Journal of Medicine*. 2009;361(3):245–254.

49. *Factor V Leiden*. National Library of Medicine (U.S.). http:// www.omim.org/search?index=entry&sort=score+desc%2C+ prefix_sort+desc&start=1&limit=10&search=Factor+V+Leid en. Accessed December 30, 2015.

50. *Antithrombin III*. National Library of Medicine (U.S.). http:// omim.org/entry/613118?search=Antithrombin%20III&highl ight=iii%20antithrombin. Accessed December 30, 2015.

51. Kaur H, Grover S, Kukreti R. Concept of pharmacogenomics and future considerations. *CNS Neuroscience & Therapeutics*. 2013 Oct 1;19(10):842–844.

52. Payne PW. For Asians only? The perils of ancestry-based drug prescribing. *Race, Pharmaceuticals, and Medical Technology*. 2008:585–588.

53. Wolpert CM, Powell JD, Haynie K, Kittles R, Royal CD. Genetic ancestry testing and identity: exploring the relationship. [Abstract]. (Ethical, Legal, Social, and Policy Issues in Genetics 2383T). Presented at the 64th Annual Meeting of the American Society of Human Genetics, October 21, 2014, San Diego, CA.

54. Francke U, Dijamco C, Kiefer AK, et al. Dealing with the unexpected: consumer responses to direct-access BRCA mutation testing. *Peer J*. 2013;1(e8).

CHAPTER 16

CHRONIC CARE PERSPECTIVES

Virginia McCoy Hass • Gerald Kayingo

Chronic conditions are the leading causes of illness, disability, and death in the United States today. In 2010, almost 52% (160 million) of all Americans had at least one chronic condition such as diabetes, heart disease, or asthma.[1] Diabetes alone affects more than 29 million people in the United States.[2] Almost 50 million Americans are disabled by a chronic condition. By 2030, this is expected to grow to 171 million people.[3] In addition to the personal burden of disease, the costs to the U.S. health care system are staggering. Eight percent of Medicare beneficiaries have two or more chronic conditions.[1] National health expenditures in 2013 were 17.4% of the U.S. gross domestic product ($2.9 trillion). It is projected that by 2024, health care spending will rise to 19.6% of the U.S. gross domestic product.[4] In 2010, chronic illness accounted for more than 86% of U.S. health care expenditures.[1]

Although chronic illnesses affect individuals of all ages, they are most prevalent in older people.[5] There are more than 40 million people aged 65 and older in the United States.[6] This population is expected to double by 2060, representing more than 20% of the U.S. population.[7] The average person in this age range has two or more chronic conditions, many of which are associated with physical or mental disability. A threefold or greater increase in the disabled elderly population is predicted by the year 2050.[8] The burden of chronic illness falls disproportionately on poor individuals, educationally disadvantaged people, and ethnic minorities.[9] *REACH 2010* reported a substantially higher prevalence of health-risk factors (e.g., obesity, cigarette smoking) and selected chronic conditions (diabetes, cardiovascular disease, hypertension, hyperlipidemia) among ethnic minorities in the United States compared with national estimates.[10] Additionally, age and socioeconomic stress factors interact synergistically to increase risk. These figures highlight an urgent need to redesign our health care system and adapt new models of care that will ensure better access, high-quality, affordable, and coordinated care for chronic diseases.

A NEED FOR COORDINATED, PATIENT-CENTERED CARE

Despite recent changes in health care policies such as the Affordable Care Act, the U.S. health care system remains fragmented and poorly organized to meet the challenges of chronic illness care. Care is not patient centered, and it often leaves patients feeling incapable of meeting the day-to-day challenges of living with a chronic condition. In fact, "over 50% of people with chronic illness do not receive modern, evidence-based care."[11] As described in the 2001 Institute of Medicine report, *Crossing the Quality Chasm: A New Health System for the 21st Century*, the "current health care system cannot do the job," and "merely making incremental improvements in current systems of care will not suffice."[12]

Beginning in the mid-1990s, a number of organizations around the country started addressing these challenges. The MacColl Institute of Healthcare Improvement, under the direction of Ed Wagner, MD, MPH, developed a new systematic model for chronic illness care. This model has been introduced and evaluated in a variety of clinical settings nationwide. Data suggest that a more systematic, proactive, patient-centered and evidence-based approach to care keeps patients with chronic illnesses healthier for a longer period of time.[13–15] In the Chronic Care Model (CCM), the health needs of patients are effectively and timely met. In this model, care delivery can be safe, equitable, and efficient for both patients and providers while morbidity and mortality related to chronic illnesses are reduced.

Another major development in the coordination of care has been the implementation of the patient-centered medical home (PCMH) concept. The PCMH is a health care model in which a team of health professionals work collaboratively to provide high levels of care coordination and integration as well as quality and safety on an ongoing basis.[16,17] In the PCMH, health care is coordinated across all elements of the broader health care system. Coordination of care is associated with reduced emergency department visits, hospitalizations, and readmissions for patients with complex care needs, such as older adults.[18,19] Over the past 7 years, 11,296 primary care practices have transformed into the PCMH model.[20]

PATIENT–CLINICIAN PARTNERSHIPS AND TEAM-BASED CARE: A PARADIGM SHIFT IN CHRONIC DISEASE MANAGEMENT

Chronic disease management requires patient–clinician partnership and a team-based approach. The patient–clinician partnership requires collaborative care, self-management education, self-efficacy support, and effective communication. In team-based care, patients are active members of the teams that manage their chronic illness. Patients should be part of the decision-making process, they should be able to communicate their preferences and choices, and they should have easy access to their clinics and providers. To improve outcomes and patient satisfaction, clinicians should provide effective self-management support and improved

communication among all members of the health care team. This requires innovative solutions such as coordination of care through health information technology, evidence-based practice, a population-wide approach, and continuous quality improvement initiatives.[21]

The CCM identifies six essential elements needed to improve chronic care within the community and health system. Community factors include resources and policies; health system factors include health care organizations, patient self-management support, delivery system design, decision support tools, and clinical information systems.[13] The goal of the model is "Promoting effective change in provider groups to support evidence-based clinical and quality improvement across a wide variety of health care settings."[1] This goal is accomplished through "productive interactions" between a "prepared, proactive practice team" and an "informed, activated patient," which in turn will lead to improved health outcomes.[13-15] The CCM was developed to promote integrated change with components directed at:

- Influencing provider behavior
- Better use of nonphysician team members
- Enhancement of information systems
- Planned encounters (interactions linked through time to achieve specific goals)
- Patient self-management
- Modern self-management support

The CCM incorporates additional themes within the context of the model's elements: (1) patient safety (Health System), (2) cultural competency (Delivery System), (3) care coordination (Health System and Clinical Information Systems), (4) community policies (Community Resources and Policies), and (5) case management (Delivery System Design).[22] Fig. 16.1 illustrates the relational concepts of the Chronic Care and PCMH models.

ELEMENTS OF THE CHRONIC CARE MODEL

The *community* creates the context in which health care is delivered. Community programs can support or expand a health system's ability to care for chronically ill patients. The health care system can enhance care for its patients by forming partnerships to support and develop interventions that fill gaps in needed services and by avoiding duplication of effort.[22]

Health systems can create an organizational culture and mechanisms that promote safe, high-quality care. Ideally, this culture: "1) visibly supports improvement at all levels of the organization, beginning with the senior leader; 2) promotes effective improvement strategies aimed at comprehensive system change; 3)

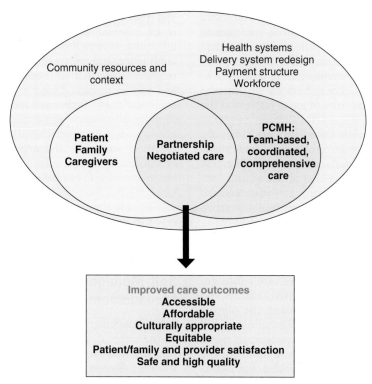

FIG. 16.1 ■ Model for chronic care in the patient-centered medical home.

encourages open and systematic handling of errors and quality problems to improve care; 4) provides incentives based on quality of care (e.g., pay-for-performance, provider incentives); and 5) develops agreements that facilitate care coordination within and across organizations."[22]

All people make decisions and engage in behaviors that affect their health, and this is no less true for people with chronic illness. These behaviors constitute *self-management*. The outcomes of chronic illness depend largely on the self-management decisions patients make. Effective *self-management support* prepares patients and their caregivers to manage their health and health care by (1) emphasizing patients' central role in managing their health; (2) using strategies that include assessment, goal setting, planning, problem solving, and follow-up; and (3) organizing resources to provide sustainable self-management support.[22]

Improving the health of people with chronic illness requires the creation of a system that is proactive and focused on promotion of health. This objective is accomplished through design of *delivery systems* that ensure effective clinical care and self-management support. This design increases the use of nonphysician team members by defining roles and distributing tasks based on efficient use of team

members' skills. In a proactive delivery system, there are planned interactions that support evidence-based care. Approaches to these interactions may include (1) longer visits (not necessarily more frequent), (2) an agenda, (3) regular follow-up by the team, and 4) clinical case management services for patients with complex needs. Health literacy and cultural competency are two important concepts in health care. Effective delivery system design includes the ability to respond effectively to the diverse cultural and linguistic needs of patients.[22]

Decision support is essential to the delivery of high-quality, evidence-based care that incorporates patient preferences. In a delivery system with effective decision support, evidence-based guidelines are embedded into daily clinical practice through reminders, feedback, standing orders, and other methods that increase their visibility at the time that clinical decisions are made. Furthermore, these guidelines and information are shared with patients to encourage their participation. For more complex patient care, specialist expertise is integrated into the delivery of primary care.[22]

Effective chronic illness care requires information systems that ensure access to vital data on both individual patients and patient populations. *Clinical information systems* may be electronic or paper based and are used to organize patient and population data to facilitate care. At the individual level, information systems provide reminders to patients and providers and facilitate individual care planning. At the population level, information systems identify related subpopulations for targeted care and aid monitoring the performance of providers, the practice team, and the care system.[22]

These six elements combined support *productive interactions* that are the core of chronic disease management. Note that "interaction" is used deliberately to move away from the idea that all encounters are clinical visits. Phone calls, emails, self-management classes, and support groups are all examples of strategies demonstrated to be effective in improving patient–clinician communication.[23-26] Half of the productive interaction is a *prepared, proactive practice team*. To have productive interactions, we need a different kind of team. Also, effective care coordination within health care teams and across facilities and community resources means rethinking the players on the team, their roles, and using all members to full capacity. In addition to the PA, physician, or nurse practitioner, new team members can be added or the roles of existing team members expanded. For example, with enhanced training medical assistants can help with previsit planning, reconcile medications, participate in quality improvement projects, and provide health coaching for patients.[27] Registered nurses (RNs) are ideally suited for direct patient care and leadership roles in PCMHs, based on their education in patient care and family and systems theory. Data show that use of RNs in team-based primary care to provide episodic and preventive care and chronic disease management and to oversee clinical operations such as staff supervision and quality improvement, resulted in improved patient outcomes, productivity, and reduced cost.[28] Seventy-one percent of physician visits involve medication management, including evaluation of therapeutic efficacy, adverse drug events, and potential drug interactions.[29] Studies have demonstrated a correlation between the risk of adverse drug events and nonadherence and complexity of the medication regimen.[30,31] This is an opportunity to use the untapped potential of clinical pharmacists to optimize complex therapeutic regimens. Clinical pharmacists perform comprehensive therapy reviews, resolve problems with medications, support adherence and self-management, and recommend economical therapeutic alternatives.[32] In addition to having the right mix of health care professionals, the team must have decision support tools, clinical information systems available at the point of service, and the resources necessary to deliver high-quality care. A crucial member of team-based care,

and the other half of the productive interaction, is an *informed, activated patient (and caregiver)*. An informed, activated patient has the knowledge, skills, confidence, and motivation to self-manage care. This requires more than the traditional patient teaching and will be discussed later in this chapter. There is evidence that, with appropriate self-management support, almost any patient can become a relatively effective self-manager.[33-36] Productive interactions are recognizable by the presence of (1) assessment of self-management skills and confidence as well as clinical status; (2) collaborative definition of problems; (3) collaborative setting of goals and problem solving; (4) the development of a shared care plan; (5) tailoring of clinical management by stepped protocols and guidelines; and (6) planned, active, and sustained follow-up.[22]

Self-Management and Self-Management Support

Self-management and self-management support are at the core of the clinician–patient encounter. All patients manage their day-to-day lives and health, whether they do it effectively or otherwise. In the context of chronic illness, self-management becomes particularly important. Research regarding the effectiveness of patient education tells us that providing information alone is not enough. That is, providing information in the absence of self-management support does not change health outcomes.[24,37,38] This has been described by Bodenheimer[34,36] as the "50% rule"; half of patients are unable to repeat back what they are told by a physician, half do not understand how to take their medications and take them incorrectly, and half of patients leave a clinical visit without understanding what the physician said.[39-41] The lifelong work of patients managing chronic illness encompasses three sets of tasks. The first set entails medical management of the illness, such as diet, medications, regular follow-up, and laboratory tests. The second set includes adaptation of life roles and behaviors, such as modification of work or recreational activities to fit functional capacity. Finally, the third set involves coping with the emotional aspects of chronic illness, which can include depression, anger, and fear. Self-management programs, therefore, must include all three sets of tasks required to effectively manage chronic illness.[42]

The components of effective self-management support are (1) providing information; (2) intensive, disease-specific skills training; (3) encouraging healthy behavior change; (4) teaching patients both action-planning and problem-solving skills; (5) assisting patients with the emotional aspects of having a chronic illness; (6) encouraging patients to become "informed and activated"; and (7) providing ongoing and regular follow-up.[43] Current evidence demonstrates that follow-up has the greatest impact on health outcomes and that follow-up need not be a clinic encounter. Strategies such as web-based programs, email, telephone calls, and peer support are all effective.[18,20] A meta-analysis of 31 randomized controlled trials (RCTs) testing the effect of self-management education on hemoglobin A_{1C} in adults with type 2 diabetes demonstrated that the effect of education wanes after 3 months and that sustained follow-up closely correlated with improved glycemic control.[25,26,44] A meta-analysis of eight RCTs testing the effect of changing provider–patient interactions and provider counseling style on patient diabetes self-care and diabetes outcomes showed that interventions aimed at improving patient self-efficacy were more successful in improving outcomes than interventions aimed at provider behavior.[35]

MOTIVATIONAL INTERVIEWING AND ACTION PLANNING

Miller and Rollnick[45] define motivational interviewing as "a directive client-centered counseling approach for initiating behavior change by helping clients to resolve ambivalence." It is beyond the scope of this chapter to instruct the reader in all the aspects of motivational interviewing. For further information, readers are referred to *Motivational Interviewing: Preparing People for Change*, 2nd ed. (p. 325).[45] Motivational interviewing is a philosophy in which a blend of patient-centered and coaching strategies, combined with understanding of what triggers behavior change, is used to guide clinician–patient interactions. The key principles of motivational interviewing are summarized in Table 16.1. Two key concepts of motivational interviewing are addressing ambivalence and recognizing resistance as a cue to the need for changing *clinician* behavior. Ambivalence can be defined as a conflict between two courses of action, each of which has potential advantages and disadvantages. Ambivalence may derive from (1) not knowing what to change, (2) not knowing how to change, (3) not believing a change needs to occur, (4) not understanding why a change needs to occur, or (5) doubt in the ability to be successful in making the change. Resistance occurs because the person is unwilling to make the change or perceives the costs associated with the change (e.g., giving up smoking) as outweighing the

TABLE 16.1 Key Principles of Motivational Interviewing

1. Express empathy.
   - Reflective listening is used to *understand* the patient's feelings *without judging*. Accurate empathy is acceptance of the patient's perspective as valid within his or her framework. It is *not* agreement or approval.
   - Acceptance facilitates change.
   - Ambivalence is normal.
2. Develop discrepancy.
   - Develop and magnify, from the patient's point of view, the discrepancy between the behavior and their long-term or larger goals.
   - The goal is to aid the patient in moving past ambivalence toward change.
   - The patient, not the health care provider, should present arguments for change.
3. Roll with resistance.
   - Resistance is a signal to respond differently; resume asking questions rather than offering answers.
   - The patient, not the provider, generates solutions.
   - An analogy is to "dance with" rather than "wrestle with" the patient.
   - Respectful of autonomy.
   - Avoids arguing for change by not directly challenging resistance.
4. Support self-efficacy.
   - The patient's belief that change is possible is an important motivator.
   - The patient, not the provider, chooses and brings about the change.
   - Self-efficacy (confidence) is a good predictor of outcomes.

Adapted from Miller WR, Rollnick S. *Motivational Interviewing: Preparing People for Change*, 2nd ed. New York: Guilford Press; 2002.

benefits (e.g., possibly avoiding future lung disease). The principles of motivational interviewing are best described as an interpersonal style that can be used in a variety of therapeutic encounters, rather than a prescribed set of techniques. Table 16.2 compares clinician behaviors that facilitate motivational interviewing with those that impede the process. Physician assistants (PAs) are in an excellent position to identify patients at risk for poor health outcomes and to use the patient-centered communication method of motivational interviewing to actively engage them in a successful behavior change process. The role is not to tell patients what to do but to listen, provide empathy, alleviate ambivalence, provide information, and serve as a change agent. Motivational interviewing strategies provide a framework for this effort, as demonstrated in Case Study 16.1. Respect of autonomy and self-determination and support of self-efficacy are key elements that contribute to success.

TABLE 16.2 Comparison of Clinician Behavior Impact on Motivational Interviewing

Clinician Behaviors That Facilitate Motivational Interviewing	Clinician Behaviors That Impede Motivational Interviewing
• Use reflective listening to understand the patient's perspective. • Express acceptance and affirmation. • Elicit and selectively reinforce the client's own self-motivational statements, self-efficacy, and resolution of ambivalence. • Assess the patient's readiness to change. • Avoid resistance by not moving forward faster than the patient. • Respect and acknowledge the patient's autonomy and freedom of choice.	• Argue that the patient must change. • Offer direct advice without the patient's permission. • Direct behavior change without actively encouraging the person to make his or her own decisions. • Use the "expert" role to keep the patient in a passive role. • Control the conversation by doing most of the talking. • Behave punitively or coercively. • Use "motivational techniques" as a means to manipulate the patient.

CASE STUDY 16.1 USING MOTIVATIONAL INTERVIEWING STRATEGIES IN SMOKING-CESSATION COUNSELING

S.S. is a 50-year-old Vietnamese man with a recent diagnosis of chronic obstructive pulmonary disease (COPD). He has a 36-pack-year history of cigarette smoking. He works as a computer programmer. He has been happily married for 27 years, with three children, ages 25, 22, and 14 years. The youngest child lives at home; the older two live nearby. He has lived in the United States since 15 years of age. He has a large extended family also living in the area. Family history is significant for gastric cancer in his mother and early death from lung disease in his father. Both of his parents smoked. S.S. is here today for a planned visit to follow up on his COPD. He also has a chief complaint of productive cough. As his primary care PA, your role is to provide information and support for health behavior change related to his lung disease and smoking.

EXPRESS EMPATHY

Empathy expression is accomplished by being nonjudgmental, with a genuine concern for the patient's well-being; allowing him to set the agenda while you ask necessary questions.[33] You can begin to raise awareness about COPD by asking him about the symptoms he is having, his tobacco use, and previous attempts to quit smoking. Encouraging the patient to talk is respectful and builds autonomy. Asking open-ended questions facilitates information gathering and explores his feelings. Reflective listening demonstrates to him that what is said is actually being heard. As the conversation continues, the goal is to develop discrepancy. Mr. S. stated he knew that his smoking was making his cough worse, and he is concerned that he will die early, as did his father, and "miss knowing my grandchildren." He has tried to quit twice before, but "just couldn't do it." Cigarettes help him relax when his work pressures "build up." Empathy is the objective identification with the affective state of another, not his or her experience. Empathy is the primary interpersonal skill for expressing caring and understanding. For example, Mr. S. wishes to quit smoking but enjoys the relaxation he gets from smoking. We do not have to smoke ourselves to understand these conflicting desires. An empathic response would be, "It would be difficult to quit smoking when it helps you relieve stress." Strategies such as affirming and elaborating further explore and reinforce self-efficacy.

DEVELOP DISCREPANCY

Developing discrepancy is a means of creating cognitive dissonance,[45] the psychological discomfort that arises from holding two conflicting thoughts in the mind at the same time. Cognitive dissonance is a powerful motivator of change. Discrepancy may be developed by asking the patient to list the benefits versus the costs of the behavior or behavioral change he or she is contemplating and then reflecting on the pros and cons while highlighting inconsistencies. Asking the patient to elaborate on discrepancies between stated goals and present behaviors that contradict those goals is a powerful means of developing discrepancy and motivating change. For example, Mr. S. continues to smoke. You state, "Mr. S., I see that you continue to smoke. What are your thoughts about how this affects your goal to live long enough to know your grandchildren?" The question is nonjudgmental and draws on Mr. S.'s own conclusions. Although it creates dissonance, it does not present an argument for change. The question is designed to facilitate the patient's "change talk" or arguments for change based on examining his risks, recognizing them, and foreseeing potential consequences.

AVOID ARGUMENT

Avoiding argument means not eliciting resistance by forcing patients to defend the behaviors they are trying to change. By avoiding argument, it is more likely that patients will see you as an ally.[45]

For example, Mr. S. states, "I've tried quitting smoking before, and couldn't do it. There's no point in trying again." Resistance is a cue to change your approach; use open-ended questions to get the patient talking. Rather than tell him many patients have to try more than once, you state, "It sounds as if you're frustrated by your previous attempts to quit smoking. What problems did you have?" This response is empathic, addresses the patient's emotional state, and asks for additional input.

ROLL WITH RESISTANCE

Rolling with resistance means going with what the patient is willing to do. This sometimes means doing nothing at that time.[45] For example, Mr. S. states, "I'm okay. My breathing isn't nearly as bad as my father's was." Rather than arguing with this statement by responding, "If you continue smoking, you will probably get worse," you can roll with the resistance by saying, "I hope that your health continues to stay good. However, keep getting regular check-ups because that may change. I'm here to help if you wish to quit smoking as time goes on." In this way, you have followed the direction set by the patient, as well as created a discrepancy. You have not scolded him and have left the door open for future conversations.

SUPPORT SELF-EFFICACY

Self-efficacy is a patient's confidence that he or she can make life changes. Self-efficacy is an important motivator for behavior change, and supporting self-efficacy is a key skill of motivational interviewing.[45] Look for opportunities to praise the efforts patients make toward positive behavior change. For example, Mr. S. comes in for a planned visit and tells you, "I've cut down on my smoking." A supportive response would be, "That's an important step to improve your health; tell me more about how you did it." Such a response congratulates and reinforces the positive change the patient has made and facilitates the discussion of any difficulties he is encountering. In this conversation, he has accepted the fact that behavior change might decrease his risk for early death and disability. As Mr. S. continues to direct the conversation, he begins to believe he can continue cutting down on his smoking and develops ideas for other ways to reduce his stress. This is the time to actively engage him in action planning. In the end, Mr. S. elicited his own arguments for change and set goals for action.

The goal of motivational interviewing is to elicit "change talk"[45] and thus facilitate goal setting. Action planning is a proven strategy for building self-efficacy while working toward goals.[46–48] The "5 A's"—assess, advise, agree, assist, and arrange—adapted from the Agency for Healthcare

Quality Research (AHQR) clinical practice guidelines,[43,44,49-51] are a patient-centered model of behavioral counseling that is congruent with the CCM. They have been frequently used to enhance self-management support and linkages to community resources. Table 16.3 outlines the 5 A's. Readiness scales measure two concepts: (1) How important is the change to the patient? and (2) How confident is the patient that he or she can do what is needed? Importance and confidence levels of 7 or higher correlate to higher probability of success. See Figs. 16.2 and 16.3 for examples of these scales. The 5 A's and readiness scales are a quick and effective way for eliciting discussions on change and determining what else needs to happen for the patient to make an even greater commitment to change. Case Study 16.2 illustrates the use of readiness scales.

TABLE 16.3 **The Five A's**	
Assess	Patients' beliefs, behavior, and knowledge
Advise	Patients by providing specific information about health risks and benefits of change
Agree	On a collaboratively set of goals based on patients' confidence in their ability to change the behavior
Assist	Patients with problem-solving by identifying personal barriers, strategies, and social and environmental support
Arrange	A specific follow-up plan

Adapted from Agency for Healthcare Quality Research. 3 brief clinical interventions. http://www.ncbi.nlm.nih.gov/books/NBK18002/.

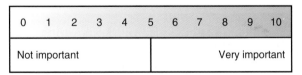

FIG. 16.2 ■ Importance scale.

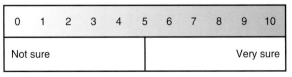

FIG. 16.3 ■ Confidence scale.

CASE STUDY 16.2 USING READINESS SCALES

In Case Study 16.1, you sense some ambivalence or resistance on the part of Mr. S. about quitting smoking. You decide to use the readiness and confidence scales to explore his ambivalence. Ask, "On a scale from 0 to 10, where 0 is not at all important and 10 is very important, how important is it for you to quit smoking?" Mr. S. answers, "Four." Rather than responding, "Why a 4 and not a 10?" which would cause him to talk about why he does not want to quit smoking, ask, "Why a 4 and not a 0?" This response elicits "change talk" because it allows Mr. S. to state reasons that he thinks it is important to quit smoking. Let him respond and then ask, "What would it take to make your answer 5 or 6?" This elicits motivating factors from Mr. S. and encourages him to think about incremental change. If he cannot come up with an answer at this moment to raise his response to 5 or 6, ask him to think about it and let you know at a follow-up visit. You are planting the seeds of dissonance to create change. The same steps are used with the confidence scale. Ask Mr. S. how confident he feels that he can quit smoking at this time.

After the patient's priorities and confidence level are identified, the next step is to facilitate action planning. Successful action plans build self-efficacy by breaking larger, long-term goals into manageable pieces. They have five basic characteristics: (1) The action to be taken is something the patient wants to do; (2) the goal is reasonable (can be accomplished in one week); (3) they are behavior specific; (4) they answer the questions, What? How much? When? and How often?; and (5) the patient's confidence level is 7 or more.[40] The steps of action planning are listed in Table 16.4. Case Study 16.3 illustrates a patient's use of the steps.

CASE STUDY 16.3 ACTION PLANNING

Ms. T. is a 47-year-old woman who is morbidly obese and has not exercised in years. During a clinic visit, she identifies two goals for improving her health: losing 60 lb and exercising daily, which she defines as walking around the park with her friend who is "very fit."

STEP 1. DECIDE WHAT SHE WANTS TO ACCOMPLISH

Ms. T.'s list includes the goal, "I want to be able to walk around the park with my friend." The perimeter of the park is 1 mile, and she currently can walk 1 block before stopping to rest.

STEP 2. LOOK FOR ALTERNATIVES TO ACCOMPLISH THE GOAL AND IDENTIFY BARRIERS

A barrier Ms. T. identifies is that she is concerned that she will not be able to get home if she walks too far. Options for reaching the goal include driving to the park before walking, taking her cell phone on her walk, and walking in front of her house.

STEP 3. DEVELOP SHORT-TERM PLAN

Ms. T.'s action plan reads, "I will walk up and down the sidewalk in front of my house for 5 minutes, before watching the evening news, three times per week, and my confidence level is 7." This is a specific, measurable statement of the behavior change, with a reasonable probability of success.

STEP 4. CARRY OUT THE PLAN

Ms. T. recorded her activity on a wall calendar with large date areas for writing. She noted the days she walked and the days she did not, with the reasons for not walking.

STEP 5. CHECK THE RESULTS

Ms. T. walked for 5 minutes in front of her house on 2 days during the week.

STEP 6. MAKE CHANGES AS NEEDED

As part of her problem solving, Ms. T identified that it was rainy and cold on 5 of 7 days during the week; she was concerned about being out in the weather. She decided to purchase a treadmill so that she could walk indoors on rainy days.

STEP 7. REWARD YOURSELF

Ms. T. decided that she would drink a 4-oz glass of her favorite red wine only after she had completed her walking. This turned a glass of wine into her reward.

POPULATION-BASED CHRONIC DISEASE MANAGEMENT

Population-based disease management evolved from single-payer systems in Europe and staff model health maintenance organizations (HMOs) in the United States as a strategy to improve the cost-effectiveness and quality of care to high-risk populations.[52] Population-based care is a structured approach to a subset of patients who share a particular characteristic or medical condition. Clinical information systems, such as patient registries, are used to collect outcome data. Evaluation of these data enables tracking of health outcomes.[53] Population-based care facilitates the delivery of targeted interventions to improve health outcomes within the population. Third-party payers and employers also use population data to monitor the performance

TABLE 16.4 Patient Steps for Action Planning

1. *Decide* what you want to accomplish.
   - These are the long-term goals—they will be broken into "do-able" chunks later.
   - Make a list of goals; put a star next to the one you wish to work on first.
2. Look for *alternative ways* to accomplish this goal. Think about barriers you might encounter, and include ideas for overcoming them.
   - List the options you might use to reach the goal. Ask family and friends for ideas if you are having difficulty with this.
   - Thoroughly explore each option before discarding it as unworkable.
3. Start making *short-term* plans by making an action plan or agreement with yourself.
   - This is the action plan and should be a specific, measurable *behavior or set of behaviors* that can be accomplished in 1 week and will help you move toward your goal.
   - Decide *what* you will do *this week.* The plan should contain four parts:
     a. Exactly what will you do?
        Start where you are, or start slowly. For example, "I will walk up and down the sidewalk in front of my house."
     b. How much will you do?
        Be specific. Continuing the above example, "for 5 minutes."
     c. When will you do it?
        Connecting the new activity to a favorite old one is a good way to make sure you do it. Continuing the above example, "before watching the evening news."
     d. How often will you do it?
        Setting a goal that is less than your ideal, e.g., three to four times per week, rather than daily, decreases the pressure to perform. It also gives you some time off. Continuing the above example, "three times a week."
     e. Assess your confidence level on a scale of 0 to 10. If your confidence that you can accomplish the plan is less than 7, consider modifying the plan.
4. *Carry out* your action plans.
   - This is usually the easy part if the action plan is well written and realistic.
   - Keep track of your progress by noting your activities, both when the activity was accomplished and when it was not. This record is used in the next step.
   - In the example, this might include making a log for recording activity or noting on the calendar both the days you walked and the days you did not. Be sure to note the factors that helped you accomplish your activity or that prevented you from doing it.
5. *Check* the results against the plan.
        At the end of the week, review the action plan. Did you complete it? Are you further along toward your goal?
6. Make *changes* as needed.
   - This is the problem-solving step. If you did not accomplish all the parts of your action plan, *do not give up.*
   - Identify the barriers that prevented you from achieving the steps.
   - List possible remedies to the problem (much as you did in step 2). Then pick *one* to try.
   - Repeat steps 3 to 6, modifying your action plan so that the steps are easier to achieve.
        Note that not all problems are solvable. If several honest attempts to work out a problem are not successful, it may be advisable to move on to another goal at present.
7. Remember to *reward* yourself.
   - Accomplishing your goals is a reward and builds confidence (self-efficacy). But do not wait until you reach your goal to reward yourself!
   - Rewards do not have to be expensive or elaborate. Think about healthy pleasures you can add to your life.

Adapted from Lorig K, Holman H, Sobel D, et al. *Living a Healthy Life with Chronic Conditions*, 3rd ed. Palo Alto, CA: Bull Publishing; 2006.

of providers and health care systems. The National Committee for Quality Assurance (NCQA) developed and maintains the Health Plan Employer Data and Information Set (HEDIS). HEDIS is a set of standardized performance measures used by health care purchasers and consumers to compare the performance of managed health care plans. In turn, third-party payers use HEDIS measures to evaluate health systems and providers. Health care providers also use HEDIS measures to self-evaluate the care they provide. HEDIS measures relate to many chronic conditions, such as heart disease, diabetes, and smoking, and include consumer satisfaction as well as health outcome measures.[53] These measures give health care consumers and purchasers the ability to evaluate and compare the quality of health plans and providers. The ability to obtain and apply information about patient populations and the larger population from which they are drawn allows the PA to implement practice-based learning and improvement. Case Study 16.4 illustrates an approach to population-based care.

A PA working in a community health clinic is concerned about the rate of complications among the patients who have diabetes. She knows that addressing individual health behaviors is an important part of chronic illness care, and she uses strategies such as motivational interviewing and action planning with her patients. However, she wonders if there is a systems-based problem that is impacting health outcomes and whether a more collaborative approach to care would improve outcomes. The PA works with the clinic staff and her supervising physician to develop a list of the patients seen at the clinic who have diabetes. Having read about the CCM, the PA investigates the Improving Chronic Illness Care website (www.improvingchroniccare.org) and finds a wealth of resources for implementing the CCM into practice (http://www.improvingchronicc are.org/index.php?p=Toolkit&s=244). On this site, she learns about CCM Implementation Tools and a variety of public domain electronic chronic disease registry tools. She goes to the Chronic Disease Electronic Management System (CDEMS) website (http://publichealth.hsc.wvu.edu/ohsr/services/chr onic-disease-electronic-management-system-cd ems). Using this tool, she is able to develop and customize a registry to share with her colleagues. The clinic has an electronic health record (EHR). However, the system does not provide robust tracking and report features. Therefore, data are pulled from the EHR and entered into the CDEMS to create a registry. Although the task appears daunting, the team works together to create a registry database for each patient that includes key health outcome measures for diabetes: (1) date of last foot examination, (2) date of last eye examination, (3) last blood pressure and date, (4) last HgbA$_{1C}$ and date, (5) last low-density lipoprotein (LDL) level and date, and (6) latest self-management goal and date. The PA and her supervising physician analyzed the data they had collected, compared the results with HEDIS53 targets for those measures, and identified the following trends in the clinic's population of patients with diabetes:

- 103 (76%) have a foot examination documented within the past year
- 45 (33%) have an eye examination documented within the past year
- 121 (89%) have last blood pressure at or below the target of 130/80 mm Hg
- 75 (55%) have last HgbA$_{1C}$ of less than 9.0%
- 82 (60%) have last LDL of 100 mg/dl or less
- 56 (41%) have a documented self-management goal

They realize that four of the six measures have room for improvement. As with action planning and behavior change with patients, systems change is best broken into manageable, achievable steps toward a goal. The entire clinic staff meets as a team to prioritize the list of goals. They elect to work on self-management goal setting with patients first because they see this as the indicator likely to have the biggest impact. The steps identified in reaching this goal were training all clinic staff in the CCM, emphasizing self-management support and action planning. They also decide to explore community resources to facilitate access to eye examinations for their patients to improve this health measure.

This scenario illustrates a constructive process for a health care provider to follow in implementing population-based care:

1. Observe and verify the existence of important patterns of disease.
2. Use published resources or conduct a literature review to identify health outcome goals and tools for change.
3. Identify the community resources available to facilitate health access for populations.
4. Serve as a facilitator for the communication of ideas and systems change.

THE PHYSICIAN ASSISTANT AS A MEMBER OF THE CHRONIC CARE TEAM: AN INTEGRATION OF THE PHYSICIAN ASSISTANT CORE COMPETENCIES

At the foundation of the CCM is the use of a population-based approach to care and of interdisciplinary teams in the coordination of care. Research suggests that people with chronic illnesses can be risk stratified, with interventions tailored to the risk level of individual patients and populations.[14,15] In applying such tailored interventions, the use of an interdisciplinary team plays a central role. Clearly, PAs play a key role in such interdisciplinary teams. Depending on the practice setting, the PA may provide care in group visits for patients who are in reasonable control of their condition and provide regular, planned chronic care visits for patients who are newly diagnosed or in poor control. The PA also plays an important role in providing self-management support for patients with chronic illnesses, ensuring that care fits with the patient's cultural background.

Whether caring for patients with diabetes, hypertension, congestive heart failure, asthma, or a combination of several chronic diseases, the PA, as a member of the prepared practice team, is instrumental in improving patient outcomes. To change—and by that, we mean to improve—outcomes requires fundamental practice changes. The integrated practice changes that are needed to shift into a chronic care collaborative approach are directed at influencing physician behavior, using PAs and other nonphysician team members better, enhancing information systems, and using planned encounters.

Incorporation of the CCM and implementation of PCMHs are systematic methods to decrease variation in quality of care among practitioners. The PA's role and the competencies for the PA profession integrate nicely into these models of care. It is interesting to point out is that research has shown that this variation of quality of care delivered is greater within a single practice than among health care systems.[12] This means that individual providers can indeed have a profound effect in changing practice to improve health outcomes in their patient population.

Before a discussion of how PA competencies relate to the CCM, a historical perspective in their development is warranted. In 1995, the American Academy of Physician Assistants (AAPA) initiated the first of three studies to identify the "core competencies" of the PA profession. This was in response to many calls for an increased focus on competency, one of which first occurred in the same year, when the Pew Health Professions Commission released their report—*Reforming Health Care Workforce: Policy Considerations for the 21st Century.*[54] The AAPA concluded that workforce regulation could be responsive to public expectation (safe, high-quality health care) if practice acts for the health professions focused on "demonstrated initial and continuing competence."[54] From 1999 to 2003, the Institute of Medicine (IOM) released a series of reports concerning quality of health care and patient safety. The first, *To Err Is Human: Building a Safer Health System,*[55] captured the public's attention with its estimate that as many as 98,000 people die annually in hospitals from preventable medical errors. The IOM suggested that patient safety could improve if licensing, certification, and accreditation agencies were to develop and implement specific patient safety standards.[55] In 2001, the IOM released a follow-up report, *Crossing the Quality Chasm,*[11] in which it recommended that change was needed at all levels of the health care system if quality of care was to improve. The IOM advocated for training and ongoing certification to ensure the continued competence of health care providers. In its 2003 report, *Health Professions Education: A Bridge to Quality,* the IOM advocated for a shift to a competency-based approach to education and ongoing certification.[56] The *Competencies for the Physician Assistant Profession* were first adopted in 2005 by the AAPA and revised in 2012 in response

to this report.[57,58] These competencies have also been adopted by other PA organizations such as the Accreditation Review Commission on Education for the Physician Assistant, the National Commission on Certification of Physician Assistants, and the Physician Assistant Education Association.[58,59]

The CCM was created as a response to the same marketplace pressures: (1) chronic disease emerging as the dominant health problem; (2) health care systems' poor performance measured by outcomes; and (3) societal expectation to receive safe, high-quality health care. Chronic disease is now the principal cause of disability and the consumer of 78% of health expenditures in this country.[60] It is understandable that because the Accreditation Council for Graduate Medical Education and PA profession core competencies and the CCM are driven by the same desire to improve health care outcomes for patients, they would share the same vision and principles.

The clinical role of PAs includes primary and specialty care in medical and surgical practice settings. Professional competencies for PAs include the effective and appropriate application of medical knowledge, interpersonal and communication skills, patient care, professionalism, practice-based learning and improvement, and systems-based practice, as well as an unwavering commitment to continual learning and professional growth. The physician–PA partnership works for the benefit of patients and the larger community being served. For an individual PA, these competencies are demonstrated within the scope of practice as defined by the supervising physician and appropriate to the health care setting.[58]

Physician assistants can use their medical knowledge and communication skills in the context of the CCM to provide appropriate care to patients with chronic conditions. To accomplish this, PAs:

- Incorporate evidence-based medicine guidelines into their management of patients.
- Obtain and apply information about their population of patients and the larger populations from which their patients are drawn.
- Are proactive by scheduling follow-up appointments; using planned encounters versus reactive encounters when a patient is in crisis or ill.
- Implement modern self-management support— *modern* in the sense that there is research that shows improved outcomes when using certain surveys or motivational interviewing techniques.

With the patient at the center of care, motivational interviewing is important to assess the patient's knowledge, skills, and confidence to establish measurable goals that are achievable through an action plan. Effective self-management support increases the patient's knowledge, skills, and confidence to set goals and achieve a healthier state and perhaps reduce further risk or consequences of an uncontrolled chronic condition. As an example, the physician–PA team, along with their staff, can improve a diabetic patient's health outcome by (1) offering *knowledge support*: regarding the etiology of diabetes, how diet and exercise for weight loss and medication work to counter the high sugar state, and consequences of poor control; (2) offering *skills support*: teaching how to perform a finger stick, use a glucometer, inject insulin and count calories; and (3) encouraging *goal setting with confidence assessment support*, through motivational interviewing. Patients may set goals to achieve a certain LDL level or $HgbA_{1C}$ level or state they want to exercise five times weekly. The key to goal setting is that it must be achievable, and the patient must have high enough confidence that he or she will succeed. The PA needs to give emotional support to patients with chronic conditions, focusing on care versus cure and improving patients' function and comfort. This requires interpersonal and effective listening skills. Case Study 16.1 demonstrates the motivational interview process.

Within the context of practice-based learning, PAs, along with their supervising physicians and health care managers, should assess, coordinate, and improve the delivery of health care and patient outcomes.[58] In the CCM, using clinical information systems and participating in quality improvement work are tied directly to delivery system design and health system organization. It is important for PAs to understand not only their role within the health care team but also how their practice and their patients fit into the larger health care system and the community as a whole. Accessing community resources will improve patient care and reduce duplication of effort and therefore reduce costs. Table 16.5 illustrates how the PA competencies interrelate and overlap with the concepts and framework of the CCM.

By embracing the CCM approach, which encompasses the societal, organizational, and economic environments in which health care is delivered, and applying it to their practice, each PA will exhibit and demonstrate the competencies laid out for the profession.

NEW REIMBURSEMENT MODELS

Starting in January 2015, Medicare is now reimbursing physicians, PAs, and most advanced practice nurses (APRN) for non–face-to-face care coordination for patients with two or more chronic conditions.[61-64] Some of the chronic care services covered in this payment reform include development and maintenance of a plan of care, communication with other treating health care professionals, and medication management. Examples of eligible chronic conditions include, but are not limited to, Alzheimer disease, arthritis, asthma, cancer, chronic obstructive pulmonary disease, depression, diabetes, heart failure, hypertension, and osteoporosis. To be eligible, coordination of chronic care management services must be at least 20 minutes of clinician time per month. Of note, the Centers for Medicare and Medicaid Services (CMS) has provided an exception to Medicare's "incident to" rules. This exception allows PAs and eligible APRNs to bill for incident-to services under the general supervision of a physician rather than the direct physician supervision usually required for incident-to billing. CMS requires an initial visit in which comprehensive, patient-centered plan for chronic care is established before billing for chronic care management services. Furthermore, CMS requires the use of certified EHR technology for implementation of the care plan.[65] Physician assistants now have 24/7 access to address patients' needs supported by access to the EHR. This facilitates care coordination, including safe and efficient care transitions. This reimbursement reform provides a new opportunity and incentives for PAs to provide effective care coordination for their patients with chronic complex conditions. Additionally, these reforms have enhanced the patient's ability to be active participants in their care and engage in effective self-management.

USE OF TECHNOLOGY IN CHRONIC DISEASE MANAGEMENT: NEW FRONTIERS

The advent of mHealth and PCMHs has led to a rise in the use of health technology for chronic diseases. Almost three quarters of the world's population has access to a mobile phone.[66] This explosion of mobile technology provides enormous potential for access to basic health information and improved chronic disease management, particularly in underserved areas. mHealth devices such as application software and wearable devices are showing great promise in improving patient adherence to exercise, nutrition education, smoking cessation, and weight loss programs.[67] EHRs, telemedicine, and mobile technologies are used to facilitate patient monitoring, education, adherence to care plans, and communication among members of the health care team.[68-70] Data show that implementation of EHRs and mHealth is associated with improved clinical outcomes, quality of care, and patient satisfaction.[71,72] Also, studies investigating the impact of telehealth have demonstrated significant reductions in cost and mortality. In a study of the efficacy of care

TABLE 16.5 Comparison of Competencies for the Physician Assistant Profession and the Chronic Care Model

Competencies for the Physician Assistant Profession (Excerpted from the AAPA)	Concepts within the Chronic Care Model
Medical Knowledge • Demonstrate core knowledge of established and evolving biomedical and clinical sciences, and apply it to patient care. • Provide appropriate care to patients with chronic conditions. • Demonstrate an investigatory and analytic thinking approach to clinical situations.	**Decision Support** • Promote clinical care that is consistent with scientific evidence and patient preferences. • Embed evidence-based guidelines into daily clinic practice. • Integrate specialist expertise and primary care.
Interpersonal and Communication Skills • Apply an understanding of human behavior. • Appropriately adapt communication style and messages to the context of the individual patient interaction. • Use effective listening skills, nonverbal, explanatory, questioning, and writing skills to elicit and provide information.	**Self-Management Support** • Empower and prepare patients to manage their health and health care. • Negotiate self-management action plans with patients. • Offer proven programs that provide basic information, emotional support, and strategies for living with chronic disease. • Use effective self-management support strategies that include assessment, goal setting, action planning, problem solving, and follow-up. • Emphasize patients' central role in managing their health. • Use a collaborative approach; providers and patients work together to define problems, set priorities, establish goals, create treatment plans, and solve problems.
Patient Care • Provide effective, patient-centered, timely, efficient, and equitable care. • Make informed decisions partially based on patient information and preferences. • Work effectively with physicians and other health care professionals to provide patient-centered care. • Develop and carry out patient management plans. • Counsel and educate patients and their families.	
Professionalism • Understanding the appropriate role of the physician assistant • Knowing professional and personal limitations • Respect, compassion, and integrity • Sensitivity and responsiveness to patients' culture, age, gender, and disabilities • Responsiveness and accountability to needs of patients and society	**Delivery System Design** • Define roles and distribute tasks among the team. • Incorporate concepts of health literacy and cultural sensitivity; use effective responsiveness to diverse cultural and linguistic needs. • Give care that patients understand and that fits with their cultural background.
Practice-Based Learning and Improvement • Analyze practice experience and perform practice-based improvement activities using a systematic methodology in concert with other members of the health care delivery team. • Obtain and apply information about patient population and the larger population from which patients are drawn.	**Clinical Information Systems** • Organize patient and population data to facilitate efficient and effective care. • Use patient registry and clinical information systems to share information with patients and providers to coordinate care. • Monitor performance of practice team and care system.
Systems-Based Practice • Cost-effective health care and resource allocation • Improve the delivery of health care and patient outcomes • Responsible for promoting a safe environment for patient care	**Health System** • Create a culture, organization, and mechanisms that promote safe, high-quality care; advocate for policies to improve patient care, community resources. • Encourage open and systematic handling of errors and quality problems to improve care.

AAPA, American Academy of Physician Assistants.
Adapted from American Academy of Physician Assistants. *Improving Chronic Illness Care. The Chronic Care Model.* http://improvingchroniccare.org/change/index.html; and Competencies for the Physician Assistant Profession. 2012. https://www.aapa.org/WorkArea/DownloadAsset.aspx?id=2178.

coordination using home telehealth in 4999 noninstitutionalized veterans, Darkins et al. found that the telehealth group had a 4% reduction in annual health costs versus a 48% increase in the usual care cohort. They also found a lower mortality rate (9.8% in the telehealth group vs. 16.6% in the usual care group).[73]

SUMMARY

The role of PA in chronic disease management has been widely documented.[74-76] PAs perform physical examinations, diagnose and treat diseases, order and interpret laboratory tests, coordinate care, provide patient education, perform procedures, take calls, make hospital or nursing home rounds, and provide home visits,[77] and they are increasingly being used in quality improvement initiatives.[78] PAs work collaboratively with other members of the health care team. The PA may be the primary provider and the patient care team leader in some settings. Data suggest that PA team-based care can improve efficiency and patient outcomes.[79] The role of PAs in fostering chronic disease self-management has also been reported. Ritsema and her colleagues analyzed 5-year data (2005–2009) from the outpatient department subset of the National Hospital Ambulatory Medical Care Survey and found that PAs and nurse practitioners provided health education to patients with chronic diseases more regularly than physicians.[80] Furthermore, PAs enhance care coordination by consulting with their supervising physicians on patients requiring more advanced care. The results from the 2013 AAPA Annual Survey revealed that 64% of PAs provide chronic disease management. The care provided by PAs is of high quality[78,81] and cost effective,[82] and patients are generally satisfied.[83,84] In a joint statement, the American Academy of Family Physicians and the AAPA have called for increased use of physician–PA teams for improving the quality of and access to health care in the United States.[85]

New reimbursement models, together with recent health care reforms, provide expanding opportunities for PAs in today's health care arena, including chronic disease management.

CLINICAL APPLICATIONS

1. Interpersonal and communication skills
   a. Identify a patient in your practice for whom health behavior change would decrease health risk(s) or improve control of a chronic illness.
   b. Schedule a planned encounter to discuss the health behavior.
   c. Practice the techniques of motivational interviewing and self-management support outlined in this chapter.
   d. Evaluate yourself—How did the conversation go? If you encountered resistance, consider how you could change your approach the next time. If you were successful in "rolling with resistance," keep up the good work!
2. Practice-based learning and improvement
   a. Create a registry for subpopulations in your clinical practice. These may be patients with any chronic illness.
   b. Research the HEDIS measures for the chronic illness you have identified.
   c. Analyze the health outcomes of your population based on the HEDIS guidelines.
   d. Collaborate with your colleagues and supervising physician to develop a plan for improvement based on the results of your analysis.

KEY POINTS

- The demand for health care providers who can provide systems and population-based chronic illness management as well as individual care will continue to grow as the U.S. population ages.[1-6]
- Disparities in health outcomes persist, especially in vulnerable, high-risk populations. The CCM has been demonstrated to be cost effective; improve quality of care; improve quality of life; and reduce morbidity and mortality associated with diabetes, asthma, arthritis, and depression.[13-15]
- PAs are logical collaborators as we build solutions to what seem to be intractable problems in caring for chronically ill patients. These solutions can include developing patient registries, taking ownership for a population of patients, and creating plans to improve the care for specific groups of patients.
- PAs must be able to analyze the health systems within which they work, design quality improvement plans and delivery systems that support chronic disease management, and evaluate the outcomes of such plans. Critical to the success of such projects is the ability to partner with patients and motivate behavior change.[13,14,45]

- PAs must be ready to practice within the new paradigm of the CCM and PCMH. In doing so, PAs will aid the achievement of the goals of *Healthy People 2020*: (1) attain high-quality, longer lives free of preventable disease; (2) achieve health equity and eliminate disparities; (3) create social and physical environments that promote good health; and (4) promote quality of life, healthy development, and healthy behaviors across life stages.[9] Attainment of these goals will reduce the burden and costs of chronic disease.
- Since the mid-1990s, the CCM has been implemented widely, and evidence demonstrates the model's effectiveness in improving health outcomes for patients with chronic illness.

References

1. Gerteis J, Izrael D, Deitz D, et al. *Multiple Chronic Conditions Chartbook*. AHRQ Publications No. Q14–0038. Rockville, MD: Agency for Healthcare Research and Quality; April 2014.
2. Centers for Disease Control and Prevention. *Diabetes Report Card 2014*. Atlanta, GA: Centers for Disease Control and Prevention, U.S. Dept of Health and Human Services; 2015.
3. Centers for Disease Control and Prevention. *Measuring Healthy Days*. Atlanta, GA: Centers for Disease Control and Prevention; 2000.
4. Centers for Medicare & Medicaid Services (2015). National Health Expenditure Data Fact Sheet. https://www.cms.gov/Research-Statistics-Data-and-Systems/Statistics-Trends-and-Reports/NationalHealthExpendData/NHE-Fact-Sheet.html. Accessed March 21, 2016.
5. He W, Segupta M, Velkoff VA, DeBarros KA. 65+ in the United States: 2005. Current Population Reports. http://www.census.gov/prod/2006pubs/p23-209.pdf. Accessed March 21, 2016.
6. Werner CA. *The Older Population: 2010 Census Briefs*. United States Census Bureau; 2011.
7. U.S. Department of Health and Human Services. *Aging Statistics*. Administration on Aging; 2015.
8. Jackson SA. The epidemiology of aging. In: Hazzard WR, Blass JP, Ettinger WH, et al., eds. *Principles of Geriatric Medicine and Gerontology*. New York: McGraw-Hill; 1999.
9. U. S. Department of Health and Human Services. *Healthy People 2020*; November, 2010. http://www.healthypeople.gov/2020/topicsobjectives2020/default.aspx. Accessed March 21, 2016.
10. Liao Y, Tucker P, Okoro CA, et al. REACH 2010 Surveillance for Health Status in Minority Communities—United States, 2001–2002. *MMWR Surveillance Summaries*. 2004;53(6):1–36.
11. Wagner E. The Chronic Care Model: Presentation. http://www.improvingchroniccare.org/index.php?p=The_Model_Talk&s=27. Accessed March 21, 2016.
12. Committee on Quality Health Care in America. *Institute of Medicine. Crossing the quality chasm: a new health system for the 21st century*. Washington, D.C.: National Academies Press; 2001.
13. Wagner E. Improving Chronic Illness Care: The Chronic Care Model: Model Elements. http://www.improvingchroniccare.org/index.php?p=Model_Elements&s=18. Accessed March 21, 2016.
14. Bodenheimer T, Wagner EH, Grumbach K. Improving primary care for patients with chronic illness. *JAMA*. 2002;288(14):1775–1779.
15. Bodenheimer T, Wagner EH, Grumbach K. Improving primary care for patients with chronic illness: the chronic care model, part 2. *JAMA*. 2002;288(15):1909–1914.
16. Bodenheimer T. Transforming practice. *N Engl J Med*. 2008;20:2086–2089.
17. Goldberg DG, Kuzel AJ. Elements of the patient-centered medical home in family practices in Virginia. *Ann Fam Med*. 2009;7(4):301–308.
18. Jackson GL, Powers BJ, Chatterjee R, et al. The patient-centered medical home: a systematic review. *Ann Intern Med*. 2013;158(3):169–178.
19. Rich E, Lipson D, Libersky J, Parchman M. *Coordinating Care for Adults With Complex Care Needs in the Patient-Centered Medical Home: Challenges and Solutions*. White Paper (Prepared by Mathematica Policy Research under Contract No. HHSA290200900019I/HHSA29032005T). AHRQ Publication No. 12-0010-EF. Rockville, MD: Agency for Healthcare Research and Quality; January 2012.
20. National Committee for Quality Assurance. Growth of Recognized Medical Homes. http://www.ncqa.org/. Accessed March 20, 2016.
21. Bodenheimer T, Ghoroh A, Willard-Grace R, Grumbach K. The 10 building blocks of high-performing primary care. *Ann Fam Med*. 2014;12(2):166–171.
22. Wagner EH. Chronic disease management: what will it take to improve care for chronic illness? *Eff Clin Pract*. 1998;1:2–4.
23. Wiecha J, Pollard T. The interdisciplinary eHealth team: chronic care for the future. *J Med Internet Res*. 2004;6(3):e22. www.jmir.org/2004/3/e22/. Accessed March 19, 2016.
24. Haynes RB, Yao X, Degani A, et al. Interventions for enhancing medication adherence. *Cochrane Database of Systematic Reviews*. 2005;(4): CD000011. http://dx.doi.org/10.1002/1465 1858.CD000011.pub2.
25. Lorig KR, Ritter PL, Laurent DD, Plant K. Internet-based chronic disease self-management: a randomized trial. *Med Care*. 2006;44(11):961–963.
26. Norris SL, Lau J, Smith SJ, et al. Self-management education for adults with type 2 diabetes: a meta-analysis of the effect on glycemic control. *Diabetes Care*. 2002;25(7):1159–1171.
27. Naughton D, Adelman AM, Bricker P, et al. Envisioning new roles for medical assistants: strategies from patient-centered medical homes. *Family Practice Management*. 2013;20(2):7–12.
28. Smolowitz J, Speakman E, Wojnar D, et al. Role of the registered nurse in primary health care: meeting health care needs in the 21st century. *Nursing Outlook*. 2015;63(2):130–136.
29. Hing E, Cherry DK, Woodwell DA. *National Ambulatory Medical Care Survey: 2004 Summary*. Advance data from vital and health statistics; no. 374. Hyattsville, MD: National Center for Health Statistics; 2006.
30. Brophy TJ, Spiller HA, Casavant MJ, et al. Medication errors reported to US Poison Control Centers, 2000–2012. *Clinical Toxicology*. 2014;52.8:880–888.

The resources for this chapter can be found at www.expertconsult.com.

31. Fried TR, O'Leary J, Towle V, et al. Health outcomes associated with polypharmacy in community-dwelling older adults: a systematic review. *Journal of the American Geriatrics Society*. 2014;62.12:2261–2272.

32. Smith Marie, Bates David W, Bodenheimer Thomas S. Pharmacists belong in accountable care organizations and integrated care teams. *Health Affairs*. 2013;32.11: 1963–1970.

33. Lorig K, Holman H. Self-management education: history, definition, outcomes, and mechanisms. *Ann Behav Med*. 2003;26(1):1–7.

34. Bodenheimer T. *Self-management support: is it evidence based?* Presentation to the California Academic Chronic Care Collaborative; February 21, 2007.

35. van Dam HA, van der Horst F, van den Borne B, et al. Provider-patient interaction in diabetes care: effects on patient self-care and outcomes. A systematic review. *Patient Educ Counseling*. 2003;51(1):17–28.

36. Bodenheimer T, Lorig K, Holman H, Grumbach K. Patient self-management of chronic disease in primary care. *JAMA*. 2002;288:2469–2475.

37. Gibson PG, Powell H, Coughlan J, et al. Limited (information only) patient education programs for adults with asthma. *Cochrane Database of Systematic Reviews*. 2002;(Issue 1).

38. Riemsma RP, Kirwan JR, Taal E, Rasker JJ. Patient education for adults with rheumatoid arthritis. *Cochrane Database of Systematic Reviews*. 2003.

39. Schillinger D, Piette J, Grumbach K, et al. Closing the loop: physician communication with diabetic patients who have low health literacy. *Arch Intern Med*. 2003;163(1):83–90.

40. Schillinger D, Wang F, Rodriguez M, et al. The importance of establishing regimen concordance in preventing medication errors in anticoagulant care. *J Health Comm*. 2006;11(6):555–567.

41. Roter DL, Hall JA. Studies of doctor-patient interaction. *Ann Rev Public Health*. 1989;10:163–180.

42. Griffin S, Kinmonth AL. Systems for routine surveillance for people with diabetes mellitus. *Cochrane Database of Systematic Reviews*. 1998;(1).

43. Shilts MK, Horowitz M, Townsend MS. Goal setting as a strategy for dietary and physical activity behavior change: a review of the literature. *Am J Health Promotion*. 2004;19(2):81–93.

44. Cullen KW, Baranowski T, Smith SP. Using goal setting as a strategy for dietary behavior change. *J Am Dietetic Assoc*. 2001;101(5):562–566.

45. Miller WR, Rollnick S. *Motivational Interviewing: Preparing People for Change*, 2nd ed. New York: Guilford Press; 2002.

46. Anderson R, Funnell MM, Butler PM, et al. Patient empowerment: results of a randomized control trial. *Diabetes Care*. 1995;18:943–949.

47. Bodenheimer T, Lorig K, Holman H, Grumbach K. Patient self-management of chronic disease in primary care. *JAMA*. 2002;288(19):2469–2475.

48. Lorig K, Sobel D, Stewart A, et al. Evidence suggesting that a chronic disease self-management program can improve health status while reducing utilization and costs: a randomized trial. *Med Care*. 1999;37(1):5–14.

49. California Academic Chronic Care Collaborative. *Self-Management Support*. Unpublished manuscript from the California Academic Chronic Care Collaborative Learning Session 1; February 21–22, 2007.

50. Agency for Healthcare Quality Research. *AHCPR Supported Guide and Guidelines [Internet]*. Rockville, MD: Agency for Health Care Policy and Research (U.S.); 1992–2008. Three brief clinical interventions http://www.ncbi.nlm.nih.gov/books/NBK18002/. Accessed March 20, 2016.

51. The Tobacco Use and Dependence Clinical Practice Guideline Panel, Staff, and Consortium Representatives. A clinical practice guideline for treating tobacco use and dependence: a U.S. Public Health Service report. *JAMA*. 2000;283(24): 3244–3254.

52. Lasker RD. *The Committee on Medicine and Public Health*. Improving the quality and cost-effectiveness of care by applying a population perspective to medical practice. Medicine and Public Health: The Power of Collaboration. New York: The New York Academy of Medicine; 1997.

53. National Committee on Quality Assurance (NCQA). *HEDIS—Health Plan Employer Data and Information Set*. Volume 1: Narrative. Washington, D.C.: NCQA; 2011.

54. Pew Health Professions Commission. *Reforming Health Care Workforce Regulation; Policy Considerations for the 21st Century*. Report of the Taskforce on Health Care Workforce Regulation; December 1995.

55. Kohn LT, Corrigan JM, Donaldson MS, eds. *To Err Is Human: Building a Safer Health System*. Washington, D.C.: Committee on Quality of Health Care in America, Institute of Medicine; 2000.

56. Greiner AC, Knebel E, eds. *Health Professions Education: A Bridge to Quality*. Washington, D.C.: Committee on Health Professions Education Summit, Institute of Medicine; 2003.

57. AAPA Special Article. Competencies for the physician assistant profession. *JAAPA*. 2005;18(7):14, 15, 18.

58. ARC-PA, NCCPA, PAEA, AAPA. *Competencies for the Physician Assistant Profession*; 2012. https://www.aapa.org/WorkArea/DownloadAsset.aspx?id=2178. Accessed March 21, 2016.

59. Kohlhepp B, Rohrs R, Robinson P. Guest editorial: charting a course to competency. *JAAPA*. 2005;18(7):16–18.

60. Holman HR. *Patient self-management: essential to solving the health care crisis*. Presentation at University of California, Davis, Health System; May 16–17, 2005.

61. Edwards ST, Landon BE. Medicare's chronic care management payment—payment reform for primary care. *N Engl J Med*. 2014;371(22):2049–2051.

62. Aronson L, Bautista CA, Covinsky K. Medicare and care coordination: expanding the clinician's toolbox. *JAMA*. 2015;313(8):797–798.

63. Basu S, Phillips RS, Bitton A, Song Z, Landon BE. Medicare chronic care management payments and financial returns to primary care practices: a modeling study. *Annals of Internal Medicine*. 2015;163(8):580–588.

64. Bindman AB, Blum JD, Kronick R. Medicare payment for chronic care delivered in a patient-centered medical home. *JAMA*. 2013;310(11):1125–1126.

65. Medicare program; revisions to payment policies under the physician fee schedule, clinical laboratory fee schedule & other revisions to Part B for CY 2014. https://www.federalregister.gov/articles/2013/07/19/2013-16547/medicare-program-revisions-to-payment-policies-under-the-physician-fee-schedule-clinical-laboratory. Published July 19, 2013. Accessed March 20, 2016.

66. Mobile phone access reaches three quarters of planet's population. World Bank; 2012. Jul 17, [2014-09-17]. http://www.worldbank.org/en/news/press-release/2012/07/17/mobile-phone-access-reaches-three-quarters-planets-population. Accessed March 21, 2016.

67. Milani RV, Carl JL. Health Care 2020: reengineering health care delivery to combat chronic disease. *American Journal of Medicine*. 2015;128(4):337–343.

68. Hamine S, Chaney B, Barry AE, et al. Impact of mHealth chronic disease management on treatment adherence and patient outcomes: a systematic review. *Journal of Medical Internet Research*. 2015;17(2).

69. Lim S, Kang SM, Shin H, et al. Improved glycemic control without hypoglycemia in elderly diabetic patients using the ubiquitous healthcare service, a new medical information system. *Diabetes Care*. 2011 Feb;34(2):308–313.

70. Fischer HH, Moore SL, Ginosar D, et al. Care by cell phone: text messaging for chronic disease management. *Am J Manag Care*. 2012 Feb;18(2):e42–e47.

71. Miller RH, West CE. The value of electronic health records in community health centers: policy implications. *Health Affairs*. 2007;26(1):206–214.

72. Irani JS, Middleton JL, Marfatia R, et al. The use of electronic health records in the exam room and patient satisfaction: a systematic review. *The Journal of the American Board of Family Medicine*. 2009;22(5):553–562.

73. Darkins A, Kendall S, Edmonson E, et al. Reduced cost and mortality using home telehealth to promote self-management of complex chronic conditions: a retrospective matched cohort study of 4,999 veteran patients. *Telemedicine and e-Health*. 2015;21(1):70–76.

74. Everett C, Thorpe C, Palta M, Carayon P, Bartels C, Smith MA. Physician assistants and nurse practitioners perform effective roles on teams caring for Medicare patients with diabetes. *Health Affairs*. 2013;32(11):1942–1948.

75. Everett CM, Thorpe CT, Palta M, Carayon P, Gilchrist VJ, Smith MA. Division of primary care services between physicians, physician assistants, and nurse practitioners for older patients with diabetes. *Medical Care Research and Review*. 2013. 1077558713495453.

76. Morgan PA, Abbott DH, McNeil RB, Fisher DA. Characteristics of primary care office visits to nurse practitioners, physician assistants and physicians in United States Veterans Health Administration facilities, 2005 to 2010: a retrospective cross-sectional analysis. *Human Resources for Health*. 2012;10(1):42–49.

77. Nabagiez JP, Shariff MA, Khan MA, et al. Physician assistant home visit program to reduce hospital readmissions. *The Journal of thoracic and cardiovascular surgery*. 2013;145.1:225–233.

78. Wilson IB, Landon BE, Hirschhorn LR, et al. Quality of HIV care provided by nurse practitioners, physician assistants, and physicians. *Annals of Internal Medicine*. 2005;143(10):729–736.

79. Hooker RS, Everett CM. The contributions of physician assistants in primary care systems. *Health & Social Care in the Community*. 2012;20(1):20–31.

80. Ritsema TS, Bingenheimer J, Scholting P, Cawley JF. Differences in the delivery of health education to patients with chronic disease by provider type, 2005-2009. *Preventing Chronic Disease*. 2014;11:130175.

81. Ackermann RJ, Kemle KA. The effect of a physician assistant on the hospitalization of nursing home residents. *Journal of the American Geriatrics Society*. 1998;46(5):610–614.

82. Association MGM. *Physician Compensation and Production Survey: 2010 Report Based on 2009 Data*. Medical Group Management Association; 2010.

83. Hooker RS, Cipher DJ, Sekscenski E. Patient satisfaction with physician assistant, nurse practitioner, and physician care: a national survey of Medicare beneficiaries. *JCOM*. 2005;12(2):88–92.

84. Roblin DW, Becker ER, Adams EK, Howard DH, Roberts MH. Patient satisfaction with primary care: does type of practitioner matter? *Medical Care*. 2004;42(6):579–590.

85. Family Physicians and Physician Assistants: Team-Based Family Medicine. *A Joint Policy Statement of the American Academy of Family Physicians and American Academy of Physician Assistants*; 2011. http://www.aafp.org/about/policies/all/fp-pa.html. Accessed on March 22, 2016.

CHAPTER 17

CONSIDERATIONS FOR A LOGICAL APPROACH TO MEDICATION PRESCRIBING

Courtney J. Perry • Reamer L. Bushardt

All states, the District of Columbia, the Commonwealth of the Northern Mariana Islands, and Guam permit delegated prescribing of various drugs and medical devices by physician assistants (PAs). PAs must possess foundational knowledge and be efficient in accessing pertinent, evidence-based information related to the safety, tolerability, efficacy, price, and use of prescribed medications and devices. To support effective prescribing, this chapter offers a historical perspective on prescribing, key information about controlled substances, guidance for evidence-based decision making, highlights of scientific factors related to medications, tips about safe and effective prescribing for special populations, challenges commonly faced by patients in adhering to prescribed therapies, the rationale for interprofessional collaboration with drug therapy experts, and ethical considerations. Vast and rapidly expanding knowledge about drug therapies exists, and PAs must become expert in analyzing emerging scientific data about medications and incorporate

an assessment of that evidence with preferences of patients and families in an approach to optimize health, manage illness, provide cures, and prevent disease. The right to prescribe is accompanied by a tremendous responsibility to safeguard patient safety and quality of care as well as accountability to various regulators for responsible, ethical prescribing.

HISTORY OF PRESCRIPTION WRITING

Rx is an abbreviation for the Latin word "recipe" meaning "take." Today the abbreviation Rx is used to signify a drug, procedure, or therapy prescribed by a practitioner to a specific patient in the prevention, treatment, or maintenance of his or her clinical diagnosis. A prescription drug refers to medications that require a prescription because they are considered potentially harmful if not used under the supervision of a licensed health care practitioner.

TABLE 17.1 **Classes of Controlled Substances**		
Class	**Description**	**Drug Examples**
I	• Highest potential for abuse • No currently accepted medical use in treatment in the United States • Lack of accepted safety for use of the drug or substance under medical supervision	Heroin, marijuana, cocaine, LSD
II	• High abuse potential • Currently accepted medical use in treatment in the United States (often with restrictions) • Abuse may lead to severe psychological or physical dependence	Morphine, oxycodone, methamphetamine
III	• Abuse risk less than Class I or Class II substances • Currently accepted medical use in treatment in the United States • Abuse may lead to moderate or low physical dependence or high psychological dependence	Acetaminophen combined with codeine or hydrocodone
IV	• Abuse risk less than Class III substances • Currently accepted medical use in treatment in the United States • Abuse may lead to limited physical or psychological dependence • Dependence relative to Class III substances	Chloral hydrate, phenobarbital, diazepam
V	• Low abuse risk • Currently accepted medical use in treatment in the United States • Abuse may lead to limited physical dependence or psychological dependence relative to Class VI substances	Pregabalin, small quantities of codeine, diphenoxylate with atropine

LSD, lysergic acid diethylamide.
From U.S. Food and Drug Administration. Controlled Substance Act, www.FDA.gov. §§13 Drug Abuse Prevention and Control-812-813; 1970.

Rules and regulations regarding prescribing are dictated by both federal (i.e., U.S. Food and Drug Administration [FDA]) and state governing bodies (i.e., boards of pharmacy). The drug formulary for PAs has evolved immensely in the past decade to a more extensively sophisticated formulary, the scope of which is ultimately dictated by individual state laws and supervisory agreements with a physician. The responsible use of this privilege is an essential component of prescribing. With a large selection of medications available to prescribers, the choice among agents can be daunting and must take legal, evidence-based, pharmacologic, and patient-specific factors into consideration.

CONTROLLED SUBSTANCES

Controlled substances are regulated by the Drug Enforcement Agency (DEA) based on schedule or class system. Classes of controlled substances range from Class I, which are not recognized by the federal government as having medicinal use, through Class V medications (Table 17.1). Lower classes of controlled substances have higher abuse potential. Specific regulations exist regarding each class of scheduled drugs in regard to their prescribing and oversight and should be considered in the prescription process. Among these restrictions are often the

ability to prescribe electronically or via fax, quantity supplied, refills prescribed, and expiration date.[1]

EFFECTIVE PRESCRIBING

A prescription is an order from a practitioner to a pharmacist for a medication, product, or device for a specific patient. Prescribing requires a basic working knowledge of the essential parts of a prescription. Laws and regulations regarding mandatory components of a prescription vary from state to state and are discussed next.

CONTENT OF A PRESCRIPTION[2]

• Date of issuance: Prescriptions have an expiration date. This also helps the pharmacist determine that the medication remains appropriate for the particular patient at this time.
• Name and address of the patient
• Name, address, and telephone number of the prescriber: This information is usually preprinted on the prescription.
• DEA number when prescribing a controlled substance
• Name and strength of the medication: The generic name is preferred.

- Dosage form: Many medications are available in tablets, liquids, capsules, and suppositories.
- Route of administration and directions for use: Directions for use differ based on indication. Only standard abbreviations should be used. However, to avoid errors, it is preferred that abbreviations be avoided altogether.
- Quantity supplied and refills
- Most important, a prescription should be legible and clear.

Traditionally, prescriptions were written on a prescription pad and were brought to the pharmacy to be filled. With advances in technology and a push toward more secure prescribing, this has changed in the past few decades. Written or paper copies of prescriptions are often "tamper resistant" and contain details to assist prescribers and pharmacists to know that a prescription is authentic (Box 17.1). Medicaid prescriptions are required by law to contain three tamper-resistant features as of 2008.[3] Other modes of prescribing include electronic and fax. Federal and state regulatory bodies determine which medications are appropriate for these modes of prescribing.

When writing inpatient prescriptions in the hospital, the process is much more simplified with the addition of computerized physician order entry (CPOE). This process allows providers to place orders into a computer system directly and into the chart of a patient, bypassing the need for many of the components of a prescription. These orders are directed toward a pharmacist for verification and dispensing.

BOX 17.1 TAMPER-RESISTANT FEATURES

One or more industry-recognized features designed to prevent unauthorized copying of a completed or blank prescription form

One or more industry-recognized features designed to prevent the erasure or modification of information written on the prescription by the prescriber

One or more industry-recognized features designed to prevent the use of counterfeit prescription forms

From Centers for Medicare and Medicaid Services. Tamper Resistant Prescription Law. www.CMS.gov. 2008.

---

further broken down into six steps. These steps are discussed in detail in Table 17.2.

Assessing effectiveness of a medication, step 3, in your patient is particularly challenging because it requires the review of evidence-based literature to support your management decision. Considerations should include what is the drug of choice in this disease state? Is the drug of choice safe and effective in my patient (i.e., no allergies or contraindications to use)? Does the literature supporting efficacy of this medication in a large population correlate to my patient population as well? This is referred to as a risk–benefit analysis during which you must decide that the benefit of the medication regimen in your patient far outweighs any risk of using this medication regimen (e.g., cost, adverse effects, morbidity, mortality).[4]

CASE 17.1

Ms. M. is a 28-year-old woman who presents to clinic for management of her allergic rhinitis. She has seasonal allergies and manages her symptoms of itching, rhinorrhea, and congestion with loratadine and pseudoephedrine. She is 6 weeks pregnant and wants to know what is the safest and most effective treatment for her to use during pregnancy. The management of allergic rhinitis in pregnancy does not require any controlled substances, so you will likely electronically prescribe her medication to her local pharmacy.

EVIDENCE-BASED APPROACH TO MEDICAL DECISION MAKING

The World Health Organization created a guide to good prescribing and suggests that all drug therapy decisions should consider efficacy, safety, cost, and sustainability.[4] The process of rational prescribing is

---

CASE 17.2

Step 1. Ms. M. is a pregnant 28-year-old woman with mild allergic rhinitis with itching, rhinorrhea, and nasal congestion.

Step 2. Your goal is to manage and control Ms. M.'s allergic rhinitis symptoms.

Step 3. Preferred first-line management of allergic rhinitis is an oral antihistamine with the addition of an intranasal corticosteroid or intranasal antihistamine if symptoms are severe. Decongestants can be added on for patients who are waiting for intranasal corticosteroids to take effect. Pseudoephedrine and other decongestants are not first-line options in pregnant patients because of risks to fetuses and should be avoided. Nondrug therapies are preferred in pregnant patients for the management of allergic rhinitis, and intranasal corticosteroids such as budesonide or a second-generation antihistamine such as loratadine can be considered.

Step 4. You recommend saline irrigations once to twice daily as management of allergic rhinitis for Ms. M.

Step 5. You counsel Ms. M. on the use of saline irrigations and the risk of infection when used improperly.

Step 6. Recommend that Ms. M. follow up with you in the next 2 weeks if her symptoms are not managed by nondrug therapy, and you may consider adding another agent.

PHARMACOLOGY AND THERAPEUTICS

Pharmacology can be broken down into two main topics, pharmacodynamics and pharmacokinetics. Pharmacodynamics can be easily described as the effect of the drug on the body and pharmacokinetics as the effect of the body on the drug. Recognizing basic pharmacodynamics and pharmacokinetic principles is a key concept that is needed in medication prescribing, monitoring, and management.

Pharmacodynamics

Pharmacodynamic effects of a medication are typically described in quantitative terms (e.g., blood pressure and heart rate) and are helpful in comparing the potency, efficacy, and safety of medications. The three major categories of pharmacodynamics to consider are receptor binding, chemical interactions, and dose-response relationships. Drugs are ligands that must bind to receptors via chemical interactions that affect chemical signaling and elicit a response (e.g., diphenhydramine binds histamine receptors, blocking the histamine response associated with allergies). Drugs that bind to and activate a receptor are classified as agonists, and drugs that prevent activations of the receptor are characterized as antagonists (e.g., morphine is an opioid receptor agonist used to manage pain, and naloxone is an opioid receptor antagonist used to reverse the effects of opioids). Other medications produce effects without altering cellular function or without binding to a receptor. These are defined as chemical interactions; antacids are an example, designed to neutralize the gastric pH, and do not require receptor binding to take effect. A dose–response relationship is determined using a time versus plasma concentration curve (Fig. 17.1).[5]

Pharmacokinetics

Pharmacokinetics is broken down into the ability of the body to absorb, distribute, metabolize, and

TABLE 17.2 World Health Organization's Steps to Rational Prescribing

Step	Description
1. Define the patient's problem.	Disease state Signs or symptoms of underlying disease Psychological or social problems Side effect of a drug Refill request Nonadherence to treatment Preventive treatment
2. Specify the therapeutic objective.	Goals of treatment • Manage • Prevent • Cure
3. Verify whether your preferred treatment is suitable for this patient.	Effectiveness: ability to produce an effect in *your* patient Safety: think about contraindications, drug–drug, or drug–disease interactions and allergies Convenience: route, duration of treatment, dosing schedule Cost
4. Start the treatment.	Refer to the section on effective prescribing.
5. Give information, instructions, and warnings.	Effects of the drug • Why is the drug needed? • What should the patient expect? • When should the patient expect it? Side effects • When will they occur? • How long will they last? • How serious are they? • What action should they take? Instructions • How should the drug be taken? • When should the drug be taken? • For how long should the drug be taken? Warnings regarding the drug • When to follow-up. • Confirm the patient understood. • Ask if everything is clear. • Ask the patient to repeat important information. • Field questions.
6. Monitor the treatment.	Passive monitoring: Explain what to do if the treatment is ineffective, inconvenient, or causing side effects; monitoring is done by the patient. Active monitoring: The patient must schedule an appointment for you to determine whether the treatment is effective (i.e., laboratory studies, examinations).

From De Vries TPGM, Henning RH, Hogerzeil HV, Fresle DA. *Guide to Good Prescribing: A Practical Manual.* Geneva: World Health Organization, Action Programme on Essential Drugs; 1994. http://apps.who.int/medicinedocs/pdf/whozip23e/whozip23e.pdf.

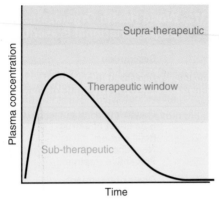

Plasma concentration (y-axis) vs Time (x-axis)

Supra-therapeutic

Therapeutic window

Sub-therapeutic

> The therapeutic window is the range of concentrations that produce a therapeutic response and can typically be defined with a peak effect. Medications with a narrow-therapeutic window typically require serum-concentration monitoring. Supra-therapeutic concentrations are those at which significant adverse effects occur in patients, and sub-therapeutic is the range of concentrations that produces lower than desired effects.

FIG. 17.1 ■ A dose–response relationship is determined using a time versus plasma concentration curve. (From Porter RS, Kaplan JL, Beers MH. *The Merck Manual Online.* Whitehouse Station, NJ: Merck Research Laboratories; 2006.)

excrete medications. All processes, when altered, can affect the efficacy and toxicity of a medication. Absorption of oral medications is determined by ionization of the drug molecule that is determined by pH changes along the gastrointestinal (GI) tract. For this reason, many drugs are better absorbed in one area of the GI tract more predominantly that in others. Medications given to patients with nonfunctioning GI tracts or those requiring administration via feeding tubes may have altered absorption and efficacy and should be considered in the drug selection and administration process. After a medication is absorbed into systemic circulation, it can be distributed to tissues and interstitial fluids to allow for effect and then is metabolized and excreted. The primary route of drug metabolism is via the cytochrome-P450 (CYP) enzyme system located predominantly in the liver. Drugs can be designated as a substrate (a drug metabolized via this enzyme), inhibitor (a drug that inhibits this enzyme), or inducer (a drug that enhances enzymatic metabolism via this enzyme) of one of the enzymes. Enzymatic inhibition as well as induction are major causes of drug–drug interactions and can result in significant alterations in drug concentration and effect.[5]

Common inducers and substrates are listed in Table 17.3. In addition to those via enzymatic pathways, drug interactions can also be classified as additive or as a result of competitive protein binding. Additive drug interactions can be defined as using two medications that cause the same effect, resulting in too large of an effect. For example, when using two antihypertensive medications together, it is imperative to monitor blood pressure to ensure you do not cause hypotension. The most common protein for a drug to bind to is albumin. Because

TABLE 17.3	**Common Inducers and Substrates**	
Type	**Drugs**	**Effects**
Inducers	Carbamazepine Phenytoin Phenobarbital Rifampin	Decreased concentration of active drugs Increased concentration of prodrugs*
Inhibitors	Cimetidine Fluconazole Ritonavir	Increased concentration of active drugs Decreased concentration of prodrugs*

*Prodrugs are drugs that are inactive upon administration and require metabolism to be activated.
From Porter RS, Kaplan JL, Beers MH. *The Merck Manual Online.* Whitehouse Station, NJ: Merck Research Laboratories; 2006.

supplies of albumin are limited in our body, using two medications that are highly bound to albumin can result in increased unbound concentration of medication and therefore increased risk of toxicity. It is important to understand the mechanism and effect of drug interactions when prescribing medications as they often require dose adjustments or monitoring.[5]

Metabolism serves primarily to prepare drugs for excretion from the body. Although there are multiple routes of drug excretion, the primary route is via the kidneys. An estimation of renal function is determined by calculating the creatinine clearance (CrCl) using the Cockroft-Gault formula (Fig. 17.2). This value is used to determine when dosage adjustments are needed in patients with poor or declining renal function because of a reduced ability to clear medications.[6]

$$\text{Creatinine clearance (mL/min)}$$
$$= \frac{(140 - \text{age}) \times \text{wt (kg)}}{\text{Serum creatinine (mg/dL)} \times 72} \quad (\times\, 0.85 \text{ for females})$$

*Weight should be calculated using ideal body weight.

Normal values for adults range from 80 to 140 mL/min, with dose adjustments needed in patients with a CrCl <50 mL/min in drugs that are cleared renally.

FIG. 17.2 ■ An estimation of renal function is determined by calculating the creatinine clearance (CrCl) using the Cockroft-Gault formula. (From Cockcroft DW, Gault MH. Prediction of creatinine clearance from serum creatinine. *Nephron.* 1976;16(1):31–41.)

CASE 17.3

Ms. M. returns to clinic in 3 weeks and says that her symptoms of allergic rhinitis have not improved. You decide to start her on loratadine, a second-generation antihistamine, to treat her rhinorrhea and itching and budesonide, an intranasal corticosteroid, to manage her nasal congestion. Antihistamines should start working right away, but the intranasal corticosteroid may not take full effect for up to 4 weeks.

Ms. M. has normal renal and hepatic function, so you do not need to alter the dose of either medication to account for reduced clearance. Loratadine is a "minor" substrate and inducer of enzymes in the cytochrome P-450 system. Typically, medications must be "major" substrates, inhibitors, or inducers to be considered likely to cause clinically significant drug interactions. Budesonide has minimal systemic absorption because it works locally in the nares, so drug interactions are not of major concern.

Loratadine is an antihistamine medication that can cause sedation. Ms. M should be cautious using other medications that can cause sedation because the drug interaction would have an additive effect.

Special Patient Populations

Pediatrics

Pediatric patients have differences in their pharmacodynamic and pharmacokinetic properties that can result in significant differences in drug effect and toxicity compared with adult patients (Table 17.4). Limitations to prescribing in pediatric patients include identifying appropriate dosing (mg/kg and dosing based on body surface area), availability of dosage forms (because many

TABLE 17.4 Alterations in Drug Properties in Pediatric Patients

Absorption	Muscle • Reduced mass and perfusion • Reduce absorption of drug • Pain on administration • Caution in pediatric patients younger than 6 years of age Skin • Thinner stratum corneum • Increased BSA-to-weight ratio • Increased absorption • Caution using topical medications in neonates and young children
Distribution	Neonates and infants have significantly larger total body water than adult patients and significantly less total body fat.
Metabolism	Neonates and infants have immature metabolism that begins to peak in childhood and then reduces to adult levels in adolescents. Neonates and infants clear medications much more slowly, and adolescents clear medications much more quickly than adult patients.
Excretion	Glomerular filtration does not fully develop until 1 year of age. Immature elimination by the kidneys can lead to accumulation of medication and toxicities.

BSA, Body surface area.
From Porter RS, Kaplan JL, Beers MH. *The Merck Manual Online.* Whitehouse Station, NJ: Merck Research Laboratories; 2006.

pediatric patients cannot swallow pills), palatability, and lack of data. Additionally, only approximately one-fourth of drugs approved by the FDA have pediatric indications.

Geriatrics

Similar to the challenges in pediatric patients, medication prescribing in geriatric patients presents its own challenges because physiologic changes in older adults can make them more sensitive to a drug's effect. Although changes in absorption are inconsequential with increasing age, alterations in metabolism and excretion are not. Hepatic blood flow is variable, resulting in an almost 40% decline in CYP-450 activity. Similarly, the glomerular filtration rate generally decreases with aging at an estimated 10 mL/min for every decade after 30 years of age, ultimately requiring dose adjustments in many patients.

Geriatric patients are also more likely to have more disease states and take more medications, which can lead to adverse effects and polypharmacy (the use of unnecessary medications). When selecting a medication for an elderly patient, it is important to consider those that are potentially inappropriate because of the risk for adverse events such as falls. A few examples of practical resources to guide appropriate prescribing in elderly patients include the Beers List,[7] Screening Tool of Older People's Prescriptions (STOPP) and Screening Tool to Alert to Right Treatment (START) criteria, and the Anticholinergic Drug Burden Scale. Examples of medications on the Beers list are discussed in Table 17.5.

Obesity

Recommended dosing for drug administration is generally based on pharmacokinetic data obtained from individuals of normal weight. Fewer data are available to help guide in the appropriate dosing of medication in obese patients. Medications that are lipophilic may require adjustment of dose or frequency to avoid accumulation in fat stores; other medications may not reach a therapeutic effect in obese patients when dosed at standard recommended doses. This issue is particularly challenging in anesthesia in which inappropriate dosing can result in respiratory depression and loss of airway patency. For medications dosed based on weight, the pharmacologic properties of the drug should be considered when determining if ideal, actual, or adjusted body weight is most appropriate for use.[8]

Although data on dosing of medication in obese adults are limited, the data are even more sparse in pediatric patients, requiring careful consideration of the disease state and extrapolation from adult literature.

Pregnancy and Lactation

Previously, drugs were placed into categories to signify the safety of their use in pregnancy. The categories were A, B, C, D, and X, where a category A medication is one that is considered safe because controlled studies in humans show no risk to the fetus. Category X include medications in which animal or human studies demonstrate fetal abnormalities, and use of these agents is contraindicated in pregnancy. In 2015, the previous pregnancy labeling was changed and is now better designed to help practitioners understand the risks and benefits of medications in three areas: pregnancy, lactation, and women and men of reproductive potential.[9] Details of contents you can find in each category are described in Fig. 17.3. When choosing a medication in a patient who is pregnant or lactating, there are three main considerations: risk versus benefit, necessity of the medication, and health of the mother without the drug.

TABLE 17.5	**Common Medications Classes on the Beers List**
Drug Class	**Rationale**
Anticholinergic	Increased risk of confusion, dry mouth, constipation
Alpha blockers	Increased risk of orthostatic hypotension
Antipsychotics	Increased mortality in patients with dementia
Benzodiazepines	Increased risk of cognitive impairment and falls
Insulin and sulfonylureas	Increased risk of hypoglycemia
Opioids	Increased risk of neurotoxicity
NSAIDs	Increased risk of GI bleed

GI, Gastrointestinal; *NSAID,* nonsteroidal antiinflammatory drug. From American Geriatrics Society. 2012 Beers Criteria Update Expert Panel. American Geriatrics Society updated Beers Criteria for potentially inappropriate medication use in older adults. *J Am Geriatr Soc.* 2012;60:616–631.

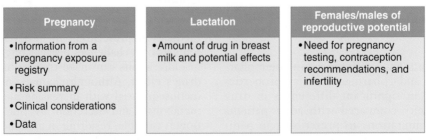

Pregnancy	Lactation	Females/males of reproductive potential
• Information from a pregnancy exposure registry • Risk summary • Clinical considerations • Data	• Amount of drug in breast milk and potential effects	• Need for pregnancy testing, contraception recommendations, and infertility

FIG. 17.3 ■ Risks and benefits of medications in three areas: pregnancy, lactation, and women and men of reproductive potential. (From Food and Drug Administration. *Pregnancy and Lactation Labeling Rule,* 2014. http://www.fda.gov/Drugs/DevelopmentApprovalProcess/Development Resources/Labeling/ucm093307.htm.)

TABLE 17.6 Examples of Medications With Practical Implications of Pharmacogenetic Research

Drug	Use	Implication
Abacavir	HIV	Safety: HLA-B*5701 allele presence correlates with high risk of hypersensitivity reaction.
Clopidogrel	Antiplatelet	Efficacy: Presence of CYP2C19*2 allele results in reduced drug levels. Safety: Reduced drug levels are associated with increased risk of cardiovascular events.
Codeine	Pain	Efficacy: CYP2D6 poor metabolizers have reduced active drug levels and therapeutic effect. Safety: CYP2D6 ultra-rapid metabolizers will have high or toxic levels and increased risk of adverse effects.
Bronchodilators (e.g., albuterol)	Asthma	Efficacy: Gly16Arg genotype for the *ADRB2* gene is associated with reduced bronchodilator response. Safety: Asthma worsening in patients on continuous bronchodilator therapy.
Mercaptopurine	Oncology	Safety: TPMT* deficiency is associated with excess toxicity.

*Thiopurine *S*-methyltransferase, an enzyme responsible for the metabolism of mercaptopurine.
From Ingelman-Sundberg,[10] Wang et al.,[11] Paré et al.,[12] Lima et al.,[13] and Stocco et al.[14]

CASE 17.4

Antihistamines and intranasal corticosteroids are considered safe for use in pregnancy and have not been associated with an increased risk to fetuses. The lowest effective dose of both should be used to minimize any exposure to fetuses. The benefit of these medications outweighs any risk and is appropriate and necessary for Ms. M.

PERSONALIZED MEDICINE AND PHARMACOGENOMICS

Typically, medications are dosed similarly in all patients even though there is a considerable inter-patient variability in drug response. Although many factors can account for changes in response to drug therapy (e.g., pregnancy, age, weight, renal or hepatic function), as discussed earlier in this chapter, genetics can also play a major role. An advancing area of pharmacotherapy is pharmacogenomics, named because of human genome projects and identification of novel biomarkers of drug response. Pharmacogenomics, a subset of personalized medicine, is the study of how inherited and acquired gene variation across the genome affects drug response. This new field of study aims to create safe and effective medications at doses that are tailored to a person's specific genetic makeup—in other words, personalized drug therapy. Pharmacogenetics, although the term is often used interchangeably, is considered a subset of pharmacogenomics and is focused on individual genes that affect drug metabolism, distribution, and response.[10]

Advances in pharmacogenomics and pharmacogenetics will allow for personalized drug therapy that will individualize therapy intensity and minimize toxicities. Most medications have not been adequately studied to assess response variation based on genes, but this is certainly one of the most up and coming areas of pharmacotherapy research. One area of study that has been particularly changed by advances in pharmacogenomics is oncology. Examples of medications with practical implications of pharmacogenetic research are discussed in Table 17.6.

BARRIERS TO PATIENT COMPLIANCE

Now that you have selected an agent for your patient with appropriate follow-up and monitoring, one of the biggest barriers you will face is patients' compliance to their medication regimens. Many factors contribute to patient compliance and are discussed in detail in Table 17.7.

CASE 17.5

Ms. M. returns to clinic 2 weeks after you prescribed her loratadine and intranasal budesonide, and although her symptoms of rhinorrhea and itching are improving, her congestion has not improved. After further discussion, you realize she is not taking the intranasal budesonide because she has a friend who developed osteoporosis from using prednisone daily, which she read was also a steroid medication. Her noncompliance is due to both a fear of drug toxicity and lack of health literacy, so you educate her

TABLE 17.7 Patient Barriers to Compliance

Barrier to Compliance	How to Overcome the Barrier
Inadequate health literacy	Use verbal and written explanations and handouts. Avoid medical jargon.
Cost of medication regimen	Avoid brand-name medications. Refer to a social worker.
Cultural differences	Language barrier: Use an interpreter. Religious differences (e.g., fasting, Jehovah's Witness and blood products): Tailor therapy to the patient's beliefs.
Previous drug therapy failure or toxicity	Acknowledge fears and stress the importance of current therapy.
Lack of motivation	Start with small, attainable goals. Explain the consequences of noncompliance. Elicit support of family members and social workers.
Complexity of medication regimen	Simplify regimens when possible (e.g., combination therapies, long-acting medications).

on the use of intranasal budesonide and inform her that it rarely has systemic side effects, as oral prednisone will, because it has limited absorption into your body and is used for a local effect in the nose. The risk of osteoporosis for Ms. M. is extremely low and unlikely. After you have acknowledged her concern regarding the intranasal budesonide, she states she feels more comfortable using it and will follow up with you in 2 weeks.

INTERPROFESSIONAL COLLABORATION WITH A PHARMACIST

Interprofessional collaboration is imperative to ensure the safest, most effective, and most thorough care of your patient. Pharmacists are medication experts who are ideal for tackling medication therapy management in both the primary and tertiary care settings, yet they are often underused. With their known roles in optimizing therapeutic outcomes and promoting cost-effective medication use, pharmacists have been cited as making positive contributions to the quality and safety of patient care. Their roles include interacting with the health care team on rounds to provide a systematic review of each medication for appropriateness, efficacy, and safety to achieve optimal safety goals; interviewing patients to assess adherence and health literacy regarding their medications; reconciling medication discrepancies on admission and discharge; providing medication counseling; and providing follow-up. Although the pharmacist's role as a provider has yet to be established legally, they still maintain an integral role on the health care team for managing and recommending pharmacotherapy regimens.

ETHICAL QUANDARIES

The ability to prescribe medications brings many potential challenges, especially when considering medications that have high abuse potential. Some ethical quandaries to consider are how to appropriately manage medication abuse and addiction, defining who your patients are, and determining what follow-up and monitoring are appropriate and expected.

Addiction, tolerance, and dependence are often used in conjunction with one another but are actually much different and must be acknowledged as such in practice. Addiction is a primary chronic neurobiologic disease state characterized by at least one of the following: impaired control over drug use, compulsive use, cravings, and continued use despite harm. Tolerance and dependence are often present in a patient with addiction, but their presence does not necessarily indicate addiction. Dependence is a state of adaptation in which abrupt cessation or dose reduction can produce withdrawal symptoms and is a natural physiologic reaction. Tolerance results when exposure to a medication over time results in a decrease in one or more of the drug's effects and leads to dose escalation. It is important to recognize the difference among addiction, dependence, and tolerance when prescribing controlled substances because continual dose escalation or symptoms of withdrawal do not always mean that a patient is abusing or addicted to a medication. Furthermore, when presented with a patient who has a history of drug abuse, you should create a formal contract with him or her that explains the circumstances under which you will continue to prescribe controlled substances to the patient. You can also present the patient with resources for problems with substance abuse. This can help manage patients who appear to be drug seeking and helps protect your license while still helping your patient.[15]

As a provider, you will encounter family, friends, and patients asking for you to provide them with prescriptions. It is important to recognize that prescriptions are from a medical provider to a patient whom he or she has examined and knows, making it illegal to prescribe medications for someone who is not formally your patient. This also means that prescribing a medication for yourself is considered ethically and legally inappropriate.[2]

Aside from prescribing drugs of abuse and dealing with the question of who is considered a patient, it is important to remember something so simple it is often forgotten. If you start a patient on a medication, it is your responsibility to follow up on his or her progress on the medication and to monitor its continued appropriateness. If a patient is unable or unwilling to follow up with you as expected, you may consider refusing to refill the prescription until she or he will.

CASE 17.6

On follow-up, Ms. M. states that her symptoms have improved and is wondering if you wouldn't mind prescribing the intranasal budesonide for her husband, who also has allergic rhinitis. Because her husband is not your patient and you are unable to assess him and take a history and physical examination, you are not legally allowed to prescribe medications for him. If he would like, he can schedule an appointment to be seen and evaluated.

CONCLUSION

Prescribing involves knowledge of laws and regulations, pharmacology, patient-specific considerations, and a great deal of responsibility. Choosing a medication can be a daunting process but can be made more straightforward when done systematically and in collaboration with a health care team, including a pharmacist, to ensure effective and safe use of medications. After you have effectively prescribed a medication, it is imperative to remember how important continued follow-up and monitoring are to the success and safety of your patient.

KEY POINTS

- Medication decision making should include evidence-based considerations of efficacy, safety, cost, and sustainability of drug therapy.
- Individualized prescribing must be considered for patients at different stages of development and for those with unique characteristics and illnesses that can alter the safety and efficacy of a medication.
- The responsible use of prescribing privileges within state and federal limitations is essential in mitigation of abuse and protection of your medical license.
- The overwhelming wealth of information required for safe and effective medication prescribing requires interprofessional collaboration with pharmacists.

References

1. Controlled Substance Act, www.FDA.gov §§ 13 Drug Abuse Prevention and Control-812–813 (U.S. Food and Drug Administration, 1970).
2. Abood RR. *Pharmacy Practice and the Law*. 7th ed. Sudbury, MA: Jones and Bartlett; 2012.
3. Tamper Resistant Prescription Law, www.CMS.gov (Centers for Medicare and Medicaid Services, 2008).
4. De Vries TPGM, Henning RH, Hogerzeil HV, Fresle DA. Guide to Good Prescribing: A Practical Manual. Geneva: World Health Organization, Action Programme on Essential Drugs, 1994. http://apps.who.int/medicinedocs/pdf/whozip23e/whozip23e.pdf. Accessed April 3, 2016.
5. Porter RS, Kaplan JL, Beers MH. *The Merck Manual Online*. Whitehouse Station, NJ: Merck Research Laboratories; 2006.
6. Cockcroft DW, Gault MH. Prediction of creatinine clearance from serum creatinine. *Nephron*. 1976;16(1):31–41.
7. American Geriatrics Society. 2012 Beers Criteria Update Expert Panel. American Geriatrics Society updated Beers Criteria for potentially inappropriate medication use in older adults. *J Am Geriatr Soc*. 2012;60:616–631.
8. Leykin Y, Miotto L, Pellis T. Pharmacokinetic considerations in the obese. *Best Pract Res Clin Anaesthesiol*. 2011 Mar;25(1):27–36. Review.
9. Pregnancy and Lactation Labeling Rule, www.FDA.gov-8.1-4 (U.S. Food and Drug Administration, 2014).
10. Ingelman-Sundberg M. Pharmacogenetics: an opportunity for a safer and more efficient pharmacotherapy. *J Intern Med*. 2001;250:186–200.
11. Wang L, McLeod HL, Weinshilboum RM. Genomics and drug response. *N Engl J Med*. 2011;364:1144–1153.
12. Paré G, Mehta SR, Yusuf S, et al. Effects of CYP2C19 genotype on outcomes of clopidogrel treatment. *N Engl J Med*. 2010;363:1704–1714.
13. Lima JJ, Blake KV, Tantisira KG, Weiss ST. Pharmacogenetics of asthma. *Current opinion in pulmonary medicine*. 2009;15(1):57–62. http://dx.doi.org/10.1097/MCP.0b013e32831da8be.
14. Stocco G, Cheok MH, Crews KR, et al. Genetic polymorphism of inosine triphosphate pyrophosphatase is a determinant of mercaptopurine metabolism and toxicity during treatment for acute lymphoblastic leukemia. *Clin Pharmacol Ther*. 2009;85:164–172.
15. Consensus statement of American Pain Society, American Academy of Pain Medicine, and the American Society of Addiction Medicine, 2001.

The resources for this chapter can be found at www.expertconsult.com.

The faculty resources can be found online at www.expertconsult.com.

CHAPTER 18

COMPLEMENTARY AND INTEGRATIVE HEALTH

Susan LeLacheur

CHAPTER OUTLINE

NATURAL PRODUCTS

MIND–BODY PRACTICES

ADDRESSING COMPLEMENTARY AND INTEGRATIVE HEALTH IN CLINICAL PRACTICE

CLINICAL APPLICATIONS

KEY POINTS

Complementary and integrative health refers to the incorporation of practices and techniques to gain or maintain better health but fall outside of the realm of traditional Western medicine. Patients and practitioners use complementary practices to supplement conventional medicine. *Integrative medicine* refers to the conscious and coordinated combination of conventional and complementary practices. Another commonly used designation is *alternative medicine*, which refers to practices and systems of care used in place of conventional medicine. According to the National Center for Complementary and Integrative Health (NCCIH, formerly the National Center for Complementary and Alternative Medicine), a center within the National Institutes of Health (NIH), about 34% of Americans use some form of complementary health approach,[1] and more than 50% of Americans use a dietary supplement[2] based on the National Health Statistics Report. The NCCIH dropped the term *alternative* from its name to reflect the facts that much of what was once considered alternative is joining the mainstream in a variety of health care settings and that most of its use in this country is in conjunction with medical care.

The mission of the NCCIH, established in 1998 within the NIH, is to "define, through rigorous scientific investigation, the usefulness and safety of complementary and integrative health interventions and their roles in improving health care." It provides a coherent approach to researching various complementary products and techniques as well as providing a clearinghouse for evidence-based information

on both the efficacy and potential dangers of complementary products and techniques.[3] The NCCIH considers complementary health approaches in two major categories, natural products and mind–body practices. The former includes herbs, vitamins, minerals, and special diets, and the latter refers to a broad range of therapies such as yoga, chiropractic manipulation, acupuncture, and guided imagery.

In addition to these broad categories, there are whole systems of care such as traditional Chinese medicine, Ayurvedic medicine, naturopathy, and homeopathy that hold an approach to healing that is very different from that of conventional Western medicine. Patients and practitioners may subscribe entirely to one of these traditions or may use practices from another system of care as a complementary technique. For example, traditional Chinese medicine conceives illness as a disharmony within the body and between the body and the world around it. Balance between the opposing and complementary forces, yin and yang, promotes the free flow of energy (qi) through the body, promoting good health. There is not the same distinction between mind and body as there is in the Western conception of health, and a particular type of imbalance will lead to both physical and mental or psychological consequences. Acupuncture, tai chi and qi gong (both exercise and movement practices), and various herbal formulations are all used to gain and maintain this balance. Of course, this system, which dates back thousands of years, is far richer and more complex than can be described here. Another ancient system is Ayurvedic medicine

(Sanskrit for "science of life") developed in India that uses a variety of techniques and remedies. As with traditional Chinese medicine, Ayurvedic medicine is based on an Eastern worldview that is very different from that of empiric Western science. Other examples include homeopathy in which very small doses of a particular toxin or irritant are used to prevent or heal the ailment it causes.

Given the common and increasing[1] use of many practices outside the realm of traditional Western medicine, clinicians must have a basic understanding of some of the more commonly used therapies and techniques and be able to access the relevant scientific evidence in regard to their safety and efficacy. As with other therapeutic realms such as physical therapy, occupational therapy, and dentistry, the physician assistant (PA) must be acquainted with commonly used complementary modalities and prepared to advise patients. Having open conversations with patients on their use of complementary therapies can serve to improve the patient–provider relationship. Discussion of patient's use or potential use of complementary and integrative medicine also creates the basis for relaying information on current research.[4]

Research on the expansive array of complementary and integrative practices and products has been difficult for a number of reasons. For natural products, there are two major problems, both related to funding. Because most of these products are widely available and account for approximately two thirds of the $33.9 billion of out-of-pocket expenditures for complementary health in the United States,[3] there is little incentive for manufacturers and marketers to engage in robust research. In addition, because there is no available patent for most plant-based and herbal remedies, there are not the same economic forces as exist in the far more tightly controlled pharmaceutical market. In addition to the fiscal difficulties, there is little standardization in terms of formulation and potency of most products both in research and in the public marketplace.

The Dietary Supplement and Health Education Act of 1994 classifies vitamins, minerals, botanicals and amino acids as nutritional supplements that can be marketed without proof of safety or efficacy. Marketers may not claim an undocumented (and Food and Drug Administration [FDA]-approved) clinical indication but may make claims that the product supports or enhances normal function. For example, a particular supplement may be said to "support bone health" but not to "treat osteoporosis."

For mind–body practices, there is the additional difficulty in conducting good research trials: Accounting for the placebo effect is complicated. Although

it is simple to use an inert substance in place of an herb, it is more difficult to design an effective sham procedure for something such as acupuncture and to ensure blinding throughout a study.[5] That said, the data on complementary and integrative practices are increasing. In the following pages, we will review some of the most commonly used products and practices and the available research.

CASE STUDY 18.1

Your patient is a 23-year-old woman who is pregnant for the first time. She has been experiencing a lot of morning nausea and was told by her grandmother that she should try chopping fresh ginger and boiling it for 15 minutes to make a tea. She asks if this is safe during early pregnancy. Her only current medication is a prenatal vitamin.

You quickly check on the NIH's website (see "Resources") and find that not only is ginger safe in pregnancy but also is likely effective. You let her know that she might try the ginger tea but to call if she continues to have difficulty. At your next visit, she states that she is no longer experiencing nausea, and the ginger tea was very helpful.

CASE STUDY 18.2

Your patient is a 48-year-old man with HIV infection previously well controlled on a single tablet regimen of elvitegravir, cobicistat, emtricitabine, and tenofovir disoproxil. His most recent laboratory test results showed an increase in viral RNA. You question him on adherence and he states he has not missed any doses and takes the medication with food as directed. His only other medication is bupropion 150 mg twice daily for depression, a dose that has been unchanged for several years. You ask about over-the-counter medications or other supplements. He reluctantly admits that, on the advice of a friend, he had started taking St. John's wort to see if this natural remedy might allow him to discontinue his antidepressant. His intent was to start reducing his dose of bupropion after taking the herb for a month or two.

You check on the NIH's website and find that hypericin, the active ingredient in St. John's wort, has many drug–drug interactions, including a likely reduction in the activity of cobicistat used in his HIV medication to boost the activity of elvitegravir to levels sufficient to control his HIV with a once-daily dose. You explain this to your patient, and he agrees to discontinue the herb and to review his psychiatric medication with his psychiatrist.

NATURAL PRODUCTS

The use of special diets for health maintenance or to manage disease is common and in constant flux. There is ongoing controversy regarding the efficacy of various approaches, but the overall recommendation for most Americans is to maintain a healthy weight; consume more fruits, vegetables, and whole grains; and reduce sugar and salt.[6] The Healthy People 2020 goals include increasing the total intake of vegetables (from a 0.77-cup equivalent for the years 2001 to 2004 to a 1.14-cup equivalent per 1000 calories) and reducing the percent of total daily calories from added sugars (from 15.7% for the years 2001 to 2004 to 10.8%).[3,7] The DASH (Dietary Approaches to Stop Hypertension) diet, which includes a combined total of 8 to 10 servings of fruit and vegetables daily, has been shown to reduce hypertension and improve lipid levels.[8,9] The need for vitamin and mineral supplementation depends on the overall quality of the diet and the presence of specific health conditions.

The use of natural products other than vitamin or minerals is widespread; 17.7% of adults use them, according to the 2012 survey.[3] Plant-based products are generally considered to be safe in small quantities, but concentrated forms and large doses may have adverse effects. Some of these products may interact with prescribed medications or otherwise cause harm, so it is critical for PAs to find out what products a patient uses and be able to offer guidance. The NCCIH offers online reference materials, and we will cover several of the more commonly used products here. Review the NCCIH website[3] or one of the other resources listed for products not listed or for further information.

Aloe vera is a succulent plant that contains a viscous gel often used for a variety of skin conditions and found in a multitude of products. It is sometimes used orally for constipation and a variety of other conditions. Although the plant does contain a laxative, it is hard on the kidneys, and the FDA required aloe to be removed from laxative products in 2002 because of safety concerns. Aloe vera can reduce blood sugar when used orally, but the same safety concerns must be considered. Rodent studies of oral aloe vera have shown clear evidence of carcinogenesis. In humans, this risk is unknown, but it can cause diarrhea and abdominal cramping and can reduce the absorption of medications.

As a topical therapy, aloe vera can increase circulation and control bacteria and thus may promote healing. Studies of this effect have, however, been mixed, and it may actually reduce healing in some situations, particularly deeper wounds. It is likely safe and effective for minor burns and abrasions.

Black cohosh or snakeroot is a plant whose root is formulated into teas or tinctures. Research on its most common use of relieving the symptoms of menopause, particularly hot flashes, has been mixed and is ongoing. There do not appear to be any significant interactions with medications. People with any form of liver dysfunction or who take other medications that may harm the liver should avoid black cohosh. There have been several cases of hepatitis in women taking black cohosh, though the relationship is unclear.

Chamomile is a flowering plant used for anxiety, sleeplessness, and upset stomach. The flowering tops are made into a tea or tincture. It is also a common ingredient in topical therapies for ulcers and abrasions. Early studies on the topical use of chamomile indicate that it may be effective for minor skin irritations and for mouth ulcers. There are not yet any conclusive data regarding its efficacy as an oral agent. It does not appear to have any major interaction with medications, and its only known harmful effect is allergic reaction in some individuals.

Cinnamon is widely used in the United States as a flavoring agent in sweets and curries and is certainly safe when taken in small doses. There is some research on its potential beneficial effects on diabetes and heart disease, but there is not yet any clear evidence of its utility for these conditions. Cinnamon contains coumarin, also found in warfarin, but there are no data on its effect on clotting. However, because of its potential effects on clotting those with clotting disorders or on warfarin, patients should be advised against consuming large quantities of cinnamon. Similarly, the potential effect of lowering blood glucose should be considered for those on medication for diabetes.

Cranberry is widely used in food and beverages. Its most common use is in preventing urinary tract infections. Current research demonstrates that it may be effective in preventing bacteria from adhering to the epithelium off the urinary tract, but cranberry has not been shown to have any role in the treatment of an established UTI. A more recent potential use for cranberry is in reducing the ability of *Helicobacter pylori* to survive in the stomach. Some preliminary research supports the possibility of this effect. It may also serve to reduce dental plaque. There are no documented adverse effects of cranberry, but it should be used with caution in those taking warfarin or aspirin.

Echinacea is widely used to stimulate immune function and to treat or prevent colds and influenza. To date, research has not clearly supported this indication, although studies continue. There is some indication that people with asthma and atopy are more likely to have allergic reactions to echinacea, but it seems to have no other significant adverse effects. Echinacea may interact with caffeine and with medications metabolized by cytochrome P450, CYP 3A4 such as some statin medications, estrogen, some antiretroviral drugs, and macrolide antibiotics.

Ephedra (ma huang) is used in the East to treat colds and congestion. In the West, it was previously used in products for weight loss and for athletic performance. In 2004, the FDA banned the use of ephedra in dietary supplements because of the very high rate of adverse events. Ephedra can cause seizures, gastrointestinal distress, high blood pressure, stroke, arrhythmia, and heart attack. Herbal teas and traditional Chinese remedies may still contain ephedra. It has some efficacy for short-term weight loss, but this effect cannot be balanced against its many adverse effects. One should never combine ephedra with other stimulants, including caffeine.

Garlic is, of course, an everyday ingredient for cooking. As a supplement, it may be effective for cardiovascular disease and in the prevention of certain cancers. Current research indicates some effect in lowering blood pressure and a possible effect on cholesterol levels. Studies on cancer prevention are ongoing, but no current data confirm its utility for this indication. Garlic may also be an effective topical antifungal agent (0.6% ajoene gel).

Oral garlic interacts with antiplatelet medications, increasing the risk of bleeding, and with most protease inhibitors, reducing their activity. Garlic decreases levels of isoniazid, used in treating or preventing tuberculosis, as well as some antiretroviral medications (nonnucleoside reverse transcriptase inhibitors and some protease inhibitors). Garlic is otherwise safe for most people.

Ginger, commonly used in cooking, is helpful to treat nausea. It can be used fresh, generally coarsely chopped and boiled to make a tea, or in powdered form. Placebo-controlled trials of ginger for nausea in early pregnancy have shown a positive effect. The results of studies using ginger for nausea related to surgery are mixed. Ginger may also be efficacious in treating menstrual pain and for osteoarthritis, although results for this use are also unclear. The data on drug interactions are unclear, but ginger is likely safe at lower doses for most patients. It may reduce clotting and blood sugar, so use caution recommending ginger to those on diabetes medication or anticoagulants.

Ginkgo biloba is an ancient tree found originally in China whose leaves and seeds have been long used there for a variety of conditions, mostly those involving mental function. It seems to have some effect in improving circulation and reducing clotting. Smaller studies showed some beneficial effect in Alzheimer disease and dementia, but a large study (>3000 participants) conducted by the NIH showed no difference in cognitive function between those on ginkgo and placebo after 6 years.[3] Research on ginkgo for anxiety disorders and depression as well as for premenstrual syndrome and hypertension has not yet demonstrated a consistent effect.

Those with seizure disorder should not take ginkgo because it may induce seizures. It may also increase the risk of serotonin syndrome for those taking serotonin reuptake inhibitors (SSRIs). It may also increase the risk of bleeding in those taking Coumadin or other blood thinners. Be cautious in using ginkgo along with any medication metabolized through the liver. The nuts of the ginkgo tree have shown some toxicity and carcinogenesis in animal studies.

Ginseng is a root made into capsules, tablets, or teas used to treat or prevent colds and flu. Smaller studies have shown a substantial effect for respiratory infections,[3,10] but the data remain inconclusive in larger trials. It may also have the effect of reducing blood sugar in those with diabetes. Ginseng is the subject of many current research studies for these uses as well as for improving cognitive function in those with Alzheimer disease. Some have attributed the mixed research results on ginseng to variable dosing in different preparations.

Side effects include gastrointestinal, sleep disturbances, headaches, and allergic reactions. It has potential drug interactions with angiotensin-converting enzyme inhibitors, calcium channel blockers, and anticoagulants.

Goldenseal is widely used in the United States as an immune booster and for respiratory infections. Although there is some evidence that one of its components, berberine, may have some beneficial effect, there is no evidence that the currently available preparations are effective. It has many potential interactions with a wide variety of medications including antibiotics and antivirals. Breastfeeding women should avoid goldenseal because it may cause or exacerbate jaundice in infants.

Kava root is formulated into teas or tinctures to improve mood and well-being. There are no data regarding its effectiveness, yet there are numerous reports of significant adverse effects, including liver damage and central nervous system (CNS) effects. Kava interacts with most medications that affect the CNS.

Milk thistle is an herb used for its effect on protecting the liver from damage by toxins or infection. Studies by the NIH have not shown any significant effect on the disease process of patients with chronic hepatitis C, although it did show some effect in reducing the symptoms of the disease. Milk thistle may also be helpful in managing diabetes and hyperlipidemia. Some patients may have an allergic response to milk thistle, particularly those with ragweed allergies.

Saw palmetto is a small palm used to relieve symptoms of prostatic hypertrophy and for prostate cancer. To date, placebo-controlled studies have not confirmed this effect, but studies are ongoing. It is generally safe but may interact with anticoagulant medications, increasing their effect.

St. John's wort is widely used for depression, obsessive-compulsive disorder, and premenstrual syndrome. Research on its use has had mixed results, but larger studies have shown no significant effect. It has significant interactions with many medications, including many used to treat HIV and antidepressants.

Tea tree oil comes from an Australian tree long used by the aboriginal people. Topical tea tree oil is likely effective to fight bacterial and fungal infections. In vitro studies have given preliminary data confirming its antibacterial properties, and smaller studies have supported its activity as an antifungal and antiacne agent. It can cause irritation when used in higher strengths. It should not be taken internally, but the topical use of diluted forms is considered safe.

Turmeric is a widely used herb that also has a history of use in Ayurvedic and Chinese medicine for a variety of ailments. Turmeric is taken medicinally for intestinal ailments and for its potential antioxidant and immune-boosting properties. There are also some data indicating that turmeric may be helpful in treating osteoarthritis. Data on these effects are mixed, but turmeric is certainly safe in its normal culinary use and in usual doses as a supplement.

Valerian is a bitter root used for insomnia as a tea, capsule, or tincture. There are several studies indicating it may be helpful and others showing no effect. Valerian should not be combined with sedative medications but is otherwise considered safe.

Yohimbe is used to improve sexual function in men and for anxiety and depression. It has many potential side effects, including tachycardia, tremor, hypertension, hyperglycemia, anxiety, and agitation. It has drug interactions with some antidepressants and antihypertensives. It is available in prescription form as yohimbine, and clinicians should review the prescribing information of this product before recommending for or against its use.

CASE STUDY 18.3

You are treating a patient for chronic low back pain that has been controlled but not resolved with physical therapy and medication. She asks about acupuncture. You check the NIH Center for Integrative Medicine's site as well as the Cochrane database and find that results of various studies are mixed. You discuss this information with your patient, and she decides to go ahead. You help her to find certified local acupuncturist. She returns to see you after 2 months of acupuncture treatment. She states that she is feeling much better and has been able to reduce her pain medication.

CASE STUDY 18.4

A 74-year-old man with Parkinson disease diagnosed 5 years ago comes to you in hopes of getting help with his movement disorder as well as cognitive function. He has read about brain implants that can be helpful, but his past medical history of cardiopulmonary disease make him a poor surgical risk. His wife has been taking classes in tai chi. She asks if this might benefit her husband. You review the information available at the NIH Center for Integrative Medicine's website and find that there is research demonstrating some benefit to balance and stability in people with Parkinson disease. Data on its effect on cognitive function are inconclusive, but it appears to cause no harm. After 3 months of tai chi, his balance and movement are somewhat improved, but his cognitive function has continued to decline.

MIND–BODY PRACTICES

The effect of the mind on the body and the body on the mind is clear. We know that exercise, for example, improves sleep.[11] Ongoing research into the physiology of empathy, meditation, and other mental techniques is showing neurologic effects of these practices, although it is not yet clear how these changes manifest in terms of physical or mental health. Nonetheless, many are using these practices and find them to be very helpful. For the most part, they are very safe when the practitioner or teacher is well trained.

Acupuncture is, as noted earlier, an ancient technique used widely in China and Japan. It involves the (generally painless) insertion of thin needles into specific points on the body intended to improve the flow of energy called *qi* (pronounced "chi"). Controlled clinical trials of acupuncture involve the insertion of needles in points that are not true acupuncture points and have had mixed results.[3] That said, many patients find acupuncture to be helpful, and much may depend on the skill of the practitioner. Nonphysician acupuncturists must be licensed in most states.

The *Alexander technique*, developed by F.M. Alexander, an Australian actor, is a gentle technique of postural realignment. Alexander found he frequently lost his voice when performing. He experimented with the position of his head and neck and developed a system of reeducating the body in its poise and movement. Teachers of the technique work with students to improve their body position. It has shown some positive effect for people with chronic neck pain[12] and is currently in research for patients with Parkinson disease. Alexander teachers may practice without credentialing but are usually certified by the American Society for the Alexander Technique (AmSAT).

Biofeedback uses electronic sensors to provide the individual feedback on his or her pulse, breathing, and blood pressure to bring these processes under conscious control. It is a training, in which the patient learns the technique, rather than a treatment. Biofeedback has demonstrated efficacy for female urinary incontinence, anxiety, chronic pain, hypertension, and many other conditions.[13] Practitioners should be certified by the Biofeedback Certification International Alliance.

Chiropractic manipulation is a well-established treatment in the United States, dating back to the 19th century and with an estimated 3% to 11% of individuals having seen a chiropractor during the past 12 months.[14] Chiropractors adjust the alignment of the spine and other structural components of the body with the goal of treating a wide variety of clinical complaints. It is likely effective in treating back and neck pain, but research yields mixed results.[15] The skill and training of the practitioner are key to successful treatment. Chiropractic physicians are licensed to practice in all U.S. states and territories. In addition, most states require practitioners to pass the National Board of Chiropractic Examiners examination.

Qi gong and *tai chi* are linked; both are practices based in Chinese medicine in which gentle body movements are combined with mindfulness techniques and a focus on breathing. Qi or chi is the same energy flow that, as conceived in traditional Chinese medical practice, is modulated by acupuncture. The exercises of both of these techniques are designed to improve the flow of energy and improve health and well-being. Data indicate that tai chi is helpful for patients with parkinsonian movement disorder and for fall reduction. There is no currently accepted standard of training or certification.

Yoga is by far the most commonly used of the mind–body practices in the United States.[1] Swami Vivekananda introduced yoga when he first came to the United States to give the opening address to the Parliament of Religions in 1893. Yoga developed in the ancient spiritual traditions of India. As practiced in the United States, yoga is a series of movements and postures, generally with coordinated breathing patterns, used more for physical than spiritual benefit.

Research on yoga is suggestive of a significant benefit in reduction of pain, anxiety, depression, and blood pressure. It is safe but, as with any exercise, might require some modification for those with certain medical conditions and can cause harm if practiced improperly. Certification exists for teachers at various levels but is not required to teach yoga.

ADDRESSING COMPLEMENTARY AND INTEGRATIVE HEALTH IN CLINICAL PRACTICE

Practitioners can assume that approximately one in three patients use products and practices other than traditional medicine to maintain or improve their health. PAs must specifically ask about alternative products and practices. Even clinicians who are well versed in integrative medicine frequently encounter the use of integrative therapies with which they are unfamiliar, so it is important to become familiar with good resources from which current and accurate data can be obtained.

Patients present with use of, or interest in, not only a wide variety of products and practices but with an even wider variety of preconceptions. Using a patient-centered approach, the clinician must first discover what therapies the patient is currently using, as opposed to therapies in which he or she is expressing interest. Patients understand that PAs may not be experts in the area but appreciate an open attitude and a commitment to help in gathering further information.

Much in the realm of complementary and integrative health lacks good scientific evidence, but most are low risk. PAs should familiarize themselves with substances known to have interactions with medications, such as St. John's wort, as well as those known to have significant adverse effects, such as ephedra. If there is no harmful effect, a trial of a supplement or practice is reasonable and its effect evaluated after a period of weeks or months. For practices and products for which research has demonstrated efficacy, PAs may feel safe in recommendations and referrals.

CLINICAL APPLICATIONS

1. Take a moment to reflect on the following. What were your beliefs about illness when you were a child? Where did those beliefs come from? What did your family of origin believe about the causes of illness and how they should be treated? What are your beliefs now?

2. Have you ever used some form of complementary and integrative health care? Think about the reasons why you did. What modality did you choose and why that particular one? What was your experience? Did the existence of quantitative research play a role in your decision to use the alternative? Did you or would you share this information with your health care provider? Why or why not?

KEY POINTS

- It is every PA's responsibility to become knowledgeable about complementary and integrative health modalities, as well as where to locate reliable research and information.
- It is imperative that PAs are able to establish open and effective provider–patient relationships that will enable patients to discuss complementary and integrative health usage, questions, and concerns.
- Be nonjudgmental, be open minded, and make no assumptions concerning complementary or integrative modalities, the patient's use of these modalities, and complementary or integrative health providers.

ACKNOWLEDGMENT

The editors and author would like to acknowledge Emily White-Horse, the author of this chapter in the previous editions.

References

1. Clarke TC, Black LI, Stussman BJ, Barnes PM, Nahin RL. Trends in the use of complementary health approaches among adults: United States, 2002–2012. *National Health Statistics Reports*. 2015.
2. Stussman BJ, Black LI, Barnes PM, Clarke TC, Nahin RL. Wellness-related use of common complementary health approaches among adults: United States, 2012. *National Health Statistics Reports*. 2015.
3. U.S. Department of Health & Human Services. National Center for Complementary and Integrative Health. https://Nccih.Nih.Gov/. Accessed March 25, 2016.
4. Faith J, Thorburn S, Tippens KM. Examining CAM use disclosure using the behavioral model of health services use. *Complement Ther Med*. 2013;21(5):501–508. http://Dx.Doi.Org/10.1016/J.Ctim.2013.08.002. Accessed March 25, 2016.
5. Vickers AJ, Cronin AM, Maschino AC, et al. Acupuncture for chronic pain: individual patient data meta-analysis. *Arch Intern Med*. 2012;172(19):1444–1453. http://Dx.Doi.Org/10.1001/Archinternmed.2012.3654. Accessed March 25, 2016.
6. U.S. Department of Health and Human Services, Office of Disease Prevention and Health Promotion. 2010 Dietary guidelines. http://Health.Gov/Dietaryguidelines/2010/. Accessed March 25, 2016.
7. U.S. Department of Health and Human Services. Healthy People 2020. http://Www.Healthypeople.Gov/. Accessed March 25, 2016.
8. Sacks FM, Svetkey LP, Vollmer WM, et al. Effects on blood pressure of reduced dietary sodium and the dietary approaches to stop hypertension (DASH) Diet. DASH-Sodium Collaborative Research Group. *N Engl J Med*. 2001;344(1):3–10.
9. Lopes HF, Martin KL, Nashar K, Morrow JD, Goodfriend TL, Egan BM. DASH diet lowers blood pressure and lipid-induced oxidative stress in obesity. *Hypertension*. 2003;41(3):422–430.
10. Mcelhaney JE, Goel V, Toane B, Hooten J, Shan JJ. Efficacy of cold-fx in the prevention of respiratory symptoms in community-dwelling adults: a randomized, double-blinded, placebo controlled trial. *J Altern Complement Med*. 2006;12(2):153–157.
11. Reid KJ, Baron KG, Lu B, Naylor E, Wolfe L, Zee PC. Aerobic exercise improves self-reported sleep and quality of life in older adults with insomnia. *Sleep Med*. 2010;11(9):934–940. http://dx.doi.org/10.1016/J.Sleep. Accessed April 14, 2010.
12. Macpherson H, Tilbrook H, Richmond S, et al. Alexander technique lessons or acupuncture sessions for persons with chronic neck pain: a randomized trial. *Ann Intern Med*. 2015;163(9):653–662. http://Dx.Org/10.7326/M15-0667. Accessed March 25, 2016.
13. Frank DL, Khorshid L, Kiffer JF, Moravec CS, Mckee MG. Biofeedback in medicine: who, when, why and how? *Ment Health Fam Med*. 2010;7(2):85–91.
14. Cooper KL, Harris PE, Relton C, Thomas KJ. Prevalence of visits to five types of complementary and alternative medicine practitioners by the general population: a systematic review. *Complement Ther Clin Pract*. 2013;19(4):214–220. http://Dx.Doi.Org/10.1016/J.Ctcp.2013.06.006. Accessed March 25, 2016.
15. Parkinson L, Sibbritt D, Bolton P, Van Rotterdam J, Villadsen I. Well-being outcomes of chiropractic intervention for lower back pain: a systematic review. *Clin Rheumatol*. 2013;32(2):167–180. http://Link.Springer.Com/Article/10.1007/S10067-012-2116-Z#Page-2. Accessed March 25, 2016.

The resources for this chapter can be found at www.expertconsult.com.

CHAPTER 19

GERIATRIC MEDICINE

Freddi Segal-Gidan • Gwen Yeo

This chapter provides an overview of geriatric medicine oriented to beginning clinicians, including basic information and clinical perspectives that are useful to health care providers (HCPs) in approaching the social and medical complexities associated with care of older persons. The health care of older adults in the United States presents clinicians with numerous challenges. In addition to complex medical conditions, many older patients present with social, spiritual, economic, and political challenges. When these challenges are successfully met, however, PAs caring for older patients in any setting can experience enormous satisfaction and provide an important contribution to the well-being of both patients and society.

Our society is growing older just as our medical care has become more sophisticated at an ever-increasing cost. By the year 2030, projections are that one in five Americans will be 65 years of age or older, and there will be twice as many people 65 years of age and older as there were in 2000. This huge increase began in 2011 when the first cohort of baby boomers reached age 65 years.[1] These older Americans will also be increasingly diverse, with 40% of them belonging to one of the minority populations by midcentury. Medical practices are experiencing the effects of this increase in the older population just as many also experience a changing medical reimbursement system and uncertainty about the structure of medical care in the future. Physician assistants (PAs) are providing an increasingly important role in general geriatric care, specialty care, and long-term care. The challenge to all PAs is to provide competent, cost-effective, functionally oriented, ethnically competent health care to each older person in their practice.

GERIATRIC CARE

Chronic Conditions

There are some significant differences in providing appropriate geriatric care that require PAs to make a clear shift in the goals they usually have in patient care.

Because most of the health conditions older adults present with are likely to be chronic rather than acute, it requires the provider to concentrate on *management* in most cases rather than *treatment* in the expectation that the condition will be cured. Because the chronic conditions are not time limited and additional chronic diseases are frequently added, geriatric clinicians are most often faced with trying to manage a patient's multiple conditions, which usually entail multiple medications as well. Fig. 19.1 illustrates the most common chronic diseases experienced by older adults in the United States. The goal is to help older adults maintain the highest possible function to maximize their quality of life in the context of their chronic conditions.

Functional Status

This emphasis on functional status is a critical component of good geriatric care and requires the clinician to use the measure of function as a constant tool. The two principal methods of functional assessment are determining the level of independence or dependence in performing activities of daily living (ADLs) and instrumental activities of daily living (IADLs). See Box 19.1 for a list of

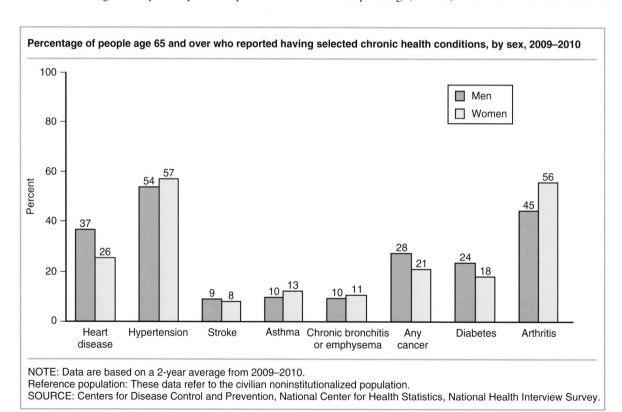

Percentage of people age 65 and over who reported having selected chronic health conditions, by sex, 2009–2010

NOTE: Data are based on a 2-year average from 2009–2010.
Reference population: These data refer to the civilian noninstitutionalized population.
SOURCE: Centers for Disease Control and Prevention, National Center for Health Statistics, National Health Interview Survey.

FIG. 19.1 ■ Chronic health conditions among the population, ages 65 years and older. (From Federal Interagency Forum on Aging-Related Statistics. *Older Americans 2012: Key Indicators of Well-Being.*)

BOX 19.1 ACTIVITIES OF DAILY LIVING (ADLs) AND INSTRUMENTAL ACTIVITIES OF DAILY LIVING (IADLs)

ADLs
Feeding
Dressing
Ambulation
Toileting and continence
Bathing
Transfer (bed, chair, toilet)

IADLs
Cooking and food preparation
Shopping
Laundry
Housekeeping
Using telephone
Managing medications
Ability to handle finances; money management
Transportation

ADLs and IADLs and Fig. 19.2 for the profile of Medicare enrollees who have limitations in either measure.

Dependence on ADLs is commonly used as a measure of eligibility for services such as nursing homes, adult day health care, or in-home support services. There are several different versions of the lists of ADLs and IADLs, but they all contain the basic activities. Scoring schemes vary from yes/no answers to questions such as, "Do you need help performing the following activities?" to five categories of dependence for each activity.[2]

In the routine clinical encounter, function needs to be a constant concern. Can a patient with diabetes see well enough to be able to self-administer insulin? Can a patient easily swallow antibiotics for pneumonia or would a liquid be easier and promote compliance? Can a patient limited by arthritis remove the cap from the medication bottle or easily remove the tablets from the office samples given him or her? The question that should always underlie any change of condition or new diagnosis is, "How does this affect

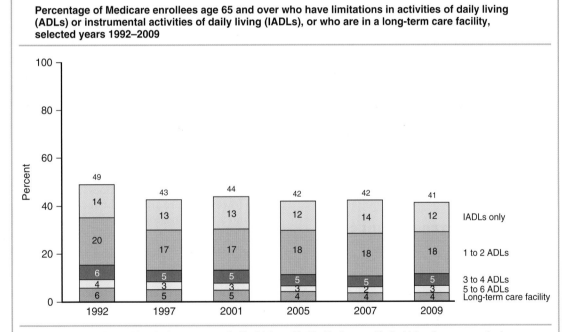

Percentage of Medicare enrollees age 65 and over who have limitations in activities of daily living (ADLs) or instrumental activities of daily living (IADLs), or who are in a long-term care facility, selected years 1992–2009

NOTE: A residence is considered a long-term care facility if it is certified by Medicare or Medicaid; has three or more beds, is licensed as a nursing home or other long-term care facility, and provides at least one personal care service; or provides 24-hour, 7-day-a-week supervision by a caregiver. ADL limitations refer to difficulty performing (or inability to perform for a health reason) one or more of the following tasks: bathing, dressing, eating, getting in/out of chairs, walking, or using the toilet. IADL limitations refer to difficulty performing (or inability to perform for a health reason) one or more of the following tasks: using the telephone, light housework, heavy housework, meal preparation, shopping, or managing money. Percents are age-adjusted using the 2000 standard population. Estimates may not sum to the totals because of rounding.
Reference population: These data refer to Medicare enrollees.
SOURCE: Centers for Medicare and Medicaid Services, Medicare current beneficiary survey.

FIG. 19.2 ■ Percentage of Medicare enrollees age 65 years and older who have limitations in activities of daily living or instrumental activities of daily living (IADLs) or who were in a facility from 1992 to 2007. (From Federal Interagency Forum on Aging-Related Statistics. *Older Americans 2012: Key Indicators of Well-Being.*)

the person's ability to manage the activities of daily living?"

Time and Perspective

Geriatric practice often differs in time and perspective in that PAs working with geriatric patients frequently need to spend more time learning and understanding their patients' medical status and personal preferences. In many cases, care of older adults includes working with family members or other caregivers, which involves additional time and a unique set of skills. Time is often the critical factor in eliciting a thoughtful and comprehensive history, especially in patients with multiple chronic conditions. Many older patients need more time to disrobe and dress again. The PA may have to work into his or her schedule driving time to a patient in a nursing home whose condition has changed or for a routine continuity-of-care visit. When an older patient who is chronically ill develops an acute condition, a prior therapeutic relationship with the patient and a clear sense of the patient's baseline are extremely important because they enable the provider to identify the subtle signs (e.g., confusion, decreased appetite, listlessness) that may often be the only clues of a new underlying disease process. Although initially the PA may need to spend more time getting to know an elderly patient, he or she will find it easier to spot acute or chronic change and be able to preempt the problem. After such a meaningful therapeutic patient–PA relationship has been established, the PA will be of enormous help in that he or she will be able to establish the contextual framework for the patient's illness, thereby significantly increasing the overall efficacy of the practice (Table 19.1).

NORMAL AGE-RELATED CHANGES

Aging is commonly viewed as the gradual loss of function and independence with increasing years. Successful aging is remaining active and functional in the physical, cognitive, and emotional realms until death.[3] The aging process depends on the complex interaction of genetics, disease, health habits (e.g., smoking and alcohol consumption), diet, and exercise over the life course. In differentiating disease from aging, it is important for PAs to have an understanding of important age-related changes that tend to occur even in those who have an active and healthy lifestyle. Common age-related changes are summarized by system in the sections that follow.

Sensory Changes

With older age, there is an increased incidence of cataracts (gradual density and clouding of the lens in the eye) and a consequent decrease in visual acuity resulting in, among other risks, an increased incidence of falls; most often, the visual acuity can be restored by surgical replacement of the affected lens. There is an age-related reduction in the ability to hear higher frequencies (presbycusis), resulting in communication difficulties if not corrected by hearing aids. When one is communicating with an older person who is known to have sensory impairment, it is important to speak slowly and clearly, sit close to the person, and make sure one's face is well lit. These simple measures can reduce confusion and anxiety and make for a more successful clinical encounter.

There also appears to be a decrease in acuity of taste with increasing age, so food tends to be perceived as bland. The clinical consequences can be a decreased appreciation for food and a loss of appetite, which can lead to significant weight loss and nutrition deficiency, and increased use of seasoning to enhance taste, such as salt or sugar, which can exacerbate underlying medical conditions and their treatment (e.g., hypertension, heart failure, diabetes). The aging skin has thinner epidermis and subcutaneous fat layers and reduced oil production. The result is increased risk with ambient temperature changes for hypothermia and hyperthermia among older adults and a propensity for dry skin (xerosis), skin breakdown, and ulcerations.

Cardiovascular Changes

The resting cardiac output does not change with age. However, there are a slight decrease in the heart rate and a compensatory increase in stroke volume. Heart rate response to exercise is decreased in older adults secondary to a decrease in the β-adrenergic response. Also, diastolic dysfunction may be seen during both rest and exercise in older adults. Systolic blood pressure tends to rise with age more than diastolic, and sustained elevations (hypertension) in either one or both increase the risk for stroke and heart disease. Decreases in vascular compliance with age contribute to positional changes in blood pressure (orthostatic hypotension), which can lead to increased complaints of dizziness, imbalance, and risk for falls.

Coronary artery disease is the most common cause of death among those 65 years and older. A well-balanced healthy diet and regular exercise have

TABLE 19.1 10-Minute Screener for Geriatric Conditions

Problem	Screening Measure	Positive Screen
Vision	Two parts: 1. Ask: "Do you have difficulty driving or watching television or reading or doing any of your daily activities because of your eyesight?" 2. If yes, then: Test each eye with the Snellen chart while the patient wears corrective lenses (if applicable).	Yes to question and inability to read >20/40 on Snellen chart
Hearing	Use audioscope set at 40 dB; test hearing using 1000 and 2000 Hz	Inability to hear 1000 and 2000 Hz in both ears or inability to hear frequencies in either ear
Leg mobility	Time the patient after asking: "Rise from the chair. Walk 10 feet, turn, walk back to the chair, and sit down."	Unable to complete task in 10 sec
Urinary incontinence	Two parts: Ask: "In the past year, have you ever lost your urine and gotten wet?" If yes, then ask: "Have you lost your urine on at least 7 separate days?"	Yes to both questions
Nutrition, weight loss	Two parts: Ask: "Have you lost 10 lb over the past 6 months without trying to do so?" Weigh the patient.	Yes to the question or weight <100 lb
Memory	Three-item recall	Unable to recall all items after 1 minute
Depression	Ask: "Do you often feel sad or depressed?"	Yes to the question
Physical disability	Six questions "Are you able to do strenuous activities such as fast walking or bicycling?" "... do heavy work around the house, such as washing windows, walls, or floors?" "... go shopping for groceries or clothes?" "... get to places out of walking distance?" "... bathe, using a sponge bath, a tub bath, or a shower?" "... dress, including putting on a shirt, buttoning and zipping, and putting on shoes?"	No to any of the questions

From Moore AA, Siu AL. Screening for common problems in ambulatory elderly: clinical confirmation of a screening instrument. *Am J Med.* 1996;100:438; and modified from Kane RW, Ouslander JG, Abrass IB. *Essentials of Clinical Geriatrics*, 3rd ed. New York: McGraw-Hill; 1994.

a tremendous positive impact on the cardiovascular changes associated with aging. A *reasonable* diet and exercise program should be strongly encouraged for persons in their advanced years. They can increase their stamina and aerobic fitness level if they exercise regularly.[4]

Endocrine Changes

Aging is associated with deteriorating glucose tolerance changes, and peripheral glucose utilization is thought to be the major factor in this phenomenon.[3] Thyroid function is generally normal in physiologic aging, although older patients tend to have low triiodothyronine (T_3) levels. There is an increase of 2% to 5% in the prevalence of hypothyroidism in those older than age 65 years, and the prevalence continues to rise with age. The clinician should consider hypothyroidism when confronted with complaints of fatigue, depression, loss of initiative, confusion, dry skin, and constipation in an older patient. Serum parathyroid hormone (PTH) increases in older adults, and this increase correlates with a decline in vitamin D levels; treatment with 1,25-$(OH)_2$-D_3 results in a decrease in PTH levels. Age-related increases in PTH are thought to be a major factor accounting for age-related bone loss, which for postmenopausal women is estimated to be 1% per year if untreated.

Immunologic Changes

There is an overall decrease in immunity with age, resulting in a greater prevalence of infections (e.g., pneumonia and urinary tract infections [UTIs]), shingles, gram-negative bacteremia, and severe episodes of influenza. Aging is accompanied by changes in both cellular and humoral immunity. The function of lymphocytes is altered with decreased proliferative capacity of T lymphocytes. Macrophage function is altered, and delayed-type skin hypersensitivity (DTH) declines. Older adults often present an atypical clinical picture, with absence of fevers, presence of hypothermia, altered eating patterns, delirium, and agitation in response to infection. They may also fail to mount a leukocytosis in response to an infection but will frequently have a left shift in the face of a normal leukocyte count. The clinical implication is that even simple illnesses in older adults need to be monitored closely and treated aggressively as indicated.

Renal Function

There is an overall decrease in kidney mass and loss of parenchymal mass over time. The total number of glomeruli decreases with age, and the renal vasculature undergoes sclerotic changes. All of these changes result in a progressively decreasing glomerular filtration rate (GFR). Concomitantly, with increasing age, there is a reduction in lean body mass, which results in decreased creatinine production. Therefore, the creatinine can continue to remain falsely low or "normal," even in the face of decreasing GFR and compromised renal function. Even the commonly used Cockcroft and Gault equation can lead to a mean underestimation of the measured creatinine clearance of 12.1 mL/min in a group of healthy patients.[5] Therefore, calculated creatinine clearances should be avoided in older adults in favor of short-duration, timed urine collections to measure the actual creatinine clearance. To avoid overmedication, any medicine excreted by the kidneys must be carefully considered for dosing and closely monitored.

Creatinine clearance = (140 − age) × Body weight in kilograms/(72 × Serum creatinine

GERIATRIC SYNDROMES

Dementia

Dementia is the most common cause of mental decline among older adults; it affects more than 5 million people in the United States and increases in prevalence with age from an estimated 11% aged 65 years and older to 32% in those aged 85 years and older.[6] The *Diagnostic and Statistical Manual of Mental Disorders* (DSM-5) of the American Psychiatric Association in 2013 incorporated dementia into the diagnostic categories of major and mild neurocognitive disorders, but the term *dementia* is still in common usage as an overall term. To meet DSM-5 criteria for major neurocognitive disorder, an individual must have evidence of significant cognitive decline (e.g., decline in memory, language, or learning), and the cognitive decline must interfere with independence in everyday activities (e.g., assistance may be needed with complex activities such as paying bills or managing medications).[7] Disability may also be seen in the following areas:

- Aphasia (language disturbance)
- Apraxia (inability to perform complex movements)
- Agnosia (failure to recognize or identify objects)
- Executive function (judgment and reasoning, problem solving)
- Visuospatial ability
- Calculation

The label *mild cognitive impairment* is frequently used for individuals with mild but measurable changes in thinking abilities that are noticeable to the person affected and to family members and friends but that do not affect the individual's ability to carry out everyday activities.[6] They may or may not progress to full-blown dementia.

Alzheimer disease (AD) accounts for an estimated 60% to 80% of all dementia cases and is characterized by progressive accumulation of the protein fragment β-amyloid (plaques) outside neurons in the brain and twisted strands of the protein tau (tangles) inside neurons; the neurons are eventually damaged and die. *Vascular dementia* is characterized by multiple infarcts in the cortical and subcortical gray matter or white matter demyelination in the cerebral cortex and in its pure form affects approximately 10% of individuals with dementia. However, it is very common in older individuals with dementia, with about 50% having pathologic evidence of vascular dementia (infarcts). In most cases, the infarcts coexist with Alzheimer pathology, which is referred to as *mixed dementia*. In recent years, other types of dementias have been increasingly recognized. These include *dementia with Lewy bodies*, which includes dementia plus parkinsonian signs, detailed visual hallucinations leading to secondary delusions, and alterations of alertness or attention, and *frontotemporal lobar degeneration*, which is typically characterized in the early stages by marked changes in personality and behavior and difficulty with producing or comprehending language. Unlike AD, memory is typically spared until later stages.[6]

As people age, they may experience such cognitive changes as slowing in information processing, where it takes longer or more repetitions to learn new information, but these kinds of changes are benign. In contrast, dementia is a progressive and disabling pathologic condition that is not considered part of normal aging.

Caregivers and patients often misinterpret initial symptoms of AD (e.g., memory loss) as normal age-related changes. The two greatest risk factors for AD are age and family history. Genetic mutations on chromosomes 1, 14, and 21 are responsible for the rare forms of familial AD that begin before age 60 years (presenile or early-onset AD). The apolipoprotein E gene *(APOE)* on chromosome 19 is the only identified genetic risk factor presently for the more commonly occurring late-onset AD.

Gradual onset and progressive decline in cognitive functioning characterize AD. Motor and sensory functions are usually spared until late stages. Memory impairment for new material is a core symptom of any dementia, and this is seen even in the earliest stages of AD. Typical cognitive symptoms of AD include the following:

- Difficulty learning and retaining new information
- Disorientation, first to time and then to include place
- Language disability, particularly word finding
- Visuospatial dysfunction (getting lost)
- Impaired judgment and reasoning

The cognitive loss with dementia initially affects the patient's IADLs and then later his or her ADLs so that eventually the patient becomes completely dependent on others. Recognition of dementia may be further complicated by the presence of depression and the need for the PA to be aware of treatable conditions that can mimic dementia by their clinical presentation (Table 19.2).

Patients with dementia commonly experience symptoms of depression, and depressed patients frequently present with cognitive complaints. Behavioral disturbances are also common in dementing illnesses and often include anxiety, irritability and agitation, delusional thinking, apathy, and sleep disturbances.

Dementia Workup

Patient and family member interviews and office-based clinical assessment are the most important diagnostic tools for dementia. This should include the following:

- A comprehensive history with special attention to the onset and rate of cognitive and functional change

TABLE 19.2 Causes of Potentially Reversible Dementias

Neoplasms	Autoimmune Disorders
Metabolic disorders	Central nervous system vasculitis, temporal arteritis
Trauma	Disseminated lupus erythematosus
Toxins	Multiple sclerosis
Alcoholism	Drugs
Heavy metals	Nutritional disorders
Organic poisons	Psychiatric disorders
Infections	Depression
Viral, including HIV	Other disorders (e.g., normal-pressure hydrocephalus)

Source: Kane RL, Ouslander, JG, Abrass IB, Resnick B. *Essentials of Clinical Geriatrics*, 7th ed. New York: McGraw Hill Education; 2013.

BOX 19.2 MENTAL STATUS SCREENING TOOLS

Folstein Mini Mental State Examination (MMSE)
Modified Mini-Mental State Examination (3MS)
Montreal Cognitive Assessment (MoCA)
Mini-Cog Screening
St. Louis University Mental Status (SLUMS)

- Use of validated screening tests of cognitive function (Box 19.2)
- Physical examination, with special attention to cardiovascular and neurologic function
- Laboratory evaluations (complete blood cell count [CBC], thyroid-stimulating hormone [TSH], Venereal Disease Research Laboratory [VDRL]) and vitamin B_{12} are recommended.[8]

Brain imaging studies (magnetic resonance imaging [MRI] or computed tomography [CT]) should be considered in patients if the following conditions apply:

- Dementia onset occurs at an age younger than 65 years.
- The condition is postacute (symptoms have occurred for <2 years).
- Focal neurologic deficits are present.
- The clinical picture suggests normal-pressure hydrocephalus (triad of onset within 1 year, gait disorder, and unexplained incontinence).

Biomarkers in cerebrospinal fluid and in positron emission tomography scans are used in research projects to identify the presence of τ- and β-amyloid that can help confirm the diagnosis of AD. They are not currently used in routine clinical assessments but have been suggested as possible future components.

CASE STUDY 19.1

Dr. C is a 76-year-old retired professor who with his wife has recently moved from his home several states away into an assisted living apartment to be closer to his adult children. He has enjoyed an active retirement, playing tennis and golf, socializing with friends, and traveling. Three years ago on a cruise ship, he had difficulty finding his cabin and then got confused scoring a golf game and became concerned about his memory. He saw his internist for evaluation and was diagnosed with mild dementia and early AD. He comes to establish care in the geriatric medicine practice where you work as a PA. Today his MoCA is 25 of 30, with ability to recall two of five words spontaneously and the other three with cueing, misnaming one animal and missing two numbers on serial subtraction. He is slightly hesitant in his answers, and there is some overall slowing to his demeanor, which could be normal for age. He has urinary frequency attributed to benign prostatic hypertrophy (BPH), systolic hypertension for 8 years, and glaucoma and wears a hearing aid in his left ear. On examination, his speech is normal, and his gait has a wide base and unsteadiness with tandem walking. Medications include timolol ophthalmic drops, donepezil, tamsulosin, 81 mg of aspirin, and vitamin D. A review of medical records includes Mini-Mental Status Examination from 3 years ago of 28 of 30, normal CBC, chemistry, vitamin B_{12}, and TSH. The report of a CT scan reads "within normal limits for age." You order a brain MRI, which shows enlarged ventricles and minimal sulci widening with the note "consider normal-pressure hydrocephalus" (NPH). He is admitted to the hospital for a lumbar drain and after 3 days of improvement in gait speed is recorded by his physical therapist. The neurosurgeon agrees he is a good candidate for ventriculoperitoneal shunt placement, which is done several weeks later. The patient does well, his gait improves, his urinary frequency improves, and there is no further cognitive decline over the next 3 years.

DISCUSSION

Memory complaints are common with increasing age, but all memory loss is not AD. This case demonstrates the importance of considering the patient as a whole and all diagnoses in the differential diagnosis. NPH, although uncommon (<1% of all dementias), is one of the few treatable causes of cognitive loss. The presentation is often subtle and easily confused with normal aging or attributed to other causes, as in this case.

Management of Dementia

Primary treatment goals for patients with dementia are to enhance and preserve quality of life and to optimize functional performance by managing cognition, mood, and behavior.[9] Working closely with the patient and caregivers to establish a trusting relationship and a therapeutic alliance facilitates management. Current recommendations are for pharmacologic therapy to be started early in the disease process, beginning with an acetylcholinesterase inhibitor and then adding an N-methyl-D-aspartate (NMDA) agonist. Acetylcholinesterase inhibitors include donepezil (Aricept), rivastigmine (Exelon), and galantamine (Reminyl). Namenda is an NMDA glutamate agonist.

Nonpharmacologic treatments, such as physical and cognitive stimulation and reminiscence therapy, are also important components. It is of critical importance that clinicians initiate discussion about long-term health and financial care plans while the patient is still in the early stages of dementia when he or she can participate in these crucial decisions. Caregivers are often subject to enormous stresses and should be referred to caregiver support groups, which have been shown to be effective in alleviating stress and preserving caregiver health. Respite care and other community resources such as dementia adult day care offer caregivers relief and help postpone patient institutionalization. Familiarity with community resources and referral to social work care management or organizations such as the Alzheimer's Association are essential components of care for patients with dementia and their families.

Delirium

Delirium, or an "acute confusional state," is a common geriatric syndrome that is often overlooked and underdiagnosed. Up to one third of all hospitalized elderly patients exhibit some level of delirium, and delirium is the leading complication of hospitalization among older adults.[10] As the number of patients of increasing age undergo surgery, the risk for postoperative delirium and prolonged postoperative confusion is increasing. Delirium is an independent risk factor for poor medical outcomes in older adults. An advanced age, history of dementia, poor functional status, and sensory impairment are known predisposing factors for delirium. The Confusion Assessment Method (Box 19.3) is a practical and useful tool for detecting delirium, particularly among institutionalized older adults.[11] Acute infection, postoperative state, acute myocardial infarction, and alcohol withdrawal are common precipitating factors. Iatrogenic delirium is extremely

BOX 19.3 CONFUSION ASSESSMENT METHOD

For a diagnosis of delirium, a patient must have:
1. Presence of an acute and fluctuating course
   and
2. Inattention
   and either
3. Disorganized thinking or
4. Altered level of consciousness

Source: Inouye SK, van Dyk CH, Alessi C, et al. Clarifying confusion: the confusion assessment method. A new method for the detection of delirium. *Ann Intern Med.* 1990;113:941.

common among older adults, and drugs with anticholinergic effects are some of the most common culprits. Other causative drugs include antihistamines, antiparkinsonism drugs, benzodiazepines, and H_2-blockers. Management of delirium includes the following:

- High index of suspicion and early identification
- Withdrawal of suspected offending drug(s), especially anticholinergics
- Treatment of the underlying cause
- Supportive care, including a well-lit, safe, and familiar environment
- Reassurance for both the patient and the family

Urinary Incontinence

Unfortunately, incontinence is frequently not mentioned by patients and is not often asked about by providers. It is all too often mistakenly assumed by patients to be a normal function of aging. In reality, it is not inevitable and is usually treatable. Urinary incontinence of one or more episodes in the past month affects about 20% of people older than age 60 years, 50% of those in institutions, and twice as many women than men.[12] One third to half of affected patients have never sought medical attention for incontinence.

The adverse effects of incontinence can be extremely troubling, resulting in skin breakdown, frequent UTI, and falls from an unsteady gait rushing to the toilet or slipping on some urine. The psychological impact of incontinence can lead to social isolation and depression. There can be tremendous stress on the caregivers, and it can result in institutionalization.[13] The economic costs can be considerable when supplies, laundry, labor, and the medical cost of managing complications are totaled. The total direct costs alone have been estimated at more than $14 billion per year in the United States alone.[14,15]

Incontinence can be classified as acute or chronic. Acute incontinence in an otherwise healthy person is usually secondary to infection or inflammation (e.g., atrophic vaginitis, urethritis). It is important to note that the differential diagnosis for acute incontinence covers a wide range of possibilities, including restricted mobility.

The principal types of chronic urinary incontinence can be categorized as stress, urge, overflow, functional, or mixed (involving more than one type).

Stress Incontinence

Stress incontinence is involuntary loss of urine, usually a small amount, secondary to increased intraabdominal pressure from a cough or laugh. Common causes are weakness and laxity of the pelvic floor musculature and weakness of the bladder outlet or urethral sphincter.

Urge Incontinence and Overactive Bladder

Urge incontinence is leakage of urine, usually a large amount, caused by the inability to delay voiding after the sensation of bladder fullness is perceived. Common causes are detrusor muscle instability, alone or associated with a local genitourinary condition (UTI, urethritis, tumor, stones), and central nervous system disorders (parkinsonism, cerebrovascular accident, dementia).

Overflow Incontinence

Leakage of urine results from mechanical forces in an overdistended bladder. Common causes are anatomic obstruction (urethral stricture secondary to BPH or cystocele), acontractile bladder (associated with diabetes or spinal cord injury), and neurogenic bladder (result of detrusor–sphincter dyssynergia associated with multiple sclerosis and other suprasacral cord lesions).

Functional Incontinence

The inability to toilet caused by impaired cognitive or physical function, environmental barriers, or psychological unwillingness (depression, anger, or hostility).

The PA's approach to incontinence should include the following measures:

- A thorough history to quantify the amount of urine lost and circumstances of the incontinent episodes sufficient to affect daily life in an alert patient

- A physical examination, including abdomen, genital, rectal, and neurologic screening and mobility and joint examination
- Laboratory assessment of urine with culture and sensitivity testing
- Other laboratory tests or referral to a specialist (gynecologist, urologist, neurologist) depending on history and physical findings

Management of urinary incontinence is usually based on the classification or type. For the most common types affecting older women—stress and urge—the nonpharmacologic, noninvasive behavioral intervention known as *pelvic floor muscle training*, or *Kegel exercises*, has been found in a majority of cases to substantially reduce or eliminate incontinence problems.[16] PAs can improve the quality of life of many of their older patients who have lost control of their urination by giving them the instructions described in Box 19.4 and then scheduling regular follow-up visits to monitor and reinforce their progress. Pharmacologic intervention with anticholinergic, antimuscarinic medications such as oxybutynin, tolterodine, solifenacin, darifenacin, trospium, and fesoterodine are commonly used for urge incontinence if the behavioral interventions are unsuccessful. The side effects that profile these agents (confusion, dry mouth, constipation, dry eyes, blurred vision) limit their tolerability in older adults.

Instability and Falls

Falls account for a significant number of cases of injury and death among older adults. Accidents are the sixth leading cause of death among older adults, and falls account for two thirds of accidental deaths.[17] Besides the acute trauma noted in patients who present in the emergency department (ED) or office, a significant number of falls with resulting soft tissue injury and psychological stress occur and are unreported. This leads to decreased independence, a reduced sense of autonomy, and for some, a fear of falling again that can be disabling.

Falls are a multifactorial problem in older adults. The intrinsic factors affecting stability and predisposing an older person to falls include the following:
- Changes in vision, including depth perception and acuity
- Decreased proprioception
- Decreased lower extremity muscle strength
- Increased postural sway
- Changes in gait, both speed and height of step
- Almost any disease process that exacerbates the expected aging changes, especially dementia, depression, cardiovascular disease, arthritis,

podiatric problems, diabetes, peripheral neuropathy, and stroke

Extrinsic factors play an important role in falls and include the following:
- Poor lighting
- Irregular surfaces (cracks in the sidewalk, short or irregular steps)

BOX 19.4 INSTRUCTIONS FOR PELVIC MUSCLE (KEGEL) EXERCISES

IDENTIFYING AND CONTRACTING (TIGHTENING) YOUR PELVIC MUSCLE

The pelvic muscle is the muscle you tighten to stop your urine flow and to keep from passing gas or, if you are a woman, to "pull up" your vagina. Women can easily feel if they are tightening this muscle by placing one or two fingers in the vagina and contracting around their fingers.

It is important to be able to contract your pelvic muscle without contracting your abdominal muscles, which could cause you to leak urine. To determine if you are tightening your abdominal muscles, place a hand on your abdomen while you tighten your pelvic muscles. If you feel your abdomen tighten, you need to practice relaxing your abdomen while continuing to contract your pelvic muscles.

PRACTICING PELVIC MUSCLE EXERCISES

First, empty your bladder. Sit or lie in a comfortable place and relax for a minute. Then tighten your pelvic muscle (without tightening your abdomen). Keep it tight for 10 seconds. Relax for 10 seconds. Repeat for a total of 15 contractions. Do these 15 contractions three times each day. If you are not able to hold the muscle tight for 10 seconds or are unable to repeat it 15 times, just do it as many times as you can. Your ability to perform the exercise will improve with time.

WHAT TO EXPECT

The benefit increases the longer you practice the exercises. Most women notice a decrease in their frequency of incontinence within 4 to 6 weeks. Studies have shown that this exercise program is effective in reducing incontinence by an average of 70% and completely eliminates incontinence in about one third of women after 6 incomplete weeks. As the exercises become familiar, you can practice them anytime, such as when you are watching television, driving, or in bed.

IF INCONTINENCE PERSISTS

If incontinence persists, there are additional treatment options of medication or surgery that you may want to discuss with your doctor.

- Slick surfaces (throw rugs)
- Furniture too high or too low
- Bathroom fixtures without support bars or at an inappropriate height

Patients who have fallen require a careful and complete medical evaluation, including assessment of orthostatic blood pressure changes, cardiovascular status, neurologic deficits (including mental status), musculoskeletal conditions, foot disorders, and sensory deficits (especially visual). A careful review of medications, particularly psychotropic agents, and nonprescription or over-the-counter (OTC) medications, along with prescription medication, is especially important for elderly patients who report a history of falls.

Fall prevention strategy requires attention to factors that can be medically or surgically corrected (e.g., cataract surgery, medication adjustment, adequate hydration). Observation of the patient arising from a chair and walking ("Get Up and Go Test") is an essential component of fall prevention and evaluation. Physical disabilities can be addressed with physical therapy and, if appropriate, assistive devices such as walkers and canes. A home health nursing evaluation or a home visit by the PA may help identify and address the extrinsic factors. Community resources such as senior centers and Area Agency on Aging (AAA) often provide information on low-cost installation of bathroom and hallway bars.

Eight key factors found to influence falls in older adults have been identified[18]:
- Postural hypotension
- Use of sedative-hypnotic medication
- Use of more than four medications
- Toilet and bathtub safety
- Environmental hazards

- Abnormal gait, transfers, and balance
- Lower and upper extremity strength and range of motion
- Foot problems

Exercise plays an important role in the prevention of falls. Studies demonstrate that even the very old (older than 80 years of age) can benefit from exercise and weight training. Low-impact programs such as chair exercise, yoga, and especially the practice of tai chi have been shown to improve balance, leading to a reduced incidence of falls.[19]

COMMON PROBLEMS IN GERIATRIC CARE

Screening and Health Promotion

Preventive health practices are an important, and often overlooked, part of caring for older adults. Cancer is the second major cause of death in people older than 65 years of age, after cardiovascular disease.[20] Leukemia and cancers of the digestive tract, breast, prostate, skin, and urinary tract increase in incidence up to the age of 84 years. PAs should take every opportunity when caring for an older patient to incorporate primary and secondary disease prevention strategies into both routine and episodic care. These include screening for common age-related diseases (hypertension, diabetes, osteoporosis, hyperlipidemia) and updating immunizations (tetanus, pneumonia, herpes zoster, influenza). Table 19.3 lists comprehensive recommendations for screening and health promotion strategies for older adults.

TABLE 19.3 Summary of Preventive Medicine and Screening Recommendations for Older Adults*

Maneuver	Evidence[†]	Recommendation (Source)	Grade[†]
		Screening‡	
Blood pressure	I	At least every 1–2 yr (USPSTF)	A
Physician breast examination	I	Annually after age 40 yr (ACS, USPSTF)	A
Mammography	I	Annually after age 50 yr (ACS) or every 1–2 yr, ages 50–69 yr (USPSTF, ACP); continue every 1–3 yr, ages 70–85 yr based on life expectancy (AGS, USPSTF)	A; C >age 69 yr
Pelvic examination and Pap smear	II	Every 2–3 yr after three negative annual examinations; can be discontinued after age 65–69 yr (ACS, USPSTF, CTF, AGS)	A; C >age 65 yr
Cholesterol	I–III	Adults every 5 yr (NCEP); less certain for older adults	B; C >age 65 yr
Rectal examination	II	Annually after age 40 yr (ACS)	C
Fecal occult blood test	II	Annually after age 50 yr (ACS)	B

Continued

TABLE 19.3 Summary of Preventive Medicine and Screening Recommendations for Older Adults*—cont'd

Maneuver	Evidence[†]	Recommendation (Source)	Grade[†]
		Screening[‡]	
Colonoscopy	II	Every 10 yr age 50–75 yr (ACS)	B
Visual acuity test	III	Periodically in older adults (various)	B
Test or inquire for hearing impaired	III	Periodically in older adults (various)	B
Mouth, nodes, testes, skin, heart, lung examinations	III	Annually (ACS, AHA)	C
Glucose	III	Periodic in high-risk groups (USPSTF)	C
Thyroid function	III	Clinically prudent for older adults, especially women (USPSTF)	C
Electrocardiography	III	Periodically after age 40–50 yr (AHA)	C
Glaucoma screening	III	Periodically by eye specialist after age 65 yr (USPSTF)	C
Mental and functional status	III	As needed; be alert for decline (USPSTF)	C
Bone mineral density (women)	III	Once after age 65 yr; then as needed (USPSTF)	C
Prostate examination and prostate-specific antigen	III	NR; symptomatic after age 50 yr; not after age 75 yr (USPSTF)	C–D
Chest radiograph	III	If needed for treatment decision (USPSTF)	D
		Prophylaxis and Counseling	
Exercise	I–II	Encourage aerobic and resistance exercise as tolerated (USPSTF, AHA)	A
Tetanus–diphtheria vaccine	I–II	1 series, then booster every 10 yr (ACP, USPSTF)	A
Influenza vaccine	I–II	Annually after age 65 yr or if chronically ill (ACP, USPSTF)	B
Pneumovax	II	23-valent at least once after age 65 yr (ACP, USPSTF)	B
Herpes zoster	I	Once after age 60 to prevent shingles and post-herpetic neuralgia.	
Calcium	II	800–1500 mg/day (various)	B
Aspirin	I–II	Men after age 50 yr, 80 yr 325 mg every day, every other day (various) (USPSTF)	C

*Recommendations on prevention and screening in older adults, summarized from this paper and other literature. Modified from Goldberg TH, Chavin SI. Preventive medicine and screening in older adults. *J Am Geriatr Soc.* 1997;45:351.

[†]Grades of evidence and recommendations adapted primarily from U.S. Preventive Services Task Force (USPSTF). Grades are those given by the Task Force except when none is available and grades are assigned by authors.

[‡]Screening recommendations apply only to asymptomatic individuals; specific clinical circumstances may necessitate different testing and treatment schedules. Where no upper age limits are listed, screening should continue until approximately age 85 years or when the patient is not a treatment candidate because of limited active life expectancy or quality.

NR, Not recommended for routine screening in asymptomatic individuals, although it may be useful when clinically indicated.

From American College of Physicians (ACP), American Cancer Society (ACS), American Geriatrics Society (AGS), American Heart Association (AHA), Canadian Task Force (CTF) of the Periodic Health Examination, National Cholesterol Education Program (NCEP), USPSTF, and the authors' interpretation of the literature.

Complications of Pharmacotherapy

CASE STUDY 19.2

Mrs. CK, an 81-year-old woman, is brought by paramedics to the ED at 4 AM after being found on the floor in the bathroom by her husband at 2 AM. She denies pain, is confused, and vital signs are normal. She has no evidence of injury or stroke, and some wheezes and rhonchi are noted on lung examination. She has a history of recent upper respiratory infection with cough for 3 days, spinal stenosis for which she has been using a cane to assist with ambulation for the past year, a history of polymyalgia rheumatica (PMR), and overactive bladder. Laboratory tests demonstrate CBC with a WBC count of 7200 mcl and a slight increase in percent lymphocytes. Chemistry is normal except blood urea nitrogen of 23 mg/dl. Urinalysis is positive for leukocytes and bacteria. Chest radiographs show a possible small infiltrate in the left middle lobe. Her husband hands you a bag with her medications, which include 1 mg of prednisone, oxybutynin, a multivitamin, vitamin D, and OTC cough and cold liquid (acetaminophen, guaifenesin, and diphenhydramine). Her husband tells you that he gave her one of his Vicodin pills earlier that evening "so she could sleep." She is admitted and is initially very lethargic, but after 48 hours of intravenous (IV) fluids and antibiotics, she is awake and fully oriented. Upon questioning, she has no recollection of the fall or being transported to the hospital, but she does recall taking the OTC cold medication "every 2 or 3 hours" for her cough. After another day in the hospital with assessment by an occupational therapist and physical therapist, she is discharged home with a 7-day course of oral antibiotics and home health physical therapy.

How could this happen? Unfortunately, this is not uncommon. Sharing of medication and mixing of prescription and OTC medications can lead to disastrous consequences for older adults. Confusion is a common reaction to both toxic medication levels and infection in older adults. In this case, a mixture of medications with sedating and anticholinergic properties in an older individual with an underlying infection (in this case, both a UTI and possible pneumonitis) resulted in delirium and a fall.

The Beers criteria[21] list of medications to avoid or use with caution in older adults is a guideline to help improve safe prescribing of medications for older adults. For appropriate prescription practices and avoidance of polypharmacy, the following recommendations have been made to HCPs by the American Geriatrics Society[2]:

1. *Obtain a complete drug history.* Be sure to ask about previous treatments and responses, as well as about other prescribers. Ask about allergies, OTC drugs, nutrition supplements, alternative medications, alcohol, tobacco, caffeine, and recreational drugs.
2. *Use e-prescribing to reduce the risk of transcription and medication errors.* Check insurance coverage, and avoid a 2% payment penalty on their Medicare Part B services.
3. Avoid prescribing before a diagnosis is made except in severe acute pain. Consider nondrug therapy.
4. Review medications regularly and before prescribing a new medication. Discontinue medications that are no longer needed, that are ineffective, or that do not have a corresponding diagnosis.
5. Know the actions, adverse effects, drug interactions, monitoring requirements, and toxicity profiles of prescribed medications. Avoid duplicative effects.
6. Consider the following for new medications: Is the dosing regimen practical? Is the new medication affordable?
7. Start long-term drug therapy at a low dose, and titrate the dose on the basis of tolerability and response. Use drug concentration monitoring when available.
8. Attempt to reach a therapeutic dose before switching to or adding another medication. Use combinations cautiously; titrate each medication to a therapeutic dose before switching to a combination product.
9. Avoid using one drug to treat the adverse effects caused by another.
10. Attempt to use one drug to treat two or more conditions.
11. Communicate with other prescribers. Do not assume that patients will—they assume you do!
12. Avoid using drugs from the same class or with similar actions (e.g., alprazolam, zolpidem).

Dizziness and Syncope

Dizziness can be classified as follows:
- Vertigo (rotational sensation)
- Presyncope (impending faint)
- Disequilibrium (loss of balance without head sensation)
- Lightheadedness

Benign positional vertigo is a common cause of dizziness among older adults and manifests as episodic dizzy spells that are usually precipitated by changes in position, such as turning, rolling over, getting into and out of bed, or bending over. These are often brief (5–15 seconds), usually relatively mild and self-limited. Presyncope is the sensation of near fainting caused by diminished cerebral perfusion; it occurs secondary to cardiac causes (arrhythmias), vascular causes (orthostatic hypotension), or vagal stimulation, which in some cases can result in syncope (micturition syncope). Syncope is defined as a sudden, transient loss of postural tone and consciousness not caused by trauma and with spontaneous full recovery. Similar to presyncope, syncope is generally caused by a reduction in cerebral perfusion. The clinical history, physical examination, and electrocardiogram have been found to be the most useful steps in evaluating syncope,[22] and they should be used in most patients to determine whether further testing is necessary.

Sleep Problems

Difficulty falling asleep, nighttime awakening, early morning awakening, and daytime sleepiness are common sleep disorders experienced by older adults. Risk factors for sleep disturbance include chronic illness, mood disturbance, lack of physical activity, and increased physical disability. Older people report an earlier bedtime and an early awakening. They also report decreased total sleep time with fragmented sleep patterns characterized by frequent arousals during the night and diminished deep sleep (stages III and IV of sleep). Consequently, older patients may report dissatisfaction with the quantity and quality of their sleep and often attribute their low energy, easy fatigability, and excessive daytime sleepiness to poor nighttime sleep.

Screening Older Patients for Sleep Problems

The National Institutes of Health Consensus Statement on the Treatment of Sleep Disorders of Older People[23] recommends that the following three questions be asked:
1. Is the person satisfied with his or her sleep?
2. Does sleep or fatigue interfere with daytime activities?
3. Do the bed partner or others complain of unusual behavior during sleep, such as snoring, interrupted breathing, or leg movements?

Although a detailed account of the diagnosis and management of sleep problems is beyond the scope of this chapter, at minimum, a thorough review of medications and medical conditions, with attention to impact on sleep, should be conducted. Older patients should be counseled about the use of OTC sleep products that often contain diphenhydramine (Benadryl), a sedating histamine that can cause confusion. Long-term usage of sedative-hypnotics in older patients should be avoided because they are associated with many adverse effects, including

secondary depression and increased incidence of falls with injury, especially hip fractures.

Depression

Depression is underdiagnosed and undertreated in older adults.[24] Late-life depression has been found to be associated with higher than expected mortality rates and persistent functional impairment.[25] Older patients tend to be more preoccupied with somatic symptoms (e.g., constipation, insomnia, pain) and report depressed mood and guilty preoccupations less frequently, so depression may often be masked. The primary symptoms of depression, including persistent feelings of a sad mood (in the absence of normal causes like recent bereavement) and anhedonia or loss of pleasure, are hallmarks of depression and are helpful in the identification of depression in most medically ill patients.

The diagnosis of major depression in older persons is complicated by the overlap of symptoms of major depression with those of physical illness (e.g., weight loss, insomnia, loss of libido, changes in bowel habits). Debilitated patients and those with serious illness may be preoccupied by thoughts of death or worthlessness. Older adults are also often taking numerous medications (e.g., beta-blockers, steroids, H_2-blockers), which can complicate the picture even further. Certain medical conditions (e.g., hypothyroidism) that commonly occur in older adults also predispose to depression. As individuals grow older, they often experience a loss of friends, family, personal function, economic resources, and social position. Any such loss (especially the death of a spouse or child) can precipitate a reactive depression that should be addressed by the HCP. To simply regard depression as a natural component of aging and to thereby dismiss it disregards the possible serious consequences.

Clearly, the identification of depression in older adults is a diagnostic challenge. Untreated depression can significantly reduce the patient's quality of life and can cause immense suffering. Depression can result in increased morbidity and mortality in patients who have coexistent medical illnesses. Development of depression in patients after a myocardial infarction, congestive heart failure, or cardiac bypass surgery has been shown to increase mortality rates. Depression can impair judgment, leading to risks not usually taken and ultimately to an accident or fall. Lack of appetite and loss of sleep can seriously affect frail older adults and exacerbate underlying disease. The withdrawal and apathy that may be the first signs of depression can result in severe social isolation and lack of self-care. Depression can

For each question, choose the answer that best describes how you felt over the past week:

1.	Are you basically satisfied with your life?	Yes/No
2.	Have you dropped many of your activities and interests?	Yes/No
3.	Do you feel that your life is empty?	Yes/No
4.	Do you often get bored?	Yes/No
5.	Are you in good spirits most of the time?	Yes/No
6.	Are you afraid that something bad is going to happen to you?	Yes/No
7.	Do you feel happy most of the time?	Yes/No
8.	Do you often feel helpless?	Yes/No
9.	Do you prefer to stay home, rather than going out and doing new things?	Yes/No
10.	Do you think you have more problems with memory than most people?	Yes/No
11.	Do you think it is wonderful to be alive now?	Yes/No
12.	Do you feel pretty worthless the way you are now?	Yes/No
13.	Do you feel full of energy?	Yes/No
14.	Do you fell that your situation is hopeless?	Yes/No
15.	Do you think most people are better off than you are?	Yes/No

1 point for each response in capital letters. 0–5 normal; >5 suggests depression and warrants a follow-up interview; >10 almost always indicates depression

FIG. 19.3 ■ Geriatric Depression Scale Short Form.

precipitate a downward spiral of biologic and social events, ultimately leading to morbidity and death.

Depressed older patients with comorbid physical illness, who live alone, who are male, or who are alcoholic are at high risk for suicide. Persons aged 65 years and older represent fewer than 13% of the population but account for 25% of suicides. Older depressed patients are more likely to attempt suicide, more likely to commit suicide violently (firearms and hanging), and more likely to succeed compared with younger counterparts. "Psychological autopsy" studies have shown that older adults who commit suicide were often suffering from a major depression. The vast majority had seen a primary care physician within 1 month of the act. Therefore, the need for frequent screening of older adult patients for depression cannot be overemphasized. The short form of the Geriatric Depression Scale (GDS) is a rapid and effective tool for screening older adult patients for depression.

Steps in the diagnosis of depression in older adult patients include the following:

- A quick review of medications for possible depressive adverse effects (e.g., steroids, beta-blockers, benzodiazepines)
- A social history focusing on recent changes in finances, living circumstance, new diagnosis of disease, and loss of friends or family

- Screening with the short form of the GDS (Fig. 19.3)
- Focused history and physical examination for the early manifestations of disease or a change in existing disease
- Screening of TSH to rule out hypothyroidism as appropriate

It is important to note older adults who immigrate to the United States from other countries are at increased risk for depression. This is especially true if they come to live with younger family members and find themselves isolated at home most of the time while the others in their household are at work or if they come as refugees after having experienced traumatic events in their homeland. The availability of the GDS in multiple languages (www.stanford.edu/~yesavage/GDS.html) provides a tool that can help the PA when there is a lack of a common language for communication. One common difficulty in diagnosing depression among older immigrants is that the symptom complex may not be the same as those described in American psychiatric literature. Depressed Asian older adults, for example, especially those from China or Southeast Asia, and Hispanics, have been found to be much more likely to present with somatic symptoms such as loss of appetite, sleep disturbances, and even headaches or stomachaches and to not reveal feelings of sadness or dysphoria.

In many cultures, there is a stigma around having a diagnosis of depression.

After depression has been diagnosed, appropriate treatment should be pursued. If necessary, referral to a psychiatrist or other therapist who specializes in the treatment of older adults should be considered. Ideally, a therapist who is culturally and linguistically appropriate to the patient's background will make the referral easier and chance of success more likely. Depression is usually a treatable disease and should not be regarded as a hopeless circumstance to be endured and hidden. Antidepressant medication and psychotherapy have both been found to benefit older depressed patients.[26]

Older Women's Health

Currently, U.S. women can expect to live into their 80s and beyond. Many of the health risks that characterize these later years of life for women can be attributed to postmenopausal changes. Physiologic aging of the woman accelerates after menopause, especially in the genital tract. The ovarian follicular estrogen (estradiol) diminishes dramatically in postmenopausal women, and estrone—a low-potency estrogen derived from androstenedione—takes over as the major estrogen. Progesterone, derived mainly from the adrenals, also diminishes. The genital organs undergo atrophy, resulting in sclerotic ovaries; a smaller, atrophied uterus; a pale, foreshortened, narrow vaginal canal (sometimes causing dyspareunia); and the loss of acidic vaginal pH, causing increased vulnerability to infection. Hormone replacement therapy (HRT), estrogen alone or combination of estrogen and progesterone, has been shown to be associated with a slightly increased risk of thromboembolic disease (blood clots and stroke) and breast cancer, as well as reduction in colon cancer and bone loss.[27] HRT is currently recommended for a limited time for the treatment of troubling postmenopausal symptoms (hot flashes, vaginal dryness).

Hormonal changes caused by menopause also result in accelerated osteoporosis, so that, by age 75 years, one third of women and, by 85 years, half meet criteria for osteoporosis. Recommendations include regular monitoring of bone density and use of estrogen agonists (Evista) or bisphosphonates.[28] Increased levels of cholesterol, triglycerides, and low-density lipoprotein and decreased levels of high-density lipoprotein secondary to ovarian failure increase older women's predisposition to heart disease.

SEXUALITY AND AGING

CASE STUDY 19.3

AW is an 86-year-old widowed woman who was the primary caregiver for her husband who had Lewy body dementia and died at home 2 years ago. She had been married since 18 years of age; was very devoted to her husband; and at the time of his death, she was so distraught that her daughter moved back home for several months for fear that her mother was going to harm herself. By the end of the first year, AW was doing better, playing bridge with friends again, and decided to move from her home to a condominium in a retirement community. Two months ago, she met another resident in her complex, a 72-year-old gentleman who has been divorced twice. They spend every day together, are very affectionate with one another, and are the stars of weekly dance party. You are a PA with the medical group that provides care for many of the retirement complex residents. AW comes in for her flu shot and asks to speak with you, saying she has never dated and needs some advice.

As life expectancy increases, it is important to recognize that continued sexual activity is an essential component of old age in promoting satisfactory relationships and good quality of life. Many older patients maintain sexual interest and capacity as long as they have their health, a healthy partner, and a good relationship with that partner. Normal change in sexual function in men is manifested in the following ways:

- The need for more time for arousal
- The need for more time for reaching orgasm
- Less rigid and fewer erections
- Orgasms that last for a shorter time than when they were younger
- Less force of ejaculation and less volume of ejaculate

Older women are often more concerned about their appearance and their desirability. Although some women retain multiorgasmic capacity throughout life, postmenopausal hormonal changes result in physical and psychological changes for many. In addition, older women are often primary caregivers for their aging partners and are often greatly burdened by caregiver stress syndrome. Because women tend to outlive their male counterparts, they may have difficulty finding good partners and meaningful relationships.

Often, there is a generational difference between the HCP and older adult patients that may cause some discomfort for both parties in discussing issues of physical intimacy. The provider should approach the issue with an open-ended question that allows the patient to choose to participate and voice concerns or questions. For example, during the review of systems, the PA could ask, "Are there any sexual or relationship issues or questions you would like to discuss this visit?" A sensitively elicited sexual history; a focused physical examination as directed by the history, diagnosis, and treatment of sexually transmitted diseases when present; and offering overall guidance and support continue to remain important components of care of the aging patient.

Prostate Disease

Benign prostatic hypertrophy is one of the most common conditions among aging men. It affects three of four men older than age 60 years and accounts for more than 4.4 million office visits annually in the United States. Although one of the more common surgical procedures among older adults, with improved medical treatments, the number of surgeries for BPH has declined in recent years.[29] A nonmalignant enlargement of the epithelial and fibromuscular components of the prostate gland that may result in irritating (frequency, urgency, nocturia) or obstructive (hesitancy, intermittency, weak stream, incomplete emptying) urinary symptoms is almost universal among older men. If left untreated, it can result in significantly diminished quality of life in older men. Treatment options include lifestyle modification (avoidance of caffeine, decrease in late evening fluid intake), avoidance of problematic medications (e.g., anticholinergic drugs), and treatment with appropriate medications such as α-adrenergic antagonists (e.g., doxazosin, terazosin, tamsulosin) and 5α-reductase inhibitors (finasteride). Surgery is reserved for patients who have severe symptoms that are refractory to medical treatment or for patients who are unable to tolerate the adverse effects of medication.

Prostate cancer is a cancer of old age. Its incidence increases with age and is rare in men younger than 40 years of age. Autopsy studies in which the entire prostate was examined have revealed histologic evidence of prostate cancer in 30% of men older than age 50 years and 80% of men older than age 80 years. Prostate cancer usually arises in the peripheral zone of the prostate and remains asymptomatic in most patients, especially in the early stages. Currently, there is no direct evidence that early detection decreases mortality rates from prostate cancer. Most men with prostate cancer die with the disease, not from it. Serum prostate-specific antigen (PSA) is a nonspecific test, with elevations in PSA occurring in BPH and prostatitis and transiently in response to conditions such as ejaculation and prostatic massage or even a digital rectal examination. The U.S. Preventive Services Task Force, the American College of Physicians, and the Canadian Task Force on the Periodic Health Examination have recommended *against* routine PSA screening for prostate cancer.[30–32]

Acute bacterial prostatitis is characterized by fever, chills, dysuria, and a tense or tender prostate as seen in older men with indwelling urinary catheters; an infectious agent is not identified in 80% of cases. Treatment includes antibiotics, and hospitalization may be required in severe cases. *Chronic bacterial prostatitis* presents classically as recurrent bacteriuria, and continuous low-dose antibiotic suppressive therapy can be considered for patients with frequent symptomatic relapse.

UNIQUE ISSUES IN GERIATRIC CARE

Elder Abuse

Evaluation of older adult patients cannot be considered complete unless the issue of elder abuse and mistreatment has been addressed. The term *elder mistreatment* denotes acts of omission or commission that result in harm or threatened harm to the health or welfare of an older adult. Abuse can be physical abuse (including sexual abuse), emotional abuse, intentional or unintentional neglect (including self-neglect), financial exploitation, abandonment, or a combination of these. Neglect is the most common type of mistreatment. It is estimated that between 2% and 10% of older adults experience abuse, and it appears to be increasing.[33] It can occur in the homes of older adults or their relatives or in institutional settings and is found among all socioeconomic strata and ethnic populations. Poverty, dependency of older adult persons for caregiving needs, functional disability, frailty, and cognitive impairment are some of the risk factors for elder abuse, along with family stress and conflict.

All states have some type of mandatory reporting requirements in which health and social service providers are required to report suspected cases of elder mistreatment to adult protective services. Primary care providers are in a unique position to detect elder abuse. Clues include patients who look ill-dressed with poor personal hygiene; are malnourished, listless, or apathetic; are brought to the clinic or the ED by someone other than the caregiver; present with fractures or bruises in various stages of healing, unexplained bruises, or unusual bruises (e.g., bruises in inner arms or thighs); have cigarette, rope, or chemical burns; or have facial lacerations and abrasions or marks occurring only in areas of the body usually covered by clothes. Evidence that material goods are being taken in exchange for care or that personal belongings (house, jewelry, car) are being taken over without consent or approval, as well as reports of being left in unsafe situations or of inability to get needed medication, can be indicators of underlying abuse. Astute PAs who maintain a heightened suspicion for potential elder abuse can identify cases by a careful history and a discerning physical examination, as well as by watching for subtle changes in the physical and psychosocial status of the patient.

Medicare and Medicaid

Medicare is the federal health insurance program for Americans aged 65 years and older and people younger than 65 years with permanent disabilities; 95% of older Americans have Medicare coverage. As such, it influences much of geriatric care (e.g., how long and in what circumstances Medicare pays for certain services, such as physical therapy or home health care). All of the authorization for Medicare coverage must be made by physicians. Unless an older adult is enrolled in a Medicare Advantage Plan, such as a health maintenance organization or preferred provider organization, his or her coverage is organized by the following parts of the original Medicare:

- Part A of Medicare helps pay for inpatient care in the hospital and medically necessary care in a skilled nursing home or home health care for a maximum of 100 days after a minimum 3-day inpatient hospital stay, hospice care, and medically necessary home health care for homebound patients.
- Part B helps cover 80% of many medically necessary outpatient care costs after a deductible is met. Beginning in 2011, it also covered most preventive services given by providers who accept assignment, meaning that the provider agrees to charge only what Medicare allows.
- Part D helps pay for prescription medications if the Medicare enrollee joins one of many drug plans offered by different companies, with varying deductibles and copayment options.

In general, Medicare is complicated and often confusing to both the provider and patient alike. It does not cover many of the costs of health care older adults use, such as vision care by nonphysicians and glasses, hearing aids, care in assisted living homes, and long-term custodial care in nursing homes. Many older Americans also have supplementary insurance (called MediGap insurance) to help pay for the copayments and deductibles not covered by Medicare for outpatient care, and some also have long-term care insurance to help cover the costs of nursing homes and long-term in-home care.

PAs may be reimbursed for health care provided in outpatient offices or clinics without the requirement of "direct physician supervision" (interpreted as the supervising physician being onsite). PAs are also reimbursed in the hospital, surgical, and skilled nursing home settings. The rate of reimbursement in outpatient settings, first-assist in surgery, hospital care, and skilled nursing care is 85% of the rate of reimbursement for a physician. An excellent resource for the details of the latest legislation is the American Academy of Physician Assistants, Department of Government and Professional Affairs, 2318 Mill Road, Suite 1300, Alexandria, VA, 22314; phone: 703-836-2272.

Medicaid is a federal and state health insurance program for low-income people aged 65 years and older, as well as those who are blind or with certain disabilities. People who have both Medicare and Medicaid coverage are called *dual eligibles*. Medicaid covers many of the costs not covered by Medicare, such as long-term custodial care in nursing homes. Reimbursement rates are generally lower for Medicaid than Medicare and vary considerably from state to state. Different states call their Medicaid programs by various names (e.g., MediCal in California).

Ethnogeriatrics

Just as the United States as a whole is becoming more diverse, the cultural heterogeneity among older Americans is growing rapidly. As mentioned earlier, the numbers of older adults in the five major ethnic minority categories (American Indian or Alaska Native, African American, Asian, Pacific Islander, and Hispanic) are growing even more rapidly than the rapidly exploding numbers of older adults in general. Within and between each of the minority populations, as well as among those considered the majority, are vast differences in characteristics that affect health care encounters. These include acculturation level and age at immigration, religion, culturally related beliefs about causes and treatments of medical conditions, expectations and trust of HCPs based on historical experiences, and who has the authority and responsibility to make decisions about an elder's health care. Rates and risk factors for specific diseases also vary considerably by ethnic and racial population.[34] Although it is beyond the scope of this chapter to provide a detailed discussion of ethnogeriatric topics PAs are likely to face, it is important to remember some basic principles:

- Each older patient from a background other than non-Hispanic white may or may not fit the profile of the population that one might expect.

- Trained interpreters in person or by phone or video are needed for every encounter with an older patient who is limited English proficient; ad hoc interpreters (family members, friends, or untrained staff) increase the likelihood of medical errors and reduce the effectiveness of crucial communication. Children should never be used as interpreters in a medical setting. Documents such as consent forms should be translated into the patient's native language if the patient does not read English.
- Showing culturally appropriate respect to older adults is extremely important in building a therapeutic relationship, especially because in many cultures, older adults are held in high esteem.
- It is always important to try to understand older patients' perspectives (sometimes called the "explanatory model") of their own illnesses and integrate these perspectives into the management plan to increase the likelihood of their adherence to the plan.
- Family caregivers are major members of the health care team, especially in cultures in which there is a strong expectation that adult children should care for their parents. In some cases, the decisions and preferences of the children may not be the same as the parents, so the parents' choices should be obtained.

For more information and resources on ethnogeriatrics, see the Stanford Geriatric Education Center's websites at http://sgec.stanford.edu and http://geriatrics.stanford.edu.

Social Support and Caregiver Support

A supportive social network has been found to be a major factor in maintaining the health of older adults. For those without available family nearby or who are otherwise isolated, social support may mean having important connections with friends and neighbors or through faith communities or other community resources, such as senior centers. PAs can help to foster these connections by encouraging their older patients to interact with others or by facilitating social work interventions to connect them with important community resources. If social work services are not available, PAs can encourage the connections themselves.

In some cases of dependent older adults, the family caregiver is the major source of social support, as well as physical and instrumental support. Support of the caregiver, then, is a major part of geriatric care, especially when older adults have dementia or other debilitating conditions. It is not unusual for the cause of institutionalization of an older patient to be the illness of the caregiver after long periods of extreme stress from caregiving. PAs need to monitor the stress level and health condition of primary caregivers as part of the care of their geriatric patients and help them get the health, respite, or support services they need in order to continue providing the support.

Some communities have specific programs for support of caregivers who are caring for dependent older adults. They may include respite programs for someone else to care for the elder while the caregiver has some time to take care of their own needs, sometimes subsidized by public funds; support groups; and instructional programs on caring for dependent older adults. The Family Caregiver Alliance of the National Center on Caregiving has a wealth of information and materials available for caregivers (http://www.caregiver.org).

End of Life

Death and dying are a part of caring for aging adults. The majority of deaths occur in persons older than age 65 years, most in hospitals, but increasingly more in nursing homes and at home.[35] Discussions with patients about their wishes for care at the end of life and designation of a surrogate decision maker if the patient is unable to make his or her wishes known are encouraged. Patients should be routinely questioned about completion of advanced directives (power of attorney for health care [POAHC] and physician/medical orders for life-sustaining treatment [POLST/MOLST]), and copies should be placed in their medical records. When appropriate, discussion of and referral for palliative care and hospice should occur.

CASE STUDY 19.4

Mrs. A is a 76-year-woman female with chronic obstructive pulmonary disease (COPD) caused by a lifelong history of asthma who was recently moved from the intensive care unit after being extubated and is transferred to the step-down unit for rehabilitation with the goal of returning home. She is a widow and lives in her own home with her adult daughter, a recovering addict recently diagnosed with bipolar disorder, whom she supports. Mrs. A is obese and has diabetes, a history of paroxysmal atrial tachycardia, and macular degeneration. This is her third hospitalization in the past year for exacerbation of COPD, usually in association with a viral illness. At a family meeting with her two adult daughters to discuss her discharge plan, Mrs. A states, "I never want to be intubated again. I'd rather die." You are the PA working with the hospitalist. You inquire about her advanced health care directive and learn that it was written 10 years ago and has not been updated since her husband died. The daughter who lives with Mrs. A becomes tearful and agitated, escalating into a confrontation between the daughters over their mother's increasing care needs and who will make decisions. The social worker agrees to work with Mrs. A and her daughters to complete a new advanced directive and develop a postdischarge care plan. The social worker arranges for a psychological evaluation that confirms Mrs. A retains capacity to make her own decisions. The team recommends discharge home to a palliative care program that can provide medical care for Mrs. A, honors her request for care with no further intubation, and supports the daughters in caring for their mother during this last stage of life.

COMMUNITY RESOURCES AND SERVICES

A major part of geriatric primary care is knowing the important health-related support services available for older adults in the community, knowing when they are indicated to support the maintenance of older patients' functional status and quality of life, and then helping older adults access the services they need. Because a truism in geriatrics is that it is by nature a multidisciplinary enterprise, to be a successful provider is to be a team player. Unfortunately, in many medical settings, the other members of the geriatric team (e.g., social worker, psychologist, chaplain, home care nurse, therapists) are employed by other organizations and are less accessible for coordination of care than the medical provider might prefer.

This section describes some of the major types of services primary care providers should be familiar with in their local communities. Keeping current contact information (phone numbers, website addresses, brochures) of such resources in the office directory can be a useful means of dealing with common geriatric situations, such as the need for posthospitalization care for an older widow who lives alone, the mild depression and growing isolation of a retiree, or the increasing stress and fatigue of an older woman trying to care for her husband with mild dementia. In addition to the resources discussed here, there are hundreds of others that would be valuable in helping older patients improve or maintain their health and quality of life.

Information and Referral Services

A logical place to start for most community resources is one of the agencies organized to (1) maintain current listings of services older adults need and (2) provide the appropriate information to older adults or their advocates. To find the local equivalents of the services listed in this section, the PA can consult an Information and Assistance (I&A) service in one of two agencies.

Area Agencies on Aging plan and coordinate services for older adults in every corner of the United States. One of the requirements imposed by the Older Americans Act, which created the AAAs, is that they maintain I&A services for the region they cover, usually including one or more counties. Unfortunately, AAAs frequently have some other official designation, such as Department on Aging or Senior Services Council, and they may be associated with a governmental or private nonprofit agency, but one can usually find the phone number for the local AAA or its I&A through the listings in the front of the telephone directory under "Senior" or "Aging" services. They can also be located on the Internet by search engines.

Another excellent source of I&A services is the local *multipurpose senior center*, which is available in almost every town or suburb of any size. Most senior centers offer among their services a comprehensive I&A department that has up-to-date information on services older adults need, such as housing, home health care, transportation, home-delivered meals, and nursing homes, for the particular area they serve.

If these resources are difficult to locate, the national Elder Care Locator has information on services in all communities. It can be reached by calling 800-677-1116.

Case Management or Care Coordination

An important role within the geriatric team is coordinating the myriad of fragmented health and social services and agencies a frail older adult with multiple problems might need. A *case manager* or care coordinator not only deals with medical services but also assesses needs and helps to arrange for transportation; in-home assistance (e.g., home-delivered meals and homemaker services); assistance with business affairs; and, if needed, more supportive housing such as assisted living. They also follow up to see that the services are delivered and are satisfactory. Unfortunately, case managers are not yet available in all communities and to all older residents, but they are increasingly part of community-based long-term care services designed to provide alternatives to institutional care for frail older adults. Private case management programs are also growing in many areas.

Multipurpose Senior Centers

It is safe to say that the lives of millions of older adults across the nation are enhanced by participation in their local senior centers, which typically offer a wide range of programs at no or low cost for healthy independent older adults. Programs provided in a center for older adults who live in the community enable older adults to do the following:

- Take classes in subjects such as fitness (frequently ranging from armchair exercises to yoga to aerobics), music of various types, languages, financial management, and self-management for chronic disease.
- Eat a nutritious, low-cost lunch subsidized with Older Americans Act funds.
- Learn about and take advantage of special services or programs for senior citizens, such as travel and tours, hypertension screening, and assistance with tax forms.
- Visit with friends in an attractive, upbeat environment that encourages older adults to be active and stay involved with the world.

Physician assistants would do well to become acquainted with the staff and activities in the local senior center so that patients can be referred there for a wide range of health-related support services, including nutrition, fitness, health screenings, health education, health insurance assistance and counseling, and antidotes to depression for older adults who are isolated and lonely.

Day Care and Day Health Care Programs

Just as multipurpose senior centers are important health centers for generally healthy, independent older adults, day care (sometimes called "social day care") and day health care programs serve a similar function for frail older adults. Both usually offer programs for movement-impaired or cognitively impaired older adults who need assistance, and the programs are typically offered 5 days a week. Both are designed to provide respite for the family caregivers of frail older adults, frequently enabling adult children to keep frail older adults in their homes when both children and their spouses work outside the home. Some day centers also accept older adults who are incontinent. Both models typically offer transportation, and the cost is usually figured on a sliding scale. Programs commonly include music, arts and crafts, current events, and a nutritious lunch. In addition, the day health care programs provide nursing, social work, and physical and occupational therapy services on the basis of assessed need. For older adults at risk of institutionalization, these centers are extremely important resources that can help maintain their lives at home for much longer than would otherwise be the case because the staff can monitor changes in their health and functional status on a daily or weekly basis and can keep the PA informed about problems, such as reactions to medications or acute confusion that might signal an infection.

In-Home Care

Many patients prefer to remain at home as long as possible, and because this desire often represents the option that both supports the patient's highest quality of life and is the most cost-effective, the goal of geriatric care is often to keep a patient at home. There is great comfort in being in familiar surroundings and, if possible, being cared for by family and friends. To that end, the PA should know about a variety of resources available to assist patients who prefer to be at home but need professional and other types of support that cannot be provided by the informal support system.

The *home health care* industry has become extremely sophisticated and offers a wide range of services to homebound elderly persons. In-home care through home health agencies should be considered as a possible resource to prevent nonacute hospitalization or placement in a skilled nursing facility. The services provided vary, depending on the agency, and can include physical therapy; occupational therapy; social work to evaluate and coordinate assistance with financial, social support, and mental health resources; hospice care for dying patients and their family members; and skilled nursing support. Skilled nursing care can include IV hydration, IV antibiotics, wound care, management of medication, follow-up of office assessment, fecal disimpaction, placement of urinary catheters, drawing of blood for laboratory assessment, pain control, and a nursing assessment of the patient's condition. The skilled nursing care and affiliated services provided by home health agencies can be extremely important in maintaining continuity of posthospitalization care for older patients.

The role of the PA in home health care includes the following:

- Evaluating the patient medically and recommending a course of treatment
- Documenting the need for the services provided by the home care agency
- Acting as a liaison for the agency to monitor care and outcomes and provide support for the staff if medical questions arise
- Understanding the resources and financial constraints involved in recommending home care and ensuring that all parties understand the scope of needed services and the cost

Although most PAs in practice know and work with home health agencies, older patients can often profit from less skilled and more varied support at home.

In many cases, the prevention of institutionalization depends on the availability of someone to assist the elder with ADLs and IADLs at home. This assistance, referred to as *personal care* or *homemaker or chore services*, can often be provided by the same home health agencies that furnish skilled professional care or home care companies that focus exclusively on nonmedical in-home care. The advantages of going through an agency are that workers are screened and bonded for security, workers may have some training, and substitutes can be provided if a worker is absent. The disadvantage is that the services obtained through a home health care agency may be more expensive than those arranged privately. Some communities maintain registries of names of possible assistants.

Home-delivered meals are provided in most communities on a sliding fee scale for older adults medically certified as homebound through Older Americans Act funds, but there may be a waiting list to receive such services. Other in-home services, such as *home repairs and renovations* for wheelchairs, are frequently also available; the best source of information is a case manager or an I&A service.

An especially important service for frail or at-risk older adults who are living alone is an *alert system*. These are electronic monitors that can be attached to clothing or worn around the neck so that an older adult who has fallen or otherwise has an emergency can easily contact a central switchboard, which then summons assistance as needed. The private systems that are widely advertised on TV tend to be much more expensive than those run in many communities through a local hospital or other health care agency. Communities also frequently have volunteer programs to provide *friendly visiting or telephone reassurance* on a regular basis for homebound older adults at risk for isolation.

Senior Housing

Many choices of housing are especially designed for older adults and provide all degrees of support needed. When PAs are included in the process of recommending or deciding on residential options, it is imperative that they know the differences between levels of care so that the support available in the living environment can be matched to the level of care needed. The most important principle to use in those decisions is that of *the least restrictive environment*, meaning that older adults need to be given the option of living in the type of environment that allows them the most freedom possible while giving them the support they need. The major options available in most communities are described as follows:
- Continuing care retirement community
- Retirement or senior housing

- Board and care
- Assisted living
- Nursing home or convalescent hospital

CONCLUSION

Caring for older adults can be both challenging and extremely rewarding. Geriatrics, based on team care, is ideally suited to PAs with broad-based clinical medicine skills and knowledge. There is tremendous value in learning to differentiate what is "normal" and "expected" and comparing it with the physical manifestation of disease and its varied presentations with age. The geriatric population often offers students and clinicians the opportunity to observe findings associated with aging and disease processes that challenge stereotypes and sharpen the clinical learning process.

Students may struggle with the fundamentals of the history, physical examination, and diagnosis, as well as the options for treatment. However, medical care is more than ascertaining the correct diagnosis and treatment. Working with older adults enables the PA student to struggle with the social, emotional, and cultural challenges inherent in working with the medically complex person. Also, patients benefit tremendously by being in the care of a provider who takes the time to get to know the person behind the disease and to provide care that takes into account the physical, psychological, social, functional, and spiritual components of need. For the student to avoid the challenge of treating older patients because they are too complex, too hard to talk with, or simply too difficult is to lose an essential learning experience that cuts across all medical disciplines to the core of the health care experience, which is to make a difference and help patients find meaning in their lives amid the challenges generated by their illnesses.

CLINICAL APPLICATIONS

- Summarize age-related changes for each body system that are common in elderly patients.
- Identify four steps in assessing the medication status of elderly patients.
- List eight common causes of reversible dementia in older adults. Which cause is the most common?
- Describe how you would teach pelvic muscle exercises to a patient with incontinence.
- List eight components of a safety assessment of the home environment of an elderly patient.
- Identify community resources commonly used by older adults.

KEY POINTS

- Geriatrics emphasizes function, preventing functional decline, and maintenance of optimal function as goals.
- Aging is not a disease. Differentiating normal or expected changes of age from disease is often not easy.
- Polypharmacy requires frequent review of all medications (prescribed and OTC) with an attempt to reduce the number of medications and dosages to minimize risk of adverse drug reactions and interactions.
- Cognitive decline is not normal but is increasingly common with age, requiring a high index of suspicion and assessment for reversible causes.
- Good geriatric care requires familiarity with the presentation and management of geriatric syndromes and common chronic conditions by HCPs.
- Knowledge about community resources and services available for older patents is an essential part of geriatric medicine.

References

1. Federal Interagency Forum on Aging-Related Statistics. *Older Americans 2012: Key Indicators of Well-Being. Federal Interagency Forum on Aging-Related Statistics.* Washington, DC: U.S. Government Printing Office; July 2012.
2. Reuben DB, Herr KA, Pacala JT, et al. *Geriatrics at Your Fingertips: 2015.* 17th ed. New York: The American Geriatrics Society; 2015.
3. Banks WA, Willoughby LM, Thomas DR, et al. Insulin resistance syndrome in the elderly: assessment of functional, biochemical, metabolic, and inflammatory status. *Diabetes Care.* 2007;30:2369.
4. Buchner DM. Physical activity and prevention of cardiovascular disease in older adults. *Clin Geriatr Med.* 2009:25661.
5. Malmrose LC, Gray SL, Pieper CF, et al. Measured versus estimated creatinine clearance in a high functioning elderly sample: MacArthur Foundation study of successful aging. *J Am Geriatr Soc.* 1993;41:715.
6. Alzheimer's Association. *2014 Alzheimer's Disease Facts and Figures.* Chicago: Alzheimer's Association; 2014.
7. American Psychiatric Association. *Diagnostic and Statistical Manual of Mental Disorders.* 5th ed. Arlington VA: American Psychiatric Publishing; 2013.
8. Knopman DS, DeKosky ST, Cummings JL, et al. Practice parameter: diagnosis of dementia (an evidence-based review). Report of the Quality Standards Subcommittee of the American Academy of Neurology. *Neurology.* 2001;56:1143–1153.
9. Segal-Gidan F, Cherry D, Jones R, et al. Alzheimer's disease management guideline: Update 2008. *Alzheimers Dement.* 2011;7:e51.
10. American College of Physicians. *Delirium.* Philadelphia: American College of Physicians; 2007.
11. Fong TG, Tulevaev SR, Inouye SK. Delirium in elderly adults: diagnosis, prevention and treatment. *Nat Rev Neurol.* 2009;5(4):210–220.
12. Tennstedt SL, Link CL, Steers WD, et al. Prevalence of and risk factors for urinary leakage in a racially and ethnically diverse population of adults. *Am J Epidemiol.* 2008;167:390.
13. Thom DH, Haan MN, Van Den Eeden SK, et al. Medically recognized urinary incontinence and risks of hospitalization, nursing home admission and mortality. *Age Ageing.* 1997;26:367.
14. Stothers L, Thom D, Calhoun E. Urologic diseases in America project: urinary incontinence in males: demographics and economic burden. *J Urol.* 2005;173:1302.
15. Thom DH, Nygaard IE, Calhoun EA. Urologic diseases in America project: urinary incontinence in women—national trends in hospitalizations, office visits, treatment and economic impact. *J Urol.* 2005;173:1295.
16. Kegel AH. Physiologic therapy for urinary incontinence. *JAMA.* 1951;146:915.
17. Centers for Disease Control. http://www.cdc.gov/nchs/fastats/deaths.htm. Accessed April 3, 2016.
18. Tinetti ME, Baker DI, McAvay G, et al. A multifactorial intervention to reduce the risk of falling among elderly people living in the community. *N Engl J Med.* 1994;331:821.
19. Liu H, Frank A. Tai chi as a balance improvement exercise for older adults: a systematic review. *J Geriatr Phys Ther.* 2010;33:103.
20. Sahyoun NR, Lentzner H, Hoyert D, Robinson KN. *Trends in Causes of Death Among the Elderly.* Hyattsville, MD: National Center for Health Statistics; 2001. Aging Trends; No. 1.
21. Criteria for Potentially Inappropriate Medication Use in Older Adults. *J Am Geriatr Soc.* 2015;63(11):2227–2246.
22. Kenny RA. Syncope in the elderly: diagnosis, evaluation and treatment. *J Cardiovas Electrophysio.* 2003;149(suppl 7):S74–S77.
23. Consensus Statements [Internet] NIH. *National Institutes of Health (US). Office for Medical Applications of Research.* Bethesda, MD: National Institutes of Health; 1977–2002.
24. NIH Consensus Conference. Diagnosis and treatment of depression in late life. *JAMA.* 1992;268:1018.
25. Denihan A, Kirby M, Bruce I, et al. Three-year prognosis of depression in the community-dwelling elderly. *Br J Psychiatry.* 2000;176:453.
26. Zeiss AM, Breckenridge JS. Treatment of late life depression: a response to the NIH consensus conference. *Behav Ther.* 1997;28:3.
27. Rossouw JE, Anderson GL, Prentice RL, et al. Writing Group for the Women's Health Initiative Investigators. Risks and benefits of estrogen plus progestin in healthy postmenopausal women. Principal results from the Women's Health Initiative randomized control trial. *JAMA.* 2002;288:321.
28. U.S. Department of Health and Human Services. Bone Health and Osteoporosis: A Report of the Surgeon General. Rockville, MD: U.S. Department of Health and Human Services, Office of the Surgeon General; 2004.
29. Wasson JH, Bubolz TA, Lu-Yao GL, et al. Transurethral resection of the prostate among Medicare beneficiaries: 1984 to 1997. For the Patient Outcomes Research Team for Prostate Diseases. *J Urol.* 2000; 164(4):1212–1215.

30. Wolf AMD, Wender RC, Etzioni RB, Thompson IM, et al. American Cancer Society guideline for the early detection of prostate cancer: update 2010. *CA Cancer J Clin*. 2010;60:780–798.

31. Moyer VA. Screening for prostate cancer: US Preventive Services Task Force recommendation statement. *Ann Intern Med*. 2012;157:120–134.

32. Carter HB, Albertsen PC, Barry MJ, Etzioni R, Freedland SJ, Greene KL, et al. Early detection of prostate cancer: AUA guideline. *J Urol*. 2013;190:419–426.

33. O'Brien JG. The mistreatment of older adults. In: Arenson C, Busby-Whitehead J, Brummel-Smith K, eds. *Reichel's Care of the Elderly: Clinical Aspects of Aging*. 6th ed. New York: Cambridge University Press; 2009.

34. Yeo G. How will the U.S. health care system meet the challenge of the ethnogeriatric imperative? *J Am Geriatr Soc*. 2009;57:1278.

35. Miniño AM. *Death in the United States, 2009*. Hyattsville, MD: NCHS data brief, no. 64; 2011. National Center for Health Statistics.

The resources for this chapter can be found at www.expertconsult.com.

CHAPTER 20

END-OF-LIFE ISSUES

Barbara Coombs Lee

You matter because you are you. . . . You matter to the last moment of your life, and we will do all we can, not only to help you die peacefully but also to live until you die.

—DAME CICELY SAUNDERS

This chapter is designed to serve as an introduction to some of the issues that may be encountered when working with terminally ill patients and those with advanced disease. It offers a broad perspective on topics commonly encountered as patients begin to anticipate the end of their lives.

Medical decisions are simpler throughout most of one's life. When you are young, you get vaccinations. When you have an infection, you take an antibiotic. When you have a cold, you rest. But as multiple medical problems develop, the situation becomes more complex. With the advent of modern medicine, many patients now face treatment options that offer little or no benefit. The treatments may be painful, and they may be burdensome to both the patient and his or her caregiver. There comes a time when the patient or family must weigh the benefits of a treatment against the burdens because the goals of care shift as the patient's condition changes.

We live in a society that attempts to deny death. No one wants to admit he or she, too, will die someday. Although we know everything is impermanent, we want permanence; we expect permanence. Our natural tendency is to seek security. We do not like change. We do not like that our bodies change shape. We do not like that we age. We are wary of wrinkles. And most notably, we are afraid of the unknown death brings.

TRUTH TELLING

Medicine is a moral enterprise grounded in a covenant of trust. Historically, patients innately trusted their health care providers (HCPs) to act in their best interests and did as they were told. When medicine began to move away from such a paternalistic approach, patients were faced with a new dilemma. Were HCPs divulging the full story or just enough information to prompt the patient to act as the HCP desired? Medicine cannot be a public-service calling without the virtues of humility, honesty, intellectual integrity, compassion, and effacement of excessive self-interest.[1]

One of the central issues in end-of-life care has been controversy over what the terminally ill patient should be told about his diagnosis and prognosis. In the Hippocratic tradition, the standard of practice in many cultures has been to refrain from telling patients about their impending death. This approach has been used in Japan, Eastern Europe, and many Latin American countries.[2]

In 1961, a survey examined physicians' attitudes toward disclosing a cancer diagnosis to their patients. Eighty-eight percent of respondents usually followed a policy of *nondisclosure*. The same study, repeated in 1979, showed that 98% of physicians now usually followed a policy of *disclosure*.[3] During this period, paternalism gave way to patient self-determination. The HCP no longer had final say in the patient's care; rather, it was the patient himself or herself, now operating on principles of autonomy and informed consent. Improvements in cancer treatment options, improved survival rates, fear of malpractice suits, altered social attitudes about cancer, and the increased recognition of communication as an effective means of enhancing patients' understanding and compliance also aided this shift in disclosure practices.[4]

There may be times when cautious or limited disclosures are necessary. But to maintain trust, the whole truth should be divulged in a manner appropriate to the patient's circumstances. Information about a serious illness or impending death should be shared or offered to patients, even if they do not specifically request the information. Patients have legal and moral rights that must be respected. The question must no longer be "Should we tell?" but rather "How do we share this information with the patient?"[5]

HELPING PATIENTS MAKE INFORMED DECISIONS

Focus. End-of-life care should focus on the patient's life and current experience. Too often death is seen as a failure of treatment, not a natural event. This deprives patients of the opportunity to enter what Kübler-Ross calls "the final stage of growth." Too often physicians either withdraw from patients in the terminal stage of illness or encourage them to continue intensive therapies and not "give up."

Self-determination. Individuals vary in their tolerance for pain and suffering. Only patients can determine whether they are suffering or are suffering too much. They should receive state-of-the-art comfort care accordingly. Providers should prescribe opioid analgesics generously for pain and breathlessness. Patients should control the dose and frequency of administration. Symptoms such as hiccups, nausea, diarrhea, itching, and fatigue can be oppressive and should not be disregarded.

Autonomy. Decisions about end-of-life care begin and end with the autonomous patient. The answer to the question "Who should decide?" is "The patient decides." Even very ill patients usually retain decisional capacity. Loved ones and providers should avoid inadvertently usurping decisions when communication becomes difficult. If patients are no longer capable of decision making, their known wishes or their values and end-of-life priorities still dictate decisions.

Personal beliefs. Patients should feel empowered to make decisions based on their own deeply held values and beliefs, without fear of moral condemnation or political interference. Law and policy should not place the provider's moral beliefs above the patient's or protect providers who withhold vital information about treatment options. Dying patients should not be subject to subtle or overt suggestions that their choices are wrong or immoral.

Informed consent. Patients must have comprehensive, candid information in order to make valid decisions and give informed consent. Patients should receive encouragement to exercise a "BRAIN" process assessing the:
Benefits
Risks
Alternatives, their own
Insight into what these mean to them
Nothing (The consequences of doing nothing before giving consent to procedures and treatment).

Four crucial questions often go unasked or incompletely answered when a patient consents to disease-specific treatment:
1. What is the chance it will prolong my life?
2. By how much?
3. What are the side effects?
4. What are the alternatives?

Providers should not withhold information about legal alternatives. This deprives the patient of crucial information to give informed consent.

Balance. Patients should feel empowered to make decisions on the basis of their own assessment and the balance between quantity and quality of life. Patients may reject treatment because of unacceptable side effects or extraordinary demands on their precious time and energies.

Saying "no" to burdensome treatment may mean saying "yes" to the joyful experiences of life for as long as possible.

PLANNING FOR DEATH

In 2013 (the most current information available at this writing), 2,596,993 people died in the United States.[6] Death can occur unannounced at any given moment. Although many Americans will live well past 70 years of age, finally succumbing to heart disease, cancer, or stroke, not everyone shares this fate.[7] Some of the cases that shaped American attitudes toward dying involved young adults. Karen Ann Quinlan was only 21 years old when she had a cardiopulmonary arrest and fell into a persistent vegetative state. In *In the Matter of Quinlan*, the Supreme Court of New Jersey ruled that her family could remove her from a ventilator. This landmark ruling led to the prevalence of ethics committees in medical institutions and to the creation of advance directives.[8] Nancy Cruzan was only 25 years old when she fell into a persistent vegetative state after being involved in a car accident. In its landmark decision, the Supreme Court of the United States paved the path for surrogate decision making in the removal of artificial nutrition and hydration.[9] Terri Schiavo was 26 years old when her heart stopped. She, too, fell into a persistent vegetative state and, in 2005, became one of the more than 300,000 Americans withdrawn from artificial food and fluids.[10] Brittany Maynard was a 28-year-old healthy newlywed when she developed terminal brain cancer and made the choice to move to Oregon to take life-ending medication under Oregon's Death with Dignity law.[11] The sagas of these four young women illustrate the importance of planning and sharing values and priorities for the end of life with family and friends.

When thinking about the end of life, personal values about quality of life need to be considered. What makes living meaningful must be carefully weighed. Urge patients to talk with loved ones about their views and to choose someone to speak for them if they become unable to speak for themselves.

A patient's right to refuse medical intervention is well established in medicine and law. Patients and families of unconscious patients routinely choose to stop or not start ventilators, artificial nutrition and hydration, and antibiotics. Patients voluntarily stop eating and drinking (VSED). Do not resuscitate (DNRs) orders are being replaced with orders to Allow Natural Death (AND). Either one can prevent the distress that futile attempts at cardiopulmonary resuscitation (CPR) can bring. Surrogate decision makers may elect for palliative or terminal sedation.

The purpose of completing end-of-life documents is to make intentional decisions and express them in writing. Completed documents, discussed and shared with family and friends, lay the foundation for decision making in line with a person's values and priorities at the end of life.

Sectarian health care directives. Some religiously affiliated health care institutions may decline to honor expressed health care choices that conflict with their doctrine and beliefs. An individual may specify in advance that admission to a religious facility does not imply consent to particular care mandated by its ethical, religious, or other policies.[12] If the facility declines to follow the preferences in an advance directive, a prepared advance directive addendum directs that the patient be transferred to a hospital, nursing home, or other institution that will agree to honor the instructions set forth in the directive.

Lesbian, gay, bisexual, transgender (LGBT) families. The LGBT community faces additional challenges at the end of life. Until recently, the partners of LGBT patients were routinely not allowed to participate in the medical treatment decisions of their loved ones or even visit them in the hospital. In 2014, in the case of Ob*ergefell et al. v. Hodges, Director, Ohio Department of Health, et al.*, the U.S. Supreme Court granted constitutional protection for same-sex marriage.[13] It remains to be seen how this right will play out at a local level with end-of-life decision making and respecting surrogate decision making established by these marriages.

ADVANCE DIRECTIVES

It is prudent for adults to complete an advance directive for health care (AD). Regardless of age and health status, none can predict when an event might leave a person unable to speak for himself or herself. If patients are not able to make or communicate decisions about medical treatment, a written record of their intentions for end-of-life care is invaluable.

Advance directive is a generic term used for documents that traditionally include a living will and the appointment of a health care agent. These documents allow individuals to provide instructions relating to their future health care, such as when they would want to receive all medical treatment available or when they would want to stop or decline life-sustaining medical treatments.

The living will portion of an AD allows the patient to specify which kinds of treatments and care are desired if he or she were permanently unconscious or terminally ill and unable to speak for himself or herself. The second part, often referred to as the *durable power of attorney for health care*, allows the appointment of someone to act on the patient's behalf in matters concerning his or her health care when the patient is unable to speak for himself or herself because of illness or incapacitation. Please note that the person appointed to speak on behalf of the patient may be called a *health care agent, proxy, surrogate,* or *representative.*

An AD allows patients to express their wishes about decisions regarding life-sustaining treatments, including treatments and procedures a patient *does or does not* want. Statements regarding organ and tissue donation may also be included. The instructions provided in this portion of the form serve as evidence of the patient's wishes.

The durable power of attorney portion of an AD allows the appointment of an agent to speak on behalf of the patient and communicate his or her wishes when the patient is not able to do so. Appointing an agent and making sure the agent is aware of and understands the individual's values and priorities is one of the most important things that can be done. If the time comes for a decision to be made, the agent can participate in relevant discussions, weighing the pros and cons of treatment decisions on the basis of the patient's previously expressed intentions. The agent can act on behalf of a patient even when decision-making capacity is only temporarily affected. The patient need not be permanently unconscious or terminally ill but may be stuporous, delirious, or demented, for example. The degree of authority (how much or how little) the patient wants his agent to have can be defined in this document. Alternate agents can also be appointed in case the primary agent is unwilling or unable to act. Additionally, the patient may name specific individuals who are *not* to participate in decision making. If an agent is not appointed, the law in most states provides for other decision makers by default, usually beginning with the spouse and adult children and ending with the patient's physician. When physicians tend to err on the side of prolonging life, their decisions may not be consistent with the patient's desires. In extreme cases, if the patient does not have an AD, a court may be required to appoint a guardian.

Advance directives ease the burden of uncertainty on family members. They help relieve the stress and doubt associated with having to make important health care decisions on behalf of someone you care about but without clear instruction. By making wishes known in advance, patients can help guide their families and friends, who may otherwise struggle to decide the best course.

Advance directives are legally valid in every state. Each state and the District of Columbia have laws that permit individuals to sign documents stating their decisions for life-sustaining treatment if they are permanently unconscious or terminally ill. A few states provide for such instruction in the case of advanced dementia as well. The specifics of these laws vary, but the basic principle of listening to the patient's wishes is the same everywhere. The law gives great weight to any form of written directive. If the courts become involved, they usually attempt to follow the patient's stated values and preferences, especially if they are in written form. An AD may be the most concrete evidence of wishes possible. It is important to note that although it is legal to have an AD in every state, states vary in the degree to which they require adherence to the directive. Most states offer legal protection to HCPs for following, or deciding not to follow, the instructions contained in an AD.

An AD can be changed or cancelled at any time. This can be accomplished by notifying the agent or HCP, in writing, of the decision to do so. It is best to destroy all copies of the old AD and create a new one. Make sure to provide copies of the new form to the appropriate individuals. It is strongly recommended to review ADs every year and resign and redate them to indicate that the document continues to reflect current wishes.

Physician Orders for Life-Sustaining Treatment

Another health care planning document is the Physician Orders for Life-Sustaining Treatment form, more commonly known as the POLST. In some states, is it called a MOLST (Medical Order for Life-Sustaining Treatment). The POLST is designed to help HCPs honor the end-of-life wishes of their patients. They are appropriate in situations when resuscitative efforts would likely be futile and injurious to the patient. The question to ask is "Would you be surprised if the patient died within the next year?" The form documents physician orders that adhere to the patient's intentions and treatment goals and are readily accessible to emergency medical personnel, assisted living facility staff, and other caregivers. They follow a patient from home, to emergency services, and to a hospital or other facility. Not all states have POLST programs in place. Currently, 26 states have fully implemented programs, and 27 other states are developing POLST programs.[14]

Out-of-Hospital Do Not Resuscitate Orders

On average, only 5% to 10% of people who receive CPR survive.[15] Most states have some type of documentation that tells emergency medical services (EMS) personnel not to attempt resuscitation or perform heroic measures on a particular patient who has reached a point of medical futility. In states that do not have POLST programs, these documents can be called *out-of-hospital DNR orders, nonhospital DNRs, bedside DNR orders, EMS DNR orders, prehospital DNR orders,* or a *CPR advance directive.* Similar to the POLST, these documents are signed by the patient's HCP. Their intent is to prevent medical staff or EMS personnel from performing unwanted medical interventions on a seriously ill patient.

To avoid unwanted intubations or CPR during transport to or between medical facilities, patients must have appropriate state-specific forms that can be provided to those involved with their transport. Having a living will, health care power of attorney, and a DNR order in a hospital chart will *not* necessarily prevent this from occurring. The patient *must* have the appropriate POLST or out-of-hospital DNR orders to safeguard his or her wishes reliably.[16]

HOSPICE

In Latin, "hospice" means *host* and *guest* or *a place of shelter.* Hospice is a concept of care for terminally ill patients that places an emphasis on comfort and living. Modern-day hospice began in 1967 in London when Dame Cecily Saunders founded St. Christopher's Hospice. The first U.S. hospice opened in Connecticut in 1974.

Hospice care is a form of palliative care. To palliate means to "ease (symptoms) without curing the underlying disease; to moderate the intensity of."[17] Hospice provides aggressive pain and symptom management by using an interdisciplinary team consisting of physicians, physician assistants (PAs), nurses, social workers, spiritual care providers, therapists (psychiatric, art, music, physical, occupational, and speech), and volunteers. The focus of hospice is comfort-oriented care when disease-specific therapy is no longer helpful and end-of-life plans come to the fore. Living life as fully as possible is emphasized; entering hospice care does not mean all treatments must end. Hospice treatments aim to relieve the physical, emotional, and spiritual distress that often accompany a life-limiting illness. Hospice supports families while they care for their loved ones and provides grief support after the death occurs.

To qualify for hospice care, a patient must have a terminal illness. Although lung, breast, and prostate cancers are the three most common diagnoses,[18] a patient may have any diagnosis and be any age. Hospice patients must usually have a prognosis of 6 months or less. In recent years, there has been a movement within hospice to admit people with conditions that are less clearly terminal, and such admissions account for most patients with noncancer diagnoses. These diagnoses may include unspecified debility of age (a chronic "disease" diagnosis with no single major illness), dementia, and heart failure and lung disease. An HCP should refer patients to hospice when they have a prognosis measured in months versus years and when the goals of care have switched from cure to comfort. As long as the clinical criteria are met, a patient may usually be referred to hospice regardless of his or her ability to pay. Not all hospice programs require that a patient have a DNR order, but resuscitation attempts in the hospice setting are rare. Hospice is not an end to treatment; rather, it is a shift to intensive palliative care that focuses on helping the patient to live life to the fullest. It is comfort-oriented care with end-of-life closure. In general, hospice care occurs wherever a person calls home and can be either community or institutionally based.

An option authorized in some states (Oregon in 1994, Washington in 2008, Montana in 2010, Vermont in 2012, and California in 2015) is medical aid in dying. Although controversial in some forums, having the option of aid in dying provides peace of mind and may be considered by individuals who are decisionally capable, terminally ill, suffering, and determined to remain in charge of their own end-of-life experience. In the previously mentioned states, this option is available through a strict and thoughtful medical process to enable a physician to prescribe medication in a life-ending dose. Patients who decide to ingest the medication must do so themselves.

Various other end-of-life options are supported in law and medicine to enable individuals to advance the time of death if they are suffering in their dying. Competent adults or their appointed health care agents may have the power to direct the discontinuation of any medical treatment. Competent adults are permitted to refuse unwanted treatment regardless of the reason for their refusal or the nature of their illness; they need not be terminally ill. These same patients also have the legal right to stop life-sustaining medications or treatments, including voluntary stopping of eating and drinking. Although not for everyone, more people are learning about these voluntary end-of-life choices and discussing them with their families and HCPs.

HAVING THE CONVERSATION

One of the most productive ways to help patients as they approach the end of life is to encourage

TABLE 20.1 Representative Questions for Initiating the Discussion About End-of-Life Issues

Domain	Representative Questions
Goals	Given the severity of your illness, what is most important for you to achieve?
	How do you think about balancing quality of life with length of life in terms of your treatment? What are your most important hopes? What are your biggest fears?
Values	What makes life most worth living for you? Would there be any circumstances under which you would find life not worth living? What do you consider your quality of life to be like now? Have you seen or been with someone who had a particularly good death or particularly difficult death?
Advance directives	If with future progression of your illness you are not able to speak for yourself, who would be best able to represent your views and values (health care proxy)? Have you given any thought to what kinds of treatments you would want (and not want) if you become unable to speak for yourself in the future (living will)?
Do-not-resuscitate order	If you were to die suddenly, that is, you stopped breathing or your heart stopped, we could try to revive you by using cardiopulmonary resuscitation (CPR). Are you familiar with CPR? Have you given thought to whether you would want it? Given the severity of your illness, CPR would in all likelihood be ineffective. I would recommend that you choose not to have it but that we continue all potentially effective treatments. What do you think?
Palliative care (pain and other symptoms)	Have you ever heard of hospice (palliative care)? What has been your experience with it? Tell me about your pain. Can you rate it on a 10-point scale? What is your breathing like when you feel at your best? How about when you are having trouble?
Palliative care ("unfinished business")	If you were to die sooner rather than later, what would be left undone? How is your family handling your illness? What are their reactions? Has religion been an important part of your life? Are there any spiritual issues you are concerned about at this point?

From Rando TA. *Grief, Dying, and Death: Clinical Interventions for Caregivers.* Champaign, IL: Research Press Publishers; 1984. Reprint courtesy of Timothy E. Quill, MD.

them to have a conversation with their loved ones about their preferences for treatment and end-of-life wishes. This conversation should include family members, friends, HCPs, and religious or spiritual advisors—anyone in the patient's life and involved with his or her care. The conversation should be viewed as one leg of a three-legged stool: (1) naming a surrogate decision maker, (2) documenting the wishes, and (3) discussion of values and priorities.

In addition to promoting this conversation, HCPs can enable it. Set a time for the patient to meet with his or her family and friends to discuss these issues. If possible, attend the meeting to help keep the conversation going and to help address any questions or concerns that may arise. Table 20.1 lists questions that may help patients as they begin to sort out these issues, and Box 20.1 provides questions patients may ask of you as they begin to come to terms with their own mortality.

Death is an uncomfortable topic. Many people believe that if they do not talk about it, it will not happen, especially to them. In reality, death must be discussed. Discussions are most useful if a plan is in place long before crucial decisions arise.

BOX 20.1 SOME DIFFICULT QUESTIONS FROM PATIENTS

"Why me?"
"Why didn't you catch this earlier? Did you make a mistake?"
"How long do I have?"
"What would you do in my shoes?"
"Should I try long-shot or experimental therapy?"
"Should I go to a 'medical Mecca' for treatment or a second opinion?"
"If my suffering gets really bad, will you help me die?"
"Will you work with me all the way through to my death, no matter what?"

From Rando TA. *Grief, Dying, and Death: Clinical Interventions for Caregivers.* Champaign, IL: Research Press Publishers; 1984. Reprint courtesy of Timothy E. Quill, MD.

Although these conversations may seem awkward at first, they often bring families closer together. Talking about death is deeply personal; sharing beliefs and priorities with loved ones produces more intimate relationships. It takes courage to have these conversations.

STAGES OF DYING

Death is a process, not an event. Every tissue of the body participates, each in its own way and at its own pace. The living–dying interval is the period of time between the normal processes of living and the point at which death occurs. There are three stages: acute crisis, chronic living–dying, and terminal.[19]

The physical changes that occur as death nears may happen over a few hours or several days. When the changes begin, the patient is considered to have begun actively dying.

As death approaches, the patient may feel cool to the touch, and his or her skin color may change. The patient may sleep more. He or she may appear uncommunicative or unresponsive and may be difficult to arouse. Disorientation may occur. Incontinence of bowel and bladder may occur as muscles begin to relax. Congestion in the lungs and throat occurs, and as fluid intake decreases, secretions thicken, and the patient becomes unable to cough. Restlessness, such as pulling at bedding or clothing, is common. Urine output decreases. The patient's regular breathing pattern may change. Periods of rapid breaths may alternate with periods of very slow, drawn-out breaths. The time between breaths can range from 5 seconds to 1 full minute.

Emotional, spiritual, and mental changes occur leading to death. The patient may withdraw as he or she begins to let go. He or she may want to be with only very few people. The patient may talk about speaking with deceased relatives or friends. He or she may also report seeing things not visible to others. The following statements are commonly heard as a patient nears death:
Where's the map?
I'm getting ready to travel.
I want to go home.
I'm not alone.
I see (name of deceased relative or friend).
An angel is in the room.
I'll be there soon.
I know when I will die (day of week, time of day).

The patient is beginning to detach from life. Although others cannot hear or see what the patient senses, it feels real to him or her, so it is best not to challenge or contradict the experience. Although this may be unnerving, paranormal experiences are not distressing to the patient and may be comforting.

Patients have strong feelings about the care they receive as they near the end of their lives. They worry how their decisions will affect their families, both emotionally and financially. Although they want to work with their HCPs to make the best treatment decisions, they often fear these same HCPs may stop caring for them when death is near. Dying patients desire emotional and spiritual care along with good medical care. Most want to die as peacefully as possible, free from pain, suffering, and prolonged dependence. Dying patients often want to forgive others, forgive themselves, say thank you, and say good-bye. They fear a loss of control, being in pain, and being isolated from family and friends.

STAGES OF GRIEF

Grief is the mental and physical pain experienced when loss of a significant object, person, or part of the self is realized. This begins with the terminal diagnosis and includes a profound loss of future dreams and goals (realization of all of the things that will not happen).

Because aging often leads to loss of independence, strength, health, and mobility, it commonly causes grief as well. This type of grief for self can result in depressive symptoms and profound sadness, but it is separate from clinical depression. Grief for self can be a normal, healthy response to the changes and limitations older individuals experience.

In 1969, Elisabeth Kübler-Ross published a book detailing the grief process.[20] Her research identified five stages of grief: denial, anger, bargaining, depression, and acceptance. Hope can remain throughout all stages, even though what is hoped for is likely to change from hope for cure, for example, to hope for one last family gathering or hope for a peaceful death.

The grieving process is an individual process, unique to each person. There is no "right" or "wrong" way through the grieving process; there are just different ways. It is worth noting that not everyone experiences every stage of grief, and the stages may overlap, repeat, or appear in different order.

Grief is an intensely personal process and can be quite complicated. If the survivor sees the death as appropriate and timely, that understanding can mitigate the grief. We often see unresolved, morbid, or exceptional grief reactions when the significance of the loss is unrecognized or discounted. Another form of grief is anticipatory grief, which allows for major emotional reaction before an expected loss. This does not replace postdeath grief but may reduce its severity. Disenfranchised grief is experienced when a loss is suffered that cannot or is not openly acknowledged, publicly mourned, or socially supported. Chronic sorrow is grieving a loss that cannot be fully resolved because there will be an ever-present sadness that recurs with its original pain at periodic intervals. Individual psychological and cultural differences can foster one form of grief over another. A broad range of literature is available on grief and the grieving process.

EMERGING ISSUES

Emerging issues in end-of-life care include changing laws, billing regulations, and evolving standards of care. These changes bring a host of questions and points for ethical discussions. As a PA, how will you balance professional practice and empathy, your own beliefs versus the autonomy of your patient? Below you will find several emerging issues and resources to learn more.

In July 2015, the Centers for Medicare & Medicaid Services introduced two new billing codes to reimburse physicians for two 30-minute conversations with patients to discuss advance-care planning. As introduced earlier in the chapter, these conversations can have a huge impact on end-of-life comfort for patients and their families and give clear guidance for end-of-life decisions. The *Journal of the American Medical Association* (*JAMA*) stated that these conversations are "critically needed to ensure receipt of goal-concordant care."[21]

The Campaign to End Unwanted Medical treatment is a collaboration of 19 organizations that came together to confront the current state of end-of-life care and work to ensure that people receive care that is consistent with their personal goals and beliefs. The coalition works to change governmental policies at the federal level to ensure that HCPs do not have incentives to provide tests and treatments inconsistent with a person's advance directive or in violation of a DNR order of POLST. In addition, they work to educate the "public, patients, families, caregivers and providers about the rights of patients to determine how much and the types of treatments they receive ranging from all treatment options available—to their right to refuse unwanted, unnecessary or life-prolonging treatment if they so choose."[22]

In 2015, the subject of Death with Dignity laws was thrust into the public eye more than ever before. Oregon's 16 years of data and the recent passing of the End-of-Life Options Act by the State of California mean this topic will continue to be discussed at the state and national levels.[23] Currently, there is legislative action in 27 states and Washington, DC.[24]

New research means constant refining of standards for end-of-life care. For example, a recent study in *JAMA* found that chemotherapy at the end of life does not offer the expected improved quality of life. The study showed that patients in poor physical condition had no quality-of-life improvement with treatment, and those in good physical condition actually worsened with chemotherapy. Studies such as this constantly redefine optimal care for terminally ill patients.[25]

To quote Sherwin B. Nuland, "Every life is different from any that has gone before it, and so is every death. The uniqueness of each of us extends even to the way we die."[26] The truth is that every last one of us will die. Some of us will die as our lives are just getting on track, and others will die of debilitating conditions many decades from now. Few of us will have the privilege of sitting with someone as they die. But for those of us who do, it will be a defining moment in our lives; it will be one that will leave deep impressions and ultimately guide us as we venture forth in the health care profession. Working with patients as they approach the end of their lives is not for everyone. But those who discover their niche in this area will find it to be a profoundly rewarding experience.

CLINICAL APPLICATIONS

- A 60-year-old man is hospitalized after a massive stroke. His condition remains stable in the intensive care unit on a ventilator. He is unconscious, and the medical staff agrees his mental status is unlikely to improve. Options include maintaining life support and discharging him to a skilled nursing facility or turning off the machines and allowing a natural death. The family disagrees on a course of action. There is no living will or durable power of attorney. What do you do?
- During a routine office visit, an elderly patient initiates a discussion on her end-of-life wishes. What do you include in the discussion?
- A patient with stage 4 lung cancer declines further treatment and opts to allow his disease to progress to a natural death. What recommendations would you make to him to increase his chance for a good quality of life and a comfortable death?

GLOSSARY

Advance directive: Encompasses both living wills and medical durable power of attorney.

Aid in dying: A practice specifically authorized in Oregon, Washington, Montana, Vermont and California that allows mentally competent, terminally ill adults to request a prescription for life-ending medication from their physician. This medication must be self-administered.

Autonomy: The capacity of a rational individual to make an informed, uncoerced decision.

Hospice: An HCP offering comfort care for dying patients when medical treatment is no longer expected to cure the disease or prolong life. Hospice is provided wherever the person resides. The term may also apply to an insurance benefit that pays the costs of comfort care (usually at home) for patients with a prognosis of 6 months or less.

Informed consent: The communication process between a doctor and a patient that results in the patient having clear, unbiased information about treatment options in order to arrive at the decision that is best for him or her.

Living will: A term commonly substituted for advance directive or for the portion of an advance directive containing specific instructions.

Out-of-hospital do not resuscitate order: An order written by an HCP directing other providers in the out-of-hospital setting to withhold or withdraw resuscitation efforts the event of respiratory or cardiac arrest.

Palliative or total sedation: Also referred to as terminal sedation. The continuous administration of medication to relieve severe, intractable symptoms that cannot be controlled while keeping the patient conscious. An unconscious or semiconscious state is maintained until death occurs.

POLST: Physician Orders for Life-Sustaining Treatment. A medical order governing life-sustaining treatment that remains in effect across treatment settings and in the home.

Terminal, terminally: An illness for which the medical expectation is that it will cause death within the foreseeable future, usually 6 months.

VSED: Voluntary stopping eating and drinking.

KEY POINTS

- Patients act on principles of autonomy and informed consent. HCPs are almost always obligated to divulge the truth of the patient's diagnosis and prognosis to them.
- It is never too early to begin to plan and discuss treatment preferences at the end of life. It is prudent for every adult to have an AD for health care and, when appropriate in the setting of advanced disease, a POLST or out-of-hospital DNR order. Conversations with family and friends help lay the foundation for rational end-of-life decision making. These conversations can prove invaluable. Conversations should follow the three-legged stool concept: naming a surrogate, documenting wishes, and discussing values and priorities.
- Hospice provides aggressive palliative pain and symptom management to terminally ill patients, allowing them to live as fully as possible until they die.
- Dying is a process. It is a personal journey, unique to each of us.
- Working with dying patients can be a profoundly rewarding experience.

References

1. Crawshaw R, Rogers DE, Pellegrino ED, et al. Patient-physician covenant (1995). In: Beauchamp TL, Walters L, eds. *Contemporary Issues in Bioethics.* 5th ed. Belmont, CA: Wadsworth Publishing; 1999.
2. Beauchamp TL, Veatch RM. *Ethical Issues in Death and Dying.* 2nd ed. Upper Saddle River, NJ: Prentice Hall; 1996:64.
3. Beauchamp TL, Veatch RM. *Ethical Issues in Death and Dying.* 2nd ed. Upper Saddle River, NJ: Prentice Hall; 1996:69.
4. Beauchamp TL, Childress JF. *Principles of Biomedical Ethics.* 5th ed. New York: Oxford University Press; 2001:285.
5. deBlois JC, Norris P, O'Rourke K. *A Primer for Health Care Ethics: Essays for a Pluralistic Society.* Washington, DC: Georgetown University Press; 1994:27–29.
6. CDC FastStats. Deaths and mortality: preliminary data for 2013. http://www.cdc.gov/nchs/fastats/deaths.htm. Accessed November 6, 2015.
7. CDC National Center for Injury Prevention and Control. Leading causes of death reports, 1999-2007. http://webappa.cdc.gov/sasweb/ncipc/leadcaus10.html. Accessed November 5, 2015.
8. Matter of Quinlan 70 N.J. 10; 355 A.2d 647; 1976 N.J.
9. Cruzan v. Director, Missouri Department of Health, 497 U.S. 261, 278, 110 S. Ct. 2841, 111 L. Ed. 2d 224 (1990).
10. Fritz M. How simple device set off a fight over elderly care. *Wall Street J.* Dec. 8, 2005. A1.
11. People. Terminally ill 29-year-old woman. Why I'm choosing to die on my own terms. http://www.people.com/article/Brittany-Maynard-death-with-dignity-compassion-choices. Accessed March 19, 2016.

12. Sectarian Healthcare Directive, Denver, CO: Compassion and Choices. 2016. https://www.compassionandchoices.org/wp-content/uploads/2016/03/Directive_Sectarian_Healthcare.pdf Accessed December 5, 2016.

13. Supreme Court of the United States. Obergefell et al. v. Hodges, Director, Ohio Department of Health, et al. http://www.supremecourt.gov/opinions/14pdf/14-556_3204.pdf. Accessed March 20, 2016.

14. Center for Ethics in Health Care. Oregon Health & Science University. Physician Orders for Life-Sustaining Treatment Paradigm. http://www.polst.org/. Accessed March 19, 2016.

15. Mann D. Real CPR Isn't Everything It Seems to Be. http://www.webmd.com/content/article/32/1728_79637.htm. Accessed March 20, 2016.

16. Pennsylvania Department of Health. Out-Of-Hospital Do-Not-Resuscitate (DNR) Orders. http://www.portal.health.state.pa.us/portal/server.pt/community/emergency_medical_services/14138/polst_-_out-of-hospital_dnr_orders/556979. Accessed November 6, 2015.

17. Merriam-Webster Online Dictionary. http://www.m-w.com/dictionary/palliate. Accessed March 19, 2016.

18. National Hospice and Palliative Care Organization. Professional Resources: Hospice Statistics and Research. http://www.nhpco.org/sites/default/files/public/Statistics_Research/2014_Facts_Figures.pdf. Accessed March 19, 2016.

19. Rando TA. *Grief, Dying, and Death: Clinical Interventions for Caregivers*. Champaign, IL: Research Press Publishers; 1984.

20. Kübler-Ross E. *On Death and Dying*. New York: Macmillan Publishing Company; 1969.

21. Trends in Advance Care Planning in Patients With Cancer: Results From a Longitudinal Survey. *JAMA*. http://oncology.jamanetwork.com/article.aspx?articleid=2383145. Accessed March 20, 2016.

22. Campaign to End Unwanted Medical Treatment. Statement of Purpose. http://endumt.org/userfiles/campaign-principles.pdf. Accessed March 20, 2016.

23. Oregon Health Authority. Oregon's Death with Dignity Act Report 2014. https://public.health.oregon.gov/ProviderPartnerResources/EvaluationResearch/DeathwithDignityAct/Documents/year16.pdf. Accessed March 20, 2016.

24. Compassion and Choices. What You Can Do in Your State. https://www.compassionandchoices.org/what-you-can-do/in-your-state. Accessed March 20, 2016.

25. Chemotherapy Use, Performance Status, and Quality of Life at the End of Life. *JAMA*. 2016. http://oncology.jamanetwork.com/article.aspx?articleid=2398177. Accessed March 20, 2016.

26. Nuland SB. *How We Die: Reflections on Life's Final Chapter*. New York: Alfred A. Knopf; 1994:3.

The resources for this chapter can be found at www.expertconsult.com.

The Faculty Resources can be found online at www.expertconsult.com.

SECTION III

INTERPERSONAL AND COMMUNICATION SKILLS

COMMUNICATION ISSUES

Robin Risling-de Jong

"Communication between and among human beings is complex. It occurs at many levels simultaneously. Doctors, allied health professionals, and public health communications experts grapple with how best to reach their audiences most effectively."[1]

Communication skills are crucial in the effective and efficient delivery of health care. They are needed in order to build trusting relationships, to relay important and critical health information, and to negotiate best plans of care with patient shared decision making that ultimately leads to lifestyle change and treatment adherence. Communication skills are also critical in managing emotionally charged situations such as trauma and end-of-life situations. To maintain and improve a patient's health and medical care, communication skills are considered one of the most important skills students must learn and master in medicine.[2] Studies have shown that communication has the ability to not only improve patient satisfaction and safety but also contributes to improved health outcomes. Conversely, miscommunication and disregard for patient understanding and preferences contribute to health care disparities. Patient safety, satisfaction, and value hinge on progress made in communication.[3]

To help put health care communication issues into perspective for students and clinicians, this chapter focuses on five topics of discussion. These topics address patient-centered communication, health literacy and cultural competency, interprofessional communication, information technology (IT), and professionalism.

PATIENT-CENTERED COMMUNICATION

"Extensive research has shown that no matter how knowledgeable a clinician might be, if he or she is not able to open good communication with the patient, he or she may be of no help."[4,5]

The medical literature regarding patient-centered communication is often confusing because there are seemingly different terms that ultimately mean the same thing. To begin a discussion about patient-centered communication, it is prudent to first define what is meant in this chapter by patient-centered communication.

"Early work to define communication skills relevant to medical practice used the terms physician-patient communication or excellence in communication. The term patient centered communication has emerged in more recent writings on the subject."[6] Patient-centered communication can further be defined by the targeted goals and outcomes of patient interactions. To what extent these goals and outcomes are directly related to interpersonal communication is not easy to determine because of coexisting variables. Essentially, effective patient–provider communication is evaluated and measured in terms of the patient's ability to follow through with medical recommendations, self-managing chronic medical conditions, and adopting preventive health behaviors.[4]

Identifying the goals and desired outcomes for a patient's health and well-being is usually not the hardest part of the clinician–patient encounter. It is, however, the first step in the process of patient-centered communication. Standing between goals and outcomes is the ability to effectively communicate so that both the patient and provider feel good about the process and progress of health management.

There are two major communication obstacles in health care delivery that make up the majority of problematic communication. These obstacles are found in communication breakdowns and common communication barriers that hinder effective and collaborative communication. To create the best health outcomes possible for the patient, identifying where these more common areas of communication breakdowns usually occur and recognizing these barriers of communication will help promote successful encounters. Acquiring the knowledge and skills to overcome communication obstacles has far-reaching positive implications in patient and provider health outcomes satisfaction.

Communication Breakdowns

"Communication is a two-way street. Differences in knowledge, perceptions, and decisions frequently surface when people communicate. This can cause disagreement, misunderstanding, and conflict. However, the communication process is not harmed if disagreement is managed constructively."[7] According to The Joint Commission, identified areas of communication breakdown occur between ineffective or incomplete communications among clinicians, the patient, and the patient's caregivers. This takes into account forms of communication such as written, verbal, and recorded. Other areas of breakdowns include those having to do with patient education and patient accountability.[8] When are these breakdowns most likely to happen? Communication breakdowns occur across the continuum of care and often involve ambiguity regarding responsibilities.[9] Communication breakdowns result in incomplete or misunderstood diagnostic and therapeutic instructions and subsequently have a negative effect on patient mortality and morbidity. In patient referrals, quality of care often suffers from interprofessional miscommunication, which can lead to poor continuity of care, unnecessary diagnostic procedures, delayed diagnoses, polypharmacy, and increased litigation risk.[10]

Effective communication relies on the patient and everyone involved in the patient's care to be clear and in sync. The patient and the caregivers must be clear about the plan and understand their tasks and responsibilities in carrying out the plan. The degree to which this can happen influences patient safety and treatment adherence, cumulating in improved health outcomes.

Barriers of Communication

The barriers that hinder effective communication are vast. They also overlap and correspond with reasons for breakdowns in communication. Common barriers of communication are differences and competency in language, education, cultural responsiveness, and health literacy. Lack of perceived courtesy, respect, and engagement interwoven through all aspects of care are also common recurring themes in barriers to effective health care communication.

Another barrier to clinician–patient communication is patient interruptions, particularly as they relate to the time constraints of the patient encounter. The skill and art of history taking are the most important parts in the diagnostic workup of patients for practicing clinicians. An estimated 70% to 90% of a diagnosis is made from the patient's history alone.[11] Studies of clinician–patient visits, unfortunately, show that patients are often not provided the opportunity to tell their stories. This is often due to time constraints and interruptions, which compromise diagnostic accuracy. In such circumstances, the patient can perceive that what he or she is saying is not important, which leads to patients feeling reluctant about offering additional information. When patients are interrupted, the provider risks the opportunity of collecting essential information. The patient's feeling rushed or interrupted also undermines the patient–provider relationship.[4]

One of the most dangerous consequences of breaches in communication are those of medical errors. The ways in which medical errors can happen when caring for patients is not hard to understand given the potential for miscommunication as previously discussed. However, what bears specific mention is written prescriptions. Written prescriptions have often been identified as one cause for medication errors. Illegible handwriting and medication mix-ups caused by similar-sounding names of medications lead to misinterpreted dosages and incorrect medication administration.[12] Verbal instructions to patients in regard to medication use and adverse effects in place of written instructions have also been an identified culprit in medical errors. This is especially dangerous when the patient does not feel like he or she shares in the decision-making process and either does not feel capable of questioning the caregiver or is unable to reach the ear of the caregiver. Table 21.1 illustrates breakdowns and barriers to communication, any or all of which can impact patient safety and treatment adherence.

TABLE 21.1 **Overlapping Variables in Effective Communication**	
Breakdown in Communications	**Barriers to Communication**
Interprofessional communication	Language, courtesy, respect, engagement, time constraints of patient encounters
Provider–patient communication	Health literacy, language, cultural competency, courtesy, respect, engagement
Provider–patient–caregiver communication	Cultural competency, health literacy, language, courtesy, respect, engagement
Interprofessional–patient–caregiver communication	Courtesy, respect and engagement, health competency, language, time constraints of patient encounters
Incomplete or misunderstood instructions	Time constraints of patient encounters, courtesy, respect, engagement, language, cultural competency

HEALTH LITERACY AND CULTURAL COMPETENCY

Health literacy is a broad term with a specific purpose of alerting health care providers to a significant barrier to equitable access and utilization of health care. Poor health literacy is not simply a matter of one's educational level, language skills, culture, or ethnicity. There are many components contributing to poor health literacy, and health literacy is important and applicable to everyone. Ultimately, anyone who needs any type or form of health care services needs health literacy skills.[13] Many studies have shown a link between poor health literacy and poor health outcomes.[14] This equates to health disparities.

Health literacy is defined by the Institute of Medicine's report, *Health Literacy: A Prescription to End Confusion*, as "the degree to which individuals have the capacity to obtain, process and understand basic health information and services needed to make appropriate health decisions."[15] More recently, the definition has broadened to include a focus on the specific skills needed to navigate the health care system and the importance of clear communication between health care providers and their patients.[16]

Poor health outcomes caused by poor health literacy place a responsibility on health care providers to not only be cognizant of this as a major health disparity but also to remain vigilant against it in practice. Overcoming health literacy problems for improved patient outcomes is an achievable task. The first step

is recognizing the factors involved in creating the disparity with the individual or community served, and the second is implementing tools that overcome these disparities.

Common identifiable factors impeding health literacy have been illuminated in many studies. These include how information is communicated, experience with the health care system, the format of the deliverables, linguistic and cultural variables, access to health care, age, low socioeconomic status, and patient–provider relationship.[17]

Research linking ways to overcome poor health literacy and improve health outcomes is ongoing. Some ways to overcome literacy barriers have become common practices, such as printing patient information in different languages and delivering information in plain language, thereby eliminating practice-specific jargon. Strategies such as tailored and targeted health communication that enhance information relevance to the intended audience have also shown some promising benefits.[18]

Cultural respect has been demonstrated to overcome major components of health literacy having to do with ethnicity, equity, and access to care. When a clinician is respectful and responsive to health beliefs, cultural beliefs and practices, and linguistic needs, many study outcomes show remarkable efficacy in decreasing disparity and providing high-quality access to care.[19] Conversely, when patients experience a stereotype threat in the clinical settings, it can have devastating effects on health outcomes and can be considered a health disparity.[20]

It is the imperative to teach current and future clinicians the skills for acquiring cultural competency and cultural respect. Cultural competency is the ability to incorporate a set of behaviors, attitudes, and policies that come together in a system or agency or among professionals that enable effective work in cross-cultural situations.[21] Cultural competency is an important skill to possess in order to overcome barriers to health care access, patient safety issues, and overall outcomes in terms of screening, diagnostics, and treatment adherence. Attaining cultural competency begins by self-reflection, and it requires an honest, ongoing assessment of biases that can impede delivery of care caused by a lack of respect and understanding toward patients or other health professionals.[22]

INTERPROFESSIONAL COMMUNICATION

The introduction of the Triple Aim goals for reforming health care in the United States has fostered the advocacy for patient- and population-centered health care delivery using teams of professionals. The

Institute for Healthcare Improvement developed the Triple Aim framework, which seeks to improve the quality of health care through three dimensions: (1) improving the patient experience of care (including quality and satisfaction), (2) improving the health of populations, and (3) reducing the per capita cost of health care.[23]

Perhaps the most familiar entity evolving from the Triple Aim is the patient-centered medical home (PCMH). A PCMH is a patient-centered health care delivery model that is team based in order to provide comprehensive health care. PCMHs are believed to improve health outcomes, safety, and quality of care and provide a more efficient use of practice resources.

Interprofessional relations involve relaying and receiving vital clinical information from one profession to another concerning patient care. This underscores the importance of effective, efficient, and comprehensive communication practices in order to prevent adverse patient care outcomes. Communication mishaps cumulating in safety issues and medical errors arising from professionals working with other professionals is certainly not new. In fact, it remains a hot topic in the delivery of quality of care. As a result, effective communication tools and resources have been developed and implemented in health care settings that reduce adverse patient outcomes.

- TeamSTEPPS
- SBAR (situation, background, assessment, and recommendation)
- Teach Back
- Call Outs
- Check Back
- Handoffs
- Teach to Goal

Because the health care culture is transitioning from silo-based care to interprofessional team-based care, dedicated and coordinated interprofessional educational and training care strategies targeted at communication issues are being developed and put in place in all health care disciplines. Interprofessional education is a part of the physician assistant (PA) curriculum and is part of the accreditation standards for allied health professions, nursing, pharmacy, and medical schools.

At the forefront of helping programs implement and integrate interprofessional team-based, patient-centered care practices into the curriculum of health care professionals is the Interprofessional Education Collaborative (IPEC). The IPEC is a cooperative organization made up of health care disciplines involved in patient care. It promotes and encourages coordinated efforts to advance substantive interprofessional learning experiences to help prepare future health caregivers to function in a team-based model, thereby improving population health outcomes. This collaborative, representing many areas in health care, created core competencies for interprofessional collaborative practice to guide curriculum development across health profession schools.[24]

One of the identified IPEC core competencies needed to engage in safe and effective interprofessional team-based care is effective and efficient interprofessional communications. IPEC's general communication competency domain stresses the need to "communicate with patients, families, communities, and other health professionals in a responsive and responsible manner that supports a team approach to the maintenance of health and the treatment of disease."[25]

HEALTH INFORMATION TECHNOLOGY

Health informatics has expanded from the medical provider-centered use of electronic health records to public-wide availability of health information. The widespread consumer use of IT and the Internet has prompted a careful look at how health information can be used and distributed to improve access to health and health outcomes for individuals and populations. Some of the more common ways this is done is by informational websites, patient portals, social media, and telemedicine.

Multiple health care entities, public and private, use websites targeted at disease prevention and health promotion. An Internet search on any disease topic can yield vast amounts of information on the topic and deliver that information in a variety of formats: written, images, audio, and video. Furthermore, a variety of informational websites are specifically designed to effectively communicate with targeted populations to help overcome certain barriers of poor health literacy.

Websites are also used to create patient portals. The use of portals is an innovative way to enable patients to not only take responsibility for their health by being alerted to health maintenance and preventive services but also enables the patient to engage in shared decision making through interactions with health care providers. This occurs through the ability to retrieve health information via the portal at any given time and at any place in the world with Internet capability.

Online social network platforms such as blogs, forums, Facebook, and Twitter are other ways for patients and communities to build relationships and share health information. Individuals can tell their stories, relate their progress, and relay resources that others may use to overcome health issues.

Telemedicine is a way to use technology to deliver health services across distances. It can be used to remotely monitor patients, consult specialists, and assist in surgeries. It is commonly used in hospitals, surgical settings, clinics, and medical homes. Telemedicine uses two-way video, email, smartphones, wireless tools, and other forms of telecommunications technology.[26]

The speed, scope, and scale to which we are rapidly using, adopting, and adapting IT in the health arena may be both promising and fascinating, but it is not without its challenges. Social media and dedicated emerging technologies can blur the lines between expert and peer medical opinions.[27] Other challenges include making user-friendly applications; access to computers; access to the Internet; navigational ability; and how to help people synthesize, process, and deal with conflicts in information. However, one of the biggest challenges of all is in the ability to measure and evaluate the actual and direct impact of IT on health outcomes.

PROFESSIONALISM AND CONDUCT

Professionalism and conduct are communicated through any and all forms of human interactions. Common ways people communicate their intentions are through written, verbal, and nonverbal (gestures, movement, eye contact) methods. Social media serves as a major communication platform that can incorporate all three of these methods.

The American Medical Association, while recognizing the great potential of social media in disseminating important health information and building and maintaining provider–patient relationships, also cautions providers to be mindful of professionalism in its article, "Professionalism in the Use Social Media." Although geared toward physicians, this article is applicable to all health care professionals and students when engaging with patients in any form of social media relations, among which are summarized below.

- Maintain patient privacy in all environments.
- Realize that privacy may not be assured even when using privacy settings and what is posted online may never be able to be permanently erased.
- Monitor information posted.
- Maintain appropriate physician–patient relationship boundaries in accordance with ethical guidelines.
- Any unprofessional content violating professional norms posted by colleagues should be reported to the colleague and if necessary to proper authorities if the content remains posted.

- Recognize that online behavior and posts can negatively affect the person's professional reputation among patients and colleagues. This can adversely impact one's health care career by undermining public trust. Medical students should particularly heed caution.[28]

Professional conduct is an important aspect of the PA profession. Being a relatively new health profession that is scrutinized for gaining more and more responsibility for the delivery of health care, PAs cannot afford breaches of professionalism that would undermine public trust and hinder public acceptance of PAs as competent providers. Professionalism is engrained in PA training, and upon graduation, the PA is expected to conduct him- or herself in accordance with professional standards.

Physician assistants are held accountable for professionalism in all phases of training and interactions with patients and the public. Accreditation standards for professionalism state that "the curriculum must include instruction about intellectual honesty and appropriate academic and professional conduct."[29] Furthermore, the accreditation standards explain that "The role of the PA demands intelligence, sound judgment, intellectual honesty, appropriate interpersonal skills and the capacity to respond to emergencies in a calm and reasoned manner. Essential attributes of the graduate PA include an attitude of respect for self and others, adherence to the concepts of privilege and confidentiality in communicating with patients and a commitment to the patient's welfare."[29]

It is important for students and practicing clinicians to be aware of two considerations regarding the credentialing process in states, clinics, surgery centers, and hospitals. The first is that these entities ask questions of faculty, peers, and evaluators about the applicant's display of professionalism and conduct. The second is part of routine quality assurance. It is common that patients will be surveyed about their health care experiences with health care providers and staff in these settings. It is incumbent for students and practicing clinicians to be cognizant that their interactions with administration, staff, peers, and patients are at the highest level of professional conduct.

CONCLUSION

This chapter was written to explain communication issues and the various ways to handle health literacy, health IT, social media, and professionalism. The following are key points to recall about the information within this chapter.

KEY POINTS

- Communication is a complex process, and methods used to effectively communicate with patients and with other professions are continually evolving.
- Health literacy and cultural competency are essential to improved health outcomes and equal access to care.
- Health IT has the ability to overcome barriers to health care delivery systems by enabling people to interact with their health care providers over distances.
- Social media is a way to build and maintain patient relationships and guide medical care to patients and populations.
- Professional conduct is not only crucial to the individual professional but also to the PA profession as a whole in terms of public trust and acceptance.

References

1. *Health Literacy*. Bethesda, MD: National Institutes of Health (NIH). http://www.nih.gov/institutes-nih/nih-office-director/office-communications-public-liaison/clear-communication/health-literacy. Accessed December 1, 2016.
2. *The Most Important Skill in Medicine*. Medscape. http://www.medscape.com/viewarticle/764270. Accessed December 1, 2016.
3. Paget L, et al. Patient-Clinician Communication: Basic Principles and Expectations. Washington, D.C.: Institute of Medicine. 2011. http://www.accp.com/docs/positions/misc/iompatientcliniciandiscussionpaper.pdf. Accessed December 1, 2015.
4. *Impact of Communication in Healthcare*. Institute for Healthcare Communication. http://healthcarecomm.org/about-us/impact-of-communication-in-healthcare/. Accessed December 1, 2016.
5. Asnani MR. *Patient-Physician Communication*. West Indian Med J 2009;58(4):357-361. http://caribbean.scielo.org/pdf/wimj/v58n4/v58n4a12.pdf. Accessed December 1, 2015.
6. Dine CJ, et al. Feasibility and Validation of Real-Time Patient Evaluations of Internal Medicine Interns' Communication and Professionalism Skills. Journal of Graduate Medical Education, 2014;71-77. http://www.jgme.org/doi/pdf/10.4300/JGME-D-13-00173.1. Accessed December 1, 2016.
7. *Communication Among Caregivers*. Chronicle of Nursing. 2008. http://www.asrn.org/journal-nursing/376-communication-among-caregivers.html. Accessed December 1, 2016.
8. *The need for a more effective approach to continuing patient care*. Chicago: The Joint Commission. 2012. http://www.jointcommission.org/assets/1/18/Hot_Topics_Transitions_of_Care.pdf. Accessed December 1, 2015.
9. Greenberg CC, et al. Patterns of Communication Breakdowns Resulting in Injury to Surgical Patients. J Am Coll Surg. 2007; 204(4):533-40. http://www.atulgawande.com/documents/2007JACS–CommunicationBreakdowns.pdf. Accessed November 30, 2016.
10. Gandhi TK, et al. Communication breakdown in the outpatient referral process. *J Gen Intern Med*. 2000;15(9):626–631. http://dx.doi.org/10.1046/j.1525-1497.2000.91119.x.
11. Tsukamoto T, et al. The contribution of the medical history for the diagnosis of simulated cases by medical students. International Journal of Medical Education. 2012;3:78-82. http://www.ijme.net/archive/3/diagnosis-by-medical-students.pdf. Accessed December 1, 2016.
12. American Society of Hospital Pharmacists. ASHP guidelines on preventing medication errors in hospitals. *Am J Hosp Pharm*. 1993;50:305–14. https://www.ashp.org/DocLibrary/BestPractices/MedMisGdlHosp.aspx. Accessed December 1, 2016.
13. *Learn About Health Literacy*. Atlanta: Centers for Disease Control and Prevention. 2016. http://www.cdc.gov/healthliteracy/learn/. Accessed December 1, 2015.
14. Health Literacy. Rockville, MD: American Speech-Language-Hearing Association. http://www.asha.org/slp/healthliteracy/. Accessed December 1, 2016.
15. Health Literacy: A Prescription to End Confusion. Washington, D.C.: National Academies Press. 2004. https://iom.national-academies.org/~/media/Files/Report%20Files/2004/Health-Literacy-A-Prescription-to-End-Confusion/healthliteracyfinal.pdf. Accessed December 1, 2016.
16. Health Literacy Introduction. Bethesda, MD: National Network of Libraries of Medicine. 2012. https://nnlm.gov/ner/training/material/HealthLiteracyIntroduction.pdf. Accessed December 1, 2016.
17. Paasche-Orlow MK, Wolf MS. The causal pathways linking health literacy to health outcomes. *Am J Health Behav*. 2007;31(1):S19–S26.
18. Kreuter MW, Wray RJ. Tailored and targeted health communication: strategies for enhancing information relevance. *Am J Health Behav*. 2003;27(1):S227–S232.
19. *Cultural Respect*. Bethesda, MD: National Institutes of Health (NIH). http://www.nih.gov/institutes-nih/nih-office-director/office-communications-public-liaison/clear-communication/cultural-respect. Accessed December 1, 2016.
20. Burgess D, et al. Threat and health disparities: what medical educators and future physicians need to know. *J Gen Intern Med*. 2010;25(suppl 2):169–177. http://dx.doi.org/10.1007/s11606-009-1221-4.
21. Culture, Language and Health Literacy. Washington, D.C.: Health Resources and Service Administration (HRSA). http://www.hrsa.gov/culturalcompetence/index.html. Accessed December 1, 2016.
22. The Providers Guide to Quality and Culture. Cambridge, MA: Management Sciences for Health. http://erc.msh.org/mainpage.cfm?file=1.0.htm&module=provider&language=English. Accessed December 1, 2016.
23. Institute for Healthcare Improvement: The IHI Triple Aim. http://www.ihi.org/engage/initiatives/tripleaim/Pages/default.aspx. Accessed December 1, 2016.
24. About the Interprofessional Education Collaborative (IPEC). Washington, D.C.: IPEC. www.ipecollaborative. https://www.ipecollaborative.org/About_IPEC.html. Accessed December 1, 2016.
25. Interprofessional Education Collaborative Expert Panel. *Core competencies for interprofessional collaborative practice: Report of an expert panel*. Washington, D.C.: Interprofessional Education Collaborative. 2011. https://ipecollaborative.org/uploads/IPEC-Core-Competencies.pdf. Accessed December 1, 2016.

26. What Is Telemedicine. Washington, D.C. The American Telemedicine Association. http://www.americantelemed.org/about-telemedicine/what-is-telemedicine#.Vl3CGb8_wsI. Accessed December 1, 2016.

27. Health Communication and Health Information Technology. Washington, D.C.: Office of Disease Prevention and Health Promotion. 2014. http://www.healthypeople.gov/2020/topics-objectives/topic/health-communication-and-health-information-technology. Accessed December 1, 2016.

28. Professionalism in the Use of Social Media. Chicago: American Medical Association. http://www.ama-assn.org/ama/pub/physician-resources/medical-ethics/code-medical-ethics/opinion9124.page?. Accessed December 1, 2015.

29. Standards of Accreditation. Johns Creek, GA: ARC-PA. 2016. http://www.arc-pa.org/accreditation/standards-of-accreditation. Accessed December 1, 2016.

The resources for this chapter can be found at www.expert consult.com.

The Faculty Resources can be found online at www.expert consult.com.

ELECTRONIC HEALTH RECORD

Roy H. Constantine

Health informatics (also known as *health care informatics, health care informatics, medical informatics, nursing informatics,* or *biomedical informatics*) is a discipline at the intersections of information science, computer science, and health care. It deals with the resources, devices, and methods required to optimize the acquisition, storage, retrieval, and use of information in health and biomedicine. Health informatics tools include not only computers but also clinical guidelines, formal medical terminologies, and information and communication systems.[1]

Health information technology (HIT) consists of electronic methods used to manage people's health and health care.[2] Legislation requires the use of certified electronic health record (EHR) technology for exchange of health information to improve the quality of health care.[3] The terms *EMR* and *EHR* are frequently interchanged.[4] However, there is a difference. The electronic medical record (EMR) is simply an electronic version of the paper chart. The EHR shares health information across the continuum of services (e.g., physicians and laboratories). Information can follow the patient through different health care settings (e.g., clinics, hospitals, nursing homes, catastrophic events). Hurricane Katrina is an example of a catastrophic event after which medical information of displaced patients was retrievable.

The personal health record (PHR) extends the capabilities of what is being called the *virtual chart*. The PHR can stand alone or be interconnected to the EHR. Capabilities include prescription refills, appointments, insurance information, and patient education.[2] Sharing of medical data in the PHR can be influenced by patients' willingness to share their condition and sociodemographic variables, which include age, education, and severity of health and public health emergencies. Although safety-monitoring mechanisms are being implemented, patient trust will ultimately facilitate support sharing.[5]

DEVELOPMENT

The 2000 Institute of Medicine (IOM) report estimated 44,000 to 98,000 deaths occur annually in the United States because of errors. The IOM's report "Crossing the Quality Chasm" emphasized that a redesign in health care should include a focus on information technology.[6] The Leapfrog Group,[7] a voluntary program focusing on the safety, quality, and affordability of health care, and The Joint Commission,[8] an accrediting body for organizations and programs, promote the implementation of the EHR. However, they also agreed with the Food and Drug Administration that "consistency, reliability, and accuracy needed to be evaluated."[9]

In 2008, only 2% of the nonfederal general acute care hospitals had a comprehensive EHR, but 7.6% had a basic EHR.[10] In 2013, basic EHR growth had increased fivefold.[11] Larger hospitals and teaching hospitals had higher utilization of electronic record systems.[12] Adoption rates did not differ among high- and low-indigent patient populations in hospitals known as the Disproportionate Share Index Hospitals (DSH).[10]

Regional Health Information Organizations (RHIOs) were designed to enhance clinical data availability and provide Health Information Exchange (HIE).[2] A federal initiative from the Office of the National Coordinator of Health Information Technology (ONCHIT) included the development of a functional health information infrastructure.[6] The ONCHIT funded Health Information Technology Regional Extension Centers (RECs). The RECs provided assistance to primary care physicians, physician assistants (PAs), and nurse practitioners in the United States to develop their EHR system.[13] The Health Information Technology Economic & Clinical Health Act (HITECH) provided an opportunity to expand the use of HIT with grants, loans, and financial assistance.[10] HITECH funds mostly supported primary care and critical-access and rural hospitals with fewer than 50 beds.[13]

Lewis[14] notes that the decision to switch his office to an electronic system provided fantasies of a streamlined, technologically efficient, and almost functionless setting, which in reality was not the case. Practices and organizations need to use the EHR now to avoid penalties. Improved outcomes occur when emphasis is placed on better technology, integration, and privacy concerns.[15] One should consider the implementation of an EHR system in an institution with 200 or more beds to take the same time as completion of construction on a new hospital building.[9]

MEANINGFUL USE

Recent federal initiatives include the American Reinvestment and Recovery Act (ARRA), for which "meaningful use" incentives were applied in order to meet performance metrics. Assisted by the Centers for Medicare & Medicaid Services (CMS), stage I and stage II of meaningful use requirements includes the "capturing of information and the exchange of information."[16] ARRA focuses on standards, quality needs, functionality, communication, and government program links. This also includes transmitting prescriptions to the pharmacy electronically and demonstrating the capability of the EHR to electronically exchange key information.[10]

Beginning in 2016, penalties will be applied if meaningful use quality and efficiency criteria are not met. As each stage progressed, the ability to meet these criteria became more difficult.[17] With stage III, in 2017, interoperability among different health care EMR systems will allow for greater sharing of information. The concern with the advent of ICD-10 (International Statistical Classification of Diseases and Related Health Problems—World Health Organization [WHO] medical classification) is that the degree of interoperability will become limited.[18,19] Clinical information exchanges among different health care systems may not occur because of the higher requirement for mapping needed to ensure standardization in terminology.[20] Many advisory organizations, including the American Medical Association, believe that more time is necessary to build these mechanisms so that "adoption and innovation" occur.[21]

IMPLEMENTATION

Major EHR market vendors include Cerner, Eclipsys, EPIC, iMD Soft, McKesson Provider Technologies, MediTech, Misys Healthcare Systems, Philips Medical Systems, Picis, and Siemens.[9] In 2004, the military implemented the Armed Forces Longitudinal Technology Application, which is the Department of Defense's global health record.[22]

When choosing a system, it is important to look at the success of the system in the marketplace. Ideally, you would speak with other institutions that have implemented the same system and discuss customer satisfaction. Workflow implications differ for various stakeholders within institutions.[23] Approximately 30% of EHR implementations fail because of steep learning curves and loss of productivity. The development of a flexible navigation system, enhanced functionality, and the ability to complement your work will enhance usability.[24]

It is essential to secure organizational commitment when EHR implementation is going to occur. A broad group of extrinsic and intrinsic stakeholders needs to be involved in the implementation process. Change is not an easy concept. Therefore, the existence of a change management organizational culture is essential. Intentional planning that is clear and consistent with the vision and principles of the organization must be present.[25]

It is important that PAs become incorporated early in the process of EHR development. Factors that go beyond technology can hinder HIE.[26] The cultural change is even more important than the challenge with technology. Work sessions need to be created to enhance training, develop workflows, and limit complaints during the process.[27]

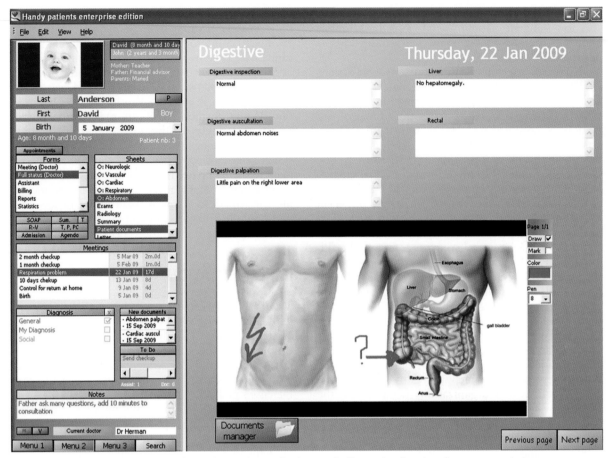

FIG. 22.1 ■ Sample of an electronic medical record. (From the Creative Commons website. http://creativecommons.org/licenses/by-sa/3.0/us/.)

Many clinicians think that EMR is a direct extension of computerized physician order entry (CPOE) and that improvements in functionality, performance, learning curves, and technology have resulted.[28] A selected group of subject matter experts (SMEs) should develop order set content. Integrating general admission order sets with disease-specific order sets improves outcomes.[29] Selected PAs with subject matter expertise strengthen the integration process. PAs who use specific order sets can incorporate evidence-based links to enhance core-measure compliance. Development of order sets will increase utilization, time, and compliance in addition to eliminating discrepancies with handwriting, signature, dating, and timing in the EHR (Fig. 22.1). A good example is in the recent development of the Surviving Sepsis Campaign Order Sets in which critical elements must be met with the first hour, third hour, and sixth hour of resuscitation (e.g., blood cultures, broad-spectrum antibiotics, lactate levels, crystalloids, possible vasopressors, and repeat lactate levels).

Mandatory elements in the EHR include a problem list, a medication list, vital signs, allergies, a smoking record, discharge documentation, a discharge summary, CPOE for medications, drug-to-drug and drug-to-allergy checks, the ability to electronically exchange key clinical information, decision support, security, laboratory test results, patient list of conditions, patient-specific education sources, and medication reconciliation. Critical value alerts can be incorporated into an EMR screening system for early recognition of potentially life-threatening outcomes. Additional functions include advanced directives, electronic surveillance, and the ability to submit electronic data to public health organizations.[12] A dedicated integrity and clinical content team becomes essential in monitoring and recommending improvements within a system.

Functionality is incorporated across services and commonly occurs in laboratory data, radiology images, and radiology reports.[10,30] Whereas laboratory data and reports are considered to be passive, writing progress notes and CPOE are considered to be active.[9] Clinical information and data should be handled at "point of care" or in "real time."[6] Device integration allows bar coding and hemodynamic data to be immediately charted.[6,9]

Physician assistant "champions" are integral in the necessary training and reinforcement during the EHR initiative. If hospital-wide implementation follows a big-bang initiative, then administrative recommendations are made to be 100% paperless. Other hospitals may want to start slowly with one service at a time being integrated into the paperless process. System failures have been noted when a paper backup is required. The prevention of work-arounds is essential with both approaches to minimize safety flaws and incidents. When too much nonessential information is populated into a note, a condition called "note bloat" occurs. Attention to the body of the content becomes unfocused, with greater focus placed on only the assessment and plan and not the note itself. Copy and pasting or copy forwarding has resulted in inaccurate information being posted and ultimately can result in a sentinel event.

BENEFITS AND BARRIERS TO IMPLEMENTING ELECTRONIC HEALTH RECORDS

Benefits to implementing an EHR immediately starts with improved legibility, dating, and timing. Greater emphasis on CPOE will perpetuate meaningful use implementation and best practice advisories. Improved encounter classifications enhance the ability to assess and review patient information with universal access in real time. Over a wide range of patient populations,[31] the quality of personal performance responses is thought to improve.[32]

Barriers to implementing an EHR immediately starts with cost, purchasing, implementation, and maintenance.[2,33] The time involved in educational training and medical record keeping continues to become more involved.[34] Failure can result if extrinsic and intrinsic stakeholders are not part of a strong interdisciplinary steering committee. The benefit to quality is still not clear, but other benefits such as "efficiency, patient engagement and health care information" are thought to exist.[35] A reluctance to embrace new technology is evident.[31] Current and precise information is essential; otherwise, the belief of "garbage in, garbage out" holds true.[32]

SECURITY

The Health Insurance Portability and Accountability Act (HIPAA) focuses on unauthorized access to patient data and improper disclosure of health information.[2] Sole providers are becoming a rarity, with authorized disclosure of this information being available to the workplace and insurance companies. Therefore, disclosure of health information is considered to be beyond the boundaries of the Hippocratic oath.[36] Hospitals need to create new relationships to control the medical record and increase this control. Legal issues include who views the medical record because multiple clinicians and institutions are involved. The privacy of the data must be secured at all times. Screens should be logged off when active use is discontinued. Warnings and alerts in the record should not be overridden, and if a safety issue occurs, appropriate reporting is necessary.[37] The incorporation of passwords and logouts is helpful.[9]

Layman[38] notes that the EHR must maintain the ethical elements of beneficence, autonomy, fidelity, and justice. If there is a breach in the EHR, the patient needs to be informed about the breach and potential harm that can occur. Ethical procedures for disclosure must be made along with a time frame. A discussion on how the breach occurred, what was breached, the consequences, and corrective action must be made. At all times, the interest of the patient must be supported.[39]

SAFETY

A critical analysis of the EHR literature focuses on distractions. The comparison is the same as texting and driving and in the hospital setting has become virally known as "distracted doctoring." Reestablishing necessary etiquette in the use of computers, tablet computers, smartphones, and mobile devices is essential in bedside communication and examination skills.[40]

The Joint Commission has stressed increased awareness of safety risks and preventable adverse events that occur with the use of electronic communication devices before a go-live period. These include:[41]

1. Examine workflow processes and procedures for risk and inefficiencies.
2. Actively involve clinicians and staff who will be affected by the technology.
3. Assess your organization's technology needs (review vendors and other organizations).

4. During the introduction of new technology, continuously monitor for problems, and address any issues as quickly as possible (workarounds or incomplete error reporting).
5. Establish a training program.
6. Develop and communicate policies delineating staff authorized and responsible for technology implementation, use, oversight, and safety review.
7. Before taking a technology live, ensure that all standardized order sets and guidelines are developed, tested on paper, and approved by the Pharmacy and Therapeutics Committee.
8. Develop a graduated system of safety alerts in the new technology.

The Joint Commission has also stressed risks associated with the EHR's ability to detect and prevent errors. These include[42]:

1. Human–computer interface (33%): ergonomics and usability issues resulting in data-related errors
2. Workflow and communication (24%): issues relating to health information technology support of communication and teamwork
3. Clinical content (23%): design or data issues relating to clinical content or decision support
4. International organizational policies, procedure, and culture (6%)
5. People (6%): training and failure to follow established processes
6. Hardware and software (6% software design issues and other hardware/software problems)
7. External factors (1%): vendor and other external issues
8. System measurement and monitoring (1%)

Suggested actions include a "culture of safety, utilization of the performance improvement process and strong leadership."[42]

As a PA, it is important to be a key member of your organization's interdisciplinary EHR team. Because "human infallibility is impossible, the only chance to keep human errors from hurting patients is by creating collegial interactive teams."[43]

CLINICAL APPLICATIONS

- How would you determine the best EHR for your organization?
- How would you monitor meaningful use metrics and content integrity?
- Discuss budget requirements, device selection, staffing, and training for your organization's EHR.
- Discuss the importance of HIPAA in the development of your organization's health information security policy.

KEY POINTS

- PAs are savvy and passionate clinicians who provide testing, training, and end-user support.
- PAs are subject matter experts who are integral in template development, clinical content, and workflows.
- In addition to the mandatory elements of the electronic health record, PAs have expertise in the integration of performance indicators, handoff communication, and the development of the legal chart.
- Avoid cutting and pasting and copy forwarding. Inaccurate data that are duplicated can result in a sentinel event.
- Focus on writing concise notes with current data. Avoid note bloat!

References

1. *Health Informatics*, Wikipedia, 2016. http://en.wikipedia.org/wiki/Health_informatics. Accessed December 1, 2016.
2. *Health Information Technology in the United States—Where We Stand.* Robert Wood Johnson Foundation, Massachusetts General Hospital, and the George Washington University; 2008.
3. Murphy EM, Oxencis CJ, Klauck JA, et al. Medication reconciliation at an academic medical enter: implementation of a comprehensive program from admission to discharge. *Am J Health System Pharm.* 2009;66:2126.
4. Ong K. *Medical Informatics—An Executive Primer.* Chicago: Healthcare Information and Management Systems Society; 2007.
5. Weitzman E. Sharing medical data for health research: the early personal health record experience. *J Med Internet Res.* 2010;12:e14.
6. Palacio C, Harrison JP, Garets D. Benchmarking electronic medical record initiatives in the US: a conceptual model. *J Med Syst.* 2010;34:273–279.
7. *About us and our mission.* The Leapfrog Group. 2016. http://www.leapfroggroup.org/about_us. Accessed December 1, 2016.
8. *DataMart*, Chicago: The Joint Commission. 2016. http://www.jointcommission.org/about_us/data_mart.aspx. Accessed December 1, 2016.
9. Friedman L, Halpern N, Fackler J. Implementing an electronic medical record. *Critical Care Clinics.* 2007;23:347.

10. *Health Information Technology in the United States—On the Cusp of Change*. Robert Wood Johnson Foundation, Massachusetts General Hospital, and the George Washington University; 2009.

11. Charles D, Gabriel M, Furukawa M. (2014, May). *Adoption of Electronic Health Record Systems among U.S. Non-federal Acute Care Hospitals: 2008-2013*. Retrieved November 27, 2015, from https://www.healthit.gov/sites/default/files/onc databrief9final.pdf.

12. Jha AK, DesRoches CM, Kralovec PD, Joshi MS. A progress report on electronic health records in U.S. hospitals. *Health Affairs (Millwood)*. 2010;29:1951–1957.

13. Maxson E, Jain S, Kendall M, et al. The Regional Extension Program Center program: helping physicians meaningfully use health information technology. *Ann Intern Med*. 2010;153:666.

14. Lewis S. Brave new EMR. *Ann Intern Med*. 2011;154:368.

15. Abraham S. Technological trends in health care. *Health Care Manag*. 2010;29:318.

16. O'Neill T. Primer: EHR Stage 3 Meaningful Use Requirements. American Action Forum. Retrieved on November 5, 2015, from http://americanactionforum.org/research/primer-her-stage-3-meaningful-use-requirements.

17. Early Results of the Meaningful Use Program for Electronic Health Records — NEJM. (n.d.). Retrieved November 15, 2015, from http://www.nejm.org/doi/full/10.1056/NEJMc1213481.

18. Lareau D. 5 EHR considerations for the ICD-10 conversion. Government Health IT. Retrieved November 16, 2015, from http://www.govhealthit.com/print/15847.

19. Jacob J. On the road to interoperability: public and private organizations work to connect health care data. *JAMA*. 2015;314(12):1213–1215.

20. Mace S. ICD-10 and EHR Fuel Clinical Documentation Improvements. *HealthLeaders Media*. March 18, 2014. Retrieved November 16, 2015, from http://healthleadersmedia.com/content.cfm?topic=TEC&content_id=302012.

21. *AMA and Others Call for Pause in Meaningful Use Program*. Chicago: American Medical Association Sept. 17, 2015. http://www.ama-assn.org/ama/pub/news/news/2015/2015-09-17-ama-calls-pause-in-meaningful-use-program.page.

22. Electronic Medical Records. Santa Monica, CA: Rand Corporation. 2016. http://www.rand.org/topics/electronic-medical-records.html. Accessed December 1, 2016.

23. *Electronic Health Records*. Agency for Healthcare Research and Quality (AHRQ). https://healthit.ahrq.gov/ahrq-funded-projects/emerging-lessons/electronic-health-records. Accessed December 1, 2016.

24. Smelcer J, Miller-Jacobs H, Kantrovich H. Usability of electronic medical records. *Int J Usability Stud*. 2009;4:70.

25. McGrath D. The sociology of change. *J Med Pract Manage*. 2009;25:105.

26. Vest J. More than just a question of technology: factors related to hospitals' adoption and implementation of health information exchange. *Int J Med Inform*. 2010;79:797.

27. Devore S, Figlioli K. Lessons premier hospitals learned about implementing electronic health records. *Health Aff*. 2010;29:664.

28. Vishwanath A, Singh SR, Winkelstein P, et al. The impact of electronic medical record systems on outpatient workflows: a longitudinal evaluation of its workflow effects. *Int J Med Inform*. 2010;79:778.

29. Munasinghe R, Arsene C, Abraham TK, et al. Improving the utilization of admission order sets in a computerized physician order entry system by integrating modular disease specific order subsets into a general medicine admission order set. *J Am Med Inform Assoc*. 2011;18:322.

30. *Health Information Technology in the United States—Moving Towards Meaningful Use*. Robert Wood Johnson Foundation, Massachusetts General Hospital, and the George Washington University; 2010.

31. Harrison J, Palachio C. The role of clinical information systems in health care quality improvement. *Health Care Manag*. 2006;25:206.

32. Holden R. Physicians' beliefs about using EMR and CPOE: in pursuit of a contextualized understanding of health IT use behavior. *Int J Med Inform*. 2010;79:71.

33. Jha A, DesRoches CM, Campbell EG, et al. Use of electronic health records in U.S. hospitals. *N Engl J Med*. 2009;360:1628.

34. Tevaarwerk G. Electronic medical records. *Can Med Assoc J*. 2008;178:1323.

35. Thompson G, O'Horo J, Pickering B, Herasevich V. Impact of the electronic medical record on mortality, length of stay, and cost in the hospital and ICU. *Crit Care Med*. 2015;43(6):1276–1282.

36. Rothstein M. The Hippocratic bargain and health information technology. *J Law Med Ethics*. 2010;38:7.

37. Sitting D, Sing H. Legal, ethical and financial dilemmas in electronic health record adoption and use. *Am Acad Pediatr*. 2011;124:31042.

38. Layman E. Ethical issues and the electronic health record. *Health Care Manag*. 2008;27:165.

39. Council on Ethical & Judicial Affairs (CEJA). Chicago: American Medical Association. 2016. http://www.ama-assn.org/resources/doc/hod/a-09-ceja-opinons-reports.pdf. Accessed May 10, 2011.

40. Papadakos P. Electronic distractions of the respiratory therapist and their impact on patient safety. *Respir Care*. 2014;59(8):1306–1309.

41. *Safely implementing health information and converging technologies* Chicago: The Joint Commission. December 11, 2008. Retrieved November 16, 2015, from. http://www.jointcommission.org/sentinel_event_alert_issue_42_safely_implementing_health_information_and_converging_technologies/.

42. *Safe use of health information technology*. Chicago, The Joint Commission. March 31, 2015. Retrieved November 15, 2015, from http://www.jointcommission.org/assets/1/18/SEA_54.pdf.

43. Nance JJ. *Why Hospitals Should Fly – The Ultimate Flight Plan to Patient Safety and Quality Care*. Bozeman, MT: Second River Healthcare Press; 2012.

The resources for this chapter can be found at www.expertconsult.com.

The Faculty Resources can be found online at www.expertconsult.com.

CHAPTER 23

PATIENT EDUCATION

Patty J. Scholting • Erin Hoffman

CHAPTER OUTLINE

BARRIERS TO PATIENT EDUCATION Patient Barriers Provider Barriers Health Literacy	**PROVIDING STRUCTURE FOR EFFECTIVE PATIENT EDUCATION** **KEY POINTS**

Patient education is an integral part of every health care interaction. It is one of the most powerful tools a health care provider can use to influence positive changes in health and wellness for patients. Whether the visit requires a diagnostic study, lifestyle changes, or a medication, the provider will offer the necessary patient education to the patient. Effective patient education provides patients with the information they need to make informed decisions regarding their health. Proper teaching must go beyond simple instructions such as how to take a medication correctly. Patient education allows us to address disease prevention, safety, nutrition, and physical activity. It also serves to manage expectations for procedures or future visits. Perhaps most important, the process of patient education creates an environment that facilitates relationship building, increases patient trust, and builds rapport between the patient and provider.[1] Patients have an expectation that they will be fully informed about their health and treatment plans. The challenge then becomes how to do so effectively.[2]

BARRIERS TO PATIENT EDUCATION

If the process of educating patients was simple and straightforward, it is likely that the prevalence of some of the most common health problems, such as heart disease and type II diabetes, would be decreasing due to the successful implementation of lifestyle modifications taught by providers. Many barriers can stand in the way of effective patient education and its ability to motivate patients to change. Many factors can adversely affect the communication

between a physician assistant (PA) and her or his patient. Age, gender, socioeconomic status, ability to learn, provider skill, and a patient's environment are just a few of the potential barriers in the patient-provider interaction. In addition, simply arming patients with knowledge is enough to create meaningful change. The provider must assess the patient's motivation and ability to implement changes.[3] This chapter is designed to help PAs understand some common reasons patient education fails to translate into positive health behavior change.

Barriers to patient education can be simplified into two categories: communication barriers and implementation barriers. An interaction with an elderly patient can illustrate both types of barriers. An older man with hearing loss may struggle to hear the provider but smile and nod anyway, indicating to the PA that he understands her message. Unfortunately, the patient will not be able to act on the PA's advice because he never heard her advice. An implementation barrier exists when the patient hears and understands the instructions but faces obstacles that may prevent him from implementing these instructions. Common implementation barriers include the inability to afford recommended medications, lack of transportation to and from appointments, or the lack of vision or dexterity needed to carry out treatment recommendations. In most patient interactions, both communication and implementation barriers are present and must be managed by negotiation between the patient and the provider. To successfully overcome them, a deeper understanding of these barriers is essential.

Patient Barriers

Most patients want to avoid the discomfort and costs associated with chronic disease, yet providers struggle to get patients to follow their advice on how to prevent or effectively manage these disorders. Motivation is a determining factor in the successful implementation of patient education and a health care plan. Some patients receive the teaching that is provided and implement it successfully; however, many do not. It is common for providers to seek innovative ways to inspire and motivate patients. In the past, fear tactics were used as the primary tool to motivate patients. Fear works for some people, but for many, it isn't enough to inspire action.[4] Fear can lead patients to develop attitudes of denial, avoidance, or hopelessness.[4]

Motivation is an intrinsic quality that is difficult to influence. The stages of change model developed by Feldman allows the provider to assess where the patient is in her willingness to implement a change in behavior.[5] Using this model allows providers to identify which patients are ready and motivated to make a change and which patients need more information and encouragement.

Feldman's stages are precontemplation, contemplation, preparation, maintenance, and relapse.[5] These stages can be applied in any situation during which a provider is asking a patient to make a behavioral change. Smoking cessation counseling is used as an example here.

A patient in the *precontemplation* stage is aware that smoking is bad for him or her but will either dismiss the problem or deny it.[5] This patient might resist change by using an example of someone he or she knows who smoked his or her whole life and never became unwell. This patient is not motivated or willing to make a change yet.

In the *contemplation stage*, the patient is more aware of the problem, may begin to articulate a desire to quit smoking, and understands some of the benefits of doing so.[5] This patient will weigh the desire to change against the perceived benefits of continuing to smoke. A patient in the contemplation stage might make a few attempts at change, but these efforts are often inconsistent and short-lived.

During the *preparation stage*, the patient is ready to commit to making a change.[5] In this stage, the patient who smokes is willing to set a quit date. The patient has not yet implemented any changes but exhibits a willingness to do so.

Patients in the *action stage* are actively engaged in executing behavioral change.[5] The patient has reached his or her preestablished quit date and is using a provider-recommended plan of action to successfully avoid smoking. This stage requires daily effort to maintain the change to avoid smoking.

When the patient reaches the *maintenance stage*, the implemented behavioral change has become a habit.[5] The patient may not need to use daily strategies to feel like he or she is able to maintain a smoke-free life. During this stage, the change begins to feel more integrated into normal life. The final stage is *relapse*, which is exactly as it sounds. This is when the patient begins to smoke again after a period of success.[5] Not all patients will relapse. Feldman's model, however, encourages both patients and providers to anticipate and plan for what will happen if relapse occurs.

Physician assistants who take the time to assess where the patient's willingness to change can tailor the message to the patient in a way that encourages him to move toward the action and maintenance stages. For example, if a patient is solidly in the precontemplation stage, the provider should not see the task as impossible and avoid the conversation with the patient about smoking cessation. Conversely, it would be premature for the provider to attempt to engage the patient in a plan of action for smoking cessation because the patient is not yet ready for this step. Instead, the PA should engage the patient in a conversation targeted at moving the patient from the precontemplation stage to the contemplation stage. The provider should use the time to understand the patient's concerns and correct any misperceptions the patient might have. The provider should always encourage the patient to let the provider know when he might want to talk about making a change. Similar provider strategies exist for each stage, which are designed to increase and encourage patient readiness for change (Table 23.1).

Patients give many reasons for their previous failed attempts to change behavior or their current unwillingness to attempt change. Common reasons include lack of time, lack of family support, level of difficulty, cost, time of high stress, and lack of resources. If two similar patients want to start an exercise program, both of whom are in the preparation stage but have similar barriers such as stressful jobs, lack of time, and no gym access, why is one successful and the other unsuccessful? Patients have belief systems that influence their faith in their ability to overcome obstacles.[6] These barrier-beliefs create rationalizations and excuses that undermine a patient's ability to succeed.[6] Ultimately, if these rationalizations and excuses are not managed by the health care provider and the patient together, the patient will give up on change. Barrier beliefs are created by the patient's past experiences and perceptions and can be divided into three distinct categories: attributions,

TABLE 23.1 **Provider Strategies**		
Stage of Change	**Patient Characteristics**	**Provider Strategies**
Precontemplation	Denies problem and its importance Is reluctant to discuss problem Problem is identified by others Shows reactance when pressured High risk of argument	Ask permission to discuss problem. Inquire about the patient's thoughts. Gently point out discrepancies. Express concern. Ask the patient to think, talk, or read about the situation between visits.

Contemplation	Shows openness to talk, read,
	   and think about the problem
	Weighs pros and cons
	Dabbles in action
	Can be obsessive about problem
	   and can prolong stage
	Understands that change is needed
	Begins to form a commitment to specific
	   goals, methods, and timetables
		Elicit the patient's perspective first.
		Help identify the pros and cons.
		Ask what would promote commitment.
		Suggest trials.
		Summarize the patient's reasons for change.
		Negotiate a start date to begin some or
		   all change activities.

Preparation and
   determination
	Can picture overcoming obstacles
	May procrastinate about setting a
	   start date for change
	Follows a plan of regular activity
	   to change the problem
	Can describe the plan in detail
		Encourage the patient to announce publicly,
		Arrange a follow-up contact at or shortly after start
		   date.
		Show interest in the specifics of the plan.
		Discuss the difference between a slip and relapse.
		Help anticipate how to handle a slip.

Action	Shows commitment in facing obstacles
	Resists slips
	Is particularly vulnerable to abandoning
	   effort impulsively
	Has accomplished change or improvement
	   through focused action
	Has varying levels of awareness regarding
	   the importance of long-term vigilance
		Support and reemphasize the pros of changing.
		Help to modify the action plan if aspects are not
		   working well.
		Arrange follow-up contact for support.
		Show respect and admiration.
		Inquire about feelings and expectations and
		   how well they were met.
		Ask about slips and any signs of wavering
		   commitment.

Maintenance	May already be losing ground through
	   slips or wavering commitment
	Has feelings about how much the change
	   has actually improved life.
	May be developing a lifestyle that
	   precludes relapse into former problem
		Help create a plan for intensifying activity
		   if slips occur.
		Support lifestyle and personal redefinition
		   that reduce the risk of relapse.
		Reflect on the long-term and possibly permanent
		   nature of this stage as opposed to the more
		   immediate gratification of initial success.

From Feldman MD, Christensen JF, eds. *Behavioral Medicine: A Guide for Clinical Practice.* 4th ed. New York: McGraw-Hill Education; 2014.

self-efficacy, and negative outcome expectations.[6] For a provider to successfully encourage patients to adhere to treatment plans, these three elements should be considered.

Attributions are the reasons a patient uses to explain her lack of success in implementing a change or a strategy.[6] It is human nature to ascribe meaning and reasoning to an undesirable behavior or outcome. These attributions can be factual, interpreted, and even implausible.[6] For example, if a patient is asked to take a medication for hypertension every day, he or she may use the following attributions to explain why he or she is unable to do so. Factual: "I cannot afford the medication." Interpreted: "Taking medication every day will be too many chemicals for

my body to handle." Implausible (or misinformed): "Lowering my blood pressure will make my heart have to work harder to get blood to my feet, so it will wear out my heart if I take this medication." The type of attribution used by the patient will direct the PA's response.

Self-efficacy is the patient's belief that she is capable of completing an action or meeting a goal.[6] Self-efficacy is often the decisive factor in determining success or failure. If one patient believes he or she can exercise on a regular basis, then that patient will overcome her busy schedule and lack of gym membership. However, if the patient does not believe she is capable of exercising on a regular basis, the barriers will prevent the patient from achieving her goal.

Many factors influence a person's self-efficacy: previous failures or successes, other people's failures or successes, other people's opinions regarding their ability to succeed, low self-esteem, or knowledge about the steps needed to achieve the goal.[6]

Negative outcome experiences are beliefs that implementing change will precipitate an undesirable outcome.[6] These outcomes could be social, physical, or monetary.[6] For example, dieters may have one of the following reasons for not dieting. Social: "My family won't eat the healthy food I make, and it is important that we eat the same foods." Physical: "I feel tired in the afternoons when I eat healthy so I have to eat more." Monetary: "Healthy food is really expensive, and the food spoils so quickly. I can't afford to do this."

Health care providers must consider these dynamics when counseling their patients. If the provider does not account for a patient's willingness to change and the patient's belief in his or her ability to make a change, the provider cannot tailor the message to the patient to give the greatest opportunity for long-term success. Without tailored education, the patient is less likely to succeed.

Provider Barriers

Physician assistants may also encounter personal barriers that can limit the potential for effective patient education. One of the most frequently cited barriers for providers is a lack of time.[7] Providers are asked to accomplish much in the brief span of an office visit. Health information is complex. When faced with limited time, PAs may provide partial information, rush the delivery of information, or choose not to provide the information at all. PAs may eliminate patient education as a part of a patient encounter because of a developed sense that education is a waste of time and does not result in appreciable change.[7] Providers who do not develop the skills to overcome patient education barriers will find patient education frustrating and perhaps even pointless.

Some PAs may think that they are not qualified to teach patients.[7] Although PAs spend much of their education learning clinical medicine, the training they receive tailored specifically to teaching and educating patients is less extensive. PAs may believe they lack detailed knowledge of rarer diagnoses and feel inadequate to teach the patient about these diseases and their management. Providers should develop a set of readily available resources to overcome this barrier.

Another barrier to effective patient communication is the tendency by some providers to speak in medical jargon.[8] Patients often feel uncomfortable interrupting a provider to say that he or she did not understand a term or phrase. Patients often simply nod and agree with the provider to hide their lack of understanding. Patients feel frustrated that they were not able to get the information they so badly need out of the encounter. Providers should monitor their own speech and ensure they are using lay terms when speaking with patients. Asking the patient to explain the concept back to the provider is an effective way to assess the patient's understanding of the information given during the encounter.

Providers are often frustrated by the difficulties patients have in recalling crucial health information provided at the visit. Even if the provider has accounted for the potential barriers to communication, research suggests that a patient will only remember a maximum of seven new pieces of information from each visit.[2] Providers commonly err by giving too much information during a single patient encounter. Less is more. Too much information overwhelms the patient, which inhibits both understanding and recall. Providers must develop the ability to prioritize information and structure the presentation of new information logically to help the patient retain the most crucial messages from the visit.[2]

Health Literacy[9,10]

Health literacy is the degree to which a patient has the ability to obtain, communicate, process, and understand health information and services to make informed health decisions.[11] Improving health literacy should begin with identifying the barriers to effective communication with a particular patient. Common health literacy barriers include:
1. The patient does not speak English.
2. The patient has never learned to read or reads poorly in any language.
3. The patient does not have sufficient numeracy to be able to manage medications or complete self-management charts.
4. The patient does not know the basics of how the body works.
5. The patient has limited education and does not understand how the scientific process is applied to diagnosis and treatment in medicine.
6. The patient does not understand statistics, probability, or the concepts of risk that are used in medical decision making.
7. The patient does not have access to a computer or does not know how to use a computer.

As PAs, it is our job to identify patients who may have health literacy struggles and provide them the information in a way that is accessible to them. Effective strategies to overcome health literacy barriers include:

1. Choose the essential information that the patient must have today, and discuss only those topics. Schedule the patient for another visit soon to give them further information. The more information you give the patient, the less likely he or she is to retain any of it. Dole it out in small pieces for easy digestion.
2. Use translators and translated materials with non–English-speaking patients. Translators (or use of a phone translation line) are required by law in the United States. Although providers occasionally use an adult friend or family member to help clarify the discussion with a limited English speaker, it is never appropriate to use a child for translation or clarification.
3. Write all patient handouts at the third grade level or below. Most commercially available word processing software includes tools for assessing the grade level of the handout. Even better educated people benefit from simple and clearly written health information.
4. Always use pictures that demonstrate the proper way to do something. Never use pictures that demonstrate the improper way to perform a skill. Patients who cannot read may confuse the two.
5. If possible, schedule a double appointment for patients who struggle with one or more health literacy challenges to allow you more time for your discussion. Use this extra time to ask the patient to explain what you have just said back to you to assess their level of comprehension.
6. Explain concepts of risk with drawings. For example, show patients what 1 in 10 means by drawing 9 people with a blue marker and one person with a red marker.
7. Ask patients if they have a computer, if they know how to use a computer, or if they have a tech-savvy friend to help them with a computer before you refer them to online education or self-management resources. Giving a URL to patients who do not have or cannot access a computer is the same as giving them no information at all.

PROVIDING STRUCTURE FOR EFFECTIVE PATIENT EDUCATION

Structure and organization are essential components to maximizing the amount of information that a patient recalls from the patient–provider interaction.[2] Although there are many models for how to structure the process of giving information to patients, most providers develop their own method and style to accomplish this task. There are key elements that should be included in the provider's approach to communication that are critical to the provider's ability to overcome barriers and work toward patient understanding and adherence. The following elements can serve as a step-by-step guide for a new provider to develop his or her process for effective patient education (Box 23.1).

1. **Introduce the patient to the topic to be discussed.** This is an important starting place. Often, providers will forge into advice and instructions without providing a context for the conversation to the patient. Providing a preview of the discussion allows the patient to establish an organizational structure for the conversation in her or his brain. It informs the patient of the purpose of the interaction and what he or she can expect from the information that will be given. It also allows the provider to be organized and thoughtful in the approach to the information. Think of this as a road map for both the provider and the patient.
2. **Assess the patient's level of knowledge and expectations.** If the PA does not assess what the patient already knows and doesn't know, he or she will be unable to tailor the message to meet the patient's needs. For example, if a PA is teaching a patient with diabetes about how many units of insulin to take for each carbohydrate unit and the patient has no understanding of carbohydrate counting, this patient education would be completely ineffective and potentially dangerous. Taking time to assess the patient's current knowledge allows the provider to identify misinformation, prioritize information delivery, and determine a starting point for teaching. A PA might ask a patient with diabetes, "Can you tell me what you have been taught about diabetes?" "How do you think the treatment will help your diabetes?" or "How does exercise affect the control of your

---

BOX 23.1   STEPS TO EFFECTIVE PATIENT EDUCATION

1. Introduce the patient to the topic to be discussed.
2. Assess the patient's level of knowledge and expectations.
3. Present prioritized information in plain language.
4. Assess the patient's understanding and reactions to the information.
5. Use collaborative negotiations and shared decision making.
6. Ask the patient to summarize the plan in his or her own words.
7. Plan for follow-up.

From Lloyd et al,[8] Matthys et al.,[12] and Elwyn et al.[13]

diabetes?" Providers under time pressure often make the mistake of skipping this step in the process.

It is also critical to understand patient expectations for the visit and for the future. If a provider fails to assess and fully address these expectations, it provides an additional barrier to the implementation of the treatment plan. The provider can simply asked the patient if he or she has *ideas* about what is wrong, if the patient has *concerns* or worries about what could happen, or if he or she has any *expectations* about what should be done at today's visit.[12] The acronym "ICE" can be used to remember ideas, concerns, and expectations.[12] Understanding the patient's perspective allows the provider to address the concerns raised. For example, a patient may report to the PA that he or she believes that elevated blood sugar levels are attributable to a new exercise regimen. If the PA is aware of this belief, he or she can take the time to educate the patient about exercise and diabetic management. If a patient confides that he or she is terrified of needles and will do anything to avoid insulin shots, the provider can evaluate other potential treatments or manage the concern if insulin is needed. Finally, if the patient has an expectation, no matter how outrageous, the provider must know about it to be able to meet it or address it. For example, if a patient with diabetes expects that he or she will eventually be cured by a pancreas transplant and assumes that other treatments are temporary, the provider can spend time educating the patient about realistic current treatments and potential future treatments.

3. **Present prioritized information in plain language.** This is the provider's opportunity to teach the patient what he or she needs to know. The goal is to provide enough information for success while avoiding so much information the patient is overwhelmed. Start with the most important piece of information first, and keep the number of items addressed small.[2,8] Speak in plain language. The patient should not need to ask the definition of a word or the meaning of a phrase. Patient understanding can be enhanced by using drawings, models, or other visual aids when appropriate.[8]

The provider should make sure all messages are specific. If the PA recommends behavior change, she should work with the patient to set goal. The he or goals set must be manageable, measurable, and tailored to the patient's current situation. For example, asking a patient to start exercising every day for 60 minutes is measurable, but it is not manageable or tailored to a patient who currently gets winded walking to the mailbox each day. Instead, the PA may start with a recommendation that the patient set a goal of walking to the mailbox twice a day for 1 week and then progress to walking to the end of the street daily the next week. Have the patient schedule return visits to assess progress toward current goals and to set new goals.

4. **Assess the patient's level of understanding and reactions to the information provided.** The best way to implement this step is to perform it concurrently with step 3. As part of providing good structure for the information, it should be presented in segments that make sense together. As the provider reaches the end of a segment, allow the patient to ask questions, offer concerns, and share her or his understanding of the information. Armed with the data garnered from these checkpoints, the provider can continually shape the subsequent education to fit the patient's specific needs. The provider can also take the time to reteach or dispel misinformation immediately if necessary.

Continuous assessment is also helpful when a patient has an emotional reaction to information presented by the PA. Some emotional reactions can stop the flow of communication and become a barrier to the effective delivery of any education that follows. For example, if the provider has recommended an MRI scan for the patient and the patient is claustrophobic, the patient may miss all further information while he or she worries about being scared during the scan. Pausing to check understanding allows the patient time to process, share those emotions, and react to the information. When the provider becomes aware that the patient has had an emotional response to a certain component of the plan, the messages can be adapted to the patient's needs, both medical and emotional.

5. **Use collaborative negotiation and shared decision making.** When students learn about patient education in clinical medicine courses, the formula for educating patients about each disease can be "one size fits all." For example, the education for an obese patient includes a healthy, calorie-restricted diet; routine exercise 4 or 5 days a week; and follow-up for success. Unfortunately, real-world application is not that simple. After providing information to the patient and taking time to check for the patient's understanding and reactions, the PA should take time to negotiate with the patient a plan of action that they both can agree on. This process allows for barriers to be addressed and managed in the planning process. The provider needs to be able to recognize that there are varied options for how to achieve a desired goal and allow for a creative, collaborative approach to common problems.[13] This creative approach allows for the

patient's preferences and ideas to be part of the plan.[13] Patients should be encouraged to share the things that they believe will make a recommendation difficult, and they should be engaged in the process of finding solutions. When patients feel invested in the decisions and the plan creation, they are more likely to adhere to that plan.[1] Treat the patient as the expert in his own health, and help him make informed decisions.

6. **Ask the patient to summarize the plan in her own words.** It is likely that a great deal of information has been shared and many new things have been discussed. This check of patient understanding is the most important. The PA gauges if the patient knows what she is supposed to do when she leaves the office. Asking the patient to speak the plan aloud also solidifies the recommendations through repetition, increasing patient retention. Providing patients with written instructions to reinforce the information also increases retention. Written information should never replace any of the above steps but should assist the patient in remembering the discussion.[1]

7. **Plan for follow-up.** Not every office visit will require follow-up. However, assisting the patient with behavior change or managing a chronic illness will require follow-up visits. These visits allow the provider to celebrate the victories and develop new strategies for challenges. Even when ideal collaboration with the patient exists, barriers may not become apparent until the patient attempts implementation. Following up allows the provider time to revisit and reinforce the goals and recommendations and to develop new shared decisions to allow for continued progress toward the patient's goals for better health. Documentation of the patient–provider interaction is an important element to effective follow-up. The documentation should be complete enough so that recommendations and goals can be easily recognized by other providers who might see the patient.

CASE STUDY 23.1

Ms. Jones (MJ) came to the clinic for a routine physical examination but has expressed that she would like to lose weight. The PA will provide guidance on how to get started losing weight.

STEP ONE

PA: Ms. Jones, I am glad that you have come to me with your desire to lose weight. I would like to talk to you a little about what you are currently doing to try to lose weight, what you have tried, and what has been hard for you. Then we can work together to come up with some goals for you to work on. Would that be okay with you?

MJ: Yes, that sounds good. I am not really doing anything right now. I wanted to talk to you first.

STEP TWO

PA: It is a good idea to get information before starting a new change. Why don't you tell me what you think are the necessary things to do to be successful losing weight?

MJ: Well, I know you need muscle to burn calories, so you need to exercise every day and eat a lot of protein.

PA: Have you tried anything before?

MJ: I tried eating only salads for a while, and I walked some. But I gained weight instead of losing any, so I must be doing something wrong. But I have never done any weight loss plans or anything like that, if that is what you mean.

PA: No, I was just wondering what types of things you had already tried. When you were eating salads, how did you choose your salads?

MJ: Salad was my only rule. So I would just pick which one sounded best. Looking back, I often picked the ones with fried chicken on it, but I figured that would be okay because I was only eating salad.

PA: Do you have any concerns or expectations about learning about weight loss today?

MJ: I am concerned that I will fail again. I am hoping to get a plan that I can do and see some weight loss come from it.

STEPS THREE AND FOUR

PA: I'd like to talk to you a little bit about the fundamental keys to success for weight loss, okay?

MJ: That seems like a great place to start.

PA: The basics are simple, but making it happen can be hard. If you are going to lose weight, you have to burn more calories than you eat. There are two ways of doing that. One is to eat less, and the other is to exercise more. Which one do think is more important?

MJ: The exercise. You need to burn a lot of calories.

PA: That is a common misconception. There is a saying that goes, "You cannot exercise yourself skinny." The exercise is there to help you toward your goal, but it is the control over your food consumption that is most important. If you are going to succeed, you need to keep track of your food in a food journal and be as accurate as you can be. Using your salad diet as an example, two salads of the same size could range in calories from 250 to 2000 calories. If you don't look up the calories, you could be undoing all your hard work with one salad. I want to make sure that I am communicating well. Could you tell me what that most important part of losing weight is?

MJ: I can't believe a salad could possibly have 2000 calories! That explains a lot! The most important part is that I need to look up my food and write it down.

PA: Excellent. You are off to a great start, but don't forget to count any calories in the beverages you drink, too. Exercise is important for everyone to do to help keep our bodies strong. Exercise can really help you increase the amount of weight you lose each week by increasing how many calories you burn. Think of exercise as the weight loss helper. You can use exercise two ways: You can use it to burn more calories so you lose more weight each week, or you can use it to give you more freedom in your diet. I recommend using it to speed up your weight loss. Can you tell me what you understand about exercise?

MJ: Oh, this seems so simple that I feel silly that I haven't asked you about this until now. Exercise can be done to help my weight loss or to give me a few more calories in my diet.

PA: Yes, and exercise is really important for everyone, not just people who are trying to lose weight.

MJ: Got it.

STEP FIVE

PA: Knowing what you know now, what changes do you think you could do over the next 4 weeks to move you toward your goal of weight loss?

MJ: Well, I think I should count my calories, write them down, and exercise every day.

PA: That is great and very ambitious. Do you think you can sustain that for 4 weeks, or should we set the goal at an easier level?

MJ: Maybe I should focus on writing all my foods down and start walking several days a week.

PA: That might be more manageable. There are apps you can use to help you count calories on your phone. I will get you a list of them. I also have a calorie-counting book here in my office that I can give you if you would prefer to use paper and pen. I would like you to be specific in your exercise goal so that you know when you have met it. Would a goal of walking 3 days a week for 30 minutes seem like a reasonable start?

MJ: Yes, I should be able to do that easily.

STEP SIX

PA: Excellent. Can you summarize our plan for today?

MJ: I am going to keep track of all the calories that I eat or drink for the next 4 weeks. I am going to go for a walk at least 3 days each week for at least 30 minutes.

STEP SEVEN

PA: I think that sounds like a great place to start. You may find that this gets hard when you get hungry or there is a special event going on. Please feel free to call my office for support whenever needed. I would like to follow up with you in 4 weeks to see how things are going. You can also call me with weekly weigh-in updates if you want support or encouragement.

MJ: That sounds great. See you in a month.

Patient education is a key component to moving patients toward better health. A provider must be aware of the potential barriers that need to be overcome in order to have effective outcomes. In an effort to manage these barriers, a provider should develop a step-by-step approach to presenting patient education in an organized and prioritized fashion. Providers should not underestimate their ability to empower, encourage, and support patients through positive changes in health.

KEY POINTS

- Patient education should be part of every office visit.
- Providers must be aware of the many barriers that can impede effective patient education.
- Providers must have a systematic approach to presenting patient education.
- Providers should involve patients in their education sessions, prioritize the information to be provided, provide the information in small chunks, and check for understanding to help the patient retain the information.

References

1. Falvo DR. *Effective Patient Education: A Guide to Increased Adherence*. 4th ed. Sudbury, MA: Jones and Bartlett; 2011.
2. Langewitz W, Ackermann S, Heierle A, Hertwig R, Ghanim L, Bingisser R. Improving patient recall of information: harnessing the power of structure. *Patient Educ Couns*. 2015;98(6):716–721.
3. Ghisi GL, et al., A systematic review of patient education in cardiac patients: do they increase knowledge and promote health behavior change? *Patient Educ Couns*. 2014;95(2):160–174. http://dx.doi.org/10.1016/j.pec.2014.01.012.
4. Ruiter RAC, Kessels LTE, Peters G-JY, Kok G. Sixty years of fear appeal research: current state of the evidence. *Int J Psychol*. 2014;49(2):63–70.
5. Feldman MD, Christensen JF, eds. *Behavioral Medicine: A Guide for Clinical Practice*. 4th ed. New York: McGraw-Hill Education; 2014.
6. Bouma AJ, van Wilgen P, Dijkstra A. The barrier-belief approach in the counseling of physical activity. *Patient Educ Couns*. 2015;98(2):129–136.
7. Bastable SB, ed. *Essentials of Patient Education*. Sudbury, MA: Jones and Bartlett Publishers; 2006.
8. Lloyd M, Bor R, Blache G, Eleftheriadou Z. *Communication Skills for Medicine*. Edinburgh; New York: Churchill Livingstone; 2009.
9. Bowen, Denise; 5 How To's for Teaching Health Literacy. Physician Assist Educ Assoc; September 2015. http://www.paeaonline.org/hows-of-health-literacy/. Accessed December 15, 2015.
10. National Institutes of Health. Health Literacy. http://www.nih.gov/institutes-nih/nih-office-director/office-communications-public-liaison/clear-communication/health-literacy. Accessed November 19, 2015.
11. U.S. Department of Health & Human Services. Centers for Disease Control and Prevention. *Learn About Health Literacy*. http://www.cdc.gov/healthliteracy/learn/index.html. Accessed December 16, 2015.
12. Matthys J, Elwyn G, Van Nuland M, et al. Patients' ideas, concerns, and expectations (ICE) in general practice: impact on prescribing. *Br J Gen Pract*. 2009;59(558):29–36.
13. Elwyn G, Lloyd A, May C, et al. Collaborative deliberation: a model for patient care. *Patient Educ Couns*. 2014;97(2):158–164.

The resources for this chapter can be found at www.expertconsult.com.

The Faculty Resources can be found online at www.expertconsult.com.

CHAPTER 24

PROVIDING CULTURALLY COMPETENT HEALTH CARE

Susan LeLacheur

CULTURAL COMPETENCE

The term *cultural competence* has a variety of definitions, but perhaps the most relevant for physician assistants (PAs) is Betancourt's 2002 definition:

Cultural competence in health care describes the ability of systems to provide care to patients with diverse values, beliefs and behaviors, including tailoring delivery to meet patients' social, cultural, and linguistic needs.[1]

This definition refers to a *system*, recognizing that no one individual can achieve the level of care needed without the integrated support of an organization in which diversity is understood and valued. Each of us can strive through our own actions and reactions to improve both our individual encounters and, to the extent we are able, the system in which we practice. This chapter focuses primarily on the individual with the understanding that we must also work with our clinical and ancillary teams to create a context that is welcoming to all.

INTRODUCTION TO CULTURALLY COMPETENT PRACTICE

The single overarching goal of culturally competent practice is to reduce medical errors by improving patient–provider communication. Communication, of course, is a two-way process, and errors can occur in either direction. For example, a provider may encounter a patient who uses a wheelchair and has slow speech who the clinician assumes to be intellectually challenged. Similarly, a financially stressed patient may encounter a clinician who appears to be of a higher social and economic stratum and assume the clinician has no understanding of the challenges of poverty. Either of these assumptions may be made fairly automatically and with little or no conscious thought, and either can lead to significant barriers in communication, regardless of the accuracy or inaccuracy of the assumption.

Assumptions about others are often based in stereotypes, categories of traits that are connected in our understanding. Stereotypes range from fairly innocuous, such as the assumption that a blue collar worker is more likely to bowl than play golf, to detrimental, such as the idea that a black man is more violent than a white man. In either case, the stereotype is based on an unsubstantiated association of unrelated traits. Stereotypes are universal and normal but can lead to bias, a consistent shift (positive or negative) in thoughts and behavior that is not substantiated by facts.

In the clinical setting, PAs and other clinicians must often make rapid judgments with regard to diagnostic and treatment decisions. Such decisions may be colored by incomplete or inaccurate assumptions based in stereotypes.[2] Because these rapid thought processes are subconscious, their occurrence cannot generally be consciously controlled, but this does not mean we are powerless.[3]

If the clinician is aware of the effect of personal bias on decision making, he or she can check any assumptions by eliciting further information from the patient. Errors in patient understanding of the illness and its treatment can be reduced by eliciting the patient's understanding of the illness and expectations of care during the encounter. In addition, the clinician can ask about social or cultural factors that may potentially influence patients' decision making during an encounter. Checking assumptions during the patient encounter helps the clinician to remove stereotypes, allowing the patient to be seen more as an individual than a member of a group (with all its attendant associations). A framework for eliciting the patient's understanding and cultural context is Kleinman et al.'s explanatory model[4]:

- What do you think has caused your problem?
- Why do you think it started when it did?
- What do you think your sickness does to you? How does it work?
- How severe is your sickness? Will it have a short or long course?
- What kind of treatment do you think you should receive?
- What are the most important results you hope to receive from this treatment?
- What are the chief problems your sickness has caused for you?
- What do you fear most about your sickness?

The busy practitioner may not have time to get all this information in a single visit, but incorporating just a few of these questions into your standard clinical history can help resolve errors in communication. The following three questions will usually allow the clinician to evaluate whether or not further discussion of the interaction between personal and cultural beliefs and the understanding and management of illness should be explored:

- What do you think your sickness does to you? How does it work?
- What kind of treatment do you think you should receive?
- What are the most important results you hope to receive from this treatment?

Although obtaining a good understanding of the patient's view of health and disease may be crucial to building rapport and improving communication in a primary care setting or other ongoing patient–provider interaction, it may not be possible in the context of emergent care. The emergency department (ED) is, however, a place where it is critical

that subconscious bias and stereotyping be avoided so that it does not influence clinical decision making.[5,6] The most rapid way to circumvent bias and improve the patient–provider interaction is through perspective taking.[7,8] Perspective taking is instantaneous; the clinician merely takes a moment to picture him- or herself in the patient's shoes, seeing the situation through the patient's eyes. The patient can no longer be seen as "other," and stereotypes fall away. The effect of perspective taking is not equal across clinicians or situations, but with practice, it can become a tool that is both quick and easy.

The basics of culturally competent practice are summarized in Box 24.1. To clarify the processes involved in improving the interaction between patient and provider, we will delve further into the rationale behind the need to reduce communication barriers and some background into the psychology behind their operation.

RATIONALE

To fully understand the importance of culturally competent practice and the steps outlined earlier, we must explore how perceived differences between individuals affect clinical decision making and, ultimately, contribute to health care disparities. Disparities in health and in health care are related to a complex web of factors. The landmark Institute of Medicine report in 2003, "Unequal Treatment," determined that although disparities in health care are influenced by many elements outside of the clinician's direct control, including the operation of health systems and legal and regulatory factors, they are largely attributable to discrimination, bias, and stereotypes on the part of health care practitioners.[9]

BOX 24.1 BASICS OF CULTURAL COMPETENCE IN PRACTICE: IMPROVING COMMUNICATION

- Check assumptions.
  - Understand bias.
  - Be aware of assumptions.
- Explanatory model
  - Check patient understanding.
  - Check patient expectations.
- Perspective taking
  - Put yourself in your patient's shoes, seeing the world through his or her eyes.
  - Check assumptions.

Bias and stereotypes are largely subconscious and can lead to errors in clinical decision making. Outward discrimination is less common but can occur without intent. For example, choosing to locate a clinic far from a bus route may discriminate against those without cars even though no discrimination was intended.

The reduction of health care disparities is a key goal of incorporating cultural competence into patient care.[10] Obviously, not all disparities in patient care are related to communication, but the improvement of communication, both conscious and subconscious, can go a long way toward resolving at least one cause of disparities. Communication also involves creating a welcoming atmosphere.

BIAS AND STEREOTYPING

The term *stereotype* was coined by Walter Lippman, a journalist, in 1922 and refers to a printing plate made to duplicate a particular type of page. He used it to refer to the tendency of people to form mental images based on preconceptions that members of a particular group are alike in certain ways.[11] These mental images make it easier to associate another person with something that conforms to the stereotype than with something discordant. In other words, congruent associations are automatic, and incongruent associations are just a little slower. The entire process is subconscious and is based in our culture, the images we see every day, and the world around us, not in our own logical thoughts or beliefs. Over the past few decades, the process of stereotyping has been evaluated through multiple techniques. Since the advent of computers, the easiest method has been to simply measure the time it takes to associate two items, words, or pictures. This process is repeated with random allocation of right and left, positive and negative associations on a wide variety of subjects. You can test your own automatic associations at Harvard University's Project Implicit, https://implicit.harvard.edu/implicit. Keep in mind that this is not a test of your values but of the way your world pulls you to automatically respond. It should be used to increase your awareness of the potential for stereotyping so that you can focus your efforts on interrupting the process through further assessment both of your patient and of your own thoughts and feelings.

Bias and stereotyping are important in clinical care because they have been shown to influence diagnosis and management in a discriminatory way. The association between a negative automatic association and reduced quality of care has been shown in computer-based patient scenarios[2] and in patient care.[12] Misperceptions can lead to misdiagnoses and inadequate or inappropriate treatment.

COGNITIVE ERRORS IN DECISION MAKING

Current psychological research considers human thought as being divided into two pathways variously called fast and slow; intuitive and analytical; or, simply, system 1 and system 2. System 1, frequently used in clinical encounters, involves pattern recognition and rapid associations.[13] System 2 thinking is a slower analytic process. Although system 1 thinking is extremely helpful in emergency situations, it must always be moderated, even by experienced clinicians, by a process of forcing oneself into system 2 thinking in order to avoid medical errors. Many errors in cognitive decision making have been described, but two are closely related to the need for cultural competence in clinical care: ascertainment bias and fundamental attribution error.[14,15]

Ascertainment bias is caused by an automatic association between two or more traits—a stereotype. For example, a man smelling of alcohol is brought to the ED unconscious. The clinician might initially conclude through system 1 thinking that his loss of consciousness was caused by alcohol but must also bring his or her system 2 thinking into action to consider the myriad of other potential causes. The stereotype must be consciously overridden to provide quality patient care. Other stereotypes, whether based on gender, race, ethnicity, or class, must similarly be recognized and consciously overridden. Otherwise they can lead to erroneous assumptions about the patient's symptoms and to faulty diagnosis and treatment.

Fundamental attribution error is related to ascertainment bias but is caused by the provider having a judgmental approach to the patient at the start. Fundamental attribution error is particularly problematic for PAs working with marginalized populations. It involves blaming the patient for the problem without full consideration of contextual factors. For example, an obese patient might be seen as being at fault for his diabetes because of a poor diet. However, the patient may have a poor diet because he has no transportation to a supermarket and is forced to buy his food at a convenience store, limiting his access to healthy food.

Reducing errors in errors in decision making is an ongoing process of combining appropriate pattern recognition with checking assumptions and carefully considering other possibilities. Cultural competence practice does not require the PA to ignore automatic associations but to evaluate them in the care of each patient as an individual.

KNOWLEDGE, SKILLS, AND ATTITUDES

In addition to managing the automatic processes of our minds, clinicians must build their knowledge of the people and communities with whom they work. Culture may be defined as the beliefs, values, norms, and customs of a particular group. Although knowledge of the culture is a help in working with individual patients, it is important to ascertain how the individual interacts with that culture. Understanding culture is just a starting point. Your patient may ascribe to some, none, or all of the group norms and values. The clinician must check her or his assumptions. For example, one cannot assume that a patient from a particular religious community follows every tenet of that religion. This is where cultural understanding can lead to stereotyping. There are also important environmental influences on behavior of both the individual and the group. Cultures shift according to time, place, and circumstance, leading to changes in behavior of individuals and of the group.

The skills involved in culturally competent practice are those used in all patient-centered care. Creating a partnership between the clinician and the patient improves both patient perceptions and understanding.[16] The clinician can make errors in assuming a patient who seems like him- or herself has similar thoughts and values as easily as in assuming one who seems different has differing thoughts and values. Effective communication requires shared language, meaning that the clinician must check the meaning behind a patient's words even when both are speaking a shared language. The clinician must also evaluate how the patient understands of explanations and instructions.

The clinician can use Kleinman et al.'s questions to obtain an understanding of the patient's view and then build a partnership based on that understanding. Another model for cross-cultural communication is the LEARN model[17]:

L: Listen to the patient's perspective.
E: Explain and share one's own perspective.
A: Acknowledge differences between the two perspectives.
R: Recommend a treatment plan.
N: Negotiate a mutually agreed upon treatment plan.

Good communication allows the clinician to focus on the patient as an individual rather than categorizing. In this way, the patient and provider can build a partnership, collaborating as a team with a shared understanding and shared goals. Perspective taking—imagining oneself in the patient's situation and then checking one's understanding—can help the clinician to better understand and empathize.

The attitudes needed for effective cross-cultural communications are exactly as you would expect—respect and sensitivity. The difficulty is that the clinician may not know how respect is expressed in a different cultural context.[18] This is where the knowledge piece can help, but one can always simply ask. Sensitivity toward the variability of customs and norms and even underlying conceptions of the world and its inhabitants and a willingness to learn can help the clinician to bridge differences.

One additional consideration in cross-cultural communication is the variability of nonverbal cues across cultures. Physical expressions of attitude and mode can be very different. The clinician must explicitly validate his or her understanding of actions as well as words.

LANGUAGE BARRIERS

One cross-cultural communication skill that requires particular attention is that of working across a language barrier. Clearly, little or no accurate patient–provider interaction can occur without a shared language. In 2000, the United States Department of Health and Human Services first published the National Standards for Culturally and Linguistically Appropriate Services (CLAS) in Health and Health Care. The goals of the CLAS Standards are to respond to the rapidly changing demography in the United States and eliminate long-standing disparities and improve the quality of health services and outcomes, as well as respond to legal and regulatory factors.[10] These standards guide both the health care system and individual clinicians in better providing care to a diverse population. The current CLAS Standards specifically relating to patient–provider communication are

- Provide effective, equitable, understandable, respectful, and quality care and services that are responsive to diverse cultural health beliefs and practices, preferred languages, health literacy, and other communication needs.
- Offer communication and language assistance.

Within the requirement that language support be offered, the Standards also offer guidance regarding the nature of that support. Medical interpreters should be trained specifically for this role. (The term *interpreter* is applied when the communication is auditory or via sign language; *translator* is the term used when communication is in writing.) A well-trained interpreter will not elaborate or simplify and will remain aloof from the interaction. It is the provider's role to manage the interaction, including the interpreter's part in the visit. Both the patient and provider should speak to each other directly with the interpreter sitting out of the line of the primary interaction. It will initially feel natural to speak to the interpreter rather than the patient, but you should do so only when there is a question about the meaning of a word or phrase (Box 24.2).

There are several potential barriers to working with interpreters. The most basic barrier is a failure to appreciate the need for an interpreter. Sometimes this occurs because the patient fails to ask for language assistance. The patient may fail to understand the potential for miscommunication across the language barrier. A patient may lack knowledge regarding the availability of interpretation services. On the provider side, interpretation services may not be offered automatically, and their availability may not be advertised.

Another barrier is the "informal" interpreter, a friend or family member asked to accompany the patient to interpret. For all the obvious patient confidentiality reasons, this situation should be avoided except when it is very clear that the patient prefers for the other person to participate in the encounter. Even when the patient would like for the friend or family member to stay, it is better to bring in a professional interpreter. Untrained interpreters are far more likely to add to or abbreviate the words of patient and provider. In addition, informal interpreters may not know proper medical terminology. Friends or family members may have a different agenda from that of the patient, through misunderstanding, a wish to "protect" the patient, or frank self-interest. On occasion, using a friend or family member for some or all of the interaction may be the best option available. When this situation occurs, the clinician must remain in control of the encounter and realize that there will be far more frequent need for clarification with and direction of the untrained interpreter.

Another potential pitfall of working across a language barrier is the reliance on partial understanding in cases of limited language proficiency on the part of either the patient or the provider. Partial understanding between the patient and provider can lead to serious, if not fatal, medication errors. In some cases, the patient will refuse interpreter services, even when one is clearly needed. They can be reluctant for a number of reasons. The provider must make every attempt to understand the cause of the patient's concern and address the problem in order to assure optimal communication.

As with all communication difficulties, a language barrier can lead to misdiagnosis and other errors in clinical decision making. On the patient side, there can be failure to understand instructions, leading to medication errors. Each health care facility is required by law to have interpretation services available. These may be provided in person or might be obtained through a telephone service. Telephone service is particularly helpful when the language needed is not a common one. Computer-assisted audio-video service is also available when interpretation is needed for the hearing impaired. With the continued improvements in technology, interpretation services will become more available for both the clinician and patient.

SPECIAL POPULATIONS

When speaking of cultural competence, most of us think of people from different races, ethnicities, and geographic locations, but there are huge cultural variations much closer to home. For example, sexual minorities, youth, the deaf community, and many others each have their own values, norms, and even language. For the more marginalized groups, it is particularly important to create a welcoming atmosphere by making it clear that they will be accepted and understood. The knowledge, skills, and attitudes we've discussed can be equally applied to any of these and a myriad of other groups. Even when working within your own culture, it is important to check assumptions, evaluate patient understanding and expectations, and negotiate a shared plan of care.

CONCLUSION

Culturally competent care is a learned skill. It will require a great deal of practice and will lead to many embarrassing moments as attempts to discern the appropriate norms fail. That said, its immediate and long-term rewards make it not only very possible but almost always preferable. Patients immediately appreciate the clinician's effort to understand and create a partnership. The patient, in turn, will become more involved in his or her own care, leading to greater satisfaction on the part of patient and clinician alike. PAs are in the perfect position to improve patient–provider communication across every kind of barrier. The basic skills are easy to learn and become automatic with practice. The results of your efforts—improving your communication, clinical decision making, and contributing to the reduction of health disparities—are crucial both to your own practice and to the nation's health.

CASE STUDY 24.1

EF is a 29-year-old woman who recently emigrated from Ethiopia. She speaks very limited English and refuses an interpreter, although the service was offered when she scheduled the appointment, and you speak no Amharic. You ask her again if she will accept interpretation services, but again she refuses. As you begin your intake history and physical examination, you discover that she has a diagnosis of HIV infection. Because you have some knowledge of the tight-knit, devoutly Christian Ethiopian community in your area, you ask if she is concerned about confidentiality. When she says yes, she is worried that any Amharic-speaking person you might bring in could lead to risk of disclosure of her status. You describe the possibility of using a telephone-based service, to which she agrees.

With the help of the telephone interpretation service, you are able to obtain a more complete history and at her follow-up appointment provide improved patient education, including the elucidation and resolution of several key barriers to medication adherence, which are critical in managing HIV.

KEY POINTS

- Culturally competent practice is essential for patient safety.
- All health care providers have some degree of bias and engage in stereotyping. Being aware of this tendency and engaging in perspective taking can mitigate the effects of bias and stereotypes.
- PAs need to work to understand the culture of the communities they serve to provide effective and safe care.
- There are special added concerns about patient safety when working with a patient who speaks a different language than the PA. All PAs should learn how to effectively use language interpreters.

References

1. Betancourt JR, Green AR, Carrillo JE. *Cultural Competence in Health Care: Emerging Frameworks and Practical Approaches.* Vol. 2004. The Commonwealth Fund; 2002.
2. Green AR, Carney DR, Pallin DJ, et al. Implicit bias among physicians and its prediction of thrombolysis decisions for black and white patients. *J Gen Intern Med.* 2007;22(9):1231–1238.
3. Dasgupta N, Greenwald AG. On the malleability of automatic attitudes: combating automatic prejudice with images of admired and disliked individuals. *J Pers Soc Psychol.* 2001;81(5):800–814.
4. Kleinman A, Eisenberg L, Good B. Culture, illness, and care: clinical lessons from anthropologic and cross-cultural research. *Ann Intern Med.* 1978;88(2):251–258.
5. Blanchard JC, Haywood YC, Scott C. Racial and ethnic disparities in health: an emergency medicine perspective. *Acad Emerg Med.* 2003;10(11):1289–1293.
6. Shah AA, Zogg CK, Zafar SN, et al. Analgesic access for acute abdominal pain in the emergency department among racial/ethnic minority patients: a nationwide examination. *Med Care.* 2015;53(12):1000–1009. http://dx.doi.org/10.1097/mlr.0000000000000444.
7. Galinsky AD, Martorana PV, Ku G. To control or not to control stereotypes: separating the implicit and explicit processes of perspective-taking and suppression [References]. In: Forgas Joseph P, Williams Kipling D, et al., eds. *Social Judgments: Implicit And Explicit Processes.* 2003. New York, NY: Cambridge University Press; 2003:343–363.
8. Blatt B, LeLacheur SF, Galinsky AD, Simmens SJ, Greenberg L. Does perspective-taking increase patient satisfaction in medical encounters? *Acad Med.* 2010;85(9):1445–1452.

9. Smedley B, Stith A, Nelson A. *Unequal Treatment: Confronting Racial And Ethnic Disparities In Health Care*. Washington, DC: National Academies Press; 2002.

10. Office of Minority Health, U.S. Department of Health and Human Services. National standards for culturally and linguistically appropriate services in health and health care: a blueprint for advancing and sustaining CLAS policy and practice; 2013.

11. Hamilton D, Stroessner S, Driscoll D. Social cognition and the study of stereotyping. In: Devine PG, Hamilto DL, Ostrom TM, eds. *Social Cognition: Impact on Psychology*. San Diego: Academic Press; 1994:292–321.

12. Van Ryn M, Burgess D, Malat J, Griffin J. Physicians' perceptions of patients' social and behavioral characteristics and race disparities in treatment recommendations for men with coronary artery disease. *Am J Public Health*. 2006;96(2):351–357.

13. Kahneman D. *Thinking, Fast And Slow*. New York: Farrar, Straus and Giroux; 2011.

14. Groopman JE. *How Doctors Think*. Boston: Houghton Mifflin Company; 2007.

15. Croskerry P. The importance of cognitive errors in diagnosis and strategies to minimize them. *Acad Med*. 2003;78(8):775–780.

16. Beach MC, Sugarman J, Johnson RL, Arbelaez JJ, Duggan PS, Cooper LA. Do patients treated with dignity report higher satisfaction, adherence, and receipt of preventive care? *Ann Fam Med*. 2005;3(4):331–338.

17. Berlin EA, Fowkes WCJ. A teaching framework for cross-cultural health care. Application in family practice. *West J Med*. 1983;139(6):934–938.

18. Beach MC, Roter DL, Wang NY, et al. Are physicians' attitudes of respect accurately perceived by patients and associated with more positive communication behaviors? *Patient Educ Couns*. 2006;62(3):347–354.

PATIENT CARE: CLINICAL ROTATIONS

CHAPTER 25

FAMILY MEDICINE

Scott D. Richards • Jennifer Feirstein

PHYSICIAN ASSISTANTS IN FAMILY MEDICINE: A BRIEF HISTORY

Family medicine, as a physician assistant (PA) specialty, cannot be discussed without first understanding the intertwined history of PAs and primary care medicine. Of all medical specialties, the roots of the PA profession are truly grounded in that of primary care. The shortage of generalist medical providers and the expansion of patients with access to care because of the enactment of Medicare and Medicaid ultimately led to the innovative development of this new medical practitioner in the 1960s.[1] The development of the PA profession was an innovative strategy to help solve the problem of an overtaxed health care system that was unable to effectively manage the influx of patients seeking primary medical services. In fact, the University of Washington MEDEX PA program, which was one of the first established PA programs, was specifically developed with the mission of training ex-military corpsmen to become primary care providers in the rural areas of the Northwest.

Physician assistants practicing in primary care medicine have had very dynamic roles and experiences over the course of the profession. Historically, the PA profession was developed with the intent of being able to extend the care offered by the physician by providing health care for simple medical problems, such as uncomplicated upper respiratory infections and musculoskeletal injuries. The intended result was that physicians would have more time in their schedules to provide health care to patients requiring chronic disease management and to evaluate more complicated medical complaints. However, as the PA profession grew and developed, many PAs in primary care started managing the full spectrum of care for acute and complicated medical cases alike.

Although the scope of practice for PAs in primary care has been greatly expanded over the past 50 years, there is a trend toward more PAs practicing in medical or surgical subspecialties. What was once a profession created as a pipeline of providers that would help solve the primary care provider shortage has become a profession that currently only has approximately 30% of its members practicing primary care medicine.

Of the primary care sub-specialties, family medicine encompasses the largest distribution of PAs. According to the 2013 American Academy of Physician Assistants (AAPA) Annual Survey, 23.3% of clinically practicing PAs practice in family medicine with or without urgent care. Although the family medicine predominance within the PA profession is starting to be surpassed by other specialties, such as surgery (26.6% of clinically practicing PAs), there are still a significant proportion of PAs who are practicing family medicine.

HISTORY REPEATS ITSELF

With the passage of the Patient Protection and Affordable Care Act (ACA) in 2010, the shortage of primary care providers in the American health care system has again been brought to the forefront. Similar to the 1960s, there has been a rapid influx of patients who have been provided with the ability to afford health care. However, there is a concern about whether there are enough medical providers to provide this access to care. Addressing this concern has brought renewed attention to the field of primary care, along with incentives for practicing primary care medicine. The ACA provides expanded funding for the National Health Service Corps, financial support for the training of primary care providers, and Medicare payment bonuses and improved Medicare physician fee schedules for primary care providers.[2] Historically, the PA profession has always been a profession that is concerned about access to care and one that identifies a need within the health care system and fills that need. Therefore, with the financial incentives for primary care providers being offered by the federal government and with the specific inclusion of PAs as designated primary care providers by the ACA, the interest and practice of primary care medicine by PAs is likely to again expand.

In addition to the historical focus on primary care medicine; PAs also have a rich history of practicing medicine in medically underserved and geographically rural areas. As the profession grew, more and more PAs started practicing in more suburban settings, and there has been less focus on providing health care in medically underserved areas. However, this too may again become the focus of the profession with the increased emphasis on the need for medical providers in these areas and as incentives from the federal government are provided. The renewed emphasis of PAs practicing primary care medicine will likely lead to great diversity in what primary care medicine looks like for PAs in different settings. PAs may practice primary care in any of the following areas:

- **Rural:** PAs practicing primary care in rural areas are often involved in the full array of health care services and may have a scope of practice more expansive than PAs in other geographic areas. Because specialists are often not easily accessible, rural primary care PAs may treat many disease states or perform many procedures that, in another area, may be referred to a specialist.
- **Suburban and urban:** PAs practicing primary care in these settings have great variance in their scope of practice. Some PAs may have a similar practice to PAs in rural areas; however, some PAs may be involved more with the coordination of health care, including more specialty referrals.

- **Federally Qualified Health Centers (FQHCs):** FQHCs receive federal funding to provide comprehensive primary care services to medically underserved areas or populations. Many community health centers (CHCs) meet criteria to be an FQHC. From 2006 to 2010, it was estimated that approximately 10% of patient visits at CHCs were to PAs, and the majority of visits were for chronic disease treatment.[3] CHCs have also significantly increased the utilization of PAs, evidenced by a 61% increase in the number of PAs, nurse practitioners, and certified nurse midwives employed by CHCs.[4] The full spectrum of primary care services provided at FQHCs in addition to the expanded hiring of PAs by CHCs is bound to shape the next generation of PAs.
- **Patient-centered medical homes (PCMH):** The PCMH is a model of holistic, patient-centered health also emphasizing accessible care committed to quality improvement and safety.[5] Increasingly, PAs will find themselves leading the health care team in PCMHs, thus expanding administrative roles of PAs in primary care. The PCMH model is discussed in more detail later in this chapter.
- **Accountable care organizations (ACOs):** ACOs are groups of health care providers or hospitals that work together to provide high-quality appropriate care at the right time with a focus on prevention of medical errors and fiduciary responsibility in providing medical care.[6] PAs are vital components of ACOs, and in primary care, this is another setting in which administrative roles may be expanded for PAs.

With the new strategies and models of care that have been and will continue to be developed in medicine, it is evident that PAs in primary care will continue to be needed to fill a void that has been present throughout the history of the profession.

THE SPECIALTY OF FAMILY MEDICINE

In 1969, family medicine shifted from the traditional generalist model of medicine to become the 20th medical specialty in the United States.[7] In effect, this shift graduated family medicine to become the newest primary care discipline and the second largest medical specialty in the United States.[8] The specialty of family medicine overlaps pediatrics, general internal medicine, general obstetrics and gynecology, primary care geriatrics, and general psychiatry. Given this overlap, it is easy to understand why family medicine is well known for a traditionally complex and large scope of practice.[9] Family medicine providers are well prepared to manage highly complex illnesses, diseases, and comorbidities and able to collect and interpret a great amount of data. This is fueled by an extensive understanding of organic medicine, behavioral health, and general health care systems, resulting in the provision of effective, patient-centered medical care at the lowest cost to the patient and health care system.[10]

Providing evaluation, treatment, and continuous care for patients from "birth to the grave," ranging from prenatal care to end-of life care, is inseparable from the family medicine approach to patient care.[11] And to further distinguish family medicine providers from others, family medicine providers are among the only medical specialists who are distributed in the same geographic proportion as the U.S. population.[12] Vital to the particular patient approach shared by family medicine providers are the assurances of patient accessibility to high-quality, evidence-based, and culturally sensitive care.[13]

In their research and exploration of family medicine clinician identity, Carney et al.[8] identified five core domains: (1) patient/family relationship; (2) patient advocacy; (3) career flexibility such as options in building a practice and practice emphasis; (4) balancing the breadth and depth of care given the comprehensive expertise needed to evaluate, treat, and follow patients with a wide array of conditions and illnesses across the lifespan; and (5) the comprehensive nature of patient care and continuity of care. Interestingly, Carney et al. also found that many family medicine providers included the importance of supporting and pursuing social justice as a principal element of family medicine. Above all else, many regard the successful establishment of a strong and effective therapeutic relationship with both patient and family as a pillar of family medicine. Particular to family medicine, the provider–patient relationship spans a patient's life cycle, continuing beyond treatment or cure, and includes the patient's family members.

A fundamental concept in family medicine is the understanding that knowledge about a patient's family is of great importance to develop holistic and effective patient management strategies and treatment plans[14]; this concept is inherent in the systems approach to primary health care, a hallmark of family medicine. Systems theory highlights the interrelationship between natural and social science in helping the family medicine provider to best understand causes and effects as related to patient presentations and outcomes. Biosciences and social sciences become intertwined into a contextual biopsychosocial framework in which the knowledge of a medical science coupled with the context of each

BOX 25.1 GUIDING PRINCIPLES OF A PATIENT-CENTERED MEDICAL HOME APPROACH

- Develop strong relationships with patients.
- Provide first contact and continuity of care.
- Incorporate a clinician-led team-based approach at the practice level, assuming responsibility for the continuous care of patients.
- Adopt a whole-person orientation in which the clinician provides for his or her patient's health care needs, including but not limited to appropriate referrals and follow-up, throughout the life span and for acute, chronic, preventive, and end-of-life care.
- Ensure coordination and oversight of care throughout complex health care systems using such tools as electronic health records to assist in identifying health care services.
- Provide enhanced access to care by incorporating expanded hours, open scheduling, and various forms of communication (e.g., phone, web based, remote communication, face to face).

patient's individual characteristics and qualities, family, and community informs the diagnosis, workup, treatment, and follow-up plan.[15]

Perhaps one of the best ways to describe the family medicine–specific approach to patients is through the well-adopted PCMH model.[16,17] The PCMH concept was initially introduced in the 1960s by the American Academy of Pediatrics (AAP) to refer to a central location for storing and accessing a pediatric patient's medical records. In 2002, the AAP expanded the definition to incorporate access to care, continuity of care, comprehensive care and family-centered, compassionate, and culturally sensitive medical care of patients. In 2007, the American Academy of Family Physicians, the AAP, the American College of Physicians, and the American Osteopathic Association developed the Joint Principles of the Patient-Centered Medical Home outlining guiding standards for the more current PCMH model (Box 25.1). The family medicine approach to the PCMH provides for the comprehensive primary care of children, adolescents, and adults, creating partnerships between individual patients and families with their personal primary care providers. At the heart of the model are the principles of quality and safety to better establish primary care clinicians and practices as strong advocates for the well-being of their patients with a goal of optimal, patient-centered outcomes via a strong, compassionate partnership among the patient, clinician, and practice.

Family medicine cannot be simply defined by practice location, condition severity, organ system, or even patient age or gender but rather by the provider–patient relationship, as well as relationships with patients' families and communities.[18] In their research on core themes in family medicine, Bradner et al.[19] identified five core attributes embraced in family medicine: (1) a deep understanding of whole person dynamics; (2) the fostering of personal growth in patients, including practices to promote behavioral change leading to improved quality of life; (3) humanizing patient experiences within the health care setting; (4) enhanced availability for and open communication with patients; and (5) a natural command of complexity.

Beyond providing for first contact and a continual relationship, another particularly common theme in family medicine is the prevention of and screening for disease, including the appropriate management of patients to prevent chronic disease exacerbations resulting in emergency room visits and hospitalizations.[10] The importance of such an approach cannot be overemphasized. Research supports that regions with more primary care providers also have improved population health with lower health care costs; lower death rates from such illnesses as heart disease, cancer, and strokes; and lower infant mortality rates.[10] And as a signal of the importance of family medicine specifically, the correlation among improved health, treatment outcomes, and lower costs was strongest from family medicine providers.[10,20] Additionally, evidence supports that family medicine outpatient encounters are equally or more complex than specialty nonprimary care specialty encounters.[21]

Family medicine providers practice a very broad breadth of care while maintaining a strong continuing relationship with patients and patients' families, bridging the boundaries between well-being and illness.[22] In addition to improved access to care for patients of all ages, strong focus on preventive care, and the early management of illness and disease processes, a family medicine approach is also concerned with reduction of unnecessary referral for specialty services and educating patients how to care for themselves whenever feasible.[10] Patient protective and cost reducing practices include rapid access to care, evidence-based care, preventive care strategies, and limiting unnecessary utilization of diagnostics and unnecessary specialty referrals. The provision of cost-effective care, not only to benefit individual patients but also to benefit the larger health care systems is a common theme among family medicine providers.

Family medicine recognizes the great importance of having knowledge of the whole patient to set the stage for a strong and continuous relationship between patient and clinicians. Such knowledge includes not only past medical and psychiatric histories but also social and financial circumstances. For family medicine providers, more utility is often gained from a medical history than "fishing for labs." Therefore, one characteristic of the family medicine approach is the incredible importance of garnering a comprehensive and accurate patient history.

THE FAMILY MEDICINE CLINICAL ROTATION

Before and throughout their family medicine clinical rotation, students would be best served to recall that the family medicine specialty is unique among specialty practices, ensuring first contact (for both acute and chronic conditions) continuity care for patients of all ages and genders frequently presenting with complex comorbidity or multimorbidity and ill-defined problems.[23] Many family medicine patients present multiple times each year and with multiple issues, complaints, and concerns at each visit.[24] And the prevalence of patients with not just comorbidity but multimorbidity is increasing.[25] It is the provider's responsibility to prioritize these problems, orchestrating the visit to ensure that patient needs are met; the student shares this responsibility.

Coordination and integration of complex medical problems and comorbidities coupled with the expertise to manage a wide range of acute, subacute, and chronic conditions in a variety of practice settings is required of family medicine providers. Many family medicine providers even include home visits as part of their practice, identifying connections between environment and illness.[26] Additionally, each patient visit, regardless of reason and setting, is an opportunity for health promotion and disease prevention for both the patient and the patient's family—an opportunity to prevent future illness; address chronic conditions; and potentially, provide care for other family members present during the visit.

Family medicine clinical rotation students should be knowledgeable about the most common acute and chronic presentations and diagnoses seen in family medicine practices. Given the breadth and comprehensiveness in family medicine, these presentations cover a wide variety of conditions and level of urgency, and students can benefit from using multiple key resources throughout their family medicine clinical rotation. Because the family medicine rotation covers such a wide breadth of patients and conditions, it is important for students to be familiar with both texts that offer in-depth coverage of pediatrics and internal

BOX 25.2 KEY STUDENT RESOURCES FOR THE FAMILY MEDICINE CLINICAL ROTATION

CLINICAL MEDICINE RESOURCES PROVIDING IN-DEPTH INFORMATION ON INTERNAL MEDICINE AND PEDIATRICS

Kasper DL, Fauci AS, Longo DL, et al., eds. *Harrison's Principles of Internal Medicine,* 19th ed. New York: McGraw-Hill; 2015.

Kliegman RM, Stanton B, St. Geme J, Schor NF. *Nelson Textbook of Pediatrics,* 20th ed. Philadelphia: Elsevier; 2016.

CLINICAL MEDICINE RESOURCES FOR THE FAMILY MEDICINE ROTATION

Esherick JS. *Tarascon Primary Care Pocketbook.* Burlington, MA: Tarascon Publishing; 2016.

Post TW, ed. UptoDate. Waltham, MA: UpToDate; 2016. http://www.uptodate .com/home/product.

South-Paul J, Matheny S., Lewis E. *Current Diagnosis & Treatment: Family Medicine,* 4th ed. Columbus, OH: McGraw-Hill Education; 2015.

PHARMACOTHERAPY RESOURCES

Gilbert DN, Chambers HF, Eliopoulos GM, Saag MS, eds. *The Sanford Guide to Antimicrobial Therapy 2015,* 45th ed. Sperryville, VA: Antimicrobial Therapy; 2015.

Hamilton RJ, ed. *Tarascon Pocket Pharmacopoeia.* Burlington, MA: Tarascon Publishing; 2016.

Prescriber's Letter. Stockton, CA: Therapeutic Research Center. http://prescribersletter.therapeut icresearch.com/home.aspx?cs=&s=PRL.

LABORATORY, IMAGING, AND PROCEDURE RESOURCES

ARUP Consult. *The Physician's Guide to Laboratory Test Selection & Interpretation.* http://www.arupconsult.com.

Ferri FF. *Ferri's Best Test: A Practical Guide to Clinical Laboratory Medicine & Diagnostic Imaging,* 3rd ed. Philadelphia: Saunders; 2015.

Pfenninger JL, Fowler GC, eds. *Pfenninger and Fowler's Procedures for Primary Care,* 3rd ed. Philadelphia: Mosby; 2010.

PREVENTIVE CARE

- Students would be well served to become familiar with the United States Preventative Services Task Force (USPSTF) recommendations for clinical preventive services. The USPSTF publishes evidence-based recommendations and guides for screening, testing, and management via an independent panel of primary care experts (http://www.uspreventiveservicestaskforce.org).

medicine as well as texts that offer more rapid access of information (Box 25.2).

The U.S. Centers for Disease Control and Prevention collects medical care utilization data regarding diagnoses made in ambulatory settings such as family medicine practices. After these data have been collected, they are presented in national health statistics reports (http://www.cdc.gov/nchs/products/nhsr.htm) and then are often used to inform medical educators on expected student competencies. For example, the Society of Teachers of Family Medicine (STFM) used such reports to develop the STFM's Family Medicine Clerkship Curriculum, which outlines both the common and serious causes of acute and chronic conditions (Box 25.3) in addition to health promotions (Box 25.4). These curricula are geared toward the entry-level clerkship student, serving as a valuable resource in preparing for the family medicine rotation.

It is equally beneficial to review the National Commission on Certification of Physician Assistants (NCCPA) Content Blueprint. The Blueprint is based on a national PA practice analysis. This analysis is subsequently used to guide the NCCPA as to the content of the Physician Assistant National Certification Exam, including the most common and important conditions and tasks covered to evidence competency as a practicing PA. The Blueprint is divided into organ systems and task areas. Task areas include history taking and performing physical examinations, using laboratory and diagnostic studies, formulating most likely diagnosis, health maintenance, clinical intervention, pharmaceutical therapeutics, and applying basic science concepts.

It is also important to note that many family providers have a practice area of emphasis or special focus.[27] A particular area of emphasis may augment a practitioner's approach to the patient. Common areas of focus include emergency medicine, geriatric medicine, obstetrics and gynecology, palliative care, hospitalist medicine, addiction medicine, occupational medicine, and psychiatry.[28]

COMMON MEDICAL PROCEDURES IN FAMILY MEDICINE PRACTICES

The types and frequency of procedures differ from one practice to another.[29] Although family medicine providers may perform a wide variety of procedures,

BOX 25.3 COMMON AND SERIOUS CAUSES OF ACUTE AND CHRONIC DISEASE PRESENTATIONS

ACUTE DISEASE PRESENTATIONS
- Cardiovascular conditions: chest pain, edema
- Comorbidity and multimorbidity: presentation and management of patients presenting with more than one chronic illness
- Dermatologic conditions: common skin rashes and lesions
- Fever
- Gastroenterologic conditions: abdominal pain
- Gynecologic conditions: abnormal vaginal bleeding, vaginal discharge, initial presentation of pregnancy
- Musculoskeletal conditions: joint injury and pain, low back pain
- Neurological conditions: headache, dementia, dizziness
- Psychiatric conditions: initial presentation of depression
- Pulmonary conditions: upper respiratory symptoms, cough, shortness of breath, wheezing
- Peripheral vascular conditions: edema, deep vein thrombosis
- Psychiatric conditions: anxiety, depression, acute psychosis, hypomania, mania, substance use, dependence and abuse
- Urinary conditions (male and female): dysuria, symptoms of prostatic disease

CHRONIC DISEASE PRESENTATIONS
- Cardiovascular and peripheral vascular conditions: chronic artery disease, heart failure, hypertension, hyperlipidemia
- Endocrine conditions: diabetes, obesity
- Musculoskeletal and rheumatologic conditions: arthritis, chronic back pain, osteopenia, osteoporosis
- Pulmonary conditions: asthma, obstructive pulmonary disease

Adapted from Society of Teachers of Family Medicine (STFM). *The Family Medicine Clerkship Curriculum,* 2015. http://www.stfm.org/Resources/STFMNationalClerkshipCurriculum.

BOX 25.4 COMMON HEALTH PROMOTION CONDITIONS FOR ADULTS AND CHILDREN/ADOLESCENTS

HEALTH PROMOTION CONDITIONS FOR ADULTS
- Cardiovascular conditions: coronary artery disease
- Endocrine conditions: diabetes mellitus, obesity
- Fall risk (for elderly patients)
- Infectious disease: sexually transmitted infections, tuberculosis, HIV, hepatitis
- Musculoskeletal and rheumatoid conditions: osteoporosis
- Oncologic conditions: breast cancer, cervical cancer, colon cancer, lung cancer, oral cancer, prostate cancer
- Psychiatric conditions: depression, substance use
- Violence: intimate partner violence, family violence

HEALTH PROMOTION CONDITIONS FOR CHILDREN AND ADOLESCENTS
- Accidental and nonaccidental injury
- Lifestyle: diet, exercise, nutritional deficiency
- Family and social support
- Growth and development
- Hearing, vision
- Immunizations
- Lead exposure
- Sexual activity
- Psychiatric conditions: depression, substance use
- Infectious disease: hepatitis, HIV, tuberculosis

Adapted from Society of Teachers of Family Medicine (STFM). *The Family Medicine Clerkship Curriculum,* 2015. http://www.stfm.org/Resources/STFMNationalClerkshipCurriculum.

depending on their setting (e.g., rural, inner city) and potential area of emphasis, it is the authors' experience that most family medicine practices tend to focus on a limited number of procedures. Fig. 25.1 lists results of a recent survey regarding types of procedures performed by family medicine providers. As noted, survey respondents reported the routine performance of a wide variety of procedures ranging from endoscopies to obstetric procedures. Given the variety among family medicine practices, some

controversy exists over expectations of what students should expect to see and perform in their family medicine training.[30] Although students should be prepared to expect a fair amount of variability among practices and preceptors, researchers and national organizations have strived to compile a standard list of expectations and required procedures for family medicine training. Table 25.1 lists the procedures students should be most prepared to perform on their family medicine rotations; the list is derived from the most recent standards and expectations for medical program graduates and family medicine residency program students[23,31] and the authors' own experiences in rural, suburban, and urban family medicine practices. The list is in addition to, not in place of, standard head-to-toe physical examination skills.

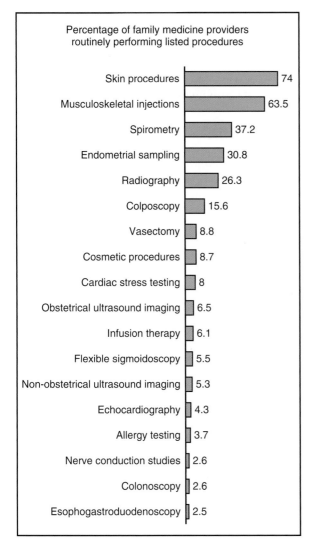

Percentage of family medicine providers routinely performing listed procedures

Procedure	Percentage
Skin procedures	74
Musculoskeletal injections	63.5
Spirometry	37.2
Endometrial sampling	30.8
Radiography	26.3
Colposcopy	15.6
Vasectomy	8.8
Cosmetic procedures	8.7
Cardiac stress testing	8
Obstetrical ultrasound imaging	6.5
Infusion therapy	6.1
Flexible sigmoidoscopy	5.5
Non-obstetrical ultrasound imaging	5.3
Echocardiography	4.3
Allergy testing	3.7
Nerve conduction studies	2.6
Colonoscopy	2.6
Esophogastroduodenoscopy	2.5

FIG. 25.1 ■ Type of procedure and percentage of family medicine provider survey respondents routinely performing procedure. (Adapted from American Academy of Family Physicians, Member census, June 30, 2014. http://www.aafp.org/about/the-aafp/family-medicine-facts/table-12.html.)

THE BENEFITS OF PRACTICING FAMILY MEDICINE

The advantages of working in family medicine, as already outlined in this chapter, include the ample opportunity to truly individualize one's medical practice. A PA in family medicine will find multiple opportunities ranging from rural to suburban to urban geographic areas and from a small, single-specialty solo provider office to a multispecialty group office, to community health centers, to hospital-owned multiclinic family medicine practices (and everything in between). Additionally,

TABLE 25.1	Core Procedures to be Expected of Family Medicine Students Based on National Standards and Experiences
Cardiac and pulmonary procedures	Electrocardiographic testing and interpretation Spirometry testing and interpretation
Dermatologic procedures	Cryotherapy, electrocautery Draining of subungual hematoma Collection of samples for cultures and fungal studies Incision and drainage of an abscess Laceration repair and wound closure Punch and excisional biopsies, excision of superficial lesion Removal of foreign bodies
Eye, ear, nose, and throat procedures	Cerumen impaction removal Epistaxis treatment, including anterior packing Fluorescein eye exam, slit-lamp examination Removal of foreign body from ear, eye, and nose Nasal swabbing for influenza, pertussis, throat culture
Gastrointestinal and colorectal procedures	Anoscopy, digital rectal examination, stool guaiac testing Nasogastric tube placement
Genitourinary procedures	Bladder catheterization Urinalysis: both dip and microscopic
Gynecologic and obstetric procedures	Collection of samples for vaginal discharge cultures and testing Endometrial biopsy Insertion and removal of intrauterine device Pap smears Wet mount and KOH evaluations of vaginal discharge
Life support and stabilization procedures	Advanced cardiac life support, pediatric advanced cardiac life support Intravenous rehydration
Musculoskeletal procedures	Initial management of simple fractures Injection and aspiration of bursa and large joints Reduction of nursemaid's elbow Upper and lower extremity splinting
Miscellaneous procedures	Glucometer testing Phlebotomy, initiation of an intravenous line
Wound care procedures	Digital block for anesthesia, topical anesthesia Wound debridement, cleaning, and closure

PAs may find themselves working in offices that focus more on *managing* care, with a lot of early patient referrals to specialists, or may practice in offices that focus on *evaluation and patient assessments* by performing numerous procedures and thorough diagnostic evaluations prior to specialist referrals. Depending on the practice, a PA in family medicine may practice very autonomously with little physician supervision or may collaborate with physicians and other team members daily in a highly team-based medical care office.

The autonomy of individualizing one's practice is complemented nicely with an attractive salary for PAs in family medicine. The 2015 AAPA Salary Report lists the median base salary of PAs in family medicine as $86,000 (range, $72,500–$110,000) with a median annual bonus of $5000 (range, $600–$23,205); this is on par with the national median annual salary of $93,800, reflective of all full-time PAs in the United States practicing in any specialty. Early career PAs are able to enter the family medicine specialty and quickly earn a salary near the family medicine median, with the median salary ranging from $80,500 (range, $72,000–$95,680) for PAs with up to 1 year of experience to $97,280 (range, $78,000–$130,000) for PAs with 20 or more years of experience. The discrepancy between the salaries of PAs who practice in family medicine or other primary care fields and PAs in medical and surgical specialties is significantly less than the discrepancies between physicians in primary care versus specialties. This in combination with the many other benefits of practicing family medicine should keep this specialty relevant within the PA profession.

Even more impactful on the attraction of medical providers to the specialty of family medicine is the more human side of medicine. One would be hard pressed to find a family medicine PA who doesn't speak to the connections and relationships that are built with their patients as one of the most rewarding aspects of this specialty. This is a specialty in which the PA can see the same patient over the course of a lifetime, from birth through childhood, adolescence, and adulthood and into advanced age. Family medicine PAs will see multiple members of the same family. They are able to understand how valued these familial relationships are and appreciate the importance of these connections on their patients' health. Often, an appointment with a long-standing patient can feel more like a visit with an old friend than a traditional medical visit. PAs in family medicine serve as the entrance point for a vast multitude of patient concerns, and thus, many patients have shared their deepest fears, saddest days, greatest triumphs, and most joyous moments with their PAs. This opportunity—to go on a body, mind, and spirit journey with the whole person against the backdrop of health care—is what embodies family medicine, and that is the reason why many PAs find this specialty to be so rewarding.

CONCLUSION

In closing, it might be of benefit to provide a sense of our own love of the practice of family medicine. Ventres[32] eloquently summed up the joys of practicing family medicine and the magnetic attraction family medicine offers to practitioners, both in what each provider contributes to and receives in return from their practice. The complex benefits of family medicine can be divided into the categories of love and faith; mystery, with a requisite tolerance for uncertainty given the breadth of practice and inherent variety of complaints, conditions, illnesses and disease processes, patient needs and desires, and challenges; place, both within and beyond the hegemony of biomedical constructs; dance, the rhythmic or not so rhythmic interaction among patient, patient's family, and provider set to the beat of pursuing the greatest well-being for our patients; and medicine, the structure and foundation of medical practice integrating the roles of counselor and guide and diagnostician and healer. Some readers may question the terms "love" and "faith" in describing the joys of family medicine; however, the pull to enter into and remain in family practice does involve a strong commitment that seems to surpass emotional, physical, and intellectual boundaries.

Given the very broad scope of practice in family medicine, bridging age, gender, organ system, and procedural domain, the family medicine specialty is both inclusive and expansive—centered on the patient–provider relationship in which patients' needs outweigh other needs and, more often than not, results in both the patient and provider sharing respect, trust, and an invitation to discuss and contemplate some of the greatest suffering and joy life has to offer. Across the lifespan, family medicine providers, knowing that they and patients are more similar than dissimilar, both navigating life's trajectory from birth to death, willingly and compassionately assist patients to navigate life's complexities and obstacles to well-being. And in so doing, they have the opportunity to achieve a greater sense of personal well-being.

Along with this knowledge, family medicine providers also share a faith in the existence of life's potential for both suffering and joy, for ill-being and well-being, for both ease and dis-ease. Such faith propels us to move forward and explore opportunities for beneficial change even in the most difficult of times. Such a worldview is, as described by Ventres,[32] both inexplicable and interdependent, transcending a simplistic biomedical model of life, suffering, and well-being. As family medicine providers, we sit with patients in both their darkest and lightest hours and are honored to do so; each patient interaction holds the potential opportunity for us to become better human beings. Surely, such a potential is founded in love and faith. Family medicine is a specialty practice that is focused on the pursuit of well-being by providing unbiased, compassionate, holistic care incorporating evidence-based practices via an approach that intertwines patient, family, and community across gender, age, organ system, and disease process, assisting patients in the pursuit of well-being from the very beginning to the end of their lives.

KEY POINTS

- The PA profession began as a strategy to manage an overtaxed health care system with a large influx of patients seeking primary medical services. This strategy has become a defining principle of the profession, with PAs fulfilling the needs of access to care for medically underserved populations, particularly in primary care specialties.
- The family medicine specialty is unique among medical specialties, incorporating pediatrics, general internal medicine, general obstetrics and gynecology, primary care geriatrics, and general psychiatry.
- Family medicine PAs embrace the relationships, patient advocacy, flexibility, and comprehensive nature of patient care that is inherent to the specialty.
- The goal of the family medicine rotation is to effectively manage both acute and chronic medical conditions, including complex multimorbidity, and to promote preventive medicine and health promotion. This is completed while prioritizing visits to address patient needs while developing strong interpersonal provider–patient relationships.
- Family medicine PAs are compassionate, highly skilled healers providing whole-person health care to the patient, family, and community.

References

1. Physician Assistant History Society, Johns Creek, GA. Timeline: 1957 to 1970, The Formative Years (2015). http://pahx.org/period02.html Accessed September 11, 2015.
2. Assistant Secretary for Public Affairs. Creating health care jobs by addressing primary care workforce needs. U.S. Department of Health & Human Services. http://www.hhs.gov/healthcare/facts/factsheets/2013/06/jobs06212012.html. Published March 23, 2015. Accessed September 12, 2015.
3. Morgan P, Everett C, Hing E. Nurse Practitioners, physician assistants, and physicians in community health centers, 2006-2010. *Healthcare*. 2015;3:102–107.
4. Proser M, Bysshe T, Weaver D, et al. Community health centers at the crossroads: growth and staffing needs. *JAAPA*. 2015;28(4):49–53.
5. Patient Centered Medical Home Resource Center. Defining the PCMH. Agency for Healthcare Research and Quality. https://pcmh.ahrq.gov/page/defining-pcmh. Accessed September 15, 2015.
6. Accountable Care Organizations (ACOs). General Information. Centers for Medicare & Medicaid Services. http://innovation.cms.gov/initiatives/aco/. Published November 27, 2015. Accessed December 7, 2015.
7. Tobbell D. Plow, town, and gown: the politics of family practice in 1960s America. *Bull Hist Med*. 2013;87:648.
8. Carney PA, Waller E, Eiff E, et al. Measuring family physician identity: the development of a new instrument. *Family Medicine*. 2013;45:708–718.
9. Collier R. Grappling with family practice complexities. *CMAJ*. 2012;184:E943.
10. Young RA, Bayles B, Benold TB, et al. Family physicians' perceptions on how they deliver cost-effective care: a qualitative study from the Residency Research Network of Texas. *Fam Med*. 2013;45:311–318.
11. Page C, Carlough MC, Lam Y, Steiner J. Reinvigorating pediatric care in an academic family medicine practice. *Fam Med*. 2014;46(2):120–123.
12. Pungo PA, McGaha AL, Schmittling GT, et al. Results of the 2010 national resident matching program: family medicine. *Fam Med*. 2010;42(8):552–561.
13. Beaulieu M, Rioux M, Rocher G, Samson L, Boucher L. Family practice: professional identity in transition. A case study of family medicine in Canada. *Soc Sci Med*. 2008;67:1153–1163.
14. Howe A. Family practice: meanings for modern times. *British Journal of General Practice*. 2010;60:207–212.
15. Taylor RB. Family practice and the advancement of medical understanding. The first 50 years. *J Fam Pract*. 1999;48:53.
16. Kahn N. The future of family medicine's role in American medicine. *Family Medicine*. 2015;47:646–648.
17. Patient Centered Primary Care Collaborative (PCPCC). *Joint principles of the patient-centered medical home*; 2007. http://www.aafp.org/dam/AAFP/documents/practice_management/pcmh/initiatives/PCMHJoint.pdf.
18. Olid AS, Zurro AM, Villa JJ, et al. Medical students' perceptions and attitudes about family practice: a qualitative research synthesis. *BMC Med Edu*. 2012; 81.

19. Bradner M, Crossman S, Gary J, Vanderbilt A, VanderWielen L. Beyond diagnoses: family medicine core themes in student reflective writing. *Fam Med*. 2015;47(3):182–186.

20. Shi L, Macinko J, Starfield B, Wulu J, Regan J, Politzer R. The relationship between primary care, income inequality, and mortality in the US states, 1980-1995. JABFP. 16(5):412–422.

21. Katerndahl D, Wood R, Jaen CR. Famil medicine outpatient encounters are more complex than those of cardiology and psychiatry. *J Am Board Fam Med*. 2011;24:6–15.

22. Flocke SA, Frank SH, Wenger DA. Addressing multiple problems in the family practice office visit. *J Fam Pract*. 2001;50:211.

23. Society of Teachers of Family Medicine (STFM). *The family medicine clerkship curriculum*; 2015. http://www.stfm.org/Reso urces/STFMNationalClerkshipCurriculum.

24. Dawes M. Symptoms, reasons for encounter and diagnoses. Family practice is an international discipline. *Fam Pract*. 2012;29:243.

25. Cordes DH, Rea DF. Workplace visits: an important place in family practice. *Am Fam Physician*. 1994;49:733.

26. Fortin M, Bravo G, Hudon C, Vanasse A, Lapointe L. Prevalence of multimorbidity among adults seen in family practice. *Ann Fam Med*. 2005;3:223–228.

27. Gutkin C. The future of family practice in Canada: The Patient's Medical Home. *Can Fam Physician*. 2011;57: 1224–1224.

28. Kondro W. The changing face of family practice. *CMAJ*. 2011;183:E1174.

29. van den Hombergh P, Schalk-Soekar S, Braspenning JC, Bottema BJ, Campbell SM, Kramer A. Are family practice trainers and their host practices any better? Comparing practice trainers and non-trainers and their practices. *BMC Fam Pract*. 2013;14: 23.

30. Nothnagle M, Sicilia JM, Forman S, et al. Required procedural training in family medicine residency: a consensus statement. *Fam Med*. 2008;40(4):248–252.

31. Dickson G, Chesser A, Woods NK, Krug NR, Kellerman RD. Family medicine residency program director expectations of procedural skills of medical school graduates. *Fam Med*. 2013;45(6):392–399.

32. Ventres W. The joy of family practice. *Ann Fam Med*. 2012;10:264–268.

INTERNAL MEDICINE

Patty J. Scholting

Internal medicine is a medical specialty that provides comprehensive health care to adult patients. This includes health prevention and the management of complex acute and chronic disease. The nature of the practice of internal medicine allows health care providers to establish a long-term relationship with patients. Providers have the opportunity to be involved in all aspects of medical care, offering patients ongoing care for many years. Medical care most commonly takes place in an ambulatory outpatient clinic but can also include inpatient care during hospitalization and in skilled nursing facilities.

Upon completing a 3-year residency in internal medicine, physicians are referred to as "internists" and practice general internal medicine. A hospitalist is a physician trained in internal medicine, whose primary focus is in caring for hospitalized patients. Subspecialists in internal medicine complete the 3-year residency and a 2- or 3-year fellowship in the area of interest, which includes 13 areas of medicine, including allergy and immunology, cardiology, endocrinology, gastroenterology, geriatrics, hematology, and oncology, to name a few.[1]

Physician assistants (PAs) with a strong interest in internal medicine may choose to broaden their knowledge base by enrolling in a postgraduate fellowship. These programs are offered by medical institutions and are commonly 12 months in duration. Upon completion of a fellowship, the PA will receive a certificate indicating the completion of the postgraduate training in internal medicine.

PHYSICIAN ASSISTANTS IN INTERNAL MEDICINE

Physician assistants in internal medicine can expect to encounter a broad range of health issues. Patients present with health conditions that are relatively simple and straightforward, but other issues can be complex and involve multisystem disease processes. Preventive medicine is an important aspect of the practice of internal medicine and includes the promotion of a healthy lifestyle and the prevention of chronic illnesses such as diabetes mellitus, cardiovascular disease, and cancer.

Practice settings for internist PAs range from ambulatory outpatient clinics, hospitals, or long-term skilled care facilities. Practicing in these different environments is advantageous because it allows the PA to follow a patient through a continuum of care. Continuity of care is essential to maintaining quality and consistency in dealing with chronic disease.[2]

Physician assistants in general internal medicine can expect an average annual base salary of $73,800 to $112,000, depending on multiple factors including years of practice and the geographic location where they practice.[3] Compensation packages and benefits depend on the institution or practice.

Physician Assistants in Internal Medicine Subspecialties

In addition to general internal medicine, PAs commonly practice in one of the 13 internal medicine subspecialties. According to the 2013 National Commission on Certification of Physician Assistants Statistical Profile of Certified Physician Assistants, of the survey respondents, 7.7% (*n* = 4178) indicated that they practiced in one of the internal medicine subspecialties.[4] Physician assistants in one of the subspecialties can expect a similar base salary as general internal medicine. This information can be accessed through the American Academy of Physician Assistant (AAPA) Salary Report, published annually by the AAPA.[3]

Internal Medicine Rotation

The general internal medicine rotation offers PA students the opportunity to expand their knowledge regarding common acute and chronic illnesses in adult patients as well as screening and preventive medicine. The rotation broadens the depth and breadth of the student's medical knowledge base about the disease process and the pharmacotherapeutics used in the management of disease. The rotation reinforces clinical skills in patient interviewing; physical examination; and interpretation of ancillary testing, case presentations, and detailed written documentation. The student benefits from working in a team-based environment while using clinical reasoning skills. The rotation assists the student in developing skills necessary to assess accurately clinical situations, develop a differential diagnosis list, and arrive at a working diagnosis. The experience may be mostly outpatient based or hospital based or a combination of both environments.

What to Expect and Know

Expectations and student responsibilities depend on the rotation site and the preceptor. Generally speaking, the PA student should have basic knowledge of a broad spectrum of acute and chronic illnesses and be a self-directed learner. The student should be able to perform a thorough patient history and comprehensive physical examination confidently. The development of a concise differential diagnosis list based on the history and physical examination will guide the student in ordering and the interpretation of appropriate diagnostic tests. The PA student will formulate an assessment, plan, and the appropriate

patient education and follow-up. Each case is presented to the preceptor by clearly identifying the patient's chief complaint, history, pertinent physical examination findings, assessment, plan, and follow-up. The presentation needs to be well organized and provide the preceptor with the essential information regarding the patient encounter. The student should be prepared to answer questions about each case as well as ask appropriate questions of the preceptor to augment the learning experience. At the conclusion of an internal medicine rotation, the student should gain broader knowledge of the pathophysiology of acute and chronic disease, improve his or her skills in developing a comprehensive differential diagnosis list, confidently order and interpret diagnostic testing, and have a solid understanding of the role of pharmacotherapeutics in the management of disease.

Clinical Environment

Practice settings for PAs in internal medicine range from outpatient clinics to hospitals, skilled nursing facilities, or a combination of all. The job of the PA in the inpatient setting is to care for patients who are typically acutely ill. It requires the PA to participate in daily rounds on the patients either independently or part of a multidisciplinary health team. Effective organizational skills are essential in managing multiple hospitalized patients. It can be helpful to develop a system for keeping patient data at your fingertips. It may be the responsibility of the PA to perform the initial complete history and physical examination on all newly admitted patients. This information must be meticulously gathered because it may affect the initial management of a patient. The role of the PA in the hospital setting may include direct communication with patients and their families. It is important for PAs to feel comfortable and confident when discussing all aspects of the management of hospitalized patients.

Many PAs in internal medicine, especially in smaller communities, care for patients residing in skilled nursing facilities. This may require the PA to round on patients and manage their care through effective communication with the nursing staff, patients, and many times, families. In certain situations, nursing home patients are transported to the outpatient clinic for routine care. A patient may not have a family member accompanying him or her or may have difficulty with verbal communication, so it is important that written orders for the nursing staff at the facility are clear and concise.

The ambulatory clinic setting requires the ability to work autonomously while using critical thinking skills in the assessment and management of disease. Time management, organizational skills, and the ability to think on your feet are vital in the outpatient clinic setting.

OTHER HEALTH PROFESSIONALS

In addition to internists, PAs work with a multidisciplinary team of health professionals in internal medicine. These individuals play a significant role in the effective care of the patient; therefore, it is important to have the ability to work well with a team. Internal medicine PAs often collaborate with primary care providers, internal medicine subspecialists, surgeons, physical therapists, pharmacists, nurses, and social workers, among others. It is essential to understand the role of each member of the health team and be able to communicate effectively with these individuals to provide the best care possible to patients.

PATIENTS AND SPECIAL POPULATIONS

Physician assistant students and PAs practicing in general internal medicine or one of the internal medicine subspecialties are exposed to a variety of adult patients with a broad range of backgrounds, medical issues, and socioeconomic concerns. Many of these patients may have multiple health conditions, which can result in functional limitations that require supportive services to assist with daily care or transportation. Decreased hearing and visual acuity can make patient–provider communication a challenge. Patients with a diagnosis of dementia are common in an internal medicine practice, and performing a history and physical examination takes time and patience. Many geriatric patients live on a fixed income, which can influence their ability to afford medications or diagnostic testing. The internal medicine environment allows providers to practice many aspects of medicine and to care for a diverse group of patients.

CHALLENGES AND REWARDS

Practicing in internal medicine comes with both challenges and rewards. Patients present with multisystem disease states that can be complex and at times overwhelming. It requires a good clinician to have excellent problem-solving skills and the insight to pursue lifelong self-directed learning. Caring for adults requires patience and empathy but is rewarded with patient trust. As a PA, the practice of internal medicine can potentially be very rewarding because of these deeply rooted patient–provider relationships that develop over time. It is common to care for different generations of the same family line. Providers in internal medicine develop relationships with patients based on trust, confidentiality, and professionalism. Patient–provider relationships are many times long standing until the end of life.

KEY POINTS

- Internal medicine is a medical specialty that provides comprehensive health care to adult patients.
- There are 13 internal medicine subspecialties that offer practicing PAs and PAs student a rich and rewarding learning environment.
- Internal medicine patients often present with complex multisystem medical conditions.
- Practice settings for internist PAs range from ambulatory outpatient clinics, hospitals, or long-term skilled care facilities.

References

1. American College of Physicians. *ACP: About Internal Medicine*. December 2015;2015(28).
2. Buckley Kimberly. Gain exposure to many specialties as a physician assistant internist. *Clinical Advisor*. 2011.
3. AAPA. *2015 AAPA Salary Report: National Findings*; 2015.
4. NCCPA. 2013 Statistical Profile of Certified Physician Assistants: an Annual Report of the National Commission on Certification of Physician Assistants. *Annual Report*. 2013.

The resources for this chapter can be found at www.expertconsult.com.

CHAPTER 27

WOMEN'S HEALTH

Erin Nicole Lunn McAdams

APPROACH TO THE PATIENT

Since the inauguration of the physician assistant (PA) profession, primary care has played a key role in training PA students. Obstetrics and gynecology (OB/GYN) are practiced by many primary care and family medicine PAs; therefore, it is an important topic of interest in PA student education. The remarkable feature of OB/GYN is that it encompasses not only the outpatient setting but also the operating room (OR), inpatient setting, and labor and delivery setting. For this reason, it is important for PA students to be educated in every facet of these realms and understand this unique area of medicine. In obstetrics, you will treat pregnant women as well as their unborn children. In gynecology, you will be able to treat women from adolescence through menopause. OB/GYN gives you the capacity to build an effective rapport with your patients that will carry them through a life span. In this setting, you will encounter acute, subacute, and chronic conditions. You will need to be fluent as a geneticist, internist, and general practitioner. You will approach most gynecologic patients in a comprehensive manner, sometimes even functioning as their primary care provider and internist. You will manage chronic conditions such as hypertension and diabetes throughout pregnancy. An understanding of genetics is important in this setting because you need to illustrate to patients the reasoning and outcomes of prenatal testing.

WHAT TO EXPECT ON CLINICAL ROTATIONS

Surgery Service

On the surgical service, you should expect to be up early preparing for cases and mentally preparing for your day in the OR. You should also read up on the cases the night before surgery to familiarize yourself with the anatomy. You may also have several postoperative patients whom you will round on before or directly after the surgical cases for the day. Common gynecologic surgeries include

312

hysterectomy (total or partial), which may be performed through a variety of different surgical approaches depending on the situation, physician preference, and patient desire (open, laparoscopically, vaginally). Know the risks, benefits, indications, and complications of these procedures. Other surgeries include myomectomy, tubal ligation, and inserting a pelvic mesh to help support the bladder or uterus.

Inpatient Service

Arrive early to round on your patients before your intern or resident arrives. This allows you to have extra time to interview your patients without any other distractions. In many academic hospital settings, you will round with your resident and again with the attending physician. If you are rounding with a private practice physician, the same rules apply: Arrive early and round on patients so you may orally present each case to the physician. This will prove to your preceptor that you have spent the extra time with the patients and have thoroughly researched their conditions.

Outpatient Service

In an outpatient service, you will rotate in a clinical setting. This may range from private practice to an instructional setting, where several providers are associated with a teaching institution such as a university hospital. In both settings, you will provide care for patients with and without health insurance. You may even care for patients who are incarcerated. Clinic days may vary with obstetrics and gynecology. You will perform Papanicolaou (Pap) tests, pelvic examinations, rectal examinations, sexually transmitted infection (STI) screens, breast examinations, measurement of fundal heights, Leopold maneuvers, and complete cervical checks for dilation; interpret ultrasound images; provide extensive patient education; and communicate appropriate routine health maintenance on a daily basis. Procedures in the office may include intrauterine device (IUD) insertions, colposcopy, endometrial biopsies, and draining of Bartholin gland abscess. Two office procedures that you should familiarize yourself with in detail are Pap tests and insertions of IUDs.

According to the Centers for Disease Control and Prevention, almost 70% of women older than 18 years of age received a Pap test within the past 3 years.[1] It is your duty to educate patients on the recommended frequency for screening. Many guidelines regarding the screening of women for cervical disorders have recently been updated, and you should familiarize yourself with them. It is important to note that many women seek care from an obstetrician or gynecologist unsure of how often they should receive such examinations. Even if women do not meet the criteria for a Pap test, almost all women should receive a complete pelvic examination on an annual basis, according to the American Congress of Obstetrics and Gynecology (ACOG). To perform a Pap test, you should have the woman lie in the lithotomy position with her feet placed gently in the stirrups. She should be wearing a gown and be covered from the waist down with a drape. You should depress the drape in the center so that from a seated position, you are able to visualize her face. You should explain all techniques to the patient before performing them. First, you should gently place the back of your gloved hand against the inside of her thigh and inform her that you will be inspecting the external genitalia. After this, you should depress the posterior vaginal introitus (again while verbalizing all of this to the patient in layman's terms) and insert an appropriately sized speculum at a 45-degree angle into the vagina. The speculum should be warmed and lubricated with water only. As you advance the speculum, continue to rotate it to a full 90 degrees. For women who have posterior placement of the cervix, you may have to apply downward pressure so the cervix comes into view. Keep in mind that this may add discomfort to the patient, and explaining that a posterior cervix is an anatomic variant may ease some of her discomfort and allow her to understand that you are not trying to cause her any unnecessary discomfort. If you are still unable to view the cervix, you should have your preceptor come in behind you. When the cervix in in view, including the os and transformation zone, lock the speculum in place and take samples as necessary while inspecting the cervix and vaginal walls. As you complete the examination, remember to unlock the speculum and gently guide it out of the vagina in the same manner in which you inserted it.[2]

Inserting an IUD can be one of the most difficult yet interesting procedures you will perform in OB/GYN practice. A few key points to learn when inserting an IUD will help you while on your rotation. First and most important, be sure that you receive consent from the patient to perform the procedure. Ensure that you and the preceptor have discussed all of the risks, side effects, and benefits of the procedure to the patient before placement. You will perform a speculum examination as described earlier. Confirm that the patient is not allergic to iodine or latex before performing the next step. If she is allergic to either iodine or latex, adhere to the institution's protocol. Clean the cervix with povidone–iodine solution, and don sterile gloves. The next step is the placement of the tenaculum. It may improve the discomfort for this segment of the examination if you have the patient take a deep inhalation and then blow out swiftly and forcefully while you place the tenaculum at the same time. This instrument is used to grip a portion of the anterior cervix and allows you to manipulate the cervix and hold it in place while you insert the IUD. Make sure not to maneuver the cervix too forcefully or excessively because this may cause a vagal response in the patient (hypotension, syncope, nausea, and vomiting). Remember to explain all steps of the procedure to the patient as you perform them. Next, measure the fundal height of the uterus with an instrument called a uterine sound. You will be able to determine the length of the uterus by the mark of iodine left on the instrument. After this, use your measuring tool on the IUD kit to properly measure to the height of the fundus. Place the IUD according to the manufacturer's directions.[3] After you have ensured proper placement, remove the tenaculum and trim the strings of the IUD, leaving 1 to 2 inches. You can trim the strings again at a later date after some time has passed and you have established that the IUD is in the proper position. Ensure the patient's comfort, and then remove the speculum.

Managing abnormal cervical cytology can be a difficult task for providers, and a diagnosis of dysplasia can also be a source of anxiety for patients. For this reason, it is essential that you understand the current guidelines and how to follow the recommended algorithms. Many women wonder how often they should obtain a Pap test. The evidence-based guidelines for the screening and management of abnormal Pap tests are formulated by the American Society for Colposcopy and Cervical Pathology (ASCCP). This body publishes guidelines based on evidence-based medicine. A few important changes to the guidelines include:

1. Co-testing for human papillomavirus (HPV) and cytology for atypical squamous cells of undetermined significance (ASC-US) every 3 years rather than every 5 years in patients with a history of an HPV-negative Pap test result
2. Patients with negative cytology without endocervical cells may be managed without annual testing.

3. If cervical cytology is unsatisfactory, then a repeat Pap test is needed even if the patient does not show the presence of HPV.
4. HPV-negative and ASC-US Pap test results are not sufficient means to discontinue screening in women older than 65 years of age.
5. In patients with ASC-US, immediate referral for colposcopy is no longer considered first-line management, and a repeat Pap test should be delayed for 1 year. If the subsequent test result is also negative, testing should resume at regular 3-year intervals.
6. Pap-only testing (cytology) without HPV is typically limited to women younger than 30 years of age. Women with dysplasia between the ages of 21 and 24 years are managed as conservatively as possible because colposcopy and other cervical procedures can damage the normal shape, length, and functionality of the cervix, thereby increasing the risk of preterm labor in future childbearing.[4]

Labor and Delivery and Postpartum

On the labor and delivery service, you may be expected to work long hours. This can include night shifts, overnight call, or weekends. Babies don't have a timeline or wait for the workday to start. If your preceptor permits it and the patient you're following hasn't delivered, remain until the fetus is delivered even if it means that you stay past your scheduled shift. This facilitates the opportunity to deliver your own patient. You should familiarize yourself with how to perform a cervical check for dilation and effacement. It is also essential to acquaint yourself with how to calculate a Bishop score so you will understand that if a patient has a score for induction of labor, it correlates to a successful vaginal delivery.[5] During postpartum rounds, you will provide similar services as you did on your other inpatient gynecology patients. You should ask in all postpartum patients about pain, bleeding to include blood clots, and flatus. Build rapport with your patients; remember their names and the names of their infants.

EXPECTATIONS FOR A SUCCESSFUL ROTATION

In an article published by the Association of Professors in Gynecology and Obstetrics (APGO), a successful rotation is built on realistic ("do") and unrealistic expectations ("do not"). We will divide these expectations based on the clinical setting.

	Do	**Do Not**
Surgery	Familiarize yourself with the surgical cases and procedures before getting started. Recall sterile field boundaries.	Don't scrub into a case if you are sick or have to leave during the surgery.
Inpatient	Get to know your patients on the service. Remember their names; if they are OB patients, know their infants' names. Get to the service before your intern and round on your patients.	Don't expect others to see your patients. Don't walk into a service and not introduce yourself even if you've seen the patient before.
Outpatient	Review the last few progress notes to familiarize yourself with the patient in order to guide treatment. Review previous lectures and read about common pathology related to OB/GYN.	Do not perform pelvic or breast examinations without a chaperone present. Don't make appointments or engagements immediately after clinic because most times you will stay the duration of your scheduled shift.
Labor and delivery and postpartum	Find a patient on the service and continue her care even if your shift is over. Make yourself accessible for any procedures and emergencies.	Don't assume that patients and other members of the health care team know you are a student. Don't leave the floor even if the service is slow because situations can and do change swiftly.

GYN, Gynecology; *OB,* obstetrics.

Interprofessionalism on Obstetrics and Gynecology

In a surgical setting, you may encounter scrub techs; preoperative, postoperative, and surgical nurses; acute care nurse practitioners (NPs); PAs; and OB/GYN physicians, anesthesiologists, and certified nurse anesthetists (CNAs). To ensure the safety of patients, you will witness any of these members of the health care team performing "time outs." This is a practiced universal protocol that will ensure the correct patient, the correct site of the operation, and the correct type of surgery to be performed.[7] All health care team members are integral to the time-out to help decrease errors and iatrogenic injury to the patient. The University of Arizona Medical Center has implemented a Safety First Program to help decrease medical errors.[8]

In an inpatient setting, you will encounter patient care assistants, floor nurses, PAs, and OB/GYN physicians. Care will be provided to patients with acute or chronic OB/GYN issues and postoperative and postpartum patients. It is important to be familiar with the patients on this service because you will likely encounter them for consecutive days or weeks. Assimilation of the health care team's mannerisms in which they care for patients allows you to become an integral member of the team and help to provide a holistic approach to any given patient.

In an outpatient office setting, you will likely work with a variety of other clinicians. This may include medical assistants (MAs), nurses, NPs, PAs, certified nurse midwives (CNMs), and OB/GYN physicians. All of these health professionals work as a team to work toward one common goal. The main objective is to aid women in the maintenance of a healthy lifestyle from adolescence through menopause. The team is also responsible for patient care during pregnancy and in the postpartum period. To provide high-quality health care, an integrated medical team is necessary to enhance favorable patient outcomes.[9] Many training programs embody this model of interprofessional education and collaborative practice to improve the understanding of roles that each specialty performs on the health care team. The New York University School of Medicine at Langone Medical Center requires OB/GYN fellows to design and integrate an interprofessional simulation into their undergraduate or postgraduate courses. The purpose of this mission is to improve students, residents, and staff members as specialists.[10]

In the labor and delivery setting, you will collaborate with patient care assistants, obstetric and neonatal nurses, CNMs, NPs, PAs, and OB/GYN physicians along with pediatricians and neonatologists. If there are known medical conditions that affect the fetal cardiac, renal, or gastrointestinal tract, you may also consult with a pediatric cardiologist, nephrologist, or pediatric general surgeon. These specialists are usually available at the time of delivery of the baby. Each member of this team is integral in caring for the mother and child to ensure they both receive the most appropriate tailored care. When a child may be born with a fetal defect or mishap, it is imperative to consider the mental health status of the mother. In this instance, it is appropriate to involve mental health specialists, grievance counselors, and social workers. These specialists are able to provide a unique set of services for the mother.

CLINICAL INFORMATION

In the OR, be familiar with common equipment used during female surgical procedures. Know the technique of scrubbing in for surgery and the properties and rubrics for maintaining sterile fields. The preoperative interview with the patient should include previous medical and surgical histories, medication allergies, and any complications while under anesthesia or former perioperative morbidities. Acquaint yourself with the anatomy before a procedure so you understand the pathology and can relate the diagnosis to the indication for surgery. Review the complications that may occur during the postoperative period and how to prevent and treat them.

Patients in the hospital setting, especially those who are postoperative, should be questioned again about flatus, abdominal distention, and postoperative pain. The reasoning for inquiring about these issues is that it may aid in the early diagnosis of postoperative complications such as an ileus caused by surgery. In postpartum patients, vaginal bleeding and the size of blood clotting should be addressed to uncover any signs of early postpartum hemorrhage and to intervene as necessary. Lactation, if desired, should also be addressed in these women as well immediately after delivery. Women admitted with complications during pregnancy after 20 weeks of gestation should be screened for symptoms of preeclampsia to include scotoma, blurry vision, headaches, hepatic tenderness, and fetal movement. Inquiring about fetal movement is a fetal vital sign in women after 28 weeks' gestation. She should perform fetal kick counts on a daily basis or if she notices a change in fetal movement. There should be at least 10 fetal kicks in a 2-hour period.[11] If a pregnant woman notes a decrease in the fetal movement, further evaluation is necessary. Patients who are admitted with pregnancy complications, especially those who are confined to bedrest for extended periods of time, should also be screened for mental health disorders such as anxiety and depression. There is a known increased risk for the development of depression in high-risk obstetric patients who have been hospitalized.[12]

In an outpatient setting, it is pertinent that the clinician obtain a full history to include the patient's complete OB/GYN history. This may include a discussion of STIs, number of sexual partners, sexual preference, history of abortion (either elective or spontaneous), and history of rape or domestic violence. The gynecologic history should also include full details about the menstrual cycle to include menarche, cycle length, amount of menstrual flow per cycle, the presence or absence of menstrual symptoms (breast tenderness, Mittelschmerz, irritability), dysmenorrhea, and the presence of intermenstrual bleeding. In older women, a history detailed with menopausal symptoms to include changes in menstrual flow, vasomotor symptoms, changes in mood lability, and vaginal dryness is helpful in determining the best course of treatment.[13] The full medical history, including chronic health conditions and disease management, is also pertinent because certain diseases in OB/GYN can lead to other comorbid conditions of major organ systems and vice versa. For example, a patient with hypertension, obesity, insulin resistance, and hirsutism may have polycystic ovarian syndrome, which may interfere with her ability to conceive. Another example is an obese woman who has a history of gestational diabetes mellitus. This places her at a 50% to 75% increased risk of developing type 2 diabetes in her lifetime.[14]

Patients in the labor and delivery settings should be educated about the stages of labor, pain management, fetal heart rate, fetal movement, and what to expect during the process of labor and delivery. As a student, you should be familiar with the physiology of labor, cervical dilation and effacement, fetal station, and the cardinal movements so you may provide this education to the patient and her family member(s). In a setting where emotions are high, it is imperative that you remain calm despite any complications that may arise. The most salient advice is to keep the patient informed of all events that are occurring and provide her with education for any procedures that may be expected so she may make appropriate informed decisions.

PROMOTION OF WELLNESS

In practicing women's health, you will encounter a number of situations when you will modify your interview and management plan to promote a healthy lifestyle. Wellness in this setting includes sexual health, diet and exercise, menstrual hygiene, conception, contraception, pregnancy, childbirth, parenting, and menopause. There are multiple resources for women online regarding many of these issues, but some sources can be ambiguous. It is ultimately up to the health care provider to sort through this information and clear up any misconceptions to provide clear indications to what is or is not evidence-based guidelines and treatment. OB/GYN treatment may include the use of complementary alternative medicine approaches, medications that have been routine practice for several decades, and new medications that have just concluded the clinical trial phase.[15] It is the responsibility of PAs and PA students to sift through this knowledge and provide a tailored treatment plan for each patient, taking into account her history and the severity of her condition and weighing the risks versus benefits of any treatments prescribed.

Sexual health is a significant issue in women's health. Alfred Kinsey, a professor at Harvard University in the 1930s, was one of the first recognized sexologists.[15] He, along with other colleagues, published a book on female sexual behavior, which was unusual for this time period because women and sexuality were still considered taboo subjects. In 1979, Helen Singer Kaplan, a sex therapist, published a book called *Disorders of Sexual Desire* that illustrated sexual dysfunction. This helped to introduce female sexual dysfunction as a medical condition and is now recognized by the *Diagnostic and Statistical Manual of Mental Disorders* (DSM-V-TR) as a group of clinical diagnoses classed into disorders associated with sexual arousal, painful intercourse, decrease in sexual desire, and orgasm.[16]

Many OB/GYN practitioners also function as primary care providers and sometimes are the only health care providers women seek on an annual basis. According to Women's Health-Prevention and Promotion, all practitioners should follow certain guidelines to promote healthy lifestyles and preventive screening measures.[17] A simple office visit is often an opportunity to discuss other health issues, including safe sexual practices; obesity; mental health disease; and other conditions that may affect gastrointestinal, lung, heart, or breast health.

Safe sexual practices should be discussed at every visit regardless of the patient's marital status. It is not correct to assume that just because a woman is married that she is in a monogamous relationship or that she is not at risk for the transmission of STIs or sexual violence. It is also essential to discuss unsafe sexual practices, including the risk of having multiple partners, unprotected intercourse and the risk of oral sex, and violent relationships. To facilitate the interview regarding these sensitive issues, it may help to open the session with a statement such as, "I am not trying to exclude any information, so I ask all of my patients these questions: Do you currently only have one sexual partner?" "Do you use condoms all of the time you are engaging in sex or only right before ejaculation?" "Do you have vaginal or anal intercourse or both?" and "Do you participate in oral sex, or what do you consider being oral sex?" This will help guide the interview in a nonjudgmental format to enhance the amount and detailed information provided by the patient. You must take into consideration your patient's perceptions about sexual behavior. You should accept that discussing matters such as sexual behavior may be uncomfortable for you and for your patient. How you respond during the interview will affect how much information she is willing to divulge. If you become too judgmental, she may shut down or seek the help of another provider. Your duty is to provide a listening ear, educate her, and provide a welcoming environment where she feels free to discuss any issues.

Obesity has become a widespread problem in the United States. According to the World Health Organization (WHO), in 2008, more than 1.4 million adults were overweight, and more than half of these persons were obese (body mass index >30 kg/m²).[18] Comorbid conditions often associated with obesity include diabetes, hypertension, coronary artery disease, and certain cancers. The WHO encourages patients to engage in physical activity 30 minutes or more in duration on most days of the week as well as limit their intakes of high-calorie foods. Health care providers in the setting of OB/GYN can aid in keeping patients accountable for these lifestyle changes and support women to make healthy decisions.

As the stigma on mental health begins to decline, many women have sought counsel from their OB/GYN practitioners to discuss a number of topics ranging from depression and alcohol abuse to domestic violence and eating disorders. Many women find comfort and encouragement from their women's health providers and thus are more open to discuss these issues in a safe environment. If needed, appropriate referrals can be made to help patients receive appropriate and timely care. If the patient is referred to a psychologist, it may still be the responsibility of the OB/GYN practitioner to prescribe medications if medically necessary. Depression can be a delicate subject but is best approached by asking open-ended questions such as, "Do you feel fidgety or restless?" "How are your stress levels at work and at home?" "Do you feel guilty about anything in your life?" "Tell me about your sleeping and eating habits." Certain questions that can help to facilitate disclosure of domestic issues may include "Do you feel safe in your home?" "How are things going at home?" or "How do you feel about the relationships in your life?"[19]

HOW TO APPROACH THE DIVERSE PATIENT

You will encounter a wide variety of sexual diversity in OB/GYN practice. Lesbian, bisexual, and transsexual patients; women with physical and mental disabilities; and patients with cultural differences are all populations you must be familiar with. It is important to keep a nondiscriminatory attitude when engaging with these populations so as to encourage them to provide the most accurate information of their health and situation. Any suspicion of judgment perceived by the patient will hinder the interview and prevent her from seeking further care. According to a study done in San Francisco in 1994, there were certain barriers that lesbians identified that hindered their care. These included providers who assumed they were heterosexual; a sense of false perception that they were not affected by STIs or HIV; and a lack of access to health care or health insurance, especially if the spouse or partner was of the same sex.[15] Of utmost importance in the lesbian population was the transition of their health from adolescence through adulthood. Studies have proven that a lack of appropriate social support from family or peers may increase the risk for lack of self-identification and mental health disorders to include depression, suicide, and substance abuse.[15] It is not unusual to see transgendered individuals in this setting. This population is at an increased risk for becoming suicidal (≈10% more likely); therefore, your attitude and judgment can have lasting negative impacts on these patients. Two crucial points should not be overlooked when treating transgendered individuals: (1) honor the patient's preferred gender and (2) respect the patient's gender identity.[20] It becomes your responsibility to be the patient's advocate and treat the patient without judgment. If the patient feels betrayed in any way, this could potentially be the last time the person ever visits a health care professional. Make sure you do not impair any relationship the patient may have in the future with other health care professionals.

Women with physical disabilities or cultural differences present a number of challenges for the OB/GYN providers who manage their care. These women may present with atypical disease symptoms or complaints or be less inclined to provide pertinent information regarding their health based on their values and perceptions.[15] Some providers do not acknowledge that women with disabilities are sexually mature and engage in sexual activity; thus, these health care providers may be disinclined to discuss these issues. According to *Healthy People 2020*, the objectives to improve health outcomes for people with disabilities include receiving intervention and services that in OB/GYN include preventive medical services such as mammograms and Pap smears.[21] It may be necessary to obtain a legal power of attorney to help guide medical decision making in the best interest of the patient for those who are medically illiterate or require a caregiver. Also, patients with cultural differences may not want to discuss sexual dysfunction with a male provider, and this factor should be recognized and respected. You should be aware that you may come across patients with specific cultural beliefs. This may include only speaking to or being treated by a female provider. Some cultural differences may also include the use of various birth control methods. Table 27.1 outlines various religious beliefs regarding contraception and sexuality according to the Family Planning Association.[22]

Another challenging patient population in OB/GYN is patients with chronic pain. In medicine, our mission is to help others and relieve them of pain. Patients with chronic pain can be distressing for any provider in any field of medicine and in the setting of this specialty may arise when treating postoperative complications, endometriosis, fibroids, or generalized pelvic pain. Chronic pain is at best manageable and not always curable. This becomes frustrating not only for providers but for patients as well because many times, there is no treatment for cure. The best way to handle patients with chronic pain is through a team-based approach.[23] This includes the involvement of the supervising physician and other health care team members such as pain specialists, psychologists, and counselors.

STUDENT AND FACULTY RESOURCES

Most medical diagnosis, testing, intervention, and treatment you will encounter during your OB/GYN rotation should be evidence based. You will find there are plenty of free resources available at your fingertips. Two such resources are the websites of the ACOG and the APGO. Both of these online sources have the most updated evidence-based medicine practices and will serve you well when you are unsure about how to manage a

TABLE 27.1 Religious Beliefs Regarding Contraception and Sexuality

Religion	Sexual Beliefs	Contraceptive Beliefs	Beliefs on Abortion
Buddhism	Avoid acts of sexual misconduct.	Conception occurs at fertilization, so oral contraceptives may or may not be an appropriate option.	Abortion is an act of murder and goes against beliefs. If there is threat to the woman carrying a fetus, then by "the most ethical choice," it may be seen as appropriate to terminate the pregnancy.
Catholicism	Monogamous relationships within a marital union	Believes in abstinence during fertile phase of menstrual cycle, otherwise known as natural family planning	Against religious moral beliefs
Hinduism	Avoid sexual misconduct.	All methods of contraception are permitted. Many Hindus choose not to use contraception until they bear a son.	Spiritual and physical life begins at conception, so abortion may not be an accepted practice.
Islam	Monogamous relationships within a marital union	Contraception as it pertains to protection of the mother such as during breastfeeding or other personal reasons	The soul does not enter the fetus until the 120th day of conception. If indicated or accepted by practice, abortion should be performed before this time.
Judaism	Monogamous relationships within a marital union	Men may not use any form of contraception. Women may use contraception that does not destroy sperm in any way (spermicides).	Consultation with a rabbi. Orthodox Jews permit abortion when the mother's life is in danger.
Sikhism	Sexual relationships should remain within a marital union.	No conclusive contraceptive method is preferred.	If pregnancy constitutes a serious threat to the woman mentally or physically or if the gestation is the result of rape, then abortion may be accepted.

Adapted from Family Planning Association. *Talking Sense about Sex,* January 2011. http://www.fpa.org.uk/sites/default/files/religion-contraception-and-abortion-factsheet.pdf.

specific condition. The ASCCP's website provides algorithms based on the current evidence regarding how to manage abnormal Pap smears. Other sources include UPTODATE and Access Medicine, which allow you to analyze and interpret the most current evidence-based medical practices.

STUDENT TIPS

While rotating in the OB/GYN setting, you should be ready to obtain as much experience as possible. Most of your days will be fast paced, and you will constantly be learning. It is important to reflect at the end of each day in order to assimilate the information from the cases you may have witnessed that day. This includes going over lecture materials and patient notes and reading about what conditions you have seen during your shift. Reading and research are also beneficial for your end-of-rotation (EOR) examinations. Working through practice questions as they pertain to OB/GYN can help to boost not only your EOR grades but also

improve the performance on your Physician Assistant National Certification Exam (PANCE).

During your OB/GYN rotation, you should have a professional attitude and come to each setting with a positive outlook. Every patient and every case are learning opportunities that will help you to become a seasoned professional. Volunteer for any procedure or patient encounter, even if you might find it challenging or uncomfortable. This will enhance your interviewing skills and give you the confidence to deal with awkward situations. You can never have too much experience, so be eager to help out wherever it is needed even if it means gathering instruments for a procedure or doing a simple blood draw. Be open and honest with your patients as well as your preceptors. This is the time for you to learn and experience, and it is understood that you do not possess all of the knowledge that you will require for this rotation. If you find yourself feeling defeated, talk with your interns, residents, or attending physician. Ensure you get feedback from your supervisors 1 to 2 weeks into the rotation so you may adjust and make improvements throughout the remainder of your time.

Be prompt, arrive earlier than your preceptor if needed, and review your patient notes or previous encounters. If you are unsure about a procedure or medication, research it. Familiarize yourself with the anatomy before any procedure so you understand complications that may arise. Be self-taught. There is only so much information that can be assimilated during this short rotation, and most of the learning will be what you decide to clarify for yourself.

To prepare for the first day of your rotation, acquaint yourself with common OB/GYN complaints, diagnoses, and treatments. A great starting place is the NCCPA's website, which helps you to understand the topics you will expected to know to pass the board examination.[24] It also gives you an idea of things that you were unable to experience on your rotation but that you will still need to understand before taking the PANCE. Understand the hierarchy of the hospital or clinic you are going to be working in by talking with other students who have encountered the same clinical site. Research your preceptors, for example, by reading their curricula vitae posted on their websites. This will provide you with an understanding of their clinical or research interests. All of these are only suggestions that may further your clinical experience and can heighten your knowledge outside of the classroom.

STUDENT COMMENTS

The University of South Alabama's OB/GYN clerkship not only teaches students academically but also emphasizes the importance of autonomy between students and patients. In OB/GYN, the interview with the patient and establishing rapport is in my opinion one of the most important factors in determining your future with patients. I feel as though the residents and attendings [physicians] provided students with the tools and confidence to be successful in this clerkship. The [rotation] also allowed students to be a part of the team in labor and delivery, [outpatient] clinic, and gynecologic surgery to provide the students with the most experience possible.

C.P., PA student, University of South Alabama, class of 2015

PHYSICIAN ASSISTANT ROLES IN OBSTETRICS AND GYNECOLOGY

The scope of practice varies widely for PAs in the field of OB/GYN, as do the roles of PAs in OB/GYN in any given state. States where PAs are allowed to perform autonomous vaginal deliveries include New Jersey, New Mexico, and West Virginia; however, there are extra qualifications that most states require for a PA to obtain to perform independent vaginal deliveries. These privileges are delegated by the state and local hospitals where the PA practices. In the surgical setting, PAs assist in gynecologic surgeries and cesarean sections and assist in or perform vaginal deliveries. Although some PAs practice female health only in a general practice setting, others work in a surgical, hospital, or specialty practice setting. In a clinical setting, PAs work with women during their prenatal, intrapartum, and postpartum care. They are able to read and interpret ultrasounds; perform routine Pap smears and culture collection; counsel patients regarding appropriate contraceptive practices; and perform IUD insertions, endometrial biopsies, and colposcopies. With the number of insured patients on the rise and the subsequent decline in access to health care because of the newly passed health care reform, the door has opened for PAs in the field of OB/GYN. Practices that employ PAs find that patients are able to be seen in a timelier manner and receive the same level of care as before health care reform. There are currently about 1500 PAs that practice in OB/GYN. To obtain more information on the scope of practice of PAs in OB/GYN, you can visit www.paobgyn.org or the American Academy of Physician Assistants' website.[25]

WHEN TO REFER

Part of practicing as a mid-level provider is knowing how to set your own boundaries. Go with your gut feelings. If you have doubts about a patient's diagnosis or feel uncomfortable about a situation, you should first seek advice from your supervising physician. Build a good relationship with your future supervisor, and keep an open line of communication. If you have a question or if there is a threat or danger to the patient's life, you should immediately inform your supervising physician so that specific and appropriate assistance with the patient's diagnosis, testing, intervention, and treatment can be clarified. Other possible reasons to refer to your supervising physician may include a high-risk pregnancy, previous high-risk pregnancies, to discuss operative benefits and side effects, or if you feel uncomfortable about discussing an impending unfavorable diagnosis such as fetal demise or cancer.

SPECIAL CHALLENGES

Each specialty in medicine has its own advantages and disadvantages. In OB/GYN, especially smaller practices, practitioners may have unpredictable hours. They may take calls or may get behind schedule because of emergency deliveries or surgeries.[26] Another difficult situation is approaching a patient with a devastating diagnosis. For example, explaining to a patient that she has ovarian or breast cancer, that there is fetal demise, or that her child has a genetic malformation is difficult. These conversations are best prefaced with words of humility and caring. In a patient who has cancer, you may introduce the conversation with "I regret to inform you" or "Your results did show that you have cancer. I would like to be here to support you through this new diagnosis." In a patient with a miscarriage, you may present the topic by saying, "I'm sorry for your loss. I hope you will come to me with any questions or concerns about what has happened" or "I'm here to help you emotionally and physically through this very distressing time." It is always desirable to show empathy and care for the patient's well-being physically, mentally, and emotionally. Issues dealing with death can present a multitude of troubling feelings for patients. You can refer them to outside resources and support if you are unable to provide these services or if the patient requests them. Two services, Compassionate Friends and SHARE Pregnancy and Infant Loss Support, are notable resources that are available to any patient struggling with fetal loss.[27,28] There are also cancer support groups in most communities that provide invaluable support and encouragement to women diagnosed with cancer.

REWARDS OF WORKING IN OBSTETRICS AND GYNECOLOGY

What is more rewarding than being able to experience the birth of a new life and the joy it brings to all involved in the event? You will experience joy such as this that you may never experience in any other field of medicine. There are other benefits to working in this specialty as well, including building patient rapport and being able to follow women from adolescence through menopause. You will perform a similar role to a primary care practitioner in this setting, allowing you to build fundamental and long-lasting relationships with your patients.

CONCLUSION

I hope that you find your OB/GYN rotation challenging and rewarding. The field of women's health encompasses many other fields of medicine and demands much studying and professionalism. There is nothing more exciting than delivering a baby, and there is nothing more despairing than delivering the diagnosis of cancer. You will experience these and other aspects of medicine and humanity in OB/GYN, and it will teach you how to develop realism and empathy for your patients.

KEY POINTS

- As in every rotation patient communication is paramount in order to successfully treat OB/GYN patients.
- Interprofessional relationships and team cooperation will facilitate patient safety and your success during the OB/GYN rotation.
- A good understanding of the patient's needs and what the attending physician physician expects of you will help make you a good provider, especially in situations that present OB/GYN challenges.

References

1. *Cervical Cancer Screening Rates*; September 2014. Available from: http://www.cdc.gov/nchs/data/hus/2013/084.pdf. Accessed September 2015.
2. *Bates Guide to Physical Examination and History Taking*. 11th ed. Vol. 1. Philadelphia, PA: Wolters Kluwer; 2013.
3. *Mirena Insertion Steps and Removal Instructions*; April 2015. Available from: http://www.bing.com/search?q=mirena&form=IE11TR&src=IE11TR&pc=LNJB. Accessed November 2015.
4. *2012 Updated Consensus Guidelines for the Management of Abnormal Cervical Cancer Screening Tests and Cancer Precursors*; January 2012. Available from: http://www.asccp.org/Portals/9/docs/ASCCP%20Updated%20Guidelines%20%20-%203.21.13.pdf. Accessed October 2015.
5. *Frequently Asked Questions Labor, Delivery, and Postpartum Care*; January 2012. Available from: http://www.acog.org/-/media/For-Patients/faq154.pdf?dmc=1&ts=20151125T0942134029. Accessed October 2015.
6. *The Obstetric s and Gynecology Clerkship: Your Guide to Success*; November 2014. Available from: https://www.apgo.org/binary/ObGynClerkshipGuidetoSuccess.pdf. Accessed September 2015.
7. The universal protocol for preventing wrong site. wrong procedure, and wrong person surgery: guidance for health care professionals; 2015. Available from: http://www.joint commission.org/assets/1/18/UP_Poster.pdf. Accessed October 2015.
8. *Committed to Quality and Safety*; 2015. Available from: http://www.aha.org/advocacy-issues/initiatives/quality.shtml. Accessed November 2015.
9. *A Team Approach to Hospital Care May Improve Outcomes*. February 2010. Available from: http://www.medscape.com/viewarticle/717448. Accessed October 2015.
10. *Simulation Fellowship in OBGYN*; 2015. Available from: https://www.med.nyu.edu/obgyn/educational-programs/fellowship-training-programs/simulation-fellowship-obgyn. Accessed November 2015.
11. *Kick Counts*; 2015. Available from: http://americanpregnancy.org/while-pregnant/kick-counts/. Accessed November 2015.
12. Byat N, et al. Depression and anxiety among high-risk obstetric inpatients. *Gen Hosp Psychiatry*. 2013;35(2):112–116.
13. Gass M, Rebar R. The Menopause.*Glob. libr. women's med.*, (ISSN: 1756-2228); 2008.
14. Rice GE, Illanes SE, Mitchell MD. Gestational diabetes mellitus: a positive predictor of type 2 diabetes? *Int J Endocrinol*. 2012;2012:721653.
15. *Women's Health: A Primary Care Clinical Guide*. 4th ed. Boston, MA: Prentice Hall, 2012.
16. American Psychiatric Association. (2013). *Diagnostic and statistical manual of mental disorders* (5th ed.). Arlington, VA: American Psychiatric Publishing.
17. *Women's Health Prevention and Promotion*; 2005 March. Available from: http://www.nihcm.org/pdf/WHOverview05.pdf. Accessed November 2015.
18. *Obese and Overweight Fact Sheet*; 2015 January. Available from: http://www.who.int/mediacentre/factsheets/fs311/en/. Accessed October 2015.
19. *How to Ask Domestic Abuse Screen*; 2015 January. Available from: http://domesticabuse.stanford.edu/screening/how.html. Accessed November 2015.
20. *Primary Care Protocol for Transgender Patient Care: Transgender Patients*; 2015. Available from: http://transhealth.ucsf.edu/trans?page=protocol-pateints. Accessed November 2015.
21. *Healthy People 2020: Disability and Health*; 2014. Available from: http://www.healthypeople.gov/2020/topics-objectives/topic/disability-and-health. Accessed November 2015.
22. *Family Planning Association: Talking Sense about Sex*; 2011 January. Available from: http://www.fpa.org.uk/sites/default/files/religion-contraception-and-abortion-factsheet.pdf. Accessed October 2015.
23. Debar L, et al. A primary care-based interdisciplinary team approach to the treatment of chronic pain utilizing a pragmatic clinical trials framework. *Transl Behav Med*. 2012;2(4):523–530.
24. *NCCPA Blueprint*; 2015. Available from: http://www.nccpa.net/ExamsContentBPOrgans. Accessed November 2015.
25. *Physician Assistant in Obstetrics and Gynecology*. Available from: http://www.paobgyn.org/docs/WhatIsAPABrochure. Accessed November 2015.
26. *Challenges in Obstetrics and Gynecology*; 2013 September. Available from: http://www.drugs.com/conferences/challenges-obstetrics-gynecology-13698/. Accessed November 2015.
27. *Pregnancy and Infant Loss*; 2015. Available from: http://www.compassionatefriends.org/Online_Support/pregnancy_and_infant_loss.aspx. Accessed October 2015.
28. *Welcome to SHARE Pregnancy and Infant Loss Support*; 2015. Available from: http://nationalshare.org/. Accessed November 2015.

PEDIATRICS

Jonathan M. Bowser

HISTORY

Pediatrics gained recognition as a distinct medical discipline in the United States in the mid-19th century as an appreciation of the burden of infant mortality and awareness of the unique vulnerability of children to certain diseases increased. Before that, the medical concerns of children were viewed as the domain of internal medicine or obstetrics/gynecology, and there was little consideration given to the unique development and physiology of children. The first hospital dedicated to the treatment of children was the Children's Hospital of Philadelphia, founded in 1855. Abraham Jacobi, a German immigrant who is considered by many to be the father of American pediatrics, established the children's clinic at New York Medical College in 1860. In 1876, an emerging leader in pediatric medicine, Job Lewis Smith, was appointed Clinical Professor of the Diseases of Children at Bellevue Hospital in New York City. Lewis authored a textbook, *Treatise on the Diseases of Infancy and Children*, which was adopted by virtually all medical schools until the late 1890s.[1]

The decline in infant mortality rates seen in the 20th century is one of the great public health success stories of modern times. In 1900, mortality rates in the first year of life approached 30% in some U.S. cities. By the end of the 20th century, infant mortality rates had declined by 99%, with fewer than 0.1 death per 1000 live births. In the early part of the 20th century,

improvements in infant mortality were largely due to public health measures, including milk hygiene, clean water, and improved sanitation. In 1912, the Children's Bureau was formed within the Department of Labor and played an important role in improving maternal and infant welfare in the first half of the century. The discovery and widespread use of antibiotics, fluid and electrolyte replacement therapy, and safe blood transfusions were also critically important factors in improving infant mortality rates by midcentury.

The latter half of the 20th century saw continued improvements in medical care and public health measures, including great strides in perinatal and neonatal medicine, precipitous declines in vaccine-preventable illnesses, and improved access through the implementation of Medicaid in 1965. In 1994, with funding from the U.S. Department of Health and Human Services, Health Resources and Services Administration, Maternal and Child Health Bureau, the first edition of *Bright Futures: Guidelines for Health Supervision of Infants, Children, and Adolescents* was published with the goal of ensuring that all children in the United States could look forward to a bright future, regardless of race, religion, or socioeconomic factors (https://www.health ypeople.gov/2020/tools-resources/evidence-based-resource/bright-futures-guidelines-for-health-supervision-of) . With release of the third edition in 2008, the American Academy of Pediatrics (AAP)'s

Bright Futures: Guidelines for Health Supervision of Infants, Children, and Adolescents became recognized as the standard for recommendations on preventive care of children. In 2010, the Patient Protection and Affordable Care Act was passed into law and included a provision that all children receive the standard of preventive screenings and services, as recommended in the third edition of the AAP's *Bright Futures Guidelines*.

In 1930, the AAP formed when the pediatric section of the American Medical Association (AMA) broke away. The American Board of Pediatrics was founded in 1933 with the goal of raising standards of pediatric care in the United States. The first pediatric board examination was administered in 1934. In 1965, Henry Silver, MD, and Loretta Ford founded the nurse practitioner (NP) profession by creating a pediatric nurse practitioner (PNP) program at the University of Colorado. Three years after the first physician assistant (PA) program was founded at Duke University in 1965, Dr. Silver created the Child Health Associate program at the University of Colorado School of Medicine. This program, based on the PA model, offered specialty training in pediatrics and was the first PA program to confer a master's degree.[2]

PEDIATRIC ROTATIONS

All Physician Assistant students are assigned to a required pediatric rotation/experience during their clinical year. A key purpose of this chapter is to prepare students for this experience. Pediatric clinical rotations take place in a wide range of settings including ambulatory experiences in group and private practices, community health centers, public health settings and school based clinics. Hospital-based pediatrics experiences are found in children's hospitals,academic health centers, community hospitals, and charity-funded settings andspecialty hospitals. What all of these rotations and experiences have in common is that the care of pediatric patients also includes involvement with their families, their cultural environment and their socioeconomic status—which includes their access (or lack of access) to health care. Table 28-1. provides online resources on pediatric topics. The sections in this chapter provide detailed clinical information which will be useful across the pediatric experience.

WELL CHILD VISITS AND IMMUNIZATIONS

The periodic evaluation of a well child is the cornerstone of pediatric primary care practice. From birth through adolescence, the growth and development of children is a complex and variable process that requires frequent monitoring and preventive intervention. The AAP's *Bright Futures* guidelines recommends no fewer than 10 scheduled well-care visits between birth and age 2 years and yearly visits through adolescence. Even with this frequency of visits, pediatric PAs are challenged to cover all of the necessary tasks in each 15- to 30-minute visit. At each well-care visit, the pediatric patient must be evaluated for disease and screened for problems with nutrition, growth, and development, and appropriate counseling should be delivered on prevention and health promotion. Particularly in the early childhood years, immunizations are a key feature of every well-child visits. Frequently changing and updated, the American Academy of Pediatric's recommended schedule, Bright Futures can be accessed at www.aap/en.us. For children with developmental disabilities or chronic illness, extra time should be planned for the well-care visit.

The approach to the physical examination of the child depends on the age, verbal capacity, and cooperativeness of the patient. With preverbal children, typically birth through age 2 or 3 years, careful observation of the child for developmentally appropriate behaviors, including interactions with the caregiver, is an important component of the examination and should be accomplished before approaching or touching the child. Children often develop stranger anxiety beginning between 6 and 12 months of age and persisting until age 2 or 3 years. It is important to develop strategies for examining a child who is quite apprehensive. Use a soothing, calm voice and slower movements. It may be helpful to approach at eye level rather than from above, and with most children in this age group, it is best to perform most elements of the physical examination with the child in the caregiver's lap. The sequence of the examination is best approached case by case, and the PA should take advantage of opportunities unique to this age group. For example, with a sleeping infant, auscultation of the heart and chest with a warmed stethoscope may yield excellent results without waking the child. The most invasive examinations such as the ear and throat examination should be reserved to the end of the examination for this age group. It is important to prevent the child from moving while the otoscope tip is in the auditory canal; therefore, take extra care that the child is properly restrained either against the caregiver's shoulder or chest. If the caregiver is not able to effectively hold the child, the ear examination is probably best done on the examination table with the child restrained on his or her side by a caregiver. The knee-to-knee position is helpful for examining

TABLE 28.1 Useful Web Resources While on Pediatric Rotation

Immunization schedules: CDC	http://www.cdc.gov/vaccines/schedules/hcp/child-adolescent.html
Vaccine concerns or refusal: AAP	https://www.aap.org/en-us/advocacy-and-policy/aap-health-initiatives/immunization/Pages/communicating-parents.aspx
Oral health: AAP and Smiles for Life Resources	http://www2.aap.org/commpeds/dochs/oralhealth/index.html http://www.smilesforlifeoralhealth.org
Mental health: SAMHSA and AACAP resources	http://www.samhsa.gov/children http://www.aacap.org/aacap/families_and_youth/Family_Resources/Home.aspx
Early childhood literacy: AAP Toolkit	https://littoolkit.aap.org/Pages/home.aspx
Developmental screening: ASQ and AAP	http://agesandstages.com http://pediatrics.aappublications.org/content/118/1/405.full
Periodic health screenings: AAP	https://www.aap.org/en-us/Documents/periodicity_schedule_oral_health.pdf
Adolescent psychosocial interview: HEEADSSS	http://contemporarypediatrics.modernmedicine.com/contemporary-pediatrics/content/tags/adolescent-medicine/heeadsss-30-psychosocial-interview-adolesce?page=full
Secondhand smoke: CDC	https://www.cdc.gov/tobacco/basic_information/secondhand_smoke/
Pediatric mental health screening and resources for primary care: AAP Task Force on Mental Health, Algorithms for Primary Care	https://www.aap.org/en-us/advocacy-and-policy/aap-health-initiatives/Mental-Health/Pages/Primary-Care-Tools.aspx?nfstatus=401&nftoken=00000000-0000-0000-0000-000000000000&nfstatusdescription=ERROR%3a+No+local+token
Adolescent confidentiality laws: AAP	http://pedsinreview.aappublications.org/content/30/11/457

AAP, American Academy of Pediatrics; *ASQ,* Ages & Stages Questionnaires; *CDC,* Centers for Disease Control and Prevention; *HEEADSSS,* Home, Education/Employment, Eating, Activities, Drugs and Alcohol, Sexuality, Suicide and Depression, Safety; *SAMHSA,* Substance Abuse and Mental Health Services Administration.

the oropharynx of young children. The provider should sit facing the caregiver with his or her knees close together, forming a "table" on which to lay the child. The caregiver initially holds the child on the lap facing him or her and then lays the child back so that the child's head lies in the lap of the provider. The examination of the oropharynx is generally viewed as invasive by most small children, so this examination position is helpful in reducing their anxiety.

An alternative to the knee-to-knee position in an apprehensive child is to lay the child on the examination table with a caregiver holding the child's arms above his or her head with the elbows positioned against the ears so the child's head cannot move side to side. Many young children will clench their teeth together to prevent the tongue blade from entering their mouths. Because young children do not have a second molar, it is very effective to slide a tongue blade, held on its side, into the mouth between the teeth and buccal mucosa and then turn the blade so it is flat when it is at the back of the teeth and move it through the gap between their mandible and maxilla directly onto the base of the tongue. This will elicit a gag reflex and allow an opportunity for a quick look at the child's pharynx.

CASE 28.1

A 19-month-old boy is in the clinic for a well-child care visit. As you enter the examination room, the child begins screaming and struggling in his mother's arms. When you attempt to get closer to the child, he begins to kick his legs, trying to crawl up higher in his mother's arms. The mother seems frustrated and is having difficulty holding him. What strategies might help you complete a physical examination on this boy?

Preschool-aged children (aged 3–5 years) are generally cooperative and curious and may engage in the visit without protest. It is often helpful to engage the child in conversation or tell a story while performing the examination. Allowing the child to hold the stethoscope or other diagnostic equipment, demonstrating the examination techniques on yourself, an older sibling, or a doll, and encouraging engagement of the parent or other caregivers are strategies that can help alleviate apprehensiveness. When possible, attempt to make the examination fun for the child using toys or games. Some children may have unpleasant memories associated with previous visits or anxiety about immunizations or other painful procedures. Unusual reticence or avoidance at this age warrants additional investigation to determine if the child is reaching age-appropriate developmental milestones or has been the victim of child abuse. Most children develop modesty around age 4 or 5 years, so the provider should expect some reluctance to remove the gown or clothing. This is an excellent opportunity for the provider to engage the child and caregiver in a discussion around teaching the child appropriate interaction with adults that protect the child from becoming a victim of sexual abuse.

School-aged children (5–10 years) are typically easy to engage in conversation, and the PA will find few barriers to performing a thorough and thoughtful evaluation in this age group. It is very important to establish rapport with children in this age range while appreciating that modesty is very important to many school-aged children. Allowing the child to disrobe out of sight of others and offering appropriate gowning and draping can help to develop trust and maintain modesty. An important component to the pediatric well visit that begins in this age range is the assessment of school performance or any school-based concerns. Addressing school performance issues and any school-based social concerns early and directing caregivers to resources may be helpful in preventing self-esteem and school avoidance issues in the future. See Table 28.1 for resources.

The approach to an adolescent (11–18 years) is similar to that taken with an adult patient with some important caveats. The visit should be scheduled for an appropriate amount of time, usually 30 to 40 minutes. Anticipate taking an extensive psychosocial history and spending some or all of the patient interview with the caregiver out of the room. It is appropriate to take a past medical history, family history, and general social history with the caregiver present. Providers should develop a strategy for asking caregivers of adolescents to leave the room, increasing the possibility that the adolescent will be more candid in his or her responses. One option is to advise the caregiver that there are interview questions for the adolescent that are typically asked privately and would the caregiver be willing to wait outside the room and be brought back into the room for the physical exam. The HEEADSSS (home, education and employment, eating, activities, drugs and alcohol, sexuality, suicide and depression, safety) psychosocial inventory is a guiding tool frequently used to collect information related to the sensitive adolescent psychosocial interview.[3] It is important for providers to develop an approach to validating the perspectives of adolescents through reflective listening.[4] This takes some practice and patience. After conducting the patient interview around less intrusive questions such as general past medical history, it may seem less intimidating to an adolescent to begin the interview questions about sexual behaviors, tobacco use, recreational drug use, and so on with questions about acquaintances or friends' behaviors in these domains and then narrow the questions to how the patient feels about these behaviors and what behaviors he or she is engaging in. Be thoughtful about the amount of information that is provided to adolescents regarding risky behaviors at each visit because the goal of the visit should be building rapport and trust. Additional visits can be scheduled as needed to revisit concerns that are identified. Encourage healthy choices in tobacco use, alcohol, sexual behaviors, recreational drug use by helping them articulate life goals that might be unattainable if unhealthy choices are made.

CASE 28.2

A 13-year-old girl is in the clinic because of her mother's concerns that for the past 3 months the teen has been ditching school once or twice a week, and her grades are falling. This has led to several family arguments, and the parents are "at their wit's end" trying to deal with the situation. What approach(es) would you use to evaluate the teen and her family? What advice would you offer the family?

AMBULATORY PEDIATRICS

In the typical outpatient pediatric clinic, the PA student will be expected to perform an appropriate history and physical examination and to develop an assessment and detailed treatment plan for newborns, infants, children, and adolescents. Preventive care is such an important facet of general pediatric practice that it is critical to the success of the rotation that, in addition to a good foundational knowledge of common pediatric disorders and their presentations, the PA student arrives prepared with a good understanding of pediatric developmental milestones and up-to-date recommendations for preventive screening, immunizations, and nutrition, diet, and exercise. Table 28.1 contains resources for health screening and health promotion tools.

During the pediatric rotation, the PA student is expected to acquire some very important skills that are specific to pediatrics. The ability to evaluate children for appropriate development at any age is of fundamental importance to general pediatric practice. In infants and young children, development should be evaluated by considering language, motor, and personal-social domains. There are several validated child development evaluation instruments in common usage (see Table 28.1). Child development should be considered from a biopsychosocial model, recognizing development as an interaction among biological, psychological, and social factors.

CASE 28.3

The parents of a 2-year-old boy are in clinic with concerns about his behavior. Specifically, they are concerned that he has frequent tantrums that involve screaming and hitting others. This has been an issue at his preschool, and the caregivers there have asked the parents to seek the advice of their pediatric provider. Are there any specific history questions or screenings that might be helpful in assessing this child? What advice might you provide to the parents for handling his behaviors?

CASE 28.4

A 6-month-old girl is in clinic for her well-child care visit. The parents are very concerned that she isn't sitting without their help yet. They report that her older sister was sitting unassisted by age 5 months, but this daughter will slump to the side when they try to sit her up unless they hold her hands to keep her steady. What assessment and advice would be appropriate for this child and her parents?

There is significant variety in a pediatric rotation. As an example, in a typical day in the outpatient pediatrics setting, one might see a newborn, 9-month-old infant, 14-year-old adolescent, and 2-year old twins, all for well-child care, in addition to acute care visits for fever in a 2-year-old child, vomiting and diarrhea in a 6-year-old child, parental concerns about obesity in a 9-year-old child, and acting out and school performance in a 13-year-old teenager.

One should expect to develop strategies for engaging parents who are concerned about vaccines or refuse to vaccinate, discussing secondhand smoke exposure, providing advice regarding parental nutritional concerns, and screening and referring for behavioral and mental health concerns.

CASE 28.5

A 3-day-old girl comes to the clinic today to establish care. Her mother is accompanied by the infant's maternal grandmother, who is opposed to vaccination. The grandmother states that she has read extensively on the subject of immunizations and is certain the government is using vaccination to poison the population. The infant girl didn't get a hepatitis B vaccine at birth because of the grandmother's disapproval. How might you approach this situation?

CASE 28.6

A 12-month-old boy is being seen in clinic for well-child care, accompanied by his father. He has not had a physical or immunizations since the age of 4 months because of issues with his medical insurance. His examination reveals he is growing well and does not have any developmental delays. What vaccines should he receive today? When should he return for the next set of vaccines?

Learners on a pediatric rotation should be knowledgeable about the signs and symptoms of common pediatric disorders and have resources available to determine the best patient management. They should be familiar with the types of pathogens that circulate at various times of the year and, if possible, have a resource for identifying when specific pathogens are circulating in the local community.

Upper respiratory disease frequently seen in the pediatric population includes viral upper respiratory infections, acute otitis media, croup, and pharyngitis. Common lower respiratory disease includes community-acquired pneumonias, asthma, and bronchiolitis. Gastrointestinal complaints are frequently encountered in the pediatric population, and they always necessitate an evaluation of hydration status. Rashes are a common pediatric complaint with a broad differential diagnosis and are often confusing for the novice clinician. Consultation with a more experienced clinician on the team is usually helpful in arriving at a diagnosis for a skin complaint. Fever is often a concerning symptom for the caregiver of a child. Although fever guidelines are not uniformly followed by all community-based pediatric providers, guidelines are available and quite useful in determining the most appropriate workup for a febrile child.[5]

CASE 28.7

A 7-month-old girl is in the emergency department (ED) for 3 days of fever. She has a temperature of 103.4°F rectally. She has had a cough and runny nose for the past 5 days. Her past medical history indicates she is usually a healthy child, and her vaccinations are up-to-date. In the ED, her rectal temperature is 102.8°F. The remainder of her vital signs are normal except for a heart rate of 130 beats/min. Her examination does not reveal a source of infection. How would you manage this patient?

CASE 28.8

A 4-year-old girl has been brought to the urgent care clinic with a 4-day history of cough and runny nose and a fever of 101°F. Her past medical history indicates that she is a generally healthy child with up-to-date vaccinations. Her examination does not reveal any focus of infection. Her father requests that she receive antibiotics to make her better sooner. You don't believe antibiotics are indicated. How would you discuss this with the parent?

CASE 28.9

A 10-year-old boy is in the clinic after an ED visit for an asthma exacerbation. He has had a history of asthma diagnosed at age 7 years and uses fluticasone, 44 mcg, 2 puffs twice a day, and an albuterol metered-dose inhaler, 2 puffs every 4 hours as needed for a rescue treatment. What history will help you assess his level of asthma control? Are there any interventions that might help avoid another ED visit?

HOSPITAL PEDIATRICS

Students performing clinical rotations in inpatient pediatrics will have the opportunity to work on a team of providers in the care of more acutely ill children. The inpatient team generally consists of an attending provider, residents at varying levels of training;

other medical trainees; and depending on the type of pediatric service, social workers, pharmacists, and other health professionals. The attending provider is a licensed health care provider who has completed all training and leads the team in the care of their assigned patients. Pediatric residency is a 3-year program in the United States; therefore, the residents on the team will be designated as first year, second year, and third year, depending on how much training they have completed. Other medical trainees on the team may consist of PA students, medical students, and NP students.

The duties of the team include daily rounds on all patients assigned to the team's service, performing admission history and physical examinations, writing hospital orders, developing discharge plans, and night and weekend call, and the team may even perform procedures. All of these activities are performed by hospital-based PAs.[6] PAs are viewed as important contributors to quality patient care in the hospital settings, and opportunities for PAs to work as hospitalists are growing.[7] For students who are interested in pursuing careers as hospitalist PAs, the Society of Hospital Medicine offers Fellow and Senior Fellow in Hospital Medicine designations via application after 5 years of hospitalist experience.

There are several groups of patients within the pediatric population that require special consideration.

FOSTER AND ADOPTED CHILDREN

The growing number of foster and adopted children, both domestically and internationally, has introduced a new area of specialized health care. Currently, more than 400,000 children are in foster care in the United States.[8] Children from international adoptions are at increased risk for chronic and previously undetected medical conditions, lack of immunization, developmental concerns, and emotional and behavioral issues. Therefore, these children require a specialized approach when they present to primary care. The AAP Committee on Early Childhood, Adoption, and Dependent Care publishes guidelines for the complete evaluation of foster and adoptive children.[9]

NEWBORNS

The neonatal period, defined as the first 4 weeks of life, is a time of tremendous physiologic change for the infant. To successfully navigate the complex transition from intrauterine to extrauterine life, a neonate must adapt to changes in cardiovascular, pulmonary, gastrointestinal, hepatic, renal, endocrine, and immune function. Early and frequent evaluation of well newborns is critical to ensuring safe transition through the neonatal period. Premature infants present a unique set of challenges to practicing PAs. The perinatal history, including the reason for premature delivery, if known; gestational age at birth; and hospital course, including supplemental oxygen and other supportive care are all important factors in determining the approach to the "ex-preemie." Infants born at or before 32 weeks' gestation or those born at very low birth weight (<1500 g) are at higher risk for complications of prematurity.

FAILURE TO THRIVE

Failure to thrive (FTT), characterized by physical growth that is less than that of same-age peers, is associated with poor developmental and cognitive outcomes. Although FTT can be secondary to organic causes, such as congenital or metabolic diseases, in the United States, the majority of FTT is attributable to psychosocial factors, such as poverty, poor parent–child bonding, or environmental stress from abuse. The appropriate treatment of a child with FTT requires a thorough evaluation of the child's overall health, nutritional status, home environment, and caregiver–child interactions.[10] Hospitalization may be indicated in severe cases.

ORAL HEALTH

The burden of oral diseases and disorders in the pediatric population is significant. Dental caries, a preventable, vertically transmitted infectious disease, is the single most common chronic childhood disease. Striking disparities in dental disease, by income and other measures, exist in children. Although many children have a medical home, far fewer have a dental home, and there is a great need for medical providers to fill gaps in the prevention and treatment of oral disease. In 2011, the Institute of Medicine released two reports on oral health, *Advancing Oral Health in America* and *Improving Access to Oral Health Care for Vulnerable and Underserved Populations*. These reports made specific recommendations for the enhancement of the role of nondental health care professionals in improving oral health care in the United States.[11,12] In 2014, the U.S. Preventive Services Task Force issued recommendations for primary care medical providers to apply fluoride varnish to all children younger than the age of 5 years, regardless of oral health risk factors.[13] Screening for oral disease and preventive treatment with fluoride are now accepted as essential components of the medical care of children.

CASE 28.10

A 16-month-old boy is in the clinic for his 15-month-old well-child care visit. He is growing well, and his development is on target. In collecting a diet history, you learn that he is taking three 8-oz bottles of whole milk and two 8-oz bottles of apple juice every day, including one bottle of milk at bedtime. The parents have not yet identified a dentist and were not aware that they could start brushing his teeth. His examination does not reveal any pathology. What advice is appropriate for the parents of this child?

DEVELOPMENTAL DISABILITIES

Children with special health care needs related to developmental disabilities encompass a broad spectrum of severity and needs. At one end of this spectrum are children with mild disabilities, who are educated in regular classrooms and receive minimal ancillary services. At the other end are children with severe disabilities, who have significant comorbidities and require health care services from a team of medical specialists and other professionals. Specific categories of developmental disability include intellectual disabilities, communication disorders, learning disabilities, cerebral palsy, and autism spectrum disorders.[14]

BEHAVIORAL AND MENTAL HEALTH DISORDERS

Disorders of behavior, such as attention deficit disorder, and mental health conditions, such as anxiety, depression, and bipolar disorder, are commonly encountered in the pediatric setting. Testing using validated instruments and referral to qualified specialists are important steps in the evaluation of children with behavioral and mental health conditions. Mental health is a critical and often underappreciated part of a child's overall health. Mental health issues in children can adversely impact school performance, psychosocial development, and physical health. Appropriate management may necessitate involvement of school or child-care officials and state and local agencies.

CHRONIC DISEASE

With the exception of several commonly occurring conditions, chronic illness in childhood is quite rare. Common chronic conditions include allergic disorders (asthma, eczema, and allergic rhinitis), childhood caries, congenital heart disease, and neurologic conditions (seizure, cerebral palsy, and other neuromuscular disorders). Chronic conditions, such as arthritis and diabetes mellitus, occur frequently in adults but are relatively rare in children. The care of children with chronic disease should be managed by multidisciplinary teams with particular attention paid to psychological support of the child and caregivers.

For any provider starting out in pediatrics, there is some basic knowledge that will prove helpful with all patients. The resources listed in Table 28.1 are a good reference for attaining this knowledge. Providers should know the expected health screenings of pediatric patients by age so that opportunities for well-child care are not missed. It is important to screen for developmental milestones at each well-child care visit, and providers should understand the validated tools for these screenings. Caregivers often ask questions around diet and other anticipatory guidance items, and pediatric providers need to have a working repository of this information. An excellent resource for this is available from *Bright Futures*. Finally, the Harriet Lane handbook is very helpful for normal vital signs by age, pediatric dosing of medications, and a variety of other pediatric patient information.

Table 28.1 provides web links for resources that will be useful on a pediatric rotation.

KEY POINTS

- A knowledge of normal childhood developmental milestones is essential for PAs in pediatric practice.
- The most current immunization schedule—as recommended by the American Academy of Pediatrics—should be integrated into well child visits to assure prevention of pediatric and other infectious diseases.
- PAs who are caring for children must be skilled in differentiating expected versus concerning childhood behaviors and providing effective counseling to caregivers.
- Pediatric PAs require a toolbox of skills related to developing rapport with younger patients to maximize the value of the office visit.
- Opportunities are expanding for PAs to work in hospital and outpatient settings.

References

1. Cone TE. *History of American Pediatrics*. Boston: Little, Brown; 1979.
2. Glicken AG, Merenstein G, Arthur MS. The Child Health Associate Physician Assistant Program - an enduring educational model addressing the needs of families and children. *J Physician Assist Educ*. 2007;18(3):24–29.
3. Klein DA, et al. HEEADSSS 3.0: the psychosocial interview for adolescents updated for a new century fueled by media. *Contemp Pediatr*. 2014:1–16.
4. Goldenring JM, Rosen DS. Getting into adolescent heads: an essential update. *Contemp Pediatr*. 2004;21(1):64–90.
5. Baraff LJ, Bass JW, Fleisher GR, et al. Practice guideline for the management of infants and children 0 to 36 months of age with fever without source. Agency for Health Care Policy and Research. *Ann Emerg Med*. 1993;22(7):1198.
6. Society of Hospital Medicine (SHM). *2005–2006 SHM Survey: State of the Hospital Medicine Movement*. Philadelphia: Society of Hospital Medicine; 2006.
7. Ottley RJX, Agbontaen JX, Wilkow BR. The hospitalist PA: an emerging opportunity. *JAAPA*. 2000;13(11):21–28.
8. Child Welfare Information Gateway. *Foster care statistics 2014*. Washington, DC: U.S. Department of Health and Human Services, Children's Bureau; 2016.
9. Jones VF, High PC, Donaghue E, et al. Comprehensive health evaluation of the newly adopted child. *Pediatrics*. 2012;129(1):e214–e223.
10. Frank D, Silva M, Needlman R. Failure to thrive: mystery, myth and method. *Contemp Pediatr*. 1993;10:114–133.
11. *Advancing Oral Health*. Institute of Medicine; 2014. http://www.hrsa.gov/publichealth/clinical/oralhealth/advancingoralhealth.pdf. Accessed June 17, 2016.
12. *Improving Access to Oral Health Care for Vulnerable and Underserved Populations*. Institute of Medicine; 2014. http://www.nationalacademies.org/hmd/~/media/Files/Report%20Files/2011/Improving-Access-to-Oral-Health-Care-for-Vulnerable-and-Underserved-Populations/oralhealthaccess2011reportbrief.pdf. Accessed June 17, 2016.
13. U.S. Preventive Services Task Force. *Prevention of dental caries in children from birth through age 5 years: U.S. preventive services task force recommendation statement*; 2014. Rockville, MD. http://www.uspreventiveservicestaskforce.org/Page/Document/RecommendationStatementFinal/dental-caries-in-children-from-birth-through-age-5-years-screening. Accessed June 6, 2016.
14. Boyle CA, Boulet S, Schieve L, et al. Trends in the prevalence of developmental disabilities in US children, 1997–2008. *Pediatrics*. 2011;127(6):1034–1042.

CHAPTER 29

BEHAVIORAL SCIENCE AND MEDICINE: ESSENTIALS IN PRACTICE

Marci Contreras • Michelle Buller • Jill Cavalet

Similar to many physical disorders, mental and behavioral disorders are the result of a complex interaction among biological, psychological, and social or environmental factors. Physician assistants (PAs) must realize that the concept of mental health includes an amalgam of subjective well-being, perceived self-efficacy, autonomy, competence, intergenerational dependence, and self-actualization of one's intellectual and emotional potential.[1]

Behavioral medicine skills are imperative for the practicing PAs in any specialty field, not just primary care. The goal of this chapter is to help PA providers and students understand the interrelationship among psychological, physical, social, and cultural issues of patients.

In this chapter, the following elements are introduced:
- A brief history of mental illness
- Common myths and stigmas regarding the psychiatric patient
- The importance of empathy and building rapport with patients
- Strategies in approaching psychiatric patients
- Skills necessary for managing mental health needs of patients
- Models to better understand concepts in behavioral medicine
- Treatment and screening tools for specific disorders
- Suggestions on how we might accept challenges in the future

HISTORY OF MENTAL ILLNESS

Throughout history, many cultures have viewed mental illness as a form of religious punishment or demonic possession. In ancient Egypt, Greece, and Rome, mental illness was categorized as a religious or personal problem. During the Middle Ages, mentally ill individuals were believed to be possessed or in need of religion. Negative attitudes toward mental illness persisted into the 18th and 19th centuries in the United States, leading to stigmatization of mental illness and unhygienic (and often degrading) confinement of mentally ill individuals. A movement toward *deinstitutionalization* became popular in many countries, which forced the closure of many asylums and institutions because of mistreated patients, bad management and poor administration, lack of resources, lack of staff, lack of training, and inadequate quality assurance protocols.[2]

MYTHS AND STIGMAS ATTACHED TO PSYCHIATRIC ILLNESS

1. Assume the patient is psychotic, violent, or dangerous.
2. Suspicions that the patient is "faking" symptoms or seeking attention
3. "There is nothing you can do as a provider if symptoms are severe."
4. Psychiatric illnesses usually do not exist in children and adolescents, but if they do, then unfortunately, they are "ruined for life."
5. Psychiatric disorders are not "real" medical illnesses.
6. The patients are just plain "crazy."
7. Depression equates to "mentally weak" (or lazy) or some character flaw. "They just need to snap out of it."
8. Addiction is the result of a person having "no willpower."
9. Psychiatric illness is probably the product of nurture versus nature, and thus bad parenting was involved.
10. Assume the psychiatric patient is or will become a criminal. (However, mental health issues do exist in correctional institutions and do present a definite health disparity; this is discussed in a separate chapter.)

AWARENESS OF YOUR OWN BIASES

What is your personal philosophy on life? How does this balance with your professional life?

When PAs vow to care for the lives of others they are confronted with their own humanity and provided a grave responsibility as a health care provider. They must be mindful of their physical, emotional, and spiritual health in order to be effective clinicians who focus on the well-being of others.

EMPATHY AND RAPPORT

Everyone makes choices and engages in behaviors that affect their health, whether positive or negative. The key to success in dealing with even challenging or "difficult" patients is to put aside disagreement or any negative judgment and imagine what it must be like from their perspective. The power of empathy allows for an alliance with the provider and patient, which not only increases patient satisfaction but also helps improve patient outcomes.[3] Although empathy is not generally considered a therapeutic tool, in the realm of behavioral medicine, it is one of the most powerful clinical tools to support and encourage healthy behaviors.

THE PHYSICIAN ASSISTANT–PATIENT ENCOUNTER

The Approach to the Patient

The initial psychiatric interview is one of the most important components of a psychiatric diagnostic evaluation. It is a crucial skill that can be learned and developed over time. The encounter begins with nonverbal communication during the very first meeting of a patient in an outpatient clinic or inpatient hospital unit. The PA must observe the patient's behavior and body language both before and during the encounter. The best way for a provider to begin gathering information from a patient is to start with open-ended, nonfocused questions.

Identifying Information

When documenting the psychiatric patient encounter, begin with identifying information similar to any other medical record. Include the patient's name, age, marital status, race or ethnicity, gender, occupation, and referral source.

For example, Jane Doe is a 45-year-old single white woman with a history of paranoid schizophrenia who was admitted involuntarily for suicidal ideation. It is important to identify the source of the information whether it is the patient, a family member, a friend, or other. Reliability of the source must be included as well.

Chief Complaint and History of Present Illness

The chief complaint is a brief statement using the patient's own words and states the reason for presentation. For example, "I don't know why I am here; the sheriff brought me into the hospital." As in any medical history, the history of present illness outlines the current symptoms and identifies reasons leading up to patient presentation. The description of the patient's illness must be balanced in the documentation so as to not include extraneous details but rather lead to a pointed diagnosis and treatment plan. If the patient's condition is chronic, begin with the most recent onset of the episode. Inquire about the course of illness, including aggravating and alleviating factors. Elicit any triggers or stressors that precipitated this episode, such as work, school, legal, medical, financial, or interpersonal problems. Document symptoms, severity, and associated factors for each diagnosis. For the psychiatric history, it is extremely important to quote the patient's own words, especially if hallucinations or delusions are present. In considering a diagnosis, inquire and document pertinent positive and negative symptoms to construct the appropriate differential diagnosis.

Past Psychiatric History

This section should encompass the first psychiatric onset of symptoms and further review in detail any past or current diagnoses. Past pharmacologic treatments should be well documented, including details of medication doses, length of trial, reason for discontinuation, and response to the medication. Previous hospitalizations should also be included, with dates, lengths of stay, and reasons for admission. Inquire about past (or present) suicidal behavior (ideation, intent, plan, attempts) and self-harm behaviors (cutting or burning for relief of distress). Finally, obtain patient information regarding past visits to psychologists, counselors, and psychiatrists.

Social History

It is important to learn details about the patient's personal and social life. Review the patient's developmental history, home environment, relationships with parents and siblings, academic and behavioral performance in school, highest level of education, legal issues, traumatic events, past and current employment, marital or relationship status, sexual history, children, religion, hobbies, diet and exercise, and any military service.[4] Learn about the patient's support system. Discover the patient's expectations and if there are any safety concerns. The PA must establish whether the patient has an addictive personality or history of substance use, including caffeine, tobacco, alcohol, or illicit drug use. Additionally, have there been any consequences because of substance misuse such as legal issues? It is important to note the patient's history of seizures or delirium tremens because it could indicate recurrent behavior and withdrawal symptoms. Discuss with the patient previous attempts for treatment, such as rehabilitation or self-help groups and whether they were found valuable.

Family History

Many psychiatric illnesses have a genetic predisposition.[5] Family history should include any mental illness, hospitalizations, or suicide in family members. Family history of suicide attempts is a significant risk factor for suicide in psychiatric patients.[5] Document the family history of substance abuse and medications that have worked for family members. If a medication has worked for a family member with the same disease, there is an increased chance it will be efficacious for the patient.[5]

Past Medical History

Although the priority may be focused on the psychiatric history, the clinician should detail a comprehensive past medical history as well. Certain comorbidities have increased risk for mental illness, including seizures, traumatic brain injuries, episodes of unconsciousness, and other central nervous system disorders. Other conditions may affect mental health such as diabetes, metabolic syndrome, hepatic or renal disease, or reproductive dysfunction.

Psychiatric Review of Systems

It is good medical practice to screen for other psychiatric illnesses. Major depression is one of the most common mental illnesses, with a worldwide lifetime prevalence of approximately 12%.[1] The PA should be aware that in most countries, the majority of cases of depression go unrecognized in primary care settings and that in many cultures, somatic symptoms are very likely to constitute the presenting complaint.[6] An excellent screening tool for major depressive disorder is to use the classic mnemonic SIGEMCAPS (Box 29.1).[7] If the patient admits to five of nine symptoms, this should give the PA reason to suspect a major depressive disorder.

The psychiatric review of systems should also include screening for history of mania, psychosis (hallucinations or delusions), anxiety (generalized, panic,

---

BOX 29.1 SIGEMCAPS

Sleep changes: insomnia or hypersomnia
Interest: loss of interest (anhedonia) in activities
previously enjoyed; lack of motivation
Guilt: feelings of guilt or hopelessness or worth-
lessness
Energy: lack of energy; fatigue is a common com-
plaint
Mood: depressed, sadness
Concentration: difficulty concentrating, up to
memory loss
Appetite: change in appetite may include an
increase or decrease, which may lead to weight
gain or weight loss
Psychomotor: retardation or agitation
Suicidal ideation: preoccupation with death

---

social), obsessions or compulsions, posttraumatic stress disorder, substance use disorders, personality disorders, eating disorders, attention or impulsive symptoms, and cognitive impairments. For example, when screening for bipolar disorder, ask the patient if (at any point in his or her life) for more than 4 to 7 days, felt on "top of the world" and not his or her *usual* self. Consider other disorders that may have overlapping symptoms. For example, a patient might have concerns about attention deficit hyperactivity disorder because she or he has problems concentrating or concerns with Alzheimer disease because he or she is experiencing memory loss. However, it is important to note that depression and anxiety may also include these symptoms.[6]

Mental Status Examination

The mental status examination (MSE) is an important clinical assessment tool in which the provider may determine the patient's state of mind through observation and open-ended questioning under several domains including appearance, behaviors, speech, mood/affect, thought content, thought process, perception, cognition, insight and judgment. Information on the MSE can be found in Box 29.2. The clinician should be careful to not misinterpret low education level, poor language skills, impaired vision, or cultural diversity.

Physical Examination

A physical examination is rarely done in the psychiatric assessment unless in the emergency department or an inpatient setting. However, vital signs should always be obtained in every patient. A focused neurologic examination should also be considered. For patients taking antipsychotic medications, clinicians should perform an Abnormal Involuntary Movements Scale (AIMS) to assess extrapyramidal side effects such as dystonia, akathisia, or tardive dyskinesia.

Assessment and Impression

The psychiatric assessment includes a brief summary of all pertinent data to formulate a diagnosis and to support the criteria for any diagnoses. This summary should include the differential diagnoses along with results of diagnostic studies and a safety assessment.

Example: "Mr. Smith is a 47-year-old male with a history of major depressive disorder, severe, who is admitted for suicidal ideation. He has had a low, depressed mood for 2 months. This is accompanied by anhedonia, decreased concentration, insomnia, decreased appetite, and 10-lb weight loss. He has thoughts of wanting to hurt himself by overdosing. He stopped his medication 6 months ago, which was Prozac 80 mg/day. He had been taking Prozac for 5 years when originally diagnosed and has not had any episodes of depression from that time until now. This has impacted his life significantly, including avoiding going to work, marriage problems, financial difficulties, and isolation from friends. He has expressed some anxiety but doesn't meet criteria for any other psychiatric disorders."

Plan and Treatment

The treatment plan should encourage preventive strategies such as sleep hygiene, tobacco cessation, diet and exercise, caffeine modification, abstaining from alcohol or illicit drugs, and weight management strategies. The psychiatric provider plays an important role in medication management; therefore, knowledge of pharmacotherapy is essential. Options include initiating a new medication, tapering, or leaving the dose unchanged. Always assess for drug interactions and educate the patient of potential side effects.

For appropriate therapy (and continuity of care), it might be necessary to obtain previous records or communicate with the patient's current primary care provider or therapist. In this case, you will need to discuss with the patient reasons for his or her consent. Referrals to other specialists or therapists may be necessary.

Any counseling that a PA may provide is more supportive; therefore, document any brief psychotherapeutic intervention performed. Validation of feelings and behaviors is important throughout the entire patient encounter. It is important to assess the patient's expectations as well as her or his long- and short-term goals of treatment. Examples of a patient's goals may include mood stabilization; medication compliance;

BOX 29.2 MENTAL STATUS EXAMINATION

APPEARANCE AND BEHAVIOR
This is a general description of the patient's appearance. Observe and document whether the patient looks her or his stated age. Note the patient's eye contact, attire, and facial expressions. Scars, tattoos, or other noteworthy findings may also be included. Describe the patient's behavior. Is the patient cooperative, guarded, agitated, hostile (especially if brought involuntarily), disinterested, or suspicious?

MOTOR ACTIVITY
This can be normal, slowed, or increased. Are there any signs of abnormal movements, unusual or sustained postures, pacing, restlessness, or tremor? Extrapyramidal side effects of antipsychotic medications may be noted such as tardive dyskinesia (lip smacking or tongue protrusion).

SPEECH
Note the fluency, language content, rate, volume, and tone of the patient's speech.

MOOD AND AFFECT
Mood is subjective and includes what the patient says he or she feels (e.g., happy, sad, euphoric, depressed, fearful, anxious, or irritable). Affect is objective and is the patient's outward expression of inner experiences observed by the clinician. Affect can be measured in terms of quality (measure of intensity), quantity range (restricted, normal, labile), appropriateness (affect correlates to the setting), and congruence (with patient's described mood). Examples of affect include dysphoric, euthymic, irritable, angry, tearful, restricted, flat (severely restricted), full, labile, expansive, or congruent with mood.

THOUGHT CONTENT
There are several components of thought content. *Obsessions* are intrusive, repetitive thoughts. *Compulsions* are ritualized behaviors that patients feel compelled to perform to reduce anxiety. *Delusions* are false beliefs. Delusions can be either *bizarre*, meaning they could never occur in reality, or *nonbizarre*, meaning the thoughts are not out of the realm of possibility. Common delusional themes include *persecutory, grandiose, erotomanic, jealous,* or *somatic*.

Ideas of reference is the belief one is the subject of attention by others or that he or she is receiving special messages, such as through media. *Paranoia* can be *soft* (mild suspiciousness) to *severe* (worrying about cameras, microphones, or the government monitoring them). *Suicidality* must be ruled out. The patient may have none or may have suicidal ideation that could be passive or active. If present, further probe whether the patient has a plan, intent, or access to a means to end her or his life. *Homicidal ideation* must also be identified and whether it involves a particular victim, plan, or intent. In this case, the clinician is obligated to notify the proper authorities.

THOUGHT PROCESS
This component describes how the patient's thoughts are formulated, organized, and expressed. Ask yourself if the patient's ideas logically connect from one to the next. Keep in mind, however, that a patient can have a normal thought process with significantly delusional thought content.

A normal thought process can be described as linear, logical, or goal directed. The following are examples of abnormal thought processes:
- *Circumstantial* is the addition of many irrelevant details that impede the patient's ability of getting to the point, but the patient eventually does.
- *Tangential* is the patient responding to the question without actually answering it. The thoughts go off onto a tangent and do not come back around to the point.
- *Loose associations or thought derailment* is a lack of logical connection between the content. The patient may construct sentences, but the sentences do not make sense in sequence.
- *Flight of ideas* shift abruptly, but the sentences are logically connected, unlike those in loose associations. Flight of ideas often occur in a manic state and accompanied by rapid, pressured speech.
- *Perseveration* is repeating the same word or phrase or focusing on an idea with an inability to progress to other topics.
- *Thought blocking* is an abrupt halt in the train of thought so that the patient is unable to complete the thought. *Thought insertion* is the belief that someone or something is putting thoughts into his or her head. *Thought withdrawal* is the belief that someone or something is removing thoughts from his or her brain.
- *Broadcasting* is a belief that thoughts can be heard by others.
- *Neologism* is the invention of new words or phrases (or condensing several words).
- *Word salad* is a collection of words that do not make sense.
- *Clang associations* are using words that rhyme.

PERCEPTUAL DISTURBANCES
This category can be subdivided into *illusions* and *hallucinations*. *Illusions* are a misperception of actual stimuli. *Hallucinations* are a false sensory perception without a stimulus. To evaluate this, you may ask the patient if he or she has ever heard sounds or someone talking when no one else is there. Further inquiry can be made regarding when they occur, how often, and if it is uncomfortable for the patient (ego dystonic). Additionally, does the patient hear words, commands, or conversations or recognize the voice?

Continued

BOX 29.2 MENTAL STATUS EXAMINATION—cont'd

Auditory hallucinations are the most common. *Nonauditory hallucinations* (those involving the other senses) may indicate a neurologic or substance intoxication or withdrawal etiology. *Visual hallucinations* may involve shapes of people and occur commonly in delirium and dementia. *Tactile or somatic hallucinations* may consist of a burning sensation or feeling like something is crawling on the skin. This is common with cocaine intoxication or delirium tremens. *Olfactory hallucinations* of unusual smells may be indicative of temporal lobe epilepsy or other seizure etiology.

Depersonalization is feeling like one is standing outside one's own body observing what is happening. *Derealization* is feeling that one's environment has changed, such as not feeling real or not present.

COGNITION
Assessing cognition includes:
- Alertness: The patient is alert, drowsy, somnolent, comatose, or other.
- Orientation: Assess whether the patient is oriented to person, place, and time.
- Concentration: This can be assessed through serial 7s or spelling "world" backwards.
- Memory: Recent memory, or *immediate* recall, is the ability to repeat three objects that were just stated. *Short-term* memory is evaluated by asking the patient to recall the three words after 3 to 5 minutes. *Long-term* memory is assessed by the patient's ability to recall historical information, from months to years ago.
- Calculation: This can be assessed by serial 7s or other examples such as asking the number of nickels in a dollar.
- Fund of knowledge: Ask the patient to list the last five presidents or current events.
- Abstract reasoning: Ask the patient to interpret proverbs or similarities.

INSIGHT
Insight is a patient's conception and understanding of his or her current state or illness. Assess whether the patient realistically understands his or her illness and expresses a need or desire for treatment.

JUDGMENT
A patient's ability to make decisions and act on them demonstrates that he or she can use problem-solving skills and good judgement. You can ask a patient the following questions: What would you do if you found a stamped, addressed envelope on the sidewalk? What would you do in a movie theater if you smelled smoke?

Adapted from Fadem B. *Behavioral Science in Medicine,* 2nd ed. Philadelphia: Wolters Kluwer; 2012; and Sadock B, Sadock V. *Kaplan & Sadock's Synopsis of Psychiatry: Behavioral Sciences/Clinical Psychiatry,* 11th ed. Philadelphia: Wolters Kluwer; 2015.

and optimal social, familial, or occupational functioning. Determine a follow-up plan, noting that the patient is welcome to contact the office with questions or schedule an earlier appointment if needed.

Crisis Management

Patients at risk for suicide require a safety plan that may include voluntary or involuntary admission to an inpatient unit. If outpatient, the PA must first work with the patient to identify warning signs of suicidal ideation such as thoughts, images, and mood or behavior change. The patient may use internal coping strategies without the need to contact someone for support. Patients can be further educated to make a list of things that might distract their mind from stressors. "Mood charts" are another tool patients may use to track mood, anxiety, irritability, weight, hours slept, and medications taken. Developing a support network of people or social settings that provide distraction and assistance can also serve an important role for patients. Patients should be equipped with contact information and resources for professionals or agencies such as psychiatric providers, primary care physicians, local mental health clinics, urgent care, national suicide prevention hotlines, or simply dialing 911. Providers should ensure that the patient's environment is safe upon discharge. Patients who experience suicidal ideation should have restricted access to lethal means of harming themselves. In this case, the provider should assess whether there is a responsible person who can ensure the patient's safety and adhere to the treatment plan.

DIAGNOSTIC AND STATISTICAL MANUAL OF MENTAL DISORDERS, 5TH EDITION

The American Psychiatric Association has published the *Diagnostic and Statistical Manual of Mental Disorders,* 5th edition (DSM-5) as a guide in the diagnosis of mental disorders. The DSM classifies mental disorders with associated criteria designed to facilitate more reliable diagnoses. Reliable diagnoses are essential for guiding treatment recommendations, identifying patient groups for clinical and basic research, and documenting public health information such as morbidity and mortality rates. This information is valuable not only to PAs but also to all health care professionals associated with various aspects of mental health care.

Please see the end of this chapter for additional resources on specific mental disorders and access to the DSM-5.

CASE STUDY 29.1

A 32-year-old female presents to the primary care office indicating that she has been "feeling down" for the past several months and does not feel like doing much of anything. For the past year, she had been working 80 hours per week, dealing with daily difficulties and conflicts working in a busy attorney's office. She found work to be increasingly stressful, which led her to take a leave of absence. She has now been on long-term disability leave for at least the past 4 months. During her visit, she further indicates she has "no joy left in life." She does not continue with any hobbies she previously enjoyed. She sleeps approximately 14 hours each day and constantly feels guilty and hopeless. She complains of extreme fatigue and inability to concentrate and is unable to follow through with any one particular task. She has been very forgetful recently, which concerns her because her grandmother had Alzheimer disease. She admits to a loss of appetite and a 15-lb unintentional weight loss in the past 3 months. She is married and has three children. Her marriage is described as "excellent," and she indicates her husband is very supportive. She has, however, had a significant decrease in sexual interest. In general, her health has been excellent except for a "panic attack" she had at 19 years old. Both her mother and father were alcoholics, but she admits to drinking alcohol only on social occasions. She denies smoking or drug use. Her physical examination is unremarkable.

DISCUSSION

The diagnosis in this patient is major depressive disorder (MDD). The criteria for MDD according to the DSM-5 are as follows:

A. *Five (or more) of the following symptoms have been present during the same 2-week period and represent a change from previous functioning; at least one of the symptoms is either (1) depressed mood or (2) loss of interest or pleasure. Note: Do not include symptoms that are clearly attributable to another medical condition.*

1. *Depressed mood most of the day, nearly every day, as indicated by either subjective report (e.g., feels sad, empty, hopeless) or observation made by others. (Note: In children or adolescents, can be irritable mood.)*

2. *Markedly diminished interest or pleasure in all, or almost all, activities most of the day, nearly every day (as indicated by either subjective account or observation.)*

3. *Significant weight loss when not dieting or weight gain (e.g., a change of more than 5% of body weight in a month), or decrease or increase in appetite nearly every day.*

4. *Insomnia or hypersomnia nearly every day.*

5. *Psychomotor agitation or retardation nearly every day*

6. *Fatigue or loss of energy nearly every day.*

7. *Feelings of worthlessness or excessive or inappropriate guilt nearly every day.*

8. *Diminished ability to think or concentrate, or indecisiveness, nearly every day.*

9. *Recurrent thoughts of death (not just fear of dying), recurrent suicidal ideation without a specific plan, or a suicide attempt or a specific plan for committing suicide.*

B. *The symptoms cause clinically significant distress or impairment in social, occupational, or other important areas of functioning.*

C. *The episode is not attributable to the physiological effects of a substance or another medical condition.*

Note: Must distinguish grief from a major depressive episode (MDE). (It is useful to consider that in grief the predominant affect is feelings of emptiness and loss, while in MDE it is persistent depressed mood and the inability to anticipate happiness or pleasure.)

For further diagnostic criteria, see the DSM-5 as referenced at the end of this chapter. Coding and recording procedures are based on severity and several other specifiers.

EXPECTATIONS OF PHYSICIAN ASSISTANT STUDENTS ON PSYCHIATRIC CLINICAL ROTATIONS

Eliciting a psychiatric history. Students completing a psychiatric rotation should become proficient in eliciting a psychiatric history from a new patient or an interim history from an established patient.

Presenting. Students should have an opportunity to present history or examination findings to a preceptor. Similar to all rotations, a concise but accurate presentation is preferred.

Documenting. Students may document findings in the patient's chart. Examples may include the history, MSE, physical examination, and progress notes.

Ordering diagnostics. Although there are no confirmatory diagnostic studies for any of the psychiatric illnesses, diagnostic tests may still be warranted. For example, levels of anticonvulsant medications used for bipolar disorder need to be monitored. Complete blood counts are required for clozapine administration. Toxicology screens are helpful when considering comorbid substance abuse. Obtaining laboratory studies to rule out medical conditions that may present with psychiatric symptoms is equally important.

Medical evaluations. On occasion, students completing a psychiatric rotation may be involved in evaluation, treatment, or follow-up of medical conditions, particularly if the setting is on an inpatient unit.

Psychiatric consultations. Students may be involved in completing consultations on patients who are on a medical inpatient setting and have a need for psychiatric assessment. The evaluation of the patient would again be the same as an initial psychiatric assessment.

Psychopharmacology. Knowledge of common medications used in the management of psychiatric illness is essential. Common categories include antidepressants, mood stabilizers, anxiolytics, and antipsychotics.

Patient Populations Seen on a Psychiatric Rotation

There are opportunities to work with patients of all ages and unique practice settings, including behavioral health facilities, rural and public hospitals, private practice, jails and prisons, emergency departments, addiction medicine, Veterans Affairs, geriatric units, and pediatric settings.

Special Considerations During This Rotation

Students on a psychiatric rotation need to be mindful of safety regulations, especially on inpatient units. Students should be aware that patients on these units should not have access to certain items such as belts, shoelaces, and sharp objects. As in any medical setting, encountering a hostile, violent, or psychotic patient requires awareness of safety protocols. Finally, students should be familiar with the voluntary or involuntary commitment guidelines for inpatient hospitalization.

Other Members of the Team for This Discipline

Students may come into contact with those who are also seen in the medical model of training, including attending physicians, interns, or fellows. Social workers play an integral role in the evaluation and treatment of patients with psychiatric illnesses. Follow-up and coordination of community services are the primary functions. Occupational and recreational therapy are important components of an inpatient psychiatric setting. Nurses and case managers are also encountered. Finally, mental health workers and psychiatric technicians provide services on inpatient units, including individual or group therapy, assistance with activities of daily living, and medical documentation.

MOTIVATIONAL INTERVIEWING

Physician assistants must be mindful to not separate physical health from mental health because behavior certainly influences decisions on exercise, adequate sleep, eating a proper diet, avoiding excessive alcohol, smoking cessation, safe sex practices, wearing a seatbelt or helmet, compliance with certain medical treatments, and a host of many other choices (or behaviors) that one may make. The PA must also consider how interpersonal relationships and culture may play a role in a patient's behavior. Certainly, age, gender, and genetics as well as socioeconomic factors and demographics influence the prevalence of a disease. The potential for stress in a patient's life and his or her ability to cope are significant signs in prognosis.

Motivational interviewing (MI) is a client-centered approach of promoting behavioral change in an interpersonal context by exploring and resolving ambivalence to a decision. MI has been used in situations of alcohol misuse, smoking, diet, diabetes control, pain management, screenings, sexual behavior, chronic disease, physical activity, and medical adherence. In MI, the provider works collaboratively with the patient to help explore any ambivalence. Understanding barriers and obstacles on both sides of the decision needs to be take place for a positive change to occur.

Traditionally, medical providers have often taken a paternalistic approach in which the clinician identifies an unhealthy behavior, tells the patients what to do, and expects the patient to follow through. This approach is not always effective and may even result in patient dissatisfaction and failure to follow up. MI uses the opposite approach in which the provider is to help the patient find the motivation and reason for the change; thus, change becomes much more likely.

The first step in MI is to assess where the patient is regarding her or his readiness to change and capacity to make that change. It is important to remember that this is the patient's readiness, not the provider's. The provider's role is to be reflective, supportive, and empathetic such that patient resistance is reduced and "change talk" starts to develop. A critical part of any patient encounter is to build rapport and attempt to understand how the patient feels about things. The clinician should attempt to identify the patient's motivators rather than making assumptions about what they might be.

The next component of MI is to understand the patient's perceptions regarding the change and further explore the expected outcome of different courses of action. If the patient is ready to proceed, the provider can help formulate realistic, achievable goals that are connected to a behavior change plan. MI works by activating a patient's own motivation for change and adherence to treatment by exploring and resolving ambivalence. The provider interview is critical in helping the patient activate this self-motivation, and the approach used in the interview has a profound influence. There are four components to successful motivational interviewing:

1. **Empathy**
2. **Discrepancy.** Discrepancy is the clinician's perception of patient behavior and whether or not it matches the patient's goals and values (which are powerful internal motivators). Using discrepancy in MI helps the patient see how behaviors and values are linked and how an unhealthy behavior might be in direct opposition to a value. For example, a patient who is a heavy smoker *(behavior)* says that he cares deeply for his family *(value)*. Through MI, he realizes that his smoking is compromising the health of his family *(a behavior–value mismatch)* and decides that he is ready to quit smoking.
3. **Reflection.** Reflecting what was said back to the patient shows that the provider hears what is being said and cares about the patient's situation, which is a very effective way to decrease resistance.
4. **Supporting self-efficacy.** When a patient starts to use "change talk," assurances of ability and empowerment can signal support and help build deep commitment in the patient.

To be successful, patients need to develop their own reasons for making changes. When patients indicate a desire to change and then begin resisting, it usually means the provider is doing something wrong, such as pushing a decision or arguing with the patient's assessment. The patient may be feeling threatened with a loss of choice. As a reminder, MI is dialogue about the client's ambivalence, and the interview helps explore both sides of the issue.

As mentioned earlier, patient resistance is best met with clinician reflective listening. In reflective listening, the clinician is making a hypothesis statement on what he or she believes the patient is trying to say. This clarifies and amplifies the person's own experience and meaning through statements that prompt the patient to elaborate, such as:

- "It sounds like you . . ."
- "So, you're feeling . . ."
- "You're wondering if . . ."
- "It seems to you that . . ."
- "So, this is what I hear you saying . . ."
- "To sum it up . . ."

A clinician can do a brief assessment during MI by using the "importance and confidence ruler." The patient is asked to answer the following two questions with a value between 1 and 10 (1 is not at all important, and 10 is extremely important): (1) How *important* would you say it is for you to make a change? and (2) How *confident* (regarding self-efficacy) would you say you are that if you decided to take action, you could do it? (Are you sure that if you decided to make a change in this area of your life you could do it? How ready are you to consider making this change?) For change to occur, a patient must believe that the change is important and have the confidence to make it happen. This tool allows the clinician to see if the two conditions are met and to identify the area that might be lacking. For example, if a patient says the change is very important but has low confidence for making the change, this will be seen in the patient's responses, and the clinician will be able to help the patient work on confidence.

When done correctly, motivational interviewing can have a tremendous impact on patients' lives and the choices they make, which in turn affects other people's lives as well.[8]

THE ROLE AND FUTURE PHYSICIAN ASSISTANTS IN PSYCHIATRY

It seems that psychiatry is one of the last fields of medicine that PAs have entered; however, it can be an extremely fulfilling field. According to the National Institute of Mental Health (NIMH), neuropsychiatric disorders are the leading cause of disability in the United States, with depression taking the lead.[9] Currently in the United States, there is a huge demand for mental health care providers because of decreasing numbers of physicians and other providers being lured into other subspecialties. There is an increase, however, in public funding for mental health services, increasing insurance coverage as well as reimbursement for PAs. PAs are instrumental in filling this gap to enhance quality health care with a team-based approach. Being well trained in psychiatry is a skill that is valuable in any aspect of medicine. Even rural family practice PAs need to be competent in mental health because of the shortage of specialty providers in those areas.

CLINICAL APPLICATIONS

- What is the goal of MI? Or how might one resolve ambivalence?
- How can PAs adjust to meet the need of other cultures not "born American"?
- Do a "self-check." Explore your own biases and review your own personal coping mechanisms.

KEY POINTS

- A comprehensive assessment of the patient, including a psychiatric history and mental status exam, is essential in formulating an appropriate diagnosis and treatment plan.
- Crisis management of suicidal, homicidal, or psychotic patients requires a careful examination and documentation, utilizing appropriate resources or services to determine safety and a plan of care.
- Expectations of the student psychiatric rotation are similar to others in medicine, with a focus on history taking, presenting, documentation, and psychopharmacology.
- Motivational interviewing is a client-centered approach that has been successful in patients with disorders such as substance use, obesity, pain management, and treatment adherence.
- The physician assistant must be mindful of his or her own physical, emotional, and spiritual health in order to be an effective clinician.

References

1. World Health Organization (WHO). Mental Health Gap Action Programme (mhGAP): Scaling up care for mental, neurological, and substance use disorders. Retrieved via http://www.who.int/topics/mental_health/en/. Accessed December 4, 2015.
2. Novella EJ. Mental health care and the politics of inclusion: a social systems account of psychiatric deinstitutionalization. *Theor Med Bioeth*. 2010;31:411–427.
3. Blatt B, et al. Does perspective-taking increase patient satisfaction in medical encounters? *Acad Med*. 2010;85:1445–1452.
4. Fadem B. *Behavioral Science in Medicine*. 2nd ed. Philadelphia, PA: Wolters Kluwer; 2012.
5. Sadock B, Sadock V. *Kaplan & Sadock's Synopsis of Psychiatry: Behavioral Sciences/Clinical Psychiatry*. 11th ed. Philadelphia, PA: Wolters Kluwer; 2015.
6. American Psychiatric Association. *Diagnostic and Statistical Manual of Mental Disorders*. 5th ed (DSM-5). Arlington, VA: American Psychiatric Publishing; 2013.
7. Tallia AF, Cardone DA, Howarth DF, Ibsen KH. *Swanson's Family Practice Review: A Problem-Oriented Approach*. 5th ed. Philadelphia, PA: Elsevier; 2005:368.
8. Miller W, Rollnick S. *Motivational Interviewing: Preparing People for Change*. 2nd ed. New York: Guilford Press; 2002.
9. National Institute of Mental Health (NIMH). U.S. DALYs Contributed by Mental and Behavioral Disorders. http://www.nimh.nih.gov/health/statistics/disability/us-dalys-contributed-by-mental-and-behavioral-disorders.shtml. Accessed November 22, 2015.

The resources for this chapter can be found at www.expertconsult.com.

CHAPTER 30

SURGERY

Bri Kestler

In cognitively demanding fields, there are no naturals. Nobody walks into an operating room straight out of a surgical rotation and does world-class neurosurgery.

MALCOLM GLADWELL

HOW DO PRACTITIONERS IN A SURGICAL PRACTICE APPROACH THE PATIENT?

Whenever a surgical practitioner approaches a patient, the questions in the back of his or her mind include "Will this patient benefit from surgery?" "Is surgery the most appropriate next step?" "Is this patient a surgical candidate?" These questions are answered after a history and physical examination have been performed. Even though the practitioner may have a large amount of information on the patient because he or she has been consulted by a primary care provider or other specialist, it is always necessary for the surgeon to perform his or her own history and physical examination. The last thing the practitioner wants is to find out that the information he or she has been provided by someone else is incorrect. This could lead to the cancellation of surgery or an increased risk of surgical complications.

Will this Patient Benefit from Surgery?

Surgery is not always a guaranteed cure or help; sometimes a surgery can leave a patient in worse pain or increased disability. A wise surgeon once said, "It takes 10 years for a surgeon to learn how to cut and another 10 years to learn when NOT to cut." If the risk of complications, which can include postsurgical neuropathies, scar tissue damage, loss of function, or increased need for further surgeries, is greater than the surgical benefit to the patient, surgery may not be warranted. PAs can ensure that this question is answered by having a thorough and frank conversation with the patient, informing him or her of the risks, benefits, and alternatives to surgery and allowing the patient to take an active role in determining his or her treatment course. When a patient believes that a surgery is forced on him or her; the risks, benefits, and alternatives were not clear; or the urgency of the situation was inflated, it can lead to a mistrust of the surgical team and potentially a longer recovery because the patient does not trust the postsurgery instructions and becomes noncompliant with them. The best task a surgical physician assistant (PA) can perform is to be a staunch patient educator and ensure that the patient has made an informed decision.

Is Surgery the Most Appropriate Next Step?

In a trauma or emergency situation, this question is very easy to answer because the patient's life or limb may be in jeopardy, but when the patient has a chronic disorder that has been treated for the past 15 years, the answer may be more difficult to come by. A thorough history and physical examination can elicit information about the length and quality of the patient's previous treatment(s). This helps the PA to identify patients who have participated in a proper pharmacologic therapy and are still deteriorating and those who have not undertaken appropriate first-line treatment. Because of the increased risks of surgery over pharmacologic therapy, all efforts to ensure that the lowest risk treatment is administered first should be made.

Is this Patient a Surgical Candidate?

At this point, you have determined that your patient would benefit from surgery and that surgery would be the most appropriate next step; now you wonder if the patient is a surgical candidate. Will the patient recover from surgery, or will he or she even be able to survive the surgery itself? Does the patient have a known reaction to anesthesia medications, or does the patient have an electrolyte imbalance that may lead to cardiac arrest on the surgical table? A patient may have a carotid stenosis of 80% and be symptomatic, but if he or she has had radiation therapy to the neck, the surgical wound has a lower chance of healing; therefore, the patient may not be a candidate for a carotid endarterectomy. Likewise, if a patient is septic and having failure of multiple organs because of bacterial endocarditis, an attempted valve replacement may be fatal.

WHAT DO PHYSICIAN ASSISTANTS IN SURGERY TYPICALLY DO ON A DAILY BASIS?

There is a wide variety of surgical PAs; some stay in the hospital, assisting on cases and rounding on the inpatients, and others perform in-office procedures and see patients in a clinical setting for surgical consults and postoperative follow-up appointments. We will explain all aspects so surgical PA students are familiar with them.

Hospital Operations

If a surgeon's patient is posted for the first case of the morning, then it is usually the PA's job to ensure that the patient has arrived at the hospital on time and is advancing through the preoperative clearance requirements. Some hospitals allow patients to come to the hospital a few days early to get their preoperative laboratory studies drawn and meet with the anesthesiology staff. This allows for the day of surgery requirements to proceed faster. If the patient has not been precleared, he or she will have to have blood drawn and usually electrocardiography and potentially chest radiography performed before meeting with the anesthesiologist. The anesthesiologist will perform an independent history and physical examination to confirm that the patient is a surgical candidate from the clearance requirements. The anesthesiologist will identify the proper type of anesthesia, whether it includes epidural, moderate, or general, as well as the best method for oxygenation, such as an endotracheal tube or a laryngeal mask airway. If the anesthesiologist identifies a reason why the surgery should be canceled or delayed, he or she will inform the surgeon and operating room (OR) staff.

After the anesthesiologist has cleared the patient, the PA will verify that all the preoperative information is correct and perform a preoperative history and physical examination. Discussing the risks, benefits, and alternatives again with the patient in a thorough manner will guarantee the patient is able to provide informed consent and allow the patient to decline the surgery if he or she has had a change of heart. The patient will provide his or her consent for the surgery, and then either the surgeon or the surgical PA (depending on the policies of the hospital) may sign the surgical site. The signature should be legible and in an area that is visible to the OR staff but not directly over the expected incision line.

The PA can then make a quick stop by the assigned OR for the first case and confirm that all specialized instruments are available, equipment representatives have arrived and will be aiding in equipment identification and acquisition, and all supplies are available. Information on patient positioning, potential blood-borne pathogen status (hepatitis- or HIV-positive patients), and operative procedures can be offered to the OR staff so that everyone is aware of the specific needs of the surgeon and patient.

While the patient is finishing up the preoperative clearance and being moved into the OR, the surgical PA can then begin to make rounds on any patients who are in the hospital. These patients may include those who are awaiting surgery, are postoperative, or have been readmitted for surgical complications or previous surgical patients receiving additional treatment in the hospital. Rounding occurs whenever there is a free moment. You may not be able to see all your patients before starting your first case of the day. Typically, a surgical PA will start with the patients in the intensive care unit (ICU) or critical care unit and then proceed to the lesser acuity floors. Rounding on patients involves reading the notes of all other providers involved in the care of the patient, reviewing current laboratory tests and imaging, identifying any new diagnoses, and confirming appropriate treatment. All of these aspects are required to complete a detailed progress note on the patient. In addition to completing a progress note on the patient, the surgical PA

identifies patients who are appropriate for discharge home. Patients who are going to be discharged home require a discharge summary and medication reconciliation to be completed, and the surgical PA usually completes these. Patient education regarding follow-up appointments, proper medication administration, recovery restrictions, rehabilitation exercises, and wound care instructions need to be provided by a member of the surgical team before discharge home.

The surgical PA is frequently in contact with the OR staff over the course of the day. By calling into the OR to see if the patient is there and ready for positioning and draping, the surgical PA can make every effort to not delay the operation start time and waste the time of the OR staff. After it has been confirmed that the patient is in the room, the PA should head to the OR and assist in positioning the patient on the OR table. Patient positioning takes multiple people because anesthesiology staff needs to protect the airways and lines, and OR staff need to pad bony points on the patient to lessen the risk of skin breakdown and neurologic complications. The surgeon needs the best access to the area of surgical interest.

During surgery, the PA is the surgeon's extra hands. The goal of the surgical assistant is to provide the surgeon with the best surgical view. This can involve retracting tissue, suctioning blood, or repositioning light sources. Tension and countertension during retraction are the hallmarks of surgery. The surgical PA is supposed to know the surgeon's next four steps in his or her head so he or she can preemptively ask for instruments the surgeon will need and have the area prepped before the surgeon needs it.

Surgical scopes of practice vary among surgeons, specialties, and hospitals. Some surgeons may be very comfortable with their PAs' abilities and allow them extensive procedural leeway, but other surgeons limit the amount of primary surgical processes that their PAs can perform. The amount of work you see one surgical PA do may be very different from the amount of work that another surgical PA does. Just plan on taking it all in, and use that information to determine if you would like to work in a surgical specialty. When the surgery is over, there is more paperwork that needs to be completed, including an operative note, medication reconciliation, and postoperative orders, and nonpaperwork items such as talking to the family of the patient. The surgical team may divide and conquer these tasks. For instance, the surgeon may dictate a detailed operative note and talk to the family while the PA completes a postoperative note and completes the orders.

Another aspect of working in a hospital are surgical consults. Consults can come from the emergency department (ED) or from another specialty in the hospital. The ED may consult you on a patient who was found to have appendicitis, which requires that you admit the patient to your service (meaning you are the primary for that patient) or you contact the patient's primary care provider and ask that she or he admit the patient, meaning you could then act as consultant, schedule the patient for surgery, and follow the patient through her or his hospital course. An alternative scenario is an oncologist consulting you for placement of a power port in a patient who requires chemotherapy. For this type of consult, you don't have to admit the patient or act as the primary provider, but you need to write a consult note, schedule the patient for surgery, and follow the patient postoperatively. Consults can come at any time of the day, and some PAs take calls that require them to see the consults on the nights or weekends that they are on call. Every surgical practice is different, and call schedules are unique to each individual surgical PA. Call shifts usually correlate to late surgery coverage as well. If a surgery is running later than the PA's normal shift, some practices have a late PA who will scrub in to relieve the PA who is ready to head home; most of the time this is also the on-call PA. Just like call schedules, a late PA or late coverage is unique to each surgical group; sometimes the late coverage may be a physician rather than another PA, but it is seen as a way to keep the late nights more equally dispersed among the surgical PAs.

Clinic Operations

Some aspects of hospital operations can carry over into a surgical clinic, especially if the surgical practice also performs in-office procedures. These may include procedures performed under local anesthesia such as a lesion biopsy, removal of a tunneled catheter or incision and drainage of an abscess, or even procedures using moderate sedation. With moderate sedation, an anesthesiology practitioner will administer the short-acting anesthesia medications and monitor the patient's vital signs and response to the medications. Patients undergoing moderate sedation procedures still need a full workup performed by the anesthesiology practitioner and proper preoperative laboratory studies with a postoperative recovery time. Because the moderate sedation medications are not given in the dosages and do not have the long-term affect as the general anesthesia, the recovery time is significantly reduced. These patients cannot drive home under their own accord, but they do not have effects of drowsiness or sleepiness for as long a period as general anesthesia patients.

Clinic patients may range from consults by other providers, presurgical clearance workups, postoperative checks, and disease surveillance appointments.

WHAT WILL I BE EXPECTED TO DO DURING THE SURGERY ROTATION?

Hospital Operations

The majority of a PA student's surgical rotation will be in a hospital setting; as such, the expectations revolve around operative patients. Students will be expected to preround on their assigned surgical patients before the resident rounds on them. This requires that the PA student arrive at the hospital very early in the morning. The first surgery of the morning usually starts at 7:30 AM, and depending on the size of the patient census and number of students on the service, sometimes an arrival time of 4:30 to 5:00 AM is necessary. The morning goal of every surgical PA student should be to have performed a focused history and physical examination, reviewed laboratory work and recent imaging, and completed a detailed progress note on each of her or his assigned patients before meeting with the services resident for the morning. The residents, interns, and students will round on the patients as a team before the attending surgeon arrives at the hospital, at which time another team rounding session will occur with the surgeon. During each rounding, the student should be prepared to brief the resident and attending on the status of each patient.

Hospital patients can be broken up into three categories: preoperative patients, postoperative patients, and medical patients. Preoperative patients include those who are scheduled for surgery. They may be trauma patients who have to have other medical therapy completed before undergoing surgery (e.g., stabilization of blood pressure or correction of electrolyte imbalances), or they may be patients who have inflammation or infection (systemic or at the site of incision) that needs to be addressed before surgical correction. Postoperative patients are those who have just undergone a surgery and are recovering and patients who have already been discharged from the hospital after the initial surgery and have returned because of complications such as infection, wound dehiscence, or failure of the surgery. Medical patients include those who are being treated for a medical condition that doesn't warrant surgery, but if the treatment fails, these patients may become surgical candidates. Sometimes surgery services are consulted on patients known to them because of yearly surveillance for existing conditions because they may be admitted to the hospital for other conditions, and the admitting doctors would like the surgical team to offer assistance with their care. An example of a medical patient is a patient who is admitted for chronic constipation by a gastroenterologist, who then consults the surgeon because the patient has a known abdominal aneurysm. In this case, the surgeon can offer advice if other procedures need to be performed and follow the patient's hospital course.

A PA student ought to include the items listed in Table 30.1 in her or his brief oral presentation of each surgical patient.

It is important for a PA student to check on her or his assigned patients multiple times throughout the day because this allows the PA student to read what other services wrote, be proactive about any requests from those services, identify any complications, and initiate early treatment for those complications.

In addition to rounding on assigned patients, the PA student may be asked to take admits from the ED or a doctor's office or consults from other providers. This requires the student to obtain a detailed history and physical examination surrounding the surgical diagnosis, write a consult note, and present the consult patient to the resident or attending physician for finalization of the assessment and plan. These consults may require a lot of time and effort, especially if the patient has multiple diagnoses requiring

multiple care providers or if the patient has an extensive surgical history. An important part of the consult note is identifying any aspect of the patient's history that may complicate the intended surgery or cause an increased risk of postoperative complications. A patient who has had multiple abdominal surgeries is at an increased risk for abdominal adhesions, which would complicate the surgery by requiring the surgeon to perform a greater amount of dissection in the abdominal cavity. This extensive dissection could lead to an increased risk of bleeding and bowel perforation, as well as increased anesthesia time.

When in the OR, there may not be a great number of tasks for the PA student to perform, but there are plenty of places for the student to help. If there are quite a few other students with the surgical service, the students may need to take turns scrubbing into cases. When a PA student is allowed to scrub into a case, he or she will take on the role of observer more than any other role. There may be a few instances when a PA student can provide some retractor support, cut suture tails, or suction the surgical field. Other surgeons may be at ease with a student maneuvering

TABLE 30.1 Important Items to Include When Presenting a Patient

Preoperative Patient	Postoperative Patient	Medical Patient
What procedure the patient is scheduled for and when?	Days status post and from what procedure	Why is the surgical team following the patient?
Brief overview of the patient's hospital course to date	Brief overview of the patient's recovery to date	Brief overview of the patient's previous clinic visits with any surveillance studies
Any issues the patient was having (e.g., if something has kept the patient from having the procedure) or that have come up overnight	Any complications or issues the patient has been having (e.g., wound issues, ileus, nausea)	Any current complaints
Physical examination (focusing on any previous abnormalities noted and their resolution or deterioration)	Physical examination (focusing on the vital signs, surgical incision, and complete examination of the organ system involved in the surgery)	Physical examination (focusing on the organ system involved with the patient's chronic disease)
Current laboratory studies (to include results from early morning laboratory draws and pending laboratory studies such as cultures) with information on any trends (e.g., monitoring blood urea nitrogen and creatinine in a patient with kidney disease); current imaging with radiologist readings (if available)	Current laboratory studies (to include results from early morning laboratory draws and pending laboratory studies such as cultures) with information on any trends (e.g., monitoring hemoglobin and hematocrit after acute blood loss); current imaging with radiologist readings (if available)	Current laboratory studies and imaging that are associated with the patient's chronic disease
Quick review of other providers on the patient's care team assessment and plan (e.g., physical therapy, nephrology, infectious disease)	Quick review of other providers on the patient's care team assessment and plan (e.g., physical therapy, nephrology, infectious disease)	Review of the admitting doctor's planned course of treatment with additional input provided by other consulting services
Identification of any potential consults	Identification of any potential consults	Identification of when the patient may become a surgical candidate

around laparoscopic cameras, suturing incisions, or conducting first-assistant duties. The bottom line is that the level of hands-on experience that a PA student receives depends on the number of residents and students on the surgical service, the willingness of the student to be involved, and the comfort of the surgeon. If a PA student is not scrubbing into the case, he or she can help the rest of the OR team by pulling up radiographs of the patient, getting gowns and gloves for personnel who are scrubbing in, helping to transfer the patient onto the OR table, and answering phone calls and pages for the scrubbed-in surgical team. After surgeries are completed, the PA student may volunteer to write the operative note and postoperative orders, help transfer the patient on a stretcher, and follow the patient to the postanesthesia care unit (PACU).

Clinic Operations

In-office procedures may allow PA students to obtain more procedural practice because these procedures are generally lower acuity with less of a chance of serious complications. Even small procedures, such as suture removals or wound dressing changes, can provide PA students with the ability to hone their manual dexterity and should be volunteered for at any chance.

The bulk of time spent in the surgery clinic will be used in seeing patients for scheduled visits. Very similar to the way in which hospital patients can be categorized, clinic patients can be broken into preoperative patients, postoperative patients, and surveillance patients.

Preoperative patients include those referred by other providers for a surgical workup (see the first part of this chapter) and those who have already been identified as surgical candidates who need preoperative laboratory work or imaging or need to be scheduled for surgery with the hospital OR scheduling staff. At the end of the visit with the referred preoperative patient, the PA student should be able to determine if the patient (1) requires surgery and should be scheduled appropriately with surgical clearance laboratory testing or imaging ordered, (2) does not require surgery or is not a surgical candidate but should return for follow-up surveillance appointments, or (3) does not require surgery or is not a surgical candidate and does not need any additional appointments with the surgical clinic. Regardless of the disposition of the patient, it is appropriate to inform the referring doctor's office of the assessment and plan for each patient.

Postoperative patients will return to the surgical clinic multiple times after procedures so their recovery process can be monitored. It is very important to perform a detailed interview, specifically asking about recovery limitations, medications, and therapies, to identify the patient's compliance level. Identifying a noncompliant patient early in the recovery period can allow the PA student to provide additional patient education that may save the patient from any serious complications. A focused but thorough physical examination, with emphasis on the surgical wound integrity, sensation, and infection status, should be performed on every postoperative patient. The PA student can also discuss health maintenance and prevention topics with the postoperative patient to ensure that additional chronic diagnoses are treated and monitored by the appropriate providers.

Surveillance patients can include those who have a disorder that may require surgical correction at some point but not immediately (i.e., patients with peripheral artery disease and mild symptoms) or patients who have had a procedure performed and require monitoring of its efficacy (i.e., patients with an implanted pacemaker that require generator checks). These surveillance appointments can range from a few weeks for those with increasing symptoms to a few years for those with stable surgical corrections. The PA student should be responsible for interviewing the patients, paying special attention to questions that would elicit responses consistent with disease progression, such as an increase of pain and decrease of range of motion for a patient who will need a knee replacement. Comparison of previous laboratory or imaging results may need to be performed by the PA student, and discussing any new diagnoses or recent hospitalizations or surgeries with the patient can provide additional information for the patient's medical records.

WHICH CLINICAL ENVIRONMENTS MAY I WORK IN DURING THE SURGERY ROTATION?

As stated previously, a surgical PA student could work in the hospital, taking consults, seeing ED patients, and performing surgeries or procedures in the OR, or at the bedside and following the progress of the surgical services in-hospital patients. The PA student could also work in the surgical practices clinic, seeing referred patients for surgical identification, performing preoperative clearances and postoperative recovery checks, and performing well yearly or biannual follow-up visits as required. Likewise, clinic responsibilities may include lower acuity procedures performed in the office.

WHICH OTHER TYPES OF HEALTH PROFESSIONALS WILL I WORK WITH DURING THE SURGERY ROTATION, AND WHAT CAN I LEARN FROM THEM?

The surgical team may consist of all or a combination of the following people: attending surgeon, physician assistant, fellow, fifth-year (chief) resident, junior resident, intern, and student(s).

Attending Surgeon

In most academic centers, the attending surgeon is an experienced staff member who has the ultimate responsibility for the surgical team's patients. He or she is responsible for the training of the fellows and fifth-year surgical residents and frequently teaches the more difficult and complex surgical techniques and decision making to this group. Attending surgeons often have particular areas of clinical interest (e.g., oncology, intensive care, trauma, burns, gastrointestinal disorders) and are commonly involved in research. The attending surgeon participates in the training of students on the surgical rotation as well and is called on to personally operate on the more difficult surgical cases that require experienced judgment.

Fellow

A graduate of a surgical residency, a fellow has elected to continue studies in a subspecialty (e.g., vascular, trauma, cardiac, neurosurgery). Each fellowship lasts between 1 and 3 years, during which time an intense training regimen prepares the fellow to practice in the chosen specialty. Much of this training is spent in the OR, learning and performing specialty procedures. Many fellowships include a specialized opportunity to conduct research activities.

Fifth-Year (Chief) Resident

The fifth is the last year of residency for most general surgery programs, although some extend to 7 years. The fifth-year resident is responsible for the overall day-to-day patient care provided by the team. He or she performs the most complicated operations with the attending surgeon, instructs junior residents in the OR, and provides consultation on the care of newly admitted patients and complicated cases.

Junior Resident

The junior resident is the workhorse of the residency staff. This person is responsible for the minute-to-minute care of the patient as provided by the surgical team. The junior resident does a large volume of the service's operating and is responsible for the training of the second-year resident and intern. A resident in the second year of training along with the intern does much of the admitting and discharging of the service's patients. Additionally, the second-year resident usually serves extended rotations in the ED and ICU to hone emergency care, triage, and surgical intensive care unit (SICU) skills.

Intern

The first-year resident, or intern, is a recently graduated medical student and a new arrival on the surgical service. He or she is responsible for the brunt of the everyday tasks required for patient care and routine orders, admissions, discharges, consults, night calls, intravenous (IV) lines, tubes, laboratory tests, and radiologic studies. Interns are engaged in learning the basic surgical skills and techniques required for general patient care. They are excellent sources of information for PA students, and because of the great burden of tasks thrust on them, interns commonly allow PA students to learn by doing.

Student

Medical and PA students are a valuable part of the surgical team in that students provide the additional staff required to efficiently operate a large-volume service. While constantly observing, students help manage the day-to-day needs of their assigned patients, including history and physical examination, starting IV lines, drawing blood specimens, inserting chest tubes, casting, wound care, ED duties, patient assessment, patient transport, dressing changes and wound care, and monitoring response to treatment. In addition, PA and medical students learn basic surgical techniques such as suturing and knot tying; inserting monitoring lines; and first, second, and third assisting in surgery. After adequate observation and performance of techniques monitored by senior team members, the student's motto should be, "I will do that for you."

Anesthesia Team

Anesthesiologist

The anesthesiologist is an MD or doctor of osteopathy (DO) who is responsible for evaluating the patient for anesthesia and, in coordination with the operating team, for providing safe conduct of the patient through the chosen anesthetic technique.

Anesthesiologists care for the patient through-out the recovery room period and into the SICU if required. Many have particular expertise in pain management.

Certified Registered Nurse Anesthetists

Certified registered nurse anesthetists (CRNAs) train in nurse residency programs to perform many of the same tasks as an MD or DO anesthesiologist. Deeply versed in anesthetic practice, CRNAs provide qual-ity care, often without the direct supervision of an anesthesiologist, and are used by many surgeons for uncomplicated surgical procedures. Limitations on CRNA practice are dictated by hospital and state regulations and vary from institution to institution and from state to state. CRNAs are similar to the PAs of the anesthesiology world.

Anesthesiology Assistants

These are individuals who attend a training pro-gram to conduct anesthesia but who are not phy-sicians or CRNAs. Several training programs are available in the United States, although only a handful of states have regulations or laws that allow administration of anesthesia by anesthesiology assistants (AAs). AAs perform anesthesia practice under the supervision of a licensed anesthesiologist and are valued members of the anesthesia team, on which they are used.

Operating Room and Recovery Team

Postanesthesia Care Unit or Recovery Room Nurse

The PACU nurse is trained in assessing and treat-ing patients in the immediate postoperative period, including maintenance of hemodynamic and car-diopulmonary stability, pain management, and crisis intervention when necessary. Such professionals are invaluable sources of guidance and information on postanesthesia patient care.

Operating Room Director

Usually a veteran registered nurse (RN), the direc-tor controls the overall activity of the OR and is responsible to the chief of surgery (a surgeon) and the hospital's director of nursing. The OR director represents the OR to other hospital departments, manages the department's fiscal requirements, and oversees the management of OR personnel. He or she can set the tone for a favorable climate for PAs in the OR.

Operating Room Supervisor

Also usually an RN, the OR supervisor manages the day-to-day activities in the OR and makes important policy decisions in conjunction with the OR director. The supervisor is responsible for problem solving, overall procedure and OR staff scheduling, instru-ment purchases, and staff training.

Circulating Nurse (Circulator)

The circulator supervises the general activity of each individual in the OR, including assessing patients in the holding area before bringing them into the OR and transporting patients to the recovery area after surgery. Patient safety, also the responsibility of the circulator, centers on appropriate positioning of the patient on the OR table and preparation of the patient by scrub preparation of the skin before the incision. The circulator assists the scrub nurse in assembling the supplies and instruments required for the opera-tion and in accounting for all sponges, needles, and instruments before and after each operation. Cir-culators provide additional supplies for the opera-tive field when required. They receive and connect the various tubes and wires coming from the sterile field (e.g., suction tubes, laparoscopic equipment, and electrocautery wires) to the appropriate devices. They operate and troubleshoot nonsterile equipment and prepare tissue specimens received from the sur-geon for transport to the pathologist for analysis.

Scrub Nurse or Registered Nurse First Assist

Scrub nurses assist the surgeon by providing all instruments, sutures, and supplies required for the smooth execution of each procedure. Scrub nurses anticipate the needs of the surgeon and first assis-tant by understanding each step of a procedure and by monitoring the progress of the operation, often handing the appropriate instrument to the surgeon without prior request. In addition, the scrub nurse occasionally assists in retracting tissues, cutting sutures, sponging blood from the field, and operat-ing the suction. A well-trained and experienced scrub nurse often performs certain portions of the proce-dure without direct supervision by the surgeon. One of the scrub nurse's primary responsibilities is know-ing the locations and counts of all items in the ster-ile operative field before, during, and after surgery, ensuring that nothing has been left in the wound. The scrub nurse is an invaluable source of informa-tion on the conduct expected of the PA or medical student in the OR and the skills required at the OR table. Also, a scrub nurse who has worked frequently with a given surgeon may have invaluable information regarding that surgeon's preferences and dislikes in the OR.

Certified Surgical Technologist or Scrub Tech

Although not an RN or LPN, the certified surgical technologist (CST) is trained by an American Medical Association–approved center and meets rigid certification examination criteria to perform a wide variety of functions in the OR. Many of these responsibilities parallel those of the scrub nurse, although many large institutions do not allow CSTs to circulate during surgery. CSTs often assist the surgeon while scrubbed and fill an important position in the operating suite.[1]

WHICH CLINICAL INFORMATION DO THE PHYSICIAN ASSISTANTS AND PHYSICIANS ON THE SURGERY ROTATION ALWAYS WANT TO KNOW ABOUT THEIR PATIENTS?

As mentioned previously, a thorough history, both medical and surgical, will always be wanted. A physical examination is also a requirement. Any allergies to medications, anesthetic agents, or latex or complications of prior anesthesia are paramount.

WHICH SPECIAL POPULATIONS OF PATIENTS MAY I SEE ON THE SURGERY ROTATION?

All types of patient populations require surgery, whether they are elective procedures or lifesaving requirements; PA students in a surgical rotation will see patients from all walks of life. Patients who are referred for elective procedures usually go through the surgical practices clinic and receive prior approval for the procedure through their insurance companies. Emergency surgeries are performed based on the patient's status, not his or her insurance coverage.

WHAT ARE THE SPECIAL CHALLENGES OF SURGERY?

Surgery can be very reactive at times, and it is this reactivity that creates hectic and packed schedules. The surgical rotation is full of long days and even longer nights in the hospital setting. PA students need to be there before everyone else to round on

their patients and then may need to stay after the last surgery is completed to check up on their assigned patients or perform last-minute admits or consults. You may be packing up to head home after a long day of surgeries, just to get called back into the OR by the resident because an emergency or critical patient came in. All surgical practices have a call schedule, and some PA programs require their students to take calls, usually overnight, at least once, during their rotations. Call can be luck of the draw sometimes, with some students not seeing a single patient but others' call pagers never seeming to stop. Rather than seeing call time as a negative, embrace all the experience you will receive because there are usually fewer people around, which means you could get some prime surgical practice. One of the fastest ways to get time in the OR is to volunteer for call and night and weekend shifts.

Specifically for the surgery rotation, you will run into a barrage of information. The Physician Assistant National Certifying Examination (PANCE) and other end-of-rotation exams can ask questions about any surgical specialty and most PA students do not have the luxury of rotating with a multitude of services. This creates a need for independent research and study time for surgical PA students. Try not to focus on studying just what you see or even the specialty you are rotating with; instead, study every organ system and the surgeries involved with each.

Blood, guts, and bodily fluids can be additional challenges for surgical PA students. Surgeries tend to be messy, and a variety of bodily orifices and fluids will be seen, felt, and even smelled. If you know you have a weak stomach or are prone to vomiting or passing out in response to these, let your resident know because he or she can help ease you into the OR and offer additional tips and tricks for coping. Make sure you stay hydrated and eat when you can; sometimes surgeries last longer than expected, and your white coat's pockets can be a great place to stash snacks for in between surgeries. Don't lock your knees when you are standing at the OR table, and if you start feeling faint, back away from the table and let someone know. The last thing you want to do is try to be tough and then pass out onto the sterile field.

WHAT ARE THE SPECIAL REWARDS OF SURGERY?

There can be immediate satisfaction with surgeries when they correct the problem relatively quickly. A fractured femur can be set, coronary arteries can be bypassed, and a portion of bowel can be resected. These all correct an issue immediately. The majority of surgeries will leave the patient feeling better or relieve symptoms that she or he has been living with for many years. Visiting with these patients in a postoperative setting can be very rewarding because you were a part of the team that improved the patient's medical situation.

SCRUBBING AND GOWNING AND GLOVING

Five-Minute Scrub

Before performing a surgical scrub with a medicated scrub brush, ensure that you remove all jewelry, do not wear artificial nails or nail polish, prewash your hands and arms if they are visibly dirty, and clean subungual areas with a nail cleaner.[2]

1. Start timing. Scrub each side of each finger, between the fingers, and the back and front of one hand for 2 minutes.
2. Proceed to scrub the arm, keeping the hand higher than the arm at all times. This helps to avoid recontamination of the hands by water from the elbows and prevents bacteria-laden soap and water from contaminating the hands.
3. Wash each side of the arm from the wrist to the elbow for 1 minute.
4. Repeat the process on the other hand and arm, keeping hands above the elbows at all times. If the hand touches anything at any time, the scrub must be lengthened by 1 minute for the area that has been contaminated.
5. Rinse your hands and arms by passing them through the water in one direction only, from the fingertips to the elbow. Do not move the arm back and forth through the water.
6. Proceed to the OR, holding your hands above your elbows.
7. At all times during the scrub procedure, care should be taken not to splash water onto surgical attire.
8. When in the OR, your hands and arms should be dried using a sterile towel and aseptic technique before donning gown and gloves.[2]

Subsequent scrubs of the day can be shortened to a total of 2 minutes with a medicated scrub brush and water, or the PA student can use alcohol-based handrub preparations.

Alcohol-Based Handrubs

1. Put approximately 3 pumps of handrub in the palm of your left hand using the elbow of you other arm to operate the dispenser.
2. Dip the fingertips of your right hand in the handrub to decontaminate under your nails for 5 seconds.

3. Smear the handrub on your right forearm up to your elbow. Cover the whole skin area by using circular movements around your forearm until the handrub has fully evaporated.
4. Repeat steps 1 to 3 on the other hand and arm.
5. Put approximately 3 pumps of handrub in the palm of your left hand using the elbow of you other arm to operate the dispenser.
6. Cover the whole surface of your hands up to the wrist, rubbing palm against palm with a rotating motion.
7. Rub the back of your left hand, including the wrist, moving the right palm back and forth, and then repeat on the other side.
8. Rub your palm against palm back and forth with your fingers interlinked.
9. Rub the thumb of the left hand by rotating it in the clasped palm of the right hand and vice versa on the other hand.
10. When the hands are dry, sterile surgical clothing and gloves can be donned.[2]

Assisted Gowning and Gloving

The arms are extended at a 90-degree angle in front of the body, and the gown is placed over the shoulders by the scrub nurse. The fingers are partially extruded through the wrist cuffs so that the cuff end rests just below the thumb (Fig. 30.1).

The right glove is placed first. The fingers are slightly abducted, and the hand is gently inserted into the glove as the scrub nurse circumferentially expands the wrist cuff. The scrub nurse then expands the left glove's wrist cuff. With the right hand, the wearer gently pulls the edge of the cuff toward the body and places the left hand into the glove (Fig. 30.2).

All surgical gowns have a wraparound tie at the waist that prevents the back of the gown from becoming unfastened. On disposable gowns, the paper "handle" is carefully handed to the circulating nurse while the person wearing the gown turns in a circle. The wearer gently pulls the tie from the paper handle without touching the paper handle and ties the front of the gown. For nondisposable gowns, the wraparound tie must be given to a sterile person.[1]

Self-Gowning and -Gloving

The gown is carefully removed from the sterile field and is gently shaken, well above the floor, to loosen the folds and fully extend the gown. The hands are placed into the armholes, and the circulating nurse or another OR staff member pulls the gown onto

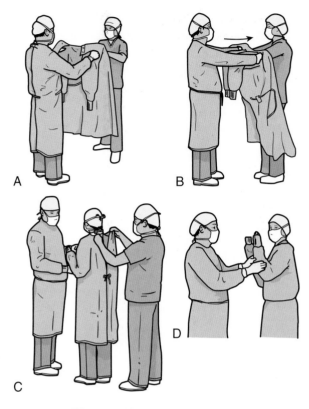

FIG. 30.1 ■ (A-D) Assisted gowning.

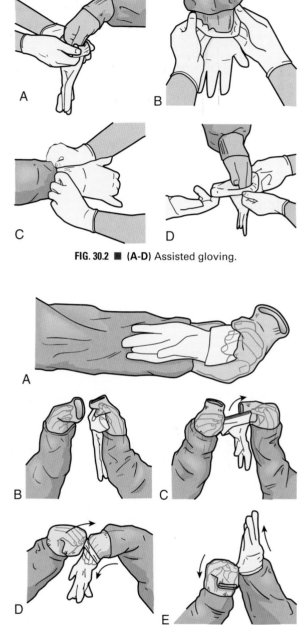

FIG. 30.2 ■ (A-D) Assisted gloving.

FIG. 30.3 ■ (A-E) Self-gloving.

the wearer's shoulders and fastens the gown from behind. The hands are not placed through the wrist cuffs but remain within the sleeve of the gown itself. The gown's cuffs may be used like mittens to manipulate the fingers and hands into the first glove without touching the glove with the bare hand (Fig. 30.3).[1] The rest of the gown is tied as previously mentioned.

KEY POINTS

- PA students will only get out what they put into the surgical rotation.
- Surgical PAs work alongside a multitude of different providers and OR personnel, and PA students can learn something different from each one.
- The OR works the best when the team is strong; find out how you can make the team better.
- Surgical PAs are not only beneficial to the patient in the OR but also during postoperative follow-up appointments. Don't slack on your responsibilities as a patient educator in all your duties.
- Have fun, be professional, and treat every person you come into contact with courteously and with kindness and compassion.

References

1. Sullivan EM. Surgery. In: Ballweg R, Sullivan E, Brown D, Vetrosky D, eds. *Physician Assistant: A Guide to Clinical Practice*. 5th ed. Philadelphia, PA: Elsevier Sanders; 2013:356–409.

2. WHO Guidelines on Hand Hygiene in Health Care: First Global Patient Safety Challenge Clean Care Is Safer Care. Geneva: World Health Organization; 2009:13. Surgical hand preparation: state-of-the-art.

The resources for this chapter can be found at www.expertconsult.com.

The Faculty Resources can be found online at www.expertconsult.com.

EMERGENCY MEDICINE

Tamara S. Ritsema

HOW DO PRACTITIONERS IN EMERGENCY MEDICINE APPROACH THE PATIENT?

Emergency medicine practitioners have one overarching goal for each patient: to answer the question: "Does my patient have a threat to life, limb, or sight today?" Emergency departments (EDs) are structured to provide lifesaving services to patients in acute need. Determining which patients are in acute need, however, can be less than obvious. A woman with a classic presentation of gastroesophageal reflux may have a myocardial infarction. A man with a complaint of a mild cough and a low-grade fever may have a pulmonary embolus. Someone with a very concerning facial droop may simply have a Bell's palsy rather than the stroke she feared when she saw her face in the mirror.

The purpose of the ED workup is to provide the correct disposition for each patient. Your preceptor will perform a focused history and physical examination followed by clinical investigations designed to determine whether the patient is "sick" or "not sick." To an emergency medicine physician assistant (PA) or doctor, "sick" means there is a possibility the patient will die today. Although a patient vomiting repeatedly from a hangover may appear sicker than a new atrial fibrillation patient who complains of generalized fatigue, in reality, the new atrial fibrillation patient is sicker and demands a more careful workup. Each patient is evaluated to see if she needs hospitalization or whether her concerns can be safely worked up on an outpatient basis after discharge.

Emergency medicine practitioners do not necessarily make a diagnosis for the patient in the ED. The goal is to provide lifesaving care and then to send the patient to the most appropriate environment for the rest of his care. For example, patients with hypotension from severe sepsis will be admitted to the intensive care unit (ICU) regardless of the source of the infection. If the source of the infection can be determined in the ED, that is certainly helpful to the medical staff. However, not knowing the source does not preclude the emergency medicine team from providing appropriate initial care and handoff to the medical team. Patients with multiple traumatic wounds will be taken to the operating room or transferred to the nearest trauma center even if the staff in the ED do not have time to characterize all the injuries.

When you are seeing the patient, keep these questions in mind:

- Does the patient appear seriously ill?
- Is the patient unable to participate with my history and physical examination?
- Does the patient have vital signs that indicate she may be dying?
- Does the patient, although well-appearing now, have symptoms that are consistent with a life-threatening pathology (e.g., chest pain, unilateral weakness)?
- Does the patient appear to be dangerous toward me or any other member of the staff?

If the answer to any of these questions is "yes," you should seek help from your preceptor sooner rather than later. No one will criticize you for seeking help early. If the patient is not as sick as you feared, you will simply be instructed to continue with your assessment and be ready to present the patient to your preceptor in a few minutes.

Finally, a word about honesty. Experienced emergency medicine practitioners know to listen carefully, sympathetically, and respectfully to the patient but to also be a bit suspicious about elements of the patient's story that potentially don't make sense. Did she really break her jaw by falling out of bed, or is it more likely that she is the victim of domestic violence? Why does this patient's opiate pain medication always seem to be "stolen" from his car only a few days after his last prescription was written? Could he be selling the pills or so addicted that he is taking far more than the prescribed dose? Is it possible that my 16-year-old female patient with nausea is pregnant despite her denying sexual activity?

WHAT DO PHYSICIAN ASSISTANTS IN EMERGENCY MEDICINE TYPICALLY DO ON A DAILY BASIS?

Physician assistants in emergency medicine have great variety in the level of responsibility they carry. Some PAs in rural EDs are the sole provider in the ED and are responsible for all aspects of care for all patients, with physician supervision at a distance. Other PAs work solely in the urgent care or fast track parts of the ED, seeing primarily patients with more minor complaints. Many PAs see all types of patients under the supervision of board-certified emergency physician. The supervision can be quite close for less experienced PAs or quite general for more experienced PAs, depending on the laws of the state, the regulations of the hospital, the requirements of the Department of Emergency Medicine, or the preference of the supervising doctor working with the PA that day.

That said, emergency medicine PAs have the opportunity to see a wide range of medical and surgical conditions. It is not unusual for a PA to simultaneously care for an oncology patient, an orthopedic patient, a cardiology patient, and a psychiatry patient. Sometimes one patient can have issues from all of these specialties! PAs evaluate patients from the beginning, determine what testing they need, carry out the testing, interpret the results, and provide an appropriate treatment. A typical shift might include a pelvic examination, suturing a laceration, transferring a patient to an ICU, interpreting an electrocardiogram, reading a chest radiograph, and dealing with eight complaints of abdominal pain. In all cases, the PA's role is to determine whether the patient is sick and to provide stabilizing or curative treatment.

WHAT WILL I BE EXPECTED TO DO ON THIS ROTATION?

After seeing a few patients with your preceptor to understand how things work at the particular ED, you will typically be sent to see patients on your own. You will be expected to obtain a relevant focused history and an appropriate examination from the patient. Typically, preceptors will ask students to avoid performing pelvic, rectal, or breast examinations so that a patient does not have to undergo these examinations more than once. You should defer these examinations until after you have presented the patient to your preceptor. After you have seen the patient, you should think about what you would like to do for the patient (further evaluation or treatment) and get ready to present the history and physical examination findings and your plan to your preceptor. You will watch for your patient's results to come back and present them to your preceptor along with your recommendations for the next step as the patient goes through his or her ED workup.

In the setting of a busy ED, you can be of great help to the team by keeping up with your patient's laboratory and radiology results, by learning where supplies are and being willing to help collect supplies for procedures, and by helping patients with comfort needs when you have a spare moment. Review the principles of sterile technique before the rotation so that if you are fortunate enough to be asked to assist with a lumbar puncture, chest tube, or central line that you will not contaminate the field or impair the PA's ability to do her or his job.

WHICH CLINICAL ENVIRONMENTS MAY I WORK IN DURING THIS ROTATION?

In emergency medicine, you will likely be primarily working in the ED. You may work sometimes in an urgent care or fast track unit or on an observation unit.

WHICH OTHER TYPES OF HEALTH PROFESSIONALS WILL I WORK WITH ON THIS ROTATION, AND WHAT CAN I LEARN FROM THEM?

Key staff in the ED include emergency nurses, emergency medical technicians (EMTs), and social work staff. Emergency nurses often have a wealth of experience and knowledge to share with a PA student—simply ask them! EMTs who bring the patients to the ED have crucial information about how they found the patient and which interventions have already been performed. Try to speak directly with the EMTs when they arrive with the patient to hear the story firsthand. Social workers provide key information about resources for your patient. Does your patient need assistance with food, medications, housing, and so on? A social worker can provide assistance far beyond what a PA or a doctor can in this situation. You can learn from them by reviewing their recommendations for the patient.

WHICH CLINICAL INFORMATION DO THE PHYSICIAN ASSISTANTS AND PHYSICIANS ON THIS ROTATION ALWAYS WANT TO KNOW ABOUT THEIR PATIENTS?

- Vital signs are vital! Make sure you have a full set on each patient and that vital signs are updated after interventions. Vital signs are one of the primary ways we determine if a patient is sick or not.
- What happened to this patient to bring him here today? You need to get a clear story in sufficient detail to help us determine if the story matches the examination we see in front of us. Try to understand why the patient came *today*, particularly if the patient has had symptoms for a while. Did the symptoms get worse today? Did the patient's spouse get sick of his complaining and force him to come? Did she run out of pain medication or albuterol treatments? What made *today* different?
- Has the patient ever had the same set of symptoms before? If yes, what was the diagnosis, and how did she do with treatment? This will keep you from making the same mistakes over and over again with the same patient.
- Is the patient's tetanus shot up-to-date? Get this information on every patient with a cut or a wound.
- Obtain medication, allergies, alcohol, and substance abuse history.

WHICH SPECIAL POPULATIONS OF PATIENTS MAY I SEE ON THIS ROTATION?

First, a high percentage of patients seen in the ED have psychiatric illness. Patients with acute psychiatric illness are seen for their depression, mania, or psychosis. In these patients, it is obvious that they have a psychiatric illness. However, patients who present with other complaints may also have a contributing psychiatric illness. Patients with depression, obsessive-compulsive disorder, borderline personality disorder, and anxiety disorder are more likely than those without psychiatric disease to come to the ED for general medical concerns. A patient complaining of tingling paresthesias all over his body may have hyperventilation from his anxiety disorder. A patient with fatigue may have depression. Be vigilant to look for signs of psychiatric illness in each patient. However, never forget that even the most psychotic patient can also have appendicitis, a myocardial infarction, or a cellulitis. Psychiatric illness does not preclude a serious medical condition that needs to be addressed.

Second, you will see patients with serious chronic illnesses that require repeated hospitalization. Every ED has a group of patients who simply have difficult-to-manage illnesses and who come through the ED to receive initial treatment and placement onto a hospital floor. These patients often know exactly what they need from the emergency staff. Listen to what they have to say, and consider it as you make your care plan.

Third, you will see the "frequent fliers." These are patients who come to the ED regularly, often for complaints that really do not require emergent medical care. Some of these patients have diagnosed or undiagnosed psychiatric issues, some are looking to get prescriptions for controlled substances, some are trying to escape a troubled home or an abusive spouse, and some are simply lonely or bored. When you notice that someone is a "frequent flier," try to understand why she keeps coming back and to determine if there is a way to better meet the patient's needs outside the ED. Occasionally, your preceptor may seem callous about one of these patients. You may be concerned about the patient's complaint of abdominal pain, only to be informed by your preceptor that the patient has come in for this same pain three times per week for the past 4 years. Early discharge for this patient, after life-threatening pathology has been excluded, means that someone with a more acute illness can be seen more quickly and reinforces the message to the patient that the ED is not the proper environment in which to seek care for chronic conditions.

WHAT ARE THE SPECIAL CHALLENGES OF EMERGENCY MEDICINE?

The biggest challenge in emergency medicine is to correctly decide who is sick and who is not. Everyone who practices emergency medicine has missed a serious diagnosis. Being able to see patients efficiently and not miss serious pathology is difficult. Those who choose emergency medicine as their specialty need to be able to live with the possibility that their actions or inactions can have serious consequences in the life of another person.

It can be hard not to become cynical about the next patient you see when the previous three patients had trivial complaints that did not require a visit to the ED or the last two patients you saw lied to you about an important part of their health history. Witnessing trauma and death can be challenging. No one knows better than an emergency medicine PA how one distracted driver or poor decision can change a person's life forever. Those who practice emergency medicine often have to give bad news: "Your son died," "You've had a stroke," or "The tumor has spread." Doing so without becoming callous requires professionalism and humanity.

WHAT ARE THE SPECIAL REWARDS OF EMERGENCY MEDICINE?

There is no greater reward in medicine than visibly saving someone's life. Restoring a patient's good looks with a nicely done laceration repair, making a rare diagnosis, working smoothly with your team to get the patient promptly to the catheterization laboratory, reducing a dislocated joint, and reassuring a terrified patient that she does not have the disease she worried about make the days fulfilling and fun.

WHAT RESOURCES MIGHT BE HELPFUL TO ME ON THIS ROTATION?

It is extremely important to review your first-year materials for all clinical procedures. Pay special attention to sterile technique. In addition, review Basic Life Support (BLS), Advanced Cardiovascular Life Support (ACLS), and Pediatric Advanced Life Support (PALS) before starting in the ED. Go back and study up on how to read radiographs, particularly chest and long bone radiographs. Review your general medicine notes on conditions that often have an urgent presentation such as asthma, cholelithiasis and cholecystitis, coronary artery disease, Crohn disease, depression causing suicidal thoughts, diabetes, chronic obstructive pulmonary disease, heart failure, infections, orthopedic complaints, and so on. Remember your differential diagnosis lists for common presentations such as chest pain, headache, abdominal pain, and dyspnea. Study your trauma lecture again, focusing on the primary and secondary survey of the patient. Know the primary and secondary survey questions by memory. Review the workup and treatment of sepsis.

KEY POINTS

- The primary focus of emergency medicine is to determine who is seriously ill and who is not and to provide lifesaving procedures as needed. Learning to establish which patients are seriously ill takes years of training and experience.
- Students should always perform complaint-focused assessment of the patients in the ED and not attempt to perform a complete head-to-toe history and physical examination. If you are concerned that a patient may have a life-threatening illness, you should get help for that patient immediately.
- Students starting on their emergency medicine rotation should review all cardiac life support curricula, sterile technique, clinical procedures, and the acute presentations of common illnesses to prepare them for their placement.

CHAPTER 32

ELECTIVE ROTATIONS

A. CARDIOLOGY

Sondra M. DePalma

CARDIOLOGY AND APPROACH TO THE PATIENT

Cardiology is the internal medicine specialty of heart and vascular diseases and treatments. The primary goals of cardiology are to reduce morbidity and mortality and improve quality of life. This is accomplished by stabilizing patients with life-threatening emergencies, treating acute conditions, managing chronic diseases, and providing primary and secondary disease prevention. Methods of prevention and treatment include lifestyle modification, medication management, endovascular procedures, and minimally invasive surgeries.

The main emphasis in cardiovascular care is evidence-based medical practice. At the same time, cardiology practitioners must attend to patient preferences, comorbidities, and socioeconomic barriers to optimal health. Therefore, cardiology is dedicated to evidence-based medicine, guideline-directed medical management, patient-centered care, a team-based approach to health delivery, and performance and process improvement to enhance health care and patient outcomes.

PHYSICIAN ASSISTANTS IN CARDIOLOGY

Physician assistants (PAs) in cardiology enjoy a complex, challenging specialty with opportunities to improve patient and population health. Cardiology PAs work in clinic- and hospital-based settings and practice autonomously and in collaboration with health care professionals. They diagnose diseases, treat acute illnesses, manage chronic conditions, and perform and interpret diagnostic tests and procedures. Specific clinical duties depend on the practice setting and type.

Common inpatient duties include hospital rounds, admission histories and physical examinations, cardiology consults, discharge coordination and summaries, pre- and postcardiac procedure management, and critical care management. PAs in cardiology also perform cardiopulmonary resuscitation, supervise and interpret exercise and pharmacologic stress tests, and perform or assist with other diagnostic studies and invasive procedures.

Usual outpatient duties include cardiology consults, acute care visits, chronic disease management, medication management and titration, disease prevention, and care coordination. Cardiology PAs in clinics also supervise and interpret exercise and pharmacologic stress tests, interpret electrocardiograms and ambulatory telemetry monitors (e.g., Holter monitors and event recorders), interrogate and program implantable cardiac electronic devices, and manage disease-specific clinics (e.g., heart failure and anticoagulation clinics).

Physician assistants in the inpatient and outpatient cardiology settings may also be involved in nonclinical duties. Opportunities to participate in research and clinical trials are available. PAs in cardiology may also be involved in quality- and performance-improvement projects, education, and management of cardiovascular service lines.

PHYSICIAN ASSISTANTS IN CARDIOLOGY SUBSPECIALTIES

As the knowledge, technology, and complexity of treatments have advanced, subspecialties within cardiology have developed. PAs have the chance to work in general cardiology or specialize in
- **Invasive or interventional cardiology,** which focuses on coronary and peripheral artery revascularization as well as structural and valvular endovascular repair
- **Electrophysiology,** which specializes in the diagnosis and management of arrhythmias and conduction abnormalities with medication, ablation, and implantable cardiac electronic devices
- **Heart failure management,** which involves the diagnosis and treatment of cardiomyopathies and other causes of heart failure, management of mechanical circulatory support, and heart transplantation
- **Pediatric cardiology,** with an emphasis on treatment of congenital heart defects and inherited cardiovascular diseases in children
- **Adult congenital cardiology,** the management of adults with medically treated or surgically corrected congenital heart defects
- **Preventive cardiology,** including management of hypertension, dyslipidemia, and the cardiometabolic syndrome

THE CARDIOLOGY ROTATION

A rotation in cardiology is beneficial for students considering a career in the specialty or in internal medicine, family medicine, emergency medicine, hospital medicine, critical care, vascular surgery, or cardiothoracic surgery. A cardiology rotation prepares PAs to manage many of the diseases commonly seen in adult medicine. Hypertension, dyslipidemia, coronary artery and peripheral arterial disease, atrial fibrillation, and heart failure are frequently encountered in clinical practice, and their incidences are expected to increase with the aging of the American population.

What to Expect and Know

Student responsibilities and expectations depend on the clinical setting and subspecialty of the cardiology rotation. Students often assist with obtaining histories and examinations, performing prerounds in the hospital, formulating treatment plans for acute and chronic diseases, and educating patients. Students may observe or assist with diagnostic tests, invasive procedures, and cardiopulmonary resuscitation.

Students should be able to perform a cardiovascular-focused history and physical examination. A problem-focused history with attention to cardiovascular symptoms, risk factors, and family history is important to assess risks and form differential diagnoses. A cardiovascular-focused physical examination and appropriate diagnostic testing are necessary to make an accurate diagnosis. Specifically,
- The history of present illness should include the characteristics of symptoms as well as aggravating and ameliorating factors. It is also important to know if symptoms are stable or worsening to determine if a condition is chronic, exacerbated, or unstable.
- An important aspect of the social history includes whether a patient uses tobacco (a risk factor for atherosclerotic cardiovascular disease), alcohol (a risk factor for cardiomyopathy and arrhythmias), or cocaine (a risk factor for coronary vasospasm and atherosclerotic disease). It is also helpful to know if a patient's work, home, or social environments expose them to pollutants (e.g., tobacco or other air pollutants) or a sedentary lifestyle that could increase cardiovascular risks.
- The family history should document whether or not any first-degree relatives (i.e., parents, children, or siblings) had premature (men before 55 and women before 65 years of age) cardiovascular disease or sudden cardiac death.
- A cardiovascular-oriented examination should include a general assessment; evaluation of vital signs; auscultation for murmurs, adventitious heart sounds, and bruits; auscultation of lung sounds; palpation of pulses and apical impulse; and other examinations based on differential diagnoses or abnormal findings. Auscultation with the patient lying on his or her left side, seated and leaning forward, or while performing Valsalva maneuvers may accentuate and differentiate murmurs. Assessment

of jugular venous pressure, edema, and ascites is important in suspected heart failure. A general evaluation of the integumentary system for pallor, cyanosis, and diaphoresis is important to determine if a patient is hemodynamically unstable; the presence of lower extremity pallor or ulcers may indicate peripheral arterial disease; and Janeway lesions or Osler's nodes may be signs of bacterial endocarditis. A retinal evaluation may reveal findings consistent with arterial disease, or the presence of Roth's spots may indicate infective endocarditis.

- Knowledge of concepts and interpretation of electrocardiograms is helpful.

In addition to performing an appropriately thorough evaluation, cardiology PA students are often expected to review the results of recent laboratory and diagnostic studies. During daily hospital rounds, it is helpful to obtain the results of tests performed during the previous 24 hours. In patients with chronic diseases, it is useful to evaluate and document the most recent cardiovascular studies and their major findings.

During a cardiology rotation, students should improve their knowledge of cardiovascular physiology and pathophysiology. Students will develop a greater understanding of noninvasive diagnostic tests, including electrocardiograms, ambulatory telemetry monitors, transthoracic and transesophageal echocardiograms, exercise and pharmacologic stress testing with and without myocardial perfusion imaging, and cardiac computed tomography and magnetic resonance imaging. Students may also learn about invasive angiography (Fig. 32A.1) and angioplasty, percutaneous valve replacements, electrophysiology studies and cardiac ablations, left atrial appendage occlusions, and implantable cardiac electronic devices. Finally, students will appreciate the cardiology lexicon of acronyms and abbreviations (Table 32A.1).

Clinical Environment

In cardiology, PAs have the opportunity to work in diverse clinical environments and may practice in outpatient clinics, hospitals, or acute and long-term care facilities. Within hospitals, PAs perform evaluations and provide care in the emergency department, inpatient units, critical care and intensive care units, and perioperative units. PAs may also assist with tests or procedures in catheterization and electrophysiology laboratories. Additional environments may be encountered through home health and telemedicine.

Each environment is unique and provides important learning opportunities. Therefore, students should try to gain experience in a variety of clinical settings. Preceptors can often assist students in obtaining opportunities in areas other than the primary rotation assignment.

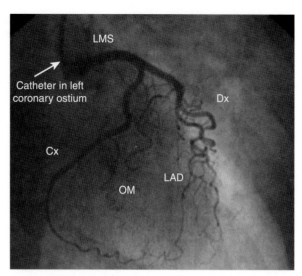

FIG. 32A.1 ■ Angiogram demonstrating the left coronary artery anatomy in the left anterior oblique view. The left coronary artery arises from the proximal ascending aorta as the left main stem (LMS). This bifurcates into the circumflex artery (Cx) and the left anterior descending artery (LAD). Branches of the LAD are the septal arteries that supply the septum and the diagonal arteries (Dx). Branches of the Cx are called obtuse marginals (OMs). The Cx is dominant. This artery is free from disease. (Reprinted with permission from Goyal D, Karim R, et al. Cardiac catheterization. *Medicine* 2010;38(7):390–394, Copyright © 2010, Elsevier, Inc.)

Other Health Professionals

Cardiology relies on a team of health care specialists, including physicians, PAs, nurses, and allied health professionals (Table 32A.2). Cardiology PAs often collaborate with primary care providers, internal medicine specialists, hospitalists, intensivists, cardiothoracic surgeons, and vascular surgeons. Because cardiology involves chronic disease and medication management, PAs may also work with case managers, social workers, dieticians, and pharmacists. In interventional cardiology and electrophysiology, interaction with medical device representatives is also common.

Patients and Special Populations

The array of patients seen in cardiology is as varied and diverse as the cardiology subspecialties. PAs in pediatric cardiology treat newborns, children, adolescents, and young adults. Some patients with congenital disorders will transition to adult cardiology and are followed through their lifespans. Pediatric and adult congenital patients may have difficulties with sports, employment, travel, body image, and interpersonal relationships. The majority of cardiology patients are adults, and many are elderly. Older patients often have multiple comorbidities, and health care management

TABLE 32A.1 Cardiology Abbreviations and Acronyms

AAA	abdominal aortic aneurysm	LAD	left anterior descending artery
ACS	acute coronary syndrome	LM	left main artery
AF (A Fib)	atrial fibrillation	LVAD	left ventricular assist device
AFI	atrial flutter	LV	left ventricle
AMI	acute myocardial infarction	MI	myocardial infarction
AO	angiography	MPI	myocardial perfusion imaging
AS	aortic stenosis	MR	mitral regurgitation
ASD	atrial septal defect	NSTEMI	non–ST-segment elevation myocardial infarction
ASCVD	atherosclerotic cardiovascular disease	OM	obtuse marginal branch or artery
BMS	bare metal stent	PAC	premature atrial contraction
CAD	coronary artery disease	PCI	percutaneous coronary intervention
CHF	congestive heart failure	PFO	patent foramen ovale
CRT	cardiac resynchronization therapy	PM	pacemaker
Cx	circumflex artery	PTCA	percutaneous transluminal coronary angioplasty
DES	drug-eluting stent	PVC	premature ventricular contraction
EF	ejection fraction	RCA	right coronary artery
EKG or ECG	electrocardiogram	RVR	rapid ventricular rate or response
EP	electrophysiology	STEMI	ST-segment elevation myocardial infarction
EPS	electrophysiology study	SVT	supraventricular tachycardia
EST	exercise stress test	TAVR	transcatheter aortic valve replacement
HFpEF	heart failure with preserved EF	TEE	transesophageal echocardiogram
HFrEF	heart failure with reduced EF	TTE	transthoracic echocardiogram
IABP	intraaortic balloon pump	VSD	ventricular septal defect
ICD	implantable cardiac defibrillator	VT	ventricular tachycardia
LAA	left atrial appendage	UA	unstable angina

TABLE 32A.2 Cardiology Personnel

Providers	Nurses (LPNs and RNs)	Allied Health
Cardiologists	Hospital	Cardiovascular technologists
Residents and fellows	Clinic	Invasive technologists
Advanced practice providers	Chronic disease management	Electrophysiology technologists
Physician assistants	Cardiac rehabilitation	Nuclear medicine technologists
Advanced practice registered nurses (nurse practitioners and clinical nurse specialists)	Transitional care	Sonographers
	Home health	Cardiac device specialists
		Exercise physiologists
		Clinical pharmacists
		Dieticians

LPN, Licensed practical nurse; *RN,* registered nurse.

may need to account for fixed incomes, cognitive deficits, and problems with mobility and travel.

CHALLENGES AND REWARDS IN CARDIOLOGY

Cardiology requires the ability to make critical decisions and manage complex patients with multiple comorbidities, which can be challenging. Unpredictability, life-threatening emergencies, and the death of patients are stressful. PAs providing chronic disease management and end-of-life care can experience feelings of sadness and futility. In addition, it can be challenging to meet the needs and expectations of both patients and families.

Despite its challenges, cardiology provides an abundance of rewards. Great satisfaction can be garnered from improving the health and quality of life of patients with cardiovascular diseases. In addition, many PAs enjoy the variety within cardiology, still-evolving technologies and therapies, the ability to practice in a specialty with reliance on evidence-based medicine and a focus on outcome improvement, and the opportunity to work in a specialty with dedication and commitment to team-based care.

HELPFUL RESOURCES

Many resources are available to complement the cardiovascular knowledge acquired in PA school. In addition to textbooks and medical journals, many evidence-based guidelines provide information regarding appropriate care. Reliable information can also be obtained from online sources and clinical applications (apps) for smart phones and portable electronic devices.

A regular resource used by cardiovascular clinicians is the American College of Cardiology's (ACC's) collection of online evidence-based guidelines, peer-reviewed journal articles, self-assessment continuing medical education, clinical toolkits, practice solutions, and evidence-based, peer-reviewed apps. The ACC is a professional organization dedicated to improving cardiovascular health, and its collection of resources can be accessed at www.acc.org.

The American Heart Association (AHA) maintains evidence-based resources for cardiovascular professionals. Numerous guidelines, policies, and publications, including the most recent cardiopulmonary resuscitation recommendations, are available at http://www.heart.org. The AHA also maintains useful patient education and resources.

Several other cardiovascular societies and their resources include:
- Heart Rhythm Society: http://www.hrsonline.org
- National Lipid Association: http://www.lipid.org
- Heart Failure Society of America: http://www.hfsa.org
- Association of Physician Assistants in Cardiology: http://www.cardiologyPA.org

Physician assistant students may find the following textbooks provide a good foundation of cardiovascular knowledge:
- *Current Diagnosis & Treatment: Cardiology*
- *Clinical Cardiology Made Ridiculously Simple*
- *Rapid Interpretation of EKGs*

SUMMARY

A cardiology rotation provides valuable knowledge and clinical skills for PAs whether they practice in adult medicine or cardiology. The approximately 2500 PAs practicing in cardiology[1] enjoy a varied, challenging, and rewarding career in which they can improved morbidity, mortality, and quality of life. An upsurge of opportunities for PAs in cardiology is expected because of the aging population, ongoing advancements in cardiovascular treatments and technologies, and the cardiovascular community's commitment to team-based care.

KEY POINTS

- The prevention, diagnosis, and treatment of cardiovascular disease significantly improve health and quality of life, decrease morbidity and mortality, and reduce health care expenditures.
- Cardiology is a diverse specialty consisting of subspecialties; hospital- and clinic-based practice; invasive and noninvasive procedures; prevention, acute treatment, and chronic disease management; research; and quality and performance improvement.
- PAs are medical providers who are known to provide high-quality, cost-effective cardiovascular care.[2,3]
- As the U.S. population ages and further advancements are made in cardiovascular treatments and technologies, cardiology will continue to grow and offer a wide range of opportunities for PAs.

References

1. American Academy of Physician Assistants. https://www.aapa.org/WorkArea/DownloadAsset.aspx?id=2902. Accessed January 10, 2016.
2. Krasuski RA, Wang A, Ross C, et al. Trained and supervised physician assistants can safely perform diagnostic cardiac catheterization with coronary angiography. *Catheter Cardiovasc Interv.* 2003;59(2):157–160.
3. Virani SS, Maddox TM, Chan PS, et al. Provider type and quality of outpatient cardiovascular disease care: insights from the NCDR Pinnacle Registry. *J Am Coll Cardiol.* 2015;66(16): 1803–1812.

B. DERMATOLOGY

Johnna K. Yealy

CHAPTER OUTLINE

APPROACH TO THE PATIENT

TYPICAL DAY

EXPECTATIONS OF THE STUDENT

CLINICAL SETTINGS

TEAM MEDICINE

ESSENTIAL CLINICAL INFORMATION TO BE OBTAINED FROM EACH PATIENT

WHAT ARE THE SPECIAL REWARDS OF DERMATOLOGY?

WHAT ARE THE SPECIAL CHALLENGES OF DERMATOLOGY?

KEY POINTS

Dermatology became a medical subspecialty at the end of the 18th century; however, many concepts regarding early dermatologic disorders were first described more than 2000 years ago by Hippocrates. When confronted with a dermatologic complaint, you may recall the old adage "If it's wet, dry it, and if it's dry, wet it." This treatment approach was first ascribed to Hippocrates. In fact, in the third century BC, the *Hippocratic Collection*, also known as the *Corpus Hippocraticum*, described the anatomy and physiology of the skin and various cutaneous manifestations of systemic disease.[1] He noted, for instance, that clubbed nails are associated with underlying pulmonary disease and that urticaria is associated with swollen joints.[1,2] Hippocrates exerted that physicians should do the opposite to the body of what was inflicted by the disease, such as applying a drying agent to a moist area and applying emollients to a dry area. He treated superficial skin tumors by curettage and cautery using a curette similar to that used today.[3]

Today dermatology is a highly sought after medical specialty, attracting the best and brightest medical students to 4-year residency programs across the United States. It is a varied specialty that requires knowledge of internal medicine, dermatopathology, microbiology, clinical dermatology, surgical care, oncology, cosmetic care and laser treatment, allergic care, rheumatology, and preventive medicine. Dermatology is a growing specialty area for physician assistants (PAs). According to the 2013 American Academy of Physician Assistants' annual survey, currently 3.3% of PAs identify themselves as "dermatology" PAs.[4]

APPROACH TO THE PATIENT

The skin is the largest organ system and the most visible, which is both an advantage and disadvantage for providers who examine the skin. On the one hand, the pathology is often readily visible to the naked eye; on the other, a student may be overwhelmed by the variety of normal variants in the skin and miss key or subtle signs of skin disease.[5] When approaching a dermatologic patient, the physical examination should be completed after a brief patient interview but before detailed history is taken. Many cutaneous lesions are so characteristic that the diagnosis will announce itself during the physical examination. Often the patient will present a history that is inconsistent with the diagnosis or related to his or her own interpretation of the origin of the lesion, which may mislead the provider assessing the patient.[6] Therefore, a quick visual inspection before detailed questioning will lead the provider down one of two paths: (1) biopsy to establish a diagnosis or (2) diagnosis and treatment.

When conducting a skin examination, it is essential to perform a complete examination during the visit. The ideal examination includes evaluation of the skin, hair, and nails as well as the mucous membranes of the mouth, eyes, nose, nasopharynx, and anogenital region. Patients often present with complaints concerning a single lesion that is worrisome to them or more often to their spouse, which are actually benign. Many patients have never had a skin cancer screening examination but are focused on the initial complaint, not knowing they have other, more concerning lesions. A baseline skin cancer screening examination allows changes from the original skin exam to be documented, establishing a time line for concerning skin changes. After the visual examination has been completed, then a more thorough history of present illness and review of systems should occur. The history of present illness should document the following:

1. History or evolution of the skin lesion: when (onset), where (site of onset), symptoms (pain/itch), how it spread (pattern or evolution of spread), how the individual lesions have changed, provocative factors (heat, cold, sun, exercise, travel, drug ingestion, pregnancy, season), and previous treatment (topical or systemic, over-the-counter or home remedies)
2. Constitutional symptoms: acute illness or syndromes, including headache, fever, chills weakness, or joint pain, versus chronic illness syndromes, including fatigue, weakness, anorexia, weight loss, and malaise
3. Recent exacerbation of chronic illnesses
   Further information to collect includes:
4. Past medical history: operations, illnesses, allergies, medications, habits (smoking, alcohol or drug use), and atopic history (asthma, hay fever, eczema).
5. Family medical history: of particular importance are history of psoriasis, atopy, melanoma, xanthomas, and tuberous sclerosis
6. Social history, particularly occupation, hobbies, exposures, and travel
7. Sexual history: history of HIV risk factors, blood transfusions, intravenous drug use, and sexual activity

After the physical examination, history of present illness, and review of systems are complete, then the dermatology provider will develop a differential diagnosis and formulate a treatment plan. The final diagnosis is often confirmed by a biopsy.

Physician assistant students will find that dermatology providers are very specific in their documentation of skin changes and lesions. The student should be able to apply the MAD approach for describing skin lesions: M for morphology, A for arrangement, and D for distribution. *Morphology* includes the type, size, shape, color, elevation, and margination of the lesion(s). When describing the type of lesion, the student should be aware that there are primary and secondary changes in the skin (Table 32B.1 and Fig. 32B.1). The *arrangement* of lesions may be single, grouped, arciform, annular, serpiginous, and so on (Table 32B.2). The *distribution* of lesions may be localized, disseminated, or in other recognized patterns, which should always be assessed and documented. Distribution of lesions often predicts diagnosis (Fig. 32B.2). By being observant and specific in the description of the lesions, the examiner will often make the diagnosis without further unnecessary testing. Many skin diseases have pathognomonic descriptions. For instance, when reviewing medical documentation, "grouped papules or vesicles on an erythematous base" is clearly herpes to any trained medical provider.

It is important to be precise in describing the location of the lesions because many biopsies result in a diagnosis of a cancerous lesion, which will require further excision. By the time results are received, the biopsy site will be well healed and render the excision site difficult to establish without a detailed documented location. For instance, rather than recording "nose" as the biopsy site, the subsequent surgical excision would be better guided by documentation that the biopsy was obtained from the left ala of the nose or the nasal bridge.

TYPICAL DAY

Dermatology PAs have busy days filled with a wide variety of patients and complaints. Dermatology PAs provide preventive, acute, chronic, complex medical, emergency, procedural, surgical, cosmetic, allergic, and follow-up care to patients of all ages. These clinics are very fast paced. Generally, a single provider, not participating in surgical procedures, will see 40 to 50 patients per day, scheduled every 5 to 15 minutes. Dermatology PAs do not typically take calls or provide hospital consultations; therefore, night and weekend duty is limited. Depending on the complaint, the patient will require a full physical skin examination, biopsy or procedural treatment, or prescription. Preventive care consists of skin examinations for follow-up of skin cancer patients or

TABLE 32B.1 Common Morphology of Skin Lesions

Type	Description
Primary Lesions	
Papule	Solid, palpable lesion <5 mm in diameter
Nodule	Solid, palpable lesion >5 mm in diameter
Macule	Flat, nonpalpable lesion <10 mm in diameter
Patch	Flat, nonpalpable lesion >10 mm in diameter
Plaque	Plateau-like lesion >10 mm in diameter; may be a group of confluent papules
Vesicle	Circumscribed, elevated lesion containing serous fluid, <5 mm in diameter
Bulla	Circumscribed, elevated lesion containing serous fluid, >5 mm in diameter
Wheal	Transient, elevated lesion caused by local edema; also known as a "hive"
Petechiae	Minute hemorrhagic spots that cannot be blanched by diascopy
Telangiectasia	Dilated, small, superficial blood vessels
Secondary Lesions	
Crust	Hard, rough surface formed by dried sebum, exudate, blood, or necrotic skin
Scale	Heaped-up piles of horny epithelium with a dry appearance
Pustule	Vesicle or bulla containing purulent material
Erosion	Defect of the epidermis; heals without a scar
Ulcer	Defect that extends into the dermis or deeper; heals with a scar
Shape	Round, polygonal, polycyclic, annular (ring shaped), iris, serpiginous (snakelike) or umbilicated or pedunculated (on a stalk), verrucous (irregular, rough and convoluted)
Color	Pink, red (erythematous), purple (violaceus), white, tan, brown, black, blue, gray, or yellow; uniform in color or variegated (multicolored)
Elevation	Dermal, subcutaneous
Margination	Well defined or ill defined, coalescing

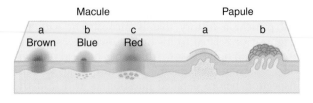

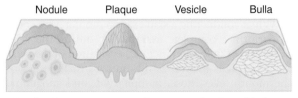

FIG. 32B.1 ■ Primary lesions. (From Longo DL, Fauci AS, Kasper DL, et al. *Harrison's Principles of Internal Medicine*, 18th ed. New York: McGraw-Hill; 2012. **http://www.accessmedicine.com**. Copyright The McGraw-Hill Companies, Inc. All rights reserved.)

TABLE 32B.2 Arrangement, Distribution, and Other Identifying Skin Lesion Terms

Arrangement	Grouped or disseminated: grouped lesions are further defined as herpetiform (grouped vesicles), arciform (partial ring or bow shaped), annular (round), reticulated (net shaped), linear (straight line), serpiginous (snakelike)
Distribution	Isolated single lesion or localized to one body area, localized to one regional area, generalized or universal
Other Descriptors	
Palpation	Consistency: soft, firm, hard, fluctuant or nonfluctuant, or sandpaper
Temperature	Warm, hot, or cold
Mobility	Mobile (freely movable) or nonmobile
Tenderness	Tender or nontender
Number	Single or multiple; disseminated lesions are further defined as scattered discrete lesions
Lichenification	Thickened skin with distinct borders
Macerated	Swollen and softened by an increase in water content
Confluence	Confluent or nonconfluent
Pattern	Symmetric, sun-exposed, sites of pressure, intertriginous areas, follicular, random or following Blaschko skin lines

initial skin examinations for at-risk patients. The next patient may require acute care, with a complaint of a bleeding or growing lesion that requires a quick skin biopsy. A patient with psoriasis on systemic biologic therapy needs complex medical and chronic care to

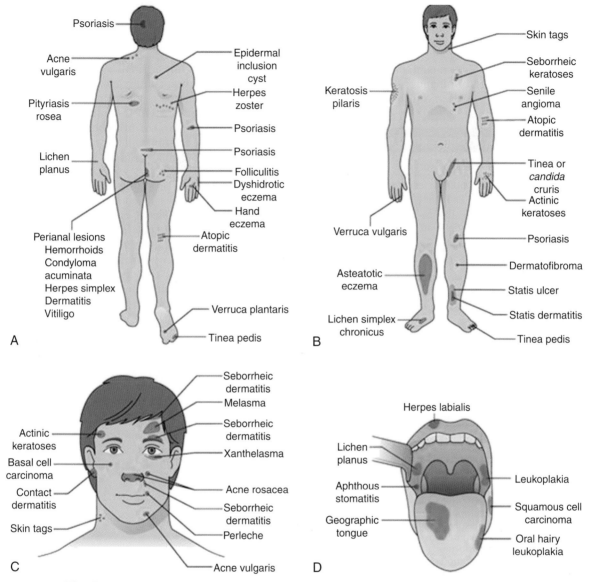

FIG. 32B.2 ■ A–D, Distribution of lesions and diagnosis. (From Kasper DL, Fauci AS, Hauser SL, et al. *Harrison's Principles of Internal Medicine*, 19th ed. New York: McGraw-Hill; 2015. http://www.accessmedicine.com. Copyright McGraw-Hill Education. All rights reserved.)

assess for complications from the medication, review of laboratory test results, and adjustment of therapy. Another patient may present for surgical excision of a cyst or skin cancer. Clinics that provide cosmetic care include patient slots for cosmetic injections or education regarding a chemical peel. If the clinic provides allergy testing, then the next patient may require education, setup of allergy patch testing, application of the patch, or interpretation of patch results. When the dermatology PA is not engaged in direct patient care, she or he will follow up on numerous biopsy

and laboratory results and likely complete documentation. Very rarely, a PA may perform a consultation on a hospitalized patient.

Many PAs are employed specifically for their surgical skills. Their days include excision of skin cancers or cysts, closure of complex excisions of skin cancers, participation in Mohs micrographic surgery, suture removal, and follow-up care of surgical patients. Dermatology providers also perform a number of specialized diagnostic techniques and reference special signs and tests that the PA student may not have used on other rotations. Specialized signs and tests include the Darier sign, Auspitz sign, Nikolsky sign, photopatch test, and Koebner phenomenon (Table 32B.3). Diagnostic tests include diascopy, potassium hydroxide preparation (KOH prep), scraping and smears, Wood's light examination, acetowhitening, and biopsy. Table 32B.4 summarizes these diagnostic tests.

TABLE 32B.3 Special Signs and Tests

Sign or Test	Description
Darier sign	Rubbing a lesion causes an urticarial flare
Auspitz sign	Pinpoint bleeding after scale is removed
Nikolsky sign	Pushing a blister causes further separation of the dermis
Photopatch test	Documents photoallergy
Patch test	Demonstrates hypersensitivity reaction
Koebner phenomenon	Minor trauma leads to new lesions at site of trauma

TABLE 32B.4 Diagnostic Techniques

Technique	Description
Diascopy	A glass slide or diascope is pressed against the skin. Blanching indicates intact capillaries; extravasated blood (purpura) does not blanch.
Potassium hydroxide preparation (KOH)	Microscopic examination of skin scrapings mounted in KOH, which dissolve keratin and cellular material but does not affect fungi, is performed. The method readily identifies dermatophyte infection.
Scrapings and smears	Blunt and sharp instruments facilitate specimen collections. Various staining techniques and visualization methods bring out certain characteristics of the lesion or responsible pathogen (Tzanck smear, dark-field microscopy).
Wood's light	Examination used to assess changes in pigment or to fluoresce infectious lesions.
Acetowhitening	Examination using acetic acid to facilitate the examination of warts.
Biopsy	May be excisional, incisional, shave, or punch and is indicated if diagnostic or pathologic confirmation is necessary.

EXPECTATIONS OF THE STUDENT

Generally, students are expected to perform a quick inspection and generate a description of the patient's skin complaint. Only a small amount of time will be allowed for patient interview. Unlike on a family practice or internal medicine rotation, where the student may be given 10 to 15 minutes with a patient before presentation to the preceptor, the student in the dermatology rotation will typically only have 3 to 5 minutes to make an assessment and report back to the preceptor.

Dermatology is a procedurally heavy medical discipline. Cryotherapy is a common treatment. Skin biopsies (shave, deep shave, and punch) are obtained in the majority of patients. Treatments may consist or electrodessication, and curettage or excision, skin scraping, and microscopy are also common. Initially, students will observe the doctors and PAs as they perform these procedures, but by the end of the rotation, students will likely be performing these procedures themselves.

To get the most out of their time on the dermatology rotation, PA students should know the material in Tables 32B.1 and 32B.2 of this chapter. Students should also review the American Academy of Dermatology's basic curriculum for medical students. This curriculum is available on their website at https://www.aad.org/education/basic-dermatology-curriculum. Each module has been peer reviewed and is based on the best available evidence. Clinical vignettes and questions within each module provide a practical framework for learning.

CLINICAL SETTINGS

Dermatology clinics are generally located in the outpatient clinic setting. These clinics may be in a free-standing building or located in a medical center professional building. Dermatology clinics that offer a larger percentage of cosmetic and laser services may include a spa-like suite or waiting area as well as procedure rooms. Dermatology clinics that focus primarily on medical dermatology appear more like traditional clinics. Most clinics include a surgical suite or minor procedure room. Dermatology clinics that provide Mohs micrographic surgery have more elaborate surgical rooms as well as a laboratory to process the pathology and a specialized waiting area for patients who are in the middle of Mohs procedures. Rarely, a student on a dermatology rotation might participate in a hospital consultation, which may be needed on any inpatient ward.

TEAM MEDICINE

The dermatology PA cannot provide care without his team. Clinic nurses, medical assistants, dermatopathologists, doctors of other specialties, pharmacists, and estheticians are all essential team members. The clinic nurse or medical assistant is usually the first person to interview the patient, getting her or him set up for the examination and providing valuable input to the medical provider regarding the patient's history and complaint. The clinic nurse or medical assistant is also be responsible for assisting during procedures and providing patient education. Many clinics have a dedicated nurse or medical assistant for each provider to enable the doctors and PAs to evaluate large number of patients and to efficiently perform procedures.

To accurately diagnose many skin diseases, the PA will send a skin biopsy to a dermatopathologist. A dermatopathologist is a medical doctor who specializes in both dermatology and pathology. She or he reviews biopsies in the laboratory and provides a written pathology report rendering a diagnosis. The report may also include information to guide treatment options for the patient. Patients with certain types and locations of skin cancers may require Mohs micrographic surgery. In this case, they may be referred to a dermatologist who has advanced training in this surgical technique. The closure of the surgical site may require advanced plastic surgical techniques, many of which are performed by the dermatology PA.

Often, the dermatology provider will refer patients to other specialists. Plastic surgeons and general surgeons often perform excisions of skin cancers that are too large to be removed in the office setting. Plastic surgeons also operate on cancers that are in cosmetically or functionally sensitive areas. Oncologists manage the medical care of patients diagnosed with melanoma. Rheumatologists may be consulted to treat lupus, psoriatic arthritis, or other systemic illnesses identified by the dermatologist. Patients with recurrent urticaria or dermatitis may be referred to an allergist for testing and treatment recommendations.

Clinics that provide cosmetic care may employ multiple estheticians to assist in skin care treatments, facial peels, and laser treatments. Each state dictates different educational requirements for estheticians. All states, except Connecticut, require these skin care specialists to complete a cosmetology or esthetician program and obtain a license. Many entry-level estheticians receive further training on the job, especially if they work with chemical treatments.

Pharmacists work closely with dermatologists to ensure that patients receive appropriate medical therapy. Dermatologists prescribe a wide range of specialized medications that may interact with other medications. Pharmacists can assist in identifying these interactions and work with dermatologists to arrive at the best treatment for the patient. Everyone who prescribes isotretinoin (Accutane) must be familiar with the U.S. Food and Drug Administration's iPledge program. Isotretinoin is a proven teratogen; therefore, female patients taking this medication for cystic acne must demonstrate that they are using two forms of effective birth control to prevent pregnancy. Prescribers and dispensers of isotretinoin must be registered with iPledge and must prove that the patient is not pregnant each time they prescribe or dispense the medication.[7]

ESSENTIAL CLINICAL INFORMATION TO BE OBTAINED FROM EACH PATIENT

Dermatology providers always want to document certain key pieces of history at each visit. Any history of skin cancer is important to note. After a diagnosis of squamous cell carcinoma, patients have a 44% to 50% cumulative risk of developing another nonmelanoma skin cancer in subsequent years.[8] A personal or family history of melanoma is significant. Melanoma is the most common type of cancer in young adults in the United States ages 25 to 29 years and the second most common in the 15- to 29-year-old age category. Patients with familial melanoma are estimated to account for 10% to 15% of all patients with melanoma. Having a first-degree relative with melanoma doubles the risk for the patient to get melanoma, and having three or more first-degree relatives with melanoma increases the risk 35- to 70-fold.[8] A history of occupations or habits that resulted in significant sun exposure is important to note. Farmers, construction workers, postal carriers, lifeguards, and people in other occupations with increased sun exposure have an increased risk for skin cancer. Patients who live close to the equator or at higher elevations are at increased risk for skin cancer as well.

The ability of the skin to tan should be documented through the Fitzpatrick skin phototypes scale. The current scale denotes six different skin types, skin color, and reaction to sun exposure that ranges from very fair (skin type I) to very dark (skin type VI) depending on whether the patient burns or tans at the first average sun exposure. The two main factors that influence skin type are (1) genetic disposition and (2) reaction to sun exposure and tanning habits. The Fitzpatrick scale has a proven diagnostic and therapeutic value to assist in the prediction of sun damage and risk of skin cancer in a patient.[9]

Previous history of solid organ or hematologic malignancy requiring radiation therapy should be noted, as should a history of organ transplantation. Radiation therapy and immunosuppression are both risk factors for skin cancers. For patients who present with an appearance of allergic dermatitis, it is important to note their occupational and recreational exposures, as well as any medications they may be taking. Patients mistakenly believe that a new exposure has caused their allergy, not realizing it is often a medication or product to which they have been exposed for months to years.

As with any specialty, there are list of medications that the dermatologist provider will prescribe frequently. The use of topical medication is much more extensive in dermatology. In particular, topical steroids are a mainstay of dermatologic therapy. Students should familiarize themselves with the side effects of long-term or highly potent topical steroids and be able to educate patients regarding proper steroid use.

WHAT ARE THE SPECIAL REWARDS OF DERMATOLOGY?

Dermatology can be very rewarding. Physical appearance is highly correlated with psychological well-being. Many dermatologic conditions, if improperly treated or left untreated, can lead to significant disfigurement. Cystic acne does not have to result in lifelong scars. Providing appropriate treatment and preventing disfigurement are immensely satisfying. Seeing a teenager regain her confidence because of improvements in her appearance is a joy. Patients with chronic conditions, such as psoriasis or rosacea, often report that their conditions have been minimized or dismissed by other providers. These patients are enormously grateful to hear that effective treatments are available to them. Early detection of melanoma, a disease that carries a high mortality rate if not found and treated early, can be lifesaving. Other rewards include working as part of a highly functioning team to see so many patients and the Monday to Friday work hours.

WHAT ARE THE SPECIAL CHALLENGES OF DERMATOLOGY?

Dermatologic practice can be frustrating in that patient expectations for treatment and cure are not always realistic. Many chronic skin conditions can be well controlled but not cured. They required ongoing treatment and may flare even when patients perfectly adhere to the treatment regimen. Cosmetic treatments, although often improving the patient's appearance, will never make the patient look like a supermodel. These frustrations can be minimized with good patient education. Setting treatment goals and describing realistic outcomes during the initial visit are vitally important. Dermatology PAs see many patients each day, and each visit is short, which can make the patient encounter challenging. The dermatology PA must learn effective communication techniques so that patients know their concerns are heard while still moving patients through efficiently.

Dermatology can also be challenging because of the large number of possible diagnoses. Although common pathologies are common, the list of uncommon diagnoses is extensive and requires constant study to keep clinical knowledge up-to-date. Often, the diagnosis presents itself clearly on the first visit, and treatment can be initiated without waiting for confirmatory laboratory tests or radiographs. Many dermatology providers enjoy seeing new and different patients on a daily basis. However, for those who enjoy developing long-term patient relationships, there are chronic diseases, such as psoriasis or lupus, that require intense medical management and result in long-standing patient–provider connections.

KEY POINTS

- Dermatology is a fast-paced specialty. Dermatology PAs see up to 50 patients per day
- In dermatology, it is often useful to take a brief history, then perform the physical examination, and then take a more detailed history based on what you have seen
- Students in dermatology need to know the terminology for morphology, arrangement and distribution of skin lesions prior to starting their rotations
- Before beginning the dermatology placement, review procedures for biopsy and the Fitzpatrick skin phototypes scale.

References

1. Pusey W. *The History of Dermatology*. Vol. 1. Springfield, IL: Charles C Thomas; 1933.
2. McCaw, I. A synopsis of the history of dermatology. *Ulster Med J*. 1944; 13(2):109–122
3. Liddell K. Choosing a dermatologic hero for the millennium: Hippocrates of Cos (460–377 BC). *Clin Exp Dermatol*. 2000:86–88.
4. American Academy of Physician Assistants. *2013 Annual Census*. Alexandria: AAPA; 2013.
5. Longo DF. *Harrison's Principles of Internal Medicine*. 18th ed. New York: McGraw-Hill; 2012.
6. Wolff KJ. *Fitzpatrick's Color Atlas and Synopsis of Clinical Dermatology*. 5th ed. New York: McGraw-Hill; 2005.
7. Isotretinoin safety notice, iPledge program, U.S. Food and Drug Administration. https://www.ipledgeprogram.com. Accessed December 12, 2016.
8. Goldsmith C. *Skin Cancer*. Minneapolis, MN: Twenty-First Century Books; 2011.
9. Sachdeva S. Fitzpatrick skin typing: applications in dermatology. *Indian J Dermatol*. 2009:93–96.

C. ORTHOPEDICS

Hannah Huffstutler

This chapter will introduce the student to the intricacies of the practice of orthopedic medicine. There are many types of musculoskeletal diseases that students will become familiar with, and the following information is designed to be a prelude to what might be experienced on the orthopedic rotation. Students should recognize that they have the responsibility for being on time or early (preferred) to the rotation, dress appropriately, and prepare for what might be encountered on any given day by independently reading about disease processes that can be encountered on the rotation.

APPROACH TO THE ORTHOPEDIC PATIENT

The basic principles of orthopedics include tightening things that are loose, loosening things that are tight, and repairing things that are broken.[1] Patients seek the advice from an orthopedist when disorders of the musculoskeletal system are affecting their mobility and quality of life. Treatment of musculoskeletal disease requires patience on the part of the practitioner and patient, and recovery is hardly ever instantaneous.

The musculoskeletal system is composed of numerous muscles, bones, ligaments, and joints. Quite often, patients present with more than one musculoskeletal complaint. When assessing patients in any age group (pediatric, adult, or geriatric), the ultimate goals are narrowing the problem list and figuring out whether the ailment is traumatic, inflammatory, degenerative,

or pathologic. With this in mind, it is important to determine if there are any associated injuries and to isolate the area of interest by asking the patient to take one finger and point to where it hurts the most. A thorough and accurate history and physical examination can diagnose 80% to 90% of orthopedic ailments.[2]

PHYSICIAN ASSISTANTS' DAILY TASKS IN ORTHOPEDICS

Typical orthopedic practices have a variety of providers who address various aspects of musculoskeletal disease. These providers can include general orthopedists and those with subspecialty training in spine, hands, feet, and sports injuries. Physician assistants (PAs) may work with one or more of these providers. Orthopedic PAs may be strictly clinic based or divide their time between the clinical setting and the operating room (OR). Clinic and scheduled surgery days usually alternate during the week. However, in the case of an emergent surgery, scheduled appointments may be delayed or canceled. Duties on clinic days range from assisting in triaging patients; diagnosing and treating new patients and postoperative patients; performing in-office procedures; documenting preoperative history and physical examinations; contacting appropriate equipment representatives for operative cases; applying dressings and casts; administering injections; answering hospital, patient, and pharmacy calls; and seeing hospital consults. One main task during clinic hours is confirming that all paperwork for the following surgery day is finalized and equipment representatives are aware of the services required. Surgery days include early rising to match the history and physical examination findings to the correct patient and to verify the correct orthopedic procedure, correct implant (if appropriate), and correct side to be operated upon. The physician will also review these items to ensure the appropriate procedure is being done; this includes signing the site to be operated on and ensuring that any supporting materials and hardware is present.

When the patient is brought into the OR, PAs aid the certified registered nurse anesthetist (CRNA) and circulating registered nurse in moving the patient from the stretcher to the operating table. The CRNA and anesthesiologist work together to provide appropriate anesthesia for the patient. This may include regional blocks, spinal anesthesia, minimal sedation, moderate sedation, deep sedation, or general anesthesia if needed.[3] Occasionally, the patient may only require a digital block, in which case the surgeon or PA may administer the block. When the desired level of sedation is accomplished, PAs may help to pad all bony prominences, shield the patient with a lead apron, and apply a tourniquet to the operative extremity if necessary. The circulating nurse will begin prepping the operative area. Finally, the time has come to scrub for the case. It may be necessary to wear a lead apron and neck cover if radiology will be used during the surgery. A mask and protective eyewear should also be worn. Scrub using the 5-minute scrub technique. (Refer to Fig. 30-1 in Chapter 30 for explanation of proper surgical scrub techniques.)

During any surgical case, the PA's main goal is anticipating the next step, such as positioning, retracting, suctioning, suturing, and applying a dressing. When a sterile dressing has been applied, the CRNA extubates (if applicable) the patient, and PAs assist the CRNA, circulating nurse, and scrub technician in moving the patient from the operating table to the stretcher. The patient is transferred from the OR to the postanesthesia care unit, and the PA typically writes the postoperative orders. Postoperative orders include transfer orders, antibiotics, fluids, diet, pain control, consults (e.g., physical therapy, internal medicine), and dressing changes. Between or after all cases, PAs round and discharge inpatients.

EXPECTATIONS OF THE STUDENT

During an orthopedic rotation, students may work with a physician or one or more of the PAs within the group. Students must be willing to learn the clinic's routine, including triaging, performing and documenting history and physical examinations, presenting patients, removing sutures and staples, applying dressings and casts, and writing prescriptions. Common splints and casts are illustrated in Figs. 32C.1 through 32C.10. Students are also responsible for recognizing and performing common orthopedic tests as displayed in Table 32C.1 as well as recognizing the Salter-Harris classification shown in Fig.32C.11.

On surgery days, the primary job of the student will most likely be acting as a second assist. Duties include positioning, retracting, suturing and stapling, and applying appropriate dressings. When rounding, the student will be expected to assist with dressing changes and write appropriate progress notes.

CLINICAL SETTINGS

Throughout the rotation, students may strictly remain in a clinical environment or divide time between clinical and surgical settings. Surgery locations include hospital and outpatient centers. Patient stability, complexity of the surgery, and availability of required equipment determine whether a surgery is performed at the hospital or surgery center. Outpatient centers contain far fewer ORs and staff and typically do not have overnight stay capability.

TEAM LEARNING FROM HEALTH PROFESSIONALS ON THE ORTHOPEDIC TEAM

There are many opportunities to work interprofessionally during an orthopedic rotation. The clinical setting is comprised of several professions. These include nurses, physical therapists, occupational therapists, orthotists, and cast technicians. The nurses aid in triaging, phlebotomy, drawing up injections, and answering and directing patient and pharmacy phone calls. An orthopedic clinic may include professionals such as physical therapists or occupational therapists who are vital to patient progress. Their main goals are to provide relief and restore mobility.[4] Orthotists are allied health professionals trained to fabricate and fit patients with a variety of braces, boots, and orthotic prostheses to alleviate pain and provide patient comfort.[5] Patient care in the office setting also provides an opportunity to work with home health agencies that can include coordinating services such as wound care and intravenous (IV) antibiotic administration.[6]

The hospital setting provides opportunities to learn from other health professionals, including scrub technicians, CRNAs, circulating registered nurses, radiology technicians, floor nurses, discharge managers, and

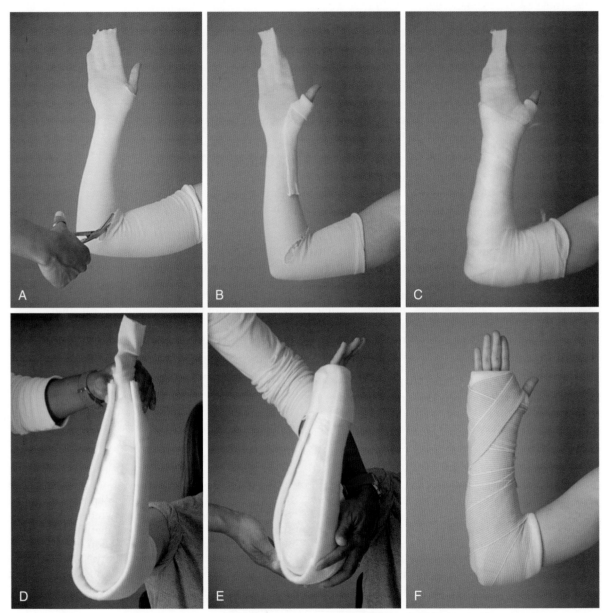

FIG. 32C.1 ■ **A–F,** Upper extremity sugar tong splint. (From Rynders SD, Hart JA. *Orthopaedics for Physician Assistants*, 1st ed. Philadelphia: Elsevier Saunders; 2013.)

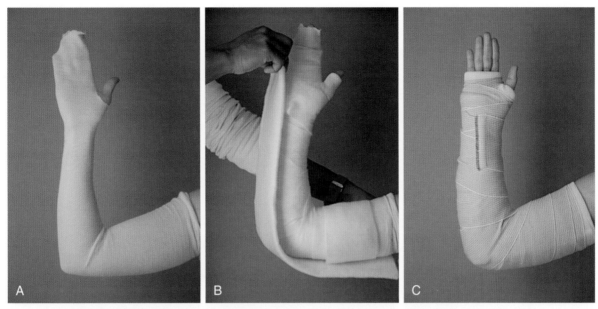

FIG. 32C.2 ■ **A–C,** Upper extremity long arm posterior splint. (From Rynders SD, Hart JA. *Orthopaedics for Physician Assistants*, 1st ed. Philadelphia: Elsevier Saunders; 2013.)

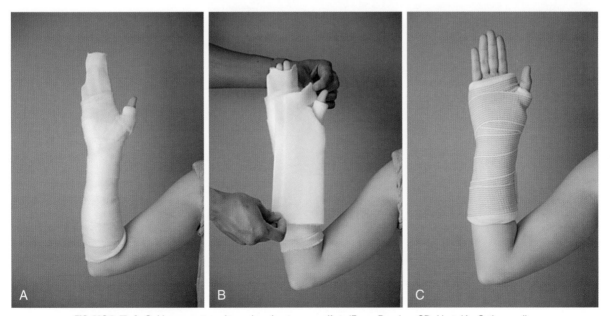

FIG. 32C.3 ■ **A–C,** Upper extremity volar short arm splint. (From Rynders SD, Hart JA. *Orthopaedics for Physician Assistants*, 1st ed. Philadelphia: Elsevier Saunders; 2013.)

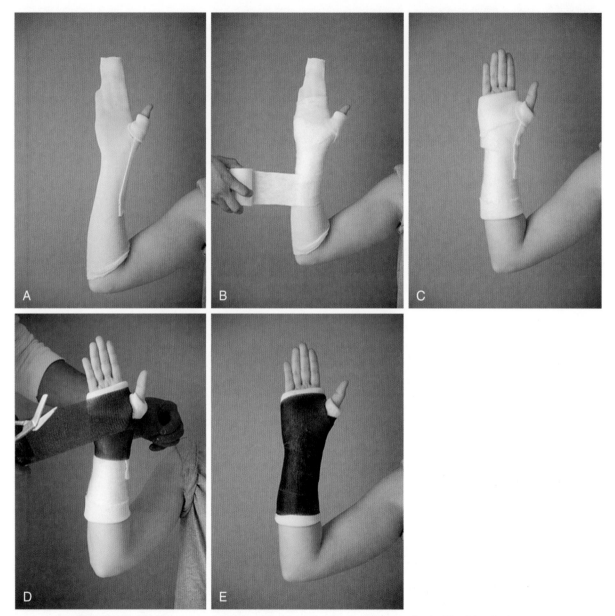

FIG. 32C.4 ■ **A–E,** Short arm cast. (From Rynders SD, Hart JA. *Orthopaedics for Physician Assistants*, 1st ed. Philadelphia: Elsevier Saunders; 2013.)

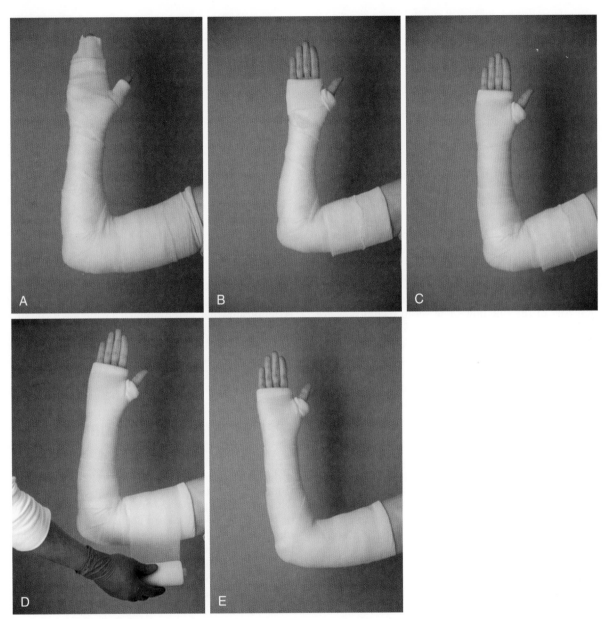

FIG. 32C.5 ■ **A–E,** Long arm cast. (From Rynders SD, Hart JA. *Orthopaedics for Physician Assistants,* 1st ed. Philadelphia: Elsevier Saunders; 2013.)

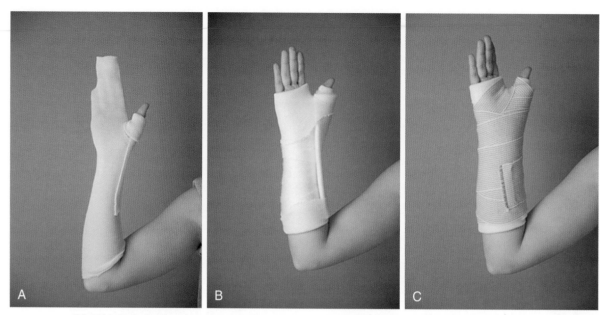

FIG. 32C.6 ■ **A–C,** Thumb spica cast. (From Rynders SD, Hart JA. *Orthopaedics for Physician Assistants*, 1st ed. Philadelphia: Elsevier Saunders; 2013.)

prosthetists. The scrub technicians, CRNAs, circulating registered nurses, and radiology technicians are a vital part of the OR flow. The scrub technicians are responsible for setting up the OR before the cases and typically know step-by-step surgical procedures. The CRNAs are responsible for providing anesthesia and sedation for the patient. The circulating registered nurses are responsible for the time-out before the incision and obtaining any necessary equipment and supplies needed during the case.[2] Discharge planners are responsible for making sure patients are released to a facility where they will benefit most and with any tools needed for recovery (e.g., crutches, wheelchair, bedside commode).[7] If a patient is in need of prosthetic services postoperatively, the prosthetist will visit the bedside and place a stump shrinker on the operative limb(s). The prosthetist will continue to monitor the patient's progress until she or he is ready to proceed with fitting of the prosthesis. Prosthetists serve a special purpose in the orthopedic world. Not only do they provide means of completing a patient physically, but they also guide the patient through the process mentally, spiritually, and emotionally.[8]

CLINICAL INFORMATION PHYSICIANS AND PHYSICIAN ASSISTANTS ALWAYS WANT TO KNOW ON THIS ROTATION

While on the rotation, students need to know that it is important to take a thorough history for several reasons. First, it is important to know if a specific injury is associated with the chief complaint. Second, it is important to know if the patient's past medical history is significant when determining if a patient is a safe surgical candidate. Finally, it is important to know if the patient has ever been treated for the chief complaint in the past, by whom, and if surgery was required. When rounding, always know if any events occurred overnight and the neurovascular status of the operative extremity.

SPECIAL PATIENT POPULATIONS

Orthopedics can cover patients of any age group from pediatric to geriatric patients. Although it may vary from practice to practice, a portion of the patients who are treated have sports-related injuries. Many of the patients are young athletes, but others are middle-aged adults playing pick-up games. Other patient populations commonly seen in orthopedic practices include those who have had injuries in the past and have progressed to posttraumatic arthritis and those who have developed osteoarthritis without a trauma history.

WHAT ARE THE SPECIAL CHALLENGES OF ORTHOPEDICS?

There are many challenges in the specialty of orthopedics, not the least of which is to be able to elicit a specific complaint in some patient populations. As previously stated, we typically ask the patient to take

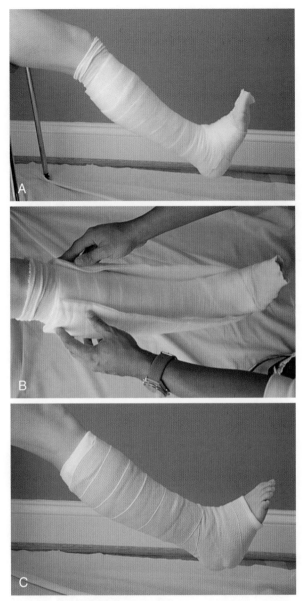

FIG. 32C.7 ■ **A–C,** Lower extremity sugar tong (ankle stirrup or U) splint. (From Rynders SD, Hart JA. *Orthopaedics for Physician Assistants*, 1st ed. Philadelphia: Elsevier Saunders; 2013.)

one finger and point to the most painful area to narrow the differential diagnosis. Another challenge is helping patients to understand that most orthopedic problems are not cured instantaneously. Musculoskeletal injuries require time to heal. Healing occurs faster and to a better degree if the patient adheres to the evidence-based guidelines for treating his or her specific problem. Patient compliance can be difficult when the ailment impedes the ability to perform activities of daily living or removes the person from a sport or pastime he or she enjoys.

Obesity is a challenge in most medical and surgical disciplines and especially in an orthopedic practice. Excess weight impacts patient mobility and sleep patterns and plays a role the development, progression, and recovery of musculoskeletal injuries.[9] Infection is yet another challenge in orthopedics and can occur in a suture line or an open fracture site, to name a few. An open fracture requires surgery in stages, and osteomyelitis (infection within the bone) can be a complication. It is difficult to cure and requires long-term IV antibiotics. It is

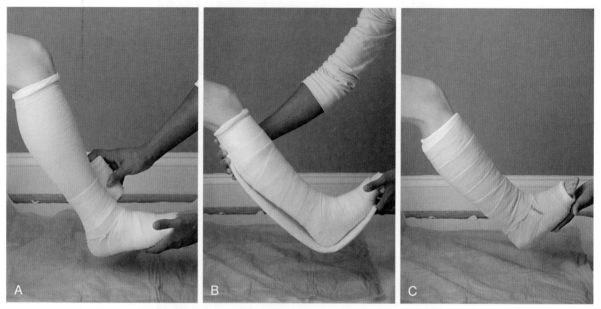

FIG. 32C.8 ■ **A–C,** Lower extremity posterior leg splint. (From Rynders SD, Hart JA. *Orthopaedics for Physician Assistants*, 1st ed. Philadelphia: Elsevier Saunders; 2013.)

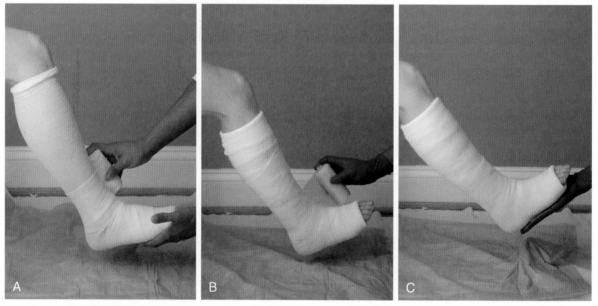

FIG. 32C.9 ■ **A–C,** Short leg cast. (From Rynders SD, Hart JA. *Orthopaedics for Physician Assistants*, 1st ed. Philadelphia: Elsevier Saunders; 2013.)

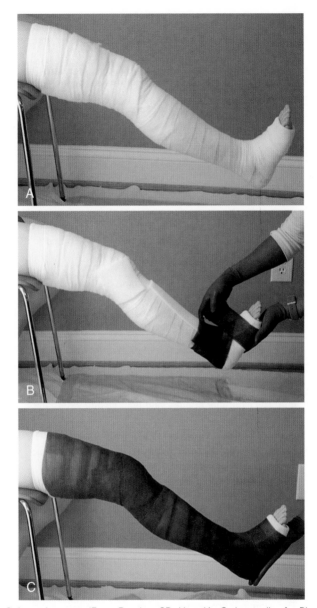

FIG. 32C.10 ■ **A–C,** Long leg cast. (From Rynders SD, Hart JA. *Orthopaedics for Physician Assistants*, 1st ed. Philadelphia: Elsevier Saunders; 2013.)

cumbersome for the patient to endure side effects of the antibiotics as well as the possibility of developing nonhealing wounds. Nonhealing wounds may lead to various types of closures, including use of negative-pressure wound therapy in which foam is attached to a suction machine and changed every other day.[10,11]

WHAT ARE THE SPECIAL REWARDS OF ORTHOPEDICS?

The rewards of orthopedic medicine are centered on restoring function and strength. Patients are able to resume their daily activities, thereby improving their quality of life.[6]

TABLE 32C.1 Common Orthopedic Tests

Structure Tested	Orthopedic Test	Procedure	Rationale
Shoulder	Hawkins	Passively forward flexing the shoulder to 90 degrees and internally rotating with the elbow flexed	Impingement is indicated by pain.
	Neer	Internally rotating the shoulder, fully passively forward flexing the shoulder, and stabilizing the scapula	Impingement is indicated by pain.
	Supraspinatus stress test	The shoulders are abducted at 90 degrees with the thumbs pointing downward; downward resistance is applied by the examiner.	A rotator cuff abnormality (e.g., impingement or tear) is indicated by weakness or pain.
	Drop arm sign	The patient holds the arms with the shoulder abducted to 90 degrees with the thumbs down.	A rotator cuff injury is indicated by the inability to the hold arm in this position.
Wrist	Tinel test	The examiner taps over the palmar surface of the wrist.	Carpal tunnel syndrome is indicated by paresthesia in median nerve distribution.
	Phalen test	The examiner flexes the patient's wrists and holds this position for 1 minute.	Carpal tunnel syndrome is indicated by paresthesia in median nerve distribution.
	Finkelstein test	The thumb is clasped into the palm, and the wrist is passively ulnarly deviated.	De Quervain tenosynovitis is indicated by pain.
Knee	Lachman test	The patient is supine with the knee at 30 degrees of flexion. The examiner places one hand slightly superior to the knee to stabilize the thigh and uses the other hand to apply anterior pressure to the proximal tibia.	An ACL injury is suspected with increased anterior translation compared with the unaffected side.
	McMurray test	The patient is supine. The examiner holds the medial heel with one hand and places the other hand on the ipsilateral knee with the thumb along the medial joint line. The examiner applies valgus force and externally and then internally rotates the lower leg.	A meniscal injury is suspected with a palpable or audible click.
	Apley test	The patient is prone; the knee is flexed at 90 degrees.	
	Anterior drawer test	The patient is supine with the knee flexed to 90 degrees. The examiner grasps the tibia below the joint line with the thumbs on either side of the patellar tendon. The examiner pulls forward on the tibia.	ACL injury is suspected with increased anterior translation compared with the unaffected side.
	Posterior drawer test	The patient is supine with the knee flexed to 90 degrees. The examiner grasps the tibia below the joint line with the thumbs on either side of the patellar tendon. The examiner applies posterior force on the tibia.	PCL injury is suspected with increased posterior translation compared with the unaffected side.
	Valgus stress test	The patient is supine with the knee flexed to 30 degrees. The examiner applies valgus force.	MCL injury is suspected with medial opening and pain.
	Varus stress test	The patient is supine with the knee flexed to 30 degrees. The examiner applies varus force.	LCL injury is suspected with lateral opening and pain.
Ankle	Anterior drawer sign	The patient is seated with the leg hanging off the examination table. The tibia is stabilized with one hand, and the foot is translated anterior with the other hand.	ATFL injury is suspected with the suction sign or pain.
	Tinel sign	The examiner taps over the posterior tibial nerve.	Tarsal tunnel is indicated with paresthesia radiating to the foot.
	Thompson test	The patient is prone with the feet hanging over the end of the examination table. The examiner squeezes the affected calf.	Achilles tendon rupture is suspected if the plantarflexion reflex is absent.
Lumbar spine	Straight-leg raise test	The patient is supine. The examiner raises the patient's leg to the point of pain or 90 degrees.	Compression or irritation of the sciatic nerve is indicated if radicular symptoms are reproduced on the affected side.

ACL, Anterior cruciate ligament; ATFL, anterior talofibular ligament; LCL, lateral collateral ligament; MCL, medial collateral ligament; PCL, posterior cruciate ligament.
Adapted from Ballweg R, Sullivan EM, Brown D, et al. Physician Assistant: A Guide to Clinical Practice, 5th ed. Philadelphia: Elsevier Saunders; 2013; and Rynders SD, Hart JA. Orthopaedics for Physician Assistants, 1st ed. Philadelphia: Elsevier Saunders; 2013.)

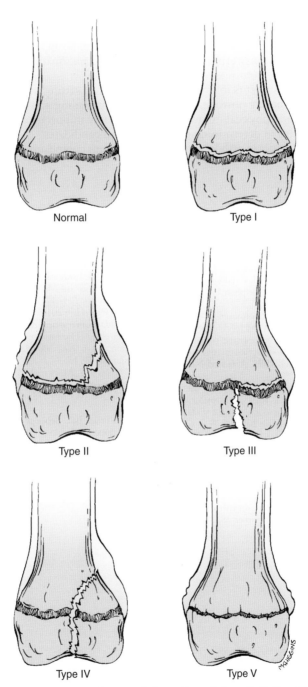

FIG. 32C.11 ■ The Salter-Harris classification. (Adapted from Ballweg R, Sullivan EM, Brown D, et al. *Physician Assistant: A Guide to Clinical Practice,* 5th ed. Philadelphia: Elsevier Saunders; 2013.)

References

1. Southlake Orthopaedics Sports Medicine and Spine Center. Physicians. https://southlakeorthopaedics.com/physicians/ekkehard-bonatz-md-phd/. Accessed November 20, 2015.
2. Ballweg R, Sullivan EM, Brown D, et al. *Physician Assistant: A Guide to Clinical Practice*. 5th ed. Philadelphia, PA: Elsevier Saunders; 2013.
3. American Society of Anesthesiologists. Continuum of depth of sedation: definition of general anesthesia and levels of sedation/analgesia. All standards, guidelines & practice parameters. http://www.asahq.org/quality-and-practice-management/standards-and-guidelines Published 1995. Accessed November 25, 2015.
4. McNalley TE, Standaert CJ. Chapter 258. Physical therapy and rehabilitation. In: McKean SC, Ross JJ, Dressler DD, Brotman DJ, Ginsberg JS, eds. *Principles and Practice of Hospital Medicine*. New York, NY: McGraw-Hill; 2012.
5. Mann JA, Chou LB, Ross SK. Chapter 8. Foot and ankle surgery. In: Skinner HB, McMahon PJ, eds. *Current Diagnosis & Treatment in Orthopedics*. 5th ed. New York, NY: McGraw-Hill; 2014.
6. Centers for Medicare & Medicaid Services. What's home health care & what should I expect? https://www.medicare.gov/what-medicare-covers/home-health-care/home-health-care-what-is-it-what-to-expect.html. Accessed November 28, 2015.
7. Department of Health and Human Services. Centers for Medicare & Medicaid Services. Discharge Planning. https://www.cms.gov/Outreach-and-Education/Medicare-Learning-Network-MLN/MLNProducts/Downloads/Discharge-Planning-Booklet-ICN908184.pdf. Accessed November 29, 2015.
8. Uustal H. Lower limb amputation, rehabilitation, & prosthetic restoration. In: Maitin IB, Cruz E, eds. *Current Diagnosis & Treatment: Physical Medicine & Rehabilitation*. New York, NY: McGraw-Hill; 2015.
9. Anadacoomarasamy A, Caterson I, Sambrook P, Fransen M, March L. The impact of obesity on the musculoskeletal system. *Int J Obes*. 2008;32:211–212. http://dx.doi.org/10.1038/sj.ijo.0803715.
10. Halawi MJ, Morwood MP. Acute management of open fractures: an evidence-based review. *Orthopedics*. 2015;38(11):e1025–e1033. http://dx.doi.org/10.3928/01477477-20151020-12.
11. Hoffman BL, Schorge JO, Schaffer JI, et al. Chapter 39. Perioperative considerations. In: Hoffman BL, Schorge JO, Schaffer JI, et al., eds. *Williams Gynecology*. 2nd ed. New York, NY: McGraw-Hill; 2012. http://accessmedicine.mhmedical.com/content.aspx?bookid=399&Sectionid=41722331. Accessed November 29, 2015.

The resources for this chapter can be found at www.expertconsult.com.

D. ONCOLOGY

Debra S. Munsell

CHAPTER OUTLINE

FOR THE STUDENT

DEMOGRAPHICS

CANCER DISPARITIES

CANCER PREVENTION

PATIENT CARE

CANCER CARE

CANCER CARE IN THE TWENTY-FIRST CENTURY

GOALS OF TREATMENT

CLINICAL APPLICATIONS

KEY POINTS

FOR THE STUDENT

The approach to the workup of an oncology patient is determined by the setting in which the patient presents. Many large comprehensive cancer centers have sections or divisions specifically designed to evaluate and treat cancers of one body system, such as gynecologic or urologic cancers. Other cancer centers treat only adult or pediatric malignancies. Some oncologists practice in hematology and oncology settings, and some treat only solid tumors. You can find clinicians practicing the care of cancer patients in outpatient and inpatient settings and clinicians who treat only patients who need radiation therapy. Whatever the setting, it is important to know which type of setting you will be working in and to plan accordingly.

The daily practice of an oncology physician assistant (PA) varies depending on the setting. Clinicians treating cancers of a hematologic origin (leukemia, lymphomas) may participate in all aspects of care, ranging from the initial presentation of the patient and diagnostic procedures (bone marrow aspiration) through multidisciplinary treatment planning, management of acute and chronic issues relating to the malignancy, and care of the patient after treatment. Surgical clinicians are similarly involved with patient care. The clinical practice may dictate that the PA assist in all aspects of the surgical treatment, or the practice may prefer the PA to manage the patient in the clinical setting. Many surgical PAs manage the postoperative care of patients and provide a link among multiple members of the health care team. Similarly, radiation oncology clinicians provide care for individuals undergoing radiotherapy and are invaluable in providing continuity of care for these patients.

In general, a student rotation in oncology includes an initial orientation to the types of malignancies treated. Many oncologists request that the student have internal medicine and surgical rotation experience before an oncology rotation. This experience will allow the student to feel more comfortable in dealing with the often complex oncologic patient. The student should contact the preceptor before the first day of the rotation for instructions. Ask about the type of practice and the student role in patient care. This is the time to find out the general layout of the facility and, the hours of operation. Professional dress, including a white coat, is required unless explicitly expressed. Basic physical examination tools, including a reflex hammer, penlight, stethoscope, and eye chart, are needed. The preceptor may suggest specific reading material or texts appropriate to the setting. A good general text for students is *Clinical Oncology: Basic Principles and Practice*, 4th edition, by Neal and Hoskin. The preceptor may recommend other texts or materials for you to review.

The oncology field, similar to other specialties, has a unique medical language and set of approved abbreviations. Obtain a list of approved abbreviations before beginning documentation; this will augment learning the new terminology. Of paramount importance is to grasp the tumor, node, and metastasis (TNM) staging system for the particular cancers treated in practice (Table 32D.1). Oncologists stage tumors and cancers at the time of diagnosis. Depending on the type of malignancy, specialized staging systems may be used. Students should become familiar with the TNM staging used in the practice. Tumor staging is the method oncologists use to communicate the severity of the malignancy based on the origin, size, and spread of the malignancy. Staging

TABLE 32D.1	Tumor, Node, Metastasis Staging
Primary Tumor	**T**
TX	Primary tumor cannot be
T0	evaluated
Tis	No evidence of primary tumor
T1, T2, T3, T4	Carcinoma in situ
	Size and extent of the tumor
Regional Lymph Nodes	**N**
Nx	Regional nodes cannot be
N0	assessed
N1, N2, N3	No regional nodal involvement
	Degree of nodal involvement (number, location)
Distant Metastasis	**M**
MX	Distant metastasis cannot be
M0	evaluated
M1	No evidence of distant metastasis
	Distant metastasis

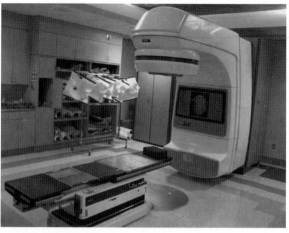

FIG. 32D.1 ■ Linear accelerator. (From Abeloff M. *Clinical Oncology*, 3rd ed. Philadelphia: Elsevier Churchill Livingstone; 2004.)

is also used to plan treatments and estimate prognosis. Participation in clinical trials is based on tumor staging.

Students will be exposed to new medical treatments and equipment on the rotation. Fine-needle aspirations, bone marrow biopsies, ultrasound-guided biopsies, and other diagnostic procedures are some of the studies students may observe on oncology rotations. Surgical oncologists may be using state-of-the-art stereotactic equipment in the treatment of brain tumors. A rotation in radiation oncology will allow you to observe external-beam radiotherapy administered by linear accelerators or proton beam therapy delivered in specialized treatment centers (Fig. 32D.1). You may witness a team of surgical oncologists and radiation oncologists deliver brachytherapy treatment or implant radioactive "seeds."

After orientation, students may be asked to perform history and physical examination, observe or assist in surgery, and follow the patients during inpatient therapy. Students may also have the opportunity to observe the roles of other members of the multidisciplinary team. Learning about all of the treatments given to cancer patients will enable the student to fully appreciate the personal struggles these individuals incur. As a student gains comfort in the role, additional tasks may be assigned.

The general oncologic rotation typically begins in the clinic or office setting. This is where evaluation and diagnosis occur. If the malignancy is treated surgically or with radiotherapy, the student will also observe those treatment areas. Inpatient treatment areas for chemotherapy are an additional setting where the student may observe and participate.

Students should take every opportunity to observe anyone involved in cancer care, including radiation dosimetrists, speech-language pathologists, child-life therapists, nutritionists, pathologists, radiologists, audiologists, clergy members, social workers, and hospice team members. Often these practitioners participate in multidisciplinary care conferences and are willing to share their role in cancer care with students. Other members of the team may include nurses, fellow students, and administrative staff. It is important for you to arrive on time (or a little early), introduce yourself, and make a point of getting to know the routine of the setting. Remember that you are a guest in the practice. Valuable lessons in patient care can be learned when communicating with all members of the team.

When approaching a patient with a malignancy, it is important to remember that this is a very stressful and profoundly life-changing time for the patient. Consider each patient as an individual with a malignancy, not a disease entity. It is important to obtain as much history from the patient as possible. A very thorough history, including an in-depth family and social history, will give the treatment team valuable information for use in treatment planning. Special attention to past medical history of malignancies and their treatments should be noted. Carefully note any surgical procedures, including cryotherapy and Mohs micrographic surgery, that the patient has undergone. Information of this nature is crucial to determining the treatment plan. Past history of radiation therapy of any type should be recorded, including when received, for what condition, the anatomic region (s) included, and the number of treatments. In the past, enlarged tonsils and thymus glands were treated with radiation, and years later, these individuals developed various cancers, including cancer of the thyroid. Family history of any malignancies should be recorded in detail, including the type of cancer and the relationship to the patient. Note the results of any genetic testing the patient or family member may provide. Careful attention to the patient's psychological state will assist the team in management of treatment and any complications. Address any signs of psychological distress or suicidal ideation urgently.

During the treatment phase, the student will learn the acute and chronic signs of treatment toxicities and tumor responses associated with the patient's particular malignancy and any signs of impending emergencies. The astute student will review this material daily. After treatment, patients will return for evaluation on schedules determined for their particular malignancies. Students may initially feel more comfortable interviewing these patients before approaching a newly diagnosed patient. Note all posttherapy complications and document weight gain or loss, pain, and any other changes since the previous visit. Always include an evaluation of psychological status.

The type of oncology practice determines the patient population. Many practices treat adults or pediatric patients only. Other practices see a variety of populations. For instance, cancers of the head and neck generally affect people older than 50 years of age, but head and neck malignancies can affect infants through adults. Some practices treat only breast cancer, a predominantly female cancer, with a low percentage of male patients. Urologic cancer practices may have a higher percentage of older male patients, with a lower percentage of pediatric and female patients.

The field of oncology is both challenging and rewarding. You will be caring for vulnerable patients and their family members. You will be challenged by the immense amount of knowledge that you must assimilate in a short period of time. You may experience the sorrow of caring for a patient who has not responded to therapy. You may experience the thrill of sharing the news that a patient has reached the 5-year mark without a recurrence of disease. A rotation in the field of oncology is a rollercoaster ride of adventure and reward. You will find that you gain much more than education about cancer care; you may develop a love for the care of patients with cancer.

Cancer is a collection of diseases in which abnormal cells divide without control. Cancer cells can invade nearby tissues and can spread throughout the bloodstream and lymphatic system to other parts of the body.[1] The collection of diseases commonly called cancer has been in existence for centuries. The Greek physician Hippocrates (460–370 BC), often referred to as the "father of medicine," is credited with the first use of the term *karkinos*.[2,3] Legend has it that he applied the term *karkinos* to lesions because "the disease has the veins stretched on all sides as the animal the crab has its feet."[2,3] Galen, another Greek physician, used the Greek term *oncos* (swelling) to describe tumors.[2,3]

Egyptian papyri from 300 to 1500 BC refer to breast tumors. The oldest specimen of a human cancer was found in the remains of a female skull dating to 1900 to 1600 BC (the Bronze Age).[2,3] Findings in mummified skeletal remains of Peruvian Incas more than 2400 years old show abnormalities that are suggestive of malignant melanoma.

The earliest documented cancer treatment is noted in the Edwin Smith Papyrus, which describes conditions consistent with breast cancer treated with the "fire drill" (cauterization).[2,3] Suggested in the papyrus is the removal of surface tumors (surgery). These writings also reveal the use of compounds of barley, pigs' ears, and other local material for the treatment of stomach and uterine cancer.[2] Scottish surgeon John Hunter (1728–1793) advocated the surgical removal of tumors that were mobile on examination.[2,3] Advances in pathology after the discovery and use of the microscope and radiography have led to the modern treatments we currently use in the treatment of cancer patients. Cancer therapy today includes many therapies besides surgery, chemotherapy, and radiation. Not only does cancer affect the physical aspect of the patient, but it also affects social, emotional, and spiritual aspects. PAs can develop a challenging and rewarding career in cancer therapy, a career that stimulates intellectual curiosity and rewards the soul. The oncology PA can choose to subspecialize in the surgical, radiation, or medical treatment of any cancer type. Opportunities also exist for PAs in clinical cancer research. The field of oncology care is a growing field that combines the use of specialized medical knowledge and skills with intuitive and compassionate interpersonal skills. It allows the PA to provide primary care in a specialized setting.

DEMOGRAPHICS

Cancer is currently the cause of death in one out of four people in the United States.[4] The American Cancer Society projects new cases of cancer will reach 22 million worldwide within the next

40 years.[4] Cancer as a cause of death in the United States is second only to heart disease.[4] Oncology is a field that cares disproportionately for the aging population. The risk for developing cancer increases with age, with most cases affecting adults who are middle aged and older. The population of the United States age 65 years and older is expected to increase substantially by 2050, to approximately 83.7 million.[5] Progress against cancer is being recorded. In the United States, the overall cancer death rate has been on the decline since the 1990s.[4] Cancer survivorship is increasing, and living beyond the diagnosis and treatment of cancer is expected to reach 19 million individuals by the year 2024.[4] Cancer patients are surviving longer because of positive trends in early diagnosis, as well as innovative cancer therapies. As cancer survivorship increases, the role of PAs in the care of these patients will change.

Cancer survivors reenter the health care system with specific needs not previously addressed. These patients are often returned to their primary caregivers after definitive therapy. Treatment sequelae, increased risks of second malignancies, and psychosocial issues need to be considered when evaluating cancer survivors. These sequelae range from skin changes to life-changing physical disabilities.

Physician assistant students need to have increased knowledge of cancer biology and cancer treatments to care for the increased numbers of survivors who will seek medical care.

The economic impact of cancer is staggering. The *Journal of the National Cancer Center* projects the costs of cancer care will be $173 billion by the year 2020.[6] This estimate includes hospital and outpatient care, inpatient care, and prescription medication. The economic cost of cancer care touches all Americans. Lack of access to medical care and lack of access to health care coverage are major problems for the United States. Ethnic minorities and under- and uninsured individuals are more likely to be diagnosed with late-stage cancer. The combination of an increasingly aging population, lack of access to health care, and health care disparities drives the financial burdens of cancer care.

CANCER DISPARITIES

The Nation Cancer Institute defines cancer health disparities as "adverse differences in cancer incidence, cancer prevalence, cancer death, cancer survivorship and burden of cancer or related health conditions that exist among specific population groups in the United States."

Cancer health disparities are noted to affect African Americans, Asian Americans, Hispanics, American Indians, Alaskan Natives, and underserved whites. These groups all have a high incidence of lack of access to health care.[7] They also are more likely to have a low socioeconomic status. African Americans continue to have higher incidence and mortality rates from the most prevalent cancer types than whites.[7] Black women are more likely to die from breast cancer, although white women have an increased incidence of the disease. African American women also have the highest rates of death from cervical cancer. African American men have the highest incidence rate for prostate cancer and the highest incidence of death. Much of the disparity can be attributed to low socioeconomic status and lack of access to health care.

Public health researchers and clinicians can work toward reducing these disparities by recognizing them and implementing strategies to actively target these populations for early diagnosis and treatment.

CANCER PREVENTION

The role of the PA is particularly suited to practicing cancer prevention because PAs are trained to be proficient in primary care. Cancer prevention can be practiced in any setting from pediatrics to geriatrics, women's health, and internal and family medicine and any subspecialty, including oncology. Primary cancer prevention includes educating patients on modifiable risk factors and avoidance of environmental hazards and assisting them in identifying any inherited risks for cancer. Well-known modifiable cancer risk factors include the use of tobacco products; infection with the hepatitis B and C viruses, Epstein-Barr virus, and human papillomavirus (HPV); *Helicobacter pylori*; and exposure to ionizing radiation. Diets high in fruits and vegetable have been associated with a possible decreased incidence of some upper digestive tract cancers (mouth, esophagus, stomach).[8] Alcohol use has also been loosely associated with an increased risk of development of certain mouth, breast, and colorectal cancers.[8] Obesity and a lack of physical activity are also included in the list of modifiable factors that have been associated with the possible development of cancer (postmenopausal breast, esophageal, pancreas, and colorectal).

Chemoprevention is the use of "natural or synthetic compounds to interfere with early stage carcinogenesis."[8] There is a robust and growing field of research devoted to the identification of chemopreventive substances. The use of aspirin and cyclooxygenase-2 (enzymes that produce prostaglandins) inhibitors has been investigated as one method of chemoprevention for colon and breast cancer. Many other substances such as vitamins C and D, calcium, and multivitamin supplements have been investigated, with no evidence of benefit with regard to cancer prevention.[8]

PATIENT CARE

The first visit a patient makes to his or her health care provider is critical in the establishment of a trusting, caring provider–patient relationship. These patients are experiencing a myriad of emotions ranging from acceptance to shock, disbelief, and denial. The initial visit for cancer treatment is often frightening for the patient. Patients seeking care have often had a preliminary diagnosis given to them by the referring health care provider and are confused. Others may have done independent research before the initial visit with the oncologic specialist. It is important to acknowledge the patient's knowledge level and anxiety; this will help establish a good foundation for the remainder of the visit.

The initial setting of the visit should be a room that is comfortable for the patient and any accompanying guests. Ideally, the initial comprehensive history should be taken from patients before they have been asked to change into an examination gown. This allows the patient to remain clothed and comfortable while sharing the detailed information. The patient's wishes regarding the presence of guests should be elicited and upheld. Often patients need the support of others during these sessions, and many find that someone else remembers important treatment information best. Allowing the patient to record the conversations may also be helpful.

A comprehensive history pertinent to the chief complaint must be recorded. For instance, if a patient presents with the preliminary diagnosis of colon cancer, a comprehensive review of the gastrointestinal system should be performed. In addition to organ- or disease-specific site questions, questions regarding anorexia, pain, insomnia, nausea, vomiting, unexplained weight loss, bruising, fatigue, hair loss, constipation, diarrhea, depression, and masses or lesions that are slow to heal should be asked. Often these somewhat vague symptoms are the initial signs of malignancy. Included in the initial examination should be a comprehensive review of all systems to ensure a comprehensive review of the patient's status. Many times the review of systems will reveal other areas of concern. The patient's general health status and any specific medical conditions must be taken into account before the development of a definitive treatment plan. Family history, social history, and medical history should be recorded, specifically detailing any personal or immediate family history of cancer. Some cancers are known to occur in familial patterns, and others besides the patient may be at risk. Patients with a personal history of cancer are more likely to develop another. A thorough social history should be elicited. This should include a tobacco and substance abuse history, as well as a history of alcohol use. The patient's occupation and prior exposure to environmental agents should be recorded. Specific questions regarding prior radiation exposure must be asked because many individuals were treated with external-beam radiation for acne before the 1970s. The social history should include questions regarding the social support available to the patient during cancer therapy. Decisions regarding a definitive treatment plan should include all aspects of the patient's life. Financial and social support may need to be arranged for the patient. Do not neglect to address the psychological status of the patient. Depression and suicidal ideation should be addressed before treatment planning.

All medications the patient is currently taking must be recorded. Significant reactions between medications and cancer therapies will be avoided if this is done. Include all complementary and alternative therapies that the patient is using because many common complementary and alternative remedies may affect medications. Many patients use complementary and alternative therapies for the treatment of conditions ranging from allergies, depression, menopausal symptoms, and various cancers.[9] These treatments are often not considered "medication," and patients do not report their use. The cytochrome P450 system (CYP450) is highly active in the metabolism of herbal treatments and chemotherapy drugs. Investigation is ongoing in the field of herbal–chemotherapy drug interactions. Some herbal compounds decrease the activity of CYP enzymes, and others increase the activity of these proteins.[9] St. John's wort, commonly used to treat depression, is known to induce one CYP450 enzyme and inhibit three others. Concomitant treatment with St. John's wort and docetaxel could lead to subtherapeutic levels of the chemotherapeutic drug. This drug is often prescribed for breast, lung, stomach, head and neck, and prostate cancers. Garlic, often used for hyperlipidemia and hypertension, can induce clotting problems and is reported to inhibit certain CYP450 enzymes, making this treatment dangerous with dacarbazine.[9] Other herbal supplements, such as green tea and nettle, interfere with the CYP450 enzyme system, decreasing the efficacy of bortezomib, which is used to treat multiple myeloma. Black cohosh, sometimes used for menopausal symptoms, may increase the toxicity of doxorubicin and docetaxel and interfere with the action of tamoxifen. Saw palmetto, often used for prostate health, increases the anticoagulant effects of warfarin. Ginkgo biloba, taken to improve memory, interacts with anticoagulants, including aspirin, warfarin, ticlopidine, clopidogrel, and dipyridamole. Grapefruit juice is another substance that has a significant impact on the efficacy of certain chemotherapeutic drugs.[9] Oncologists are aware of the ongoing research involving the interactions of herbal supplements and chemotherapeutic agents and advise against the use of these substances during treatment. Careful attention to detail at the initial patient visit will alert the clinician to any impending medical or cancer-related emergencies (Box 32D.1). Familiarity with the signs and symptoms of oncologic emergencies is essential for PAs practicing in any field of oncology.

The field of oncology is growing rapidly. Cancer research is rapidly discovering novel treatment options for many types of cancers. The population in the United States is aging, and with that aging comes an increase in the number of patients diagnosed with cancer. Patients are surviving initial therapy for cancers and are living longer, with an increased risk for developing additional malignancies. There will continue to be a need for caring, well-trained PAs in oncology.

TIP BOX

- Cancer patients are often sensitive to odors. Wear scents, hairspray, soaps, lotions, and perfumes *sparingly*.
- Have an outlet for your frustrations—a hobby or interest that refreshes you when times are tough.
- You are a vital part of the health care team, and you will need respite care; take periodic "mental health days" to restore your focus.
- Cancer patients are similar to all other patients—they respond to genuine signs of caring such as a smile, a handshake, or a hand gently placed on a shoulder.

Physician assistants have been accepted as vital participants in the cancer care team. Patients and physicians both appreciate the role that PAs play in the care of patients with cancer. There will be

---

BOX 32D.1 ONCOLOGIC EMERGENCIES

Spinal cord compression
  Increased intracranial pressure with herniation
  Superior vena cava obstruction
  Seizures
  Hypercalcemia
  Hypernatremia
  Tumor lysis syndrome
  Disseminated intravascular coagulation
  Venous thromboembolism
  Neutropenic fever

---

steady, rewarding growth of PAs who choose to work in oncology.

In a recent comprehensive analysis of the supply and demand for oncology services through 2020, the American Society of Clinical Oncologists (ASCO) predicts a shortage of oncologists and recommends the increasing use of PAs to meet the increasing demand for oncology services.[10]

CANCER CARE

Recent advances in technology and medicine have vastly improved the quality and practice of cancer care. Many institutions have adopted a multidisciplinary approach to cancer therapy. This method organizes care in disease-specific sites, offering patients the expertise of all clinicians who may be involved in their care. For instance, a new patient with head and neck cancer may initially be evaluated by the head and neck surgeon for staging. The patient may then be scheduled for consultations with the medical oncologist, radiation oncologist, audiologist, nutritionist, physical therapist, speech pathologist, and dental oncologist. All of these disciplines would be housed together in close proximity for patient convenience and optimal communication among the treating teams. The teams ideally meet regularly to jointly discuss the new patients and optimize available therapies. The value of a team approach to cancer care lies in the individual treatment plans initiated for each patient. The PA working in such a multidisciplinary setting has the advantage of participating in comprehensive care.

For many years, surgical treatment of solid tumors was considered standard of care. The objective of cancer therapy is to offer the patient the treatment modality that will offer the best likelihood of cure, and this initial treatment was often surgical in nature. Innovations in cancer detection and imaging now allow clinicians to diagnose cancer at earlier stages, opening the door to advances in medical and radiation oncology. Early-stage cancers may now be treated primarily with chemotherapy, radiation therapy, or a combination of the three modalities. PAs have a long history of practicing in the surgical suite, and many surgical oncology subspecialties employ PAs in both the clinical and operating room settings. If the treatment plan initially calls for radiation or chemotherapy, the surgical team may still be involved in obtaining appropriate biologic specimens for diagnosis.

Medical oncologists are specialty-trained physicians who use systemic therapies to treat cancer. These oncologists traditionally relied on chemotherapeutic agents to treat malignancies, but innovations in cancer care now make use of other systemic agents in addition to chemotherapy. Biologic therapy—the use of the body's own immune system to fight cancer—is a relatively new concept in cancer care. Biologic response modifiers (BRMs) are substances produced in the human body in small amounts and can now be produced in a laboratory setting. These laboratory-produced BRMs are now being used to stimulate the body's response to disease or infection, with promising results. Vaccines (therapeutic and prophylactic) have also been developed for use in cancer therapy. Examples of prophylactic vaccines are the hepatitis B vaccine and Gardasil, the vaccine being used to prevent infection with two of the strains of HPV associated with cervical cancer.

Cancer treatment vaccines, designed to treat malignancies that have already developed, are more difficult to design and produce. Sipuleucel-T is a vaccine approved to treat some cases of metastatic prostate cancer.[11] Melanoma, breast cancer, leukemia, and pancreatic cancer are among the malignancies currently being investigated in clinical trials for treatment with tumor-specific vaccines.[9] This advancement in care is just one example of the progress being made in the care of cancer patients. Practitioners in medical oncology often offer adjuvant or concomitant therapy along with radiation oncology and surgical resection. Palliative therapy for patients whose malignancies are not responding to conventional therapy is often provided by the medical oncology service.

Radiation therapy, the use of ionizing radiation to treat cancer or other benign disease, is a relatively new field compared with surgical and medical oncology. Patients undergoing radiation therapy are treated by a team of experts who are trained in the biology of cancer and the effects of ionizing radiation. The team consists of the radiation oncologist, the medical physicist, the dosimetrist, radiation technologists, and nursing personnel. Recently, many radiation oncologists have discovered the utility of including a PA in their practice. The PA serves a unique role, assisting the team in caring for the patient while undergoing specialized radiation therapy. Radiation therapy, similar to chemotherapy and surgery, has sequelae of treatment that are often troubling and life threatening for the patient. The PA is often the clinician who evaluates and treats the side effects of therapy and educates patients about their progress. Similar to chemotherapy, radiation therapy is often used palliatively in cancer care.

Rapid increases in technology have given clinicians many new diagnostic and treatment options for malignancies. The field of oncology is a rapidly growing field, with innovative therapies being introduced daily. PAs who choose to practice in oncology can have a rewarding and intellectually stimulating career, a career that will allow them to influence positively the lives of their patients.

CANCER CARE IN THE TWENTY-FIRST CENTURY

Cancer care is rapidly changing. Care of patients in the future will be quite different from the care received in the past 100 years. Initially, surgery was the only hope of cancer patients. To this option was added radiotherapy followed by basic chemotherapeutic drugs, drugs that acted to kill the malignancy but also harmed viable tissues. As cancer researchers used advances in technology, the field of cancer medicine has evolved. The National Cancer Institute now lists many different modalities of therapy.[11] In addition to ultraprecise surgical procedures, many of which are now performed robotically, targeted, refined radiotherapy is given for a variety of malignancies. These refined radiotherapy fields treat the cancer and spare viable tissues, resulting in fewer treatment sequelae. Standard chemotherapy agents continue to be used and combined with other agents. Cancer patients of today and those in the future may be treated with immunotherapy, targeted cancer therapy, hormone therapy, stem cell transplants, or precision therapy along with standard therapies in any number of combinations.

Immunotherapy—using the body's own cells to treat a malignancy—has several forms. Monoclonal antibodies are used to treat certain lymphomas. These antibodies are designed to bind to targeted tissues, causing an immune response that kills the cancer cells. Another type of immunotherapy involves stimulating the body's own T cells to fight the cancer. This approach is referred to as *adoptive cell transfer*.

Breast cancers and melanomas are two of the malignancies under investigation for the use of this unique therapy. Cytokines (interferons and interleukins) also play a role in current cancer therapy for melanoma and renal cell carcinoma.

Treatment vaccines are in development for many malignancies.

Targeted therapy is the term for cancer treatment that targets the changes in malignancies that guide cell growth, division, and metastasis. Monoclonal antibodies and small-molecule drugs are the agents used for this type of treatment. Signal transduction inhibitors, such as the epidermal growth factor receptor inhibitor cetuximab, are used to treat patients with lung and colorectal cancers. These targeted therapies are designed to aid the immune system in destroying abnormal cells, stop them from growing, and stop body signals that tell the body to develop new blood vessels. Without a blood supply, the tumor is starved. These targeted therapies are referred to as *angiogenesis inhibitors*. The drug bevacizumab is currently being used to treat patients with glioblastoma refractory to treatment and metastatic colorectal cancer.

Other targeted therapies deliver toxic substances to cells with the intention of cell death. Some therapies target the natural death process in cells (i.e., apoptosis), and others target hormones that are needed by certain cancers to grow. The role of targeted therapies in the treatment of many types of cancers is an area of intense growth. For some malignancies, hormone therapy is used. Hormones are used traditionally in breast and prostate cancers. Stem cell transplants, used primarily in individuals with leukemia and lymphoma, are reserved primarily to restore stem cells damaged by previous treatment.

Precision medicine is a promising new area of cancer therapy research. Often referred to as personalized medicine, these proposed treatments would be based on the genetic makeup of the individual tumor. In certain patients with chronic myelogenous leukemia, a certain oncogene can be identified, the *BCR-ABL* oncogene. These individuals may be treated with the targeted gene therapy such as imatinib, one of the tyrosine kinase inhibitors.

GOALS OF TREATMENT

The goal of cancer therapy is to offer the patient the best option for cure. This option must include consideration of the patient's performance status. The patient must be aware of the risks and benefits of the treatment plan and must be an integral part of the discussion. The PA is often the clinician who will manage the treatment effects and advise the patient of his or her treatment options. The PA should fully inform all patients about their diagnosis, treatment options, and survival expectations. Informed consent must include any adverse effects of the treatment modality (Table 32D.2). Giving patients this information allows them to participate fully in their care, empowering them to be involved in their treatment. If the intent of treatment is palliative, inform patients of all options, and allow them to choose those options that they believe are appropriate to their beliefs and lifestyle. Patients must be reassured that clinicians will not abandon them if they seek palliative care and that their symptoms and needs will be fully addressed at all times. Address issues of pain management at every patient visit. PAs can play a vital role in the appropriate management of cancer-related pain (Box 32D.2). Discuss quality-of-life issues with all patients undergoing cancer care, whether curative or palliative.

Perform regular evaluations of the patient with cancer to monitor treatment effects and response to treatment. Early recognition of impending complications or lack of response to treatment will allow the clinician to halt or revise the treatment plan to improve the outcomes. The patient, family, and significant others should all be included in the treatment plan from the beginning. It is important to address all questions regarding the diagnosis and treatment options. All parties involved must clearly understand survival issues to give the patient and the family time to prepare social, spiritual, and financial concerns.

TOP 20 CLINICAL PROBLEMS

1. Management of cancer pain
2. Breast cancer
3. Lung cancer
4. Colorectal cancer
5. Leukemia
6. Lymphoma
7. Bioimmunotherapy for malignancies
8. Treating the long-term cancer survivor
9. Cancer screening and early detection
10. Development of cancer vaccines
11. Melanoma
12. Cutaneous malignancies
13. Prostate cancer
14. End-of-life care of cancer patients
15. Complementary and alternative care in the treatment of cancer
16. Childhood cancers
17. Brain tumors
18. Myelodysplastic syndromes
19. Ovarian cancer
20. Pancreatic cancer

TABLE 32D.2 Common Complications of Cancer Therapy

Chemotherapy	Surgery	Radiation Therapy	Bioimmunotherapy
Nausea, emesis	Disfigurement	Fatigue	Fatigue
Fatigue	Loss of function	Osteoradionecrosis	Severe flulike symptoms
Photosensitivity	Pain—immediate and long term	Mucositis of involved mucosal surfaces	Slowed mentation
Extravasation of chemotherapeutic agent	Postoperative complications	Development of radiation-induced second malignancies	Reactions at injection sites
Anemia	Changes in sexual function, desire	Alopecia in radiated area	Short-term hematologic changes
Mucositis of involved mucosal surfaces	Changes in fertility	Skin changes (atrophy, telangiectasia, ulceration)	Appetite changes
Thrombocytopenia	Psychological changes, depression	Changes in sexual function, desire	Altered taste
Neutropenia		Changes in fertility	
Alopecia		Psychological changes, depression	
Skin changes		Anemia	
Changes in sexual function, desire		Neutropenia	
Changes in fertility			

BOX 32D.2 MAJOR REASONS FOR THERAPEUTIC INADEQUACIES IN THE MANAGEMENT OF CANCER PAIN

PATIENT BARRIERS

Limited expectations regarding the ability to provide pain relief

Excessive concern about addiction, tolerance, and the toxicities of opioids

Legitimate concern that more pain signifies progressive tumor

HEALTH CARE PROVIDER BARRIERS

Inaccurate perceptions of the patient's pain intensity

Failure to determine the cause of pain and apply specific therapy

Lack of knowledge regarding opioid equivalencies and pharmacology

Excessive concern about addiction, tolerance, and the toxicities of opioids

Excessive concern regarding the regulatory oversight of opioids

From Abeloff M. *Clinical Oncology,* 3rd ed. Philadelphia: Elsevier Churchill Livingstone; 2004.

CLINICAL APPLICATIONS

1. Review your patient population with regard to risk factors for cancer. What cancer types are most prevalent in your community? Develop a list of the most prevalent cancer types noted, and then develop a plan to address the risk factors associated with these cancers with all of your patients.
2. Review your patient population, and identify the individuals who are cancer survivors. Develop a plan to address their needs regarding follow-up, sequelae of treatment, possible recurrence, and second primaries.
3. Identify an issue such as cancer prevention or cancer awareness that is lacking in your community. Develop a plan to address this issue that includes a cross-section of the community, especially including persons or populations at high risk. Make this issue a permanent part of your health education discussions with patients.

KEY POINTS

- There is a continuous and increased demand for practitioners in the field of oncology.
- PAs are well suited to the practice of oncology.
- There is a wide variety of clinical and research opportunities for PAs interested in caring for patients with malignancies.
- Current investigation is being conducted in the use of complementary and alternative therapies as adjunct treatment for malignancies.
- Rapid advances in cancer research are allowing more people to sustain a good quality of life while undergoing therapy and as cancer survivors.

References

1. MD Anderson Cancer Center Patient Information. http://www.mdanderson.org. Accessed August 19, 2011.
2. Moss RM. Galen on cancer: how ancient physicians viewed malignant disease. http://www.cancerdecisions.com. Accessed August 19, 2011.
3. Rare Cancer Alliance Cancer History. http://www.rare-cancer.org/history-of-cancer.php. Accessed August 19, 2011.
4. American Cancer Society. *Cancer Facts and Figures 2011*. Atlanta: American Cancer Society; 2011.
5. U.S. Census Bureau News. http://www.nia.nih.gov/sites/default/files/nia-who_report_booklet_oct-2011_a4__1-12-12_5.pdf. Accessed August 19, 2011.
6. Erickson C, Salsberg E, Forte G, et al. Future supply and demand for oncologists. *J Oncol Pract.* 2007;3:79.
7. *American Cancer Society's Guide to Complementary and Alternative Cancer Methods*. Atlanta: American Cancer Society; 2000.
8. American Academy of Physician Assistants. 2011 AAPA Physician Assistant Census Report. http://www.aapa.org. Accessed August 19, 2011.
9. National Cancer Institute Cancer Topics. http://www.cancer.gov/cancertopics. Accessed August 19, 2011.
10. FDA approves zelboraf for melanoma. http://www.cancer.org/Cancer/News/fda-approves-zelboraf-for-melanoma. Accessed August 19, 2011.
11. Singh BH, Gulley JL. Therapeutic vaccines as a promising treatment modality against prostate cancer: rationale and recent advances. *Therapeutic advances in Vaccines*. 2014 Sep;2(5):137–148.

The resources for this chapter can be found at www.expertconsult.com.

E. OTHER MEDICAL SUBSPECIALTIES

Lillian Navarro-Reynolds • Kate Sophia Bascombe

This chapter aims to prepare students for clinical rotations in medical subspecialties, including rheumatology, endocrinology, neurology, pulmonology, nephrology, infectious disease, and gastroenterology.

HOW DO PRACTITIONERS IN MEDICAL SUBSPECIALTIES APPROACH THE PATIENT?

Typically, a patient is referred to one of these specialists by his or her primary care provider (PCP) for assistance with a condition that is out of the scope of the PCP's practice or has been unsuccessfully managed in primary care. At times, a patient will seek specialist care independently. The specialty care provider will review the reason for referral and the patient's medical history to decide if the referral is appropriate. In some cases, the consultant will decide the patient would be best managed within another speciality or that the case is outside her or his particular expertise.

In the introductory consultation, it is important for the specialty team to take a full history and perform a complete physical examination. The patient and the referring provider will often have formulated their own differential diagnoses, which may be outlined in a referral letter or medical records.

In the initial consultation, the patient might find her- or himself repeating a history or undergoing a physical examination that was already done in the primary care setting. In the majority of cases, the patient is happy to be listened to and reexamined. The specialist provider will integrate her or his physical examination findings, history gathered, and past medical records to develop a differential diagnosis and formulate a plan for further evaluation and management.

Specialists may also refer a patient to a more specialized provider (a subspecialist) within their field or to an academic medical center. Patients may benefit from seeing doctors who have significant experience with rare conditions or difficult procedures. For example, some thyroid tumors would benefit from biopsy but may be located very close to a blood vessel. A less experienced provider will be appropriately reluctant to attempt a fine-needle biopsy. The patient might be referred to a center where anatomically challenging biopsies are routinely done by experienced staff. The training of a gastroenterologist includes hepatology, but in many urban or academic settings, diseases of the liver, such as hepatitis C, are managed by a hepatologist who has undergone additional specialized training and manages a large panel of these patients.

PRIMARY CARE PROVIDER–SPECIALIST RELATIONSHIP

A PCP will either refer a patient to be seen one time for a procedure or treatment recommendation or for the specialist to take over ongoing management of a condition. It is essential to maintain clear communication between the PCP and the specialist provider. For the safety of the patient, this communication must continue for as long as the specialist is providing care. Poor communication can have potentially life-threatening consequences. For example, a cardiologist may not be aware of recent changes in a patient's medication. She might notice the patient's blood pressure is elevated and decide to adjust the blood pressure medication. Without the most up-to-date records, she might prescribe a medication the patient is already taking or a medication that adversely interacts with a new medication. It is up to all parties providing patient care to inform each other of changes in management in a timely manner. Patients who are referred to an endocrinologist for poorly controlled diabetes are often taking a long list of medications and find it challenging to remember all of the drug names and doses. PCPs can help ensure that specialists have the current list

at the time of the visit to ensure the best care for the patient.

WHAT DO PHYSICIAN ASSISTANTS IN MEDICAL SUBSPECIALTIES TYPICALLY DO ON A DAILY BASIS?

Physician assistants (PAs) are often the first point of contact for patients in medical subspecialties and have a great deal of responsibility. It is the job of the PA to do a full and thorough history and examination of the patient being evaluated by her team and from this assessment develop differential diagnoses, initiate appropriate investigations, and start management. Having requested testing, a PA will then evaluate the results; communicate them to the patient; and develop a management plan, often in consultation with the supervising physician. The extent to which a supervising physician is involved in this process depends on the complexity of the patient, the experience and expertise of the PA, and the preferences of the physician.

WHAT WILL I BE EXPECTED TO DO IN THIS ROTATION?

As a PA student, you will be expected to take a full history from the patients being evaluated by your team and perform appropriate physical examinations. To gain the most from your rotations, you need to develop a good list of differential diagnoses and how you would want to test for these disease processes. After developing this list, you should then present the patient to your supervising clinician for feedback and guidance with how you will continue the care of the patient. You should also generate a reasonable management plan. Be familiar with the most commonly used medications in your specialty, including dose, route of administration, potential side effects, and drug interactions.

As you gain experience as a student in a clinical setting, you might have the opportunity to preform or assist in procedures under appropriate supervision. When you become more familiar with the clinical setting in which you are working, start to anticipate the needs of the medical team and offer assistance. Volunteer your assistance to gather laboratory and radiology results. Pull together supplies which you know may be needed for procedures. Anticipating the needs of your supervisors will help you to build experience and credibility and will make you a valued asset to the team. Regularly taking initiative may also garner you a job offer at the end of your rotation.

WHICH CLINICAL ENVIRONMENTS MAY I WORK IN DURING THIS ROTATION?

In medical subspecialties, you will be working in a private outpatient office or in a practice within a hospital. You may provide consultation to patients hospitalized on other services and manage some inpatients on your own service. You also might liaise with other hospital departments such as surgery, radiology, or other medical subspecialties to coordinate care for your patient.

WHICH OTHER TYPES OF HEALTH PROFESSIONALS WILL I WORK WITH ON THIS ROTATION, AND WHAT CAN I LEARN FROM THEM?

A number of professionals are invaluable to the specialist health care team, and it will benefit you to spend time with them early in your rotation. In endocrinology, seek out certified diabetes educators to learn about management of patients with type I diabetes or the challenges of adhering to a diabetic diet. In a renal practice, there will be dialysis nurses with expertise in the electrolyte testing your patients routinely undergo as well as how to advise patients on management of their diet and fluid intake based on these results. A wound care nurse will have a wealth of information on the sometimes overwhelming choices available in dressings, which packing material to choose, and what signs they are looking for when they monitor a wound for healthy tissue growth and infection resolution. Introduce yourself to the respiratory therapists to better understand ventilator settings. Ask the smoking cessation team how best to approach this complicated and common addiction. In many specialties, particularly gastroenterology, infectious diseases, and neurology, the services of a registered dietician (RD) can be very helpful to the patient and the medical team. Consider sitting in with an RD as she counsels a patient on how to make complicated dietary changes or how to appropriately take medications with specific foods.

WHICH CLINICAL INFORMATION DO THE PHYSICIAN ASSISTANTS AND PHYSICIANS ON THIS ROTATION ALWAYS WANT TO KNOW ABOUT THEIR PATIENTS?

The primary role of the examination becomes the testing of the hypothesis derived from the history."
William Landau

An excellent workup of the patient starts with a thorough and appropriate clinical history because this guides everything from there. Certain areas of the clinical history need to be more detailed, depending on the speciality that you are in. This section provides a good place to start with an emphasis on speciality-specific information to remember when interviewing patients on your rotations. It is important to remember that these are specifics that should *enhance* but not *replace* the general medical history.

SUBSPECIALTIES

Neurology

When interviewing a patient in neurology, always consider the questions: "Where is the lesion?" (e.g., brain, spinal cord, peripheral nervous system) and "What is the lesion?" (e.g., does it have a vascular, infectious, malignant, compressive, or degenerative cause?). A detailed history enables development of anatomic and pathologic differential diagnoses, which then informs your physical examination and choice of investigations.

Every neurologic history should start with the age, sex, and handedness of the patient. If a patient has experienced seizures or blackouts or is presenting with possible dementia, then obtaining a history from a family member or close friend can be invaluable. Take care to clarify patient descriptions that can be ambiguous. In particular, words such as *dizziness, numbness,* and *weakness* can mean very different things to different patients. Your supervising physician or PA will want to see evidence that you have explored thoroughly exactly what the patient means by these words. Box 32E.1 lists some common

---

BOX 32E.1 COMMON NEUROLOGIC PRESENTATIONS

Headache
Dizziness or vertigo
Change in gait
Seizures
Tremor
Dysarthria
Dysphasia
Confusion
Memory impairment
Limb weakness
Involuntary movement or tremor
Change in taste or smell
Altered hearing
Change in personality
Sensory disturbance

neurologic presentations with which you should be familiar. Think about how you would thoroughly explore the history of these presentations and go on to investigate them.

Patients may not use medical terms correctly; therefore, you need to be careful in taking the patient's claim of a "stroke" or "migraine" as a confirmed diagnosis. Be sure to ask specifically about birth history and childhood development; this may require confirmation from family members. Ask if the patient has any neurologic conditions in the past that he or she no longer experiences (e.g., epilepsy).

Medications and drugs can cause many neurologic symptoms. A detailed history of all drugs ever taken, including recreational, complementary, herbal, and alternative therapies, is essential. Drugs commonly used in general practice, internal medicine, and surgery can have neurologic side effects. For example, a patient may have myopathy as a result of taking a statin or ataxia as a side effect of lithium. When taking a family history, use a genogram, and annotate it with illnesses and cause of death. Depending on the background of the patient, consider inquiring about consanguinity.

The social history of a patient undergoing a neurology assessment should include details of his or her diet. Is the patient a vegan or vegetarian? Does the patient take supplements or have a known deficiency? A detailed travel and sexual history is also important because of the neurologic effects of HIV and syphilis. Alcohol can cause widespread neurologic damage. Ask about the patient's living environment and any support structures required. This helps to not only gauge how well the patient is coping but also helps the team prepare for discharge planning. Always ask whether the patient drives, and try to ascertain how essential it is to his or her everyday living and job.

Neurologic symptoms can cause untold anxiety. Always assess what the patient's ideas, concerns, and expectations about her or his illness and treatment are at the initial interview. This enables a clear and open discussion around what to expect and how things will move forward. It also provides that opportunity to address concerns. If a patient has significant concerns that are not discussed early on in care, he or she might have difficulty accepting the diagnosis and retaining the information or advice you and the rest of the team provide.

Rheumatology

Rheumatology is a specialty that focuses on musculoskeletal conditions as well as systemic autoimmune conditions. As a result, it incorporates the vast majority of the body's systems, and detailed clinical histories are paramount. Box 32E.2 details some of the key points that should be considered when taking a musculoskeletal history.

There is a substantial genetic component to all rheumatic diseases, and it is always important to consider the interaction between genetics and the environment. It is therefore essential to obtain both a strong family and social history. Careful consideration should also be given to any current or previous pregnancies and any lung, liver, endocrine, hematologic, or dermatologic diseases because of the extensive systemic involvement of rheumatologic diseases.

As with taking a history from a patient in any specialty be sure to elicit any "red flag" symptoms. Those that need particular attention in rheumatology include pain preventing sleep, loss of appetite, unintentional weight loss, visual loss, blurred vision and temporal headache, loss of bladder or bowel control, and rapidly progressing symptoms. Equally, all of the following signs are red flags: inability to weight bear; red, hot joint; upper motor neuron signs; bilateral change in limb strength or reflexes; saddle anaesthesia; temperature above 100°F (38°C); and painful swelling.

The rheumatologist's perspective on routine blood tests are detailed in Table 32E.1. A rheumatology text will be useful to review blood tests that are more specific to this discipline, such as antinuclear antibody, rheumatoid factor, and anti-CCP antibodies.

Modern rheumatologic practice makes substantial use of immunosuppressive therapies, including glucocorticoids and disease-modifying antirheumatic drugs (DMARDs). Before initiating these

---

BOX 32E.2 KEY POINTS IN MUSCULOSKELETAL HISTORY

Pain: OLD CARTS (or other pain mnemonic such as SOCRATES)
Affected joint(s): acute or chronic onset, pattern of fluctuation
Stiffness: time of day
PMHx, previous trauma, FHx
Swelling or deformity
Impairment to ADLs
    Systemic symptoms

ADL, Activity of daily living; *FHx,* family history; *OLDCARTS,* onset, location or radiation, duration, character, aggravating factors, reliving factors, timing, and severity; *PMHx,* past medical history; *SOCRATES,* site, onset, character, radiation, associated factors, time, exacerbating/relieving factors, severity (pain history).

medications, it is critical to ensure that patients do not have a subclinical infectious process that will be unmasked by the immunosuppressant. Patients should always be screened for tuberculosis and hepatitis B and C. Prevention of infectious disease is also critical. Before the initiation of immunosuppression, patients should be vaccinated for all vaccine-preventable illnesses, particularly influenza and pneumonia. Patients also must be educated on the importance of trying to avoid infections through handwashing and avoidance of ill people. Finally, patients taking DMARDS need to be followed closely to assess for hematologic changes caused by the medications. See the specific monitoring instructions for the DMARD you intend to prescribe and educate your patients on the importance of this follow-up.

Infectious Diseases

Physician assistants in infectious diseases largely work in the outpatient setting but are also part of the infectious disease team that offers expert consultation to many other specialists caring for patients with infectious complications of disease. A PA working in infectious diseases should be familiar with the presentation, pathophysiology, treatment, and management of bacterial, viral, fungal, and parasitic infections. Examples of the kinds of viral infections that you might come across include human immunodeficiency virus, herpes simplex virus, hepatitis C virus, influenza, cytomegalovirus, and Epstein-Barr virus.

Bacterial and mycobacterial infections that are managed by the infectious disease team can include pneumonias, endocarditis, meningitis, colitis, nephritis, cystitis, and various sexually transmitted infections. Fungal infections can include *Cryptococcus* and histoplasmosis affecting the pulmonary tree, skin, or cerebrospinal fluid. There may also be the need to provide a workup and management of patients with fever of unknown origin (FUO) or a case of FUO in which it is proves difficult to identify the source.

The basic principles of history taking apply to a rotation in infectious disease. In addition to the standard questions, the immune status of the patient should be considered: How often is the patient becoming infected? How severe are the infections? Are they multidrug-resistant infections? A standard medical interview should always include a medication history, but in infectious diseases, you need to pay particular attention to adherence to the dosing schedule of any antibiotics or antiretroviral agents. Treatment for tuberculosis in particular is very poorly tolerated. To what degree have adverse medications reactions affected the patient's adherence to the regimen? Is it worth considering the patient for a directly observed treatment program?

HIV management requires some specialized history. Find out how long the patient has been diagnosed with HIV, which antiretroviral the patient has been prescribed (if any), and whether the patient is managing to afford and take them. What is the patient's most recent CD4, count and when was it tested? Does the patient know his or her current viral

TABLE 32E.1 Investigations in Rheumatology

Hematology	Most systemic rheumatologic diseases are associated with a normocytic normochromic anemia. Anemia can be result of drug therapy. Inflammation will raise the platelet count, but conversely, this can drop because of SLE.	
CRP and ESR	ESR is very nonspecific. CRP is a more direct measure of inflammation.	
Biochemistry	Renal function	Needs regular monitoring in patients with any vasculitis; regular creatinine monitoring for patients taking cyclosporins
	Liver function	Monitoring in patients taking methotrexate or sulfasalazine
	Immunoglobulins	Poly- or monoclonal (e.g., in myeloproliferative disorders such as myeloma)
	Uric acid	Gout
	Muscle enzymes	Elevated in those with inflammatory muscle disease
	Bone profile (including calcium, corrected calcium, albumin, total protein, alkaline phosphatase)	Markers of bone turnover can be used to determine response to treatment for osteoporosis; also used to investigate Paget disease or bone metastasis
Urinalysis	In any patient with suspected connective tissue disorder for blood and protein	

CRP, C-reactive protein; *ESR*, erythrocyte sedimentation rate; *SLE,* systemic lupus erythematosus.

load? Inquiry needs to be made into whether the patient is or has suffered with any opportunistic infections. There is a considerable psychosocial element to be considered for patients who are HIV positive or diagnosed with AIDS. This should be addressed and done so sensitively. Is the patient sexually active? Is he or she using protection? Has the patient informed his or her partner(s) of the diagnosis?

When working in infectious diseases, it very important to consider any isolation protocols that may be in place to protect patients, staff, and visitors Generally, there are two types of isolation: protective isolation (otherwise known as reverse barrier nursing) and source isolation. The former is a physical separation for the protection of a patient from pathogens carried by others (e.g., a patient with neutropenia sepsis). This may include the use of a room with positive or negative pressure. The latter is to prevent the spread of infection from a patient to others. Again, a positive- or negative-pressure room may be used for isolation. You should familiarize yourself with the signs used to indicate when isolation is required and what forms of personal protective clothing (PPC) is required and available e.g., gowns, gloves, eye shields, face masks for those needing to enter the patient's room.

Table 32E.2 outlines some common presenting complaints that are worth considering prior to starting an infectious disease placement.

Endocrinology

With any medical history, it is important to start at the beginning of the story. One of the most common conditions (Box 32E.3) managed in endocrinology is diabetes, both type I and type II. (Before your rotation, read up on the important differences between these two diseases.) Start by finding out when and how the patient was first diagnosed with diabetes. How have the patient's blood sugar, blood pressure, and lipid control been from the time of diagnosis? Discover what the patient already knows about diabetes and diet and exercise recommendations. Does the patient's check her or his blood sugar at home? Has the patient's made any lifestyle changes, and does the patient have an idea of the changes that need to be made? Be specific; you want to know what the patient's day looks like. Make sure you and your patient have a similar definition of a "healthy diet." What does the patient's portion size look like? Discuss the patient's meal content and snacks. Does the patient eat after dinner? If so, how much and how often? How active is the patient? How much alcohol does the patient drink, and is the patient aware of how alcohol affects glucose levels? The social history

TABLE 32E.2	**Common Infectious Disease Presentations and Potential Detail to Elucidate**
Sore throat	Is there any associated difficulty in swallowing, difficulty in or noisy breathing (stridor), or lymph node enlargement
Fever	Duration and pattern are very important. Is the patient drenching through night clothes? Does the fever respond to taking antipyretic drugs (e.g., acetaminophen or NSAIDs)? Has there been any recent travel?
Headache	Does the patient have any meningitic symptoms (e.g., nuchal rigidity or photophobia) to suggest a cerebral infection or bleed? Was it rapid onset or the worst headache of the patient's life?
Rash	Is it blanching? Duration and distribution of the rash: Does it wax and wane? Is there any history of atopy? Ascertaining if there have been any recent changes to the patient's drugs is also useful.
Diarrhoea	Has any suspicious food been consumed? Recent antibiotics? Any family history of IBD or cancer of the GI tract? Any recent travel?

GI, Gastrointestinal; *IBD,* inflammatory bowel disease; *NSAID,* nonsteroidal antiinflammatory drug.

BOX 32E.3 COMMON CONDITIONS ASSESSED AND MANAGED IN ENDOCRINOLOGY

Type II diabetes mellitus
Type I diabetes mellitus
Hashimoto thyroiditis
Graves disease
Multinodular goiter
Thyroid cancer
Pituitary tumors
Diabetes insipidus
Adrenal disease

---

is very important because it directly impacts your management plan.

Think about the comorbidities that are increased with diabetes and modifiable risk factors. Always ask specifically about alternative, herbal, and over-the-counter (OTC) medications because many are advertised on TV and online that that claim to "cure" diabetes. Find out about family history of diabetes, autoimmune disease, and heart disease.

Always review the patient's last hemoglobin A1C (Hgb A1C), lipids, blood pressure, and weight. Be familiar with the medications the patient is taking and look to see that the patient is up-to-date on her or his fundoscopic examination, diabetic foot examination, and urine microalbumin testing. Patients with diabetes will be seen every 3 to 6 months depending on how well their blood sugars are controlled. Be familiar with what is routinely covered in these visits. Also discuss with your supervising clinician the Hgb A1C target for the individual patient because this is not a "one size fits all" prescription.

Ask the patient about his or her medical knowledge. Is the patient educating him- or herself using online resources? There are times when virtual resources or online forums are useful and appropriate. Patients with chronic disease can be troubleshooting experts and have good insight into their limitations. In particular, people who use insulin pumps can offer peer support and ideas for dealing with unique challenges of blood sugar control in type I diabetes. Conversely, there is a lot of difficult-to-interpret and even false information on the Internet! Becoming familiar with the sources your patient uses can facilitate productive discussion of the content.

You will likely see patients with thyroid disease, including hypothyroidism, hyperthyroidism, and thyroid cancer. Be familiar with the symptoms of hyper- and hypothyroidism so you can tailor your history to pick up clues as to whether the patient is currently symptomatic or on the correct dose of thyroid hormone replacement.

Many conditions have nonspecific symptoms and can be difficult to diagnose. For example, a patient might be referred to an endocrinologist for evaluation of her adrenal function. She might be feeling tired, and a random cortisol level may have been "low." It is up to the endocrinologist to do further specialized testing such as an adrenocorticotropic hormone (ACTH, Cortrosyn) stimulation test. Blood cortisol levels are measured before and after a synthetic form of ACTH is given by injection. This testing is best done under the care of a specialist because staff and equipment to perform the test and interpret the results might not be available in general practice. With other endocrine disorders such as pituitary tumors or other hormonal disease, enter the consultation having reviewed the patient's records, and have a broad differential diagnosis in mind. Ask system questions, looking for symptoms of the disease that can rule in or out each item on your list. When you present to your preceptor, your differential diagnosis should be clear, and through the history you have gathered, your preceptor should be able to narrow the differential diagnosis further. Before starting this rotation, do some reading on the hormones of the pituitary gland and the feedback loop to glands and organs these hormones target.

Pulmonology

In pulmonology, you will see patients with difficult-to-manage respiratory diseases (Box 32E.4). As with all of the other specialties, you will gather a thorough history with special interest and detail given to the risk factors particular to the patient's disease or presentation. Always ask about smoking history because it is a risk factor for multiple conditions in pulmonology (and many other specialities) that can be very frustrating and challenging to manage for both the patient and health care provider. Ask about or review the medical records for documentation of immunization status, particularly pneumonia and yearly influenza vaccines.

If you are seeing a patient who has a pulmonary embolism, it will be important to have a clear idea of her risk factors for developing this condition. This will help the team formulate a plan with the aim of decreasing the risk of a repeat event. Is there a history or possibility of cancer? Is she taking hormone replacement therapy or estrogen-containing contraception? Is there a family history of coagulopathy? Has she had a prolonged period of immobility? Is she pregnant? Start to think about possible consequences of the pulmonary embolism. Will she need an echocardiogram to look at right heart size and function? Do some reading on anticoagulation therapy options and the monitoring this might require.

If you are seeing a patient with asthma, ask if he has had previous hospital admissions, intensive care unit admissions, or intubation. A patient who has a

---

BOX 32E.4 COMMON CONDITIONS ASSESSED AND MANAGED IN PULMONOLOGY

Pneumonia: Review the many types.
Pulmonary embolism
COPD
Emphysema
Bronchiectasis
Pulmonary hypertension
Tuberculosis
Pulmonary fibrosis: Always consider environmental exposure risks.

COPD, Chronic obstructive pulmonary disease.

history of these interventions needs to be monitored closely, and the team might have a lower threshold for repeat admission. How often does he need to take oral steroids? Again, this detail lets you and the team know how severe the asthma is. Ask about medication adherence. Does the patient remember to take preventive inhalers, or does he only use them when symptoms are present? Can he afford his prescribed medications? Show empathy when discussing this issue; acknowledge that taking multiple medications can be expensive and that your patient might have other priorities for his funds (e.g., food and shelter, gas to get to work).

If your patient is being evaluated for pneumonia, what are her risk factors for aspiration? These might include a history of stroke, dementia, alcohol abuse, or quadriplegia. You will also want to know if she has a history of HIV or possible exposure to tuberculosis. Are there results of a previous sputum culture you can gather that will help the team make an educated guess as to the most appropriate antibiotic or first-line treatment?

Nephrology

Renal failure has varied clinical presentation. When approaching a renal patient, consider the signs and symptoms of decline in renal function. Has the patient had nausea, malaise, fluid retention, pruritus, or fatigue? What is her current fluid status? All renal patients, but particularly those on dialysis, should have a very careful assessment of their fluid balance. Sometime this requires an '"input–output" chart, potentially with the use of an indwelling catheter. Does the patient know what signs and symptoms to look out for to tell whether he or she is "too wet" or "too dry"?

When interviewing a renal patient, always be sure to ascertain the stage of the patient's disease. The potassium status of renal patients should be carefully monitored, and patients should be educated about what symptoms may occur with hyperkalemia. Is the patient currently undergoing dialysis? When does she dialyze? When was her last dialysis treatment? Has she been put on the transplant list, or is this something that has been addressed as a potential option for the future. If so, when would that time be? Has she had a transplant? How is she coping with her antirejection medication?

Similar to other patients with chronic disease, renal patients typically take multiple medications. Every potential opportunity should be used to assess whether the patient is managing to take all the medications and taking them at the right time It is also important to ascertain if the patient knows what each medication treats and how to manage if she or he misses a dose or takes too many tablets by accident.

Renal failure can be acute, chronic, or acute on chronic. When possible, look for previous and most recent renal blood results, and observe the trend. Typically, acute renal failure is secondary to a circulatory dysfunction or urinary tract obstruction. When interviewing a patient with renal failure, be sure to inquire about any personal history or urinary tract infections (UTIs); family history of polycystic kidney disease; and use of medications, especially analgesics such as nonsteroidal antiinflammatory drugs. Ask about pruritus, nocturia (including any accidents), lethargy, anorexia, and nausea. Investigations of particular benefit for the renal workup include blood urea nitrogen (BUN), creatinine, estimated glomerular filtration (eGFR), albumin-to-creatinine ratio, red blood cells, glucose, and microalbuminuria. Urine should be obtained for dip testing, microscopy, cultures, and sensitivities. Assess the metabolic function of the kidney with calcium and phosphate levels. If there are any concerns with regards to systemic causes of renal disease, then the erythrocyte sedimentation rate and serum electrophoresis can be useful. Before progressing to further imaging such as computed tomography or magnetic resonance imaging, simple ultrasonography of the renal tract can detect abnormalities.

Hematuria (blood in the urine) can originate from anywhere in the renal tract. Hematuria associated with pain on urinating (dysuria) is likely to be caused by a UTI. Painless hematuria is more concerning for malignancy or glomerulonephritis. Is there concomitant hypertension, edema, or oliguria? If so, you should consider nephritic syndrome. Proteinuria tends to be discovered on a urine dipstick. Always repeat to exclude a false-positive result. Excessive protein excretion in the urine is a sign of tubular or glomerular disease, which has numerous causes. Oliguria can be a normal physiologic response to the environment, so a thorough history is important. Polyuria can also be caused by high intakes of fluid, but diagnoses such as diabetes insipidus and diabetes mellitus should always be considered.

Renal calculi (stones) can develop anywhere along the urinary tract from the kidneys to the urethra. Kidney stones are incredibly painful, and after you have witnessed a patient with a renal calculi and his or her restlessness, you always remember it. However, remember that patients can be asymptomatic with renal calculi. Staghorn calculi can often be asymptomatic but can lead to acute renal failure if bilateral. Renal calculi are common, with an equal lifetime risk for both men and women. When considering renal calculi or managing a patient with recurrent occurrences, consider the risk factors, which include diet,

---

BOX 32E.5 INTERVIEWING A RENAL PATIENT

Change in urinary flow: both the physical act of passing urine and how it appears
Any pain
Fluid status
Medications: those the patient is taking and those the patient should avoid. Is the patient compliant?
Recent blood work
Recent imaging
On dialysis? Last dialysis? Schedule of dialysis.
Future planning: Is the patient they on a transplant list? Should he or she be?

BOX 32E.6 COMMON CONDITIONS ASSESSED AND MANAGED IN GASTROENTEROLOGY

Inflammatory bowel disease: Crohn disease, ulcerative colitis
Irritable bowel syndrome (generally to confirm diagnosis) and make initial treatment recommendations
Colorectal cancer
Carcinoma of the pancreas
Nutritional disorders or chronic diarrhea
Fecal incontinence
Gastrointestinal malabsorption: celiac disease
Hepatitis A, B, and C
Cirrhosis
Esophagitis
Barrett esophagitis
Gastroesophageal malignancy
Achalasia
Esophageal varices
Hiatal hernia
Gastritis

---

obesity, chronic dehydration, positive family history, and use of some medications. Ask about previous stones and the effectiveness of treatments used in previous episodes.

Box 32E.5 summarizes the key questions and areas of inquiry you should make when interviewing a renal patient.

Gastroenterology

Gastroenterologists care for patients with problems of the gastrointestinal tract from the mouth through the anus. They care for patients with minor illnesses such as gastroesophageal reflux to much more serious conditions such as colorectal cancer, pancreatitis, and chronic hepatitis. Gastroenterology PAs play a critical role in extending the services offered by a gastroenterologist. Some gastroenterology PAs even perform endoscopy on their own.

When interviewing a patient in the gastroenterology clinic, always assess the frequency and type of stools. Does the patient have bloody stools? Dark and tarry stools? Pale stools? Assess the type, location, and character of any abdominal pain. Determine whether the patient is at risk for hepatitis because of travel, tattoo placement, sexual habits, history of incarceration, or intravenous drug use. Ask about family history of malignancy and autoimmune disease. Make sure to inquire about what OTC treatments a patient has tried for her or his symptoms because nearly all gastroenterology patients have tried to treat themselves before presenting for medical care. Review the results of any tests performed in the primary care setting for the patient.

Many patients are referred for possible colorectal cancer or for colon cancer screening. As with other subspecialties, start at the beginning by gathering your own history. Pay particular attention to the relevant "red flags" of unintentional weight loss, dysphagia, persistent indigestion, unexplained iron-deficiency anemia, rectal bleeding, and changes in bowel habit. When did the symptoms start, and how have they progressed? What are the patient's diet and bowel pattern like in general? Does she or he have a personal history of other cancers? Gather a family history with specific attention to colorectal cancer and polyps. Have a look at the patient's medical record and review the blood tests and screening that have been done in the primary care setting.

If you are interviewing a patient with a history of inflammatory bowel disease, ask about frequency of oral steroid use and previous surgeries. When was the patient diagnosed? What medications have been tried, and what were the outcomes? Ask about weight loss and the patient's diet. It is also useful to know if a female patient is using contraception or would like to become pregnant. Look up her most recent laboratory test result, and be ready to present these to your supervising clinician. Find out when her most recent colonoscopy was done and what the results were.

Box 32E.6 outlines the common conditions assessed and managed in gastroenterology. Some of the conditions, such as irritable bowel syndrome and gastritis, can be initially managed in the primary care setting. When the symptoms persist after a trial of the first-line treatment or are out of the scope or experience of the primary care team, the patient is referred on.

WHICH SPECIAL POPULATIONS OF PATIENTS MAY I SEE MEDICAL SUBSPECIALTY ROTATIONS?

Endocrinology

The bulk of the patients in this rotation will likely either have diabetes or thyroid disease. It is important to understand and empathize with the challenges of having diabetes. It is a disease in which the patient must agree to actively participate in disease self-management or face serious complications. It is up to the provider to help the patient understand the treatment options and demonstrate understanding and empathy of the challenges of making the significant life changes that are often required. I often tell people, "If we all followed diabetic lifestyle recommendations we would be a lot healthier. Lifestyle changes are not easy to make, but please tell me what support you need. I will do what I can to help you."

Neurology

Neurology can be a very rewarding specialty but is also very emotionally challenging. You will encounter patients with incurable diseases such as motor neuron disease and brain tumors. These diagnoses are life changing not just for the patient but also for all those around them. Making sure that patients and families are aware of the help and support available for them is essential. The diagnosis of a serious chronic disease such as Parkinson disease or myasthenia gravis also raises a lot of questions with regard to time scale of progression and expected impact on quality of life. Conditions such as epilepsy and multiple sclerosis can carry with them a large amount of stigma in the community. Try to help arm patients with ways of explaining their condition and direct them to useful support groups. In pediatric neurology clinics, you will encounter families dealing with diagnoses that mean their children will lead significantly different lives than their peers. In these situations, you have two to three patients to consider—the child and his or her parents.

Pulmonology

In pulmonology, you will likely see a population that is at increased risk of aspiration pneumonia such as persons with learning disabilities or quadriplegia or patients who have had strokes. Aim to learn as much as you can about decreasing the risk of readmission to these special populations. What support and education for both the patient and the caregivers can be offered by the inpatient and outpatient multidisciplinary teams?

In the majority of patients with bronchiectasis, the underlying cause is cystic fibrosis. Ask the medical team you are working with about social support groups (often virtual) available to this young population.

Patients with chronic obstructive pulmonary disease and type 2 respiratory failure present a potentially interesting challenge. Find out what the patient's optimal oxygen saturation is, and reflect on how you might approach a patient who does not want to keep an oxygen mask on or has an altered mental status secondary to hypercapnia. Many of the patients under the care of pulmonology smoke cigarettes. This is a challenging addiction and source of frustration to health care providers, patients, and family members. Become familiar with smoking cessation approaches and resources such as 1-800-QUIT-NOW

Nephrology

When rotating on nephrology, it is important to keep in mind the unique challenges patients on hemodialysis face. Their entire lives must be structured around treatment for their disease. Hemodialysis is administered three times per week, and patients often find themselves feeling exhausted and ill after the treatment. The dietary recommendations are very strict and can be difficult to follow. Patients are sometimes also on a renal transplant list, which is in itself very stressful. Dialysis nurses and transplant team members are good people to go to for more information and understanding of these specific challenges.

Gastroenterology

Many of the patients you see in gastroenterology will have been referred for assessment of possible cancer. Reflect on how you will discuss their concerns without providing false reassurance. You might also see young patients with chronic, sometimes embarrassing disease. Patients with ulcerative colitis or Crohn disease will likely have episodes of urgent, sometimes bloody stooling. They might have a temporary ileostomy at a relatively young age. Imagine how these conditions might impact the life of a young adult starting a new career or relationship. Consider the implications to social activities such as exercise or athletics. An ileostomy can be embarrassing for anyone but particularly distressing for someone who is at the age when their peers are starting families or balancing work and friends. There is a lot of potential for self-limitation because of the risk of embarrassment. Consider the questions that patients might ask themselves: How will they deal with swimwear or even light summer-clothing? Will they be able to have children? With chronic disease, there is often increased risk of depression; find out how these patients are coping and be prepared to offer support and treatment.

Infectious Diseases

Having a long-term infectious disease can carry with it a great deal of stigma and may lead to social isolation. It can have an impact on all areas of a patient's life, including her ability to form relationships. As a result of this, consider the increased potential that your patient is suffering with depression. Support groups and social network links can provide connections with people who are in a similar situation and can empathize.

Patients with certain infectious diseases be a risk to others. It is important to discuss the patient's occupation, living arrangements, and sexual behaviors to help prevent the patient from infecting other people. Occasionally, the legal system may need to be involved to protect the public health. Try to manage conversations about infection of others with sensitivity and respect while still communicating the seriousness of the situation to the patient.

WHAT ARE THE SPECIAL CHALLENGES OF MEDICAL SUBSPECIALTIES?

The primary challenge of working in a medical subspecialty is keeping open communication with the primary care team and staying current with the patient's comprehensive medical status. A specialist is often the one to tell a patient that he or she has an incurable illness, a potentially greater challenge if the PCP has not previously advised the patient of this possibility. Giving bad news can be especially difficult if the patient has viewed the specialist as potentially holding the "cure" for the illness. It is essential to continue to treat the patient as a whole rather than focusing solely on the particular disease you are assigned to manage.

WHAT ARE THE SPECIAL REWARDS OF MEDICAL SUBSPECIALTIES?

The biggest reward of specialty practice is helping a patient and the primary care team establish the proper treatment for an illness. Many times, the specialist has approaches for management that the PCP may not have considered. Rendering a firm diagnosis, even if the prognosis is grim, is very helpful to the patient. Patients can make better decisions for themselves if they know what they are facing. As an endocrinology PA, I found helping patients to take control of their diabetes incredibly rewarding. I enjoyed providing patient education and treatment recommendations and watching the pride that patients feel when they play an active role in improving their diabetes control and his quality of life.

WHAT RESOURCES MIGHT BE HELPFUL TO ME ON THIS ROTATION?

Ask you preceptor for a reference for a specialty text. Your preceptor may even have one she or he can loan you for the month. Ask students who have previously done this clerkship which references they found most helpful.

The Centers for Disease Control and Prevention (CDC) has a wealth of resources you can use before, during, and after your infectious disease rotation (http://www.cdc.gov). It is advisable to review the diseases that require submission of notification to the CDC of their confirmation (http://wwwn.cdc.gov/nndss/document/NNC_2015_Notification_Requirements_By_Category.pdf).

KEY POINTS

- Taking a medical specialty elective can allow you to explore a specialty that you might wish to practice. It can also prepare you for your board examination.
- A strong relationship between the specialist and the PCP is essential for providing safe and high-quality care for each patient.
- Listen closely in the first few days of the rotation to understand which questions your preceptor always asks and which information is most crucial to obtain for each type of patient you see.
- Take opportunities to learn from other types of specialist health providers such as RDs, dialysis nurses, respiratory therapists, and wound care specialists. They have much to teach you.

F. OTHER SURGICAL SUBSPECIALTIES

Daniel T. Vetrosky • Jennifer B. Wall

Just as a patient is referred by a primary care provider (PCP) or independently seeks the help of a medical subspecialist so too are patients who require specific surgical intervention. Many patients are referred to a general surgeon, typically for bowel, thyroid, breast, or hernia surgery. Others may need the expertise offered by a surgical subspecialist. Physician assistants (PAs) are now commonplace in nearly all surgical subspecialties. The need for PAs in the subspecialties continues to grow as resident work hours decrease and fewer surgical residency spots are available. According to the American Academy of Physician Assistants, approximately 25% of all PAs work in one of the surgical subspecialties listed in Box 32F.1.

This chapter focuses on how surgical subspecialties other than general surgery and orthopedic surgery approach the patient and how students can get the most out of a surgical subspecialty rotation.

HOW DO PRACTITIONERS IN SURGICAL SUBSPECIALTIES APPROACH THE PATIENT?

After a referral from a PCP is accepted, the introductory consultation establishes the basis for determining the appropriateness of the referral and the intervention needed. The approach to the patient being seen is specific to the surgical subspecialty and the patient disease or disorder. However, certain aspects of the patient evaluation are consistent throughout surgical and medical subspecialties; these include a thorough history and physical examination. Despite their subspecialty training, surgical specialists depend on evaluating the disease or disorder by first having knowledge of the patient's overall health. Review of the patient's past medical history, surgical history, any complications with past anesthesia, surgical recovery history,

BOX 32F.1 SURGICAL SUBSPECIALTIES

Anesthesia
Bariatric surgery
Burn surgery
Cardiothoracic surgery
Colon rectal surgery
Head, ear, nose, and neck surgery
Neurosurgery
Ophthalmology
Orthopedic surgery
Pediatric surgery
Plastic and reconstructive
Surgical oncology
Surgical intensive care
Transplant surgery
Trauma surgery
Urology
Vascular surgery

From American Association of Surgical Physician Assistants.
http://www.aaspa.com.

current medications, and allergies to medications or latex are integral to a surgical evaluation. After these factors are known, the specialist can assess the diagnostic studies necessary to determine the type of surgery, the specific approach, any other specialties that need to be involved, and adjuvant treatment necessary to achieve the expected outcome.

PRIMARY CARE–SURGICAL SPECIALIST RELATIONSHIP

If a patient is deemed a candidate for subspecialty surgery, it is common that the surgeon will request a thorough review from the referring PCP to perform a risk stratification evaluation. The surgeon is seeking advice from the PCP regarding what the risks to the patient are if the patient has the recommended surgery. When risk factors are identified, the PCP can provide interventions to help reduce the overall surgical risk.

As mentioned in Chapter 32E, the PCP–surgical subspecialist relationship depends on collaborative management of the patient. Surgeons may admit a patient to his or her service and seek assistance from the PCP or a hospitalist to manage the patient's medical problems. Alternatively, surgical subspecialists can serve as consultants for patients admitted to the PCP or hospitalist service. Both teams then round on the patient with their respective focus. As hospital systems become progressively more compartmentalized, effective communication among the teams is essential. The PA should strive to ensure that each team understands who has responsibility for each aspect of the patient's care.

WHAT DO SURGICAL SUBSPECIALTY PHYSICIAN ASSISTANTS DO ON A DAILY BASIS?

Depending on the model of the surgical subspecialty, PAs will typically divide their time among the clinic, hospital wards, intensive care units (ICUs), operating rooms (ORs), and outpatient surgical facilities. In other models, PAs work solely as the first assistant in the OR or on the hospital floor. When choosing a subspecialty surgery rotation, ensure you fully understand the preceptor's model of the practice so that the experience fits your expectations.

Physician assistants are often the first practitioner seen in a surgical subspecialty clinic, and similar to the PAs in the medical subspecialties, they have a great deal of responsibility. It is incumbent on them to perform a thorough history and physical examination, develop differential diagnoses, and determine the most salient diagnostic tests and interventions the patient might need. All of this information is then relayed to the surgeon, and the surgeon and the PA and patient work together to choose the best approach to the patient's problem.

By performing the first evaluation, the PA can establish a trusting relationship with the patient from the start. This relationship will be the basis for continuity of care. When the patient sees the PA work closely with the surgeon to develop the plan, the patient's trust in the PA is augmented. After all, the patient has sought out the surgeon for relief from his or her unique and often complex ailment. It is the role as the subspecialty PA to know every detail about the patient that the attending surgeon needs, including the appropriate history, physical examination findings, and specialty testing results. Surgical PAs must perform these duties while conducting themselves in a professional and caring manner.

Often a PA is the comforting face to a patient on hospital rounds or during frequent clinic visits. Many times the surgeon's time is best served starting an operation while the PA ties up any loose ends for the service. The PA and the surgeon work together to most efficiently accomplish the tasks needed to provide optimal patient care.

WHAT WILL I BE EXPECTED TO DO ON THIS ROTATION?

For most students, a surgical subspecialty rotation is an elective. However, this is not the time to coast. Rather, integrate your internal medicine, general surgery, and critical care knowledge to get the best experience from your surgical elective. You will have the opportunity to work with physicians and PAs who have the deepest knowledge and skill sets unique to their field. Use the rotation to refine your knowledge of this specialty area, always asking yourself, "How can I apply this expertise to my everyday practice?"

As a PA student, you will be expected to work up new patients by performing complete histories and physical examinations on your patients. You will then concisely present your findings, differential diagnoses, proposed laboratory or radiologic testing, and potential surgical intervention to the team. You will be expected to round on the hospitalized patients before the attending physician or chief resident arrives on the ward in the morning and present their preoperative or postoperative progress to the team. You may be asked to write daily progress notes and perform oral presentations as well. You most likely will accompany the attending physician, the resident, or the intern to the OR and may be asked to assist with the procedure as an observer, second assistant, or first assistant. In this setting, it is essential that you have reviewed the surgical procedure before the surgery so you can answer all questions the surgeon will inevitably ask. You may also be asked to assist in composing the postoperative orders, as a student exercise, while a resident or attending physician writes the orders. The surgeon who performed the procedure typically writes the operative note. You will work each day with the surgical team, which consists of the surgeon, anesthesiologist, nurse anesthetist, PAs, scrub nurse (or technician), circulating nurse, perioperative nurse, postoperative recovery room nurse, surgical ward nurse, and in some instances pharmacists. It is your job to assist the team to provide safe patient care, understanding your student role and remaining helpful to the overall team.

WHAT CLINICAL INFORMATION DO PHYSICIAN ASSISTANTS AND PHYSICIANS ON THIS ROTATION ALWAYS WANT TO KNOW ABOUT THEIR PATIENTS?

As has been emphasized throughout this book, a thorough history and physical examination are expected in all specialties. The more experience you gain during a given surgical rotation, the more you will know what specific laboratory studies, medications, and tasks you are expected to perform. For each specialty, you will be expected to have reviewed the correlating anatomy, physiology, pathophysiology, and common pharmacology as they relate to their practice. Consider how you would investigate symptoms and presentations in a concise and thorough manner. Keep

in mind that patients may not use medical terms when describing their complaints or symptoms. Asking the same question in a different manner or asking the patient what he or she means by a certain term can help clarify what the patient is experiencing.

Whether documenting or providing an oral presentation on the hospital ward or ICU, get into the habit of presenting the following items:
- Postoperative day number
- Antibiotic day number
- Overnight events (with insight of nurse)
- Trajectory of the patient: same, better, or worse
- Rated pain; type of pain medication provided and amount
- Pertinent system-based review of systems (always includes attention to nausea, vomiting, bowel movement, flatus, urination, oral intake, diet status, mobility status, chest pain, dyspnea, extremity swelling or pain)
- Pertinent PE and specialty testing
- System-based assessment and plan

SURGICAL SUBSPECIALTIES

Cardiovascular and Thoracic Surgery

Specific questions regarding cardiac, pulmonary, and vascular symptomatology should be emphasized during the patient history. Even if the cardiologist or primary care physician has recorded these areas of questioning, it is preferred practice to ask his or her again. Every cardiothoracic and vascular history should begin with age, gender, and onset of symptoms. This should be followed by the PPQRST questions: provocative, palliative, quality, radiation, severity, and timing of the symptoms. Box 32F.2 lists some common cardiothoracic and vascular symptoms and presentations you should become familiar with during this rotation.

Family members can be helpful when patients cannot remember if they have been diagnosed with a prior myocardial infarction, abdominal aortic aneurysm, or chronic obstructive pulmonary disease. They can also let you know if the patient has had any diagnostic testing and where it was performed.

A typical daily routine of a cardiovascular and thoracic surgery PA includes ward and ICU rounds, as well as first assisting in the OR. Common ward procedures include insertion of central venous catheters (CVCs) and Swan-Ganz catheters, inserting and removing chest tubes, removing pacing wires, and maintenance of postoperative sternal and leg wound complications. Common operations include coronary artery bypass grafting, valve procedures, and aneurysm repairs in which PAs serve as the first

BOX 32F.2 COMMON CARDIOTHORACIC AND VASCULAR SYMPTOMS AND PRESENTATIONS

Chest pain
Shortness of breath
Extremity pain
Rapid heart rate
Rapid breathing
Wheezing
Cough
Pale or blue lips or extremities
Syncope
Extremity cramping
Extremity swelling
Anxiety or feelings of impending doom
Cold extremities, numbness, or tingling
Weight loss or gain
Tearing back pain

BOX 32F.3 COMMON NEUROSURGICAL SYMPTOMS AND PRESENTATIONS

Headache
Dizziness or vertigo
Change in gait
Seizures
Paresthesias
Dysarthria
Dysphasia
Confusion
Memory impairment
Limb weakness
Involuntary movement/tremor
Change in taste or smell
Altered hearing
Change in personality
Sensory disturbance
Changes in vision or loss of vision

assistant; endoscopic leg vein harvesting is usually performed autonomously by a PA.

Physician assistants entering this rotation should have an understanding of cardiovascular risk factors, heart anatomy and physiology, electrocardiogram interpretation, shock, Swan-Ganz readings including cardiac output, systemic vascular resistance, cardiac index, end-diastolic volume index, and central venous oxygen concentration. Additionally, students should review therapeutics, including vasopressors and inotropes.

Neurosurgery

A clinical rotation in neurosurgery focuses on cerebrovascular diseases such as ischemic and hemorrhagic stroke; central nervous system malignancies; and malformations of the brain, spinal cord, and spine. Every neurosurgical patient history should begin with age, gender, and handedness (to determine brain dominance for language); drug history, including use of nonsteroidal antiinflammatory drugs, anticoagulants, and aspirin and last dose; detailed pain medication history; family history (particularly of cancer); and social history, including place of work and exposures to toxins and radiation. The onset of specific neurologic or neurovascular symptoms should be ascertained followed by the PPQRST questions. If a patient cannot answer questions because of dementia, delirium, aneurysm, stroke, or cognitive decline, family members and friends should be questioned. Box 32F.3 lists common neurosurgical symptoms and presentations that will be helpful for you to review before starting the rotation.

If you are concerned about brain pathology, you should inquire about loss of strength, sensation, coordination, hearing, vision, and coordination; history of running into walls; word-finding difficulties; slurring of speech; new onset of seizures; behavioral and personality changes; new onset or changes in headaches; and inability to care for oneself.

If you are concerned about spinal pathology, inquire about the type of pain the patient has; the distribution and severity of pain; the pattern of pain radiation; the effects with sitting, standing, walking, or bending; loss of balance; noticeable muscle atrophy; frequency of dropping items; decline in handwriting; bladder or bowel incontinence; impairment of daily living; use of assistive devices; exercise regimen; and prior conservative interventions, including physical therapy, steroid injections, and chiropractic interventions, as well as a thorough pain medication history.

Before starting this rotation, practice the following physical examination skills: Mini-Mental State Exam, cranial nerve examination, eye examination (including fundoscopy), dermatomal sensory examination, a rated muscular strength and deep tendon reflex examination, and cerebellar and gait assessment.

Take advantage of every opportunity on this rotation to review computed tomography and magnetic resonance imaging (MRI) with senior team members and radiologists. Repeated review of brain images will help you decipher subdural versus epidural hemorrhages, parenchymal versus intraparenchymal bleeds, and cystic versus cancerous lesions. Detailed review of spine MRIs will clarify where spinal cord or nerve impingement originates from to reinforce your physical examination findings.

Ear, Nose, and Throat Surgery

A clinical rotation in ear, nose, and throat (ENT) surgery, also known as otolaryngology—head and neck surgery, focuses on diseases and malignancies involving the ears, nose, sinuses, and upper alimentary tract (throat). ENT surgeons and PAs are also trained experts in voice disorders and airway management. The specialty offers a wide scope of practice, crossing the fields of oncology, neurotology, sinus, facial plastic, microvascular, endocrine, and vascular surgery. Every ENT patient history should begin with age, gender, and specific ENT complaint. The onset of ENT symptoms should be ascertained and followed by the PPQRST questions. Box 32F.4 lists common ENT surgery symptoms and presentations. Review these thoroughly before starting the rotation. Keep in mind that questioning family members can be helpful when investigating snoring, sleep apnea, and hearing disorders.

When on an ENT rotation, try to see as many types of ENT surgeries as possible. Common surgeries include tonsillectomy, rhinoplasty, endoscopic sinus surgery, myringotomy tube placement, resection of head and neck cancers, and cochlear implant placement. Some ENT surgeons may perform microsurgery or reconstructive plastic surgery depending on their training and practice. Additionally, some surgeons specialize in pediatric hearing and language disorders.

Common procedures performed by experienced ENT PAs include removal of foreign bodies of the ear or nose, mastoid cavity cleansing, rigid nasal endoscopy, nasal electrocautery, fiberoptic laryngoscopy, nasal packing or removal, removal of tubes, and I&D of peritonsillar abscesses.[2]

Recognize that sometimes a thorough ENT workup may require further specialty referrals to gather all necessary information before determining if surgery is necessary. Audiology, sleep medicine, pulmonary, speech therapy, allergy, ophthalmology, and neurology are all common collaborative services that may be involved with the ENT patient.

Urologic Surgery

A clinical rotation in urologic surgery focuses on disorders and malignancies of the male and female genitourinary tract. Every urologic surgery patient history should begin with age, gender, and specific genitourinary complaint. The onset of the complaint should be ascertained, and the PPQRST questions should follow. Box 32F.5 lists common urologic surgery symptoms and presentations. Consider how you would investigate these symptoms and presentations

---

BOX 32F.4 COMMON EAR, NOSE, AND THROAT SURGERY SYMPTOMS AND PRESENTATIONS

Headache or facial pain or pressure
Dizziness or vertigo
Tinnitus
Dysphagia
Hearing loss
Sinus pain
Rhinorrhea or postnasal drip
Sore throat
Snoring (obstructive sleep apnea)
Hearing and language problems
Hoarseness
Change in taste or smell
Coughing and sneezing
Changes in vision or loss of vision

BOX 32F.5 COMMON UROLOGIC SURGERY SYMPTOMS AND PRESENTATIONS

Frequency
Hesitancy
Decreased size of urinary stream
Stress, urge, mixed, and functional incontinence
Pneumaturia (air passed with urine)
Erectile dysfunction
Dysuria
Painful erection
Gross painless hematuria
Microscopic hematuria
Recurrent urinary tract infections
Kidney stone
Male infertility
Urgency
Nocturia
Flank pain
Fever and chills
Penile or vaginal discharge
Enuresis

---

in a concise and thorough manner. Keep in mind that questioning family members can be helpful when investigating kidney stones and urinary incontinence.

Key physical examination components include testing for CVA tenderness and abdominal, rectal, groin, and male genitalia versus female pelvic examinations. This rotation will likely allow for student skill training in traditional Foley, coudé, and straight catheterization.

Common procedures performed by experienced urology PAs include first assist OR duties, including nephrectomy, prostatectomy, orchiectomy, transurethral procedures, and stents. Office procedures include transrectal ultrasound volume studies, cystoscopy, postvoid residual evaluations, and complicated catheterization.[3]

Plastic and Reconstructive Surgery

A clinical rotation in plastic surgery may focus solely on the cosmetic surgery, typically done in a private practice setting, or integrate reconstructive surgery, commonly found in the hospital setting (Box 32F.6). A cosmetic surgeon focuses on elective esthetic surgery, and plastic surgery is dedicated to the reconstruction of facial and body defects caused by trauma, burns, disease, and congenital defects. Common surgeries performed for cosmetic purposes include breast augmentation, rhinoplasty, liposuction, blepharoplasty, and facelifts. In comparison, the most common reconstructive surgeries include tumor removal, complicated laceration repair, maxillofacial surgery, scar revision, hand surgery, skin grafting, and flap surgery. PAs working in academic settings may find that often the surgical residents are more commonly found in the OR while the PAs are working on the floor, performing needed procedures on the hospital wards and discharging patients. Private plastic surgery PAs are usually involved in all areas of clinic, wards and OR settings. Pediatric reconstruction surgery is its own specialty that focuses on congenital defects, including cleft lip and palate, craniofacial conditions such as craniosynostosis and Pierre Robin syndrome, obstetric brachial plexus injury, genital reconstruction, facial trauma, and hand reconstruction.

Physician assistants working in plastic and reconstruction surgery need to have a clear understanding of wound healing, skin graft and flap recovery,

---

BOX 32F.6 COMMON PLASTIC AND RECONSTRUCTIVE SURGERY PROCEDURES

Deep inferior epigastric artery perforator (DIEP) flap procedure breast reconstruction after mastectomy
Female breast reduction versus augmentation
Male breast reduction (gynecomastia)
Carpal tunnel syndrome
Hand or finger fracture repair
Panniculectomy versus abdominoplasty
Scar revision (facial, trauma, burn)
Brachial plexus repair
Skin grafts (split vs. full thickness)
Flaps (free vs. local)
Skin cancer lesion removal and reconstruction

---

vascular flow patterns, nerve innervation, dressing and product resources, hand radiograph interpretation, and pain management.

When evaluating a patient for elective surgery, it is essential to determine if the patient is a good surgical candidate. Factors such as smoking and likelihood of compliance with postoperative care are assessed to determine the likelihood of a successful procedure. Because these cases are not emergent, team members can work with patients and their PCPs to optimize modifiable risk factors to safely perform procedures.

Be ready to perform sensory and motor testing of the face and extremities; a proficient hand examination; and isolated nerve, tendon, and muscle testing, as well as recognition of early infection and septic joints. Common procedures you may observe or perform include debridement, complicated suturing, and application of complicated dressings.

Students should use this rotation to evaluate every wound possible and follow it through its healing continuum. Learning how to address wound complications is a great skill to have regardless of which specialty you ultimately practice. Of course, observation and practice of suturing techniques is a staple of this rotation. Often, if you inquire, OR nurses will provide you with near expired or expired suture to practice suturing and knot tying at home. You can purchase skin suturing models and an instrument pack easily online.

Trauma Surgery

A clinical rotation in trauma surgery offers a broad learning environment addressing acute injuries of the head, neck, chest, abdomen, and extremities (Box 32F.7). Trauma teams usually include general surgeons, vascular surgeons, orthopedic surgeons, and neurosurgeons. Hospitals in the United States are categorized according to the resources they have available to deal with trauma. The highest level of care is offered at level I trauma centers. The lowest designation is a level V trauma center. Most students rotating on a trauma service are placed in level I and II centers, which are typically large academic medical centers with extensive resources.

Physician assistants working on trauma teams need to be able to work along large teams in an organized, thorough, and calm manner. They have a clear understanding of fluid resuscitation, blood products, electrolyte balance, shock, advanced trauma life support protocols, therapeutics, critical care concepts, and radiographic interpretation. They must also harbor astute judgment. Typically, trauma PAs work alongside surgical residents and often provide continuity for the trauma team.

The history in trauma patients can be complicated. Often the history and physical examination are performed simultaneously. Review the primary and secondary survey for trauma by the American College of Surgeons. When patients are unable to provide history, obtain it from bystanders, family, paramedics, police, or anyone one else with knowledge of the patient. Try to obtain the time of the patient's last meal and if the patient has exposure to toxins. This information is key for patients who may require emergent surgery and will better prepare anesthesiology for potential complications. Key physical examination components also include the Glasgow Coma Score and neurologic, skin, abdominal, musculoskeletal, spinal, motor, sensory, and rectal examinations.

Procedural skills performed by experienced trauma PAs include chest tube insertion, pneumothorax needle decompression, FAST (focused assessment with sonography for trauma) exam, wound debridement, application of complicated dressings including negative-pressure wound therapy (NPWT), wound closure, insertion of CVCs and nasogastric (NG) tubes and removal thereof, airway management, and at times endotracheal tube insertion.

Burn Surgery

A clinical rotation in burn surgery may or may not be combined with a trauma or plastic surgery placement. Burn centers are usually housed within level I trauma centers (although not all level I trauma centers have a burn center). Burn physicians have a background in general surgery and may also be board certified in other subspecialties, including trauma, plastic surgery, or critical care. PAs on the burn service often serve in the clinic, hospital floors, ICU, and operative settings. Because patients usually have long-term needs, PAs also may collaborate with burn foundations and survivor support groups within the community to aid their patients. Burn service providers not only care for pediatric and adult patients with

burn injuries (Box 32F.8) but commonly also care for patients with complicated skin diseases that require a high degree of wound expertise and unique skin coverage interventions (Box 32F.9).

Physician assistants on this service are skilled in deciphering burn depth (first to fourth degree), with astute knowledge of Parkland resuscitation, shock intervention, critical care concepts, recognition of compartment syndromes, airway management, ventilation management, acute kidney injury, infectious complications, complicated wound management, wound care products, and pain management. Common procedural skills include debridement, split- and full-thickness skin grafting, escharotomy, fasciotomy, application and troubleshooting NPWT, and placement of CVC and NG tubes.

To best prepare for this rotation, one should review the definitions and characteristics of first-, second-, third-, and fourth-degree burn wounds; be able to determine burn size by the "rule of 9s"; and understand the Parkland formula for burn resuscitation, burn shock, third spacing, blood products, electrolyte management, sepsis, and wound infection versus colonization.

Students should strive to follow patients over their hospitalizations from the emergency department or trauma bay, resuscitation, operations, and discharge to the clinic setting. Students should observe and assist in every dressing change possible. Students can usually be helpful in the OR by holding limbs, providing hemostasis, and participating in dressings. This rotation will also

---

BOX 32F.7 COMMON TRAUMA PRESENTATIONS

Motor vehicle collision
Pedestrian struck by motor vehicle
Fall
Penetrating trauma
Blow to the abdomen
Rupture or burst injury of a hollow organ
Blunt cardiac injury
Traumatic amputation
Neck injuries (vascular vs. spine)
Fractures
Assault
Trauma associated with burns

BOX 32F.8 COMMON BURN MECHANISMS

Scald
Flame
Chemical
Inhalation of flame, steam, or chemical
Friction (road rash)
Abuse (child, elder, or domestic)

BOX 32F.9 COMMON COMPLICATED SKIN DISORDERS AND DISEASES TREATED BY BURN SERVICES

Stevens-Johnson syndrome
Toxic epidermal necrolysis
Graft versus host disease (cutaneous)
Purpura fulminans
Pemphigus
Fournier gangrene

allow extensive exposure to pain management. Integrative team models are crucial to both trauma and burn teams, usually consisting of physical therapy, occupational therapy, respiratory, speech, nutrition, clinical pharmacy, social work, psychology, and case management. Make good use of the knowledge of these teams to optimize your learning experience.

WHAT ARE THE SPECIAL CHALLENGES OF SURGICAL SUBSPECIALTIES?

One of the challenges common to all surgical subspecialties is maintaining consistent and open communication with the referring physicians and interdisciplinary team members. The referring physician will often suspect that a patient has serious disease, but the burden of rendering the final diagnosis may end up with the surgeon. The referring physician needs to be informed of the final diagnosis because she or he will be taking care of the patient after surgical intervention is finished.

A challenge for PAs in the surgical subspecialties is trying to be everywhere at once. The more skills and knowledge the PA obtains, the more demands are placed on the PA. It is essential in any surgical practice to be able to effectively delegate workload within your team. PAs can help manage the workload by collaborating with their surgeons to develop protocols for their teams and provide knowledge to students and residents about "how we do things here" to allow for these learners to be an effective part of the team.

WHAT ARE THE SPECIAL REWARDS OF SURGICAL SUBSPECIALTIES?

Practicing a surgical subspecialty gives the PA the opportunity to develop specialized procedural skills that most other PAs do not have. Being able to perform complex suturing, first assisting, debriding, and performing many types of procedures while keeping the patient calm and comfortable is very satisfying. Another reward of practicing a surgical subspecialty is seeing patients recover from a debilitating disease or malignancy and knowing that you had a hand in helping them. Perhaps the most rewarding aspect of surgical practice is the bond of trust established between your patients and yourself. Providing support to patients going through traumatic procedures will endear you to them forever. These patients will remind you that you have helped them improve their quality of life.

Mastering procedural skills in the surgical subspecialties is also immensely personally rewarding. These skills are harbored usually by a very small subset of professionals. Patients and nonspecialist providers are commonly immensely grateful for the unique service you offer, reinforcing your pride in your career choice. In addition, the small number of surgical providers in a hospital allows for development of a real sense of community. Networking opportunities within surgical societies and discovering leadership opportunities within your specialty can also add to longevity and job satisfaction.

WHAT RESOURCES MIGHT BE HELPFUL TO ME ON THESE ROTATIONS?

The most important resource is your ability to be curious. Go to the Internet and look up the particular subspecialty organization. Learn all you can about their organization, including its mission and goals. Ask your preceptor for any texts related to the subspecialty that you could read during breaks or at night. Look up the procedure that you will do the following day, and most especially, know your anatomy! You will be asked during the procedure, "What is this muscle?" and "What is the name of this fascia? Best of luck to you all!

KEY POINTS

- Be prepared to perform a thorough history and physical examination on each patient, paying special attention to the previous surgical and anesthesia history
- Students on these rotations will be expected to do whatever is most helpful to the team, even if that work is sometimes not very glamorous.
- Review general anatomy before the start of the rotation and review the anatomy for the surgeries you will see the night before the procedure.
- Know the patients you are following well and be prepared to present their cases concisely.

References

1. American Association of Surgical Physician Assistants. *Surgical PA Specialties*; 2015. Retrieved from http://www.aaspa.com/page.asp?tid=99&name=Surgical-PA-Specialties&navid=35.

2. American Association of Surgical Physician Assistants. *Head and Neck Surgery*; 2015. Retrieved from http://www.aaspa.com/page.asp?tid=121&name=Head–Neck-Surgery&navid=18.

3. American Association of Surgical Physician Assistants. *Urology*; 2015. Retrieved from http://www.aaspa.com/page.asp?tid=130&name=Urology&navid=18.

SECTION V

PROFESSIONALISM

CHAPTER 33

PROFESSIONALISM

William C. Kohlhepp • Anthony Brenneman

Trust between the patient and clinician is central to the therapeutic relationship. Without this requisite level of trust, patients will not reveal information about themselves nor will they follow treatment recommendations.[1-3] Trust builds from the belief that the clinician possesses expert knowledge (that will be applied to the benefit of individuals and society) and will avoid self-interest while acting on behalf of those served. Growing from that public trust, a level of autonomy to self-regulate is afforded to medicine. However, the autonomy extended to the profession must be in balance with medicine's priority of advancing the public welfare. This combination of commitment to service, the possession of a specialized body of knowledge, and the ability to self-regulate are the key components of professionalism.[4]

Some have questioned whether the shared body of medical knowledge and participation in a supervised practice qualifies physician assistants (PAs) for consideration as professionals.[5] Others have clearly demonstrated that PAs should be considered as professionals. Soon after PAs began to practice, Tworek[6] applied the standards of professionalism to PAs and concluded that those in the occupation had become professionalized. Picking up that distinction later, Gianola[7] concluded that the evolution to the modern role of PAs has resulted in our becoming a full profession.

Thus, when the four leading PA organizations adopted the Competencies for the Physician Assistant Profession,[8] they followed the lead of our physician colleagues and included professionalism as one of the six "general competencies."

Recognition as a profession brings with it opportunities and responsibilities. In recent years, a variety of pressures resulting from changes in the health care delivery system have made it more difficult for medicine to live up to those responsibilities. As a result, the professional tenets of medicine have been called into question.[2,4] A return to professionalism depends on clearly defining the term and identifying ways to foster and assess this competency. Lessons for PAs can be learned from the physician experience.

UNDERSTANDING THE IMPORTANCE OF PROFESSIONALISM

Early in the history of medicine, the promises of the Hippocratic Oath grounded medicine and instilled in physicians a strong commitment to service. As attention later shifted to the science of medicine, the specialized knowledge associated with medicine became the central focus. Consequently, the understanding of and commitment to the service responsibilities diminished with significant consequences to the overall impression of physicians as professionals.[1]

Compounding the consequences of that shift in focus, the business aspects of medicine also began to impact medicine's image. Some have suggested that medicine used its significant knowledge base to find ways to manipulate the market to increase the demand for services, dramatically increasing costs for health care. In this scenario, physicians were thought to have put their own economic interests above the needs of patients and society—an action that goes against the precepts of professionalism.[4,9]

As health care costs escalated, government and insurer involvement in health care increased with resulting tighter controls over medicine. Precertification and utilization review efforts by the government and insurers reduced the ability of health professionals to make autonomous medical decisions. Credentialing efforts by insurers that evaluated the performance of health professionals adversely impacted self-regulation efforts. As constraints over decision making and self-regulation have increased, the influence of medicine has decreased, and the image of physicians as professionals has been affected.[4,9]

With changes in the health care system challenging the professionalism associated with medicine, today's clinicians must understand what it means to be a professional and must be willing to abide by the expectations that result. However, questions have been raised concerning the uniform existence of that understanding of and commitment to professionalism. Despite a commitment to teaching clinicians in training about professionalism, these efforts have been hampered by a lack of universal agreement on the definition of professionalism.[10,11]

The goal of teaching professionalism is to assist students with developing a professional identity. The process requires a dual focus on exploring through explicit curricula the definition of professionalism and the traits associated with professional behavior as well as teaching students to participate in experiential learning activities that include a component of reflection on professional behaviors.[12]

After 2 years of observations during medical school interviews, as well as class discussions and exercises, Hafferty[13] voiced concerns about the existence of the core values central to professionalism. He noted that medical students might feel less of an obligation to be bound by the expectations set forth in a code of ethics. He also suggested that they might not feel a need to ascribe to the values outlined in professional oaths that are generally part of most medical school graduations. He also observed that even White Coat Ceremonies, despite all their symbolism, seem to fail to remind medical students of the values and obligations of professionals.

Reinforcing the tenets of professionalism during medical education is critical because there is a strong link between what is learned about professionalism in medical school and what one exhibits later in practice. In a landmark study, Papadakis and colleagues[14] at the University of California–San Francisco School of Medicine conducted a case-control study that compared medical school graduates who were disciplined by the Medical Board of California with control participants matched by medical school graduation year and specialty. Of the graduate physicians disciplined by the Medical Board, 95% experienced a violation associated with a professionalism lapse. When compared with control participants, the physicians who experienced professionalism lapses during medical school were twice as likely to later experience an adverse medical board action while in practice.[14] Recognizing the importance of responding to those early lapses, many strategies for dealing with professionalism lapses have evolved, including remediation assignments, remediation contracts, professionalism mentoring, stress management or mental health intervention, and community service.[15]

ELEMENTS OF THE PHYSICIAN ASSISTANT COMPETENCY OF PROFESSIONALISM

Recent efforts to define professionalism have shifted from the sociologic definition to a focus on values associated with professionals. The most commonly appearing elements identified in a recent literature search included a number of ill-defined concepts, such as "altruism, accountability, respect, integrity, ethic[ism], lifelong learn[ing], honesty, compassion, excellence, self-regulating, service," that provide little guidance to clinicians who aspire to professionalism.[16]

Van de Camp and colleagues[17] provide an understandable overarching structure that brings together key values with service delivery concepts. The latest model includes four areas of professional behavior: toward the patient, toward other professionals, toward the public, and toward oneself. The authors note that their behavior-based focus intentionally avoided the use of vaguely understood elements that have been associated with professionalism. Another improvement in the recent model is that it included elements that grew from the models of competency developed by the Accreditation Council on Graduate Medical Education in conjunction with the American Board of Medical Specialties.[18,19]

The Competencies for the PA Profession incorporate nearly all of the top 10 constituent elements of professionalism mentioned most frequently in the literature and fit well into the structure outlined by Van de Camp and colleagues[17] (Box 33-1). In addition, a number of other, less frequently mentioned elements are included.

BEHAVIOR TOWARD THE PATIENT

Values: Respect, Compassion, and Integrity

Respect, compassion, and integrity are the hallmarks of being an admirable PA. Professionalism first and foremost involves respect for one's patients, meeting them as equals no matter the situation. It requires a commitment to truly caring for and about another human being. Respect for others (e.g., the patient's families, coworkers, physicians, nurses, residents), as stated in the American Board of Internal Medicine's Medical Professionalism Project,[20] is the essence of humanism, and humanism is central to professionalism and fundamental to the collegiality of medical providers. Compassion, similar to respect, embodies the ideals of a caring practitioner. Similar to the Norman Rockwell pictures of the kindly physician caring for the young child and demonstrating concern for the parents, we are charged with providing that same compassion in all of our interactions with our patients and others. We must treat each person as an individual, not allowing lifestyles, beliefs, idiosyncrasies, or family systems to influence or shape our respect or compassion. This unconditional compassion for patients serves as the foundation for another key element needed in patient

---

BOX 33.1 PHYSICIAN ASSISTANT COMPETENCIES

PROFESSIONAL BEHAVIOR TOWARD THE PATIENT

- PAs must prioritize the interests of those being served above their own.
- PAs must demonstrate a high level of ethical practice.
- PAs must demonstrate a high level of sensitivity and responsiveness to a diverse patient population, including culture, age, gender, and disabilities.
- PAs are expected to demonstrate respect, compassion, and integrity.

PROFESSIONAL BEHAVIOR TOWARD OTHER PROFESSIONALS

- PAs are expected to demonstrate professional relationships with physician supervisors and other health care providers.

PROFESSIONAL BEHAVIOR TOWARD THE PUBLIC

- PAs are expected to demonstrate responsiveness to the needs of patients and society.

- PAs are expected to demonstrate commitment to ethical principles pertaining to provision or withholding of clinical care, confidentiality of patient information, informed consent, and business practices.
- PAs are expected to demonstrate accountability to patients, society, and the profession.
- PAs must demonstrate adherence to legal and regulatory requirements, including the appropriate role of the PA.

PROFESSIONAL BEHAVIOR TOWARD ONESELF

- PAs are expected to demonstrate commitment to excellence and ongoing professional development.
- PAs must know their professional and personal limitations.
- PAs must practice without impairment from substance abuse, cognitive deficiency, or mental illness.
- PAs are expected to demonstrate self-reflection, critical curiosity, and initiative.

From Physician Assistant Competencies (2005).[8] Structure adapted from Van de Camp K, Vernooij-Dassen M, Grol R, Bottema B. How to conceptualize professionalism: a qualitative study. *Med Teach.* 2004;26:696.

care, empathy. Compassion and empathy are essential elements of a positive relationship with patients. Faced with a compassionate and empathetic clinician, patients are more likely to follow treatment plans and to be satisfied with the care received.[21]

Integrity is the base from which respect and compassion grow. The definition of integrity is to be forthcoming with information and to not withhold or use that information for power.[22] Integrity requires that we admit to our errors; use resources appropriately; and exercise discretion, especially in areas of confidentiality. In addition to these three, there are other humanistic values that foster positive relationships with patients. These include accountability, taking responsibility, punctuality, being organized, politeness, courtesy, patience, positive demeanor, and maintaining professional boundaries.[23] These qualities demonstrate our respect and compassion for ourselves, our patients, their families, and our fellow health care providers.

Primacy of Patient Welfare

Altruism is central to professionalism, but the concept is both controversial and difficult to understand. Definitions of altruism include a focus on actions that benefit others and are voluntary without promise of external rewards.[24]

Arguing that the actions of health professionals are not altruistic, critics note that health professionals experience both external and internal rewards from their efforts. They note that the knowledge and skill applied by health professionals often bring wealth, status, and power to those individuals. The critics also point to the internal rewards gained (the gratitude from patients served, satisfaction from being involved in the lives of those patients, feeling good about growing knowledge and skills, and the satisfaction of curiosity, the acquisition of wisdom, and attainment of the respect of colleagues for those achievements). Those who believe the actions of health professionals are indeed altruistic counter that although those rewards do accrue, they follow the service, are secondary to them, and are not conditions that are set before services are delivered. Those proponents also remind us that health professionals attempt to deliver the highest quality service even when no reward is anticipated.[25]

It seems logical then that gaining rewards through service does not invalidate altruism for health professionals. However, what is equally clear is that clinicians must avoid conflicts of interest that result from financial or organizational arrangements.[1] For example, referral decisions cannot be influenced by managed care agreements that return bonuses when visits to specialists fall below projections.

In addition to meeting the needs of patients, altruism means advocating for patients. Some have even suggested that the PA acronym should stand for "patient advocate." In this environment of pre-authorization before the use of diagnostic studies or treatment modalities, it often takes a lot of effort to assist patients in understanding the system and overcoming the obstacles it presents. Another dimension of altruism relates to making yourself available to patients even if it means your personal plans might be affected.[26] Wilkinson believed that the responsibilities of meeting such an expectation were lost in the broader term of altruism, which led this dimension to be characterized as "balance availability to others with care for oneself."[23]

Ethical Principles and Practice

Ethical components are evident in approximately 25% of all clinical decisions that occur in the inpatient setting. In outpatient settings, estimates of the involvement of ethical components have ranged from 5% to 30%.[27,28] The ethical components result from value judgments regarding the consequences of decisions made by the decision maker and fulfillment of the rights of others. Usually, the ethical aspect is not explicitly considered because it is a garden-variety ethical conflict for which universal agreement on the resolution exists. To develop skills in applying ethical principles, PAs should make a habit of recognizing the presence of ethical dilemmas that surface even when they are a minor component of the decision making (see Chapter 34 for further exploration of ethics).

Sensitivity and Responsiveness to a Diverse Population

The U.S. Census Bureau highlights dramatic changes in our country's ethnic makeup over the next 45 years. For example, the portion of the population identified on the census as "White alone, not Hispanic" is expected to drop from the current level of 63% to 44% by 2060.[29] As a result of these changes, health care professionals will be practicing in an increasingly diverse cultural environment and will be called on to provide services to individuals from cultures other than their own. In addition, increasing attention is focused on existing racial/ethnic disparities in health care delivery that are affecting outcomes.[30]

The success of the health care encounter depends primarily on accurate and effective communication between patient and clinician. Failures of communication can result from differences in language, culture, and perspectives regarding health. Communication between patient and clinician affects "patient satisfaction, adherence to medical instructions, and health outcomes."[31] It is clear that the education of health professionals must address cultural competence (see Chapter 38 for further exploration of health disparities).

BEHAVIOR TOWARD OTHER PROFESSIONALS

Professional Relationships With Physicians and Other Health Care Providers

The physician–PA team relationship is fundamental to the PA profession and enhances the delivery of high-quality health care. In its 1998 report, the Pew Health Professions Commission highlighted the relationship between PAs and physicians, noting, "The frequent consultation, referral, and review of PA practice by the supervising physician is one of the strengths of the PA profession. The characteristics of this relationship are also considered to be the elements of professional relationships in any well-designed health system."[32]

Team practice is an essential component of the effort to improve the quality of health care. The Institute of Medicine (IOM) has called for a campaign of "Cooperation among Clinicians." Effective teams require that team members work together with clear goals and expectations. Leadership, communication, and conflict management are key to that clarity. Matching the roles and training of team members to the tasks at hand will promote cohesiveness in interdependent teams.[33] (See Chapter 7 for further exploration of the physician–PA relationship.) Mounting consensus exists that a failure of teams to establish a culture of professionalism can lead to disruptive behaviors that can result in medical errors adversely impacting patient safety.[34]

BEHAVIOR TOWARD THE PUBLIC

Responsiveness to Patient Needs and the Needs of Society

At first glimpse, this principle seems straightforward, without need of explanation—"I will be responsive to the needs of my patients." Similar language is used in the Hippocratic Oath, as well as in the Guidelines for Ethical Conduct for the PA Profession,[35] but are we responsive, and do we act on those needs? For instance, is being responsive to your patients simply filling that antibiotic prescription or casting a broken arm? Or is it the aforementioned plus actively listening and being "in the moment" with your patient

instead of thinking about the next item on the review of systems. Do your actions speak louder than your words when meeting with your patients? Will they say you are responsive to their needs even if they do not get what they think they need (e.g., an antibiotic for a 2-day history of a sore throat), or will they say you are distracted, not listening, and ultimately not caring or responsive about them as individuals? Common lapses in the responsiveness to patients include a failure to meet responsibilities, a failure to maintain appropriate relationships within the health care environment, and an inability to practice self-improvement. Some more serious lapses have been reported, including cheating, felonies, falsifying information, and forging prescriptions.[15]

In the same way, we need to be responsive to society's needs. On the surface, this again seems clear, that we devote a part of our time to serving society (e.g., working in a free clinic or homeless shelter).[36] However, it also includes monitoring our actions and the impact they have on society. It is being responsive and working with local, state, and national leaders to address health care needs, whether through access to health, coverage for care, or developing healthy lifestyle programs. It is advocating for individuals who have no health insurance by working at the state and national levels to change or effect policy. We bring to light the individuals of society who have little voice in how they receive health care. We are given a white coat to wear when we graduate from a PA program that tells those around us that we have specialized knowledge. Even when we are not "officially" wearing the white coat, we are still health care providers and, as such, must always be ready to respond to society at large or to those immediately beside us.

Accountability to Patients, Society, and the Profession

Accountability includes commitment, dedication, duty, legal and policy compliance, self-regulation, service, timeliness, and work ethic.[23] The inclusion of accountability demonstrates that after the white coat is placed on the new professional, it remains on at all times. We cannot choose to be timely in care of patients sometimes and not at other times, just as we cannot be committed to the profession part of the time. By being accountable to the profession, society, and our patients, the profession itself will be better able to provide care, advance its status, and drive changes needed for the future of health care.[4]

Examples of accountability include coming to class on time, participating in class, completing assignments, arriving to work on time, and meeting deadlines. It also means being accountable to the profession by paying your dues on time, keeping your licensure up-to-date, complying with state filing laws, and accepting and performing under state practice laws as currently stated. Additionally, accountability to society includes reporting errors. The importance of this responsibility is well documented in the IOM's *To Err Is Human*, which quantifies the cost to society, patients, and the profession if errors go unreported.[37] It also involves reporting poor behavior in peers, practicing medicine in an ethical and responsible manner, being aware of your own limits, and identifying developmental needs and ways to improve.

There is much overlap between responsiveness to society, patients, and the profession and accountability, but each has distinct attributes as well. We must constantly strive to be responsible (in many ways an inward approach) and accountable (an outward approach) to how we practice medicine, participate in our community, and interact within our profession.

Adherence to Legal and Regulatory Requirements

State laws and regulations dictate who may practice as a PA, the medical services a PA may perform, and the requirements for supervision. It is the responsibility of each PA to make sure that you have a valid and current state license and have met any additional state requirements before you begin to practice. It is your responsibility to ensure that everything you do is within the limits of your state law and regulations.[38] (See Chapter 35 for further exploration of the adherence to legal and regulatory requirements.)

BEHAVIOR TOWARD ONESELF

Commitment to Excellence and Professional Development

Excellence has been defined as "a conscientious effort to exceed ordinary expectations and to make a commitment to lifelong learning."[20] Professionals must also be committed to lifelong learning, maintaining our medical knowledge, and the provision of quality clinical care. As a profession, we must strive to keep all our members competent and to ensure appropriate mechanisms are in place to accomplish this goal.[39]

Not only is professional development the ongoing maintenance of a current certificate, the maintenance of continuing medical education, or the learning of new procedures, but it also goes beyond self and out to the profession as a whole. We are committed to maintaining and advancing our knowledge, and by this standard, we are also committed to "work collaboratively to maximize patient care, be respectful of one another, and participate in the process of self-regulation, including remediation and discipline of members who have failed to meet professional standards."[16] We also have an obligation to participate in these processes by volunteering for review boards, working on educational and standard-setting processes, and accepting external review of everything that we do.

Examples of excellence and professional development include, but are not limited to, mastering techniques (whether new or already learned), developing and setting goals, teaching self and others, and helping to develop or maintain a climate that fosters professionalism. Wilkinson defines this as having a commitment to autonomous maintenance and continuous improvement of competence.[22] Professional development also extends to working on local, state, or federal levels to promote the profession and access to health care; giving back to society, which helped educate us through being our patients, care receivers, and teachers; and teaching the next generation of care providers by mentoring new students and demonstrating professionalism first hand.

Demonstrate Self-Reflection, Critical Curiosity, and Initiative

A key part of lifelong learning is the ability to reflect on performance in practice. Self-reflection starts with the identification of an incident that challenged one's values, beliefs, or understanding. Learning from the incident involves accessing resources to increase understanding followed by considering how the situation might have been handled differently. In many situations, things are made more challenging by the complexity and uncertainty that is an ever-present part of caring for patients. Often, it leads to making plans for future learning.[40]

Another aspect of lifelong learning is self-assessment, which involves assessing one's strengths, identifying areas for additional learning, and then showing initiative to pursue appropriate learning experiences.[41] Self-regulation is a hallmark feature of professionalism, and self-assessment is essential to that process.[42]

Know Professional and Personal Limitations

One specific aspect of self-assessment is to know one's limitations. During the process of patient care, PAs may be challenged by situations in which they may need to judge whether or not they possess the knowledge and skill necessary to address the patient's needs. The quality of care delivered and patient safety depend on the PA engaging in effective self-assessment. Simply put, it is essential that you know what you do not know and know where to get help. With the physician–PA team, immediate access to assistance is built in to the patient care delivery model.

Practice Without Impairment

When identifying strengths and weaknesses in the self-assessment, one needs to be aware of any limitations from impairment. Such assessments also extend to being aware of impairment in other members of the team. Impairment has been defined as "any physical, mental, or behavioral disorder that interferes with the ability to engage safely in professional activities."[43] Other conditions that may ultimately result in impairment include fatigue, stress, and burnout. It is a professional obligation to ensure the public that its practitioners are capable of practicing safely. It is the responsibility of the PA to self-identify or for colleagues to intervene. A key goal is to remove the PA from practice either temporarily or permanently, which may ultimately mean placing the profession ahead of personal and professional relationships.

FOSTERING PROFESSIONALISM

Professionalism has been identified as the most difficult of the six competencies to foster and assess.[2] Despite these challenges, 30 years of focused attention has resulted in much progress being made in developing policies and procedures around professionalism, curricula that explicitly focus on professionalism, and methods of assessing lapses in professionalism.[15]

Many methodologies are currently in use to teach professionalism, including courses, workshops, problem-based learning, flipped classroom, role playing, simulated patients, and trigger films.[44-46] Professionalism can best be taught when students see positive examples of this competency modeled by their instructors and clinical preceptors. Conversely, what is learned in the classroom can be undermined by the "hidden curriculum," when unprofessional practices by preceptors are observed by students in clinical settings.[2,47]

Powerful symbolic tools can be used to reinforce the importance of professionalism in clinical practice. The White Coat Ceremony, with its imagery of putting on the white coat, can be used to remind students of the need to incorporate professionalism into their patient interactions.[2] Similarly, the graduation oaths taken by students signify entry into the profession of medicine with an associated commitment of the graduate to adopt the tenets of professionalism.

A number of effective ways to assess professionalism exist, including one-on-one counseling, role playing, case simulation review, peer assessment, objective structured clinical examinations (OSCEs), critical incident reports, and learner-maintained portfolios. To date, the most effective assessment tool is having preceptors directly observe student behavior in real-life clinical situations. However, the 360-degree evaluation shows promise as a tool for effectively evaluating professionalism, and multiple methods should always be used when assessing professionalism.[44-49] Another way of thinking about assessing professionalism is along a continuum similar to "Bloom's taxonomy." One progresses from basic knowledge or knowing (does the student know and understand the principles of professionalism?) through to advancing levels of doing (can the practitioner use all he or she has learned and advocate for the patient in complex systems?). With this continuum in mind, Hawkins and colleagues show how assessment activities can be appropriately targeted. For example, knowing can be assessed through testing methods or discussions and doing through chart review.[50] Areas that remain difficult to assess and do not have clear methodology for assessment include self-assessment (can the student or clinician self-assess and correct over time?); lifelong learning (does it occur, and how often); advocacy (for patients, families, and the profession); balancing availability and care for oneself; and advancing knowledge at many levels, not just medicine.[18] It remains incumbent on all PAs, whether in the learning phase or during practice, that every effort to assess, advance, and reflect on professionalism and all that it means is done regularly because by doing so, we advance ourselves, our practice, and our profession.

CONCLUSION

With the defining of competencies for the PA profession, the competency of professionalism is receiving increased attention. In fact, the National Commission on Certification of Physician Assistants has revised the certification maintenance process to include the completion of self-assessment modules. PAs are reminded of the importance of developing a "professional self," one that maintains a commitment to practicing in accordance with the values of medicine, particularly caring for the patient, and not just focusing on knowledge and skills. Success in learning about professionalism depends on recognizing that the purpose of such education is to reinforce the public, collective promise to make a priority the patient's interest and that such endeavors require hard work and focused attention over one's career.[51] Caring for the patient means focusing on the needs and welfare of that patient rather than the PA's self-interest.[52,53]

CLINICAL APPLICATIONS

- Think of a time when a "professional" treated you with unprofessional behavior. How did that make you feel, and how could the situation have been handled more appropriately?

- Discuss with a classmate how you might handle a clinical encounter when a patient requests something that you feel morally opposed to. Which of the Physician Assistant Competencies concerning professionalism might apply to this situation?
- Think about areas in your own professional development that might need to be worked on and how you might approach these areas in a positive manner.

CASE STUDY 33.1

Your daughter is scheduled to graduate from high school this afternoon. As you are completing morning rounds and are preparing to sign out to a colleague, one of your long-time patients enters the emergency department (ED) with substernal chest pain. The ED physician believes that a workup for acute myocardial infarction (MI) is warranted. You enter the ED and find another PA from your practice preparing to evaluate the situation. You know the PA to be competent and conscientious, so you plan to get home to assist in preparations for the event. When you see the patient to reassure him that he is in good hands, he pleads with you to stay and oversee his care. Apprehensively, he says, "I will feel so much better if you are here."
- Which of the four areas of professional behavior does this situation illustrate?
- What are your thoughts on an appropriate course of action?

This case is used with permission from the American Board of Internal Medicine's Project Professionalism.[20]

CASE STUDY 33.2

An unscheduled follow-up office visit awaits you. You learn that the patient whom you are seeing for the first time is returning because her urinary symptoms have not resolved. During your interaction with the patient, you discover that the electronic medical record contains an inaccurate reference to a pelvic examination that was documented as having been done during the earlier examination by a PA colleague. On further questioning of the patient, you determine that a pelvic examination was not done, and the patient was apparently treated on the basis of a cursory history by that PA.
- Which of the four areas of professional behavior does this situation illustrate?
- What are your thoughts on an appropriate course of action? Would your course of action change if the person involved was your supervising physician?

This case is used with permission from the National Commission on Certification of Physician Assistants' Foundation's *Concepts in PA Excellence: Exploring Ethics.*[54]

KEY POINTS

- Professionalism is incorporated throughout the training and professional careers of all health care providers.
- It is incumbent on each member of the PA profession to uphold and foster the tenets of professionalism as described in the Competencies for the Physician Assistant Profession.
- Professionalism embodies behavior toward the patient, behavior toward other professionals, behavior toward the public, and behavior toward oneself.
- Being part of the profession means always being aware that you will be recognized as a PA no matter what the situation is, whether in the role of a care provider or in everyday activities.
- Society grants different groups the privilege and status of a profession, but if the tenets are not upheld, society has the right to remove that status.

ACKNOWLEDGMENT

The authors recognize the contributions of the late Paul Robinson to the initial version of this chapter.

References

1. Swick HM. Toward a normative definition of medical professionalism. *Acad Med*. 2000;75:612.
2. Cohen JJ. Professionalism in medical education, an American perspective: from evidence to accountability. *Med Educ*. 2006;40:607.
3. Swick HM, Bryan CS, Longo LD. Beyond the physician charter: reflections on medical professionalism, perspectives in biology and medicine. *Perspect Biol Med*. 2006;49:263.
4. Cruess RL, Cruess SR, Johnston SE. Renewing professionalism: an opportunity for medicine. *Acad Med*. 1999;74:878.
5. Hooker R, Cawley J. *Current Status: A Profile of the Profession in Physician Assistants in American Medicine*. St. Louis: Churchill-Livingstone; 2003:67.
6. Tworek RK. Professionalization of an allied health occupation: the physician's assistant. *J Allied Health*. 1981;10:107.
7. Gianola FJ. Mortality, professionalism, and clinical ethics. *Perspect Phys Assist Educ*. 2004;15:135.
8. Accreditation Review Commission for Education of the Physician Assistant (ARC-PA), American Academy of Physician Assistants (AAPA), National Commission on Certification of Physician Assistants (NCCPA), Physician Assistant Education Association (PAEA, formerly Association of Physician Assistant Programs). Competencies for the Physician Assistant Profession (website). http://www.nccpa.net/Uploads/docs/PACompetencies.pdf. Accessed March 25, 2016.
9. Sullivan WM. What is left of professionalism after managed care? *Hastings Cent Rep*. 1999;29:7.
10. Woodruff JN, Angelos P, Valaitis S. Medical professionalism: one size fits all? *Perspect Biol Med*. 2008;51(4):525–534.
11. Birden H, Glass N, Wilson I, Harrison M, Usherwood T, Nass D. Defining professionalism in medical education: a systematic review. *Med Teach*. 2014;36(1):47–61.
12. Cruess SR, Cruess RL. Teaching professionalism—why, what, and how. *Facts Views Vis Obgyn*. 2012;4(4):259–265.
13. Hafferty FW. What medical students know about professionalism. *Mt Sinai J Med*. 2002;69:385.
14. Papadakis MA, Hodgson CS, Teherani A, Kohatsu ND. Unprofessional behavior in medical school is associated with subsequent disciplinary action by a state medical board. *Acad Med*. 2004;79:244.
15. Ziring D, Danoff D, Grosseman S, et al. How do medical schools identify and remediate professionalism lapses in medical students? A study of U.S. and Canadian medical schools. *Acad Med*. 2015;90(7):1–8.
16. Van de Camp K, Vernooij-Dassen M, Grol R, Bottema B. How to conceptualize professionalism: a qualitative study. *Med Teach*. 2004;26:696.
17. Van de Camp K, Vernooij-Dassen M, Grol R, Bottema B. Professionalism in general practice: development of an instrument to assess professional behavior in general practitioner trainees. *Med Educ*. 2006;40:43.
18. Accreditation Council on Graduate Medical Education. Common Program Requirements-IV.A.5: ACGME Competencies (website). https://www.acgme.org/acgmeweb/tabid/429/ProgramandInstitutionalAccreditation/CommonProgramRequirements.aspx. Accessed March 25, 2016.
19. Hawkins RE, Weiss KB, American Board of Medical Specialties. Maintenance of Certification Program (website). http://www.abms.org/About_Board_Certification/MOC.aspx. Accessed March 25, 2016.
20. American Board of Internal Medicine. Medical professionalism and the physician charter (website). http://abimfoundation.org/what-we-do/medical-professionalism-and-the-physician-charter. Accessed March 25, 2016.
21. McGaghie WC, Mytko JJ, Brown WN, Cameron JR. Altruism and compassion in the health professions: a search for clarity and precision. *Med Teach*. 2002;24:374.
22. National Board of Medical Examiners. Embedding professionalism in medical education: assessment as a tool for implementation (website). http://www.nbme.org/PDF/Publications/Professionalism-Conference-Report-AAMC-NBME.pdf. Accessed March 25, 2016.
23. Wilkinson TJ, Wade WB, Knock LD. A blueprint to assess professionalism: results of a systematic review. *Acad Med*. 2009;84:551.
24. Piliavin JA, Charng H. Altruism: a review of recent theory and research. *Annu Rev Sociol*. 1990;16:27.
25. Racy J. Professionalism: sane and insane. *J Clin Psychiatry*. 1990;51:138.
26. Cruess R, McIlroy J, Cruess S, et al. The professionalism mini-evaluation exercise: a preliminary investigation. *Acad Med*. 2006;81:S74.
27. Connelly JE, DalleMura S. Ethical problems in the medical office. *JAMA*. 1988;260:812.
28. Kollemorten I, Strandberg C, Thomsen BM, et al. Ethical aspects of clinical decision making. *J Med Ethics*. 1981;7:67.
29. U.S. Census Bureau. U.S. interim projections by age, sex, race, and Hispanic origin (website). http://www.census.gov/population/projections/data/national/2014.html. Accessed March 25, 2016.
30. Betancourt J. Cross-cultural medical education: conceptual approaches and frameworks for evaluation. *Acad Med*. 2003;78:560.
31. Betancourt J, Green A, Carrillo JE, Park E. Cultural competence and health care disparities: key perspectives and trends. *Health Affairs*. 2005;24:499.
32. The PEW Health Care Commission. *Charting a Course for the Twenty-First Century: Physician Assistants and Managed Care*. San Francisco: University of California San Francisco Center for the Health Professions; 1998.
33. Leavitt M. *Institute of Medicine Committee on Quality of Health Care in America. Crossing the Quality Chasm: A New Health System for the 21st Century*. Landover, MD: National Academies Press; 2001.
34. Shapiro J, Whittemore A, Tsen LC. Instituting a culture of professionalism: the establishment of a center for professionalism and peer support. *Jt Comm J Qual Patient Saf*. 2014;40(4):168–177.
35. American Academy of Physician Assistants. Guidelines for Ethical Conduct (website). https://www.aapa.org/workarea/downloadasset.aspx?id=815. Accessed March 25, 2016.
36. Hilton S, Slotnick H. Proto-professionalism: how professionalisation occurs across the continuum of medical education. *Med Ed*. 2005;39:58.
37. Kohn LT, Corrigan JM, Donaldson MS, eds. *To Err Is Human: Building a Safer Health System*. Washington, DC: National Academies Press; 1999.
38. American Academy of Physician Assistants. *From Program to Practice. A Guide to the PA Profession*. Alexandria, VA: American Academy of Physician Assistants; 2007.
39. ABIM Foundation, ACP-ASIM Foundation, European Federation of Internal Medicine. Medical professionalism in the new millennium: a physician charter. *Ann Intern Med*. 2002;136:243.
40. Stark P, Roberts C, Newble D, Bax N. Discovering professionalism through guided reflection. *Med Teach*. 2006;28:25.

41. Westberg J, Jason H. Fostering learners' reflection and self-assessment. *Fam Med*. 1994;26:278.

42. Eva KW, Regehr G. Self-assessment in the health professions: a reformulation and research agenda. *Acad Med*. 2005;80:S46.

43. American Medical Association. PolicyFinder Database: H-95.955, Physician impairment (website). http://www.ama-assn.org/go/policyfinder. Accessed March 25, 2016.

44. Ber R, Alroy G. Teaching professionalism with the aid of trigger films. *Med Teach*. 2002;24:528.

45. Stephenson A, Higgs R, Sugarman J. Teaching professional development in medical schools. *Lancet*. 2001;357:867.

46. Khandelwal A, Nugus P, Elkoushy MA, et al. How we made professionalism relevant to twenty-first century residents. *Med Teach*. 2015;37(6):538–542. http://dx.doi.org/10.3109/01421 59X.2014.990878. Epub 2015 Jan 16.

47. Duff P. Teaching and assessing professionalism in medicine. *Obstet Gynecol*. 2004;104:1362.

48. Stern DT. *Measuring Medical Professionalism*. Oxford, England: Oxford University Press; 2006.

49. Stern DT, Papadakis M. The developing physician—becoming a professional. *N Engl J Med*. 2006;355:1794.

50. Hawkins RE, Katsufrakis PJ, Holtman MC, Clauser BE. Assessment of medical professionalism: who, what, when, where, how, and … why? *Med Teach*. 2009;31:385.

51. Brody H, Doukas D. Professionalism: a framework to guide medical education. *Med Educ*. 2014;48:980–987.

52. Hafferty FW. Professionalism—the next wave. *N Engl J Med*. 2006;355:2151.

53. Orr R, Pang N, Pellegrino E, Siegler M. Use of the Hippocratic oath: a review of twentieth century practice and a content analysis of oaths administered in medical schools in the U.S. and Canada in 1993. *J Clin Ethics*. 1997;8:377.

54. Lombardo P, Cohn R, Goldgar C. In: *Concepts in PA Excellence: Exploring Ethics*. Duluth, GA: National Commission on the Certification of Physician Assistants Foundation; 2006.

The resources for this chapter can be found at www.expertconsult.com.

The faculty resources can be found online at www.expertconsult.com.

CHAPTER 34

CLINICAL ETHICS

Jason Lesandrini • Kevin Michael O'Hara • Emily Joy Jensen

CHAPTER OUTLINE

Every clinical and public health decision has ethical components that are at times difficult to recognize and process. As John Glaser noted, there are "no ethics free zones."[1,2] In the context of clinical care, ethical awareness is as essential as pathophysiology to bring about a successful patient outcome. For the physician assistant (PA), the stage is set for complex ethical dilemmas given their role in decision making and leadership. Also, being a dependent practitioner embedded within a complex health care team is apt for ethical dilemmas or uncertainty. Given the ubiquitous nature of ethical issues, all clinicians must familiarize themselves with ethical analysis and decision making. The study and application of ethics are not reserved for the ivory tower or owned by an ethics consultation services: Significant and complex ethical conundrums emerge in all clinical settings with great frequency, and thus each provider will need to have a foundation in moral reasoning to assist in achieving excellent patient care. This chapter provides that foundation and is germane for PAs at all levels of their career.

CHAPTER ORGANIZATION

This chapter constructs a foundation in ethics by introducing relevant historical and contemporary ethics cases alongside the methods of clinical ethics analysis. The organization of this chapter is unique in that we deliver the majority of ethics learning objectives through case-based reasoning. Our approach is functional for the study and application of clinical ethics. This case-based methodology relies less on formal theories, although we will discuss them intermittently throughout. Our goal is to provide practicing clinicians with a general understanding of some common ethical issues one might see in a variety of practice settings. Through this broad survey, we hope to provide a foundational understanding of certain ethical terms, principles, and theories that are generalizable to other situations. Given this textbook's diverse readership, the case studies presented highlight issues for the PA as a student, educator, clinician, and leader.

WHAT IS ETHICS?

Clinical ethics is the field of study and applied practice toward ethical issues that arise in the practice of medicine.[3] Those practicing ethics specialize in areas such as business, policy, and bioethics. The specialty of bioethics focuses on moral dilemmas as they intersect with biology and the policies and practices of medicine. Encompassed within this broad field are ethical queries within the areas of clinical, public health, and research. This text is predominately focused on clinical ethics but introduces public health and research ethics.

Ethical uncertainties and dilemmas are ubiquitous regardless of clinical setting or specialty. When a clinician is asked to identify bioethical cases, she or he might turn to visible and often deliberated end-of-life issues. This period in the life course engenders ethical issues such as futility, the right to refuse, surrogate decision making, and physician-assisted suicide. Additional oft-mentioned ethical dilemmas such as conflict of interest, decision-making capacity, and informed consent are equally visible. However, many of the more prevalent ethical issues are less palpable. These include ethical questions such as How much time will you spend with a patient? Should you prescribe a less effective treatment because it does not require insurance company prior authorization or costs less? Will you penalize patients who are late, unvaccinated, or nonadherent with a treatment plan?

THEORIES AND PRINCIPLES

The literature on theories of clinical ethics is vast, ranging from applications of standard ethical theories, such as consequentialism to virtue and newer interpretations of narrative ethics. Although these established theories are often useful and valuable to ethical decision making, our preference is to think about ethics cases in a more comprehensive manner using values, principles, concepts, or ethical considerations that factor in the care of patients. This is different from the theory-based approach that most authors use that focuses on a central value or values. Many of our readers are well aware of the "four principles" of health care ethics[3]: autonomy, nonmaleficence, beneficence, and justice. However, we believe that focusing on only principles is too narrow for clinical ethics. Thus, throughout our case presentations, discussion, and analysis, we invoke a larger array of principles, theories, concepts, and values. This method provides readers with a broader depth of knowledge of ethics and practical application in addressing ethical issues.

METHODOLOGY

To assist with decision making and resolution of complex ethics cases that arise during the daily care of patients, many individuals have developed frameworks and case analysis methodologies.[4–9] Our preference in methodology is a hybrid that includes three methods.[5,6,10] The core of our method is the approach developed by Kladjian et al.,[10] which views ethics cases with a reasoning process similar to all clinical encounters (Fig. 34.1).

This methodology provides a systematic process that readers can use to address ethical conflicts or uncertainties they face in their daily practice. We

---

1. State the problem or concern plainly

2. Gather and organize data
   a. Medical facts/indications
   b. Quality of life
   c. Patient's goals and preferences
   d. Context

3. Ask: Is the problem ethical? If so, what is the ethical question?

4. Ask: Is more information or dialogue needed?

5. Determine the best course of action, and support it with reference to one or more sources of ethical value, e.g.,

   Ethical principles: Beneficence, nonmaleficence, respect for autonomy, justice
   Rights: Protections that are independent of professional obligations
   Consequences: Estimation of the goodness or desirability of likely outcomes
   Comparable cases: Reasoning by analogy from prior cases
   Professional guidelines: AMA Code of Ethics, AAPA, ACP Ethics Manual, BMA Handbook
   Conscientious practice: Preserving the personal and professional integrity of clinicians

FIG. 34.1 ■ Clinical ethics reasoning.

will use the following case to illustrate our preferred methodology.

Mrs. Roberts is a 68-year-old woman with metastatic colon cancer that has spread to her liver and lungs. She is bedridden and is currently residing in her daughter's home. She recently was hospitalized for a severe case of pneumonia. The patient is unable to speak for herself because she also has end-stage dementia. The critical care PA approaches the patient's next of kin, her daughter Regina, about resuscitation status. Regina states resoundingly, "I want her to be resuscitated no matter what."

Mrs. Roberts never completed an advance directive and has no other living family members. The providers are concerned with resuscitating Mrs. Roberts when they state, "CPR [cardiopulmonary resuscitation] cannot bring Mrs. Roberts any clinical benefit." The clinical staff believe that resuscitation is futile and do not want to perform it. The surrogate wants CPR performed.

The first step in the process is to identify clearly the ethics problem or concern. As others have pointed out, getting clear on the presenting ethical issue is often part of the battle. In the case of Mrs. Roberts, the ethics problem is that the clinical team believes that CPR should not be initiated, and the family disagrees.

The next step in the process requires the individual to gather and organize data. In this step, we rely on another methodology to look at the broad array of facts that one needs to consider. The method is from Jonsen, Siegler, and Winslade and looks at gathering data (Fig. 34.2). Each section of "facts" looks at a different aspect of the patient's care and how it might impact the ethical decision-making process. Medical indications asks the reader to look at diagnosis, prognosis, treatment options, and goals of care of any clinical encounter. Patient preferences ask the reader to look at the clinical encounter from the patient's viewpoint, considering whether the patient can make decisions or if unable, whether he or she previously stated any preferences or whether he or she has a surrogate to make the decision.

The next step in the process asks whether the issue is really an ethics problem or concern and, if so, what the ethics question is. Mrs. Roberts' case is a classic ethical issue surrounding futility or appropriateness of initiating CPR. The ethics question is likely, given the providers' obligation to not cause unnecessary harm and to provide interventions that will benefit the patient is in conflict with the surrogate decision maker's right to decide on behalf of his or her loved one.

Next, the reader should consider whether more dialogue is needed or whether more information should be sought. In our case, perhaps the clinicians should seek outside input on the success rates of CPR in patients in Mrs. Roberts' condition. Or perhaps more dialogue with the patient's daughter is needed to determine her level of understanding.

At the crux of any ethics case, a decision will have to be made, and that decision should be based on ethics values, concepts, principles, and so on. Thus, after gathering sufficient information through chart review and meeting with the clinical team and family, an ethics recommendation should be made based on values. In the current case, one could recommend that CPR should not be performed based on the principle of nonmaleficence, claiming that starting CPR would only cause the patient unnecessary harm.

AMERICAN BIOETHICS HISTORY

This section analyzes several noteworthy moments in recent United States history that informed clinical ethics. These historical accounts are particularly useful because several illustrate ethics beyond the PA and patient encounter. This extension includes ethical dilemmas in the research and public health space. It is little surprise that many of our bioethical historical accounts took place in the 1960s and 1970s, when we find a frustrated community reaction to a dramatic technological change in the hands of physicians who practiced medicine in a paternalistic fashion. The United States is a fascinating place to study bioethics given the country's unique health economy, history of social inequality, and biotechnology growth over the past several decades.

"God Squad": An Early Ethics Committee

In 1961, a committee was formed in Seattle to determine which patients would be hooked up to a new machine designed to filter blood for those with end-stage renal disease.[11] This committee was charged with the difficult task of deciding who would receive this early and expensive form of hemodialysis. Given economic and dialysis equipment constraints, the committee would ask themselves who should be chosen and on what basis. This charge was undertaken by a committee of seven non–bioethics-trained citizens— a lawyer, minister, banker, housewife, state government official, labor leader, and surgeon—selected by the King County Medical Society.[11] They decided on factors such as gender, number of dependents, marital status, education, income, and emotional stability alongside clinical factors. Many criticized the committee of using subjective criteria and allowing for "values" to creep into what some may have claimed was a clinical decision. It was famously said, "The Pacific Northwest is no place for a Henry David Thoreau

Medical indications	Patient preferences
1. What is the patient's medical problem? Is the problem acute? Chronic? Critical? Reversible? Emergent? Terminal? 2. What are the goals of treatment? 3. In what circumstances are medical treatments not indicated? 4. What are the probabilities of success of various treatment options? 5. In sum, how can this patient be benefited by medical and nursing care, and how can harm be avoided?	1. Has the patient been informed of benefits and risks, understood this information, and given consent? 2. Is the patient mentally capable to make the requisite decision? 3. If mentally capable, what preferences about treatment is the patient stating? 4. If incapacitated, has the patient expressed prior preferences? 5. Who is the appropriate surrogate to make decisions for the incapacitated patient? 6. Is the patient unwilling or unable to cooperate with medical treatment? If so, why?
Quality of life	**Contextual features**
1. What are the prospects, with or without treatment, for a return to normal life, and what physical, mental, and social deficits might the patient experience even if treatment succeeds? 2. On what grounds can anyone judge that some quality of life would be undesirable for a patient who cannot make or express such a judgment? 3. Are there biases that might prejudice the provider's evaluation of the patient's quality of life? 4. What ethical issues arise concerning improving or enhancing a patient's quality of life? 5. Do quality-of-life assessments raise any questions regarding changes in treatment plans, such as forgoing life-sustaining treatment? 6. What are plans and rationale to forgo life-sustaining treatment?	1. Are there professional, interprofessional, or business interests that might create conflicts of interest in the clinical treatment of patients? 2. Are there parties other than clinicians and patients, such as family members, who have an interest in clinical decisions? 3. What are the limits imposed on patient confidentiality by the legitimate interests of third parties? 4. Are there financial factors that create conflicts of interest in clinical decisions? 5. Are there problems of allocation of scarce health resources that might affect clinical decisions? 6. Are there religious issues that might affect clinical decisions? 7. What are the legal issues that might affect clinical decisions? 8. Are there considerations of clinical research and education that might affect clinical decisions? 9. Are there issues of public health and safety that affect clinical decisions? 10. Are there conflicts of interest within institutions or organizations (e.g., hospitals) that may affect clinical decisions and patient welfare?

FIG. 34.2 ■ Box method. (From Jonsen AR, Siegler M, Winslade WJ. *Clinical Ethics: A Practical Approach to Ethical Decisions in Clinical Medicine,* 7th ed. New York: McGraw-Hill Medical; 2010.)

with bad kidneys,"[12] given his lack of employment, children, and religion. These concerns around the use of what some deemed inappropriate criteria led to the group being called the "God squad."

Tuskegee Study

The Tuskegee study was implemented in 1932 and remains one of the more sobering ethical violations of human experimentation in U.S. history. Tuskegee was an observational study of 399 subjects infected with syphilis matched with 200 similar but noninfected control subjects.[13] A variety of morbidity outcomes were measured with the plan to follow study participants until death. As the history of Tuskegee unfolded, it is important to understand that those enrolled in the study possessed little capacity to avoid the undue influence the researchers had over them.

Most of the research participants were illiterate, poor, and African American.[14]

By 1947, penicillin was recognized as the highly successful treatment for syphilis.[13] Despite this accessible information, the Tuskegee research team did not discontinue the study or transition to a study design that provided scientific value given the new treatment paradigm. The ability of these study participants to make autonomous decisions was further impacted by coercive practices from the research team. There are reports stating researchers made false claims of therapeutic benefit enticing participants to follow up.[14] These follow-up visits even included lumbar punctures. The study continued until 1972 when popular media and public outcry influenced public health officials.[13] In addition to the men who died of untreated syphilis, 40 wives and 19 children contracted syphilis.[14] The Tuskegee study illustrates how vulnerable communities are at risk for unethical human subject research. These communities are also at risk for unethical practice in busy clinical settings where these often-complicated patients may receive less comprehensive medicine. Many of the contemporary cases presented in this chapter highlight examples of this concern.

Common ethical dilemmas in human-subject research include unacceptable risk-to-benefit ratios, a lack of independent review and informed consent, and invalid research with low scientific value.[15] The Tuskegee study failed in each of these areas. For example, given the state of knowledge surrounding untreated syphilis and the known benefits of penicillin, the participants should have received updated informed consent. Moreover, the risk-to-benefit ratio and scientific value should have called for the cessation of the study. Second, the study design lacked oversight, accurate data collection, and overall low validity that contributed to low scientific value.[14]

Beecher Papers

In 1966, Dr. Henry K. Beecher published a landmark article titled "Ethics and Clinical Research" in the *New England Journal of Medicine*. In his paper, he reviewed 22 human-subject studies and found that many of the studies had many of the aforementioned common ethical research concerns.[16] Frequent ethical concerns included a lack of informed consent, proper study oversight, and study methods without validity or scientific utility.

Through Dr. Beecher's work, we realize that the Tuskegee study was not unique and that ethical dilemmas were prevalent throughout a variety of clinical questions, research settings, and study populations. These findings are germane to the clinical setting as well. One theme throughout Beecher's paper is how researcher bias can create unethical and invalid outcomes. Clinicians are also subject to bias, which influences the lens through which they view patient history, develop treatment plans, and deliver informed consent.

Belmont Report

The Beecher paper was one of several professional and popular publications expressing similar concern over the state of U.S. human-subject research during the 1960s and 1970s. The National Commission for the Protection of Human Subjects of Biomedical and Behavioral Research was formed out of the National Research act of 1974.[17] The commission produced a summary document titled the "Belmont Report" that established ethical principles necessary for acceptable human-subject research. The major themes were respect for persons, beneficence, and justice. This report helped articulate the ethically relevant goals of research that differ from goals in a PA and patient interaction. The Belmont report contributed to the movement that led to institutional review board requirements. These review boards have several charges, including ethical analysis of human-subject research.

Quinlan Case

Throughout the era in which the Dr. Beecher and the Belmont papers were authored, we saw innovative and paradigm-shifting technological change in medicine, including critical care and mechanical ventilation. Some of these changes created ethical questions for which little precedent existed. We see similar unprecedented technological developments today with deep brain stimulation, reproductive technology, and genetic testing.

In 1975, Karen Quinlan, at the age of 21 years, consumed alcohol along with a benzodiazepine or barbiturate at a party. This led to a prolonged respiratory suppression, resulting in her sustaining a brain injury. Ultimately, Karen would be diagnosed as being in a persistent vegetative state. At the hospital, she was placed on a ventilator and nasogastric tube for nutrition. Karen experienced decorticate posturing while in this vegetative state. We now know that recovery from this state is very unlikely. The family had little help and was concerned about her suffering, which led to a request for withdrawal of ventilator support in the fall of 1975.[18,19]

The physicians caring for Karen feared criminal and malpractice repercussions and did not follow through with the family's request for ventilator cessation.[19] This issue went before a lower court, which expressed uncertainty as to what Karen would have wanted in this situation given lack of advanced directives and allowed for the continuation of the ventilator. Ultimately, in 1976 the New Jersey Supreme Court heard the case and found that the family of a dying incompetent patient can decide what a dying patient would have wanted, provided the surrogate can establish this preference according to state-specific standards for evidence. However, the hesitant clinicians and Catholic hospital were reluctant "to kill this patient."[18]

The Quinlans, in conjunction with the clinical team, made the decision to wean Karen off the ventilator. The family was unaware that this slow process might result in the return of respiration. As a result, Karen resumed breathing without assistance but continued in this persistent vegetative state.[18] She spent the next 10 years in a nursing home in a vegetative state. The family did not think they had all the information to decide on a weaning process versus immediate cessation of ventilation.

This simplified historical account of Karen Quinlan highlights several areas in which ethical discourse has and continues to contribute significantly toward the practice of medicine. First, how do we define death? Second, what is considered extraordinary medical action in the setting of a persistent vegetative state? Third, how can we be confident that a substitutive judgment made by the surrogate reflects the preferences of the patient for whom the decision is being made?

CASES

Case Study 34.1 SHARED DECISION MAKING

DECISION-MAKING CAPACITY

Ms. Smith is a 26-year-old woman with a medical history significant for a developmental disorder with an unknown etiology, manifesting in an intellectual disability (IQ between 60 and 80). She presents to the clinic with her husband today complaining of difficulty conceiving. This is her third time presenting to the clinic over the past few years. Primary conception guidance was given to the patient and her husband during the previous two visits, but the patient never followed up. Ms. Smith denies any family history of conceiving or any other concerns. The patient asks the PA directly for Clomid, as she states, "I need help conceiving." The risk factors of using medication are discussed with her and her husband at length, as the patient is at high risk for complications. In addition,

she is informed that a strict regimen must be maintained when using these medications; failure to do so increases her chances of having an adverse outcome. The patient states, "I don't care about these risks. Just give me the medications." The PA attempts to follow up for understanding and why she does not care, and the patient provides no response. Should the PA prescribe the medication?

This case hinges on whether the patient has decision-making capacity regarding the proposed or requested intervention. Decision-making capacity is a set of cognitive abilities that a patient possesses. The components of decision-making capacity include the ability to understand the information, evaluate the risks and benefits of the proposed plan, use reason to weigh the decision, and communicate a decision (Fig. 34.3).[20–22]

It is key that all understand that capacity is decision specific, so in the case of Ms. Smith, she may not have the ability to make a decision regarding Clomid, but that does not mean she lacks capacity for other medical decisions. Each decision must be assessed separately. This is not to claim that a formal check box approach to decision-making capacity is best. Rather, this process for checking a patient's capacity is often an internal dialogue for the PA that gauges the patient's cognitive abilities.

It is also important to mention that mental illness or psychiatric disorder does not automatically eliminate the possibility for a patient to have decision-making capacity. Studies have shown that patients with numerous mental illnesses maintain the set of cognitive abilities required to possess decision-making capacity.[22,23] There may be parts of the information that Ms. Smith cannot understand (e.g., she may be unable to comprehend that one risk or benefit of taking Clomid is the increased chance of having twins or triplets), but simply because she is developmentally disabled does not mean she lacks capacity.

In terms of the ethical decision-making framework discussed earlier, capacity is the essential ethical concept and the ethical appropriateness of providing the patient the medication hinges on whether she has capacity. If she does, we believe it would be ethically permissible to provide her with the medication even though there are increased risks to providing the drug. If it is determined that the patient lacks decision-making capacity, it may be ethically permissible to refuse to provide the medication until further conversations could be had with her authorized decision maker. The case is particularly ethically complex because, if the patient does not have the capacity to make the decision regarding the medication, her surrogate—in this case, her husband—could be authorized to consent to it.

INFORMED CONSENT

Mrs. Garcia is a 46-year-old Argentinian woman with a past medical history of hepatitis C. She

Ability	Questions to ask[7,20-23]
Understand	Please tell me in your own words what you know about a) the nature of your condition; b) the recommended treatment (or diagnostic test); c) any other possible treatments that could be used.
Evaluate	Please tell me in your own words what you know about a) the potential benefits from the treatment; b) the potential risks (or discomforts) of the treatment; c) the risks and benefits of any other possible treatments; d) the potential risks and benefits of no treatment at all.
Reason	1. Tell me how you reached the decision to accept (reject) the recommended treatment. 2. What were the factors that were important to you in reaching the decision? 3. How did you balance those factors?
Communicate	Can you tell me what your decision is?

FIG. 34.3 ■ Decision-making capacity.

moved to the United States from Argentina 15 years ago with her children. Her husband works full time while she has cared for her three children and their home, speaking primarily in her native language. Her family has heard of new medications that are curing hepatitis C and want Mrs. Garcia to begin treatment. Her primary care physician makes a referral to a local hepatology office. Mrs. Garcia, Mr. Garcia, and their eldest daughter arrive at the appointment. Upon initial intake survey with the medical assistant, they refuse interpretation services, and the family states that the patient is a fluent English speaker. After the patient and family are roomed, the hepatology PA again recommends the presence of an interpreter during this appointment. The PA has a concern that the in-depth discussion that is required to educate about the benefits and risks of hepatitis C treatment will not be fully understood by the patient. The family and patient continue to refuse interpretation services because they can "understand English." The PA agrees because of time constraints.

After reviewing Mrs. Garcia's past medical history and laboratory study results, the PA decides the appropriate medication regimen. The PA then attempts to have a conversation with the patient and family about treatment options, medication compliance, adverse effects, and risks and benefits of the proposed hepatitis C treatment course.

Throughout the interaction, the PA makes a concerted effort to ensure the patient understands by trying to engage in direct dialogue with the patient. The patient often looks to her husband and daughter for reassurance and understanding. The daughter interprets portions of the interaction and states: "We all understand." However, the PA has a concern that the patient may be agreeing to treatment without shared decision making that is necessary for informed consent to treatment. The patient states, "I am willing to do anything to be cured of hepatitis C." Has Mrs. Garcia provided adequate informed consent about her hepatitis C treatment? Should the PA agree to provide the medication to treat the patient's hepatitis C?

Informed consent is the practical application of respect for the patients' autonomy.[6] When a patient seeks medical treatment, he or she is seeking expert advice about diagnosis; treatment options; and depending on patient preference, recommendations on treatment. Seeking medical treatment is rooted in trust. The patient trusts the provider will avoid causing harm and will act for the greatest benefit of the patient. The process of informed consent requires mutual participation, good communication, and mutual respect between the provider and the patient. The provider should explain the nature of the patient's problem, recommend a course of treatment and provide reasons for the recommendation, propose options for alternative therapies, and explain the benefits and risks of all options. The goals are for the patient to understand the information, assess treatment choices, and agree or disagree with the provider's recommendation.[6]

A provider needs to ensure that informed consent is obtained with every medical decision or intervention. As a provider, you have an obligation to have a conversation with your patient. The information the PA provides should be presented in an educationally, linguistically, and culturally accessible manner. This will assist the PA in assessing the patient's decision-making capacity. Mutual participation between the patient and provider is necessary to discuss the medical problem and recommend and discuss options. To contribute her or his part of the relationship, the PA should disclose all necessary information about the disease, prognosis, recommended intervention, and choices. Finally, after determining that the patient understands and has decision-making capacity and the provider discloses necessary information, the provider should ensure that the patient has voluntarily decided to accept or reject the therapeutic option recommended. Following these steps will ensure the patient has provided informed consent for each clinical scenario.

In this case, the PA provides his opinion about the nature of the patient's problem: hepatitis C treatment to cure the patient. He has a lengthy discussion about the course of treatment, risk, and benefits, but because of the refusal of an interpreter, the interaction was without what the PA perceived as mutual participation. The PA is unsure if the patient has an understanding of her options or if she has other questions about the risks, benefits, and possible adverse effects of the new hepatitis C medications. Because of the uncertainty on behalf of the PA, we believe the patient did not provide informed consent. It would be ethically permissible to wait to provide her with the hepatitis C medication until informed consent was obtained. One option would include the PA's requiring the presence of a trained medical interpreter to facilitate a conversation with the patient. This conversation could work toward fulfilling the criteria for ethically appropriate informed consent. Suggesting Mrs. Garcia to return to the clinic for a second appointment to continue the process would be advisable. This ensures that the patient voluntarily agrees to the treatment and that she will be able to follow the plan of treatment rather than what appears to a lack of understanding or mere agreement with her family's decisions. Mrs. Garcia and her family trust that the PA will provide only the best care. However, that trust does not ensure the patient knows or can recognize signs or symptoms of the drugs' adverse effects.

SURROGATE DECISION MAKING

Mr. Johnson is a 77-year-old man who presented to the hospital after being found with altered mental status in a local mall. He arrives at the hospital, and the clinical team begins their workup. Upon their review of his electronic medical record, they determine that he was recently diagnosed with esophageal cancer, and initial imaging studies suggest metastatic disease present in several bones and both his liver and brain. Before any further review can be done, Mr. Johnson has a cardiac arrest and is unresponsive for at least 20 minutes. Mr. Johnson is subsequently admitted to the intensive care unit (ICU) for further workup. While in the ICU, he continues to decline and requires escalating levels of care (i.e., increased pressor and ventilator support). The medical team feels reasonably confident that Mr. Johnson will not survive this hospital admission, perhaps not even the next few days. On day 3 of the patient's admission, his wife arrives and meets with the medical team. The team informs her of her husband's status and that "he will not" leave the hospital alive. The patient's wife demands that the medical team pursue all aggressive measures. When the medical team asks her, "Why do you think he would want that?" she replies, "I want my husband to live." How should the provider proceed?

There are three standards that health care providers should ask surrogates to adhere to when making a decision on behalf of another individual: the patient's expressed wishes, substituted judgment, and best interest. When surrogates make decisions on behalf of another individual, we are in essence asking them to stand in the shoes of the patient for the time being and make a decision as they believe the patient would. Thus, the first standard asks the surrogate to consider the patient's clearly expressed wishes from the past and whether they cover the current situation. For example, if Mr. Johnson had stated that he would not want to be placed on breathing machine, regardless of the circumstances, the surrogate should consider whether these wishes would apply in the current situation. In this setting, some have called the surrogate more of an information provider rather than a decision maker because the surrogate is providing information to the medical team regarding the patient's wishes.

If a patient's wishes are unknown, then a surrogate should switch to making a decision based on substituted judgment. A concept borrowed from the legal realm, substituted judgment requires the surrogate to consider the patient's past goals, values, and behaviors to make an inference about what the patient might want in the current context. For example, a patient may have lived her life running every day, enjoying the interactions of others, seeing real value in the ability to interact with her family, and so on. From these life experiences and past behaviors, surrogates are asked to make an inference about what the patient would want in the current state given this information.

If the above two are not applicable (i.e., a patient whom the surrogate is unaware of any relevant past behaviors, values, or goals or has no expressed wishes), then the surrogate should switch to a best interest standard of decision making. This standard requires the surrogate to take a more disconnected approach to decision making and consider what a reasonable person might want in the given circumstances. The surrogate should consider what a reasonable individual might perceive about the treatment plan.

In the current situation, the wife's language should give the providers pause because she appears to make decisions for her husband from her own standpoint and not based on the patient's preference. The medical team should work with her to understand whether the patient had ever clearly expressed preferences regarding the end of life, and if not, how a substituted judgment or best interest standard may apply. It may be helpful to the clinical team to consult their local ethics consultation service to assist with the decision-making process. The ethics consultation service can work with the clinical team and patient's family to determine if the patient ever discussed his disease with any other clinical providers. In addition, they can help explain to the team and wife what this preference means in this context.

It is likely given the progress of the patient's disease that some of his previous health care providers have discussed these issues with him and, if not, that the patient has exhibited behaviors in the past that one could use to infer about what he might want now. This is not to say that all interventions should be offered; rather, a medical team should offer those that they see as clinically appropriate and consistent with his goals, values, and behavior.

ADVANCE CARE PLANNING

Ms. Arnold is a 67-year-old woman who presented to the hospital after being found unresponsive. The emergency department physicians believe the patient has sustained a severe stroke and admit her to the neurologic ICU. Upon neuroendovascular workup, the patient is found to have had an aneurysm. She is placed in a medically induced coma given the severity of the aneurysm. Susan, the patient's surrogate decision maker, arrives at the hospital later that day with Ms. Arnold's advance directive. The documents specify that Susan will be the patient's health care power of attorney and will have all the rights afforded to her as such. In addition, the patient has completed a living will that specifies that she does not want to be intubated. Susan presents the paperwork to the PA and asks

that the patient be immediately taken off the ventilator. The ICU team is concerned with Susan's decision making but understand that the patient indicated that she did not want to be placed on a breathing machine. They are particularly concerned because the patient has a reasonable chance of regaining normal functioning, but it will take a significant amount of time to determine her prognosis and for her to recover. Should the medical team follow the surrogate's request to follow the advance directive and take the patient off the ventilator?

Advance directives are written or oral statements patients make during a time of capacity regarding the preferences and wishes for treatment during a period of incapacity. There are generally two types of advance directives: living wills and health care agent appointments. Living wills are documents in which a patient records his or her future treatment preferences. Most living wills specify interventions that a patient would or would not want in a future health state (e.g., ventilation, surgery). Most living wills specify certain medical criteria that need to be met before the treatment preferences are activated. For example, some states require that treatment preferences are conditioned on the patient's imminent death or that the patient is in a certain neurologic state (e.g., permanently unconscious).

Health care agent appointments designate individuals whom the patient wants to make decisions for him or her in the event the person cannot make the decisions him- or herself. Usually, patients select a decision maker whom they can trust to make decisions that the patient would consider authentic and reflective of his or her values, goals, and life.

Of the two documents, health care agent appointments are more flexible in that the person designated can accommodate the particularities of a certain clinical picture. However, living wills often make blanket statements (e.g., "I do not want to be placed on a ventilator") but fail to accommodate the nuances of patient preference or clinical care.

Ms. Arnold's case is particularly interesting because we do not know the specifics of her advance directive. Assuming that her directive is similar to the majority of living will documents, it is unlikely that her treatment preference section would address a fixable condition. If her treatment preferences were tied to particular clinical scenarios (e.g., terminal disease), then it is reasonable to conclude that the directive would not apply. This is not to say that the directive could not inform the decision making of the surrogate and medical team but only that it would not dictate treatment in the sense that one generally believes living wills to do so.

LIMITS TO PATIENT CHOICE

Mr. Thomas is a 64-year-old veteran who is a new patient at the practice, coming in today for his wellness visit. He has a history of diabetes, congestive heart failure, and obesity. He had scheduled an appointment with Dr. Robertson, but she called in sick today. Thus, Mr. Thomas's appointment has been moved to the PA's schedule. The PA is Tim Nguyen, a 45-year-old Asian American man who is new to the practice but has worked in health care for more than 15 years. Mr. Thomas presents to the office and learns of the change in provider for today. He is visibly upset but knows the appointment has to proceed. He goes through with the appointment, meeting with PA Nguyen for about 15 minutes. All of his questions are answered, and he leaves the examination room in what appears to be a good mood. On the way out to schedule a follow-up visit, Mr. Thomas requests to speak with the office manager. He explains to her that under no circumstance "should I ever be scheduled to see Nguyen again. I have no desire to have anyone from the East take care of me. I fought them for a reason, and don't have any desire to interact with them." The office manager can see that Mr. Thomas is extremely agitated. She does not know whether she should honor his request.

Most legal and ethics scholars agree that capacitated patients have a right to refuse recommended treatment. This right derives from the principle of autonomy that can control what providers do to them. Having this right does not entail that a patient can request or demand treatment from a provider, including choosing a provider for discriminatory reasons. Most would agree that patients are free to find providers based on their preferences (e.g., a patient may prefer a female PA to a male PA), but allowing patients to choose based on discriminatory reasons does not appear to give clinicians their due (i.e., meet the principle of justice). Furthermore, allowing such behavior to continue in a medical practice undermines the patient-provider relationship.

The challenge in the case of Mr. Thomas is that it appears that his decision to not allow PA Nguyen to care for him is based on a history that has significant consequences for the patient; that is, the patient created a frame of reference for those individuals from Eastern Asia as antagonistic and believes they are not here to help him. A clinician in this setting should attempt to understand Mr. Thomas and see if something could be done to facilitate building a relationship with the PA. If nothing can be done to repair or establish the relationship and the clinicians do not believe that having PA Nguyen treat Mr. Thomas will have a significant clinical impact on Mr. Thomas or endanger PA Nguyen, then they should inform him that they cannot honor his request. Mr. Thomas does have the opportunity to seek another provider who can fit his needs, but the practice should not in general honor request for providers based on discrimination.

CASE STUDY 34.2 PATIENT PRIVACY AND CONFIDENTIALITY

PRIVACY

A PA student is working in a rural part of Oklahoma during a family medicine rotation. Mr. O'Neil is scheduled for an appointment regarding starting an insulin pump. The PA student meets with the patient, and he is reluctant to start using the pump. The student explains to the physician that the patient thinks his life will be substantially altered (i.e., he will not be able to do all the things he wants in his life) and is against it completely. The physician enters the room and has a brief conversation with Mr. O'Neil and then states, "Listen, you know Kathy and Bill; they both have insulin pumps, and they are doing really great. Living the lives they want without any significant impediments. You should ask them." Mr. O'Neil acknowledges that he does know Kathy and Bill and tells you that he will speak with them about their insulin pumps. The PA student leaves the room feeling uncomfortable about the interaction. The student knows that working in a small town, everyone likely knows everyone, but the student is unsure if this general knowledge extends to individuals' health care problems and conditions. In addition, the PA student has also seen Kathy and Bill and knows them to be open and wonderful people. They would likely be more than willing to talk with Mr. O'Neil about using an insulin pump.

Privacy in health care is a fundamental element of the patient–clinician relationship and is ensconced in one the most significant pieces of health care legislation since the early 1990s: the Health Insurance Portability and Accountability Act (HIPAA). This makes sense because being able to trust one's health care provider hinges on the ability of being able to conceal information from others outside of that relationship.[24] For example, if I do not trust that my provider will keep health care information about me private (i.e., keep the information from outside intruders), I will be reluctant to provide truthful information, and this will have an impact on the provider's ability to care for me. But the right to privacy of health information is not absolute. It is widely recognized that health care providers have to share information with insurance companies and other clinicians to ensure appropriate care.

In the current case, it appears that the physician has violated Kathy's and Bill's privacy, and one could easily dismiss this case as relatively straightforward. But it would be too naïve of the reader to assume that this case is anything but straightforward. More than likely, these types of scenarios are all too common for rural health care providers, given the intimate relationships that smaller communities often have among their members. Although the providers should do everything they can to protect Kathy and Bill's privacy and thus not disclose information about the clinical conditions to Mr. O'Neil, there is a counterbalancing concern that he receives the best clinical care, which includes insulin via a pump. In this setting, the providers should discuss with Mr. O'Neil that other individuals have used insulin pumps before and not had a significant impact on their daily lives, leaving the "who" in general terms. Then the physician or PA could offer to Mr. O'Neil the ability to speak with patients who have used an insulin pump. At that point, the providers could approach Kathy and Bill and ask if they would be willing to talk with someone who has concerns regarding the use of an insulin pump. Failing to do so, as the case elucidates, violates the trust that patients put in their providers and chips away at the foundation of the patient–provider relationship at large.

CASE STUDY 34.3 CONFIDENTIALITY, PEDIATRICS, AND SEX

Miss Scott is a 16-year-old patient who presents to her pediatric PA for an annual physical examination. She raises several questions about safe sex. Being a consummate clinician, the PA inquires about Miss Scott's sexual history. The patient seems relieved the topic is broached and reports no sexual experiences outside of kissing a boyfriend. However, she is worried about losing her boyfriend if she does not have sex with him. She is concerned about being viewed as a prude or disinterested and thinks she will have sex with him even if she does not feel ready. The PA provides counsel and empowerment alongside proper screenings that reveal an absence of physical or structural abuse from the boyfriend. The PA offers to involve the patient's parents in this conversation, and she refuses. Should the PA discuss this issue with her parents despite her refusal? How might the PA's response change if some form of abuse is suspected or if the couple had sex already?

The PA must be aware of federal and state laws as they relate to confidentiality, sexual activity in a minor, and mandatory reporting requirements. There are more than a few variations on the law. For example, two 16-year-olds having sexual intercourse may or may not be considered illegal and may or may not be considered child abuse depending on the state. Furthermore, some states give clinicians the option to inform a child's parent or guardian if their child is seeking sexual health services provided the clinician believes it is in the child's best interest.

Clinicians working with pediatric patients must consider their relevant legal and ethical obligations in advance of these often complicated issues. The clinician should have a family discussion at the start

of the patient relationship to clearly establish when the clinician will breach confidence. This discussion allows the parent or guardian and child to proceed with greater autonomy because they are aware of what is private. It should be noted that what is agreed during this conversation creates a duty that the clinician should follow throughout the patient relationship.

The ethics of this case favor maintaining patient confidentiality. This would differ if the family had a group discussion with the clinician at the onset of the relationship in which a different expectation was agreed on. There is a duty for the clinician to maintain confidentiality. Failure to do this erodes the trust that is essential for quality clinical outcomes and proper diagnosis. Trust is of particular importance for the pediatric population because they often fail to connect behaviors with consequences because of developmental stage and need the guidance of adults, including clinicians.

CASE STUDY 34.4 ETHICAL PRACTICES IN END-OF-LIFE CARE

CARDIOPULMONARY RESUSCITATION AND DO NOT RESUSCITATE ORDERS

Mr. Brown, a 78-year-old man with mild dementia and a recent diagnosis of stage 4 pancreatic cancer, is admitted to the hospital after a ground-level fall with a displaced intertrochanteric hip fracture. Mr. Brown has emphasized to his family and physicians in the past that he does not wish for any extreme measures to keep him alive, and a do not resuscitate (DNR) and a do not intubate (DNI) order are on his chart. The orthopedic surgery team recommends open reduction and internal fixation to provide palliative fixation of the hip to alleviate pain for the patient. The family requests that the surgical and anesthesia team uphold the patient's wishes. They come to an agreement to complete the procedure under local anesthesia via nerve block and conscious sedation with no intubation. The family also requests that the surgical team not invoke an automatic suspension of DNR during surgery. The surgical and anesthesia team have reservations about agreeing to this request because they do not wish the death of a terminally ill patient to be considered a surgical death. Is it unethical to go against the explicit request of the family and patient to uphold the DNR order and initiate CPR in the operating room (OR)?

Cardiopulmonary resuscitation is a set of techniques designed to restore circulation and respirations in the event of acute cardiopulmonary arrest. It was developed in the 1960s by surgeons at Johns Hopkins and then endorsed by American Heart Association. It has become standard practice to perform CPR on all patients even though it was intended for transient and easily reversible conditions in otherwise healthy individuals.[6] The chance of survival to hospital discharge for in-hospital CPR in older people is low to moderate (11.6%–18.7%) and decreases with age.[25] Research has been done looking at the suffering and poor outcomes of CPR. Many patients have become educated of these outcomes, leading to advance directives and discussions with their surrogates about their end-of-life care. In the 1970s, the DNR order was established by many hospitals.[6] The order applies specifically to the decision to not initiate CPR and should not affect other decisions in the patient's treatment.

In modern medicine, confusion exists among providers about what the order means precisely. DNR does not mean do not treat other conditions that require interventions used commonly during CPR or Advanced Cardiovascular Life Support (e.g., vasopressors, cardioversion, intubation). Nor does it mean to withhold treatments that benefit the patient (e.g., dialysis, ICU transfer, surgery). DNR must be separated from other end-of-life decisions, and each decision must be discussed with the patient or surrogate. It is vital for the provider to clarify the goals of care early in the interaction. Communication is key— between patients and surrogates, between providers, and with nursing staff providing direct care.

In this case, the patient has stated in the past that he does not want any extreme measures to continue life, but his family and the medical team do not want his end of life to be of poor quality and filled with pain. The decision to undergo a palliative surgery is made to increase his quality of life. However, the surgical team and the family disagree on intraoperative CPR. The surgical and anesthesia team favor suspension of the DNR because of multiple arguments, including surgery puts a patient at increased risk for cardiac instability, and arrests in the OR are considered reversible because of the experienced team and equipment readily available. Surgical teams believe they should not be prevented from treating potentially reversible situations because then they will have the death of a terminally ill patient considered a surgical death.[6] When examining the opposing side, the key is that suspension of DNR order in the OR ignores the patient's rights. As medical providers, PAs must be advocates for patient rights. The PA on the primary team should recommend further discussion to occur between the family and the surgical and anesthesia team. The final decision about the intraoperative code status needs to be defined explicitly, and if disagreements occur, it is ethically permissible for the surgeon or anesthesiologist to withdraw from the case. The individual withdrawing from the case would have to appropriately transfer care to a peer or to another hospital. The family can also request a different surgeon and anesthesiologist to review the case and even request to be transferred to a different facility. Ultimately, if the DNR should stand and the patient go to the OR for surgery, if the patient has a cardiac arrest, he should not be resuscitated.

MEDICAL FUTILITY

Miss Black is a 28-year-old woman with multisystem organ failure after pulmonary embolism status post living related kidney transplant from her father. In an attempt to save her life, she was urgently placed on extracorporeal life support (ECLS), continuous veno-venous hemofiltration (CVVH), and mechanical ventilation with sedation.

On a nurse's neurologic examination, a new finding of right pupil nonreactivity is noted. The PA for the primary team repeats the exam and orders a STAT computed tomography (CT) scan of the head. CT findings show diffuse cerebral edema, and a neurologist is consulted. The neurologist notes that the patient has a diffuse anoxic brain injury with a poor prognosis with no likelihood of meaningful recovery. The neurologist states that further measures, including mannitol, steroids, and hypertonic saline or comparable therapies, will be medically futile in reversing brain swelling and will not treat the underlying process. Any further treatment will only prolong the inevitable herniation and eventual brain death. The family insists on providing all possible interventions in hope of a full recovery. The PA repeatedly explains that a full recovery is not possible, and the patient will remain in an unconscious state until her death in the hospital. The family remains insistent even in light of the treatment team's opinion that no intervention will change the outcome. Should the medical team continue with treatment as the family wishes or follow the recommendations of the neurologist?

Medical futility is the belief that interventions are unlikely to benefit the patient and would be medically ineffective,[6] that is, "that in evidence-based reasoning there is no reasonable expectation that the usually intended outcomes of a clinical intervention will occur."[26] What is more important is that this concept must be specified to be clinically useful.[27] In specifying the concept, one must focus on either goals or clinical evidence. In the case of Miss Black, the goals of treatment from the clinical standpoint differ from the goals of the family. One party to the discussion sees the goal as reversing the clinical process and restoring her to consciousness. The other party believes the goal is return her to her previous baseline function. Often, the appropriate goals and who gets to set them is the crux of futility cases.

There may also be an issue regarding what are acceptable levels of clinical evidence. The neurology team may argue that of the last 100 cases, only once did the interventions reverse the process. Thus, there is virtual certainty that the intervention will not work.[28] However, the family may see this one case as sufficient evidence to pursue the aggressive measures.

There is consensus that providers have no obligation to provide interventions that are physiologically futile (i.e., the intervention will not work at all), but most cases are not about physiologic futility. Rather, most futility cases focus on what are acceptable goals or what is the acceptable rate of success or failure.

Providers should be careful not to use "futility" as a trump card that closes down conversations between the clinical team and the patient or family. These types of cases require more communication between the clinical team and patient and family and often can be resolved on amicable terms with communication.

In the case of Miss Black, if the communication does not lead to resolution of the futility dispute, we believe that the providers would be ethically justified in withholding the intervention. We believe that further interventions would cause harm to Miss Black that is not warranted by the benefits she can receive (i.e., she cannot achieve any clinical benefits from the intervention).

HASTENING DEATH

Mrs. Jones is an 84-year-old woman with chronic obstructive pulmonary disease (COPD). She has been hospitalized three times in the past year for COPD exacerbations requiring aggressive treatment. On this admission, she has also developed pneumonia, her pulmonary function has deteriorated, and she has become debilitated. With decision-making capacity, she decides with the support of her family and medical treatment team that home hospice is her best option. She requests increased opioid dosage to ease pleuritic pain and relieve anxiety related to her respiratory status. She is prescribed 30 mg of OxyContin twice a day and 10 mg of immediate-release oxycodone every 4 hours as needed, but she is still complaining of 6 of 10 pain. The family administers the medication as needed to relieve her pain when she is home. They notice she is in a lot of pain and contact the hospice program about increasing her dosage. The hospice program sends out a nurse to assess the patient, and it is agreed that the family can increase her dosage. A new nurse arrives 3 days later to check in on Mrs. Jones. She notices the amount of pain medication being given to the patient and is concerned that the team is now just participating in the patient's death. She contacts the PA on call with her concerns. She suggests decreasing the dosage. The family is upset and asks for assistance. The case is put up for review at the hospice ethics committee to discuss whether the increased pain medications are really just the hospice participating in the patient's death.

Hospice and palliative care play a vital role in the quality of life of dying patients. This case displays the potential of hastening of the dying process by treating pain with opioids. Many providers believe that administering increased dose opioids in efforts to relieve pain may entail respiratory depression and increase the risk of dying.[6] However, a recent literature review showed that in the studies that have been performed, there was no statistically significant difference in patient survival with the higher opioid doses used or with an increase in the doses administered in the last days of life.[29] Undermedicating a patient in pain is an ethical dilemma itself. There is a fine balance and finesse that must be found in the treatment of pain in each terminally ill individual.

Relevant to the discussion is intentional versus unintentional hastening of death. The case examines if the person administering the medication is intentionally hastening the dying process or if the goal is to bring relief to the patient and death is an unintended result. The latter is otherwise known as the doctrine of double effect. The essential components of the doctrine of double effect are (1) the action must be either morally good or indifferent; (2) the bad effect must not be the means by which one achieves the good effect; (3) the good effect must be at least equivalent in importance to the bad effect; and (4) the intention must be to achieve only the good effect, with the bad effect only being an unintended side effect.[29] If the palliative intention is primary and medication doses are considered rational, then the action is ethical. If the medication is given with the primary objective to hasten death, this action would constitute euthanasia, which is not legal anywhere in the United States. Euthanasia, as defined by American Medical Association (AMA) policy, is the administration of a lethal agent by another person to a patient for the purpose of relieving the patient's intolerable and incurable suffering, resulting in the death of the patient.[30]

The ethical debate in recent years has been if a physician may respond to a competent terminally ill patient's request to assist in dying by administering a lethal drug or prescribe potentially lethal medications to be self-administered to cause death. The principal difference here is who administers the lethal drug. Self-administration of a prescribed lethal medication or combination of medications is known as physician-assisted suicide or dying, but euthanasia occurs if the provider administers the lethal medication directly.[30]

In this case, the hospice PA must weigh the ethical dilemma to treat the patient's pain with the increased dosage of pain medication, which may possibly lead to respiratory depression and death, or return to the previous regimen of pain medication that is increasing patient suffering at the end of life. We believe that the PA should continue the current pain regimen for this patient to decrease her suffering at the end of life. The PA would not be intentionally causing death when alleviating her pain but allowing her inevitable death to be without pain. It would be ethically justified to increase the pain regimen, if the patient needs it, if the end goal is to relieve pain and not to intentionally hasten the dying process.

TRANSPLANT

Ms. Thomas is a 34-year-old woman with end-stage liver disease secondary to alcohol abuse. She has been an alcoholic for 14 years, and she admits that the alcohol intake has increased since the death of her husband in a motor vehicle accident 6 years ago. Her last drink was 2 months ago, and she has been enrolled in substance abuse relapse prevention therapy twice weekly for the past month per the recommendation of the transplant team. She is a single mother of 8-year-old twin girls with a supportive family at her bedside.

Ms. Thomas is admitted with an upper gastrointestinal bleed, anemia, and acute kidney injury requiring hemodialysis. Her Model for End-Stage Liver Disease (MELD) score is now 40, meaning that her 3-month mortality risk without a transplant is greater than 70%. The inpatient transplant team expedites a workup for liver transplant. Clinically, she is determined to be a liver transplant candidate based on imaging, laboratory study results, and nutritional and functional status. She has the social support necessary after a social worker meets with her supportive parents in their early 60s who admit to ignoring her addiction in the past but vow to be the support necessary for her to survive. A psychiatrist evaluates the patient individually and with her family to assess the patient's risk of recidivism. After much discussion, the transplant committee determines that she is a candidate because of her age and having young children, and she will be listed for cadaver donor liver transplant with the caveat to complete the required substance abuse relapse prevention therapy after the transplant. Is it ethical to transplant this patient given her alcohol addiction and recent relapse?

Organ donation has changed the face of medicine and has saved many end-stage organ disease patients from the brink of death. The first organ transplant was kidney transplant between twin brothers in 1954. Vast improvements have shaped transplant medicine since that time. Some of the biggest issues in transplant today continue to be that donors and viable organs are a scarce resource. As of December 2015, more than 120,000 people are in need of a lifesaving transplant, and on average, 22 people die each day waiting for a transplant.[31] Measures have been taken to increase the donor pool, and with these changes, many ethical issues arise with changes in transplant.

In the United States, the United Network for Organ Sharing is the government-supported private organization that manages organ allocation. The country is divided into regions, and each region has an Organ Procurement Organization that supervises the distribution of organs. These groups help ensure that the choice of organ donation is 100% voluntary by the donor or surrogate.[6] Each transplant institute oversees its own list and determines who should and should not be listed for transplant based on set criteria and the in-depth discussion of an interdisciplinary team. The discussion of the interdisciplinary team often has subjective components that tap into the committee members' values. Because of this, an individual who is not a candidate at one transplant center may be accepted and listed at another transplant center.

In the case of Ms. Thomas, the ethical issue boils down to the decision of the transplant committee regarding what would be just. Would justice require that Ms. Thomas receive the organ, or would justice require that someone else on the transplant list receive the organ? Justice in its most rudimentary form requires that each person is given her or his due and that when treating similar cases, they are treated similarly.[32] In this case and many other transplant-related cases, transplant committees are tasked with weighing the risks and benefits of transplanting each patient and determine what it would mean to give everyone his or her due (i.e., the patient, the program, and the community at large). The choice to provide Ms. Thomas with the gift of organ donation is a difficult one because of her recent history of alcohol consumption. A 6-month abstinence from alcohol is usually required before acceptance to the liver transplant list and is applied worldwide. The two main objectives of the 6-month rule are (1) to challenge motivation and identify patients who can remain abstinent and (2) to evaluate for the possibility of improvement in liver function to not require a transplant.[33] The validity of the 6-month rule has been debated for many years; however, it is still the recommended and accepted practice. Ms. Thomas would likely not live to her 6-month abstinence date; therefore, it is more beneficial for her to be listed and undergo a transplant. From the opposing view, justice will be lost for those who have followed the 6-month rule to be listed and for those who may die waiting for a liver that Ms. Thomas may be allocated. Patient age, family dynamic, and intensive transplant workup play large roles in this case. Ultimately, denying a transplant of anyone requires compelling reasons. Often listing or not listing decisions weighs heavily on the members of a transplant committee. In this scenario, although it is a difficult decision because of the patient's age and young children, we believe it is ethically permissible to list Ms. Thomas and complete liver transplant. Although justice is about giving each person his or her due, it is not always focused on the past. Justice can be achieved by thinking about what one will do in the future—in this case, what Ms. Thomas can achieve with her organ transplant. The medical transplant team should have her enter into a contract that she will complete relapse counseling, consider a group program, and maintain sobriety for life. Doing so helps balance the scales of justice but with a more forward-looking perspective. This agreement also will help with future discussions among the patient, family, and medical team if the patient is unable to follow through on the treatment plan.

CASE STUDY 34.5 ETHICAL PRACTICES AT THE BEGINNING OF LIFE

PREGNANCY

Mrs. Jackson is a 32-year-old woman currently 20 weeks pregnant with her first child. She is 10 years status post living related kidney transplant from her mother because of kidney agenesis. She had an uncomplicated postoperative course. Her transplant kidney has been functioning well, and she has had no complications. This pregnancy has required years of planning with her physicians and modification of her medications. She and her husband attend the 20-week ultrasound appointment, and they are told the baby has anencephaly. The fetus will likely not survive the pregnancy. The transplant team and obstetrician advise her to terminate the pregnancy because of the risk to her kidney and health. Mrs. Jackson and her husband are both adamant about continuing the pregnancy and do not believe in termination. Her creatinine level has already increased despite optimization of her medications that are safe for pregnancy. Is it ethical for the provider to help sustain the pregnancy when it puts the patient at risk of harm?

Advances in modern medicine allow pregnancy to be closely monitored and fetal diagnoses to be made early in pregnancy. With new developments in medicine, new risks to patients and fetus arise. Constantly weighing the risks versus benefits of every intervention is vital to maintaining an ethical medical practice. One example of advancement in prenatal care is prenatal ultrasonography. It has opened up a window to examine, diagnose, and treat fetuses when anomalies are present, and with this ability, ethical dilemmas arise.

When examining this case, the 20-week ultrasound revealed a birth defect that will undoubtedly result in the death of the fetus. The pregnant patient choosing to risk her health for a nonviable fetus is concerning. The providers involved must ensure that the patient is well informed before making any decisions. When patients receive devastating news about their health or the health of their unborn children, they may not understand the consequences of their decisions. It would be justified to allow the patient to return for a future appointment and counseling after she has had time to discuss this new diagnosis and what it means to her future. The patient and her husband should return to the office to continue the discussion, during which the medical team clearly outlines the risks of carrying the pregnancy and the patient explains the reasoning for her decisions. The provider's obligation to help this patient and reduce harm is beneficence. Terminating the pregnancy would allow the patient to restart transplant medications that were held for pregnancy and likely improve her health.

On the opposing side, developing an understanding of why the patient does not believe termination is an option can assist the provider in making informed decisions with the patient. Whether religious beliefs or moral standards or attachment to the fetus are factors shaping the patient's decisions, if the medical team understands her reasoning, it helps with accepting her choice and respecting autonomy. If the patient is well informed of the risks and understands that the fetus will not survive and continues to choose not to terminate, it is ethically permissible to maintain patient autonomy and continue the pregnancy while optimizing care of the patient.

PERINATAL PERIOD

Ms. Johnson is a 28-year-old woman who presents to the hospital 38 weeks pregnant with uterine contractions. Upon examination and reviewing her medical record, the PA and obstetrician realize that the fetus is in transverse position. Contractions become closer together, and the fetus begins having heart decelerations on fetal monitoring. The medical team determines that operative intervention is indicated. The PA attempts to obtain informed consent from Ms. Johnson for an emergency cesarean section. The patient refuses surgery based on religious grounds. The PA and physician have separate conversations with the patient about the medical necessity of the procedure for the life of her child and her safety. They both deem Ms. Johnson to have decision-making capacity and is informed of the risks; however, she continues to refuse intervention. Is it ethically permissible to perform a forced C-section on Ms. Johnson?

The obstetrician in this case is experiencing a conflict regarding the mother's decision. Pregnancy is an interesting time in which there are multiple lives involved with only the mother making the decisions. The medical team working with pregnant patients must constantly evaluate the health of both individuals.

In the United States, patients have the right to refuse any procedure, and pregnancy does not abdicate that right. Women refuse C-sections for various reasons, including religious beliefs, fear of their own health or death, psychiatric disorders, attitude toward labor, and lack of understanding. Providers must work with pregnant patients to ensure that competency is present when discussing labor and birth and understand their goals and reasoning behind those goals. This is often difficult because the physician participating in care at the clinic leading up to labor may not be the physician on call when the patient is in active labor. Birth plans are one helpful tool in this brokerage. However, a birth plan should not be seen as a binding contract but more as an outline to guide decisions.[34]

The American Congress of Obstetricians and Gynecologists (ACOG) Ethic Committee has considered this issue of maternal autonomy among many other ethical issues in the perinatal period. The ACOG states:

> Pregnant women's autonomous decisions should be respected. Concerns about the impact of maternal decisions on fetal well-being should be discussed in the context of medical evidence and understood within the context of each woman's broad social network, cultural beliefs, and values. In the absence of extraordinary circumstances, circumstances that, in fact, the Committee on Ethics cannot currently imagine, judicial authority should not be used to implement treatment regimens aimed at protecting the fetus, for such actions violate the pregnant woman's autonomy.[35]

Respecting the autonomy of Ms. Johnson would be respecting her decision because of her religious beliefs and not perform the C-section. Although we are sympathetic to the concerns of the clinical team and their desire to save two lives, the repercussions of not allowing for autonomous patients to make their own decisions is too severe to not allow Ms. Johnson to choose how her child enters this world. Hill sums this up nicely, when she states:

> All health care professionals in maternity care should be working together towards a goal of healthier mothers and babies; but this they will not do by coercing and deceiving women, overriding their competent refusal to consent and detaining them unlawfully. Although fetuses clearly have interests that should be protected, this must not be at the expense of competent women's autonomy and self-determination.[34]

CASE STUDY 34.6 PROFESSIONALISM IN PATIENT CARE

PROFESSIONAL MISREPRESENTATION AND PRECEPTOR–STUDENT CONFLICT

A PA student is on her third rotation in a busy emergency department. The student's PA program stipulates that she must perform several procedures during this rotation. Among these procedures is laceration repair with suturing. This 4-week rotation is more than 50% completed, and the student has not yet sutured. Two patients required laceration repair last week, but they did not consent to have a student perform the procedure despite assurances the student would receive proper tutelage. The PA student expresses concern about this requirement, and the PA preceptor suggests she present herself as a member of the health care team, avoiding the "student" language. Later that same day, the

PA preceptor presents the student to a patient in the fast track area stating, "Ma'am, my colleague will close up this laceration for you." The student expresses unease about how she was introduced, but the preceptor pushes her to complete the procedure and get in line with the busy patient flow expected in the emergency department setting. The student is unsure how to proceed.

This is a common scenario for postgraduate and student trainees. We focus on ethical dilemmas raised for the preceptor and student separately. First, the PA preceptor must recognize the limited agency of the student. The evaluation power of the preceptor along with knowledge and often age gaps create a significant power asymmetry. Mindful of this, preceptors have a duty to guide students down a moral pathway that includes affording the PA student an opportunity to express ethical concerns. Second, all clinicians have a duty to maintain patient autonomy and avoid dishonesty. This duty is crucial because it allows patients to share in decision making in turn receiving medical care in line with their values. Failure to identify who is performing a procedure violates the principle of patient autonomy along with hospital policy and the law. This patient cannot make an informed decision to move forward with the laceration repair because she does not have all the information available. It is possible if the patient was aware a student was performing the laceration repair, she would not provide consent.

What is the PA student's ethical responsibility in this setting? Students must have a real awareness of the serious ethical and legal ramifications of professional misrepresentation. Both ethical and legal perspectives tell us the student should advise the patient that she is a student despite pressure from the preceptor. If the preceptor makes the student uncomfortable following this decision, the PA program should have a well-defined pathway for the student to raise concerns about a preceptor.

DISAGREEMENT WITH A SUPERVISING PHYSICIAN

A PA has been employed at a solo physician gynecology practice for 5 years. These two clinicians have maintained a productive professional relationship during this time. The PA practices with significant autonomy and manages a large panel of patients. Within the past year, a biological female and long-time patient of the practice started transitioning to his male gender. This patient has long identified as a man and, after careful consultation with a psychiatrist and internist, was diagnosed with gender dysphoria and began the transition with appropriate hormone therapy. Even though the patient identifies as a male, he still has health issues that require ongoing care by a gynecologist or someone trained in women's health.

The supervising physician became aware that the PA was providing gynecologic medicine for this patient with gender dysphoria who is undergoing female-to-male transition and took issue. A meeting was called, and the supervising physician informed the PA that this practice was for women only, and the PA needed to advise the patient with gender dysphoria to seek care elsewhere. The PA was surprised at this recommendation and protested that it was discriminatory. There was a debate for some time, but ultimately, the supervising physician stated, "This is an order. I do not want you caring for that patient." The patient in question has a follow-up visit next week for a routine examination and Pap smear. The PA met with several professional mentors, and they discussed several possible actions, including continuing to treat the patient, resigning from the practice, and continuing the debate with threats of resignation.

First, we consider the most ethical approach for the PA. One could argue that this highly competent and autonomous PA should continue to see the patient. However, the PA swore an oath to partner with a supervising physician. Additionally, the PA has a legal obligation as a dependent practitioner. If the PA breaks this legal obligation, the consequence could be severe. The PA could lose his or her license, impacting all of his or her current patients, future patients, and the PA's family and dependents. Thinking about this ethics case in terms of all the people who could be harmed looks at it from the theory of utilitarianism that hinges on the principle of doing the greatest amount of good for the greatest number. In this scenario, if the PA lost his or her license, it would impact a significant number of patients and others. In addition, within the structure of patient and provider, the PA has an ethical obligation to do no harm. Although the PA cannot treat the patient, the PA does have an obligation to secure a smooth transition to someone who can treat the patient. Doing no harm includes not only securing proper medical care for the patient but also protecting other transgender patients from discrimination. The American Academy of Physician Assistants' (AAPA's) ethical guidelines make particular note that gender discrimination is unethical practice.[36] The PA should consider a professional transition and report this discriminatory practice to the proper state medical board.

A STUDENT'S CONSCIENTIOUS OBJECTION TO ABORTION SERVICES

A PA student is in the midst of his obstetrics and gynecology rotation. This women's health private practice provides abortion services that are legal and considered a component of reproductive health in this region. On any given day, a patient might receive abortion counseling, a termination procedure, or follow-up care. The PA student is of a religion that considers abortion immoral, and the student refuses to participate in any of the aforementioned abortion-related visits, including counseling sessions. What allowances should be made for this student with a conscientious objection to abortion?

Although a PA does not have an obligation to perform an abortion in the United States, this does not mean a PA does not have a duty to manage complications or offer referrals and counsel related to abortion. This issue is not novel and has been addressed by a variety of ethicists and professional organizations such as the International Federation of Gynecology and Obstetrics. This organization has published a document that states that trainees cannot decline training in a procedure being performed for medically indicated purposes to which they cannot or do not object even though the same procedure can be used for medical indicators to which they object.[37] This implies that there should be mandatory training, for instance, in the management of abortion complications. Current AAPA ethical guidelines state: "PAs have an ethical obligation to provide balanced and unbiased clinical information about reproductive healthcare."[36] This requires clinicians to have basic knowledge of surgical and medical abortion and the skill set to discuss this often emotional and sensitive topic. In many cases, it is unethical to conscientiously object to an educational activity when it is unlikely the student could receive this standard of medicine skill from an alternative method such as simulation. One could argue that counseling through this difficult time is not easily learned through simulation and is best in real life under the tutelage of a preceptor. Managing the complications of abortion does not require the trainee to prescribe abortion medication or be present for surgical abortion. However, the student should participate in the management of complications and counseling of reproductive options.

In this case, we face conflicting principles given the PA has a duty to his religion but also toward his profession and patient. The autonomy of this clinician's future patients and his ability to do no harm depend on his medical education and ability to discuss these reproductive health options and manage their complications. It is doubtful this often emotional and complicated counseling session could be learned exclusively through simulation. The PA student would not have to be present or involved in an actual abortion to develop this skill set.

This is but one example of conscientious objection. Other examples include physical examinations on people of opposite gender, clinician-assisted suicide, and ritual circumcision. When this issue emerges for a PA student, there is not always a clear precedent on how to proceed. Additional guidance could be obtained from the relevant professional association and university resource.

TABLE 34.1 Print Resources in Clinical Ethics

Books	Journals
Principles of Biomedical Ethics by Beauchamp and Childress	Journal of Clinical Ethics
Clinical Ethics: A Practical Approach to Ethical Decisions in Clinical Medicine by Jonsen, Siegler, and Winslade	American Journal of Bioethics
Resolving Ethical Dilemmas: A Guide for Clinicians by Lo	Hastings Center Report
	Journal of Hospital Ethics
	HEC Forum
	Cambridge Quarterly of Health Care Ethics

TABLE 34.2 Ethics Committee and Ethics Consultation Resources

National Center for Ethics in Health Care, http://www.ethics.va.gov	Encyclopedia of Bioethics
Core Competencies for Healthcare Ethics Consultation	Improving Competencies in Clinical Ethics Consultation: An Education Guide, 2nd Edition
Handbook for Ethics Committees by Post et al.	

ETHICS CONSULTATION AND RESOURCES

The entire field of clinical ethics is beyond the scope of an introductory chapter. As a result, we provide readers with resources for further guidance and information. There are several high-quality bioethics journals and textbooks that students might be interested in reading to further their understanding of these complex issues (Table 34.1).

Professional associations provide further resources for ethical matters. The American Society for Bioethics and Humanities is the U.S. professional home for those in clinical ethics practice and research. The AAPA and AMA produce ethics guidelines that contain guidance to many specific scenarios such as clinician participation in sterilization and abortion services.[36] Although helpful, these guidelines are not exhaustive. It is useful to consult them for guidance on a particular ethical issue with the understanding that they are often from the perspective of the profession.

In addition, both local and professional ethics committees and consultation services can be useful. The integration of ethics committees and ethics consultation services into acute care has been substantial in the past 15 years. These ethics services were spawned by many factors, including a Joint Commission requirement that hospitals have a mechanism to address ethical conflicts and uncertainties. Thus, a clinician may find it appropriate to request an ethics consult when faced with an ethical dilemma or uncertainty. Ethics committees and their respective ethics consultation services are often interdisciplinary and at some locations include a trained ethics consultant. The consultation service often uses a systematic process to address ethical questions similar to the ones described earlier. For more information about ethics committees and consultation, see Table 34.2.

KEY POINTS

- The development of clinical ethics was influenced by many historical sources, including research, technological development, and legal culture.
- The specialty of bioethics focuses on moral dilemmas as they intersect with biology and the policies and practices of medicine.
- Using a systematic method to address ethical issues is useful and can provide clarity to complex and diverse scenarios.
- The number of ethical issues a PA encounters is vast and requires a sufficient level of ethics knowledge to address.
- The use of ethics resources is helpful in developing appropriate guidance in ethical situations. This includes the use of ethics committees and ethics consultation services.

References

1. Hamel R. Strengthening the role of ethics in turbulent times. *Health Prog*. 2010;91(3):60–61.
2. Glaser JW. Hospital ethics committees: one of many centers of responsibility. *Theor Med*. 1989;10(4):275–288.
3. Beauchamp TL, Childress JF. *Principles of Biomedical Ethics*. 6th ed. New York: Oxford University Press; 2009.
4. Ashcroft RE. *Case Analysis in Clinical Ethics*. Cambridge; New York: Cambridge University Press; 2005.
5. Fletcher JC, Boyle R. *Fletcher's Introduction to Clinical Ethics*. 3rd ed. Hagerstown, MD: University Pub. Group; 2005.
6. Jonsen AR, Siegler M, Winslade WJ. *Clinical Ethics: A Practical Approach to Ethical Decisions in Clinical Medicine*. 7th ed. New York: McGraw-Hill Medical; 2010.
7. Post LF, Blustein J. *Handbook for Health Care Ethics Committees*. 2nd ed. Baltimore: Johns Hopkins University Press; 2015.
8. Zoloth L, Rubin S. The Ethics Practice Case Consultation Methodology. In: Force ASfBaHCET, ed. *Improving Competencies in Clinical Ethics Consultation: An Education Guide*; 2009.
9. Bioethics GUCfC. The Georgetown University Center for Clinical Bioethics Ethics Workup. In: Force ASfBaHCET, ed. *Improving Competencies in Clinical Ethics Consultation: An Education Guide*; 2008.
10. Kaldjian LC, Weir RF, Duffy TP. A clinician's approach to clinical ethical reasoning. *J Gen Intern Med*. 2005;20(3):306–311.
11. Alexander S. They decide who lives, who dies. *Life*. 1962.
12. Sanders D, Dukeminier Jr J. Medical advance and legal lag: hemodialysis and kidney transplantation. *UCLA Law Review*. 1967;(357):15.
13. CDC. *The Tuskegee Timeline*; 2013. http://www.cdc.gov/tuskegee/timeline.htm. Accessed April 3, 2016.
14. Jones JH. *Tuskegee Institute. Bad blood: the Tuskegee syphilis experiment*. New York: Free Press; 1981.
15. Emanuel EJ, Wendler D, Grady C. What makes clinical research ethical? *JAMA*. 2000;283(20):2701–2711.
16. Beecher HK. Ethics and clinical research. 1966. *Bull World Health Organ*. 2001;79(4):367–372.
17. United States National Commission for the Protection of Human Subjects of Biomedical and Behavioral Research. *The Belmont report: ethical principles and guidelines for the protection of human subjects of research*. Bethesda, MD: The Commission; 1978.
18. Quinlan J, Quinlan J, Battelle P. *Karen Ann: The Quinlans Tell Their Story*. Garden City, NY: Doubleday; 1977.
19. McFadder R. Karen Ann Quinlan, 31, dies; focus of 76 right to die case. *New York Times*; 1985.
20. Appelbaum PS. Clinical practice. Assessment of patients' competence to consent to treatment. *N Engl J Med*. 2007; 357(18):1834–1840.
21. Appelbaum PS, Grisso T. Assessing patients' capacities to consent to treatment. *N Engl J Med*. 1988;319(25):1635–1638.
22. Ganzini L, Volicer L, Nelson WA, Fox E, Derse AR. Ten myths about decision-making capacity. *J Am Med Dir Assoc*. 2004;5(4):263–267.
23. Dastidar J, Odden A. How do i determine if my patient has decision-making capacity? *The Hospitalist*. 2011.
24. Association AM. Opinion 5.059-Privacy in the context of health care. AMA's Code of Medical Ethics. http://www.ama-assn.org/ama/pub/physician-resources/medical-ethics/code-medical-ethics/opinion5059.page?. Accessed April 3, 2016.
25. van Gijn MS, Frijns D, van de Glind EM, B CvM, Hamaker ME. The chance of survival and the functional outcome after in-hospital cardiopulmonary resuscitation in older people: a systematic review. *Age Ageing*. 2014;43(4):456–463.
26. Brett AS, McCullough LB. When patients request specific interventions: defining the limits of the physician's obligation. *N Engl J Med*. 1986;315(21):1347–1351.
27. McCullough LB, Jones JW. Postoperative futility: a clinical algorithm for setting limits. *Br J Surg*. 2001;88(9):1153–1154.
28. Trotter G. Mediating disputes about medical futility. *Camb Q Healthc Ethics*. 1999;8(4):527–537.
29. Lopez-Saca JM, Guzman JL, Centeno C. A systematic review of the influence of opioids on advanced cancer patient survival. *Curr Opin Support Palliat Care*. 2013;7(4):424–430.
30. American Medical Association. *End of life care policy*; 2015. http://www.ama-assn.org/ama/pub/physician-resources/medical-ethics/about-ethics-group/ethics-resource-center/end-of-life-care/ama-policy-end-of-life-care.page? Accessed April 3, 2016.
31. Sharing UNfO. UNOS. https://www.unos.org/; 2015. Accessed April 3, 2016.
32. Schmidtz D. *Elements of justice*. Cambridge; New York: Cambridge University Press; 2006.
33. Rustad JK, Stern TA, Prabhakar M, Musselman D. Risk factors for alcohol relapse following orthotopic liver transplantation: a systematic review. *Psychosomatics*. 2015;56(1):21–35.
34. Cahill H. An Orwellian scenario: court ordered caesarean section and women's autonomy. *Nurs Ethics*. 1999;6(6):494–505.
35. Ethics ACo. ACOG Committee Opinion #321: Maternal decision making, ethics, and the law. *Obstet Gynecol*. 2005;106(5 Pt 1):1127–1137.
36. American Academy of Physician Assistant. *Guidelines for Ethical Conduct of Physician Assistant Profession*; 2013. https://www.aapa.org/WorkArea/DownloadAsset.aspx?id=2147486552. Accessed December 20, 2016.
37. FIGO Committee for the Ethical Aspects of Human Reproduction and Women's Health. Ethical guidelines on conscientious objection in training. *Int J Gynaecol Obstet*. 2015;128:89–98.

The resources for this chapter can be found at www.expertconsult.com.

CHAPTER 35

MEDICAL MALPRACTICE AND RISK MANAGEMENT

Earl G. Greene III

A physician assistant's (PA's) medical practice deals in a world of gray. There are few clinical situations a PA encounters that clearly and unequivocally present themselves so that a ready diagnosis and treatment plan can be implemented. The vast majority of patient encounters will result in the most common "gray" component of your practice: the differential diagnosis. Through a differential diagnosis, the PA sorts out the "grays," ultimately arriving at a workable diagnosis and treatment plan.

In this world of "grays," a significant percentage of PAs are now being exposed to the black and white world of the law. Although legal matters affect a PA's practice in multiple ways and on a daily basis (Health Insurance Portability and Accountability Act [HIPAA], medical coding and billing, insurance contracts, business contracts, employment contracts, office and equipment leases), there is one area of the law that can have a significant and profound professional and emotional impact on a PA: involvement in a medical malpractice lawsuit. In the event a PA gets sued for professional malpractice, she or he will experience firsthand the very uneasy juxtaposition of law into medicine. For perhaps the first time, the PA will encounter attempts by legal professionals to take the gray world of medicine and subject it to the black and white world of law. This process, and often the result, can be a very unnerving experience. Unquestionably,

it will enhance a PA's understanding of the law even if as a fairly unwilling participant in several legal processes, including written and oral discovery, depositions, and, perhaps, a trial. Such experiences will leave a marked impact, both professionally and personally, and may even change the PA's practical and emotional approach to clinical practice.

The purpose of this chapter is simply to highlight some basic legal concepts a PA will encounter in the event of involvement in a medical malpractice lawsuit. Suggestions are also made for some risk management principles that may lessen the likelihood of involvement in a medical malpractice lawsuit.

WHAT IS MEDICAL NEGLIGENCE?

As a general proposition, "medical malpractice" can be defined as follows: In rendering professional services, a PA has failed to use the ordinary and reasonable care, skill, and knowledge ordinarily possessed and used under similar circumstances by members of the PA profession engaged in a similar practice in the same or a similar locality.[1,2]

Although several legal theories may form the basis of a medical malpractice lawsuit against a PA, the most common theory is one based on negligence. The concept of negligence is not unique to a medical malpractice lawsuit. The same basic principles of negligence apply equally to a lawsuit or claim involving the occurrence of an automobile accident, a premise liability event (i.e., a slip and fall case), or even a dog bite case. To recover on a negligence claim, the person bringing the claim or the lawsuit (the "claimant" or, in the case of a lawsuit, the "plaintiff") must establish against the person who is being sued or against whom the claim is brought ("the defendant") four components of a negligence claim:

1. The existence of a duty running from the defendant to the plaintiff
2. The breach of the duty by the defendant
3. Injuries sustained by the plaintiff
4. Proof that the injuries were legally caused by the breach of duty

Duty

The first element a plaintiff must establish in a medical negligence lawsuit is the existence of a duty. This duty arises out of the PA–patient relationship. After that relationship has been established, a PA must possess and bring to that relationship that degree of knowledge, skill, and care that would be exercised by a reasonable and prudent PA under similar circumstances. The knowledge, skill, and care established by a profession and as required to be rendered in any patient–PA encounter comprise the "standard of care." In a medical malpractice lawsuit, a plaintiff must show that the defendant PA failed to exercise the applicable standard of care by commission or omission. That is, the plaintiff establishes a breach of the standard of care by the PA doing something that should not have been done or by failing to do something that should've been done. "Good faith" or "best intentions" have no place or meaning in a medical malpractice lawsuit. Instead, the PA will be judged on whether or not conformance occurred with an acceptable and recognized "standard of care."

Breach of Duty

The second element of medical negligence a plaintiff must prove is that of "breach of duty." A plaintiff establishes this element by proving the PA failed to act in accordance with the applicable standard of care. Of course, before a plaintiff can establish that a breach of the standard of care occurred, the plaintiff must first establish what constitutes the standard of care. In most cases, the existence of a standard of care must be proved through the use of expert witnesses. That means the plaintiff must retain as a witness another PA qualified to testify as to the standard of care owed by the PA being sued. An expert witness

must testify that, based on that expert's knowledge, education, training, and experience, a specific standard of care exists concerning the alleged act of malpractice committed by the PA being sued. Furthermore, the expert must also testify as to the manner in which the PA breached the standard of care. After the plaintiff establishes in a lawsuit both the existence of a standard of care and its breach, the PA may also use expert PA witnesses or the PA's own testimony to demonstrate that no such breach of the standard of care occurred. Although the vast majority of cases rely on expert witness review and testimony to establish the standard of care and a breach thereof, some medical malpractice cases do arise in which the alleged breach of duty is so obvious as to be within the comprehension of a layperson, and no expert testimony is needed. Cases such as wrong site surgeries and failure to remove a lap sponge are examples that probably do not require an expert witness to establish a standard of care, or that a standard of care was breached by a PA.

Importantly, a PA is not held to a standard of "perfect" medicine. Liability for medical malpractice will not arise merely because a PA makes an incorrect diagnosis or institutes an incorrect plan of treatment. The key to determining if a breach of the standard of care occurred is examining the process used by the PA in arriving at the diagnosis or deciding on a plan of treatment and whether or not the process met the standard of care.

Causation

The third element of a negligence case a plaintiff must prove revolves around the relationship between the negligent act or omission committed by the PA and the resulting injury. The plaintiff must establish a "causal connection" between the negligent act and the injury. In legal terms, the "causal connection" is commonly referred to as "proximate cause." The concept of causation differs markedly from that of causation as used in medical terminology. In the legal sense, "causation" refers to a single, causative factor and not necessarily the major cause or even the most immediate cause of the injury. In contrast, medical causation or etiology usually refers to the major or immediate cause of an injury. Causation can often present as an elusive and difficult concept to understand for both medical professionals and juries. One way for laypeople to grasp the meaning of causation is an awareness of the "but for" test.[3] In simplest terms, if one occurrence would not have occurred "but for" another occurrence, legal causation exists. As contrasting examples, a PA participating in a surgical procedure may leave behind instrumentation resulting in an intestinal perforation with possible subsequent development of abscesses, future surgeries, or even death. The intestinal perforation would not have occurred "but for" the failure to remove the instrumentation and perform a proper count of instrumentation at the conclusion of the surgery. Legally, the failure to remove the instrumentation created the proximate cause of the patient's injuries. In contrast, a physician or PA's delay in diagnosing a patient or even delaying referral of a patient who has a highly aggressive malignant and terminal neoplasm might be considered an act of malpractice. However, depending on the stage of the tumor at the time of the initial presentation, the failure to diagnose or refer may not have legally caused the patient's ultimate outcome (i.e., death). In other words, the tumor may have been so advanced at the time the physician or PA failed to make the proper diagnosis or failed to make a proper referral that even a timely referral or proper diagnosis would not have saved the patient. In such a case, the breach of the standard of care (the delay in making the proper diagnosis or referral) did not proximately cause the patient's death. The patient already had an unavoidable death sentence even at the time of the alleged misdiagnosis.

Injury and Damages

The last element a plaintiff must prove in a medical malpractice claim is proof of damages. In general, the concept of damages encompasses the actual loss or damage sustained by the plaintiff arising from the PA's breach of the standard of care. If the plaintiff cannot prove harm, there can be no recovery.

Generally speaking, two types of damages may be awarded in a civil lawsuit: special damages and general damages. Special damages are damages that have a finite or tangible economic number attached to them. Examples of special damages are the amount of past, present, and future medical bills incurred as a result of the medical negligence; past, present, and future lost wages; future lost wages arising out of the loss of earning capacity; and in a wrongful death malpractice claim, funeral expenses. The other type of damages, general damages, are awarded for the nontangible, noneconomic injuries. These types of injuries include pain and suffering, mental anguish, grief, and inconvenience.

A third type of damage may be awarded in a medical malpractice lawsuit, but not all states or jurisdictions recognize this third form: punitive damages. Currently, 34 of the 50 states in the United States do allow awards that include the possibility of punitive damages.[4] Punitive damages are intended to make an example of the defendant PA or to punish egregious behavior. Such damages generally are given when the defendant's conduct has been intentional, grossly negligent, malicious, violent, fraudulent, or with reckless disregard for the consequences of his or her conduct. Again, not all states allow for punitive damages, so PAs must familiarize themselves with the laws of the jurisdiction where a practice is established.

OTHER THEORIES OF RECOVERY

Several other potential theories of liability may give a plaintiff a cause of action against a PA. These theories are not based on the concept of negligence. Instead, they have their own, individualized elements that must be established and proven by a plaintiff to make a recovery. The most common of these other theories are abandonment and lack of informed consent.

Abandonment

When a PA agrees to treat a patient, that PA agrees to provide a continuity of care until the patient is cured or stabilized. The patient cannot be abandoned, and the PA must provide an adequate surrogate when the PA and the supervising physician are unavailable. Many practices meet this obligation by making arrangements with a partner or nearby colleagues in the same or similar field of practice. Backup may also be provided by directing ambulatory patients to a nearby, physician-staffed hospital emergency department. Brief lapses of coverage are generally considered reasonable.

Informed Consent

Central to any PA–patient relationship is a complete and total disclosure by the PA to the patient of the risks and benefits of any proposed course of treatment—the informed consent talk. Under informed consent principles, a PA's duty to obtain informed consent is measured by information that would ordinarily be provided to the patient under similar circumstances by health care providers engaged in a similar practice in the locality or in similar localities.[5] In general, the PA must communicate to the patient information that a reasonable patient would require to make an "informed" judgment about whether to consent to such treatment. Such information includes the risks and benefits of proposed treatment, as well as available alternatives, including no treatment at all. Furthermore, as part of the PA–patient relationship, the PA also has an obligation to disclose to the patient the consequences of failing to undergo a recommended medical procedure, and the PA can be held liable for malpractice if such a disclosure is not made.

Informed consent is a process, not a form. The PA should never delegate the informed consent discussion to a coworker or referring physician. This talk represents a very important component of the overall PA–patient relationship and creates a prime opportunity for the PA to develop open and honest lines of communication with a patient. As part of the informed consent process, the PA must carefully document when, where, and what was discussed with the patient. Many specialized practices have, understandably, specialized informed consent forms. If a PA is part of a specialty practice, the PA must be familiar with the language of such forms and ensure the language accurately describes the specific risks and benefits facing the patient. The timing of the informed consent discussion is also an important component in establishing whether or not the standard of care in the giving of an informed consent has been met. There are no hard and fast rules in regard to such a time frame, but the topic must be discussed with the supervising physician to ensure a timely informed consent has been given pursuant to the dictates of the practice. Also, different people learn information in different fashions. Some people learn well by listening, others by reading, and yet others by watching. A clinical or hospital-based practice should make available to patients different mediums of information necessary to give an effective informed consent. In addition to the verbal giving of the informed consent by the PA, the patient should be given the option of reviewing written materials about the procedure or watching a video or DVD covering the informed consent topic. These latter two forms of communicating informed consent information cannot replace the personal informed consent talk the PA must have with the patient before any course of treatment. They may supplement the informed consent talk, but the standard of care requires that the PA or physician personally handle the informed consent discussion.

As a general rule of thumb, when giving the informed consent information, communicate the information to the patient that you would want to know if your spouse, parent, or child were undergoing this same procedure or treatment. Again, good communicative skills are a must in a PA practice, and the giving of a thorough informed consent talk and documenting it can go a long way toward preventing future malpractice action.

ELEMENTS OF A LAWSUIT

Despite a PA's best efforts and practice, a medical malpractice lawsuit may arise. As a side note, recent studies have indicated that although PAs do get sued for malpractice, the overall rate at which they get sued is significantly less than the rate at which physicians get sued. One such study indicated that over a 17-year period between 1991 and 2007, there was one malpractice payment for every 32.5 PAs, but there was one payment for every 2.7 physicians.[6]

Also of note are the statistics on why PAs get sued. In order, the reasons for suits are errors in diagnosis, treatment, medication, and surgery. A growing area of lawsuits, though, stems from a PA failing to make a timely referral to a specialist or physician.[6]

Just as any patient coming into a medical practice office may have fears regarding the unknown medical care or treatment that awaits that patient, many health care providers have a fear of the medical malpractice lawsuit simply because of the unknown and totally foreign concepts and procedures involved in a lawsuit. The following pages contain some basic information about the elements of a lawsuit. This information will not make you a lawyer. In fact, it won't even scratch the surface of what all is involved in a medical malpractice lawsuit, particularly in terms of the time, knowledge, expertise, and effort a medical malpractice defense attorney will put into defending a health care professional in a medical malpractice case. However, this information will provide the basics in terms of the process and terminology involved in a medical malpractice lawsuit.

Initial Filings

There is no magic to the filing of a medical malpractice lawsuit. The patient who believes an injury occurred as a result of a PA's negligence merely has to find an attorney willing to undertake representation of that patient in a lawsuit. The attorney will prepare the opening document, called a petition or a complaint, and pay the local court filing fee, and the suit is under way. The defendant must be legally served with a copy of the lawsuit. If a PA is served with a copy of a lawsuit, care must be taken to immediately get that document into the hands of the PA's employer risk manager, the office manager, the malpractice insurance carrier, or the practice's attorney. After defense counsel is engaged, that attorney will look at preliminary matters such as whether or not the lawsuit was timely filed (a statute of limitations question), if the lawsuit truly states a cause of action against the PA, or if the court even has jurisdiction over the matters alleged in the lawsuit. Any one of these issues may result in a pre-answer being filed with the court and an attempt at obtaining an early dismissal of the lawsuit. If the lawsuit cannot be disposed of on a pre-answer basis, the defense attorney will then file an answer to the lawsuit in which the allegations of the lawsuit are admitted or denied. The attorney may also raise certain affirmative defenses to the petition or complaint. Such defenses could include the absence of a PA–patient relationship, no breach of the standard of care, a lack of causation, no injuries or damages as alleged by the plaintiff, the fault of others over whom the PA had no control, or even the comparative fault of the plaintiff in causing his or her own injuries.

Discovery Stage

The next stage of the lawsuit involves discovery. Discovery primarily occurs in two forms: written discovery and oral discovery. Written discovery consists of written questions called interrogatories, a request for production of documents, requests for admissions, and subpoenas to other entities that may have information about the lawsuit (employment records, other health care providers, police reports, and so on). Interrogatories are exchanged between the parties to learn background information, not only about the parties themselves but also as to the existence of any fact witnesses, documents that will support either side's theory of the case, and identities and opinions of expert witnesses. The requests for production are used so that each party may obtain from its opponent any documents that side intends to use to prove its case. Such documents may include medical records, educational records, plaintiff's wage information and income tax returns in support of any lost wage claim, photographs, expert witness reports, and police reports.

After the written discovery has been completed, the parties to the lawsuit then engage in the oral discovery phase of the lawsuit. This discovery occurs in the form of depositions. A deposition is a sworn statement given by a party to the lawsuit, by a fact witness with knowledge about the lawsuit, by a treating physician, or by an expert witness. During the deposition, the attorneys have the opportunity to ask the witness questions about the nature and extent of that witness's knowledge of facts or opinions concerning the lawsuit. A PA who is a defendant in a lawsuit will give a deposition in that case in which the attorney representing the plaintiff will ask the PA questions about the care, treatment, and decision-making process used by that PA. Before the occurrence of that deposition, though, the PA will meet with her or his attorney to fully discuss the medical records, the care and treatment given to the patient by the PA, and the general scope of the deposition in order to fully prepare the PA for that deposition. Defense counsel will take the deposition of the plaintiff(s) and make inquiry about the plaintiff's theory as to why the PA

was negligent, conversations had with the PA, the patient's perceptions about the care and treatment given, and any injuries or damages claimed by the plaintiff. Depositions will also be taken of the expert witnesses involved in the lawsuit to determine the basis for any opinions, as well as the scope of the opinions.

Many jurisdictions use case progression standards in which the attorneys involved in the lawsuit are required to complete discovery according to specific time frames. Depending on any scheduling order or trial progression standards entered by the court, the discovery process in a lawsuit could take up to 18 months to complete from the date the suit is filed.

Settlement Talks and Mediation

After the parties complete discovery, they will be in position to know if the case should be tried or if meaningful settlement talks should occur. In regard to settlement talks, the past 15 years have seen a significant growth in alternate dispute resolution proceedings (ADR), such as mediation. A mediation is scheduled so the parties can meet with a neutral third party and over the course of several hours try to work out an amicable resolution to avoid having to take the case to trial and having complete strangers, in the form of a jury, decide the case. Of note, historically, about 85% of all civil lawsuits filed, including medical malpractice suits, do settle before trial. A 2004 study put that figure as high as 95%.[7] Settlements occur for multiple reasons but always involve a compromise of some sort by each side. However, if the parties to the lawsuit either cannot resolve the case at mediation or decide not to mediate a case, the case proceeds to trial.

Trial

Most medical malpractice trials last a minimum of 3 days and, depending on the complexity of the case, could last upwards to 2 weeks. During that time frame of the trial, the PA will be required to attend the trial on a daily basis and participate in the trial as necessary.

The trial follows a very specific order. In a civil lawsuit, the plaintiff must prove each of the four elements of negligence by a "preponderance of the evidence." This term means simply that the plaintiff must prove its case by the greater weight of evidence. The plaintiff will always go first in a trial because it maintains the burden of proof throughout the trial. Therefore, during the stages of the jury selection process, the opening statements, the case in chief, and the closing arguments, the plaintiff will always have the first opportunity to present its case. The defendant will have the opportunity to participate after each stage of the plaintiff's case. So, after the plaintiff's counsel first questions potential jurors during the jury selection process, then defense counsel have the same opportunity. After the plaintiff presents an opening statement, then the defense presents an opening statement. After the plaintiff's counsel conducts direct examination of each of plaintiff's witnesses, including the plaintiff, then defense counsel has the chance to cross-examine each witness as soon as plaintiff counsel finishes the direct examination. After plaintiff counsel finishes the plaintiff's case, then the plaintiff "rests." At that point, defense counsel presents its witnesses and evidence.

Upon the completion of all evidence, the trial judge and the attorneys collaborate on the jury instructions to be given to the jury. Counsel then make their closing arguments to the jury, again with the plaintiff's counsel going first. Upon the completion of closing arguments, the judge then instructs the jury and dismisses the jury to the jury room with the written jury instructions, and jury deliberations begin. Most jurisdictions have laws that if a jury returns a verdict within the first 6 hours of deliberations, that verdict must be unanimous. If a jury has deliberated for more than 6 hours and cannot reach a unanimous verdict, then the law will allow a jury to return a less than unanimous verdict but with no more than one or two dissenting jurors. If the plaintiff did prove all four elements of the negligence case (duty, breach of duty, injury, and causation), then the jury will make a monetary award to the plaintiff in the form of special or general damages. If the plaintiff failed to prove any one of the four elements of a negligence claim, then the jury will return a defense verdict in favor of the PA.

The losing party to a lawsuit has the right to appeal the decision to a higher court. If such an appeal takes place, it can easily add 1 to 2 years to the life of the case, and will either result in a higher court affirming the jury verdict or remanding the case back to the trial court for a new trial.

CASE STUDY 35.1

For 3 days, a cattle rancher had been moving cattle from one pasture to another. On the second day of moving cattle, he began having chest pain while working. When he was resting, taking a break, and driving to and from the pastures, there was no chest pain or other associated symptoms.

On the third day, the severity of the chest pain increased, and he began having some nausea without vomiting, shortness of breath, and diaphoresis. Around noon on the third day, he decided to go to the urgent care center, which was about 5 miles away from where he was working.

Because it was around noon, there were no other patients in the urgent care center. He was lucky in that he was taken in right away and seen by the PA on duty at the time. The physician was at lunch but had remained in the urgent care center.

The patient was a 54-year-old white man who had the classic substernal chest pain with exercise or work. On the third day, he started having associated symptoms of nausea without vomiting, diaphoresis, and radiation of pain to the left jaw and left arm. Vital signs were blood pressure of 160/98 mm Hg, pulse of 110 beats/min, respirations of 24 breaths/min, and temperature of 101.2°F. The electrocardiogram showed an ST elevation in limb lead 2. He was indeed diaphoretic and looked anxious.

The PA recognized that the patient was having a myocardial infarction (MI). He notified the physician working in the urgent care center immediately. In addition, he gave the patient an aspirin, started an intravenous line, and placed a nitroglycerin patch on the patient. The nurse called 911, and he was prepared to transport as soon as the ambulance arrived. A call was also placed to the local hospital notifying them that the patient was coming. The patient was transported to the hospital in stable condition.

Unfortunately, that night, the patient had another MI and died.

The man's wife and three teenage sons sued with the following complaints against the PA, physician, and urgent care center: (1) the PA did not follow the standards of care for treatment of an MI, (2) the PA failed to transfer the patient in a timely manner, and (3) the physician in the urgent care center did not see the patient.

During the deposition of the PA, it was determined that the standard of care in the treatment of an MI was followed. Also during the deposition, it was found that the PA saw the patient in a timely manner and the patient was diagnosed quickly by obtaining an accurate history, conducting a complete physical examination as it relates to an MI, and doing an electrocardiogram that showed an acute MI. It was determined that the patient was transferred from the urgent care center to the hospital in a timely manner. The PA was exonerated.

The patient's wife stated during her deposition that when she arrived at the urgent care center, she talked to the physician in the examination room while he was in with her husband, thereby disproving the claim that the physician did not see the patient. She also stated that her husband was transferred to the hospital in a timely manner. At the end of the physician's deposition, he was also exonerated.

RISK MANAGEMENT ISSUES

The PA did a good history and physical examination, made the correct diagnosis, consulted with the supervising physician on duty, and documented well. There was also good communication among the PA, the physician, and the patient and his wife, which was all documented. The urgent care center had called 911, and the patient was transported to the hospital in a timely manner. It was well documented that the patient was stable when transported.

The issues in a medical malpractice case were all satisfied. The appropriate documentation included the history and physical examination, the correct diagnosis, and the timely referral. In addition, there was good communication among the PA, the physician, and the patient and his wife. As a result of these factors, both the PA and physician were exonerated.

CASE STUDY 35.2

The patient was a 64-year-old white man who was walking on his treadmill at home. He was accustomed to doing so for the past several months and had no previous problems. After walking for approximately 15 minutes, he developed a sudden onset of back pain. The pain was in the right lower lumber area with radiation to the right buttocks, hip, and right posterior thigh. The pain was sharp and severe enough to cause him to stop walking. He did not have any associated symptoms of numbness, tingling, or weakness of the lower extremities and did not identify any problems with his bowel or bladder.

He took two Tylenol without relief of pain.

The next day, his son made an appointment with the family doctor but instead was seen by the PA at 11:00 AM.

The PA obtained the following:

The **chief complaint** was back pain with some radiation to the right buttocks and right leg.

History: Sudden onset of back pain with exercise with radiation to the right leg, hip, and buttocks. No relieving factors. The pain was worse with leaning and bending forward. Tylenol was not helpful in relieving the pain. No prior history of back pain.

Physical examination: The PA recorded that there was a right-sided lumbar muscle spasm. Reflexes were equal bilaterally in the lower extremities. There was some pain in the right buttocks and posterior right thigh with palpation. It was recorded that there was some difficulty with ambulation and difficulty with getting on and off the examination table.

Assessment: Right lower lumbar strain and muscle spasm with right leg sciatica.

Plan: Toradol 10 mg injection. Lortab 10/500 mg one tablet every 4 to 6 hours as needed for pain. Moist heat to the right lumbar area 4 times a day for 20 minutes. Rest for 24 hours and no treadmill. To follow up as needed.

The next day, the patient was no better. He had no relief of his pain with the treatment previously mentioned. He was again seen in the same office as the day before. He was seen by the PA covering the walk-in clinic. He was seen at approximately noon. His family physician was out of the office on both days.

The following was noted by the second PA. He first reviewed the medical record from the day before.

History: The back pain had not improved. There was no numbness, tingling, or weakness of the lower extremities. There was no abdominal pain, and there were no bowel or bladder habit changes. The pain medication did not help.

Physical examination: Basically no difference from the day before. The patient continued to have lumbar muscle spasm and sciatic notch tenderness. The reflexes were equal bilaterally. There was difficulty with ambulation and getting on and off the table.

Assessment: Right lower lumbar muscle spasm with right leg sciatica. This is basically the same diagnosis as the day before.

Plan: An injection of Toradol 10 mg IM. Add Flexeril 10 mg one tablet 3 times a day. Return as needed.

The next day the patient passed out at home. His family called 911, and he was taken to the local hospital.

In the ambulance, he was suspected of having a ruptured abdominal aortic aneurysm (AAA) by the emergency medical technician. Despite resuscitation attempts of massive fluids and cardiopulmonary resuscitation, the patient was pronounced dead 20 minutes after arrival at the emergency department (ED).

The patient's daughter, who was an attorney, filed a medical malpractice lawsuit within days after the funeral.

This case is bad and gets ugly for all of the reasons a PA or any health care provider might be sued for. The **risk management issues** include the following:

Untimely referral: Neither PA consulted with the supervising physician. To complicate matters further, they did not consult with the other physicians in the group who were in the office at the time the patient was seen. They did not refer the patient to the ED or radiology for radiographs of the lumbar spine. The office was attached to the hospital by a third-floor walkway.

It would be wonderful to diagnose a "triple A" by discussing it with your supervising physician or sending the patient to the ED and having the ED doctor call and say how wonderful you are by diagnosing an AAA or having the radiologist call and tell you that the patient has an AAA. In this case, the untimely referrals were not talking to the physician in the office at the time of the patient's visit and not referring the patient to the ED or radiology.

Inadequate history: Neither PA obtained an adequate history as it relates to back pain. The patient's brother had an aneurysm years earlier. The patient was a longtime smoker of 2 packs a day. The history of back pain was not specific. The first PA did not ask about abdominal pain. The second PA did ask about abdominal pain but failed to do an abdominal examination because there were no complaints of abdominal pain. As a general rule, all patients who are older than the age of 50 years should have an abdominal examination performed if their complaint is back pain. Even if the answer is "no" to "Are you having abdominal pain?" you should perform an abdominal examination.

Inadequate examination: The examination of the back was incomplete. A complete back examination always includes an examination of the abdomen whether there is complaint of abdominal pain or not. This is especially true if the patient is older than 50 years of age. One of the PAs may have noticed diminished or absent pulses of the lower extremities if an examination of the lower extremities had been performed. One of the PAs stated in the deposition that the patient was obese, and an abdominal examination would not have been of value. The patient was not obese. In fact, he was 5'11" tall and weighed only 143 lb.

Failure to diagnose: The failure to diagnose was due to the following: (1) inadequate history, (2) inadequate physical examination, (3) failure to refer, and (4) failure to order the proper radiographs.

Inadequate supervision: Neither PA consulted with the supervising physician or with the physician seeing patients in the office the days the patient was seen. The supervising physician stated in his deposition that the first time he knew of the patient's death was when he was served notice of the pending lawsuit. The patient was associated with the supervising physician's practice for the past 15 years.

A malpractice case could have been avoided if the PA had performed a more complete history and physical examination, consulted with an office physician, or referred the patient to the ED or radiology for further evaluation. Perhaps if an abdominal examination would have been done, there would have been the discovery of an AAA, and the patient would have been referred to the ED of the hospital that was attached to the medical office building.

Unfortunately, both PAs were sued, and the plaintiff won the case. For one PA, this was the second successful medical malpractice case against him. He was unable to obtain medical malpractice insurance coverage and was forced to find another profession.

The supervising physician was also successfully sued for inadequate supervision of a PA.

The combined monetary value of this case was more than $1 million. Both the physician and the two PAs were entered into the National Practitioner Data Bank.

CASE STUDY 35.3

P.W. has been a PA for 13 years and feels really good about his fund of knowledge regarding the PA profession and the treatment of primary care issues. He is confident in his medical care and consults with his physician as needed, and he does not hesitate to give his own recommendations. His primary care physician, Dr. J., is also confident in him, trusts his judgment, and does not "look over his back." P.W. orders testing when necessary, but he withholds testing when he believes that it is not indicated. His themes are "do no harm" and "don't put people through unnecessary testing." He has said in the past that "unnecessary testing is what is wrong with medicine today."

Mrs. G. came to P.W. for a checkup. She was a regular patient of the practice and saw P.W. for what she considered an urgent complaint. Dr. J. was gone that day from the office. Mrs. G. had a history of anemia and has her blood analyzed in the office on a regular basis. She was called by the office staff and notified that her most recent hemoglobin blood test was 11.6 g/dL. P.W. thought that this was adequate for her. P.W. said, "We will just watch it." After all, P.W. thought that she had no other symptoms and she felt good. No follow-up was made at this time, and although Mrs. G. wanted more testing, she trusted P.W. Even though Mrs. G. is 62 years old and has a family history of cancer, P.W. did not advise her to get a colonoscopy or sigmoidoscopy. He had never performed a digital rectal examination (DRE) on her, assuming that the obstetrician/gynecologist would do it during her annual examination.

Approximately 9 months later, Mrs. G. again complained of fatigue and weakness with some mild abdominal pain. P.W. thought that with her mild symptomatology and fairly sudden onset of symptoms, she had an acute viral illness. P.W. wanted her to "wait it out" and return if no better. She did return to see him, and she felt a little better. P.W. again thought that the viral illness was running its course. Two weeks later, Mrs. G. went to the ED with chest pain and shortness of breath. The emergency physician performed a full workup. A chest radiograph showed a large right lung mass, and a computed tomography scan showed multiple liver masses. A liver biopsy was ultimately performed and revealed metastatic cancer. Her attending hospital physician thought that the cancer had originated in her colon and spread to her lungs and liver. A colonoscopy in the hospital confirmed this. A general surgeon who was consulted explored her abdomen and found that most of it was filled with tumors. The surgeon informed Mrs. G. that nothing could be done at this point, and she should be placed in hospice to try to make her comfortable. She died 3 weeks later.

Two weeks after Mrs. G's diagnosis, P.W. and Dr. J. were served with a lawsuit. Dr. J. and P.W. were sued for medical malpractice. They both met with their defense attorney, and he warned them that a malpractice trial would be a long and unpleasant experience. Both of them were deposed before the plaintiff's attorney. P.W. was asked if he had ever discussed ordering a screening colonoscopy with Mrs. G. He had not. He was asked whether he was aware of a history of cancer in Mrs. G.'s family. P.W. said that he was aware of her family history. He was also asked if he had performed any screening on Mrs. G. for cancer (e.g., DRE, breast examination) or whether he had ever recommended that she get such screenings. P.W. replied no. Dr. J, as the supervising physician, was also questioned vigorously by the plaintiff's attorney and admitted that he had not seen the patient and was not aware of Mrs. G.'s condition. There were several days of depositions, and finally the defense attorney pulled P.W. and Dr. J. aside and said it was time to discuss a settlement offer. The case was settled for the limit of the policy, which was $1 million.

RISK MANAGEMENT ISSUES

Depositions are part of the discovery process, and it is important for all practitioners to be familiar with this process. The deposition gives a "preview" of a court proceeding and provides attorneys on both sides an idea of how the defendant will hold up under questioning if the suit leads to a trial. The deposition allows insight into the testimony and an opportunity to identify any differences in statements made during discovery.

Screening tests can be a controversial issue, especially in our cost-conscious society. Some practitioners order every screening test to "cover" themselves. Although this is a somewhat "safe" way to go, it is also expensive for the patient and society. Performing screening tests based on national guidelines and related to age, family history, and other identified risk factors is an effective method of limiting unnecessary testing in patient populations. In this case, P.W. *never* suggested a screening colonoscopy despite Mrs. G.'s gastrointestinal symptoms and age and his knowledge of her family history. P.W. is also liable because he never discussed the case or had his supervising physician see and evaluate the patient. However, if the screening colonoscopy had been ordered and the patient did not comply, the risk to the practitioners would have been low.

In general, age- and symptom-specific screening should be done regardless of patient symptoms. Examples are prostate-specific antigen testing, mammography, and colonoscopy as a minimum. Other screenings should be done on the basis of the patient's age, risk factors, and symptoms. If screening tests are ordered, they should be documented in the medical record. If the patient does not comply with your recommendations, you should also document this in the medical record.

RISK MANAGEMENT TECHNIQUES

Although there are no guarantees that a PA will not get sued, there are some steps that can be taken to hopefully minimize the risk of being sued.

Documentation: The importance of an accurate and thorough medical chart cannot be overstated. Some common areas of charting mistakes that are often seen in medical malpractice cases include entries that are not dated or timed, use of unapproved abbreviations or symbols, incorrect procedures for noting errors made in the chart, unsigned entries, and alterations to the chart without explanations.

There are some entries in the medical chart that must always be made, including the giving of an informed consent, all medications and test procedures administered to the patient, progress notes on changes in the condition of the patient (both positive and negative), consultations with specialists, patient compliance, patient and family education instructions given, and objective statements about the patient's condition. Items that should not be found in a medical chart include arguments with other health care providers, degrading remarks about patients or other health care providers, finger pointing in the event a mistake is made, and admissions of fault.

Informed consent: This topic has already been discussed in this chapter, but informed consent, properly given and documented, can go a long way toward preventing medical malpractice lawsuits. Many states have a statutory definition of informed consent, so PAs should make sure that when starting a practice, familiarity is made with any statutory language regarding the giving and documentation of informed consent.

Communication skills: PAs must develop exceptional communicative skills. Good rapport with a patient must be established with the very first contact with a patient. Do not wait until something bad happens to try to get to know a patient. When communicating with a patient, the PA must always talk with the patient, not at him or her. Look the patient in the eye and listen to all that is being said. Remember, the patient has been living with his or her problem for weeks, months, or years before you first hear anything about it. There can be all types of subtle clues about a patient's condition a PA can pick up from a thorough discussion with the patient. Always be cordial and friendly with the patient and the family members but remain professional.

In the event a bad outcome arises, a PA's communicative skills will be at a premium. If faced with this situation, the PA must be aware as to whether or not the state in which that PA practices has an "I'm sorry" statute. These types of statutes allow a health care professional to express words of caring or concern to an injured patient or that patient's family without those words being construed as an admission of fault or negligence on the part of the health care provider. If faced with a bad outcome situation, the PA should think ahead about what to say to a patient about a medical mistake or bad outcome before meeting with the patient or the patient's family. If possible, time should be taken to speak with a risk manager or the practice or hospital's attorney before having that tough discussion with the patient. The conversation should try to focus on the future and how any complications will be dealt with in the days, weeks, or months to come. The patient and the patient's family must be part of the conversation, including the making of any difficult medical decisions.

CLINICAL APPLICATIONS

1. Review a recent SOAP (subjective, objective, assessment, and plan) note you have written for incomplete or missing data that could lead to misinterpretation of the encounter.
2. Describe the proper way to make adjustments to the medical record when an error is made in a paper chart. How might this be handled in an electronic medical record?

KEY POINTS

- "Medical negligence" is particular to your specialty and your locale.
- All four elements of negligence must be established by a plaintiff: duty, breach of duty, injuries and damages, and causation.
- Negligence, abandonment, and informed consecovery.
- Good communicative skills are key to a safe and successful patient-oriented practice.

ACKNOWLEDGMENT

The author would like to acknowledge R. Monty Cary and James L. Cary, the authors of this chapter in the previous edition.

References

1. *Green v. Box Butte County General Hospital*; 2012. 284 Neb. 243, 818 N.W.2d 589. http://www.leagle.com/decision/In%20NECO%2020120803279/GREEN%20v.%20BOX%20BUTTE%20GENERAL%20HOSP. Accessed February 15, 2016.
2. *Murray v. UNMC Physicians*; 2011. 282 Neb. 260, 806 N.W.2d 118. http://www.leagle.com/decision/In%20NECO%2020110916265/MURRAY%20v.%20UNMC%20PHYSICIANS. Accessed March 21, 2016.
3. Manning J. Factual causation in medical negligence. *J Law Med*. 2007;15(3):337–355.
4. *LexisNexis 50 State Survey*; 2012. https://w3.lexis.com/research2/attachment/popUpAttachWindow.do?_m=bb4333d0572a799965cd81c3762a4316&wchp=dGLzVzk-zSkAb&_md-5=8603baadb5f12735759d030c9c9b8231. Accessed February 16, 2016.
5. Nebraska Revised Statute §44-2816. http://nebraskalegislature.gov/laws/statutes.php?statute=44-2816. Accessed March 21, 2016.
6. Hooker RS, Nicholson JG, Le T. Does the employment of physician assistants and nurse practitioners increase liability? *Journal of Medical Licensure and Discipline*. 2009;95(2):6–16.
7. Refo PA. The vanishing trial. American Bar Association, *Journal of the Section of Litigation*. 2004;30(2):1–4. http://www.americanbar.org/content/dam/aba/publishing/litigation_journal/04winter_openingstatement.authcheckdam.pdf. Accessed March 21, 2016.

The Faculty Resources can be found online at www.expertconsult.com.

CHAPTER 36

POSTGRADUATE CLINICAL TRAINING PROGRAMS FOR PHYSICIAN ASSISTANTS

Maura Polansky • David P. Asprey

Formal clinical training programs are available to provide physician assistants (PAs) with a postgraduate specialty educational experience using the physician residency model of training. These residency programs (sometimes called fellowships) provide graduate PAs with the opportunity to gain supervised clinical experience supplemented with structured didactic work in a specialty area of medicine that builds on the generalist training acquired in the entry-level PA program. Furthermore, the training typically provides an accelerated learning curve in part because of the formalized and structured didactic education component with clinical assignments and formal evaluations intended to support the professional development of the PAs. Most residency programs are located within teaching hospitals or larger clinics and hospitals and are available throughout the United States.

Employment opportunities and clinical roles for PAs have rapidly expanded to include positions in a wide variety of specialty areas. Postgraduate curricula are designed to build on the knowledge and experience acquired in PA school, enabling individuals to assume roles as well-prepared PAs on specialty health care teams more rapidly than those without formal training or prior specialty experience. Many postgraduate programs have pioneered the role of PAs in these specialty areas and offer experienced role models, as well as formalized instruction. Although this training is optional for PAs and only a small percentage of PAs elect to participate in residency programs, they can provide PAs an opportunity to receive formal clinical training, typically in academic medical centers, providing PAs a strong foundation in specialty practice not available as part of entry-level PA education.

HISTORY OF POSTGRADUATE RESIDENCY EDUCATION

The first postgraduate PA program began in 1971 at the Montefiore Medical Center in affiliation with the Albert Einstein School of Medicine in New York.[1] Montefiore Medical Center began employing and educating PAs to replace surgical house officers. These PA residents were trained alongside physician surgery house officers. In 1975, Norwalk Hospital and the Department of Surgery at the Yale School of Medicine established a 1-year surgical residency program exclusively structured for PAs, which combined didactic and clinical instruction. By 1980, six postgraduate residency programs were known to exist, and the number has steadily risen from there. At the American Academy of Physician Assistants (AAPA) Annual Meeting in Los Angeles in May 1988, a group of representatives of postgraduate PA residency programs met to formalize a national postgraduate PA program organization—the Association of Postgraduate Physician Assistant Programs (APPAP); bylaws were written and approved by the seven founding member programs.[2]

The exact number of PA residency programs has not been known because of the lack of a consistent means of tracking programs. The most accessible information regarding programs has been the Association of Postgraduate PA Programs (APPAP); however, membership in the APPAP is voluntary, and it is known that many other programs exist. The most recent membership roster of the APPAP dated September 2015 lists 58 programs.[3] The authors estimate that there are nearly 100 postgraduate clinical training programs in total, including APPAP members and nonmembers.

The number of PAs having undergone training in postgraduate residency programs has also been difficult to determine. The most recent published study that surveyed 42 nonmilitary programs found that enrollment was just over 100 PAs, with most programs enrolling 2 or 3 PAs each year.[4] Therefore, it is likely that only 200 to 300 PAs participate in residency training each year. Although comprehensive data regarding the number of current PA residents and graduates is limited, it seems apparent that even with the expansion of PA residency programs, the percentage of PAs training in such programs remains quite small.

Over the years, some of the most important questions asked about PA residency training have included what the potential value of such programs is for participants, what impact these programs have and will have on PA practice, and whether program accreditation will be beneficial or in some way detrimental to the PA profession. Despite these broad questions, relatively little research has been conducted regarding PA residency programs, particularly in recent years.

Program Development

The primary reasons for institutions to develop PA residency programs has included an identified need for additional training for PAs in the specialty, a need to replace physician residents or house officers, and the need to recruit additional PAs to the institution after graduation.[5-7] Given the work hour restrictions for physician interns and residents and the now well-established role of PAs in academic settings in specialized services, the desire for a formally trained PA workforce will likely remain a major factor for developing programs.

Institutions considering establishing a PA residency program can find valuable resources from the APPAP's website and at their biannual meetings. The Accreditation Review Commission on Education for the Physician Assistant (ARC-PA) Accreditation Standards for Clinical Postgraduate PA Programs are often used by programs as a blueprint for program development. In addition, institutions' own physician residency programs and local PA schools may be valuable resources to those considering starting a program. Factors to consider when making decisions about developing new programs include defining the mission and goals of the program; determining what resources are available, including clinical experts such as physicians, PAs, and other professionals in the specialty; identifying didactic materials that are already in place and determining new curriculum needed; and estimating the overall cost for developing and maintaining the program. Several programs have written about their experience in providing residency training to PAs, and reading these may be of value to those considering such an endeavor.[6-9]

Currently Available Programs

As previously mentioned, the exact number of programs is unknown, and earlier studies relied on membership data from the APPAP. The term "postgraduate" has often applied to both residency programs and academic programs that may or may not provide onsite clinical training. The use of membership data by the APPAP has its limitations because membership does not ensure consistency in the type of education offered, may be inclusive of programs not actively enrolling PAs, and may not include all available programs because membership in APPAP is optional. However, the use of APPAP membership data has provided general information regarding the scope of postgraduate education and a means of contacting programs to participate in survey research.

In 2008, Wiemiller and Somer[10] sought to identify all "postgraduate" PA programs to address the bias in prior studies of omitting programs that were not members of the APPAP. They identified 55 programs; 44 of these programs (76%) were members of the APPAP. Most programs reported enrolling one to five PAs annually. Thirty-eight percent of programs were described as adopting an "academic model," with 11.4% reporting charging tuition. Because this study sought to include all postgraduate programs, it is likely that it included academic programs offering an advanced degree or academic credit without an emphasis on clinical training. A later study, conducted in 2011, sought to identify only those programs that provided in-house clinical training for PAs at the postgraduate level.[4] Investigators surveyed 43 nonmilitary and 7 military programs meeting this criterion with active PA enrollment in early 2011. Twenty-six programs had enrolled their first PA between in 2008 and 2011, suggesting a significant growth in PA clinical postgraduate program development over this brief 3-year period.

Our understanding of the scope and characteristics of postgraduate programs is limited to data from these recent studies along with the current APPAP membership data with online information provided by programs. Therefore, while reading the following available program information, readers should consider the limitations of these data in understanding PA postgraduate residency programs.

GENERAL CHARACTERISTICS OF EXISTING PROGRAMS

Residency programs provide both supervised clinical training as well as formal didactic instruction. These are the hallmarks of residency training, consistent with the model of physician residency programs. Most PA residency programs are civilian programs located in academic health centers.[4,10] Fewer programs are located in other settings such as community or military hospitals. Most studies have reported on nonmilitary programs, and this chapter focuses primarily on these programs. Less has been published in the literature or online on military PA residency programs.

Residency programs typically provide specialty and subspecialty training, although there have been a few primary care programs such as family or rural medicine programs. The most common specialties represented in current programs include emergency medicine, general surgery and surgical subspecialties, and critical care.[3,4,10] However, a variety of medicine subspecialties, such as oncology, psychiatry, and dermatology, are available, although the numbers of these programs remain small.

Most programs are 12 months in duration, and programs shorter than 6 to 12 months are generally not considered residency programs for research purposes or by professional organizations such as the APPAP and ARC-PA. Class sizes vary among programs, from as few as 1 PA resident to 12 or more,

with most programs accepting 1 or 2 PAs annually based on published studies.[4,10] Some newer programs have developed multiple specialty tracks and larger cohorts, enrolling up to 28 PA residents.[3] Institutions may consider their PA residents as trainees, but others may classify them as staff and, in at least one case, they are part of the faculty.[7] It is generally thought that the majority of programs do require residents to be licensed to practice as a PA in the state and have them undergo hospital credentialing and privileging as they do their staff PAs.

Application Process

Given the widely available program information now online, students and other potential candidates are likely able to obtain extensive information online. Member programs of the APPAP are listed at http://www.appap.org, and links to programs' websites are available on this site. A web search of other programs can help potential candidates identify additional programs. PA specialty organizations such as the American Association of Surgical Physician Assistants may also be a valuable source of information regarding residencies in a specific specialty.[11]

Most students consider additional training while they are in PA schools. Program information is often made available to students during PA school, as part of classes on PA professional issues, during career festivals, and from brochures provide by residency programs to PA schools. However, many PA residents and students report that they do not learn about PA residency programs from their PA schools, and the majority of PA school faculty members have reported that they would not encourage students to consider attending, although the reasons for this have not been investigated.[12,13]

A residency program selection is often highly competitive, although the ratio of applicants to residency positions has not been published. Although no centralized application service is available that is like the Central Application Service for Physician Assistants (used by most entry-level PA programs), programs require completion of a program application package. The application material required typically includes a program application form, a copy of the diploma from PA school, school transcripts, a curriculum vita, letters of recommendation, and a narrative describing the candidate's interest in the residency and the specialty area. In addition, nearly all residency programs require personal interviews. Residency directors have reported using many different criteria in making admission decisions for their programs. Commonly used measures include interest in the specialty, interviews, letters of recommendation, level of motivation, academic performance, interpersonal skills, and prior elective rotations or other experience in the specialty.

Historical data indicate that the majority of enrolled residents reported that they had applied to a single residency program.[12] With the expansion of programs, including the presence of multiple programs in some specialties such as emergency medicine and surgery, it is likely that candidates now apply to multiple programs in their desired specialty when they are available.

Admission Requirements

Admission requirements are typically published online by each program. All programs required PA residents to have graduated from an ARC-PA PA program, and most require that they be certified by or eligible for National Commission on Certification of Physician Assistants (NCCPA). Although only half reported requiring state licensure in 1999, it is now thought that most programs have such a requirement.[5] Most programs do not require prior health care experiences before entering a residency program, although some programs may prefer such experience.

Clinical Settings

Most programs are located in academic settings that can provide a wide variety of patient care experiences and a diverse patient care mix. Instructors for residency programs consist of physicians and PAs but may also include advanced practice nurses. Because academic health care institutions employ a wide spectrum of other health care professionals such as clinical pharmacists, dieticians, physical therapists, and others, residents likely have frequent opportunities to learn from these professionals as well.

In recent years, programs have begun collaborating with nurse practitioners (NPs) to offer residencies programs to both PAs and NPs. Although these programs made up a small minority of PA residency programs surveyed in 2011,[4] the authors believe that more programs are now open to both PAs and NPs and anticipate this trend to continue. Current ARC-PA accreditation standards require that PA residency programs be led by a physician or PA; therefore, these interprofessional programs are not currently accredited.

Curriculum

The primary curricular content of PA residency programs is supervising clinical training. Clinical experience is focused around the program specialty, but unlike clinical employment, residencies are organized around a variety of clinical rotations, providing a spectrum of clinical experience for the PA. In addition to required clinical rotations, most programs also offer clinical electives to allow the PA resident opportunities to structure their training around their unique professional interests.[4] Physicians and PA preceptors provide both supervision and instruction during clinical training.

The number of clinical hours required by programs varies from specialty to specialty and from program to program. Data from a study of surgical PAs from 2007 reported residents enrolled in "internship model" programs worked an average of 72 clinical hours per week.[14] Wiemiller and Somer[10] found that 31% of surveyed programs reported requiring in-house call as part of their program, but Polansky et al. found that more than 60% of programs required in-house calls.[4] For accredited programs, work-hour restrictions include limiting work hours (including clinical and academic activities) to a maximum of 80 hours per week averaged over a 4-week period.[15] Other restrictions addressed by the ARC-PA accreditation standards include requiring a minimum of 1 in 7 days free from all educational and clinical responsibilities and 10 hours off from all daily duty periods, including being on call.

In addition to clinical training, residencies provide formal didactic instruction at the beginning of the residency, incorporated throughout the program, or both.[10] In a study published in 2000, residents estimated their total number of hours of didactic education associated with the residency program they attended to be 350 to 413.[13] Subsequent studies have not investigated the specific amount of time devoted to didactic work but have reported on the spectrum of didactic activities that PA residents may be required to participate in. Programs typically include lectures, conferences, required readings, attendance at patient care conferences, grand rounds, online courses, and others.[4,10] Some programs also require or provide optional opportunities for PAs to give presentations such as at journal clubs, conduct research, and write manuscripts for publication.[4,10] Many programs also involve their PA residents in teaching through instruction of PA students and other trainees.[4]

Credential Awarded

Earlier studies of PA residency programs described two models of postgraduate training, an "internship model" and an "academic model," with the later offering academic credit or a degree.[9] Currently, most programs do not award academic credit and instead award a certificate of completion for graduates.[4,10] This change is likely a result of the change in degrees awarded by PA schools, with a master's degree now being the standardized academic degree for PA schools.

During the past decade, military programs have offered a clinical doctorate degree. In 2006, the U.S. Army Emergency Medicine PA residency program was expanded from a 12-month program to an 18-month program.[16] The program worked with Baylor University in Waco, Texas, to provide academic credit for their training program that leads to a doctor of science in PA studies (DSc). Since that time, additional military programs have begun offering a DSc with six programs identified in a 2011 study.[4] No civilian residency programs are known to offer doctorate degrees.

Stipends and Fringe Benefits

Data from 2011 indicate that most programs provided an annual stipend between $40,000 and $60,000.[4] At that time, the highest educational stipend reported was between $70,000 and $79,999. Although some programs list salary or trainee compensation information online, comprehensive data on current compensation rates are not available. Benefit packages vary but generally include such items as health insurance, malpractice insurance, paid vacation time, and sick leave.[4,10]

RESIDENCY PROGRAM ACCREDITATION

Dating back to 1980, the PA accreditation agencies (the Joint Review Committee, which predated the ARC-PA) and PA educational organizations considered the possibility of establishing an accreditation process for PA residency programs as a means of ensuring educational standards were used by programs.[1] In 1991, the APPAP took the initial step in establishing standards for postgraduate programs by adopting its own set of program "Essentials," which were intended to identify the desirable elements of a PA residency program.[1] Although APPAP member programs were asked to agree to adhere to the essentials as a condition of membership, compliance with the Essentials was voluntary and was neither formally reviewed nor enforced.

A formal task force with representatives from the ARC-PA and APPAP was established in 1999 to formally consider the issue of accreditation. In 2001, representatives of the AAPA and APAP (former name of the Physician Assistant Education Association) joined the task force, with meetings

continuing until 2005. The potential implications on PA education and the profession were explored over time. Although some members of the task force identified accreditation as a means of ensuring core educational standards were met, others expressed concern about the potential for unintended consequences that could result from an accreditation process—specifically the concern that the existence of accredited programs might limit opportunities for PAs not trained in accredited programs to work in specialty practices.

After years of consideration, in March 2006, the ARC-PA voted in favor of offering optional accreditation to PA residency programs. The first version of the accreditation standards was published in 2007.[15] The first two programs were granted accreditation in March 2008, and as of fall 2015, eight programs have been accredited. A list of accredited programs is available on the http://www.arc-pa.org website.

The standards address a wide range of educational administration issues, including ensuring programs have adequate faculty and staff, funding, and patient care experiences.[15] Programs must be full time and be at least 6 months in duration, offering in-residency clinical training and didactic instruction. Programs must adhere to work-hour restrictions as used by the Accreditation Council for Graduate Medical Education. As part of the accreditation review process, the program curriculum must be reviewed by a medical review committee of experts in the discipline to determine if program objectives can be met by the established curriculum, and a site visit is conducted by the ARC-PA. If programs are found to adhere to the accreditation standards, programs would receive accreditation for a maximum of 3 years. An annual report is required each year, and programs must reapply for accreditation after 3 years to maintain their accreditation status. The ARC-PA has emphasized that accreditation is optional.

In July 2014, the ARC-PA announced that the accreditation process of residency programs would be held in abeyance, and a work group would be formed to "discuss alternative methods of recognition of educational quality for Clinical Postgraduate PA Programs."[15] Based on this decision, the ARC-PA suspended accepting new applications, although accredited programs would retain their accreditation pending the outcome of further study by the commission. The ARC-PA expressed concerns about the labor and resource intensiveness for programs in applying for accreditation as the reason for their decision to suspend the accreditation process for residency programs. As of the fall of 2015, the ARC-PA workgroup has conducted initial meetings, and it is expected that additional information on the status of residency accreditation will become available in 2016.

The issues of program accreditation and oversight have been considered by the AAPA over many years as well. In the 1980s, the AAPA established a policy endorsing a set of standards for PA residency programs. The policy was reaffirmed several times up until 2000.[1] However, in 2005, the AAPA House of Delegates adopted a new policy statement opposing accreditation for postgraduate PA programs. The position statement was revised in 2010, indicating that the "AAPA continues to have concerns about the accreditation of PA postgraduate training programs."[17] A primary concern raised in the AAPA position paper was the potential of credentialing bodies requiring postgraduate training and that accreditation increases awareness of programs and "with such awareness, the possibility of credentialing bodies preferring or requiring postgraduate training may become more of a reality." To date, no such requirements have occurred, and at the time of the writing of this chapter, the AAPA policy statement is undergoing review and will be considered at the 2016 AAPA meeting of the House of Delegates.[18]

ASSOCIATION OF POSTGRADUATE PROGRAMS

The APPAP has remained the primary organization representing PA residency programs. Over the years, the number of member programs has gradually grown from the initial 8 founding members to 58 programs in 20 specialties as of November 2015.[19] The organization states their purpose is to be a resource for PAs and PA students about postgraduate clinical PA education. The APPAP conducts biannual meetings and educational sessions for its members in conjunction with the annual AAPA and Physician Assistant Education Association (PAEA) conferences. The AAPA's website lists all member programs and provides information about each as well as a link to each program's website. The AAPA typically provides information during the AAPA conference at a booth in the exhibit hall and with sessions during the regular meeting and the Student Academy of the American Academy of Physician Assistants (SAAAPA) sessions. The Association of Postgraduate Physician Assistant Programs (APPAP) also provides awards to those who conduct research on residency training and to PA residents who conduct research during their training program. Currently, the APPAP responsibilities of membership include the expectation that programs will "adhere to sound educational principles and support other member programs in the pursuit of such

principles."[19] However, accreditation is not required for membership. The APPAP recognizes five classes of membership: Active Program Members, Provisional Program Members, Inactive Program Members, Affiliate Members, and Individual Members.[19]

The APPAP maintains informal liaisons with the AAPA, ARC-PA, and PAEA and works with these organizations on mutual goals to further the PA profession and postgraduate PA education. Additional information regarding current member residency programs, APPAP bylaws, and general information can be viewed at the website http://www.appap.org.

Resident Perceptions of Training

The most common reason PAs decided to pursue residency training appears to be to enhance their competitiveness for jobs in the specialty.[13] Another important reason is the desire of PAs to expand their current level of competency in the specialty, either to obtaining additional clinical knowledge and skills before going into practice or to enhance their ability to change specialty area. Studies of residency graduates have found a high level of satisfaction with their training, and they report being well prepared for their jobs.[14,20] One very early study found that 20% of former residents believed they were actually overprepared for their job.[21] However, as the scope of practice for PAs has expanded over the past 2 decades and because more recent studies have not investigated this issue, it is not clear if this remains a concern of some graduates. Graduates also report increased confidence and having increased autonomy after residency training.[14,20] Several reports indicate that residents would recommend their program to other PAs interested in the specialty.[1,20] The primary disadvantage reported by PA residents is the lower stipends received during training compared with PA salaries in the workplace.[14]

Included in this chapter is a report of interviews with three PAs who attended a residency. The interviews explore the PAs' perceptions of their residency experience and their reasons for electing to attend a residency program.

RESIDENCY GRADUATE EMPLOYMENT OPPORTUNITIES

Reports confirm that most graduates go on to practice in the specialty of their training, and several reports indicate that they are highly competitive candidate for these positions.[20] One study and substantial anecdotal reports found that residency-prepared PAs have a competitive edge over nonresidency-trained PAs when applying for PA positions.[14] Little objective information has been published comparing the number of employment opportunities and the salaries commanded between residency-prepared and nonresidency-prepared PAs. One study published in 2007 surveyed PAs in surgical settings, comparing graduates from surgical residencies with those who had not received such training.[14] The mean salary per hour was similar between the two groups. Although some graduates may receive higher initial compensation, no data suggest that there are long-term financial advantages to residency training.

SELECTING A RESIDENCY PROGRAM

Residents historically indicated that the way they learned about the residency program was either through information provided by the PA program they attended or from a student or residency graduate. Online information is now available for most programs. A complete list of programs that are members of the APPAP as of November 2015 is presented in Table 36.1.

Residents identify an improved ability to compete for a job in their specialty, interest in acquiring additional knowledge and skills before entering practice, and the desire for increased competence in the specialty area as the items that had the greatest influence on their decision to attend residency. Potential candidates should consider these factors while examining the program curriculum, including clinical experiences and didactic instruction provided and program goals, in selecting programs to apply to.

Because few programs are currently accredited, work hours and policies regarding selection, remediation, graduation requirements, and benefits may not be published for candidates, which is a requirement for accredited programs. However, candidates can request this information from programs to ensure a clear understanding of program expectations.

Residents and program graduates may provide a unique perspective, and they may be available to speak to applicants about their experience in the program. Because most programs require an onsite interview, candidates can meet program instructors, staff, and current residents; tour clinical sites; and learn more about the program at that time. If an onsite interview is not required, candidates may wish to consider arranging a program visit on their own to learn more about the program onsite.

TABLE 36.1 Association of Postgraduate Physician Assistant Programs Member Programs (September 2015)

Name of Program	Location	Critical Care and Trauma	
Acute Care Medicine		St. Luke's Hospital	Bethlehem, PA
University of Missouri	Columbia, MO	Mayo Clinic Arizona	Phoenix, AZ
Carolinas Healthcare System Center	Charlotte, NC	WakeMed Health and Hospitals	Raleigh, NC
Cardiology		Winthrop University Hospital	Mineola, NY
Mercer-Piedmont Heart	Atlanta, GA	**Emergency Medicine**	
Cardiothoracic		Albany Medical Center	Albany, NY
Emory University	Atlanta, GA	Albert Einstein Medical Center	Philadelphia, PA
St. Joseph Mercy Hospital	Ypsilanti, MI	Arrowhead Regional Medical Center	Colton, CA
Methodist DeBakey Heart and Vascular Center	Houston, TX	Carilion Clinic	Roanoke, VA
Critical Care and Trauma		Eastern Virginia Medical School	Norfolk, VA
Carolinas Healthcare System Center	Charlotte, NC	Johns Hopkins Bayview Hospital	Baltimore, MD
Intermountain Medical Center	Murray, UT	Kaweah Delta Medical Center	Visalia, CA
Emory Critical Care	Atlanta, GA	Marquette University—Aurora Health	Milwaukee, WI
Johns Hopkins Hospital	Baltimore, MD		

TABLE 36.1 Association of Postgraduate Physician Assistant Programs Member Programs (September 2015)—cont'd

Emergency Medicine	
New York Presbyterian–Weill Cornell Medical Center	New York, NY
Regions Hospital	St. Paul, MN
Staten Island University Hospital	Staten Island, NY
Team Health EMAPC Fellowship	Oklahoma City, OK
University of Iowa	Iowa City, IA

Family Medicine	
Carolinas Healthcare System	Charlotte, NC

Hematology/Oncology	
Mayo Clinic Arizona	Phoenix, AZ
MD Anderson Cancer Center, The University of Texas	Houston, TX

Hospitalist	
Carolinas Healthcare System	Charlotte, NC
Mayo Clinic Arizona	Phoenix, AZ
University of Missouri	Columbia, MO

Internal Medicine	
Carolinas Healthcare System	Charlotte, NC

Neonatology	
Children's Hospital of Philadelphia	Philadelphia, PA
University of Kentucky	Lexington, KY

Neurosurgery	
Texas Brain and Spine Institute	Bryan, TX

Obstetrics and Gynecology	
Arrowhead-Riverside	Colton, CA
Montefiore Medical Center	Bronx, NY

Orthopedic Surgery	
Arrowhead Orthopedics	Redlands, CA

Orthopedic Surgery	
Illinois Bone and Joint Institute	Park Ridge, IL

Otolaryngology	
Mayo Clinic Arizona	Phoenix, AZ

Pediatrics	
Carolinas Healthcare System	Charlotte, NC

Psychiatry	
Nationwide Children's Hospital	Columbus, OH
University of Iowa	Iowa City, IA

Surgery	
Bassett Healthcare	Cooperstown, NY
Capital Health–Hopewell–STARS	Pennington, NJ
Duke University Medical Center	Durham, NC
Hartford Healthcare	Hartford, CT
Johns Hopkins Hospital	Baltimore, MD
Montefiore Medical Center, Albert Einstein College of Medicine	Bronx, NY
Norwalk Hospital, Yale	Norwalk, CT
Texas Children's Hospital	Houston, TX
University of Pittsburgh Medical Center	Pittsburgh, PA

Urgent Care	
Carolinas Healthcare System	Charlotte, NC

Urology	
Carolinas Healthcare System	Charlotte, NC
UT Southwestern Medical Center	Dallas, TX
Rosalind Franklin University, Chicago Medical School	North Chicago, IL

CASE STUDY 36.1

Age: 30 years

PA school attended: University of Iowa

Were you in practice before attending a residency (if so, what specialty and how long?): No

PA residency program attended: University of Iowa Emergency Medicine

Dates enrolled in residency: June 2010 to December 2011

Q: What influenced you to attend a residency program after graduating from PA school?

A: A desire to prepare for and be capable of taking care of critically ill patients.

Q: Specifically, why did you elect to attend a residency program after graduation as opposed to getting your specialty training on the job?

A: Many of the skills taught in emergency department (ED) residency are very difficult to attain on the job, as is the approach to managing emergent patients and an entire ED. It is possible if employed in the perfect setting; however, it requires a lot of time, leaving a substantial knowledge gap over a large portion of a career.

Q: What exposure to the specialty of the residency you attended did you receive in your entry-level PA program education?

A: The director of the program and a current resident spoke to our PA class during a regularly scheduled meeting.

Q: Briefly describe the curriculum in your residency program—didactic component versus clinical experiences and so on.

A: Didactics included conference once a week for 4 hours, which covered a different topic each month. Testing occurred at the end of each month over that topic as well as general testing once a year. Clinical rotations are 1 month long; most are in the ED with off-service rotations on the trauma and burn unit, electrocardiography, radiology, the intensive care unit (ICU), and a couple of electives.

Q: What types of procedural skills did you gain experience with in your residency?

A: Airway management, central venous access, arterial line placement, venous pacing, chest tube placement, thoracentesis, paracentesis, lumbar puncture, fracture reduction and splinting, joint reduction, suturing and wound management, abscess drainage, lateral canthotomy, infant delivery, postmortem C-section, bedside ultrasound, and code management.

Q: Was there a research element in your residency program?

A: It was optional. I did publish one case study.

Q: How was your performance in the residency program evaluated? Written exams, simulation, evaluations by supervising clinicians?

A: Written exams monthly and yearly; simulations and feedback from peers and supervising clinicians.

Q: What was/were the most important knowledge and skills you acquired from your residency?

A: A mental approach to critically ill patients and airway management.

Q: Who served as your teachers in the residency? Faculty, residents, PAs, others?

A: Same faculty as the MD residents and occasionally third-year MD residents.

Q: What compensation did you receive during the residency? Were there benefits in addition to a salary?

A: Standard resident salary of about $42,000 a year with health and dental insurance as well.

Q: What was the length of your residency?

A: 18 months

Q: Approximately how many hours did you work during an average week in the residency?

A: 60 to 80+, depending on which rotation you are on

Q: How many PA residents were enrolled in your residency program?

A: Two.

Q: What job opportunities did you find were available when you had completed the residency? Do you think having attended a residency was important to your employer?

A: It seemed to make me more marketable; however, it did not guarantee the type of job I wanted.

Q: What were the most positive aspects of being a PA resident?

A: Having the opportunity to gain skills and knowledge in a dedicated setting and being able to show my MD resident and faculty colleagues that we as PAs are very capable of handling critically ill patients.

Q: What were the negative aspects of being a PA resident?

A: Residency is difficult; it's long hours with comparatively little pay and high expectations of performance and improvement constantly. It can also be frustrating after graduation because you will find that this training is still new, and there isn't a comfort level in many places of employment with letting PAs work in a true ED.

CASE STUDY 36.2

Gender: Male
Age: 31 years
PA school attended: Northeastern University
Were you in practice before attending a residency (if so what specialty and how long?): No
PA residency program attended: Norwalk Hospital/Yale Surgical Residency
Dates enrolled in residency: September 2011 to September 2012

Q: What influenced you to attend a residency program after graduating from PA school?

A: My surgical rotation at Norwalk played the biggest part in my decision. I had an absolutely amazing experience surrounded by residents. I was fortunate to be a student when residents were graduating as well as when a new group of residents were starting. The amount they learned through the year was astounding. They seemed so confident and well rounded and had an incredible fount of knowledge. I knew it would be a great opportunity to fine tune my skills and develop the practical knowledge that would be needed to be a better practitioner.

Q: Specifically, why did you elect to attend a residency program after graduation as opposed to getting your specialty training on the job?

A: I felt like a residency would give me a permanent leg up when competing in the job market. The timing was right. I knew I wanted to do a surgical specialty as a PA. I thought to myself, if a PA was going to be operating on me or even assisting, then I would hope he or she had additional training over a 4- or 6-week rotation. Then having the first-hand experience of seeing how the residents developed made me realize this was what I needed to do.

Q: What exposure to the specialty of the residency you attended did you receive in your entry-level PA program education?

A: I was a student at the site where I did my residency. I was able to see how involved the PA's were and experienced it firsthand. The PAs received invaluable training and were making sound decisions and were confident. To me, there was no downside after experiencing it.

Q: Briefly describe the curriculum in your residency program—didactic component versus clinical experiences and so on.

A: The didactic component consisted of a lecture every single morning before our day started. It also included grand rounds and tumor board at the hospital. We had multiple training programs throughout as well, from saw bone workshops to a laparoscopy training that was in depth. We also were involved with 3 weeks up at Yale University that consisted of lectures, pig labs, and cadaver labs. These were incredibly useful for building skill and confidence. We also had three elective rotations where we were able to select specialties that had piqued our interest in which we wanted to develop additional skills and to further professional connections.

Q: What types of procedural skills did you gain experience with in your residency?

A: Suturing, knot tying, all aspects of laparoscopy, trauma, chest tubes, Continuous Bladder Irrigation (CBI), any related operating room (OR) procedures, ICU management.

Q: Was there a research element in your residency program?

A: I was able to publish a research paper on my own. The requirement was for a final project. This was allowed to be a research paper or an institutional project that could be designed and implemented.

Q: How was your performance in the residency program evaluated? Written exams, simulation, evaluations by supervising clinicians?

A: We had quizzes and exams on each specialty we were on as well as a cumulative exam. We also had two simulation labs during the year. We were also evaluated routinely by our physicians and fellow PAs.

Q: What was/were the most important knowledge and skills you acquired from your residency?

A: The most important knowledge was how to manage both patients and the hospital. I felt much more confident in the entire treatment of the patient and managing from admission to discharge. OR skills such as laparoscopy and running a trauma in the ED were invaluable. But I think the nonprocedural skills like managing fluids, evaluating and stabilizing trauma, and managing ICU patients were skills that stuck and continue to give me the confidence to manage some patients that my attending physicians are sometimes not even comfortable with.

Q: Who served as your teachers in the residency? Faculty, residents, PAs, others?

A: Hospital physicians and PAs were the primary instructors for the residency. We also spent 3 weeks at Yale that were taught by faculty and staff (MDs, PAs, and so on) of multiple departments.

Q: What compensation did you receive during the residency? Were there benefits in addition to a salary?

A: $42,500. We also received a stipend for housing in the hospital that made it reasonable. Health care benefits were also included. In addition, we received 2 weeks of paid time off and 5 days reserved for interviews for our next job.

Q: What was the length of your residency?

A: 1 year

Q: **Approximately how many hours did you work during an average week in the residency?**
A: 50 to 60

Q: **How many residents were enrolled in your residency program?**
A: 12

Q: **What job opportunities did you find were available when you had completed the residency?**
A: Multiple jobs in orthopedics were available, which is what I wanted. I'm sure there would have been more, but I was looking to move to the same location with my then girlfriend, now wife, which narrowed our options.

Q: **Do you think having attended a residency was important to your employer?**
A: At first, no. I think when I interviewed for orthopedics, most of the jobs wanted an entire year of experience in the specialty. However, I spent one interview selling myself on the position I wanted, which included floating between multiple specialties in the practice. I think this is where the residency helped to sell my future employer that I could do it. They were able to look at the variety of cases and volume of cases I had done, and I was able to discuss the experience, which also helped. My future employer also had very little experience with hiring a former resident, which added skepticism. However, after employment, they have been able to see the diversity and understanding I can bring and in fact have been able to expand my role to everything I wanted, thanks to the residency background.

Q: **What were the most positive aspects of being a PA resident?**
A: The learning experience (knowledge gained) and camaraderie. My fellow residents are now my best friends. We hang out often and fly from all over the country to meet up two or three times per year. Three of us have also moved so that we can all work in the same city. I also feel like I constantly apply the knowledge I gained during the residency every day. It allows me to feel like I can manage any type of patient or condition, regardless of what specialty I currently work in.

Q: **What were the negative aspects of being a PA resident?**
A: The biggest negative was the fact that residencies for PAs are still not that popular. When interviewing, I had to spend a lot of time educating employers about what we did as residents and why we even did residencies. I think it was viewed negatively by employers before actually getting to converse with them in person during the interview. Most employers didn't count the residency as a full year of experience because the residency was in multiple specialties (general surgery). Some thought it wasn't necessary for a PA to do a residency and wondered why it was necessary that I do one. I think after interviews were

granted and conducted that the residency was looked at extremely positively, and employers understood and valued the experience. However, leading up to the interview required some explaining, and questioning wasn't always positive. However, with the increasing number of residencies and specialties and number of PAs entering residencies, I am hopeful this will improve.

CASE STUDY 36.3

Gender: Female
Age: 28 years
PA school attended: Rosalind Franklin University of Medicine and Science
Were you in practice before attending a residency (if so what specialty and how long?): No
PA residency program attended: Hematology/oncology at MD Anderson
Dates enrolled in residency: September 2013 to October 2014

Q: **What influenced you to attend a residency program after graduating from PA school?**
A: My passion in medicine is oncology. During PA school, I felt that the 6-week rotation was not sufficient to really understand the depth of the specialty. The fellowship at MD Anderson allowed the opportunity to spend valuable time learning medical, surgical, and radiation oncology in more detail. I felt this would give me confidence when working as an independent provider in a very specialized area of medicine while also allowing time to explore the subspecialties within oncology.

Q: **Specifically, why did you elect to attend a residency program after graduation as opposed to getting your specialty training on the job?**
A: Oncology has many specific subdepartments (lung, gastrointestinal, breast, genitourinary, and so on) that include separate disciplines (surgery, medical oncology, radiation oncology). The residency at MD Anderson gave me the opportunity to learn in and experience all of these areas while deciding which ones I found most intriguing. Although I ultimately chose to work in medical oncology, I have insight and have participated in many of the surgeries and procedures that my patients will be experiencing. I find that knowledge base is broader and with more depth because I completed the residency program.

Q: **What exposure to the specialty of the residency you attended did you receive in your entry-level PA program education?**
A: Minimal. During the didactic portion of school, we briefly reviewed oncology. Because of my interest in the specialty, I chose to do a 6-week clinical rotation and write my master's thesis on an oncology topic.

Q: Briefly describe the curriculum in your residency program—didactic component versus clinical experiences and so on.

A: My residency was composed of clinical work in medical/surgical/radiation oncology clinics, in patient rounding, surgical procedures, and ED coverage during the weekend. I also was expected to study outside of work, write a research paper, and complete four presentations.

Q: What types of procedural skills did you gain experience with in your residency?

A: I became proficient in bone marrow biopsies and lumbar punctures, skills that I now use in my current position. We also approached thoracentesis, paracentesis, and Omaya access.

Q: Was there a research element in your residency program?

A: A portion of the curriculum was to write a research article to be published in a journal of your choice. Additionally, we were asked to complete four lectures throughout the year, and research with faculty was always encouraged.

Q: How was your performance in the residency program evaluated? Written exams, simulation, evaluations by supervising clinicians?

A: I felt like we were evaluated on a daily basis by working with the physicians and PAs. However, the formal evaluation was a test at the end of each rotation. The format was decided upon by my preceptors. They ranged from written exams, panel questioning, and papers.

Q: What was/were the most important knowledge and skills you feel you acquired from your residency?

A: I gained numerous skills and knowledge from my residency that I have carried over into my current career. Starting my current career with a knowledge base and foundation was exceptionally helpful. I was also able to bring skills and insight that made me a valuable to my new employer. Specifically, I thought my experience in the different disciplines, emergency room, and palliative care and pain management, and procedural skills (bone marrow biopsy, lumbar punctures) were most important.

Q: Who served as your teachers in the residency? Faculty, residents, PAs, others?

A: Mostly faculty and PAs; this differed with each rotation.

Q: What compensation did you receive during the residency? Were there benefits in addition to a salary?

A: I received a salary that I thought was very reasonable. This included full benefits.

Q: What was the length of your residency?

A: 1 year

Q: Approximately how many hours did you work during an average week in the residency?

A: In the clinic and hospital, I worked 50 to 70 hours a week. I worked an additional 20 to 30 hours a week studying, completing papers or presentations, and doing research.

Q: How many residents were enrolled in your residency program?

A: One resident during my year. The board chooses one or two depending on applicants.

Q: What job opportunities did you find were available when you had completed the residency? Do you think having attended a residency was important to your employer?

A: I think that my residency experience at a world-renowned institution made me a more desirable candidate when interviewing. I did not have trouble finding a job position that I now truly enjoy after my program. However, many people did not know a lot about PA residency programs.

Q: What were the most positive aspects of being a PA resident?

A: There were numerous positive aspects about being a PA resident. One that I found to be exceptionally helpful is that the PAs and physicians look at you as someone who is there to learn and are very willing to teach. When you are in your job, the same time and effort are not often taken by superiors. Specifically, in my program, having the ability to experience all disciplines in each major area of oncology in addition to palliative care, pain management, and the ED was exceptional.

Q: What were the negative aspects of being a PA resident?

A: One of the most rewarding aspects of oncology is the relationship and trust you build with your patients. When you are changing rotations somewhat frequently, it is very hard to have that aspect. Additionally, the extended hours can become difficult.

CONCLUSION

Physician assistant residency education continues to evolve and mature as it has passed the 40-year milestone of existence. These programs can generally be considered successful in preparing graduate PAs to practice effectively in a variety of specialty areas within medicine. Considerable interest has been demonstrated by applicants to the residency programs and by institutions interested in developing new PA residency programs. PA residents in general are very satisfied with their educational experiences, believe that it has made them more competitive in the workplace, and would recommend the residency program to others.

CLINICAL APPLICATIONS

1. If you were interested in PA residency education, how would you find out about the distinctive features of each program?
2. What are some of the pros and cons associated with attending residency programs?

3. Interview two PAs working in the same specialty—one who attended a residency program and one who did not. Ask them to describe their PA careers and how they acquired the knowledge and skills related to their specialties. What similarities and differences can you identify?

KEY POINTS

- It is important to understand the history of the Post Graduate Residency Programs and how they fit in the current educational scheme for graduate physician assistants.
- A list of current residency programs is helpful for PAs wanting to either gain more knowledge in a specialty or retool for a job change.
- Characteristics of graduate PA programs vary in terms of length, stipends, didactic and clinical experiences.
- The current accreditation of post graduate programs is a developing process and is currently voluntary.

References

1. Polansky M. A historical perspective on postgraduate physician assistant education and the Association of Postgraduate Physician Assistant Programs. *J Physician Assist Educ.* 2007;18:100.
2. Association of Postgraduate Physician Assistant Programs. *Annual Meeting Minutes*; May 22–23, 1988.
3. Association of Postgraduate Physician Assistant Programs website. http://www.appap.org. Accessed December 18, 2015.
4. Polansky M, Garver GJH, Wilson L, et al. Postgraduate Clinical Education of Physician Assistants. *J Physician Assist Edu.* 2012;23(1):39–45.
5. Asprey D, Helms L. A description of physician assistant postgraduate residency training: the director's perspective. *Perspectives Physician Assist Educ.* 1999;10:124.
6. Reynolds EW, Bricker JT. Nonphysician clinicians in the neonatal intensive care unit: meeting the needs of our smallest patients. *Pediatrics.* 2007;119:361.
7. Will KK, Budavari AL, Mishark K, Hartsell ZC. A hospitalist postgraduate training program for physician assistants. *J Hospital Med.* 2010;5:94.
8. Magenis JP. Implementing postgraduate training for physician assistants in emergency medicine at a major urban academic medical center. *Am J Emerg Med.* 2013;31:983–994.
9. Hooker R. A Physician assistant rheumatology fellowship. *JAAPA.* 2013;26(6):49–52.
10. Wiemiller MJ, Somers KK, Adams MB. Postgraduate physician assistant training programs in the United States: emerging trends and opportunities. *J Physician Assist Educ.* 2008;19:58.
11. American Association of Surgical Physician Assistants website, http://www.aaspa.com Accessed December 18, 2015
12. Asprey D, Helms L. A description of physician assistant postgraduate residency training: the resident's perspective. *Perspect Physician Assist Educ.* 2000;11:79.
13. Fishfader V, Hennig B, Knott P. Physician assistant student and faculty perceptions of physician assistant residency training programs. *Perspect Physician Assist Educ.* 2002;13(1):34–38.
14. Brenneman T, Hemminger C, Dehn R. Surgical graduates' perceptions on postgraduate physician assistant training programs. *J Physician Assist Educ.* 2007;18:1.
15. Accreditation Review Commission for Physician Assistants website. http://www.arc-pa.net/postgrad_programs/. Accessed December 18, 2015.
16. Salyer SW. A clinical doctorate in emergency medicine for physician assistants: postgraduate education. *J Physician Assist Educ.* 2008;19:53.
17. Maintaining Professional Flexibility: Issues Related to Postgraduate Physician Assistant Programs. American Academy of Physician Assistants. Adopted 2005, amended 2010. https://www.aapa.org/threeColumnLanding.aspx?id=1202. Accessed December 21, 2015.
18. Personal communication with Reamer Bushardt. Accreditation of Postgraduate Training Programs Task Force Chair; November 16, 2015.
19. Martinez E. Baylor College of Medicine Physician Assistant Fellowship in Emergency Medicine. Presentation on July 28, 2015. University of Texas Medical Branch Physician Assistant Program Career Day.
20. Will K, Williams J, Hilton G, Wilson L, Geyer H. Perceived efficacy and utility of postgraduate physician assistant training programs. *JAAPA.* March 2016;29(3):46–48. Copyright © 2016 American Academy of Physician Assistants.
21. Keith DE, Doerr RJ. Survey of a physician assistant internship concerning practice characteristics and adequacy of training. *J Med Educ.* 1987;62:517.

The resources for this chapter can be found at www.expertconsult.com.

DEALING WITH STRESS AND BURNOUT

Ruth Ballweg

As part of physician assistant (PA) training, students receive extensive information about stress. PAs learn that almost all change creates stress, and most clinicians optimistically believe that stress can be "managed." Typical classroom presentations include the concepts of "good" and "bad" stress, the Holmes-Reye Stress Scale as a teaching and evaluation tool for patients, and recommended treatment plans (exercise, decreased caffeine intake, improved nutrition, meditation, and even short-term psychotherapy) for patients with stress. This chapter does not attempt to duplicate that information. Rather, the focus of the chapter is to identify and discuss the specifics of stress and burnout as they apply to PAs, recommend strategies for prevention, and suggest a range of treatment interventions.

THE DECISION TO BECOME A PHYSICIAN ASSISTANT

Ironically, whether we choose to look at it this way or not, PAs all become personal experts on stress as part of their medical education. The consideration of any medical career creates stress. The prospect of long hours; personal sacrifice; a commitment to care of patients, sometimes at the expense of family; and the recognition of the intensity of a medical career

demand serious consideration. Many PAs at some point considered becoming physicians. This consideration was at least understandable to our teachers, mentors, family, and friends. Becoming a nurse also made some sense ("You'll always have a job"). Although the Affordable Care Act has brought new visibility to the PA career, it still may not be fully understood or supported by family and friends. Historically, the admissions process for most PA programs has favored the selection of risk-taking and pioneering individuals who see the PA profession as a unique opportunity. One of the best ways to understand this is to spend time with practicing PAs who are willing to provide firsthand exposure to the PA profession.

Nevertheless, the first stress for many successful candidates to PA programs has been the job of answering the question, "You're going to become a what!?" Even the most understanding friend may still ask, "When will you be a doctor?" The most supportive friend, employer, or parent may still not understand why being a PA is a separate and different career with its own satisfactions and rewards.

EXPERIENCE OF STRESS IN TRAINING

Next come the adventure and stress of PA training. Asked about the difference between PA and physician training programs, many of the founders of PA education are quick to point out that both PA and nurse practitioner (NP) programs, although designed to train new types of primary care providers, were also intended to be a proving ground for new concepts in medical education. Problem-based learning, the use of simulated patients, videotaping to teach patient interviewing skills, and new types of clinical training experiences were used early on in PA and NP programs before their more recent appearance in medical schools. Objectives and competency-based learning also were used to make PA training extremely efficient. As a result, the curriculum of most PA programs is intended to present a large amount of information in a short time. PA program directors often say, "It's not that the material is so hard but that it comes in truckloads." Students often say the intensity of PA classroom training is "like drinking from a fire hydrant." As programs have moved to the graduate levels, PA curricula have also added significant research and management content, which places further demands on every PA student.

In addition to simple acquisition of information, the relatively short duration of PA training, compared with that of physicians, demands that PA students quickly develop a professional identity in an extremely responsible role. This rapid role transition actually accounts for much of the stress PA students' experience. Students entering the PA profession as a first career choice generally have a successful college career as a foundation for their PA training but may have had little exposure to patient care. Thus, the stress for these students is often that of developing a way of relating to patients and seeing themselves as decision makers on the health care team. People who enter PA programs as second-career students; former registered nurses (RNs); licensed practical nurses (LPNs); military corpsmen; paramedics; surgical, respiratory, radiology, or laboratory technicians; and other allied health personnel may have had identities as members of the health care team but generally find that they have to relinquish their former identities to assume their new role of PA.

Recognizing these concerns, PA program admissions committees often seek and choose applicants who are flexible, trainable, proactive, and proficient in multiple tasks. Students who are less adaptable to the extremely rapid didactic and clinical experiences required of them in PA training may become alienated from classmates who are enthusiastically moving ahead on an exciting career path.

Another unique aspect of PA training that often creates some short-term stress—but may actually decrease long-term stress—is the emphasis on sensitive issues and interpersonal skills as part of training.

Training includes extensive small-group work with faculty feedback to teach interviewing and physical examination skills. Course work is also required to include primary care topics dealing with sexuality, parenting, death and dying, cross-cultural issues, and family dynamics. In studying these topics, students are forced to confront their personal opinions and biases as they apply to interactions not only with their colleagues but also with their future patients.

Current trends in health profession education include an emphasis on professionalism and opportunities for interdisciplinary education. Giving and receiving feedback are critical skills in new educational environments. Although stressful at first, these new skills are designed to increase clarity regarding expectations and performance. As a result, minimizing misunderstanding and confusion can decrease stress.

One "solution" for stress in the didactic year is to focus on planning for the future in the clinical year. This diversionary tactic is probably most appealing for students with prior clinical experience, who may believe that they are "just putting in time" in the classroom until they can "really perform" in the clinical setting. In contrast, students with more extensive academic experience and less clinical identity may approach the clinical year with increasing anxiety. Regardless of each group's anticipatory viewpoint, the clinical year brings certain predictable stresses:

- No matter how well the program has prepared the site and used it in the past, some members of the physician, nursing, and administrative staff, in at least some sites, still will not know what a PA is or does.
- Medical students assigned the same clinical placements may not understand the PA role and may at first perceive the PA student as a threat.
- The process of relocating from site to site is disorienting. The health care system may, for the first time, appear extremely fragmented to the PA student, who may not have realized that medicine is practiced so many different ways in so many different settings.
- The demand for documentation (charting) as to both detail and timeliness is much greater than the student had expected. Electronic health record systems are still being adopted in some clinics and hospitals, and the transition to these new processes creates stress for all clinicians—but especially for students who may be called on to master an entirely new system for each rotation.
- Other health care workers question PA students aggressively about their career choice. What seem like "attacks" are often discovered to be the questions of individuals who are considering PA training for themselves or other colleagues.

- When required to make complex decisions about patient care, the student realizes how judgmental he or she has been about other health care providers in the past.

Throughout the process of didactic and clinical training, the impetus is toward greater recognition of how much there is to know. Other providers may make disparaging comments about the limited knowledge base of the new PA, with little recognition of past experience or of the serious decisions he or she may have been required to make in previous employment settings. It is important to have a ready and nondefensive answer to the questions, "What is a PA, and what is your training?" Fortunately, more and more medical students and residents are familiar with the PA concept and see PAs as allies in optimizing patient care.

The increasing cost of higher education also creates significant pressure on students, especially those who have incurred significant debt in their undergraduate years. Although PA students incur significantly less debt than medical students, it is still unclear how this debt influences the employment choices of new PAs.

There is always concern that employment choices of the higher paying procedurally based specialties will move us as a profession away from our original primary care mission. Chapters elsewhere in this book discuss negotiating for the first job; however, it is fair to say that most clinical year PA students are experiencing significant stress as they consider salaries and job responsibilities for their first PA employment.

Excellent resources on the topic of coping and stress reduction during medical training can be found on the website for the American Medical Student Association. These include self-assessment tools, as well as specific stress reduction activities (http://www.amsa.org).

Stress in Choosing the First Job

As the student approaches graduation, the job decision becomes the next developmental obsession. Students who enter PA training with a well-defined idea of their employment choices may suddenly see other variables often as a direct result of their clinical training experiences. Opportunities to pay student loans in exchange for service to specific populations (rural or underserved inner city) may significantly influence a student's employment choice.

Program faculty members describe new episodes of stress for recent graduates who face an extremely wide range of employment choices, many of which offer salaries and "perks" that have rarely been paid to practicing PAs in the past. In contrast to the employment scene in the mid-1980s, when the number of new PA jobs roughly equaled the number of new PAs entering the job market, the current market offers multiple positions for each graduate. In addition, the expanded access to care provided by health reform and the limitation on work hours for medical residents is forcing the creation of new PA jobs that never would have been considered in the past. Each graduate is now faced with the task of avoiding jobs that are inappropriate, as well as seriously considering offers that provide the best short- and long-term opportunities. The choice of the first PA job also shapes each PA's ultimate view of his or her new profession. Much of the initial stress for new PAs in their first job is directly related to the acceptance of PAs in the specific employment setting. This is a particular concern if other members of the health care team are not informed about PAs. It is difficult to adjust to a new role and employment setting while also being called on to educate administrators, nursing and medical staff members, credentials committees, and billing clerks about PA issues. This stress can be significantly reduced by negotiation of an orientation process as part of an employment contract, seeking the assistance of PA program clinical coordinators to provide technical assistance to new PA employment sites, or enlisting the assistance and support of other PAs practicing in the institution or community.

Some PA graduates believe that one criterion of the "perfect PA job" is current or recent employment of a PA at the site who has enthusiastically and proactively pioneered the PA role. Other graduates deliberately seek sites where there has not been a previous PA role model. They see the opportunity to be the "first PA" as one of great potential, stressful though it may initially be.

Educating Patients and Their Families

New graduates are often unprepared for the number of patients and health care professionals asking "What is a physician assistant?" It is important that PA programs train their students and graduates not only to expect these questions but also to regard them as opportunities. Unfortunately, some PAs stressfully view each such encounter as further proof that PAs are still not accepted and that the profession, state and national PA organizations, and PA programs are not doing their job of public education. In fact, health care consumers are frequently confused by the wide diversity of careers represented in any clinic and should be encouraged to ask about the training and credentials of those providing their care.

Relationships With Preceptors

The supervised nature of PA practice makes the relationship between PA and preceptor a potential source of both satisfaction and stress. Here again, the messages given to new PAs by PA training programs about the relationships between PAs and preceptors set the stage for collaboration or dysfunction. Similar to all other relationships, the preceptor–PA collaboration requires work. The preceptor needs to be well informed about the background and current clinical expertise of the PA. This may appropriately require frequent observation and supervision early in the employment period. In fact, little or no supervision from a preceptor at the start of a PA job, especially for a new graduate, should be seen as a "red flag."

Appropriate support from the supervising physician is one of the greatest stress relievers for a PA. Similarly, the physician may have chosen to work with the PA because of the opportunity that the relationship provides for sharing the challenges and frustrations of medical practice!

The fact that there is a formal backup for knowledge, decision making, and consultation makes the PA profession particularly attractive for many potential PA candidates. PAs however, need to learn to use this collaborative relationship for teaching and support. Each new job requires a renegotiation of this communication. An important stress reduction tool is to plan on regular case review and journal assignments in addition to whatever chart review is required by state law. Insistence on a theme of "lifelong learning" early in an employment setting fosters communication and decreases stress. The intense and emotional demands of medical practice are most easily shared with those who are there at the same time seeing the same patients. The opportunity to review individual cases and specific encounters often allows the preceptor and the PA to leave these cases at work and to make the transition to personal and family time more efficiently.

Relationships With Administrators

With health care increasingly being provided by large systems, the relationships of PAs who were primarily centered with physicians now include health care administrators. Although the physician may provide clinical supervision and oversight, the administrator may develop and negotiate jobs, supervise and evaluate personnel, and manage patient scheduling and follow-up. Thus, whereas PAs in the past were required to speak the "language of medicine," they now must also be able to speak the "corporate language of business." A lack of understanding of concepts such as productivity, quality improvement, supervisory relationships, capitation, per-member-per-month costs, and risk sharing will put a PA at a disadvantage.

In addition, the communication styles of administrators may vary vastly from PAs who are accustomed to working with physician preceptors. Notes on charts and hall-side consultations may be replaced with memos requiring written responses. Written evaluations of clinical performance may involve complicated spreadsheets and graphs. Electronic communication skills will soon be required for all providers.

Although some PAs and PA students may initially think that the best coping mechanism is to avoid the transition to administrative relationships, a better strategy would be to quickly acquire the skills to interact effectively with health care administrators in these new and evolving relationships.

STRESS ON THE JOB

On the job, PAs report a variety of stresses. Holmes and Fasser,[1] using the Health Professions Stress Inventory with a survey of 2334 PAs, found that PAs' stress levels were relatively low. The highest stresses were reported in the following areas:
- Caring for the emotional needs of patients
- Dealing with difficult patients
- Believing that opportunities for advancement on the job were poor
- Feeling ultimately responsible for patient outcomes
- Keeping up with new developments to maintain professional competence
- Trying to meet society's expectations for high-quality medical care

These stresses may be categorized into three types: patient care issues, formal professional issues, and role ambiguity issues.

Patient Care Issues

Caring for the emotional needs of patients, dealing with difficult patients, and feeling ultimately responsible for patient outcomes are patient care issues shared by the PA with other health care professionals. Because they are common concerns, the solution to these stresses is also best shared by colleagues. Family members and friends can be supportive of health care professionals, but because of confidentiality and a lack of specific shared experiences, it is difficult and sometimes even inappropriate for them to "debrief" their health care professional, family member, or friend about specific patient care incidents.

Some employment settings provide support groups for their clinicians. In addition to formal support networks, social events with coworkers effectively reduce stress. Although many PAs use other PAs for support in patient care issues, it is valuable to see all members of the health care team as part of a support network because different viewpoints may bring different insights to a situation or incident.

One of the best published resources on stress in the helping professions is Christina Maslach's *Burnout: The Cost of Caring*.[2] In reviewing patient care stresses, Maslach believes that a large part of the problem is that health care professionals, as students and as practitioners, are often so busy acquiring facts and proficiency in procedures that they do not learn the relatively simple interpersonal skills that will carry them through difficult situations and reduce stress on the job.

Surprisingly, interpersonal skills are often not recognized as a major necessity for providers. They are considered secondary to other professional skills: extras rather than essentials, the "icing on the cake" rather than the cake itself. This viewpoint is sadly in error because it trivializes an essential aspect of the relationship between the provider and recipient. It fails to recognize that both of them are human beings whose personal attitudes and feelings can affect not only the delivery of care but also how and even whether it is accepted.[2]

Recognizing that health care professionals may have been taught to deal with specific crisis situations, Maslach is concerned that it is in fact the daily encounters, producing incremental stress, for which daily "garden variety" interpersonal skills should be gained. Maslach lists three of these skills as examples:

1. **How to start, stop, and keep things going:** Just like true love, the course of helping relationships does not always run smoothly. Getting things started on the right foot often depends on how you greet the other person and whether there is any initial social talk to reduce tension and "break the ice." Similarly, bringing things to a successful halt depends on whether you interrupt the person (and how you do so), how you announce that time is up, whether you evaluate the progress that has been made, how you say good-bye, and so on.
2. **How to deal with different people:** The infinite variety of human beings is what makes working with people so interesting, exciting, and challenging. It is also what makes it so difficult at times. The approach that a practitioner uses with one client may not work with someone else because of differences in sex, age, cultural backgrounds, personality, values, attitudes, and so forth. Although practitioners often long for a single strategy that will work well with everybody, the truth is they need to have several different strategies in their hip pockets, ready to be used when appropriate.
3. **How to talk about unpopular topics:** All too often in helping relationships, what needs to be said is what one person does not want to say and the other does not want to hear. Practitioners dread these difficult moments, and it is here, more than anywhere else, that they express a need for additional interpersonal skills. The topics that are most difficult to handle are how to ask tough questions, how to discuss sensitive issues, and how to deliver bad news. Special skills training for these problems would go a long way toward alleviating the emotional exhaustion of burnout.[2]

Formal Professional Issues

Formal professional issues are potential stressors for PAs. Although significant progress has been made in many states, medical practice acts in some states can still be restrictive of PA practice. Reimbursement policies also vary dramatically from state to state and region to region. Institutions that have not previously employed PAs may need help in adapting their credentialing processes for the effective utilization of PAs. Relatively new graduates may have a poor appreciation of the rapid progress that has been made by the PA profession in removing barriers to practice. As a result, new PAs can feel helpless and hopeless. One of the best solutions is political involvement. State PA academies are always seeking the energies of PAs willing to serve on a wide range of committees, all ultimately dealing with the expansion of PA practice. Although some PAs have initially believed that they did not have either the time or the skills for such involvement, almost all PAs who have become engaged in these activities have found that the sense of "making a difference" is a strong deterrent to stress and burnout.

One stress that is more pressing for PAs than for other providers is keeping up with new developments to maintain one's professional competence. Initially trained in a primary care model with broad skills, PAs are first certified by an examination that tests primary care knowledge. Changes in the recertification process, along with the development of new "Certificates of Added Qualification" (CAQs) for PAs in some specialties, add to the stress for new graduates considering options for their developing careers.

Although it is difficult for most health care professionals to keep up with continuing developments in the medical field, PAs are among the few health care professionals who must undergo periodic recertification by examination at regular intervals. Recently, the time frame has been extended from 6 years to 10 years. Significantly, the profession is the only one in which recertification is tied directly to state registration and the right to work.[1]

Role Ambiguity Issues

Aside from the specifics of regulation, certification, and credentialing, the ambiguity of the PA profession is both the good news and the bad news. Many PAs have chosen the profession because of its limitless aspects. Other PAs are distressed by the fact that the PA career lacks precise definition with clearly delineated standards of practice, consistent legislation, and reimbursement standards throughout the country.

Trying to meet society's expectations for high-quality medical care in a time of rapid change in the health care system is both exciting and terrifying. Because it is a relatively new career, new opportunities for PAs are constantly being developed by creative and innovative members of the profession. Here, expectations are the critical factors. It is to be hoped that

- PA program applicants have researched the profession as part of their entry process into training.
- PA programs have given the students exposure to practicing PAs serving as role models and providing realistic insights into both the frustrations and satisfactions of their jobs.
- PA students in their clinical rotations have sought to achieve an understanding of the emotional context of their jobs as part of their training.
- Practicing PAs regard questions from consumers about PAs as opportunities to educate them not only about PAs but also about the variety of health care professions that exist today.

BURNOUT

We are all concerned when stress turns to burnout. Originally thought of as a syndrome characterized by emotional depletion and exhaustion, burnout is now better understood as a state and process that begin as a response to work-related stressors.[3] Holmes and Fasser[1] describe the process as moving through tedium ("the experience of physical, emotional, and mental exhaustion precipitated by stress and characterized by feelings of strain, emotional and physical depletion, and negative attitudes toward self, environment, and life") into burnout. "The cumulative effects of sustained tedium in the work environment produce tension, irritability, and fatigue, which end in a defensive reaction of detachment, apathy, cynicism, or rigidity, referred to as burnout."[1]

Personal Characteristics

Some individuals seem more prone to burnout than others. According to Maslach,[2] "burnout is more likely if the person is younger, less mature, and less self-confident; is impulsive and impatient; has no family commitments but needs other people who can provide approval and affection; and has goals and expectations that are not in tune with reality." Armstrong and colleagues[4] list four types of individuals most susceptible to burnout: "those who assume too much responsibility and feel driven to achieve goals; those who view their jobs as the major reason for living and fail to develop outside activities; those who place a heavy emphasis on completing the task regardless of the cost; and those who are truly overworked."

Identifying Burnout

One of the biggest problems with burnout is that we are least able to identify it in ourselves until it is a critical problem. Thus, we must rely on our friends, family members, and colleagues to be our "early warning systems." Similarly, we must provide this same assistance to other friends in health care. Colon[3] suggests that clinicians should always "maintain a high index of suspicion for symptoms of burnout." Complications can include depression, substance abuse, and even suicide. Appropriate and supportive referrals for assessment and treatment are particularly important.

Maslach[2] also believes that employers should be on the alert for burnout. The organization should institute standard reviews, or preburnout "check-ups," at periodic intervals (1 month after starting the job and then every 3 months or so). When such reviews are a ritualized and regular procedure for all staff, then no one person has to accept the burden of alerting you to the fact that he or she is beginning to get singed around the edges.

Assessment and Treatment

In assessing individual situations of burnout, three questions are important[2]:
- What is the individual's role?
- What roles do other people play?
- What role does the institution play?

Answers to these three questions will give some direction to a treatment plan.

On an individual level, Maslach describes the physical and psychological dysfunction accompanying burnout. "Exhaustion, illness, depression, irritability, increased use of alcohol and drugs, these are some of the personal costs."[2] Personal strategies might include a redefinition of work style and the search for a better balance between professional and private life.

In terms of patients and coworkers, interpersonal symptoms are changes in relationships with clients, such as callous and insensitive behavior. Colon[3] describes the "clues" of burnout in PAs: A classic example is when the clinician jokes about patients' illnesses, calls patients by symptoms, and becomes less trusting and less sympathetic toward them. Another sign is overall loss of concern and feeling for patients. Occasionally, however, the opposite is true: A burned-out clinician becomes too involved with patients or overidentifies with them and commits a considerably greater number of hours than required for their care.

Strategies for interpersonal aspects of burnout most often include the assistance of others in the same or similar situation to offer perspectives and solutions. In some situations, the best treatment plan might also call for the assistance of a therapist experienced in the concerns of health care providers.

Burnout at the institutional level may be the result of unrealistic workloads, barriers to practice, inefficient staffing patterns, and poor management. Maslach[2] describes the effects of burnout at the institutional level as being "reflected in high rates of absenteeism, turnover, and complaints about staff performance." Strategies for a dysfunctional employment setting include "redesigning jobs, changing organizational policies, devising explicit structures and contracts, establishing flexible leaves and support services, and improving the training programs for staff."[2]

"One of the most important aspects of burnout treatment (and prevention) is increasing an individual's sense of personal power, because it is 'powerlessness' that makes one feel most trapped." Maslach discusses "ways in which the individual exerts some active control in a situation rather than just passively acquiescing to it. The person changes the work routine, redefines goals, uses downshifts, takes breaks, seeks out positive feedback, engages in decompression activities, and so forth. All of these activities involve choice and initiative—the hallmarks of freedom and autonomy."[2] Believing that individual health care providers (PAs in this case) generally have more power than they realize, Maslach further notes that "by wiggling around in the job and finding out what can change and what cannot, the practitioner can counteract the helplessness and 'the hell with it all' attitude associated with burnout."[2]

The other well-known strategy for treating burnout is working toward the goal of reestablishing some balance in one's life. At the simplest level, this includes eating balanced meals and establishing realistic sleep and exercise patterns. Further activities include developing interests outside work and cultivating friendships and relationships away from the health care environment. Placing greater emphasis on family and leisure time has been effective for some individuals. Others have chosen to seek additional education or training as a way of expanding their horizons. Many health care providers see therapists as needed for help in balancing their lives.

CASE STUDY 37.1

Dennis is a 34-year-old paramedic enrolled in the first year of a PA program. It is now halfway through the didactic year of training. His classmates are concerned that he has become increasingly "negative" toward the program in which he is enrolled. This seems particularly unusual to them because he had been working toward getting into this specific program for longer than 5 years before admission, expanding his clinical experience, enrolling in basic science coursework to fulfill the prerequisite requirements for program admission, completing his bachelor's degree, and volunteering in community programs serving homeless people.

When his faculty advisor meets with him, Dennis says he believes that much of the coursework is either "too soft and a waste of time" or "not appropriate to what PAs need to know." He thinks that he is "not getting what he has paid for" from the program. The faculty advisor, who was also a former paramedic, suggests that he meet with some practicing PAs from similar backgrounds to find out their opinions on these issues. He provides him with three contacts, and they plan to meet again in 1 week.

The student meets with two of the graduates who are available that week. One works in a general internal medicine outpatient clinic, and the other is employed in a rural private practice. They both describe similar concerns during didactic training and independently share with him that, in retrospect, they think that their frustration during didactic training was actually more related to their own role transition. One PA says that during his didactic training, he did not really understand the broad roles that PAs are expected to play within the health care system. Therefore, he kept trying to "manage" his learning by focusing it down to specific areas (what he thought PAs "needed" to know). This strategy had worked during his paramedic career but turned out to be ineffective for a PA student. This PA suggests that the student look at the "bigger picture" and try to be less resistant and more flexible in his approach to the curriculum.

The second PA specifically wants to talk about the "softer stuff" in the curriculum. She says that she initially thought the behavioral science content of the program was totally unnecessary until she got into her clinical year. In the first week of her first rotation (general internal medicine), she was "blown away" to find out how many of her patients had some behavioral science component to their illness. Not only that, but they also expected her to be comfortable talking about these issues. Even more surprising was the fact that she had gained competency in these skills during the didactic year despite her resistance to these issues. Now she says it would almost be fun to take the behavioral science course again if only she had the opportunity.

The student returns to meet with his advisor. He reports on his contact with the graduates, and they discuss the findings. Although Dennis says he still has concerns about what he is learning, he seems much less hostile and anxious. He says that he plans to try to be more flexible about his approach to the curriculum and his own learning. He also has made plans to keep in contact with both the graduates he has met. One of them has offered her clinic to him as a potential training site. He says that he really feels good about this. The student and his advisor schedule a follow-up appointment at the end of the quarter or sooner if needed.

having trouble making decisions about even the simplest patient care issues.

The faculty advisor suggests that she needs to prioritize her concerns. If she spends too much time on future employment negotiations, she may not successfully complete the program. If she is ill from not eating, not sleeping, and abandoning her social contacts, she will probably not be able to fulfill her job responsibilities in a new employment setting. In addition, she may be at risk for board examination failure if she continues to be distracted from her learning during the remaining 3 months of training. The student says, "Of course. Why do you think I'm not sleeping!?"

They discuss a variety of strategies, including even a time-out from the program. Finally, they agree on the following actions:

- Complete any outstanding assignments as the highest priority, beginning with the copies of chart notes and patient care logs.
- Eat breakfast and lunch on a more regular schedule, attempt to reinstitute an exercise routine, and decrease caffeine consumption.
- Delay job negotiations at least until the completion of this rotation.
- Reestablish contact with at least two fellow students.
- Plan for weekly follow-up with faculty advisor.
- Consider referral for supportive therapy if not improved.
- Consider a brief leave of absence, with no penalty, if not improved.

CASE STUDY 37.2

Jo is a senior student who has only three more clinical clerkships before her graduation. She has been a strong student throughout both the didactic and clinical years but suddenly seems to be behind in submitting her written assignments, including chart notes, patient care logs, and a research paper on "the perfect PA job." Her faculty advisor contacts her and arranges to visit Jo in her clinic, a Veterans Health Administration outpatient site.

In meeting with Jo at the start of the day, the faculty advisor asks her how things are going and gets the following response: "I can't seem to get caught up. I can't sleep. I just can't do this!" She also says that she has a hard time fitting in regular meals, has totally abandoned her daily exercise routine, and has been too busy to even e-mail her fellow classmates. Further conversation reveals that Jo is also engaged in negotiations with four potential employers, all in sites where she has previously been assigned for clinical rotations. She is receiving almost daily calls from all of these sites and believes that she has to make a decision immediately. At the same time, she notices that she is

CONCLUSION

Given the complexity and intensity of the health care system within which we work, it is normal to expect that we will all be regularly subjected to significant amounts of stress. It is also important to acknowledge that we generally have anticipated this stress as part of our career choice. We may not, however, have always gauged accurately the emotional costs of pioneering what still is a relatively new career. We also may not always have recognized the importance that good interpersonal skills, strong support systems, and well-chosen jobs play in job satisfaction.

Unfortunately, it is not unreasonable to predict that everyone in health care will experience some form of burnout during his or her professional life. As Colon[3] points out, "Stress is a particularly urgent problem for PAs. Their unique position in health care delivery can intensify other stressors of medical practice. Consequently, PAs must be especially on guard against burnout: in themselves, in other PAs, in supervising physicians, and in support staff."

Although PAs are generally satisfied with their career and actively promote it to individuals choosing health care careers, we must be realistic in recognizing the sources of stress and satisfaction. It is only by recognizing those stresses and satisfactions that we are best able to evaluate our current professional and personal lives and make the ongoing choices that will sustain our health as individuals.

CLINICAL APPLICATIONS

• Begin a personal "stress" log to document your progress in the program. On a daily or weekly basis, list all of those issues and concerns that you believe are contributing to your stress. Divide your list into two categories: (1) things you can do something about and (2) things you cannot do anything about. Develop a strategy for attacking and resolving the items on the first list.

• Interview at least one preceptor to whom you are assigned in your clinical year. Ask about his or her perception of common stresses in professional practice and abilities to resolve these stresses. Discuss what involvement he or she has with colleagues for mutual support.

KEY POINTS

• Regardless of any prior clinical experience, all students experience significant stress during both the didactic and clinical phases of PA training. One reason for this is the need for the rapid assumption of an extremely responsible clinical role.
• An effective and supportive relationship with a supervising physician is one of the great "stress relievers" for practicing PAs.
• Burnout is more likely to be recognized by friends and colleagues than it is by the person experiencing it.
• Greater public acceptance of the PA role has reduced the stress levels of practicing PAs.

References

1. Holmes SE, Fasser CE. Occasional stress among physician assistants. *J Am Acad Physician Assist*. 1993;6:172.
2. Maslach C. *Burnout: The Cost of Caring*. Englewood Cliffs, NJ: Prentice-Hall; 1982.
3. Colon EA. Burnout. *Physician Assist*. 1986;10:18.
4. Armstrong M, King M, Meller B. Avoiding orientation burnout: a practical guide designed to help inservice instructors. *Nurs Manage*. 1982;13:27.

The resources for this chapter can be found at www.expertconsult.com.

PRACTICE-BASED LEARNING AND IMPROVEMENT

CHAPTER 38

HEALTH DISPARITIES

Erin Nicole Lunn McAdams • Bri Keslter • Robin Risling-de Jong

WHAT ARE HEALTH DISPARITIES?

According to *Unequal Treatment*, health disparities are the differences in the incidence, prevalence, mortality, and burden of diseases and other adverse health conditions that exist among specific population groups.[1] Disparities in health care exist even when controlling for gender, condition, age, and socioeconomic status. After decades of improvements in preventive health care and significant declines in disease mortality for many Americans, disparities in health and health care continue to persist in the United States.[2-4] As such, reducing and ultimately eliminating health disparities remains a focus of national attention.

Racial and ethnic minorities, those with disabilities, women, economically and educationally disadvantaged individuals, and medically underserved people, among others, continue to suffer a disproportionate burden of disease. The reasons for health disparities appear to be multifactorial, still poorly understood, and complex. Compelling evidence indicates that among minorities, race and ethnicity correlate strongly with health disparities. Minority populations, typically classified as African Americans, Hispanic Americans, Asian Americans, native Hawaiians and Pacific Islanders, American Indians, and Alaska natives, are much more likely to experience poorer health outcomes, decreased life expectancy, higher mortality rates, and premature deaths. These groups are also less likely to be recipients of health care services geared toward health promotion, disease prevention and early detection of disease, and high-quality medical treatments.[2-4]

The Healthy People 2020 initiative is a set of health promotion and disease prevention objectives for the nation. It endeavors to improve the health of all groups. Healthy People 2020 states if a health outcome is seen in a greater or lesser extent between populations, a disparity exists. Healthy People 2020 emphasizes that the term "disparities" refers to more than mere racial or ethnic disparities. Gender, sexual identity, age, disability, socioeconomic status, and geographic location all play pivotal roles in the achievement of good health. Thus, recognizing the impact of social determinants is crucial to understanding the definition of health disparities.[5]

There are a host of key factors, or determinants, of health disparities. These include but are not limited to insurance status, socioeconomic status, residential and geographic segregation, English as a second language, cultural and racial bias, and stereotyping.[2,3,6] Racial and ethnic minority groups comprise more than 50% of those uninsured, representing for some (e.g., African Americans, Hispanics, American Indians) two to five times that of white Americans. In its *Racial and Ethnic Disparities in Health Care Updated 2010* report, the American College of Physicians (ACP) discusses the literature regarding the poorer health status of minorities in the United States as compared with white Americans. It also reiterates much of the new literature that calls for structural changes within America's health care system to meet the needs of America's multicultural population and recognize the critical role of social determinants of health status and their contributions to health disparities. Residential segregation, lack of equal access to quality education, and obstacles to economic opportunity are equally important in determining one's health status. The ACP report suggests that the most significant variable influencing health disparities is insurance status. Insured Americans are more likely to have access to health care. It is well established that minorities are less likely to have insurance, even when adjusting for work status. Lack of insurance affects an individual's ability to participate in preventive health care measures, as well as manage chronic disease states. It is estimated that almost 32% of Native Americans and Alaskan natives are uninsured, with 31% of Hispanics uninsured compared with roughly 11% of whites uninsured. Of minorities enrolled in federal and state programs such as Medicaid and the Children's Health Insurance Program (CHIP), more are eligible for coverage but are not enrolled (e.g., lack of awareness, language barriers, complex enrollment process). Within uninsured individuals, racial and ethnic minorities are still less likely to have equal access to health care.[7]

The Patient Protection and Affordable Care Act (PPACA) was brought into public law in March 2010, with the threefold goal of increasing insurance quality and affordability, decreasing the number of uninsured Americans, and decreasing the costs of health care. To accomplish these goals, it was determined insurance coverage needed to be expanded and premium rates needed to be adjusted to allow for the largest number of Americans to qualify for federal programs or be able to purchase private insurance plans on the PPACA's exchange site. Insurers were now required to accept all applicants, regardless of preexisting conditions, and cover costs associated with a specific list of conditions. Changing the income requirements expanded Medicaid eligibility, dependents could remain on their parents' coverage longer, and children could qualify for their own policies regardless of their parents' insurance plans, all of which increased the number of Americans with access to insurance plans. To decrease the costs of health care, additional aspects needed to be addressed. After the PPACA was enforced, insurers were required to charge a premium based on age rather than medical history, and subsidies in the form of refundable tax credits were offered to households and small businesses that purchased policies via the exchange.

The PPACA has been the largest overhaul in American health care since Medicare and Medicaid in 1965 and therefore changed many standard operating procedures for hospital systems and private practices alike. Mandates were placed on these entities, requiring them to meet standards in patient care, technology, and reporting systems. With the PPACA decreasing the number of uninsured Americans, this growth of insured patients has strained an already stressed health care model, and clinicians are concerned with their ability to maintain the quality of care with the increase of patient visits.

The Office of Minority Health (OMH) was created by the Department of Health and Human Services (DHHS) in 1986 as a direct response to the landmark 1985 *Report of the Secretary's Task Force on Black and Minority Health*. This report documented health disparities among minorities and placed their disadvantaged health status on the forefront of U.S. health policy agenda. In conjunction with DHHS, OMH works to improve the health and health care of racial and ethnic minorities.[8] On January 14, 2011, the Centers for Disease Control and Prevention released its *Health Disparities and Inequalities Report, United States, 2011*. This report is the first in an anticipated series of serial, consolidated assessments highlighting health disparities by gender, race and ethnicity, income, education, disability, and additional social determinants of health in the United States. This report defines health disparities as differences in health outcomes among groups reflective of social inequalities and calls for innovative intervention strategies that incorporate social and health programs.[9]

In 2003, the Agency for Health Care Research and Quality introduced its first published report with regard to health care equality and health care disparities. The most recent report, the *2015 National Health Care Quality and Disparities Report*, was released in April 2016 and combines information on both qualities of health care and health care disparities. The release of this report was special because it also incorporated the *5th Anniversary Update on the National Quality Strategy*, which helped readers gain an overall understanding of the nation's progress in improving health care access, quality, and disparities.[10] Traditionally the *National Healthcare Quality and Disparities Report* (QDR) has focused on assessing the performance of our health care system and identifying strengths and weaknesses, as well as disparities, along three main axes: access to health care, quality of health care, and priorities of the National Quality Strategy (NQS).[10] In 2010, the NQS was established by a mandate because of the initiation of the PPACA, with the goal of supporting the general axes of the PPACA and QDR through six priorities: making care safer, person- and family-centered care, effective communication and care coordination, prevention and treatment of leading causes of morbidity and mortality, health and well-being of communities, and making quality care more affordable.[10]

Data from this report show that from 2010 to the second quarter of 2015, the percentage of people younger than 65 years of age who were uninsured at the time of report decreased from 17.5% to 10.3%. The age group of 18 to 29 years experienced the largest decline rate, and this drop was seen across all poverty status and racial and ethnic groups.[10] The quality of health care improvements was assessed by collecting data on the NQS priorities, and it was found that through 2013, across these priorities, health care quality improved by 60%. Despite this improvement, health care quality disparities continued to persist, especially among people in poor households, Hispanics, blacks, and Alaska natives. Specific disparities to improve since 2010 include patient safety, effective prevention and treatment, healthy living, and care affordability. Disparities that have shown more difficult to improve include person- and family-centered care and care coordination.

In the United States, health disparities are well documented among minority populations. In essence, health disparities are population-specific differences in the presence of disease, health outcomes, mortality rates, and access to health care. The literature continues to acknowledge that the leading disparities for preventable conditions often exist among racial and ethnic minority populations.[3,9,10] At present, research has shifted to include transdisciplinary multilevel research on the social determinants of health disparities, community-based participatory research, and public health approaches to eliminating health disparities. The literature states that innovative and creative, broad-based approaches are necessary to address the multiple complex factors that result in the disproportionate burden of certain diseases and poorer health outcomes for minority populations.[3-6,11,12]

HEALTH DISPARITIES: SCOPE OF THE PROBLEM

Health disparities in the United States extend beyond race, ethnicity, or religion. They extend the bounds of sexual orientation, age, and access to medical coverage, geographic location, and health literacy.[13] As health care providers, it is essential to lay aside our own personal biases to establish rapport and deliver effective and equitable health care. Learning to customize your interview for each patient is a skill that is not easily attained, as you will learn when you begin your clinical rotations. As a student, you should observe other health care professionals as they interact with patients. Emulate behaviors and characteristics of the providers who deliver exceptional care in a nonjudgmental environment. As you rotate through each subspecialty, practice your interviewing skills and develop your rapport building.

Sexual Orientation

How is gender determined? And are gender and sex the same entity? Many training programs and providers of medical care use these terms interchangeably without recognizing the concept that these impressions are fluid and can vary throughout a person's life. Objectively, the term *sex* refers to the differences between male or female. Most medical professionals document sex by the appearance of external genitalia. With the establishment and increased commonality of sex reassignment surgery, this becomes increasingly difficult for a provider to identify just based on phenotypic characteristics. Gender is rooted in psychosocial, cultural, and behavioral principles. There are currently no standard documentational or medical criteria for measuring sex and gender.[14] For this reason, it is a challenge for providers to inquire about sex or gender. It is overwhelmingly important to avoid biases when questioning patients about these two titles so as not to come across as abrasive or callous. Therefore, open communication between provider and patient should be encouraged. Effective communication has been proven to improve health outcomes for various chronic disease states. It is inferred that if providers have open communication with this specific population, their health outcomes will improve as well.

Gender minorities are noted to be at an increased risk for certain disorders. For example, a study concluded that lesbian, gay, and bisexual persons were at an increased risk for violence, discrimination, posttraumatic stress disorder, and depression, just to name a few. Just as communication has improved health outcomes for chronic diseases, so too should open communication about the health crises for patients of gender minorities. As of now, there are still no peer-reviewed or accepted tools to classify a patient's gender.[14] Another study looked at the use of tobacco in adolescents who identified themselves as gay, lesbian, or bisexual. These minorities were more likely than their heterosexual counterparts to smoke. Other studies have specifically addressed how to improve outcomes in adolescents who smoke, but there is currently no research that has specifically revealed how to improve health outcomes in the adolescent gender minority population. Some questions that may assist you in your determination of sex and gender include "What was your determined sex when you were born?" "Have you been attracted to or do you have intimate relationships with persons of the same or opposite sex?" "Do you contemplate changing your sexual identity, and if so, how would you change it?" You can always preface questions such as these by encouraging an open platform and explaining that you ask these questions of all your patients to not single out anyone out.

Age

Medicine is an ever-evolving entity, and there have been considerable advances in traditional standards of treatment. With this progress and the drive for offering preventive services, patient outcomes, and life expectancy have improved. By the year 2030, it is expected that the adult population over 65 years of age will increase to 71 million persons.[15] A substantial health concern in this population is the development of Alzheimer disease. This form of dementia places a large burden on the economy, families, and the health care system. It is anticipated that by the year 2050, up to 16 million older adults may have Alzheimer disease. The responsibility of health care professionals to screen and educate patients and their families may aide in discovering and preventing the progression of this debilitating disease. An effective technique thus far has been to ensure sufficient communication. Health care providers should also screen for other comorbid diseases such as diabetes and hypertension because these conditions can increase the risk for the development of Alzheimer disease. Other initiatives that have been implemented through the PPACA include the coverage for annual wellness physical examinations and the coverage of preventive services such as colonoscopy and mammography. These services expand for private paying insurance companies as well as Medicare, so that even adults who are not eligible for Medicare obtain the benefits. Two goals of covering preventive services are to ensure routine follow-up for older adults and compliance with the standards of the U.S. Preventive Service Task Force.[16] Each patient should be screened for needed routine health maintenance. This helps to create a complete and thorough medication evaluation to understand the necessary diagnostic studies each patient will need. A routine health follow-up especially for the elderly population will give you the ability to compile a proper medication reconciliation, assess for any adverse reactions to medications, and monitor the risk for developing chronic conditions.

Insurance Coverage

Per the ACP in *Racial and Ethnic Disparities in Health Care updated in* 2010, the most significant variable influencing health disparity populations is insurance status. One of the objectives of the PPACA was to limit the number of disparities in the coverage of Hispanic and black ethnicities by expanding coverage for both Medicaid and private insurance. Another objective was to expand coverage in young adults up to age 26 years of age. The bill, which passed in September 2010, increased the rate of coverage in young adults by nearly 200%. Overall, since the implementation of the PPACA, there has been a decline in the number of uninsured persons overall. However, there continues to be a significant discrepancy between the number of uninsured blacks and Hispanics compared with whites.[17] There have been numerous theories to explain the continued lack of coverage. One incongruence might exist because many Hispanics who are not covered are of immigrant status and do not qualify for insurance coverage. Nonelderly blacks have a higher rate of being uninsured for numerous reasons, but it is thought to be related to work status. Blacks have a higher rate of employment in blue collar–type jobs, which are less likely to offer appropriate or affordable health insurance. Additionally, this population has a higher rate of poverty than do their white and non-Hispanic counterparts, which ultimately makes it even more difficult to purchase a worthy and inexpensive health insurance policy.[17] Questioning patients about their insurance status and their ability to afford certain medications and diagnostic services should be considered at each visit. As a provider, you should become familiar with the drugs that are formulary and nonformulary for each type of insurance plan. This is a tool that you will learn being in a clinical setting that develops after time and exposure to the billing discipline. When you're able to determine which medications and services are covered, it becomes much easier to be an advocate for your patients.

Geographic Location

The Healthy People 2020 initiative has promised to achieve health equity, eliminate disparities, and improve the health of all groups. Its focus is to reduce the effects of chronic disease and to improve existing health care services.[19] According to Healthy People 2020, the lack of access to high-quality education, nutritious foods, affordable or reliable public transportation, and safe housing in America was found to be a qualitative factor that has been observed to have a negative impact on health outcomes. There is also a hindrance to the access of quality health care services in persons who live outside of city limits. The PPACA and other governmental alliances including the National Health Service Corps and Area Health Education Centers work together with many training programs to place medical providers in these rural areas and to expose students to populations that may have limited health status. At this time, the number of primary care providers available in the United States does not meet the demand for the current population. The aging population is living longer, which is further burdening the system for those who already lack appropriate access. The Health Resources and Services Administration has projected that there will be a deficit of around 20,000 primary care physicians by the year 2020. In anticipation of filling this gap, there has been a promotion to recruit more midlevel providers. In response, the job market for physician assistants and other midlevel providers is expected to increase by 58% from the year 2010 to the year 2020.[20]

Health Literacy

Implementing change and understanding the determinants of disease require a marketable level of literacy. Health literacy refers to the actual understanding of health services needed to make an informed decision on one's own medical state. The most common groups wherein health literacy is most prominent include older adults, men, ethnic minorities, and those of a lower socioeconomic status.[21] It is therefore part of the provider's responsibility to analyze each patient's health status and literacy level to ensure that each patient comprehends and is able to comply with recommended medical advice. There is still much research that needs to be focused in this area. As of now, most of the current analyses have focused on healthy literacy in racial or ethnic minorities and the effect it has on their health status and health outcomes. To certify that a patient understands his or her health status, it is important for providers to avoid using medical jargon during an interview. Leaving lines of communication open is also imperative to allow patients to ask questions so they may clarify understanding. Having patients repeat back to you in their own words their medications, treatment plan, and expectations allows you to assess their level of knowledge and any deficiencies that will require you to simplify the information.

CLINICAL APPLICATIONS

Perhaps a simple solution to closing the gap on health disparities is in educating providers. Starting from the foundation and moving upward may prove beneficial, and implementing this type of learning into training programs can help to expose students to the real issues they will face in clinical practice. A clear understanding that health disparities are all around us will continue to affect the way we practice medicine, no matter the specialty. If we can quickly identify patients whose outcomes are anticipated to be disadvantaged, we as providers can position ourselves to improve health status at an earlier step in the evaluation process. Realizing that health disparities don't just affect those of racial and ethnic minority will allow us to groom the next generation of health care providers and prepare them once they enter clinical practice. A full comprehension of the issues we face in our health care system will allow it to work more cohesively and effectively toward one common goal—the improvement of patient-centered care. As a student, be inspired to instill in yourself a spirit of cultural awareness, an attitude of empathetic understanding, and a service-led heart in educating and motivating your patients to improve their own health outcomes, no matter their background.

KEY POINTS

- Health care providers need to understand what health disparities encompass in order to provide unbiased care and therapy to all patients.
- Sexual orientation, age, insurance coverage or lack thereof, geographic location, ethnicity, religion, and health literacy are variables that can contribute to inadequate healthcare if not recognized.
- Be inspired to instill in yourself a spirit of cultural awareness, an attitude of empathetic understanding, and a service-led heart in educating and motivating your patients to improve their own health outcomes no matter their background.

References

1. *Patient Protection and Affordable Care Act*; 2010. Public Law No. 111–148.
2. Ramos E, Rotimi C. The A's, G's, C's, and T's of health disparities. *BMC Med Genomics*. 2009;(2):29. http://www.biomedcentral.com. Accessed September 18, 2016.
3. Dankwa-Mullan I, Rhee KB, Williams K, et al. The science of eliminating health disparities: summary and analysis of the NIH Summit recommendations. *Am J Public Health*. 2010;100(suppl 1):S12.
4. Rashid JR, et al. Eliminating health disparities through transdisciplinary research, cross-agency collaboration, and public participation. *Am J Public Health*. 1955;2009:99.
5. U.S. Department of Health and Human Services. Healthy People 2020. http://www.healthypeople.gov/2020/about/disparitiesAbout.aspx. Accessed August 26, 2016.
6. Gehlert S, Coleman R. Using community-based participatory research to ameliorate cancer disparities. *Health Soc Work*. 2010;35:302.
7. American College of Physicians. Racial and Ethnic Disparities in Health Care, Updated 2010. *Am Coll Physicians*. 2010. Policy Paper. http://www.ama-assn.org/resources/doc/public-health/acp-disparities-health-care.pdf. Accessed September 6, 2016.
8. Centers for Disease Control (CDC). Report on the Secretary's Task Force on Black and Minority Health. *MMWR Morb Mortal Wkly Rep*. 1986;35:109.
9. Frieden TR. Centers for Disease Control and Prevention. CDC Health Disparities and Inequalities Report—United States, 2011. *MMWR Morb Mortal Wkly Rep*. 2011;60(suppl):1.
10. Agency for Health Care Research and Quality. 2015 National Health Care Quality and Disparities Report and 5th Anniversary Update on the National Quality Strategy. *AHRQ*. April 2016. Publication No. 16–0015. http://www.ahrq.gov/research/findings/nhqrdr/index.html. Accessed August 13, 2016.
11. Satcher D, Higginbotham EJ. The public health approach to eliminating disparities in health. *Am J Public Health*. 2008;98:400.
12. Warnecke RB, Oh A, Breen N, et al. Approaching health disparities from a population perspective: the National Institutes of Health Centers for Population Health and Health Disparities. *Am J Public Health*. 2008;98:1608.
13. *Journal of Health Disparities Research & Practice* [serial online]. Available from EDS Publication Finder, Ipswich, MA. Accessed November 3, 2016.
14. Antin TMJ, Lipperman-Kreda S, Hunt G. *Tobacco denormalization as a public health strategy: implications for sexual and gender minorities*, November 2015. Accessed November 3, 2016.
15. Gupta VK, Winter M, Cabral H, et al. Disparities in age-associated cognitive decline between African-American and Caucasian populations: the roles of health literacy and education. *J Am Geriatr Soc*. 2016;64(8):1716–1723.
16. The Affordable Care Act and Medicare. Medicare.gov. https://www.medicare.gov/about-us/affordable-care-act/affordable-care-act.html. Accessed October 20, 2016.
17. Samantha Artiga. The Henry J. Kaiser Family Foundation. Health coverage by race and ethnicity: the potential impact of the Affordable Care Act. https://kaiserfamilyfoundation.files.wordpress.com/2014/07/8423-health-coverage-by-race-and-ethnicity.pdf. Accessed October 16, 2016.
19. Disparities. Healthy https://www.healthypeople.gov/2020/about/foundation-health-measures/Disparities. Accessed October 16, 2016.
20. Projecting the supply and demand for primary care practitioners through 2020. U.S. Department of Health and Human Services Health Resources and Services Administration. http://bhpr.hrsa.gov/healthworkforce/supplydemand/usworkforce/primarycare/. Accessed October 20, 2016.
21. Mantwill S, Monestel-Umaña S, Schulz PJ. The relationship between health literacy and health disparities: A systematic review. *PLOS ONE*. 2015;10(12):145455.

The resources for this chapter can be found at www.expertconsult.com.
The Faculty resources can be found online at www.expertconsult.com.

CHAPTER 39

PATIENT SAFETY AND QUALITY OF CARE

Torry Grantham Cobb

In late January 2001, 18-month-old Josie King turned on the hot water and climbed into a scalding-hot bathtub. She sustained second-degree burns on 60% of her body and was admitted to Johns Hopkins Medical Center. On February 22, 2001, 2 days before her planned discharge home, Josie's parents held their brain-dead daughter for the last time as she was disconnected from the ventilator. Her death was the result of severe dehydration and a narcotic overdose—a series of medical errors that occurred in one of the best medical centers in the country.[1]

QUALITY CARE MOVEMENT IN AMERICA

In 2000, the Institute of Medicine (IOM) Committee on the Quality of Health Care in America published a landmark report entitled *To Err Is Human, Building a Safer Health System*.[2] The report cited a study that estimated 98,000 people died every year in U.S. hospitals as a result of medical errors.[3] This is analogous to crashing a jumbo jet every day for a year and killing all the passengers on board. The analogy provided a stirring, concrete image for the magnitude of the death toll. Until this report, the magnitude of the medical error problem in the U.S. health care system was largely unrecognized.

A study published in 2013 reported the number of preventable deaths caused by medical errors to be significantly higher—an estimated 400,000 deaths annually.[4] If the Centers for Disease Control and Prevention (CDC) ranked medical errors as a cause of death in the United States, it would rank third behind heart disease and cancer. Furthermore, medical errors that result in patient harm but not death are estimated between 4 million and 8 million annually.[4]

In addition to the cost in human lives, preventable medical errors have been estimated to result in total costs (additional care, lost income, lost productivity, and disability) as high as $29 billion annually.[5] That number is estimated to reach $1 trillion annually when quality-adjusted life years are considered for those who die.[6] The less quantifiable toll of physical and psychological pain, reduced patient and provider satisfaction and trust, and poorer health status of communities and society is a significant outcome of medical errors as well.

Since the initial report was published in 2000, many public and private institutions have become involved in efforts to raise awareness of the problem and create tools for providers to use to detect and address medical errors in a systematic fashion.

Determining the Magnitude of the Problem

In 2002, the Agency for Healthcare Research and Quality (AHRQ), in collaboration with the University of California–Stanford Evidence-Based Practice Center, developed a collection of patient safety indicators (PSIs) to help health care organizations and hospitals assess, track, monitor, and improve patient safety.[7] These PSIs can be readily identified in hospital discharge data and are deemed potentially preventable patient safety incidents. In 2003, this set of 20 evidence-based PSIs was released to the public. As of 2016, the list has been expanded to include 25 PSIs (Box 39.1). These indicators are commonly used by health care organizations and governmental agencies to determine the magnitude of the problem.

Why Errors Occur

Historically, medical errors have been hidden from the public. The IOM reports that "The biggest challenge to moving toward a safer health system is changing the culture from one of blaming individuals for errors to one in which errors are treated not as personal failures, but as opportunities to improve."[7] The modern patient safety movement has replaced the secrecy and "blame and shame" of medical errors with a systems approach used in other high-risk industries such as airlines and nuclear power plants. This paradigm acknowledges humans as fallible and seeks to create strategies to anticipate, prevent, or catch unsafe events before they cause harm. The systems approach for safety in other industries has well-known and proven strategies, but these approaches have not been applied to medicine until recently.

The Swiss cheese model of organizational accidents developed by British psychologist James Reason is a good way to illustrate how medical errors occur (Fig. 39.1).[8] Rather than errors being the result of a single incident, they are viewed as multiple layers of fail-safes in which the holes align to produce a medical error. For example, there are several layers of protection for a patient whose provider orders the wrong dosage of a home medication in

---

BOX 39.1 AGENCY FOR HEALTHCARE RESEARCH PATIENT SAFETY INDICATORS

PSI 02 Death Rate in Low-Mortality Diagnosis Related Groups (DRGs)
PSI 03 Pressure Ulcer Rate
PSI 04 Death Rate among Surgical Inpatients with Serious Treatable Conditions
PSI 05 Retained Surgical Item or Unretrieved Device Fragment Count
PSI 06 Iatrogenic Pneumothorax Rate
PSI 07 Central Venous Catheter-Related Blood Stream Infection Rate
PSI 08 Postoperative Hip Fracture Rate
PSI 09 Perioperative Hemorrhage or Hematoma Rate
PSI 10 Postoperative Physiologic and Metabolic Derangement Rate
PSI 11 Postoperative Respiratory Failure Rate
PSI 12 Perioperative Pulmonary Embolism or Deep Vein Thrombosis Rate
PSI 13 Postoperative Sepsis Rate
PSI 14 Postoperative Wound Dehiscence Rate
PSI 15 Accidental Puncture or Laceration Rate
PSI 16 Transfusion Reaction Count
PSI 17 Birth Trauma Rate – Injury to Neonate
PSI 18 Obstetric Trauma Rate – Vaginal Delivery With Instrument
PSI 19 Obstetric Trauma Rate – Vaginal Delivery Without Instrument
PSI 21 Retained Surgical Item or Unretrieved Device Fragment Rate
PSI 22 Iatrogenic Pneumothorax Rate
PSI 23 Central Venous Catheter-Related Blood Stream Infection Rate
PSI 24 Postoperative Wound Dehiscence Rate
PSI 25 Accidental Puncture or Laceration Rate
PSI 26 Transfusion Reaction Rate
PSI 27 Postoperative Hemorrhage or Hematoma Rate
PSI 90 Patient Safety for Selected Indicators

From Agency for Healthcare Research and Quality. *AHRQ Quality Indicators: Patient Safety Indicators*, September 2015. http://www.qualityindicators.ahrq.gov/Downloads/Modules/PSI/V50/PSI_Brochure.pdf.

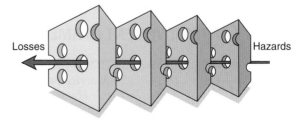

FIG. 39.1 ■ Swiss cheese model of medical errors. (From Reason J. Human error: models and management. *BMJ* 2000; 320:768. http://www.bmj.com/content/320/7237/768.full.)

the hospital. First, the order must be received by the pharmacist and not recognized as an error. Next, the nurse administering the medication must also fail to recognize the dosage error. Finally, the patient would need to accept the error as well. The model seeks ways to shrink the holes in each layer of protection, thus making the alignment less likely and resulting error less likely to occur. It also emphasizes the need to identify the root causes that make the medical errors possible.

Human Mistakes

The overwhelming majority of medical mistakes are not made because of a lack of knowledge, training, or information but rather result from faulty systems and poorly designed processes. When human errors do occur, they are made by honest, hard-working individuals who have demanding and often stressful jobs. They often occur during automatic tasks when unintentional performance lapses in an environment where faulty processes, systems, or conditions fail to catch or prevent the error.[9] The medical profession is often compared with other high-risk occupations whose members must perform under a high degree of stress with a high degree of accuracy. The difference is that medical professionals must combine complex decision making with customer interactions and automatic behaviors.[9] The training for medical providers has emphasized decision making with significantly less of a focus on customer interaction and essentially no training in how to manage risky automatic behaviors.

TYPES OF MEDICAL ERRORS

In 2001, the former chief executive officer of the National Quality Forum (NQF) coined the term "never event" to identify especially egregious medical errors (such as wrong-site surgery) that should never occur.[10] Since that time, the list of never events has been expanded to include 29 events grouped into six categories: surgical, product or device, patient protection, care management, environmental, and criminal (Box 39.2). More than 4000 surgical never events occur in the United States every year and have resulted in malpractice payments totaling more than $1.3 billion over the past 20 years.[11] Relative to the number of medical errors, never events occur infrequently. When they do occur, however, they are very likely to be fatal. Over the past 12 years, 71% of never events resulted in death.[12]

The Joint Commission has also compiled a list of events that signal the need for immediate investigation. These so-called sentinel events (that include the above never events) are defined by The Joint Commission as "unexpected occurrence[s] involving death or serious physical or psychological injury, or the risk thereof."[13] Serious injury is further defined as including the "loss of limb or function," and the phrase "or the risk thereof" includes any actions or events that would increase the risk of a serious adverse outcome if it occurred again.[13] The Joint Commission's list of sentinel events is shown in Box 39.3.

The Joint Commission's top 10 most frequently reported sentinel events (in order) in 2015 were as follows:

1. Unintended retention of foreign body
2. Wrong patient, wrong site, wrong procedure
3. Fall
4. Suicide
5. Delay in treatment
6. Operative or postoperative complication
7. Other unanticipated event (asphyxiation, burn, choked on food, drowned, found unresponsive)
8. Criminal event
9. Perinatal death or injury
10. Medication error[14]

The Joint Commission notes that the terms "sentinel event" and "medical error" are not synonymous. Not all medical errors result in sentinel events, and not all sentinel events are the result of medical errors. The Joint Commission reviews all sentinel events and mandates a root cause analysis after each.

Diagnosis Errors

In 2015, *Improving Diagnosis in Health Care* was published as a follow-up to the 2000 IOM report.[15] The new report published by the National Academy of Medicine (formerly known as the IOM) focuses on diagnostic errors, a significant but poorly addressed source of medical errors that was missing from the original 2000 report. Diagnostics errors are defined as (1) the failure to establish an accurate and timely diagnosis or (2) the failure to communicate the diagnosis to the patient. An estimated 5% of adults in the United States experience a diagnostic error each year. This equates to every American experiencing at least one error in diagnosis in their lifetime. A study by Tehrani et al. in 2013 analyzed 25 years of U.S. malpractice claims and found that the majority of paid claims were for diagnostic errors (28.6%).[16] Diagnostic errors were nearly twice as likely as other types of claims to be associated with death. The estimated 2011 inflation adjusted payout for each diagnostic error claim was $386,849.

BOX 39.2 NATIONAL QUALITY FORUM'S HEALTH CARE "NEVER EVENTS," 2011 REVISION

SURGICAL EVENTS

Surgery or other invasive procedure performed on the wrong body part

Surgery or other invasive procedure performed on the wrong patient

Wrong surgical or other invasive procedure performed on a patient

Unintended retention of a foreign object in a patient after surgery or other procedure

Intraoperative or immediately postoperative or postprocedure death in an American Society of Anesthesiologists class I patient

PRODUCT OR DEVICE EVENTS

Patient death or serious injury associated with the use of contaminated drugs, devices, or biologics provided by the health care setting

Patient death or serious injury associated with the use or function of a device in patient care in which the device is used for functions other than as intended

Patient death or serious injury associated with intravascular air embolism that occurs while being cared for in a health care setting

PATIENT PROTECTION EVENTS

Discharge or release of a patient or resident of any age who is unable to make decisions to other than an authorized person

Patient death or serious disability associated with patient elopement (disappearance)

Patient suicide, attempted suicide, or self-harm resulting in serious disability while being cared for in a health care facility

CARE MANAGEMENT EVENTS

Patient death or serious injury associated with a medication error (e.g., errors involving the wrong drug, wrong dose, wrong patient, wrong time, wrong rate, wrong preparation, or wrong route of administration)

Patient death or serious injury associated with un-safe administration of blood products

Maternal death or serious injury associated with labor or delivery in a low-risk pregnancy while being cared for in a health care setting

Death or serious injury of a neonate associated with labor or delivery in a low-risk pregnancy

Artificial insemination with the wrong donor sperm or wrong egg

Patient death or serious injury associated with a fall while being cared for in a health care setting

Any stage 3, stage 4, or unstageable pressure ulcers acquired after admission or presentation to a health care facility

Patient death or serious disability resulting from the irretrievable loss of an irreplaceable biological specimen

Patient death or serious injury resulting from failure to follow up or communicate laboratory, pathology, or radiology test results

ENVIRONMENTAL EVENTS

Patient or staff death or serious disability associated with an electric shock in the course of a patient care process in a health care setting

Any incident in which a line designated for oxygen or other gas to be delivered to a patient contains no gas, the wrong gas, or is contaminated by toxic substances

Patient or staff death or serious injury associated with a burn incurred from any source in the course of a patient care process in a health care setting

Patient death or serious injury associated with the use of restraints or bedrails while being cared for in a health care setting

RADIOLOGIC EVENTS

Death or serious injury of a patient or staff associated with introduction of a metallic object into the MRI area

CRIMINAL EVENTS

Any instance of care ordered by or provided by someone impersonating a physician, nurse, pharmacist, or other licensed health care provider

Abduction of a patient or resident of any age

Sexual abuse or assault on a patient within or on the grounds of a health care setting

Death or significant injury of a patient or staff member resulting from a physical assault (i.e., battery) that occurs within or on the grounds of a health care setting

ABO/HLA, blood group consisting of groups A, AB, B, and O/human leukocyte antigen
MRI, Magnetic resonance imaging.
From Agency for Healthcare Research and Quality. *Never Events.* https://psnet.ahrq.gov/primers/primer/3/never-events.

Medication Errors (Fig. 39.2)

Medication errors can be grouped into several categories: wrong patient, wrong drug, wrong dose, wrong route, or wrong frequency. These errors injure more than 1.5 million patients and result in billions of additional costs annually.[17] Common medication errors in the past were related to illegible prescriptions and orders (see Fig. 39.2). Fortunately, the advent of electronic medical record systems has made a significant impact.

Other medication problems stem from the lack of standardization and presence of ambiguity in

BOX 39.3 JOINT COMMISSION SENTINEL EVENTS, 2012 UPDATES

1. Any event that has resulted in an unanticipated death or major permanent loss of function not related to the natural course of the patient's illness or underlying condition or
2. Any event that is one of the following (even if the outcome was not death or major permanent loss of function not related to the natural course of the patient's illness or underlying condition):

- Infant discharge to the wrong family
- Unexpected death of a full-term infant
- Abduction of any patient receiving care, treatment, and services
- Invasive procedure, including surgery on the wrong patient, wrong site, or wrong procedure
- Unintended retention of a foreign object in a patient after surgery or other invasive procedures
- Rape or assault or homicide of any patient receiving care, treatment, and services
- Rape, assault, or homicide of a staff member, licensed independent practitioner, visitor or vendor while on site at the health care organization
- Hemolytic transfusion reaction involving administration of blood or blood products having major blood group incompatibilities
- Severe neonatal hyperbilirubinemia (bilirubin >30 mg/dL)
- Prolonged fluoroscopy with cumulative dose >1500 rads to a single field or any delivery of radiotherapy to the wrong body region or >25% above the planned radiotherapy dose
- Suicide of any patient receiving care, treatment, and services in a continuous care setting or within 72 hours of discharge

From The Joint Commission. *Sentinel Events (SE)*. http://www.jointcommission.org/assets/1/6/camh_2012_update2_24_se.pdf.

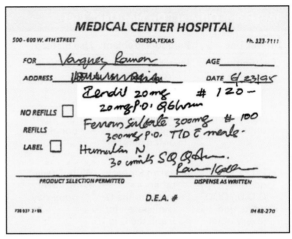

FIG. 39.2 ■ Illegible prescription. Can you discern the name of the first medication on this prescription? If you said Plendil, then you agreed with the pharmacist who filled the prescription. Unfortunately, the physician intended for the patient to get Isordil. This error resulted in a fatal overdose for the 42-year-old patient. A jury in Texas attributed the patient's death to the illegible prescription. The physician and the pharmacist each paid $225,000 in compensation to the patient's family. This was the first reported case of medical malpractice caused by illegible handwriting. (From Charatan F. Compensation awarded for death after illegible prescription. *West J Med* 2000;172:80. http://www.ncbi.nlm.nih.gov/pmc/articles/PMC1070756/.)

labeling of medications used in hospitals. For example, the epinephrine that is used in medical emergencies for cardiac arrest and anaphylaxis is packaged in the same vial with a similar label but in different concentrations. For anaphylaxis, a lower concentration of the medication should be given intramuscularly, but for cardiac arrest, a higher concentration should be given intravenously. Inadvertently giving the wrong concentration of the medication has led to fatal outcomes.[18] In an effort to decrease the risk of this medical error, some hospitals are stocking prefilled intramuscular dose syringes for anaphylaxis on their crash carts. Efforts used at the development and manufacturing level, such as removing or limiting the number of drugs that look alike or sound alike (e.g.,

Celebrex and Cerebyx), are approaches that should reduce medical errors.

Another strategy designed to reduce medication errors is the ban on the use of certain words and abbreviations when ordering medications. The "do not use" list was developed by The Joint Commission in 2004 during a 1-day summit of representatives from more than 70 professional medical organizations and special interest group.[19] The goal of the summit was to identify abbreviations, acronyms, and symbols that have the potential to cause errors and propose a method to eliminate or reduce the threat. The result was the official "do not use" list (Table 39.1). The list applies to all orders and medication-related documents that are handwritten, free texted in the computer, or on preprinted forms.

Surgical Errors (Fig. 39.3)

The NQF, a nonprofit organization that sets national priorities and goals for health care quality and safety, lists surgical events as one of the six major categories of "never events."[20] Three of the top five sentinel events reported by The Joint Commission from 2004 to 2015 were surgical events (wrong-site surgery, unintended retention of foreign body, and operative or postoperative complications).[14]

TABLE 39.1 Official "Do Not Use" List

Do Not Use	Potential Problem	Use Instead
U, u (unit)	Mistaken for 0 (zero), the number 4 (four), or cc	Write "unit."
IU (international unit)	Mistaken for IV (intravenous) or the number 10 (ten)	Write "international unit."
Q.D., QD, q.d., qd (daily), Q.O.D., QOD, q.o.d, qod (every other day)	Mistaken for each other Period after the Q is mistaken for I, and the O is mistaken for I	Write "daily." Write "every other day."
Trailing zero (X.0 mg) Lack of leading zero (.X mg)	Decimal point is missed	Write X mg Write 0.X mg
MSMSO$_4$ and MgSO$_4$	Can mean morphine sulfate or magnesium sulfate Confused for each other	Write "morphine sulfate." Write "magnesium sulfate."

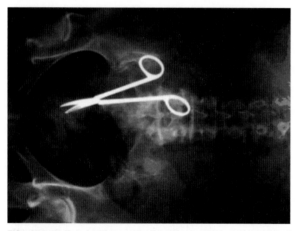

FIG. 39.3 ■ Retained surgical object. (From Associated Press. Scissors left in woman after surgery. NBCNews.com. http://www.msnbc.msn.com/id/4788266/ns/health-health_care/t/scissors-left-woman-after-surgery/#.T71khl4yeS0.)

To address surgical errors, The Joint Commission developed a universal protocol for preventing wrong-site, wrong-procedure, and wrong-person surgery.[21] Endorsed by more than 40 professional medical organizations, the protocol mandates active involvement and effective communication among all members of the surgical team. It involves a verification process, marking of the surgical site, and a time-out procedure (Box 39.4).[22]

BOX 39.4 UNIVERSAL PROTOCOL FOR PREVENTING WRONG-SITE, WRONG-PROCEDURE, WRONG-PERSON SURGERY

PREOPERATIVE VERIFICATION PROCESS
- Purpose: To ensure that all of the relevant documents and studies are available before the start of the procedure and that they have been reviewed and are consistent with each other and with the patient's expectations, as well as with the team's understanding of the intended patient; procedure; site; and, as applicable, any implants. Missing information or discrepancies must be addressed before starting the procedure.
- Process: An ongoing process of information gathering and verification, beginning with the determination to do the procedure and continuing through all settings and interventions involved in the preoperative preparation of the patient, up to and including the "time-out" just before the start of the procedure

MARKING THE OPERATIVE SITE
- Purpose: To identify unambiguously the intended site of incision or insertion
- Process: For procedures involving right–left distinction, multiple structures (e.g., fingers and toes), or multiple levels (as in spinal procedures), the intended site must be marked such that the mark will be visible after the patient has been prepped and draped.

"TIME-OUT" IMMEDIATELY BEFORE STARTING THE PROCEDURE
- Purpose: To conduct a final verification of the correct patient; procedure; site; and, as applicable, implants
- Process: Active communication among all members of the surgical or procedure team, consistently initiated by a designated member of the team, conducted in a "fail-safe" mode (i.e., the procedure is not started until any questions or concerns are resolved)

Modified from The Joint Commission. *Universal Protocol for Preventing Wrong Site, Wrong Procedure, Wrong Person Surgery.* Oakbrook Terrace, IL: The Joint Commission, 2003.)

The unintended retention of foreign objects ranked second among the most common sentinel events reported between 2004 and 2015.[14] Although the exact number cannot be determined, it has been estimated that more than 1500 cases of retained surgical objects (RSO) occur annually.[23] Studies have estimated that needles, sponges, and other surgical objects are inadvertently left in a patient's body once in every 7000 surgical procedures, with the estimate for abdominal procedures being as high as 1 in every 1000 to 1500 operations.[24,25] Strategies to prevent unintended retention of foreign objects include manual counting and intraoperative and postoperative radiographs, bar coding sponges and instruments, electronic article surveillance tags, and radiofrequency identification tags.[26]

Transition and Communication Errors

Lack of continuity of care is a well-recognized problem in health care systems. No one can provide around-the-clock coverage, so inevitably, patient care is provided by many providers. This discontinuity provides an opportunity for the inaccurate transfer of data and thus increases the risk of medical errors. The Joint Commission reports that up to 80% of serious medical errors occur as a result of miscommunication between providers during transitions of care.[27] The breakdown of communication was also reported to be the leading root cause of all sentinel events reported to The Joint Commission between 1995 and 2006. A 2015 study found that 30% of malpractice cases involved communication failures resulting in nearly 2000 deaths and $1.7 billion in malpractice costs.[28]

In an effort to reduce hand-off errors, The Joint Commission's 2006 National Patient Safety Goals require all health care providers to implement a standardized approach to handing off patients.[29] The mandate contains guidelines for this process, many of which are drawn from other high-risk industries. The following criteria must be met:
- Interactive communications
- Up-to-date and accurate information
- Limited interruptions
- A process for verification
- An opportunity to review any relevant historical data[29]

One such tool now widely used in graduate medical education is I-PASS. This tool is used for both written and verbal clinical hand-offs and has proven effective in preventing communication errors.[29,30] The information provided in the hand-off process includes:
- **I**llness severity: one-word summary of patient acuity ("stable," "watcher," or "unstable")
- **P**atient summary: brief summary of the patient's diagnoses and treatment plan
- **A**ction list: to-do items to be completed by the clinician receiving sign-out
- **S**ituation awareness and contingency plans: directions to follow in case of changes in the patient's status, often in an "if–then" format
- **S**ynthesis by receiver: an opportunity for the receiver to ask questions and confirm the plan of care[30]

A 2005 study of a computerized and structured sign-out process at an academic medical center demonstrated increased efficiency and continuity of care.[31] An investigation of sign-out protocols adapted from Formula 1 auto racing and aviation has also been shown to reduce communication errors.[32]

Traditionally, medical teams have had steep authority gradients. Fear and intimidation prevented others from expressing concerns about patient safety. The patient safety movement, however, has focused on teamwork and the leveling of responsibility to make all team members equally responsible for patient safety. A strategy originally developed by the U.S. Navy to improve communication on nuclear submarines, SBAR (situation, background, assessment, recommendation), was introduced into health care settings in 1990.[33] Since then, it has become a widely used tool to effectively communicate between caregivers. The following is an example of a telephone communication using SBAR.

Introduction

- PA Smith, this is Donna Reynolds, RN. I am calling from County Hospital about your postsurgical patient Janet Hall.

Situation

- Here's the situation: Mrs. Hall is complaining of chest pain and having increasing shortness of breath.

Background

- The supporting background information is that she had a lumbar fusion 2 days ago. About 15 minutes ago, she began complaining of chest pain. Her pulse is 122, and her blood pressure is 140/64. Her oxygen saturation was 80% on room air. She appears ashen and has increased work of breathing.

Assessment

- My assessment of the situation is that she may be having a cardiac event or a pulmonary embolism.

Recommendation

- I have started her on oxygen and would like to get a STAT EKG. I recommend that you see her immediately. Do you agree?

Health Care–Associated Conditions

In 2007, the CDC estimated that 1.7 million health care–associated conditions (HACs) occurred annually and resulted in 99,000 deaths.[34] For U.S. hospitals, the added financial burden was estimated to exceed $45 billion.[35] To address this problem and other HACs, the Centers for Medicare & Medicaid Services (CMS) initiated a new payment policy for certain hospital-acquired conditions in October 2008.[36] Initially, the CMS identified 10 categories of HAC it considers "reasonably preventable." This list was updated in 2013 to include 14 categories of HAC (Box 39.5).[37] No changes were made in 2014 or 2015. Since 2008, the CMS has refused to pay hospitals for the increased cost of care that results from preventable HACs.[36] Many states and commercial insurance companies have followed suit, thus placing further restrictions on the reimbursement of services that result from preventable HACs. The good news is that the AHRQ reports a 17% decline in HACs, from 145 HACs per 1000 discharges to 121 from 2010 to 2013. This resulted in 1.3 million fewer HACs between 2010 and 2013, saving more than 50,000 lives and more than $12 billion in health care costs.[38]

A subcategory of HACs is health care–associated infections (HAIs). In 2014, results from the HAI Prevalence Survey were published estimating 722,000 HAIs in U.S. hospitals in 2011. HAIs during hospitalizations resulted in 75,000 patient deaths. Although these numbers are better than estimated in 2007, the survey results indicate that on any calendar date, 1 of every 25 inpatients in U.S. hospitals has at least one HAI. Surgical site infections and pneumonia were the most common types of infection, with *Clostridium difficile* being the most common pathogen.[39]

PATIENT SAFETY STRATEGIES

A variety of governmental and private organizations have developed programs aimed at improving awareness and designing strategies to improve patient outcomes.

The Department of Health and Human Services National Strategy for Quality Improvement in Health Care for 2015 outlines strategies to improve the quality of care, make people healthier, and make health care more affordable. Four of the six national quality strategies outlined address problems in the health care system that can lead to medical errors. These include making care safer by reducing harm caused in the delivery of care, ensuring that patients and their families are engaged as partners in their care, promoting effective communication and

---

BOX 39.5 FOURTEEN CATEGORIES OF PREVENTABLE HOSPITAL-ACQUIRED CONDITIONS

- Foreign object retained after surgery
- Air embolism
- Blood incompatibility
- Stage III and IV pressure ulcers
- Falls and trauma
  - Fractures
  - Dislocations
  - Intracranial injuries
  - Crushing injuries
  - Burn
  - Other injuries
- Manifestations of poor glycemic control
  - Diabetic ketoacidosis
  - Nonketotic hyperosmolar coma
  - Hypoglycemic coma
  - Secondary diabetes with ketoacidosis
  - Secondary diabetes with hyperosmolarity
- Catheter-associated urinary tract infection
- Vascular catheter–associated infection
- Surgical site infection, mediastinitis, after coronary artery bypass graft
- Surgical site infection after bariatric surgery for obesity
  - Laparoscopic gastric bypass
  - Gastroenterostomy
  - Laparoscopic gastric restrictive surgery
- Surgical site infection after certain orthopedic procedures
  - Spine
  - Neck
  - Shoulder
  - Elbow
- Surgical site infection after cardiac implantable electronic device
- Deep vein thrombosis or pulmonary embolism after certain orthopedic procedures
  - Total knee replacement
  - Hip replacement
- Iatrogenic pneumothorax with venous catheterization

From Centers for Medicare & Medicaid Services. *Hospital-Acquired Conditions.* https://www.cms.gov/medicare/medicare-fee-for-service-payment/hospitalacqcond/hospital-acquired_conditions.html.

---

coordination of care, and developing and spreading new health care delivery models.[40]

A private organization created to identify problems and create solutions is the Patient Safety Movement Foundation (PSMF). The mission of the PSMF is to:
1. Unify the health care ecosystem.
2. Identify the challenges that are killing patients to create actionable solutions.

BOX 39.6 THE PATIENT SAFETY MOVEMENT CHALLENGES LIST

Challenge 1: Creating a Culture of Safety
Challenge 2: Healthcare-associated Infections (HAIs)
Challenge 3: Medication Errors
Challenge 4: Failure to Rescue: Monitoring for Opioid Induced Respiratory Depression
Challenge 5: Anemia and Transfusion: A Patient Safety Concern
Challenge 6: Hand-off Communication
Challenge 7: Suboptimal Neonatal Oxygen Targeting
Challenge 8: Failure to Detect Critical Congenital Heart Disease (CCHD)
Challenge 9: Airway Safety
Challenge 10: Early Detection of Sepsis
Challenge 11: Optimal Resuscitation
Challenge 12: Optimizing Obstetric Safety
Challenge 13: Venous Thromboembolism (VTE)
Challenge 14: Mental Health

From Patient Safety Movement. *Actionable Patient Safety Solutions (APSS).* http://patientsafetymovement.org/challenges-solutions/actionable-patient-safety-solutions-apss.

3. Ask hospitals to implement Actionable Patient Safety Solutions.
4. Promote transparency.
5. Ask medical technology companies to share the data their devices generate to create a patient data superhighway to help identify at-risk patients.
6. Correct misaligned incentives.
7. Promote love and patient dignity.
8. Empower providers, patients, and families through education of medical terminology and medical errors so they may better advocate for their loved ones.
9. Ultimately, reach the goal of zero preventable patient deaths by 2020.[41]

The PSMF has defined a set of challenges with solutions to meet these mission statements (Box 39.6).[42]

A government program that provides a comprehensive and systematic approach to hand-off communications is The Joint Commission Center for Transforming Healthcare Targeted Solutions Tool (TST).[43] This tool gives organizations a means of measuring their performance, identifying barriers to providing excellent performance, and provides them with proven solutions.

Another leading private, nonprofit organization fighting for patient safety is the Leapfrog Group (LG). The LG's goal is to save lives by reducing errors, injuries, accidents, and infections. The LG publicly reports on hospital performance via an evidence-based national tool in which hospitals voluntarily report on key indicators. The four original "leaps" endorsed by the NQF were:

1. **Computerized physician order entry (CPOE).** With CPOE systems, hospital staff enter medication orders via computers linked to software designed to prevent prescribing errors. CPOE has been shown to reduce serious prescribing errors by more than 50%.
2. **Evidence-based hospital referral (EBHR).** Consumers and health care purchasers should choose hospitals with the best track records. By referring patients needing certain complex medical procedures to hospitals offering the best survival odds based on scientifically valid criteria—such as the number of times a hospital performs a procedure each year or other process or outcomes data—studies indicate that a patient's risk of dying could be significantly reduced.
3. **Intensive care unit (ICU) physician staffing (IPS).** Staffing ICUs with intensivists—doctors who have special training in critical care medicine—has been shown to reduce the risk of patients dying in ICUs by 40%.
4. **NQF Safe Practices.** The NQF-endorsed Safe Practices cover a range of practices that, if used, would reduce the risk of harm in certain processes, systems, or environments of care. Included in the 34 practices are the three leaps above.

In 2012, the LG launched a grading system called the Hospital Safety score. All general hospitals are rated twice a year with a letter grade (A, B, C, D, F) based on patient safety.[44]

Role of the Patient

In 2002, The Joint Commission and CMS launched a national campaign advocating that patients assume a larger role in preventing medical errors by becoming active, involved, and informed participants in the health care system.[45] The program, called Speak Up, encourages patients to speak up if they have questions or concerns. The program advocates asking questions when patients and their families do not understand (Box 39.7).

The World Health Organization (WHO) is also leading the way in patient safety efforts. The program WHO Patient Safety seeks to coordinate and promote improvements in patient safety worldwide. The WHO Patients for Patient Safety program encourages consumers of health care to become partners with their health care team to make medical care safer.[46]

The American College of Physicians (ACP) also advocates for patients playing a role in their own safety.[47] The ACP summarizes the rights and responsibilities of patients as follows:

At the Appointment

Rights

- To be an active participant in discussions
- To have understandable, legible instructions and prescriptions
- To have an explanation of why a particular course of treatment is recommended

Responsibilities.

- To be open and honest about symptoms, drugs he or she might be taking, and medical history
- To voice concerns
- To speak up if he or she does not understand
- To check back on test results

At the Pharmacy

Rights.

- To receive the correct prescription
- To receive verbal and written information about how to use the drug
- To have information on drug interactions and side effects and what to do about them

Responsibilities.

- To check the prescription to make sure it is what the doctor ordered
- To remind pharmacists about other drugs or allergies
- To ask questions if necessary

At Home

Right.

- To research his or her condition using the library, Internet tools, and so on

Responsibilities.

- To know the validity of the source of health information
- To verify health information with the physician

In addition, the AHRQ provides tips to patients to help prevent medical errors (Box 39.8).[48]

Medical Error Disclosure

Since July 2001, The Joint Commission has required disclosure of adverse outcomes.[49] The Sorry Works! Coalition, founded in 2005, is dedicated to promoting apologies and full disclosure for medical errors.[50] The Sorry Works! Coalition advocates that providers and health care institutions apologize for medical errors (Box 39.9). It believes that apologies combined with up-front compensation serve to reduce the anger felt by patients and their families when errors occur. The coalition also believes that this results in fewer medical malpractice lawsuits and reduced legal costs. The approach is believed to result in expedient justice for victims (Box 39.10). The Sorry Works! Coalition believes that medial errors can be reduced through honesty and full disclosure.

During a 7-year period in which the Lexington Veterans Administration Hospital (VA) practiced the principles set forth by the Sorry Works! Coalition, the average payout for malpractice claims was $16,000, relative to the national average of $98,000. The Lexington VA reported the full disclosure reduced the number of pending lawsuits by half and reduced litigation costs from $65,000 to $35,000 per case, an annual savings of $2 million.[39]

CLINICAL APPLICATIONS

1. What is the name of the landmark report published in 2000 that launched the patient safety movement in the United States?
2. Explain the Swiss cheese model of organizational accidents.
3. What are sentinel events and never events?
4. Name two types of medical errors.
5. What are some of the strategies that have been implemented in the health care system to improve patient safety?

BOX 39.8 WHAT PATIENTS CAN DO TO STAY SAFE

The best way you can help to prevent errors is to be an active member of your health care team. That means taking part in every decision about your health care. Research shows that patients who are more involved with their care tend to get better results.

MEDICINES

Make sure that all of your providers know about every medicine you are taking. This includes prescription and over-the-counter medicines and dietary supplements, such as vitamins and herbs.

Bring all of your medicines and supplements to your provider visits. "Brown bagging" your medicines can help you and your provider talk about them and find out if there are any problems. It can also help your provider keep your records up to date and help you get better quality care.

Make sure your provider knows about any allergies and adverse reactions you have had to medicines. This can help you to avoid getting a medicine that could harm you.

When your provider writes a prescription for you, make sure you can read it. If you cannot read your provider's handwriting, your pharmacist might not be able to either.

Ask for information about your medicines in terms you can understand—both when your medicines are prescribed and when you get them:

- What is the medicine for?
- How am I supposed to take it and for how long?
- What side effects are likely? What do I do if they occur?
- Is this medicine safe to take with other medicines or dietary supplements I am taking?

What food, drink, or activities should I avoid while taking this medicine?

When you pick up your medicine from the pharmacy, ask: "Is this the medicine that my provider prescribed?"

If you have any questions about the directions on your medicine labels, ask. Medicine labels can be hard to understand. For example, ask if "four times daily" means taking a dose every 6 hours around the clock or just during regular waking hours.

Ask your pharmacist for the best device to measure your liquid medicine. For example, many people use household teaspoons, which often do not hold a true teaspoon of liquid. Special devices, such as marked syringes, help people measure the right dose.

Ask for written information about the side effects your medicine could cause. If you know what might happen, you will be better prepared if it does or if something unexpected happens.

HOSPITAL STAYS

If you are in a hospital, consider asking all health care workers who will touch you whether they have washed their hands. Hand washing can prevent the spread of infections in hospitals.

When you are being discharged from the hospital, ask your provider to explain the treatment plan you will follow at home. This includes learning about your new medicines, making sure you know when to schedule follow-up appointments, and finding out when you can get back to your regular activities. It is important to know whether or not you should keep taking the medicines you were taking before your hospital stay. Getting clear instructions may help prevent an unexpected return trip to the hospital.

SURGERY

If you are having surgery, make sure that you, your provider, and your surgeon all agree on exactly what will be done. Having surgery at the wrong site (e.g., operating on the left knee instead of the right) is rare. But even once is too often. The good news is that wrong-site surgery is 100% preventable. Surgeons are expected to sign their initials directly on the site to be operated on before the surgery.

If you have a choice, choose a hospital where many patients have had the procedure or surgery you need. Research shows that patients tend to have better results when they are treated in hospitals that have a great deal of experience with their condition.

OTHER STEPS

Speak up if you have questions or concerns. You have a right to question anyone who is involved with your care.

Make sure that someone, such as your primary care provider, coordinates your care. This is especially important if you have many health problems or are in the hospital.

Make sure that all your providers have your important health information. Do not assume that everyone has all the information they need.

Ask a family member or friend to go to appointments with you. Even if you do not need help now, you might need it later.

Know that "more" is not always better. It is a good idea to find out why a test or treatment is needed and how it can help you. You could be better off without it.

If you have a test, do not assume that no news is good news. Ask how and when you will get the results.

Learn about your condition and treatments by asking your provider and nurse and by using other reliable sources. For example, treatment options based on the latest scientific evidence are available from the Effective Health Care website. Ask your provider if your treatment is based on the latest evidence.

From Agency for Healthcare Research and Quality. http://www.ahrq.gov/patients-consumers/care-planning/errors/20tips/index.html.

BOX 39.9 THREE-STEP DISCLOSURE PROCESS

Sorry Works! is a program that needs to be administered by a team of medical, risk, insurance, and legal professionals within a medical, hospital, or insurance setting.

The Sorry Works! program is predicated on a three-step disclosure process:

- Initial disclosure
- Investigation
- Resolution

Step 1—Initial disclosure is all about empathy and reestablishing trust and communication with patients and families in the immediate aftermath of an adverse event. Providers say "sorry," but no fault is admitted or assigned. Providers take care of the immediate needs of the patient and family (e.g., food, lodging, counseling) and promise a swift and thorough investigation. The goal is to make sure the patient and family never feel abandoned. In the spirit of good customer service, pull the patient and family closer to the providers and institution.

Step 2—Investigation is about learning the truth. Was the standard of care breached or not? We recommend involving outside experts and moving swiftly so that the patient and family do not suspect a cover-up. Stay in close contact with the patient and family throughout the process.

Step 3—Resolution is about sharing the results of the investigation with the patient and family, as well as their legal counsel. If there was a mistake, apologize; admit fault; explain what happened and how it will be prevented in the future; and discuss fair, upfront compensation for the injury or death. If there was no mistake, continue to empathize ("We are sorry this happened"), share the results of investigation (hand over charts and records to patient and family and their legal counsel), and prove your innocence. However, no settlement will be offered and any lawsuit will be contested. Sorry Works! is compassion with a backbone.

From Wojcieszak D. *The Sorry Works! Coalition.* http://nneshrm.org/images/downloads/Educational_Presentations/2009_sorry_works.pdf.

BOX 39.10 SORRY WORKS! COALITION: FIVE THINGS EVERY PROVIDER SHOULD KNOW ABOUT DISCLOSURE

1. **Disclosure is good for doctors, as well as nurses, hospitals, and insurers.** An enormous and growing body of data is showing that disclosure coupled with apology (when appropriate) actually reduces lawsuits, litigation expenses, and settlements and judgments. The key is anger—disclosure and apology keep a lid on anger, whereas traditional deny-and-defend risk management strategies increase anger felt by patients and families and increase the likelihood of costly litigation.

2. **Five-star customer service, informed consent, and good communication lay the groundwork for successful disclosure.** For disclosure to work, you have to be credible. You also have to begin building positive evidence early in the process. Patients and families want to be treated with respect at all times, and they also want to see doctors and nurses treating each other with respect. Absent these feelings, disclosure after an adverse event might appear to a patient and family as a form of manipulation. "Why is Dr. McGod being nice to me now?" will be the skeptical question rolling around the heads of your patients and families. Also, procedure-specific informed consent will aid in credible disclosure discussions, especially where there was no error. Unfortunately, sending your nurse in 5 minutes before the procedure with a bunch of forms to sign does not count! You have to invest the time and energy upfront.

3. **Empathetic "I'm sorry" immediately after the adverse event.** Doctors should provide an empathetic apology immediately after an adverse event coupled with a promise of an investigation and customer service assistance such as food, lodging, phone calls, transportation, and so on. "I'm so sorry this happened Mrs. Jones . . . I feel bad for you and your family." Notice: Doctors should NOT prematurely admit fault or assign blame. Also, do *not* get defensive. Simply say you are sorry the event happened (as you should be!) and that you feel bad for the patient and family, acknowledge their feelings, promise an investigation, and take care or assist with any immediate needs of the patient and family. Show you care! Document the chart accordingly without emotion or speculation. Write down what you said, what you promised, and any questions or comments by the patient and family.

4. **Call somebody!** Call your risk manager, insurance company, defense counsel, and so on immediately after the empathetic apology with the patient and family. Inform this person of the situation and ask for assistance with an investigation that will lead to a resolution of the situation, which may include a real apology ("I'm sorry I made a mistake") coupled with fair, upfront compensation (paid for by your insurer) or more empathy if no error occurred.

5. **Train nurses and staff on disclosure!** Nurses and staff must understand their role in disclosure. No, it does not mean that nurses will be apologizing for doctors, but it does mean that nurse and frontline staff should know that it's okay for them to empathize, say "sorry," and stay connected with patients and families after the adverse event. In fact, we want the nurses and staff to take service to a new, higher level with patients and families after an adverse event. We want nurses to be part of our effort to save and restore relationships. This is so important because for far too long, nurses have literally been told to "shut up" after an adverse event and have been forced to run from their patients and families, making the doctors and hospital look guilty even if no mistake happened!

References

1. Pronovost P, Vohr E. *Safe Patients, Smart Hospitals: How One Doctor's Checklist Can Help Us Change Health Care from the Inside Out.* New York: Hudson Street Press; 2010.
2. Kohn L, Corrigan J, Donaldson M, eds. *To Err Is Human: Building a Safer Health System.* Washington, DC: Committee on Quality of Health Care in America; 2000. Institute of Medicine: National Academy Press.
3. Brennan TA, Leape LL, Laird NM, et al. Incidence of adverse events and negligence in hospitalized patients. Results of the Harvard Medical Practice Study I. *N Engl J Med.* 1991;324:370.
4. James JT. A new, evidence-based estimate of patient harms associated with hospital care. *J Patient Saf.* 2013;9(3): 122–128.
5. Johnson WG, Brennan TA, Newhouse JP, et al. The economic consequences of medical injuries. *JAMA.* 1992;267:2487.
6. Andel C, Davidow SL, Hollander M, Moreno DA. The economics of health care quality and medical error. *J Health Care Finance.* 2012;39(1):39–50.
7. Department of Health and Human Services Agency for Healthcare Research and Quality. March 2003, Revision 2 (October 22, 2004). AHRQ Pub. No. 03–R203 (website). http://www.qualityindicators.ahrq.gov.
8. Reason JT. *Human Error.* New York: Cambridge University Press; 1990.
9. Wachter RM. *Understanding Patient Safety.* New York: McGraw-Hill; 2008.
10. National Quality Forum. Serious reportable events in healthcare 2006 update (website). http://www.qualityforum.org/Publications/2007/03/Serious_Reportable_Events_in_Healthcare%E2%80%932006_Update.aspx.
11. Mehtsun WT, Ibrahim AM, Diener-West M, Pronovost PJ, Makary MA. Surgical never events in the United States. *Surgery.* 2013;153(4):465–472.
12. Agency for Healthcare Research and Quality. Never events. December 2014. https://psnet.ahrq.gov/primers/primer/3/never-events.
13. Joint Commission. Sentinel Events. 2012 Updates. http://www.jointcommission.org/assets/1/6/camh_2012_update2_24_se.pdf.
14. Summary Data of Sentinel Events Reviewed by the Joint Commission. 2/4/2016. jointcommission.org/assets/1/18/2004-2015_SE_Stats_stummary.pdf.
15. Front Matter. *National Academies of Sciences, Engineering, and Medicine. Improving Diagnosis in Health Care.* Washington, DC: The National Academies Press; 2015.
16. Tehrani A, Lee H, Mathews S, et al. A 25-year summary of U.S. malpractice claims for diagnostic errors 1986–2010: An analysis from the National Practitioner Data Bank. *BMJ Quality and Safety.* 2013;22:672–680.
17. The National Academy of Science. 2006. Preventing Medication Errors. http://www.nationalacademies.org/hmd/~/media/Files/Report%20Files/.
18. Kanwar M, Irvin CB, Frank JJ, et al. Confusion about epinephrine dosing leading to iatrogenic overdose: a life-threatening problem with a potential solution. *Ann Emerg Med.* 2010;55:341.
19. Joint Commission. 2015 Facts about the Official "Do Not Use" List (website). http://www.jointcommission.org/facts_about_do_not_use_list/.
20. National Quality Forum. Serious reportable events in healthcare 2006 update (website). https://www.qualityforum.org/Publications/2007/03/Serious_Reportable_Events_in_Healthcare–2006_Update.aspx.
21. Joint Commission. 2011 Facts about the Universal Protocol (website). http://www.jointcommission.org/assets/1/18/Universal%20Protocol%201%204%20111.PDF.
22. 2014 Joint Commission Universal Protocol www.jointcommission.org/assests/1/18/UP_Poster1.pdf.
23. Gawande A, Studdert DM, Orav EJ, et al. Risk factors for retained instruments and sponges after surgery. *N Engl J Med.* 2003;348:229.
24. Egorova N, Moskowitz A, Gelijns A, et al. Managing the prevention of retained surgical instruments: what is the value of counting? *Ann Surg.* 2008;247:13.
25. Allen G. Evidence for practice. *AORN J.* 2008;87:833.
26. Cobb TG. Iatrogenic retention of surgical objects: risk factors and prevention strategies. *J Am Acad Phys Assist.* 2010;23:33.
27. Joint Commission Center for Transforming Healthcare. 2011 Facts about hand-off communications. http://www.centerfortransforminghealthcare.org/projects/about_handoff_communication.aspx.
28. Academic Medical Center Patient Safety Organization risk Management Foundation 2015 Malpractice Risks in Communication Failures. www.rmf.harvard,edu/cbsreport.

29. U.S. Department of Health and Human Services Agency for Healthcare Research and Quality November 2015 Patient Safety Primer: Hand-offs and Signouts. https://psnet.ahrq.gov/primers/primer/9/handoffs-and-signouts.
30. Starmer AJ, Sectish TC, Simon DW, et al. Rates of medical errors and preventable adverse events among hospitalized children following implementation of a resident handoff bundle. *JAMA*. 2013;310(21):2262–2270.
31. Van Eaton EG, Horvath KD, Lober WB, et al. A randomized, controlled trial evaluating the impact of a computerized rounding and sign-out system on continuity of care and resident work hours. *J Am Coll Surg*. 2005;200:538.
32. Catchpole KR, de Leval MR, McEwan A, et al. Patient handover from surgery to intensive care: using Formula 1 pit-stop and aviation models to improve safety and quality. *Paediatr Anaesth*. 2007;17:470.
33. Hohenhaus S, Powell S, Hohenhaus JT. Enhancing patient safety during hand-offs: standardized communication and teamwork using the 'SBAR' method. *Am J Nurs*. 2006;106:72A.
34. Centers of Disease Control and Prevention. Preventing healthcare-associated infections. Retrieved from http://www.cdc.gov/washington/cdcatWork/pdf/infections.pdf.
35. Scott RD. The Direct Costs of Healthcare-Associated Infections in U.S. Hospitals and the Benefits of Prevention. 2009 Centers for Disease Control and Prevention Report (website). http://www.cdc.gov/ncidod/dhqp/pdf/Scott_CostPaper.pdf.
36. Centers for Medicare and Medicaid Services. Eliminating serious, preventable, and costly medical errors—never events (website). http://www.cms.hhs.gov/apps/media/press/release.asp?Counter=1863.
37. Centers for Medicare and Medicaid Services 2015. Hospital Acquired Conditions. https://www.cms.gov/medicare/medicare-fee-for-service-payment/hospitalacqcond/hospital-acquired_conditions.html.
38. Agency for Healthcare Research and Quality. Efforts to Improve Patient Safety Result in 1.3 Million Fewer Patient Harms: Interim Update on 2013 Annual Hospital-Acquired Condition Rate and Estimate of Cost Savings and Deaths Averted from 2010 to 2013 (Publication #15-0011-EF).

Retrieved March 26, 2016, from http://www.ahrq.gov/professionals/quality-patient-safety/pfp/interimhacrate2013.html.
39. Magill SS, Edwards JR, Bamberg W, et al. Multistate point-prevalence survey of health care–associated infections. *N Engl J Med*. 2014;370:1198–1208.
40. Agency for Healthcare Research and Quality. 2015 Annual Progress Report to Congress: National Strategies for Quality Improvement in Healthcare. http://www.ahrq.gov/workingforquality/reports/annual-reports/nqs2015annlrpt.htm.
41. Patient Safety Movement. Mission. 2016. http://patientsafetymovement.org/.
42. Patient Safety Movement. Actionable Patient Safety Solutions. 2016. http://patientsafetymovement.org/challenges-solutions/actionable-patient-safety-solutions-apss/.
43. Joint Commission Center for Transforming Healthcare. Targeted Solutions Tool for Hand-off Communications. 2016. http://www.centerfortransforminghealthcare.org/tst_hoc.aspx.
44. The Leapfrog Group. History. 2016. http://www.leapfroggroup.org/about/history.
45. Joint Commission. 2011 Facts about Speak Up™ Initiatives. http://www.jointcommission.org/facts_about_speak_up_initiatives/.
46. World Health Organization. 2011 Patient Safety. http://www.who.int/patientsafety/patients_for_patient/en/.
47. American College of Physicians. The Role of the Patient in Patient Safety. http://www.acponline.org/running_practice/patient_care/safety/patient.htm.
48. U.S. Department of Health and Human Services. Agency for Healthcare Quality and Research. 20 Tips to Help Prevent Medical Errors: Patient Fact Sheet. 2014. http://www.ahrq.gov/patients-consumers/care-planning/errors/20tips/index.html.
49. Wojcieszak D, Banja J, Houk C. The Sorry Works! Coalition: making the case for full disclosure. *Joint Commission Forum*. 2006;32(6).
50. Sorry Works! Coalition. About Sorry Works! Coalition. http://www.sorryworks.net/about.phtml.

The resources for this chapter can be found at www.expertconsult.com.

SECTION VII

SYSTEMS-BASED PRACTICE

CHAPTER 40

HEALTH AND HEALTH CARE DELIVERY SYSTEMS

Christine Everett • Justine Strand de Oliveira

HEALTH SYSTEMS

The U.S. health care system is a complex mix of contradictions. We are the envy of the rest of the world for pharmaceutical research and innovation, availability of advanced diagnostic imaging, and world-renowned specialists at academic medical centers. Yet we remain the only industrialized country without guaranteed access to health care for its citizens, with 10.4% of Americans uninsured.[1] We spend twice as much as other economically advantaged nations and have worse health outcomes. What are the historic origins of this situation?

Health care was a cottage industry from revolutionary times to the turn of the 20th century, when the Flexner report denounced many medical schools as for-profit diploma mills. With the shuttering of these proprietary schools, medicine began to evolve to a science, with resulting specialization of physicians. While Germany and other European countries created national systems of health insurance, the United States relied mostly on fee for service, although Henry Kaiser in California

and Baylor University in Dallas created mutual aid societies to assure care for patients with illnesses and injuries.

After World War II, wage freezes caused industry to seek other ways to recruit workers. Health insurance was a desirable benefit, and employer-based health insurance quickly became widespread. This had a profound and lasting effect on the U.S. health care system, tying the availability of health care coverage to employment.

In 1965, the passage of Medicare for seniors and disabled individuals and Medicaid coverage for poor individuals was a watershed event that expanded health insurance and put pressure on the system to improve access to health care. It is no coincidence that physician assistants and nurse practitioners were born that same year.

The Health Maintenance Organization (HMO) Act was passed in 1973, sponsored by Senator Edward Kennedy of Massachusetts and signed into law by President Richard Nixon. It was a move to try to control health care costs while providing a more comprehensive package of benefits for members

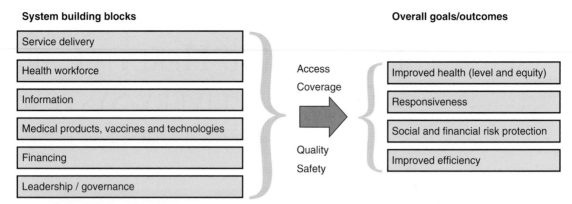

System building blocks

Service delivery

Health workforce

Information

Medical products, vaccines and technologies

Financing

Leadership / governance

Access
Coverage

Quality
Safety

Overall goals/outcomes

Improved health (level and equity)

Responsiveness

Social and financial risk protection

Improved efficiency

FIG. 40.1 ■ The World Health Organization health system framework. (From World Health Organization. *Everybody's Business—Strengthening Health Systems to Improve Health Outcomes: WHO's Framework for Action.* Geneva; 2007.)

of the HMO. The concept relied on capitation, in which the health plan is paid "per member per month," to provide a more comprehensive package of benefits but with restrictions requiring patients to go through the HMO for all care. The plans have been popular in some markets but have been the subject of backlash in others. Later approaches at health care reform would place greater emphasis on patients' experience of care (see later discussion of the Triple Aim).

In 2010, health insurance remained tied to employment; Medicare coverage was limited to people with disabilities and those 65 years of age and older; and Medicaid focused on the abject poor, pregnant women, children, and those with no financial assets requiring nursing home care. There were nearly 50 million uninsured Americans, or 16.3% of the population.[2] Bankruptcy because of catastrophic illness was burgeoning. Leaders from both parties agreed that something had to be done, but their views of the ideal solution could not have been further apart.

President Barack Obama signed the Patient Protection and Affordable Care Act (PPACA) into law in 2010 after it passed the House and Senate by the slimmest of margins. Legal challenges ensued, including a battle over the mandate that Americans purchase insurance coverage or pay a fine. The U.S. Supreme Court upheld the mandate in 2012 but ruled against the PPACA's provision requiring states to expand Medicaid to cover more low-income individuals.

The number of uninsured people dropped to 32 million in 2014, the first year of full implementation of the PPACA, a decrease of 9 million. The Gallup organization found the percentage of uninsured decreased to 11.9% in 2015, from 17.1% just before implementation of the PPACA in 2013.[3]

What Is a Health System?

A health system is made up of the people and organizations that have the primary intent of promoting, maintaining, or restoring health.[4] The World Health Organization (WHO) has provided a framework for understanding health systems (Fig. 40.1). All health systems share common functions, including preventive, diagnostic, and treatment services in a range of facilities and settings. To provide services, health systems must develop key resources, including health workforce, information, and medical technologies. A strong financial structure with effective oversight and coalition building are necessary components of any health system. All of these system building blocks are needed for a health system to accomplish its goals.

Health systems also share common goals.[4] By providing access to high-quality, safe care, health systems aim to improve the health of their members in a responsive and equitable fashion. Complementary goals include efficient provision of services and providing quality care while assuring financial stability.

Describing National Health Systems: United Kingdom, Canada, and the United States

Despite similarities in building blocks and goals, health system designs vary significantly among nations. Three questions promote understanding of a health care system: What patient population is included? Who delivers care? How is care financed? There are several common models.[5] The first is the national health service (NHS) or Beveridge model used in the United Kingdom. The second is the national health insurance model used in Canada. The third

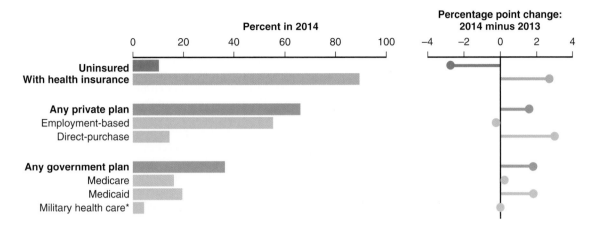

Note: Between 2013 and 2014, there was not a statistically significant change in the percentage of people covered by employment-based health insurance or military health care.
*Military health care includes TRICARE and CHAMPVA (Civilian Health and Medical Program of the Department of Veterans Affairs), as well as care provided by the Department of Veterans Affairs and the military.
For information on confidentiality protection, sampling error, nonsampling error, and definitions in the Current Population Survey, see www2.census.gov/programs-surveys/cps/techdocs/cpsmar15.pdf.
Source: U.S. Census Bureau, Current Population Survey, 2014 and 2015 Annual Social and Economic Supplements.

FIG. 40.2 ■ Percentage of people by type of health insurance coverage and change from 2014 (population as of March of the following year). (From Smith JC, Medalia C. *U.S. Census Bureau, Current Population Reports, P60-253, Health Insurance Coverage in the United States: 2014.* Washington, DC: U.S. Government Printing Office; 2015.)

is the Bismarck model used in countries such as Germany and Japan, with a mandatory insurance system financed by employers and employees through payroll deductions. Finally, there is the out-of-pocket model in which individuals pay for their care from their own funds; this is commonly used in poor nations. The United Kingdom, Canada, and the United States will be discussed as national examples for each of these (Fig. 40.2).

How Is Care Financed?

Different health system models use different approaches to financing.[5] In Beveridge models, such as the United Kingdom's NHS, health care is financed by the government through taxes. The government directly pays for care and patients do not pay out of pocket. Because there is a single payer, the government can set the cost of care and decide what services are included.

In national health insurance models such as Canada's Medicare system, there is a government-run insurance program to which every citizen contributes. Because it is a nonprofit organization without competition, there is no financial incentive for marketing or denying claims, reducing administrative costs. With a single payer, the government can determine what services will be covered and can negotiate pricing.

The United States uses a combination financial model. For military veterans who qualify, the Veterans Health Administration is similar to the Beveridge model in that it finances care through taxes. For citizens older than 65 years of age, the U.S. Medicare system is a government-run insurance program similar to Canada's. For this group, the government does set prices. However, it does not have the legal authority to negotiate for lower pharmaceutical costs, and it does require that its members pay some out-of-pocket costs called copayments. Private insurance plans that are funded through employee and employer contributions finance some employed adults and their families, similar to the Bismarck model. However, unlike the Bismarck model, many private U.S. insurance companies are for-profit organizations with high administrative costs and a profit motive. For families with low incomes, the Medicaid system is a health insurance program that is jointly funded by the federal government and the states. Unfortunately, in 2014, 32 million American citizens were uninsured and did not have access to any of these systems.[1,3,6] Any care received by the uninsured is paid for by their personal finances, so they experience the out-of-pocket model. The United States has a limited safety net system of federally qualified health centers (FQHCs), nonprofit clinics that receive federal funding to support care for underserved populations, including uninsured individuals and people living in rural areas. These clinics also receive funding from other sources, including copayments that are set according to the patient's ability to pay.

Who Delivers Care?

Health care services can be delivered directly by the government or by private companies and individuals. In the NHS in the United Kingdom, most health care is delivered by the government. Most hospitals and clinics are owned by the government, and many health care professionals are government employees. This approach removes the profit motive from individual health care providers and provides an added layer of cost control. In Canada, health care is delivered by private sector providers that are paid by the government insurance program. In the United States, there is a combination delivery system, depending on the population. Adults and children with private insurance, Medicaid, and Medicare, and uninsured people largely use private sector providers. Those in the military or Veterans Administration are served by government organizations and employees. Some uninsured people may receive services from FQHCs.

Population Served?

The final step in understanding a system is identifying the population served. *A universal system* serves all residents of a nation. The United Kingdom and Canada have universal systems.[5,7] The United States does not have a universal system; different patient populations are covered by different insurance systems. Individuals frequently move between systems, are covered by multiple systems, or are covered by none at all (see Fig. 40.2). Many adults with full-time employment and their children are covered by a private health system (Bismarck model). Adult citizens older than 65 years of age are in the Medicare system, and some poor families are covered by the Medicaid system (national health insurance model). Members of the military are served by the Department of Defense, and some veterans are served by the Veterans Administration (national health service model).

THE U.S. HEALTH CARE SYSTEM: CHALLENGES AND INNOVATIONS

It is clear that the United States has a patchwork of health systems. The U.S. health system can be conceptualized as having four levels (Fig. 40.3).[5,8] The center of the model is the individual patient. The system is defined by the characteristics of the individual and varies within his or her lifetime. The focus on the individual reflects other important forces, especially the increasing emphasis on *patient-centered* care. By encouraging clinicians to view patients as partners in medical decision making, patients begin to play a more active role in their care. The increase in patient participation reflects the move to *consumer-driven* health care.

The second level of the health system is the care team, which includes patients and their families as well as health care professionals.[5] Ideally, the types of health care providers included in the care team reflect the needs and preferences of the individual patient. These teams provide accessible, continuous, coordinated, effective care while using the skills of each team member efficiently. Although the concept of care teams is embraced, implementation of teams is far from universal and sometimes ineffective.

Teams are supported by organizations, which are the third level of the U.S. health system.[5] Health delivery organizations such as hospitals, nursing homes, and clinics provide the resources to support the work of teams. Multiple organizations may come together to form various types of *integrated systems*.

The term "integrated health system" refers to "a network of organizations that provides or arranges to provide a coordinated continuum of services to a defined population and is willing to be held clinically and fiscally accountable for the outcomes and health status of the population served."[9] A more descriptive definition of integrated systems refers to structures formed with the goals of providing high-quality, low-cost care to populations of patients in broad geographic areas, eliminating duplication of services and providing care across the continuum (referred to as "seamless" health care). Because there are multiple health systems within the United States, it is no surprise that there are multiple types of integrated health delivery systems.

Horizontally Integrated Systems

Horizontally integrated systems were created to allow private practices to increase the number of patients seen, create a centralized billing process, acquire technology such as electronic health records, implement marketing, and create more efficient call systems. In some settings, these horizontally integrated systems were configured and managed by regional hospitals as a strategy to retain community physicians in their practices but also as a feeder system for the hospital's services.

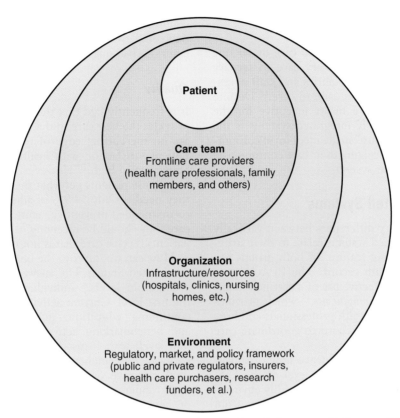

FIG. 40.3 ■ Building a better delivery system. (From Fanjiang G, Grossman JH, Compton WD, Reid PP, editors. *Building a Better Delivery System: A New Engineering/Health Care Partnership.* Washington, DC: National Academies Press; 2005.)

Some horizontally integrated systems were organized and led by physicians. These independent practice associations (IPAs) moved on to partner with insurance companies to create HMO products for their patients. Physicians and organized medicine were fond of IPAs and other structures that kept physicians in charge. A major advantage of the early IPAs was that individual physicians did not have to negotiate contracts with insurance companies.[10] Things got confusing, however, when individual practices (which were still owned by individual physicians or physician groups) joined more than one IPA and attempted to sort out the requirements of multiple insurance contracts. Practices with physician assistants (PAs) and nurse practitioners (NPs) faced additional complexities because not all insurers paid for the care they provided.

Some horizontal systems took on a more structured form by becoming integrated medical groups, buying up individual practices, and making the physicians employees. Similar to IPAs, these groups managed contracts from multiple payers and ultimately became the building blocks for the vertically integrated or virtually integrated systems, which now define large segments of the U.S. health care system.

Both IPAs and integrated medical groups rely on gatekeepers: physicians, PAs, or NPs who manage care and make referrals to specialists. These systems benefit from insurance contracts that designate them as "preferred providers," opening their doors to larger numbers of patients. In exchange, the systems give discounted rates for the care of the insurance company's subscribers. By this arrangement, only uninsured patients pay full price for health care services.

There are advantages to large medical groups. Describing the situation in California, where IPAs and Integrated Medical Groups (IMGs) are well developed, Robinson and Casalino[11] say that "small independent practices cannot stand alone in California; the advantages of belonging to a large integrated medical group or IPA are overwhelming . . . [due to] economies of scale; ability to spread the financial risk of capitation payment; reduction in the transaction costs of negotiating, monitoring, and enforcing agreements; and creation of an organizational context for continuous process innovation."

Vertically Integrated Systems

Vertical integration consolidates all care under one organizational roof, from primary care to tertiary care, and encompasses the facilities and staff necessary to provide this full spectrum of care.[10] Despite advantages for patients, a major incentive for the development of vertically integrated systems is the creation of "market share" made up of loyal consumers who are used to receiving their care continuously over time by a familiar system.

Virtually Integrated Systems

Although the primary differences between vertically and virtually integrated systems relate to their structure, the ideal unifying feature for both groups is a shared electronic health record. The PPACA provided incentives for effective use of a certified medical record through *meaningful use*,[12] which provides financial incentives for health professionals and hospitals to use the medical record to coordinate care and improve quality.

Many of the forces that influence how organizations behave occur at the fourth level of the U.S. health care system: the environment. This environment is dictated by a wide variety of policies from insurers, payors, other stakeholders, and regulators. One of the key regulatory forces that influences how organizations behave is scope of practice (SOP). SOP can influence organizational decisions regarding how PAs are incorporated into teams and what medical tasks they may perform.

Scope of practice laws are interventional laws[13] whose primary purpose is to protect the public from incompetent providers and would ideally reflect the clinical capacities of professionals to provide competent care. Although legal SOP is determined by state laws and regulations, professional SOP[14] (or professional competencies) are the services that a profession is trained and licensed to perform. Although consistency in professional competencies between states for both NPs and PAs is assured through national certification, there is considerable state variation in legal SOP within each profession.[15-18] All states require physician supervision for PA practice, with variation in requirements for physician availability to the PA and degree of physician oversight and prescribing.[19]

The Challenges

Although each type of health system results in its own challenges, having a mix of systems adds more complexity. When national health care systems in high-income countries are compared, the United States routinely ranks highest in cost but among the lowest for outcomes such as quality, access, and equity (Fig. 40.4).

Quality

It is frequently said that the U.S. health care system provides the best care in the world. It is true that we are on the cutting edge of technological advances. Patient satisfaction with health care in the United States is also high.[20] However, this satisfaction may be because patients get what they want and not what they need.[21] Only 54.9% of adults receive all of the recommended preventive, acute, and chronic illness care they should be receiving,[22,23] but about 20% of patients receive care that is not needed.[24-26]

How can we improve the quality of health care in the United States? The answer will require change at multiple levels.[8] Individual clinicians represent the first level. Current activities in this area include continuing education, guideline implementation, and benchmarking activities. Teams are the second level, with focus on task redesign and clinical pathway implementation. Organizations, the third level, improve organizational learning and quality improvement. Finally, the level of the larger system or environment highlights accreditation and payment policies (see Innovations).

Access

Access to care in the United States is less than ideal. Access to care is directly linked with having insurance, and in the recent past, as many as 22% of adults in the U.S. were without any form of insurance.[23] In 2012, 35% of uninsured adults (ages 18–64 years) and 12.9% of insured adults reported they delayed needed care at some point during the year.

Access is also related to availability of health care providers and organizations. Health professional shortage areas (HPSAs) are areas or population groups within the United States that experience a shortage of health professionals (Fig. 40.5).[27] At the end of 2015, there were more than 6000 HPSAs with primary care provider shortages, impacting more than 61 million people. Even more dramatic, more than 97 million people live in areas without sufficient numbers of mental health providers.

Cost

The United States spends more on health care than any other country despite high numbers of uninsured.[28] In 2013, the United States spent approximately $9000 per person on health care, representing

Country rankings

		AUS	CAN	FRA	GER	NETH	NZ	NOR	SWE	SWIZ	UK	US
Overall ranking (2013)		4	10	9	5	5	7	7	3	2	1	11
Quality care		2	9	8	7	5	4	11	10	3	1	5
Effective care		4	7	9	6	5	2	11	10	8	1	3
Safe care		3	10	2	6	7	9	11	5	4	1	7
Coordinated care		4	8	9	10	5	2	7	11	3	1	6
Patient-centered care		5	8	10	7	3	6	11	9	2	1	4
Access		8	9	11	2	4	7	6	4	2	1	9
Cost-related problem		9	5	10	4	8	6	3	1	7	1	11
Timeliness of care		6	11	10	4	2	7	8	9	1	3	5
Efficiency		4	10	8	9	7	3	4	2	6	1	11
Equity		5	9	7	4	8	10	6	1	2	2	11
Healthy lives		4	8	1	7	5	9	6	2	3	10	11
Health expenditures/ capita, 2011**		$3,800	$4,522	$4,118	$4,495	$5,099	$3,182	$5,669	$3,925	$5,643	$3,405	$8,508

Country rankings: Top 2*, Middle, Bottom 2*

Notes: *Includes ties. **Expenditures shown in $US PPP (purchasing power parity); Australian $ data are from 2010. Source: Calculated by The Commonwealth Fund based on 2011 International Health Policy Survey of Sicker Adults; 2012 International Health Policy Survey of Primary Care Physicians; 2013 International Health Policy Survey; Commonwealth Fund *National Scorecard 2011*; World Health Organization; and Organization for Economic Cooperation and Development, *OECD Health Data, 2013* (Paris: OECD, Nov. 2013).

FIG. 40.4 ■ Country rankings on measures of access, equity, quality, efficiency, and healthy lives. (From Mahon M, Fox B. US health system ranks last among eleven countries on measures of access, equity, quality, efficiency and healthy lives. Davis K et al. *The Commonwealth Fund* 2014 Update.)

	Number of designations	Population of designated HPSAs	Percent of need met	Practitioners needed to remove designations
Primary medical HPSA totals	6,325	61,431,084	58.92%	8,220
Geographic area	1,366	30,550,205	67.03%	3,048
Population group	1,407	29,852,966	53.62%	4,555
Facility	3,552	1,027,913	35.52%	617
Dental HPSA totals	5,189	48,245,095	40.13%	7,289
Geographic area	685	14,764,501	58.67%	1,400
Population group	1,496	32,284,398	33.07%	5,350
Facility	3,008	1,196,196	31.70%	539
Mental health HPSA totals	4,306	97,873,154	47.74%	2,690
Geographic area	1,002	83,297,306	57.55%	1,440
Population group	194	12,701,097	46.60%	320
Facility	3,110	1,874,751	18.29%	930

FIG. 40.5 ■ Designated health professional shortage areas statistics. (From Health Resources and Services Administration. *Designated Health Professional Shortage Areas Statistics. Bureau of Clinician Recruitment and Service.* Washington, DC: Health Resources and Services Administration (HRSA), U.S. Department of Health & Human Services; December 18, 2015.)

approximately 17% of its gross domestic product. Much of this cost appears to be driven by technology. U.S. residents have fewer hospital and physician visits than similar countries, but spending on diagnostic imaging and pharmaceuticals is higher.

Equity

Health equity occurs when all people are able to attain the highest level of health.[29] This occurs when there are no systematic differences or disparities in determinants of health and health outcomes. As can be seen in Fig. 40.2, the United States ranks at the bottom for equity. Disparities exist in all aspects of health, including social determinants (see Population Health), access to care, and quality of care received.[23]

Innovations

The Affordable Care Act and the Triple Aim

In 2008, Berwick, Nolan, and Whittington proposed a new approach to improving U.S. health care, which they called the Triple Aim. The three components were decreasing costs, improving the population's health, and improving patients' experience of care.[30] The third component is especially important because previous efforts at reducing costs often led to patient dissatisfaction and the perception that care was being "rationed." The Triple Aim includes the social experience of care as a key ingredient in quality.

Responding to the need to increase access to care, reduce costs, and improve health outcomes, Congress passed the PPACA in 2010 by the narrowest of margins. As with most political compromises, the PPACA satisfied no one. Those who argued for universal access to care and a single payer system decried its limited scope, and those on the other end of the spectrum objected to its mandate that everyone purchase health insurance or face fines and called for repeal. The first phase (2010) enacted changes that allowed children to stay on their parents' employer health insurance to age 26 years; eliminated lifetime limits on coverage, reducing the threat of bankruptcy due to catastrophic illness; and eliminated copayments for evidence-based preventive measures. It also limited health insurers' medical loss ratio—policy talk for administrative costs. Other changes occurred in 2014 and included the individual mandate to purchase insurance and expansion of Medicaid for low-income individuals.

The ink was barely dry on the PPACA when the legal challenges began. The first crucial test came in 2012, when the U.S. Supreme Court upheld the individual mandate but in an unexpected setback ruled against requiring states to expand Medicaid, and more than

half of states subsequently declined to do so. Despite its many shortcomings and challenges, the percentage of nonelderly Americans who were uninsured (seniors are covered by Medicare) dropped from 16.2% in late 2013 to 10.7% in early 2015[31] (Fig. 40.6).

Population Health

Health care costs are unsustainable, and despite ever-rising spending, our health outcomes are inadequate. There is growing recognition that a 15-minute clinic visit or even the totality of our efforts as a health care system will not improve the health of our nation. A new approach looking at the community as a whole holds promise. Population health looks beyond the individual to social and environmental factors that lead to health and illness, defined as "the health outcomes of a group of individuals, including the distribution of such outcomes within the group."[32] Population health focuses on social determinants of health: "access to social and economic opportunities; the resources and supports available in our homes, neighborhoods, and communities; the quality of our schooling; the safety of our workplaces; the cleanliness of our water, food, and air; and the nature of our social interactions and relationships"[29] (Fig. 40.7). From this perspective, health care accounts for only about 20% of health outcomes.

The greatest potential to improve population health requires reducing poverty and social inequity;

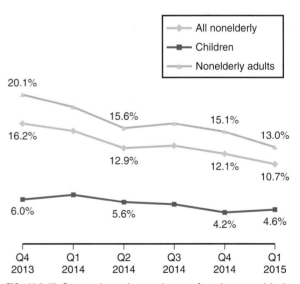

FIG. 40.6 ■ Quarterly uninsured rate for the nonelderly population by age, quarter 4 2013 to quarter 1 2015. (From National Center for Health Statistics. *Health Insurance Coverage: Early Release of Quarterly Estimates from the National Health Interview Survey, January 2010-March 2015*, August 12, 2015. http.www.cdc.gov/nchs/data/nhis/earlyrelease/Quarterly_ estimates _2010_2015 Q11 pdf.)

improving educational opportunities; and making housing, neighborhoods, and public transportation safer and conducive to physical activity. Policies that make our default decisions safe, such as using seat belts and protecting us from tobacco smoke, come next. Evidence-based preventive measures,

such as immunizations and targeted health screening, are also important. Clinical interventions and counseling have less impact than these broader approaches[33] (Fig. 40.8).

As health care providers, we must continue to provide quality, evidence-based care through positive interactions with our patients. To improve population health, we need other skills as well. Working productively in teams is a fundamental skill of PAs and is even more important in the 21st century. Also important are critical thinking and the ability to apply practice and community-based data to intervene and measure impact. We need the ability to engage with communities, listening to their wants and needs about health, rather than offering expert advice. Knowledge of the fundamentals of public health and how to interact with public health colleagues will be key. Finally, we need to advocate for policies that improve the health of our communities (Fig. 40.9).

Patient-Centered Medical Homes

Primary care is believed to be a critical part of the plan to overcome the challenges currently facing the U.S. health system. Evidence suggests primary care is an important component of effective health systems.[34,35] Unfortunately, the U.S. health system is focused on the delivery of specialty care, and many payment policies encourage delivery of care in episodes of illness rather than on prevention and coordination. This approach to care is not only inconsistent with the

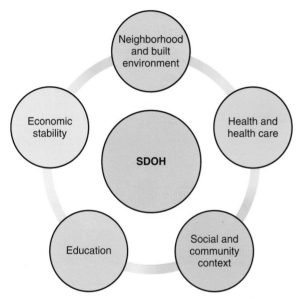

FIG. 40.7 ■ Social determinants of health. (From U.S. Department of Health & Human Services. *Healthy People 2020.* http://www.healthypeople.gov/2020/topics-objectives/topic/social-determinants-health.)

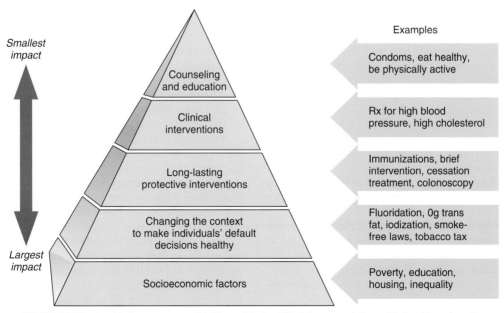

FIG. 40.8 ■ The health impact pyramid. (From Frieden TR. A framework for public health action: the health impact pyramid. *Am J Public Health* 2010;100(4):590–595.)

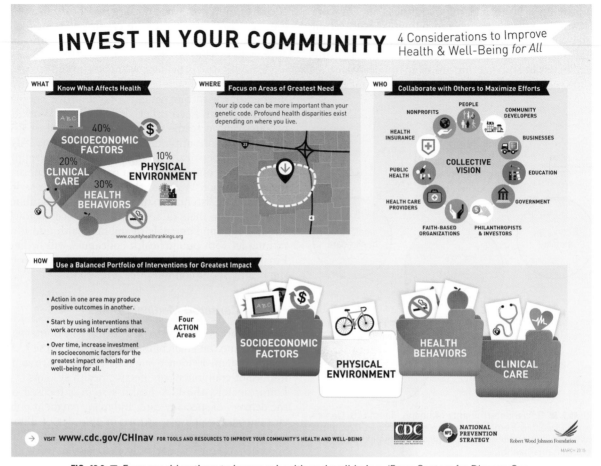

FIG. 40.9 ■ Four considerations to improve health and well-being. (From Centers for Disease Control and Prevention. *For Tools and Resources to Improve Your Community's Health and Well-Being.* http://www.cdc.gov/CHInav.)

needs of an aging population with chronic illnesses, but it is also inefficient and not fiscally sustainable.

The patient-centered medical home (PCMH) is a strategy for primary care practice redesign. Many physician groups support this approach to delivering comprehensive primary care. The PCMH is characterized by seven principles:[36]

1. **Personal physician:** Every patient has a relationship with a primary care physician.
2. **Team-based care:** A team of individuals at the practice level collectively take responsibility for the ongoing care of patients.
3. **Whole-person orientation:** The full range of patient needs are met within primary care or arranged for with other qualified individuals.
4. **Integrated and coordinated care:** Care is integrated and coordinated across all sectors of the health care system and community.
5. **Quality and safety:** There is a focus on evidence-based medicine, information technology, quality improvement, and patient involvement.

6. **Accessibility:** Enhanced access is available through expanded hours, open access, and new methods of communication with providers (e.g., email).
7. **Affordability:** Payment reform addresses value of care coordination and other services provided in the primary care setting.

Increased inclusion of PAs and NPs on primary care teams is one recommended approach to implementing team-based primary care.[37,38] Unfortunately, a recent survey suggests that a significant portion of primary care physicians believe that the increased reliance of PAs and NPs is not a positive change (Fig. 40.10).

It is unclear if PCMHs will result in improved access and quality of care while reducing costs. There is some evidence that PCMHs may improve access and reduce some costs, such as the costs associated with emergency department visits, but there is insufficient evidence on their impact on the quality of care delivered.[39] The PCMH may have limited impact because it does not have the capacity to impact the delivery of specialty care.[40,41]

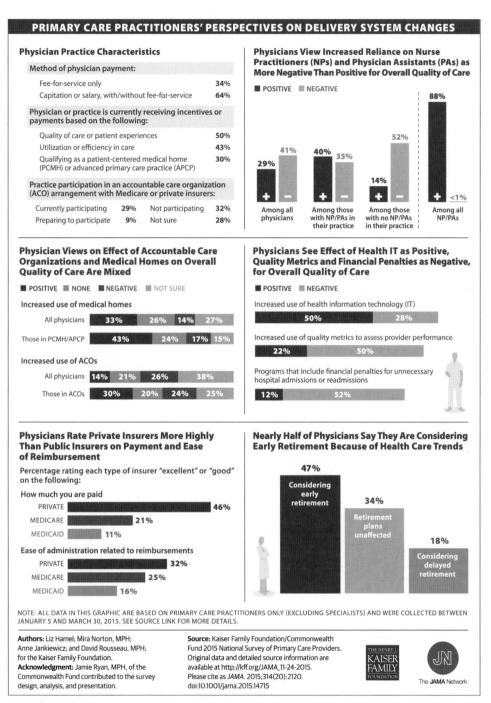

FIG. 40.10 ■ Primary care practitioners' perspectives on delivery system changes. (From Herzig SJ, Howell MD, Ngo LH, Marcantonio ER. Acid-suppressive medication use and the risk for hospital-acquired pneumonia. *JAMA*. 2015;314(20):2120.)

Accountable Care Organizations

To improve quality and reduce costs, incentives must align to reduce unnecessary care and increase efficiency across the continuum of care. Accountable care organizations (ACOs) are multispecialty organizations that agree to be accountable for the quality and cost of care for a defined population of patients.[40] The intent of this type of organization is to ensure that physicians in primary care and specialty care work together to improve the collective value of their care.[42] Little is known about the success of these organizations to date. Some report reductions in low-value services and overall costs,[43] but the jury is still out on their chance for success.

Accountable Care Communities

One of the newest trends in population health is the Accountable Care Community (ACC), first proposed by the Austen BioInnovation Institute in Akron, Ohio, in 2012. Building on successful community-based projects aimed at improving health by integrating efforts across multiple sectors, the ACC aimed to improve population health across northeast Ohio. In a model of shared responsibility, the ACC brings together clinicians and health systems, public health and other governmental organizations, industry, philanthropy and education to create a "healthier, more productive, and less illness-burdened community."[44] The ACC has several components, among them integration of medicine and public health, use of interprofessional teams, use of health information technology to track care and health status, and advocacy for policies to improve health. Several demonstration projects are under way, many funded by the Centers for Medicare & Medicaid Services' State Innovation Models.[45]

Case Study 40.1 FAMILY MEDICINE RESIDENCY

The Academic Health Center Family Medicine Clinic houses a family medicine residency, which has a mission to train primary care physicians who are skilled clinicians and leaders in transforming health care, with a special emphasis on population health. The program admits six residents a year into a 3-year program. Although the residency has regularly served as a training site for PA students, you and a PA colleague were the first PAs to join the team. You bring more than 5 years of primary care experience and enthusiasm for working in a fast-paced, stimulating academic environment and just completed your first 6 months as part of the clinical staff.

You have been well accepted by the faculty and the residents. Now that you are settled in, the plan is for the residency to engage in discussions about the appropriate role of PAs and NPs in the clinic. For example, should PAs participate in the administration and leadership of the residency? Should PAs join the faculty in interviewing medical school candidates for admission to the residency? Should PAs have faculty status within the residency? Should PAs have their own panel of patients? What happens when patients would rather see the "permanent" PAs rather than the transient residents?

1. How is your role (and your potential role) in the residency different from your prior employment in a nonacademic primary care clinic?
2. How can you affect the residents' perception of PAs and influence their choices about future employment and support of PAs in their practice setting?
3. What recommendations do you have about the residency's responsibilities for training PA and NP students?
4. What recommendations do you and your colleagues have to the residency about the best role for you right now? In 5 years? In 10 years?

KEY POINTS

- Health systems are made up of all the people and organizations that have the primary intent of promoting, maintaining, or restoring health. National health systems vary.
- The United States has a patchwork of different types of systems, depending on the population served.
- The U.S. health systems currently face the challenge of improving access and quality of care while reducing cost.
- Innovations to address these challenges include organizational innovations such as PCMHs, ACOs, and the ACC. Some of these innovations are codified in the ACC.

References

1. Smith JC, Medalia C. Health insurance coverage in the United States: 2014. In: Bureau UC, ed. Washington, DC: U.S. Government Printing Office; 2015.
2. U.S. Census Bureau. Highlights: 2010. (Accessed December 30, 2015, at https://www.census.gov/hhes/www/hlthins/data/incpovhlth/2010/highlights.html.)
3. Gallup. In U.S., Uninsured Rate Dips to 11.9% in First Quarter. Gallup, 2015. (Accessed December 28, 2015, at http://www.gallup.com/poll/182348/uninsured-rate-dips-first-quarter.aspx.)
4. World Health Organization. *Everybody's Business: Strengthening Health Systems to Improve Health Outcomes.* Geneva, Switzerland: World Health Organization; 2007.
5. Reid TR. *The healing of America: a global quest for better, cheaper, and fairer health care.* Penguin; 2010.
6. Kaiser Family Foundation. Key Facts About the Uninsured Population. Kaiser Family Found., 2015. (Accessed December 29, 2015, at http://kff.org/uninsured/fact-sheet/key-facts-about-the-uninsured-population/.)
7. Ridic G, Gleason S, Ridic O. Comparisons of health care systems in the United States, Germany and Canada. *Materia Socio-Medica.* 2012;24:112–120.
8. Ferlie EB, Shortell SM. Improving the Quality of health care in the United Kingdom and the United States: a framework for change. *Milbank Q.* 2001;79:281–315.
9. Shortell SM, Gillies RR, Anderson DA, Erickson KM, Mitchell JB. *Remaking Health Care in America, Building Organized Delivery Systems.* San Francisco, CA: Jossey-Bass; 1996.
10. Bodenheimer T, Grumbach K. *Understanding Health Policy: A Clinical Approach.* 3rd ed. New York, NY: Lange/McGraw-Hill; 1995.
11. Robinson JC, Casalino LP. Vertical integration and organizational networks in health care. *Health Aff.* 1996;15:7–22.
12. Health IT Regulations: Meaningful Use Regulations. (Accessed January 10, 2016, at https://www.healthit.gov/policy-researchers-implementers/meaningful-use-regulations.)
13. Wagenaar A, Burris S. *Public Health Law Research: Theory and Methods.* San Francisco, CA: Jossey-Bass; 2013.
14. Dower C, Moore J, Langelier M. It is time to restructure health professions scope-of-practice regulations to remove barriers to care. *Health Aff.* 2013;32:1971–1976.
15. Pearson L. The Pearson Report 2009: the annual state-by-state national overview of nurse practitioner legislation and healthcare issues. *Am J Nurse Pract.* 2009;13:8–82.
16. Wing P, Langelier M, Salsberg E, Continelli T. *The Changing Scope of Practice of Physician Assistants, Nurse Practitioners, and Certified Nurse Midwives in the Fifty States, 1992–2000.* Rensselaer, NY: Center for Health Workforce Studies, School of Public Health, University of Albany; 2002.
17. Wing P, Langelier M, Salsberg E, Hooker R. The changing professional practice of physician assistants: 1992 to 2000. *JAAPA.* 2004;17:37–40.
18. National Governors Association. *The Role of Physician Assistants in Health Care Delivery.* Washington, DC; 2014.
19. American Academy of Family Physicians. *The U.S. Primary Care Physician Workforce: Undervalued Service: American Academy of Family Physicians*; 2004.
20. Jha AK, Orav EJ, Zheng J, Epstein AM. Patients' perception of hospital care in the United States. *N Engl J Med.* 2008;359:1921–1931.
21. Fenton JJ, Jerant AF, Bertakis KD, Franks P. The cost of satisfaction: a national study of patient satisfaction, health care utilization, expenditures, and mortality. *Archives of Internal Medicine.* 2012;172:405–411.
22. McGlynn EA, Asch SM, Adams J, et al. The quality of health care delivered to adults in the United States. *N Engl J Med.* 2003;348:2635–2645.
23. Agency for Healthcare Research and Quality. *2014 National Healthcare Quality and Disparities Report.* Rockville, MD; 2015.
24. Graham ID, Logan J, Harrison MB, et al. Lost in knowledge translation: time for a map? *J Contin Educ Health Prof.* 2006;26:13–24.
25. Schuster MA, McGlynn EA, Brook RH. How good is the quality of health care in the United States? *Milbank Q.* 1998;76:517–563.
26. Grol R. Successes and failures in the implementation of evidence-based guidelines for clinical practice. *Med Care.* 2001;39:II-46–II-54.
27. Health Resources and Services Administration. Designated Health Professional Shortage Areas Statistics. Bureau of Clinician Recruitment and Service, Health Resources and Services Administration (HRSA), U.S. Department of Health & Human Services, as of December 18, 2015.
28. Mahon M, Fox B, US Health System Ranks Last Among Eleven Countries on Measures of Access, Equity, Quality, Efficiency, and Healthy Lives. *Commonwealth Fund*; 2014 Update.
29. U.S. Department of Health & Human Services. *Healthy People 2020.* Washington, DC; 2012.
30. Berwick DM, Nolan TW, Whittington J. The Triple Aim: care, health, and cost. *Health Aff.* 2008;27:759–769.
31. National Center for Health Statistics. *Health Insurance Coverage: Early Release of Quarterly Estimates from the National Health Interview Survey, January 2010-March 2015.* Washington, DC; 2015.
32. Kindig D, Stoddart G. What is population health? *Am J Public Health.* 2003;93:380–383.
33. Frieden TR. A framework for public health action: the health impact pyramid. *Am J Public Health.* 2010;100:590–595.
34. Starfield B. Public health and primary care: a framework for proposed linkages. *Am J Public Health.* 1996;86:1365–1369.
35. Institute of Medicine. *Crossing the quality chasm: a new health system for the 21st century.* Washington, DC: Institute of Medicine; 2001.
36. American College of Physicians. *Joint Principles of the Patient-Centered Medical Home (PCMH)—March 2007.* American College of Physicians online; 2007.
37. The TransforMED Patient-Centered Model. 2009. (Accessed March 28, 2011, at http://www.transformed.com/transformed.cfm.)
38. Yarnall KS, Ostbye T, Krause KM, Pollack KI, Gradison M, Michener JL. Family physicians as team leaders: "time" to share the care. *Prev Chronic Dis.* 2009;6:A59.
39. Jackson G, Lee S-Y, Edelman D, Weinberger M, Yano E. Employment of mid-level providers in primary care and control of diabetes. *Prim Care Diab.* 2011;5:25–31.
40. Rittenhouse DR, Shortell SM, Fisher ES. Primary care and accountable care — two essential elements of delivery-system reform. *N Engl J Med.* 2009;361:2301–2303.
41. Rittenhouse D, Casalino L, Shortell S, et al. Small and medium-size physician practices use few patient-centered medical home processes. *Health Aff.* 2011;30:1575–84.
42. Song Z, Lee TH. The era of delivery system reform begins. *JAMA.* 2013;309:35–36.
43. Schwartz AL, Chernew ME, Landon BE, McWilliams JM. Changes in low-value services in year 1 of the Medicare pioneer accountable care organization program. *JAMA internal medicine.* 2015:1–11.

44. BioInnovation Institute. *Healthier by design: creating accountable care communities. A framework for engagement and sustainability.* Akron, Ohio: Austen BioInnovation Institute; 2012.

45. State Innovation Models Initiative: General Information Centers for Medicare and Medicaid Services. (Accessed December 28, 2015, at https://innovation.cms.gov/initiatives /state-innovations/.)

The resources for this chapter can be found at www.expertconsult .com.

The Faculty Resources can be found online at www.expertconsult .com.

CHAPTER 41

REHABILITATIVE AND LONG-TERM CARE SYSTEMS

Kathy A. Kemle

CHAPTER OUTLINE

HOME CARE: INFORMAL CAREGIVERS	**ASSISTED LIVING FACILITIES**
HOME CARE: HOME CARE ORGANIZATIONS	**NURSING HOMES**
HOSPICE	**KEY POINTS**
MEDICAL HOUSE CALLS	

The physician assistant (PA) profession is rooted in primary care. Although increasing numbers of PAs are choosing specialty areas, 32% reported practicing in primary care (family and general medicine, internal medicine, and pediatrics) in the 2013 American Academy of Physician Assistants' (AAPA's) national census.[1] Although most medical care is delivered in outpatient offices, ambulatory care centers, and acute care hospitals, there is a growing trend for care to take place in the patient's home, fueled by a need to decrease costs and personal desire to stay in one's own home. That home may be an individual domicile, congregate housing, an assisted living facility (ALF), an inpatient hospice, or a skilled nursing or other long-term care facility. With this growth in demand, more PAs are choosing to work in nonmedical settings. In 2013, 1.4% of PA census respondents indicated working primarily in residences, with 0.9% in long-term care, 0.3% in hospice, and 0.2% in patients' homes.[1] The focus of this chapter is care delivery in these nontraditional venues. (See Table 41.1 for information on various sites of care.)

The "silvering" of the developed world is a well-established reality. This demographic shift will result in an aging "tsunami" of need for all kinds of care: medical, psychological, social, and functional. The disorders of aging do not conform to traditional medical approaches, which strive to find a single cause (diagnosis) to account for multiple symptoms. They are syndromes and thus are multifactorial, requiring a holistic approach by an interdisciplinary team. PA programs have included geriatrics and geriatric syndromes in their curricula since the 1980s. With a generalist-training model, PAs are well prepared to assume a growing role in coordinating and directing care for older adults. In addition, PA education focuses on "hands-on" clinical skills, those most readily available and needed to provide services in nonmedical environments. It incorporates a large amount of instruction in chronic disease management, a hallmark of aging and functional disability. PA education emphasizes preservation of function and independence, both of which are core values of the geriatric and disabled populations.

Most of the health care of older adults and disabled younger individuals is financed by Medicare, administered by the Centers for Medicare & Medicaid Services. Since 1998, Medicare Part B has reimbursed PA employers in all settings at 85% of the physician-allowable rate if the services are medically necessary and would ordinarily be provided by a physician. The care must be provided by PAs working with physician supervision and must be within the scope of practice allowed by state law and regulations. Supervision may be via telecommunication and does not necessarily imply the physical presence of the physician unless it is required by state law. PAs may bill any evaluation and management code except the initial comprehensive evaluation of the skilled nursing home (Part A) patient.

Table 41.2 lists the components of Medicare. Further information on reimbursement is provided in the section on each site of care.

TABLE 41.1 Sites and Types of Long-Term Care

Type or Site	Description	Payer
Inpatient rehabilitation hospital	Provide at least 3 hr of therapy per day; must make progress to continue	Medicare, Medicaid, or private insurance
Skilled nursing facility (SNF) post-acute hospital; needs therapy	PT, OT, or speech; must progress to continue	Medicare or private insurance
Long-term hospital	Handle complex care such as ventilator patients	Medicare or private insurance
Home health care	Nursing or therapy in the home; requires face-to-face encounters with a physician, NP, or PA	Medicare, Medicaid, or private insurance
Hospice	May be in the home, NH, ALF, or inpatient hospice; avoids hospitalization; usual prognosis <6 mo; concentrates on comfort	Medicare or other
Home care or personal care	ADL and IADL care in the home	Varies but usually self-pay or Medicaid
NH	Chronically ill patients who are not able to benefit from rehabilitation and need nursing care	Self-pay or private insurance; Medicaid
ALF	Institutional care; may serve small or large numbers; services vary widely, and little regulation exists; patients are usually less disabled than in NHs	Self-pay; few Medicaid
Day care	Provide limited services during day; some housed in ALFs	Self-pay; Medicaid

ADL, Activity of daily living; *ALF,* assisted living facility; *IADL,* instrumental activity of daily living; *NH,* nursing home; *NP,* nurse practitioner; *OT,* occupational therapy; *PA,* physician assistant; *PT,* physical therapy.

TABLE 41.2 Medicare Parts

Component	Covers	Eligibility	Deductible
Part A	Hospital, hospice	Aged, disabled	Yes
	Home health medical equipment		
	Nursing home rehabilitation*		
Part B	MD, PA visits	Must elect and pay premium	Yes
			Yes
	Includes house calls and nursing home visits		Yes
Part C	Medicare Advantage plans, HMOs	Must elect	Varies
Part D	Prescription drug benefit	Must elect	Varies

*Nursing home after 3-day hospital stay; initial stay is 20 days; 80 additional days with copayment.
HMO, Health maintenance organization; *MD,* medical doctor; *PA,* physician assistant.

HOME CARE: INFORMAL CAREGIVERS

The 43.5 million unpaid family caregivers are the largest source of long-term care in the United States.[2] They may provide care on a full- or part-time basis and may live with their care recipient or separately, some even at long distances. Most are women (usually wives or adult daughters), but there is an increase in the number of men serving in this role. Whereas men are more likely to assume instrumental activities of daily living (IADLs) such as handling finances, women tend to perform the "hands-on" activities of daily living (ADLs; bathing, dressing, toileting, feeding, and mobility). Women are more likely to experience emotional distress, anxiety, and depression related to their caregiving role. The majority of caregivers are middle aged (35–64 years); however, many caregivers of older adults, especially spouses, are themselves elderly. Older caregivers tend to spend more hours providing care and are more likely to have their own health concerns.

Over the past decade, with increasing numbers of care recipients with complex medical conditions, caregivers have found their roles shifting to include tasks usually considered medical or nursing, such as care of intravenous lines, injections, wound and ostomy care, and even management of home dialysis and ventilators. Sadly, many feel ill-prepared to provide this care, with about 50% reporting little or no education regarding these procedures.[1] This may account for some of the frequent hospitalizations that occur in this group of high-complexity, high-needs patients and represents an untapped opportunity to reduce costs and increase caregiver and recipient satisfaction by providing more educational support. A systematic review of interventions to prevent hospitalization of demented community-dwelling older adults in 2015 did not find significant reductions in hospitalizations in any of the studies they considered. However, the authors did note that the studies had many methodological concerns, and none addressed caregiver education or focused on medical interventions.[3]

About one fifth of the white and black populations in the United States are providing care, with slightly lower numbers of Asian and Hispanic Americans doing so. African Americans report less stress than white caregivers, and Hispanics and Asians experience more depression. One in 10 caregivers has served in the armed forces, as have their care recipients. Nine percent self-identify as lesbian, gay, bisexual, or transgender.[2] Many caregivers find great fulfillment in their roles, enjoying closer relationships with their care recipients and satisfaction from providing what they believe is the best care for their loved ones. Most caregivers are employed outside the home, which, although it adds to stress in the workplace, may actually prove beneficial as a social outlet and a means of increasing income.[4] Caregivers with higher incomes report less stress than those of more limited means.

Caregivers pay a high price emotionally and physically for their roles. Depression is the most common psychological disorder and is especially prevalent in those caring for demented persons. Elevated stress is associated with an increased likelihood of harm to the recipient. Caregivers also suffer disproportionately from increased risk for cardiovascular disease, immune system dysfunction, and elevated blood pressure. Elderly spousal caregivers experiencing stress have a markedly higher mortality rate than their noncaregiving, age-matched peers.

The monetary value of informal caregiving is difficult to assess but has been estimated to far outweigh the combined cost of home health and nursing home care. Although some support services are available,

many caregivers are unaware of their existence or how to access them. Use of support has been shown to reduce stress and depression and to delay institutionalization by as much as 1 year. As the economic contributions of informal caregivers have begun to be recognized, there has been a movement toward legislative and regulatory efforts to provide more support for individuals to remain at home. These include redirection of Medicaid dollars to informal caregivers rather than to institutions.

As primary care providers, PAs can impart an invaluable service to their caregiving patients by helping them to optimize their own health. A PA may be the only social and emotional outlet for an often-isolated caregiver. Recognizing and expressing appreciation of their efforts can be a positive incentive to continue in the role. Providing information on community support programs and assisting the family in locating respite may be important therapeutic interventions for both the care provider and recipient. (See the Resources for recommended websites for caregiver support materials.)

HOME CARE: HOME CARE ORGANIZATIONS

Home care organizations include home health agencies, home care aide organizations, and hospices.[5] Most agencies are Medicare certified and provide skilled nursing assistance. Although the enactment of Medicare in 1965 greatly accelerated growth in the industry, the changes that occurred in the 1997 Balanced Budget Act led to a decline in the home health agency sector. However, demand continues to increase, and in 2012, 4,742,500 people were enrolled in home care.[6] Medicare is the single largest payer, accounting for slightly less than one third of total payments. Other sources include private out of pocket, Medicaid, Civilian Health and Medical Program of the Uniformed Services (CHAMPUS), and the Veterans Administration. Medicaid home care expenditures vary on the basis of state eligibility rules and are oriented toward personal care activities such as bathing and dressing.

Of patients who receive Medicare home health services, most have chronic diseases that impact the ability to perform ADLs. The most common primary diagnoses in order of prevalence in 2012 were as follows: hypertension, heart disease (including congestive heart failure), diabetes, osteoarthritis and musculoskeletal disorders, malignant neoplasms, and cerebrovascular disease.[6]

Recipients generally must have a skilled nursing need and meet Medicare's definition of homebound (i.e., unable to leave their homes without great difficulty, generally only for physician office visits or to go to church). Other therapists such as physical and occupational practitioners are available without a skilled nursing need but require a physician's order. Most clients are older than 85 years of age, female, and in poor health. The increasing use of telehomecare, which uses telephone lines and Internet connections to link medical providers with homebound patients, has had positive effects on self-management of chronic illness.[7] Managed care is another source of financing for home health, usually via a negotiated prepaid rate. Most contracts are through employer-based insurance, but it is also being used by states in an attempt to reduce unsustainable Medicaid expenditures.

HOSPICE

Most medical care in the United States is delivered in the expectation or hope of attaining a cure. Palliative medicine is directed toward the relief of suffering in all of its manifestations rather than an effort to cure disease. Although those at the end of life often desire a more palliative approach, care providers should always focus on symptom management regardless of the prognosis.

Hospice is a philosophy of care that concentrates on the comfort and dignity of patients and their families. Most hospice care takes place in the home, but inpatient hospice care programs are available in some communities. Hospice may also care for patients who reside in nursing homes or ALFs. In 2007, the average length of stay on hospice varied by age and gender, with the oldest patients and women enjoying the longest length of service. Only 3% received care for at least 30 days, suggesting that the benefit is underused.[8] A 2002 survey of families revealed that longer stays were perceived as more beneficial, but even short hospice experiences were helpful.[4] By 2009, the average length of stay for the top 20 diagnoses ranged from 27 days for chronic kidney disease to 106 days for Alzheimer disease.[9] To use the Medicare Part A Hospice Benefit, patients must choose a palliative approach, although contrary to common belief, they may continue to be resuscitated in the event of a cardiopulmonary arrest. A physician must certify that the patient's life expectancy is less than 6 months if his or her disease process follows its natural progression. This requirement has contributed to the myth that hospice is only for patients with cancer because the trajectory of decline related to most neoplasms is relatively predictable, and survival in other diseases may be less well defined. However, many

TABLE 41.3 **Hospice Diagnoses in Order of Frequency in 2013**	
Diagnosis	**Patients (%)**
Malignant neoplasm	36.5
Nonmalignant diagnoses	63.5
Dementia	15.2
Heart disease, including CHF	13.4
Pulmonary disease	9.9
Cerebrovascular disease	5.2

CHF, Congestive heart failure.
From National Hospice and Palliative Care Organization. *Facts and Figures: Hospice Care in America.* Alexandria, VA: Author; 2014.

other disorders qualify, and there is no penalty for longer survival, provided the individual is declining. (See Table 41.3 for the most common hospice diagnoses.) Hospice continues to provide bereavement support of the family up to 13 months after the death of the patient.

Hospice incorporates many of the same principles as home care: physical assessment, psychosocial support, disease and symptom management, use of an interdisciplinary care team, and patient and family education. Teams include hospice nurses, the hospice medical director, social workers, clergy, and volunteers. Promotion of the dignity of individuals and their ability to live their last days and months to the fullest extent possible is the goal.

Life closure is difficult to attain when physical symptoms interfere with concentration; therefore, relief of pain and discomfort is a core skill for team members. The patient's perception of symptoms is the basis for successful management but does not always coincide with the observations of team members. Suffering incorporates pain but is also a total experience influenced by family relationships, cultural background, religious belief system, and social supports of the patient. The clinician must be well versed in medical and nonmedical means of treating these symptoms. The American Academy of Hospice and Palliative Care Medicine produces a series of self-education materials promoting best-practice approaches in palliative care. Other self-directed learning materials are also cited in this chapter.

Caring for a dying loved one is extremely rewarding but can lead to exhaustion and burnout in family members. Symptom management may become impossible to achieve in the home setting. Hospices can provide continuous care by a registered nurse until symptoms are controlled or respite care in a hospital, nursing home, or inpatient hospice setting may allow the caregivers a short vacation from their caregiving responsibilities. The hospice respite benefit is the only form of respite service covered under the Medicare program. A growing number of hospitals maintain specialized units for palliative care or palliative care consult teams using PAs as core members of an interdisciplinary team.

Few PAs are involved in hospice care, but the increasing complexity of hospice patients is beginning to increase their use. PAs mirror the practice patterns of their supervising physicians, and as more physicians become comfortable with palliative medicine, greater numbers of PAs will choose this rewarding specialty. PAs may provide a vital link between the attending physician, the patient, and the hospice agency. Changes in the reimbursement structure of the hospice benefit may also allow more hospices to employ PAs in the future.

MEDICAL HOUSE CALLS

In the early 1900s, most physician services took place in the patient's home, and diagnostic tools fit easily in the "black bag." Gradually, improvements in transportation and technologic advances led to centralized care in office-based practices, and house calls became a rare practice. Physician training became concentrated in inpatient units, so doctors had no role models in home care. Liability and safety concerns contributed to the decline. A further disincentive was poor reimbursement compared with office visits. Other reasons for the change were more personal. Clinicians may be uncomfortable with visiting certain neighborhoods or in the unfamiliar environment of another person's home. They may be unable to manage complex patients without their customary diagnostic and therapeutic tools or the immediate availability of the expertise of consultant colleagues. House calls remain an inefficient use of provider time because of the time lost in travel. House call clients often suffer from a complex array of chronic diseases, so the time devoted to care tends to be greater. However, the inefficiency of providing medical services for these patients in the office is a hidden cost to the practice and to society.

In recent years, house calls have enjoyed a resurgence of popularity. Tangible benefits of house calls are a more accurate assessment of functional status and environmental safety, a closer relationship with patients and their families (reducing liability concerns), and a better understanding of the challenges faced by both patients and their caregivers. In 2013, 343,000 home visits were billed to Medicare by PAs.[10]

Technology has advanced to allow the provider to take the office to the patient. Portable laboratory devices, electrocardiography machines, and pulse oximeters have augmented house call providers' ability to assess patients in their homes. In larger population centers, mobile services are available for diagnostic studies. The use of an electronic medical record allows the provider to record the visit and access patient materials without the need for a bulky paper chart.

Medicare reimburses for physician services provided in the home by PAs. Patients do not have to meet the stringent housebound requirement needed for home care agency visits but must simply need medical care and have difficulty accessing the physician office. Patients who reside in ALFs may receive medically necessary services in the home without other requirements because they are presumed to have transportation difficulties. Many PAs and physicians maintain a small panel of their patients whom they see in the home. Some physicians and PAs have chosen to work exclusively as house call providers and may be in solo practice or employed by companies that specialize in medical house calls.

The passage of the Independence at Home Medicare demonstration project as part of the Patient Protection and Affordable Care Act has shown the efficacy of home medical care for the highest need, most vulnerable population. This program uses home visits by medical providers to target the highest users of medical services in an effort to avoid high-cost centers such as emergency departments and hospitals. It uses a shared savings model to incentivize providers to provide excellent care at a lower cost. Beneficiaries have been very satisfied with the care, and early data show potential for substantial cost savings to Medicare, with a savings of over $25 million documented in the first year.[11] An expansion of the program is currently under consideration and should provide many opportunities for PAs as the frail population continues to increase exponentially.

CASE STUDY 41.1

Mrs. A. is an 86-year-old woman who resides in an ALF. She has diabetes mellitus II, hypertension, congestive heart failure (CHF), osteoarthritis, atrial fibrillation, and moderate Alzheimer disease. She is declining in cognition and functional status and has been hospitalized several times in the past 2 months for CHF exacerbations. The manager of the facility contacts the American Academy of Home Care Medicine, learns there is a local practice that provides home visits in their area, and arranges for

Mrs. A. to see a provider in her apartment at the ALF. A PA visits the client in her home and finds that the patient has been taking an over-the-counter nonsteroidal medication provided by her friend in the building. She explains that this medication has probably been contributing to her decompensation and assists the patient in controlling her arthritic symptoms. She reviews all of her medications and identifies two others that may be causing or increasing her cognitive decline. These medications are discontinued, and Mrs. A. enjoys 4 years of relatively good health with only one hospitalization for pneumonia. At 90 years of age, she develops a new stroke and is unable to safely eat or drink. Her daughter, who is her legal decision maker, decides to avoid artificial hydration and nutrition because "Mom would not want to live like she is now, and her greatest pleasure in life is eating." She elects to pursue comfort measures and careful hand feeding. The ALF is able to manage Mrs. A. during her final illness with the assistance of a local hospice agency recommended by the PA, and the patient dies in her home 2 months later.

ASSISTED LIVING FACILITIES

Another site of care for older and disabled adults is the ALF. Most are located in urban or suburban areas and provide assistance in ADLs. In 2006, between 600,000 and 1 million individuals resided in about 30,000 ALFs in the United States.[12] The facilities are usually funded via private payment from residents, but some are financed through state Medicaid programs and by charities. They may assist residents with medication management but are specifically prohibited from maintaining a medical director or skilled nursing services. Physicians or PAs may visit their patients in these facilities if the visit is medically necessary and if it is difficult for the patients to access the physician's office. Medicare has recognized the growing complexity of residents in ALFs and reimburses visits at the same rate as that provided for house calls. Because the growth in this industry has been exponential and the need for services is only expected to increase, it is likely that medical providers will be providing more care in ALFs.

NURSING HOMES

The mission of nursing homes has changed dramatically over the past 2 decades along with their patient populations. There are generally two types

of patients: long stays (>6 months), who usually have multiple chronic disease and functional losses, and short stays, who are there for short-term rehabilitation after an acute hospitalization. Medicare provides a 20-day fully covered period after a 3-day hospital stay for skilled nursing services or for therapy. Patients must show progress over the duration of the stay to continue to use the benefit. An additional 80 days are available with a copayment from the beneficiary. A physician, PA, or nurse practitioner must certify patients to receive this service.

A new and challenging reality is the rapid increase in the number of Americans who enter nursing homes as their final site of care. Patients require more intense medical management than ever, but physician involvement remains limited. Low reimbursement rates coupled with liability concerns have led many physicians to avoid long-term care facilities despite the rising medical intricacy of the patients housed there. According to the AAPA 2009 census, few PAs (5%) reported working primarily in nursing homes, although it is likely many see a limited number of nursing home patients as part of their practice.

Physician assistants' employers are reimbursed for visits made by PAs in nursing homes at 85% of the physician rate, provided the care is medically necessary. PAs' participation in long-term care has been shown to reduce hospitalizations to a level even lower than that of community-dwelling Medicare recipients.[13] The presence of a PA reassures nursing staff, patients, and families that a well-trained clinician is available to evaluate and manage patients' symptoms. Patients must be seen every 30 days for the first 90 days of their stay and at 30- or 60-day intervals thereafter. PAs may alternate the required visits with their physician supervisors. Acute care visits may be made at any time by the PA if warranted by the patient's medical condition. Medicare usually pays for 18 visits per year without question; however, reimbursement for additional visits may be made if documentation supports their necessity.

One exception to care by PAs is the initial comprehensive visit required for patients whose stays are covered by Medicare Part A (skilled nursing facility patients). The physician must complete this service, but if the patient needs care before the physician's assessment, the PA may see the patient and manage the acute situation. Patients admitted as self-pays or as long-term clients (International Classification of Functioning [ICF] patients) may be initially assessed by the PA. Nursing home patients must have a yearly comprehensive history and physical examination, which may be performed by either provider.

KEY POINTS

- The growth in the aged and disabled population will continue to fuel a demand for home care services.
- Informal caregivers provide most of the care of disabled persons and often experience stress as a result.
- Palliative medicine focuses on the relief of suffering in all of its forms.
- House calls are a viable option for physicians and PAs who wish to care for the vulnerable elderly and disabled population.
- Medicare reimburses for PA visits at alternative sites.
- PAs can be integral components of the care of patients in their homes, wherever those homes may be.

References

1. *2013 AAPA Physician Assistant Census Report.* Alexandria, VA: American Academy of Physician Assistants; 2013. Accessed online September 9, 2015. www.aapa.org.
2. Caregiving in the U.S. Executive Summary; AARP Public Policy Institute and National Alliance for Caregiving. June 2015. Accessed September 26, 2015.
3. Phelan EA, Debnam KJ, Anderson LA, Owe S. A systematic review of intervention studies to prevent hospitalizations of community-dwelling older adults with dementia. *MedCarem.* 2015;53(2):207–213.
4. National Association for Home Care and Hospice. *Basic Statistics for Home Care and Hospice.* Washington, DC: National Association for Home Care and Hospice; 2009.
5. Landers S, Peterson L. Trends in home diagnostic testing for Medicare beneficiaries. *J Am Geriatr Soc.* 2007;55(1):138–139.
6. Jones AL, Harris-Kojetin L, Valverde R. Characteristics and use of home health care by men and women aged 65 and over. National health statistics reports; no. 52. Hyattsville, MD: National Center for Health Statistics. 2012
7. Bowles KH, Baugh AC. Applying research to optimize telehomecare. *Cardiovasc Nurs.* 2007;22(1):5–15.
8. Caffrey C, Sengupta M, Moss A, et al. Home health care and discharged hospice care patients: United States, 2000 and 2007. *National Health Statistics Report.* 2011.
9. Medicare Hospice Data Trends. CMS.gov. Accessed online November 19, 2015.
10. The Moran Company: data prepared for the American Academy of Home Care Medicine from the Physician/Supplier Procedure Summary (PSPS) Medicare Part B summary 2008-2013. Arlington, Virginia; 2014.
11. Centers for Medicare and Medicaid Services (CMS) of the Department of Health and Human Services (HHS). *Affordable Care Act payment model saves more than $25 million in first performance year*; June 18, 2015. Washington, DC.
12. Kerr T. American Association of Homes and Services for the Aging (website). www2.aahsa.org. Updated March 6, 2007. Accessed December 4, 2011.
13. Ackermann RJ, Kemle KA. The effect of a physician assistant on the hospitalization of nursing home residents. *J Am Geriatr Soc.* 1998;46(5):610–614.

The resources for this chapter can be found at www.expertconsult.com.

CHAPTER 42

HEALTH CARE FOR THE HOMELESS

Margaret Moore-Nadler

SOCIAL DETERMINANTS OF HEALTH

Health inequality is a well-documented global issue requiring collaboration among government and non-government entities to improve human living conditions, early childhood education, and employment opportunities that create upward mobility for people living in poverty.[1-3] Families living in poverty often live in overcrowded housing and have high levels of stress, substance misuse, and domestic violence.[4,5] Reducing or eliminating social inequalities can improve global health.

HEALTH DETERMINANTS

A health determinant is based on five factors that include biology or genetics, behaviors, social and physical environments, and health services.[1] Biology or genetics cannot be altered; however, the remaining four factors are pertinent to improve the health status of humanity. The relationship between the social determinants of health and health determinants is widely recognized.[2] Therefore, improving health must focus on resolving social and personal responsibility.[6]

CATEGORIES OF HOMELESS PEOPLE

Children and Adolescents

Runaway or throwaway children and adolescents enter the foster-care system that is riddled with chronic and complex issues focused on funding, legal matters, inappropriate placement, and insufficient case management. Many of these children leave the foster-care system and become homeless. More than 3 million children were placed in protective services in 2001, and more than 900,000 were victims of abuse.[4,7,8] Young people are vulnerable and easily persuaded to use drugs and are led into prostitution by pimps and drug dealers who may physically or sexually assault the homeless youth. Homeless youth develop a deep-rooted mistrust of adults and society, are resistant to change, and are at risk for early morbidity and mortality.[9,10] The complexity of living with trauma can cause young people to become depressed, angry, or aggressive because of frequent encounters with the legal system.[7] About 5000 young people (10–24 years of age) living on the streets die from suicide (13%) or homicide (16%).[10-13]

Pregnant female adolescents present a different constellation of risk factors. They may suffer with poor nutrition, stress, depression, and substance misuse, which result in 35% to 70% of miscarriages.[9] The infant may or may not have a relationship with his or her mother, which can have lifelong implications. A study of young homeless mothers found that only half of the mothers were able to help with caring for their children, and up to one fifth of the mothers never see their children because of mental health concerns.[9]

Adults

Single homeless adults who have experienced foster care, unstable parenting, housing, or a lack of support enter adulthood without housing. Many are undereducated and live with mental illness and or substance misuse.[14] The primary cause for homelessness in single adults is related to misusing substances, which often brings them in contact with the legal system. Arrests, incarceration, and a history of felony charges often prevent them from accessing public housing.[15]

Families

Social inequality perpetuates the cycle of poverty and homelessness that causes chaotic family living, stress, depression, substance misuse, unemployment, and indifference to improving their health.[1] The cost of health care is a financial burden for families with lower incomes because they are uninsured or underinsured.[2] Uninsured and underinsured families delay seeking health care because of high out-of-pocket expenditures.[16] Rural families and individuals seeking financial, physical, or emotional stability are moving to inner cities or urban life in the hope of improving their lifestyle.[10] However, transitioning to urban living may cause a family to move in with other family members, known as doubling up. Doubling up creates a different set of health risk factors, including stress, alcohol, tobacco, illicit drug use, and physical, emotional, or sexual abuse.[10] Strengthening and empowering parenting skills can be supportive to encourage and nurture all members of the family, as well as prevent homelessness.[17]

PATIENT AND FAMILY ASSESSMENT

Therapeutic communication is vital to develop a trusting relationship with a homeless patient or family because of society and health care professionals' attitudes toward mentally ill and homeless people.[18,19] Motivational interviewing helps identify the needs and desires of the patient and helps to identify the stage of readiness to change health behaviors.[20] Providers allowing patients to share their stories can explore the history of homelessness, victimization, education, and work history.[4,17,20] Patients' freely expressing their thoughts and feeling helps to identify intellectual disabilities, developmental delays, and concerns with cognition. Moreover, determining the cultural or ethnic background is vital because of differences in perception of health and recognizing differences in metabolism.[21]

HEALTH HISTORY

Homeless people suffer a variety of acute and chronic illnesses that require medications and treatments;

however, their lack insurance or money does not allow adherence to treatment plans. Furthermore, their health status is dependent on living conditions, consumption of food and water, and sexual behaviors. Screening for communicable (tuberculosis, sexually transmitted infections) and noncommunicable (obesity, heart disease, diabetes) disease is vital while the patient is in the clinic because of transportation issues around getting to the clinic.[22]

Living on the streets or in a shelter requires homeless people to be vigilant about their personal safety and securing their belongings. Consequently, many homeless people are sleep deprived because of fear of being victimized. Sleep deprivation, stress, and loss of family or community support lead to depression, and with a lack of coping strategies, people may turn to alcohol or street drugs to cope with their stressors.[22]

Data collected in the health assessment require the physician assistant to apply critical thinking regarding the physical examination and the plan of care.[23,24] For example, will the physical examination be a head-to-toe examination that is clothed versus unclothed? How will the patient manage his or her health issue while living on the street without money or insurance to pay for additional treatments or medications? Does the patient indicate a readiness to take action toward improving his or her health status?[23,25,26]

CASE STUDY 42.1

John and Suzie were happily married with two boys, 9 and 11 years of age. One afternoon, John's employer said his son-in-law would replace John as the groundskeeper. John began to drink more heavily since the loss of his job. The loss of income was a challenge for the family to keep up with their living expenses. Eight months later, John was diagnosed with esophageal cancer. The loss of John's income and health insurance created a burden caused by out-of-pocket expenses from their savings. The family moved in with John's parents, who had a smaller house in a low-income neighborhood, and Suzie found a part-time job.

After John's surgery, Suzie arranged for home health care instead of a lengthy stay in the hospital. Suzie's long hours of caring for John began to present problems with parenting. John's cancer returned within 18 months of surgery and treatment. Suzie was unable to keep up with her job and caring for John around the clock. Exhaustion prevented much interaction with her sons, who were depressed and angry. John's parents added tension between Suzie and John because they both began to drink heavily. One day, the oldest son came home from school 4 hours late. Enraged, Suzie beat him with a broom while the youngest son and grandparents watched. The grandfather condemned the boy for upsetting his mother. The next morning, both boys were gone. Suzie notified the police, but the boys were not found. A month later, Suzie quit her job to care for John. Without an income or insurance, John's parents asked them to move out. Suzie refused to move out of the house. After John's death, Suzie was forced to move out and had did not have a place to live. Presently, the two boys have been placed in a juvenile detention center because of theft of property.

QUESTIONS

1. What social determinants might have influenced the family?
2. What did health care providers overlook when caring for John and his family?
3. Identify primary, secondary, and tertiary psychosocial and medical interventions to help each family member.
4. How could health care empower and strengthen the family unit?

KEY POINTS

- Understand the complexity of social determinants of health.
- Recognize the determinants and problems encountered by the homeless.
- Know the facets necessary for therapeutic communication.
- Recognize the history and physical examination areas needed for a complete homeless health assessment.
- Recognize the coordinated care and treatment options available for the homeless.

References

1. Ahnquist J, Wamala SP, Lindstrom M. Social determinants of health – a question of social or economic capital? Interaction effects of socioeconomic factors on health outcomes. *Soc Sci Med.* 2012;74:930–939.
2. Carey G, Crammond B. Action on the social determinants of health: views from inside the policy process. *Soc Sci Med.* 2015;128:134–141. http://dx.doi.org/10.1016/j.socscimed.2015.01.024.
3. Jia H, Moriarty DG, Kanarek N. County-level social environment determinants of health-related quality of life among US adults: a multilevel analysis. *J Community Health.* 2009;34:430–439.
4. Kilmer RP, Cook JR, Crusto C, Strater KP, Haber MG. Understanding the ecology and development of children and families experiencing homelessness: implications for practice, supportive services, and policy. *Am J Orthopsychiatry.* 2012;82:389–401.
5. Thompson RA, Haskins R. Early stress gets under the skin: promising initiatives to help children facing chronic adversity. *Future Child.* 2014;24:1–6.
6. Buyx AM. Personal responsibility for health as a rationing criterion: why we don't like it and why maybe we should. *J Med Ethics.* 2008;34:871–874.
7. Bass S, Shields MK, Behrman RE. Children, families, and foster care: analysis and recommendations. *Future Child.* 2004;14:5–29.
8. Mohajer N, Earnest J. Widening the aim of health promotion to include the most disadvantaged: vulnerable adolescents and the social determinants of health. *Health Educ Res.* 2010;25:387–394.
9. Crawford DM, Trotter EC, Hartshorn KJ, Whitbeck LB. Pregnancy and mental health of young homeless women. *Am J Orthopsychiatry Wiley-Blackwell.* 2011;81:173–183.
10. Moore-Nadler M. Promoting health and preventing illness. In: Harris J, Roussel L, Thomas P, eds. *Initiating and sustaining the clinical nurse leader role: a practical guide.* Boston, MA: Jones & Bartlett Learning; 2014:387–411.
11. Bantchevska D, Erdem G, Patton R, et al. Predictors of drop-in center attendance among substance-abusing homeless adolescents. *Soc Work Res.* 2011;35:58–63.
12. Fielding K, Forchuk C. Exploring the factors associated with youth homelessness and arrests. *J Child Adolesc Psychiatr Nurs.* 2013;26:225–233.
13. Shaw FE, Centers for Disease Control and Prevention (DHHS/PHS), 2008. Youth Risk Behavior Surveillance–selected Steps Communities, United States, 2007 and Youth Risk Behavior Surveillance–Pacific Island United States Territories, 2007. *Morbidity and Mortality Weekly Report. Surveillance Summaries. Number SS-12 (No. 1546–0738). Centers for Disease Control and Prevention.* vol. 57.
14. Gozdzik A, Salehi R, O'Campo P, Stergiopoulos V, Hwang SW. Cardiovascular risk factors and 30-year cardiovascular risk in homeless adults with mental illness. *BMC Public Health.* 2015;15:1–13.
15. Huey L. False security or greater social inclusion? Exploring perceptions of CCTV use in public and private spaces accessed by the homeless. *Br J Sociol.* 2010;61:63–82.
16. Bennett KJ, Dismuke CE. Families at financial risk due to high ratio of out-of-pocket health care expenditures to total income. *J Health Care Poor Underserved.* 2010;21:691–703.
17. Crouch C, Parrish DE. Implementing motivational interviewing in an urban homeless population: an agency–university collaboration. *Res Soc Work Pract.* 2015;25:493–498.
18. Boylston MT, O'Rourke R. Second-degree bachelor of science in nursing students' preconceived attitudes toward the homeless and poor: a pilot study. *J Prof Nurs Off J Am Assoc Coll Nurs.* 2013;29:309–317.

19. Habibian M, Elizondo L, Mulligan R. Dental students' attitudes toward homeless people while providing oral health care. *J Dent Educ.* 2010;74:1190–1196.

20. Hallgren KA, Moyers TB. Does readiness to change predict in-session motivational language? Correspondence between two conceptualizations of client motivation. *Addiction.* 2011;106:1261–1269.

21. Flaskerud JH. Ethnicity, culture, and neuropsychiatry. *Issues Ment. Health Nurs.* 2000;21:5–29.

22. National Guideline Clearinghouse. Adapting your practice: general recommendations for the care of homeless patients. http://www.guideline.gov/content.aspx?id=16325&search=health+care+for+homeless. Accessed December 1, 2015.

23. Day DB, Hale LS. Promoting critical thinking in online physician assistant courses. *Perspect Physician Assist Educ.* 2005;16:96–102.

24. Shea SS, Hoyt K. Medical decision making in emergency care. *Adv Emerg Nurs J.* 2014;36:360–366.

25. Essary AC, Stoehr J. Incorporation of the competencies for the physician assistant profession into physician assistant education. *J Physician Assist Educ Physician Assist Educ Assoc.* 2009;20:6–14. 9p.

26. Lipato T. Improving the health of the homeless: advice for physicians. *Minn Med.* 2012;95:45–50.

The resources for this chapter can be found at www.expertconsult.com.

CHAPTER 43

CORRECTIONAL MEDICINE

Robin N. Hunter Buskey

Inmates have a higher prevalence of health problems than the general population, both acute and chronic. For instance, the overall rate of confirmed AIDS cases among the nation's prison population is five times the rate of the general population. This stems in part from the communities inmates come from. More than 60% of incarcerated individuals are African American or Latino. Typically they are from an underserved urban community. By screening and treating inmates for various diseases, we take the important first step of preventing their spread into the larger community. But I believe it is also possible to make progress on eliminating disparities through corrections-based interventions.

—Vice Admiral Richard H. Carmona, MD, MPH, FACS, CCHP, U.S. Surgeon General, U.S. Department of Health and Human Services National Conference on Correctional Health Care, Austin, Texas, October 6, 2003

WORKING IN A CORRECTIONAL ENVIRONMENT

Why would a physician assistant (PA) want to work in a jail or prison? That is certainly an important question but the wrong one. The question is "Why would a PA NOT want to work in a jail or prison?" As former Surgeon General Richard Carmona observed, correctional medicine should not be quickly dismissed because it addresses public health issues that prevent the spread of disease into our communities. Furthermore, it is also an enormous opportunity to make progress on eliminating health disparities.

As the rates of incarceration have increased over the past 25 years, so have the importance and complexity of correctional medicine. For every 145 Americans, there is 1 person incarcerated. The total number of people involved in the criminal justice system is estimated at 2.3 million in custody,[1] with 10 million released annually from jails.[2]

Correctional institutions are a microcosm of society and, as such, require correctional medicine practitioners to be specialists in public health, primary care, infectious disease, and chronic disease. The correctional populations are marginalized because of racial disparities, low socioeconomic status, substance abuse, and mental health disorders. The marked health status disparities and outcomes of incarcerated populations are well documented.[3]

The opportunity to practice in correctional institutions enables PAs to rebuild lives and make a difference. Correctional health often attracts individual professionals who see this as an important role in the overall health of the community. Some of our society's sickest individuals are among incarcerated populations, and PAs working in correctional medicine need special skills and attitudes. In fact, correctional medicine is one of the cornerstones of public health in this country. PAs wanting to work in the eye of the public health storm in this country or those who want to address health disparities should consider correctional medicine as a career venue. The role and relationship between PAs and their patients are unique. The issues of race, poverty, addiction, mental illness, and economically depressed communities create enormous problems for the physician–PA health care team and present opportunities for professional satisfaction for correctional PAs.

This chapter covers the issues commonly found in correctional medicine, such as access and quality of care, staffing, and environmental, safety, and ethical issues. The chapter also assesses an array of clinical duties that correctional PAs perform, including conducting health screenings and evaluations; evaluating and managing chronic disease patients in clinics or infirmaries; conducting daily sick calls; making cell checks in segregated housing; reviewing laboratory and other diagnostic test results; developing, monitoring, and modifying individual treatment plans; and discharge planning activities.

PROVIDING HEALTH CARE IN CORRECTIONAL INSTITUTIONS

Access to Care

Providing health care in this environment requires an understanding and knowledge of governmental, bureaucratic, and paramilitary hierarchies. Many correctional health professionals are employed directly by correctional authorities. However, during the past 25 years, correctional health care models have evolved into several types. Contractual health care systems such as for-profit companies, academic medical centers, and public health agencies have assumed the administrative structure for health services in prisons and jails. Under this structure, recruiting, training, and retaining of health care professionals are often easier than when health care professionals are employed directly by the correctional authority. Having professional autonomy and judgment within organized health systems has helped to attract qualified professionals into correctional medicine. Ensuring that inmates have access to health care services is a fundamental responsibility for correctional medical professionals. It means that every inmate, regardless of where he or she is located in the jail or prison, must be able to inform health staff of his or her need to be seen, and when notified, health staff must act in a timely fashion, provide a professional clinical judgment, and ensure that ordered care is delivered. Any unreasonable barrier to inmate health service access must be removed.

What makes correctional medicine different from other venues of health care delivery is the long line of legal cases that have established incarcerated individuals' rights to health care,[4–6] addressing the responsibilities of custody officials in the health, mental health, and dental treatment of inmates. As a result of these and other court cases, correctional medicine has evolved.

Estelle v. Gamble established the concept of deliberate indifference as the test to determine whether government acted appropriately in the medical care of its inmates. As was clearly articulated, deliberate indifference is defined by prison doctors in their response to a prisoner's needs or by prison guards in intentionally denying or delaying access to medical care or intentionally interfering with the treatment he or she has been prescribed. [4]

The government must ensure that adequate medical, dental, and mental health services are provided to those whom it imprisons. To accomplish this, a responsible health authority (RHA) is established. The RHA ensures that primary, secondary, and tertiary care is provided for the well-being of the inmate population. The RHA works with custody staff to eliminate barriers that might hamper inmates from receiving these services in a timely manner. For example, one barrier might be when an officer, hostile to inmates, denies an inmate access to the sick call notification system. Training custody and health staff to recognize emerging medical or mental health needs is an important RHA role. Sometimes there are unreasonable delays in escorting inmates to see health professionals or to get to outside appointments to obtain necessary diagnostic workups. The RHA works to ensure that access-to-care procedures are flexible to accommodate the special health needs of inmates, such as chronic illness, serious communicable infections, physical disabilities, pregnancy, fragility, terminal illness, mental illness, potential for suicide, and developmental disability. Such special needs affect housing, work, and program assignments; disciplinary measures; and admissions and transfers to and from institutions. Correctional PAs and custody staff need to adequately communicate about these special needs inmates to ensure that government provides appropriate care.

What distinguishes correctional PAs from their civilian community colleagues is that they must be concerned with federal due process. The 8th Amendment to the Constitution prohibits cruel and unusual punishment, and the 14th Amendment ensures the right to due process and full protection under the law. The rights of prisoners cannot be abridged, and those with mental health problems have increased legal protections.[7] Issues such as involuntary hospitalization, transfers from prison to mental hospitals, and involuntary medication and self-harm restrictions are closely scrutinized in mentally ill inmates. Few PAs are prepared to address these thorny legal and ethical access-to-care issues and as a result do not pursue this career track.

Many PA programs offer clinical clerkships in jails, prisons, and juvenile detention centers and can provide PA students an entrance into correctional medicine; however, in general, PAs are not exposed to the complexities of correctional health care.

More PA programs need to become vested in correctional medicine and the disenfranchised populations that are served.

Clinical Autonomy

The safety of inmates, staff, and visitors takes priority in correctional institutions. Many decisions that would seem inconsequential in the free world take on greater importance in corrections. For example, the choice to issue a pair of crutches for a patient with a non–weight-bearing injury takes on a different perspective when considering the safety precautions required in a jail or prison. As a result, correctional health clinicians face a number of pressures when assessing the health needs of their patients.

Inherent in a correctional institution is the power that security staff wields, deciding on what can or cannot be permitted in the institution. Decisions about staff utilization, inmate housing, work assignments, and disciplinary sanctions for both staff and inmates are under the purview of administrative security staff. For example, hiring a PA to work in a jail takes not only the approval of the responsible physician but also that of the jail administrator. The PA must pass a detailed security screening, which, in some jurisdictions, may take several months to complete. The PA must abide by the employment rules directed by the medical authority, but he or she must also abide by the directives of security.

Sometimes there is conflict between security and medical staff over clinical decisions and actions. However, custody staff should not interfere with the implementation of clinical decisions. Qualified health professionals should direct clinical decisions and actions regarding all health care provided to their patients. Case in point: A PA orders knee magnetic resonance imaging (MRI) of a high-security-risk inmate. Security staff is reluctant to transfer the inmate to the hospital for the MRI, particularly because he is a dangerous escape risk, and policy requires three officers to transport him. The jail administrator refuses to transport the inmate because of the threat to public safety. Most civilian health staff members are not accustomed to such denials of care. In this case, the clinical decision should be tempered with cooperation and consultation with administrative security staff. How urgent is the MRI to making a clinical decision? How long has the patient been complaining of his symptoms? Is the denial of care deliberately indifferent to the inmate's medical need? The answers to these questions influence the course of action that the PA should take. More important, the successful correctional PA is one who knows how to negotiate with custody staff to achieve the goals necessary to provide the best possible care for his or her patient.

Clinical autonomy cannot be jeopardized; however, in a correctional institution, diagnostic and therapeutic orders are not issued in a vacuum. Rather, they require a coordinated effort among custodial, administrative, and health staff.

To facilitate the implementation of health care orders and decisions, most facilities hold meetings between security and health staff. Through joint monitoring, planning, and problem resolution, health, correctional, and administrative personnel can facilitate the health care delivery system. Included should be discussions on the barriers to effective treatment and care. For example, evidence-based medicine has shown that disease progression is controlled when the patient is involved in monitoring his or her disease. Patients with asthma should have peak flow meters, and patients with diabetes should have glucometers. However, custody policies often prevent such items in the housing units for fear of security breaches. Treating asthma in a correctional environment is problematic because many have inadequate ventilation systems or restrictive keep-on-person medication programs. Restricting opportunities for inmates with diabetes to self-test, self-prepare, and self-administer insulin presents additional barriers to improving disease control. Administrative problem solving, corrective actions, timetables for proposed changes, and updates on changes proposed during previous meetings are important strategies toward implementing effective patient care.

Quality of Care

Correctional PAs have to be knowledgeable in continuous quality improvement (CQI) monitoring. CQI identifies problems; proposes, implements, and monitors corrective action; and studies the effectiveness of corrective actions in addressing problems. This multidisciplinary (i.e., medical, nursing, mental health, substance abuse) structured process examines outcomes, high-risk or high-volume, or problem-prone aspects of care and ensures that established standards of care are met. CQI committees should assess processes that affect the effectiveness and efficiency of staffing, continuity of care, and quality of services.

Patient Satisfaction

Health care organizations are interested in the quality of care provided to their patients. They are interested in what their patients perceive to be quality.

Correctional health systems are no different. Patient satisfaction surveys have been conducted by health care organizations for quite some time now; however, this is a new concept in corrections and is not widely accepted by correctional administrators. After all, correctional institutions are predicated on having individuals who do not want to be there and who are mistrusted by staff. This distrustful environment does not support surveying techniques. Yet a few correctional institutions are conducting inmate-patient satisfaction surveys. For example, the Oregon Department of Corrections has been conducting patient satisfaction surveys for more than a decade and has found a positive, constructive way to implement changes in patient care.

STAFFING IN CORRECTIONAL MEDICINE

Staffing Issues

The recruiting, training, and retaining of health professionals to work in correctional health care is difficult because prisons and jails do not have medical care as the primary mission. Jails and prisons are foreign working environments for most health care professionals. Yet correctional institutions have a mandate to provide adequate and timely evaluation, treatment, and follow-up care consistent with community standards.

The numbers and types of health care professionals required depend on the size of the facility and the scope of onsite medical, mental health, dental, and substance-abuse treatment. There is a difference in the functions and responsibilities of jails and prisons. Jails detain individuals who have been accused of crimes and who are waiting adjudication by either a jury or judge. On average, jails hold detainees for about 1 year, although in some cases, jails hold individuals a few years past adjudication. The point is that after conviction and sentence have been rendered, the individual is transferred to a prison. Prisons are long-term holding facilities for individuals who have been convicted and sentenced for their crimes.

Compensation and benefit packages are generally not competitive and are a disincentive for many PAs. The security clearance process is sometimes lengthy and dissuades individuals from staying with the process, taking other jobs that may be offered. Opposition and pressure from family members is another barrier that a PA faces in taking a correctional health care position. The patient clientele are vastly different. Many are recalcitrant, ungrateful, argumentative, and even combative. Despite these drawbacks, correctional PAs find that being at the crossroad of medicine, public health, law, ethics, and criminal justice is challenging and rewarding.

To help attract health professionals, some institutions serve as clinical rotation sites for students. One such example is the Cook County Department of Corrections, Cermak Health Services, in Chicago. This site has been a clinical rotation site for area PA programs for more than 20 years. The level of morbidity and mortality in this patient population is high, and PA students often find themselves in challenging clinical situations. Clinical rotations in correctional institutions provide unique and challenging opportunities to exercise one's clinical skills and consideration for future employment.

Physician assistants generally find correctional employment working for the legal authority (the sheriff or department of corrections). Some jails and prisons contract for-profit companies, academic medical institutions, or public health agencies to provide health services. Using these models, correctional institutions can attract health staff through better compensation, faculty appointments, and continuing education opportunities.

Finding and retaining qualified health professionals to work in jails, prisons, and juvenile detention and confinement facilities is an important concern. The goal is to find professionals who are willing to establish and maintain a therapeutic relationship with inmates. Medical professionals are trained to advocate quality patient care; however, providing such services in an antitherapeutic environment is difficult.

When these two dynamics collide, conflicts about authority over health services decision making and management occur. For example, health care professionals hold to a tenet that patients should have control over the health care decisions that affect their lives. However, in correctional institutions, such autonomy creates problems for custody.

An inmate who refuses to take clinically ordered behavior-modifying medications (increasing the likelihood of disruptive behavior) or refuses to submit to a human immunodeficiency virus (HIV) blood test when a staff member has come into contact with the inmate's blood presents problems for custody. How custody responds in such situations is often not the way medical professionals would solve the problem. These frequent conflicts arising between custody and health staff require well-developed effective communication and problem-solving skills. Health professionals who do not have the skills are often co-opted and are seen as an extension of security rather than as medical professionals.

Physician assistants working in a correctional environment need to know that it is a constant balance between public safety and public health. They need to know that their environment is a paramilitary, organizational-based hierarchy and that public safety drives decision making relative to patient services. For example, administering medication to patients at a given time of day during pill call is made more complicated when the facility goes into a lockdown status (because of a breach in security, inmates are kept in their cells). The method and manner in which medication is administered may completely change to accommodate the public safety situation.

Clinical Performance Enhancement

The clinical performance enhancement process evaluates the appropriateness of a health clinician's services. The PA's clinical work is reviewed by another professional of at least equal training in the same general discipline, such as the review by the facility's medical director or chief PA. The purpose of this review is to enhance clinical competency and address areas that need improvement. It is different from an annual performance review or a clinical case conference in that it is a professional practice review focused on the professional's clinical skills.

Clinical performance enhancement reviews in a correctional environment are no different from any other institutional setting (e.g., the military or hospital). For example, treating patients with HIV must follow certain clinical guidelines regardless of setting. However, a correctional clinical performance enhancement review has an additional component in the review of one's clinical judgment by assessing how one's clinical competency affects public safety. The clinical PA may indeed be effective in managing the health care of uncooperative or even malingering inmates by gaining their trust and respect. However, if the clinical PA receives information from such inmates that public safety might be jeopardized, the clinical PA has a responsibility and duty to report it even to the point of damaging patient trust and confidence.

Staff and Inmate Safety

In January 2004, a 15-day hostage standoff between Arizona corrections officials and two inmates captivated the nation's attention. The hostage standoff ended peacefully through a negotiated surrender of the inmates and the release of a female officer. This event perpetuates the public perception that jails and prisons are dangerous places. Although that is true, it is important to remember that events such as this are not an everyday occurrence. Correctional institutions work to ensure staff safety through strict policies and procedures and by ongoing training of its staff. Staff and public safety is compromised when lapses in training or procedures occur. For example, once in Sacramento, California, a deputy U.S. marshal placed his weapon under the front seat of his vehicle before entering the jail to pick up a prisoner. When he returned with the prisoner, he forgot to retrieve the weapon. It subsequently slid back where the prisoner was sitting. The prisoner, handcuffed with his hands in front, grabbed the weapon, ordered the deputy to pull over, and escaped.[8] As this case reminds us, it is in the best interest of public safety to ensure that the health and well-being of staff are protected. When staff members forget or fail to abide by policy and procedure, harm can occur.

Risk and harm reduction create a working environment in which staff feel safe to do their work. There is no central repository for the collection of hazardous duty incidents incurred by correctional health professionals. There are no studies on inmate assaults on health staff, although anecdotally, staff members report that assaults on health staff rarely occur.

In 2001, Human Rights Watch released *No Escape*, a descriptive report on male prisoner-on-prisoner sexual abuse in the United States that outlined firsthand accounts of prisoner rape and sexual assault stories from 200 prisoners in 37 states.[9] This report reviews the conditions that contribute to prisoner rape—namely, the rapid expansion of the incarcerated population during the past 20 years; the increasing government decisions to privatize its prisons and jails; and the dismantling of prisoners' legal rights through the Prison Litigation Reform Act of 1996 (an act that made prisoner lawsuits regarding conditions of confinement and deliberate indifference more difficult). As a result of the shocking claims made in *No Escape*, Congress passed the Prison Rape Elimination Act of 2003 (PREA).[10] PREA requires "the gathering of national statistics about the problem; the development of guidelines for states about how to address prisoner rape; the creation of a review panel to hold annual hearings; and the provision of grants to states to combat the problem."[10] PREA is the first U.S. federal law passed that deals with assault on prisoners and aims to improve correctional institutions' safety.

COMMUNICABLE DISEASES IN CORRECTIONAL INSTITUTIONS

Infection Control

Correctional facilities generally have an exposure control plan that describes staff actions to be taken to eliminate or minimize exposures to pathogens.

In closed environments such as prisons and jails, it is important that health professionals maintain standard hygiene practices and precautions. They need to be aware of infection control matters and should receive orientation and annual updates to infection control policies and procedures. Facilities also have needlestick prevention programs that include the use of self-capping needles and functional sharps disposal containers.

Many correctional institutions have infection control committees that establish and maintain the exposure control plan; monitor communicable disease among inmates and staff; ensure prompt treatment for inmates and staff with infectious disease; ensure staff receive appropriate training and maintain procedures; ensure that personal protective equipment is available and used; and meet reporting requirements, laws, and regulations issued by local, state, and federal authorities.

Community-Acquired Methicillin-Resistant *Staphylococcus aureus*

A major problem occurring in many jails and prisons today is the increasing rate of community-acquired methicillin-resistant *Staphylococcus aureus* (CA-MRSA). Jails and prisons are commonly overcrowded and do not have sufficient hygienic practices with soap, water, or clean laundry. These conditions foster environments in which contagions such as *S. aureus* and CA-MRSA can be transmitted from one person to another.

CA-MRSA infections are generally mild, self-limiting minor skin infections that appear as pustules or boils.[11] Inmates often complain of "spider bites," and correctional staff too often dismiss their claims. Education is necessary for both groups so that health staff can intervene and begin treatment.

Other confounding issues complicate the matter of containing CA-MRSA outbreaks in correctional institutions. This includes comorbidities of substance abuse and mental illness, distrust of authority figures, reluctance to cooperate with health care staff, and resistance to rules of hygienic practice. These issues contribute to complicating the ability to adequately respond to self-cleanliness. Before their incarceration, many inmates were either homeless or came from home environments that did not have adequate sanitation or did not stress personal hygiene. The hygienic practices of frequent hand washing with soap and water, avoidance of picking lesions, daily showers, and limitation of the number of personal items shared with other inmates should be emphasized to all inmates.[11]

Other significant risk factors that have been found include prison occupation, gender, comorbidities, prior skin infection, and previous antibiotic use.[11] Resistance to antibiotic therapy has added to this problem. Commonly, inmates have not sought regular and consistent health care from one primary care provider. Too often when they obtained medical services before incarceration, inmates went to emergency departments and public health community clinics. This episodic approach to their health care without consistent or organized management complicates the individual's resistance to antibiotic therapy.

Another problem that complicates matters is that inmates, by nature, distrust authority and rules. When an outbreak occurs in a jail or prison, inmates are quick to blame jail administrators and health staff for the problem and not take responsibility for themselves. This distrust of authority creates a barrier to improving jail and prison conditions and eliminating the transmission of CA-MRSA.

Tuberculosis

Tuberculosis (TB) in correctional facilities is a continuous problem affecting the health status of communities at large. "Although the incident TB case rate for the general population has remained at fewer than 10 cases per 100,000 persons since 1993, substantially higher case rates, some as high as 10 times that of the general population, have been reported in correctional populations."[12]

The control of TB in correctional facilities is a multifaceted problem with no easy answers. Correctional institutions have policies on staff surveillance; however, it is difficult to maintain mandatory and periodic screening of correctional staff members. Between 2001 and 2004, the Florida Department of Corrections had one HIV-infected correctional staff member who was nonadherent with TB treatment and infected five correctional staff members over 2½ years. Four of the five cases were caused by an identical strain, indicating a probable common source.

Correctional institutions have poor ventilation and a transient population, which further complicate the control of TB. As a result, contact tracing is extremely difficult. In 2002, Kansas had a case in which a TB-infected inmate was transferred to three jails and one prison. In that process he came into contact with more than 800 individuals and was positively linked via identical-band via RFLP DNA testing to two inmates (cellmates in two different locations). In contact tracing, 318 of the 800 inmates were found—six had a negative prior tuberculin skin test (TST), and 196 inmates had no prior skin test information. Forty-one (21%) had positive skin test results.

Failure to control TB in jails and prisons is a threat to the community. From 1999 to 2000, the South Carolina Department of Corrections had a TB outbreak in which 31 prisoners and one medical student in the community's hospital subsequently developed TB. In upstate New York, there was a multidrug-resistant (MDR) TB outbreak involving several correctional facilities and a hospital. The MDR TB outbreak resulted in at least 50 health care professionals being infected and the death of one prison guard.

Latent tuberculosis infection (LTBI) is four times higher among prison inmates than in the general population. Among jail inmates, LTBI prevalence is 17 times higher than the prevalence in the general population. It is estimated that 500,000 inmates with LTBI are released nationwide every year.

Active TB is 15 times higher among jail inmates than in the general population. Two studies estimate that one third of those with active TB have been recently incarcerated.

Pulmonary TB has been reported to be as high as 3.75 times more common among foreign-born inmates and federal prisoners than among the general population.[13] Foreign-born inmates were 5.9 times more likely to have a positive TST result than U.S.-born inmates and accounted for 60% of recently diagnosed TB cases in the federal prison system.[14] Many local jails house foreign-born inmates as well. Among highly trained correctional health staff, the U.S. Public Health Service officers provide care to the majority of foreign-born inmates in federal prisons and in Immigration and Customs Enforcement, actively surveying, treating, and monitoring TB-related concerns.

Screening for TB infection is a top priority for most jails and prisons. This screening includes planting tuberculin skin tests, performing a chest radiography if positive, and then referring for treatment. Yet TB outbreaks do occur in jails and prisons because many inmates do not complete their LTBI treatment, thus creating an ideal situation to disperse the contagion.

Correctional institutions usually screen all inmates entering their facilities for TB. The Cook County Department of Corrections (Chicago), the Rikers Island Department of Corrections (New York), and the Washington, DC, jails are a few settings in which all incoming detainees receive routine radiographic screening for TB. Most jails and prisons conduct tuberculin screening tests. In addition, many facilities have TB coordinators who monitor the screening and treatment of TB among inmates (e.g., Oregon prison system, Chicago and New York jails). The high prevalence of TB in jails and prisons suggests that correctional PAs are at the forefront of this public health battle through surveillance, detection, and treatment.

Human Immunodeficiency Virus

A major portion of the HIV epidemic is seen in jails. Hammett and colleagues[2] estimate that approximately 25% of all U.S. HIV-infected persons passed through the correctional system in 1997. In 2012, the Bureau of Justice Statistics (BJS) reported that nearly one third of jail inmates had received an HIV test after admission.[15] There are no jails that conduct mandatory HIV testing, and the testing they do is less systematic than in prisons.[16]

Incarcerated women are 15 times more likely to be HIV infected than women in the general population. Black women, who bear a significant burden of the HIV epidemic, predominate in the nation's jails and prisons.

Acquired immunodeficiency syndrome (AIDS) was estimated to be three times more prevalent in prison than in the community in 2001.[17] Between 2001 and 2010, the rates for HIV/AIDS cases and AIDS-related deaths declined across all sizes of prison populations.[18] The stigma of HIV and AIDS is certainly an issue in the community, but it is even more pronounced in jails and prisons. After information about an inmate's HIV status is disclosed, it spreads throughout the institution, ostracizing the HIV-infected inmate even further in an already oppressive environment. Correctional PAs must take extra steps to protect the confidentiality of their patients' HIV status.

Screening for HIV in correctional institutions remains one of the more important public health strategies protecting community health. The potential of finding more seropositive individuals among high at-risk individuals and the potential of increasing HIV/AIDS awareness make correctional institution HIV screening a valuable resource. The Centers for Disease Control and Prevention (CDC) recommends routine testing for HIV and that a patient is to be notified that the testing will be performed unless he or she decides to opt out from the screening process.[18] Routine testing has the potential advantage to decrease any associated stigma when an inmate requests HIV testing.[18] Routine HIV testing on admission to prison may be ideal. However, in jails, this may be more problematic for a number of reasons.[19] The average jail detainee is released within 72 hours of booking, making it difficult to find an optimal time to implement routine HIV testing. In addition, many jails have limited resources to conduct such testing and may not be able to handle the

volume of inmates at the intake center or support the costs for providing such screening services.[19]

Another problem that jails face in implementing the routine HIV testing model is that when individuals are first arrested, they are stressed during the initial stages of incarceration. Issues such as addiction, potential suicide, and withdrawal from intoxication may cloud the individual's judgment, and he or she may opt out of the screening without fully understanding the benefits to such a test.[19] Also, with the open HIV testing model, the uncertainty of whether or not test results can be given to jail detainees in a reasonable time frame is an issue of concern.

There are unique barriers to the provision of health care to HIV-infected inmates in prisons and jails. Maintaining continuity of care is a major problem. A study by Bernard and colleagues[20] found a gross difference between correctional institutions and community-based HIV (CB-HIV) clinics. They analyzed 30 CB-HIV clinics against 90 correctional health professionals (representing 33 states). Approximately 43% of correctional institutions did not have access to HIV specialists compared with 93% in community-based HIV clinics. Disruption in highly active antiviral therapy (HAART) is reported in 71% of correctional institutions compared with 33% in community-based HIV clinics. Plasma HIV viral load testing is available in 65% of correctional institutions and in 87% of the community-based HIV clinics.

Health care services for HIV-infected inmates need to improve through better medication distribution schedules, better testing of CD4, viral load and genotyping needs, improved availability of HIV specialist access, and improved HIV information through peer education.[20] Improving the discharge planning of soon-to-be-released HIV-infected inmates, maintaining confidentiality, and gaining the trust of patients are other ways that the provision of health care to HIV-infected inmates can be improved.

Sexually Transmitted Diseases

The four most common sexually transmitted diseases (STDs) treated in a jail setting are syphilis, gonorrhea, *Chlamydia*, and genital herpes. The Institute of Medicine[21] has recommended that jails increase their efforts in the provision of STD screening, diagnosis, treatment, counseling and education, and partner notification. National Commission on Correctional Health Care (NCCHC) standards require that within 14 days of admission to jails and within 7 days of admission to prison, inmates are screened for STDs. However, because of the lack of health staff and resources, many correctional institutions do not adequately manage STDs; they may use "test results to diagnose and treat infections but do not routinely assess the burden of disease in their population."[22]

Syphilis

The positive test rate for syphilis is high among persons entering correctional facilities. The most high-prevention-value female cases have been found in jail settings.[22]

All persons with a positive syphilis test result should be tested for HIV because these diseases are epidemiologically linked. Patients who have latent syphilis should be evaluated for neurosyphilis. Careful evaluation and follow-up care for neonates born to syphilis-infected mothers are also recommended because mothers can transmit syphilis to their newborns.

Gonorrhea and Chlamydia

Because of their risky sexual behavior and lack of access to routine screening, jail inmates are at high risk for STDs, such as gonorrhea and *Chlamydia*. Urine testing has simplified screening techniques for chlamydial and gonococcal infections; however, because often medical staff and space are limited and there are large numbers of detainees to process, screening is not effectively accomplished. Policies that direct screening when the inmates complain of symptoms are ineffective because high rates of infected individuals do not report symptoms. For those who are tested, gonococcal and chlamydial infection rates are high.

The prevalence of *Chlamydia* among juveniles is high, mainly because of their high-risk sexual behavior. Public health departments can also provide an important service of follow-up care to adults and youths who are discharged from correctional institutions while still under treatment for *Chlamydia*.

Genital Herpes

Rapid and accurate diagnostic testing for genital herpes simplex virus (HSV) is unavailable in most correctional facilities.[22]

Treating patients with STDs in jails remains elusive and compounds a public health problem that could be remedied. Economic modeling has found that routine screening for STDs in prisons and jails is cost-effective.[15] An opportunity to improve the public's health is missed when jail health staff do not screen and treat for STDs. Along with aggressive screening, diagnostic, and treatment practices,

jail staff should use routine rapid STD screening and treatment and work with their local public health departments to ensure that contact and partner testing and counseling are accomplished.

Hepatitis

Corrections populations have high rates of hepatitis C. Estimates indicate that 12% to 39% of all Americans with hepatitis C have spent some time incarcerated. This clear and present public health threat requires consistent policies and programming. With the emergence of new treatments for hepatitis C that results in greater than 90% cure, screening, monitoring, and treatment policy development for correctional facilities are imperative for public health.

Another important strategy is vaccination. The CDC recommends that incarcerated populations receive hepatitis B vaccination. However, barriers to fully accomplishing these intervention strategies include cost; lack of staffing; and in the case of adolescents, the issue of consent.[23]

CHRONIC DISEASE IN CORRECTIONAL INSTITUTIONS

This section discusses the common correctional setting barriers to treatment of chronic diseases such as asthma, diabetes, and hypertension. Correctional PAs can play an important role in working with custody staff while advocating for patients' needs and encouraging self-management of chronic conditions among inmates.

Asthma

Data from the CDC show that a large disparity exists between minority populations and whites with asthma. Of the approximately 16 million U.S. adults with asthma in 2002, only 7.6% of whites, 15.6% of non-Hispanic multiple races, 11.6% of non-Hispanic American Indian and Alaska natives, and 9.3% of non-Hispanic blacks had the respiratory condition. Because correctional institutions have a high percentage of minorities, they will have a disproportionate burden of asthma. The CDC recommends targeted public health interventions to address these disparities.

Although asthma affects about 5% of the U.S. population, the NCCHC estimates that 8.5% of inmates have asthma.[3] The BJS, in its 2002 Survey of Inmates in Local Jails, reports that 9.9% of inmates have a current condition of asthma.

Many factors hinder asthma care in correctional institutions. Smoking restriction policies exist in a majority of correctional settings. However, some correctional institutions (except juvenile detention and confinement facilities) still permit cigarette smoking by inmates.

Other factors include environmental problems such as inadequate ventilation systems, poor temperature control, poor maintenance of air filters, and old physical structures with mold. As a result, exacerbation of asthma is high among inmates in these environments.

Many jails and prisons do not permit inmates to keep their inhalers, making it difficult for them to get timely access to their inhalers or, in some cases, timely access to urgent care. Many correctional institutions do not have adequate medication management systems that ensure medication continuity for asthmatic patients. Because of the nature of jails, where inmates bond out or are released within hours of their arrest, asthma care is episodic. Finally, inmates with asthma may be exposed to chemical means of restraint and other methods of control such as Mace, pepper spray, or Taser or stun guns. These may exacerbate their asthmatic condition.

Correctional PAs can improve the quality of life of their patients with asthma through steps that ensure appropriate categorization of patients' disease control and status as soon as they are admitted into the jail or prison. This care includes monitoring the patient's use of beta-agonist inhaler canisters during the month, offering and ensuring that patients receive flu vaccinations, and obtaining and documenting peak flow meter readings in assessing acute respiratory attacks.

One area in which correctional PAs can make a difference is tobacco control. Tobacco use before incarceration is a huge problem in this population. It is estimated that 80% of inmates used tobacco before their incarceration. Too often, inmates resume their tobacco addictions soon after release,[24] which, unfortunately, can lead to other addictive behaviors. Correctional PAs have an excellent opportunity to break the cycle by providing health education and guidance to inmates to cease tobacco use and other addictions and by referring inmates to appropriate counseling and addiction services.

Diabetes

The NCCHC estimates a prevalence of 4.8% of inmates with diabetes.[3] The BJS, in its 2002 Survey of Inmates in Local Jails, reported that 2.7% of inmates had a current condition of diabetes.

Inmates with insulin-treated diabetes should be identified within 2 hours of intake into jail; however, too often, they languish in police lockups (without any medical services) and are then transferred to jail. As a result, many do not receive health services for several hours. Rapid identification and treatment of inmates with diabetes do not universally occur.

Because inmates do not have easy access to medical staff or services, diabetic care is particularly difficult, especially with individuals with insulin-dependent diabetes. Institutional schedules such as mealtimes, pill lines, court appearances, school, and offender programming often interfere with consistent and routine diabetic care. Correctional PAs should work with their patients with diabetes and custody staff to develop flexible treatment strategies that allow inmates to work within the institutional schedule while maintaining diabetes control. This is especially true for patients with uncontrolled type 1 diabetes, who need extensive health care resources and institutional flexibility to manage their diabetes. Glucose control should be the priority. Facilities that cannot accommodate these patients' needs may not be the right place to house them. Inmates with uncontrolled type 1 diabetes should be housed in facilities with 24-hour nursing care.

The role of diet and exercise in maintaining glycemic control is well documented. Yet not all inmates with diabetes have access to daily exercise or low-fat, low-carbohydrate diets. In fact, medical nutrition is one of the most difficult factors to control in correctional institutions. Diabetic diets may be ordered, but the lack of communication or follow-through in the kitchen often results in failure to ensure that the right diet gets to the right patient. Supplemental food items in institutional commissaries are limited in heart-healthy snacks or alternatives to high-calorie, high-carbohydrate choices.

Correctional PAs can play an important role in the management of diabetes. Working with custody administration and staff, PAs can ensure that their patients with diabetes have appropriate opportunities for exercise and adequate diets and alternatives. Correctional PAs can take an active role in staff training and encouragement of patient self-management, as well as stressing the need to control carbohydrate consumption and participate in daily exercise.

Inmates' active involvement in diabetes management using self-monitoring equipment has been shown effective in the correctional setting.[17] Self-preparation of insulin remains under direct staff supervision because of security concerns.

Correctional PAs can advocate for opportunities for their inmate patients with diabetes to have a better understanding of how to control their disease through self-management and regulation. Correctional PAs can make a difference by providing annual and routine training sessions to all correctional staff on diabetes emergency care. In addition, by monitoring the status of soon-to-be-released patients with diabetes, correctional PAs can ensure that appropriate information and support are given so that follow-up in the community occurs.

Hypertension

The NCCHC estimates a prevalence of 18.3% of inmates with hypertension.[3] The BJS (2002) reported that 11.2% of inmates had a current condition of hypertension. In comparison, National Health and Nutrition Examination Survey (NHANES) data cite that 24% of the U.S. population has hypertension, and although hypertension among inmates is lower, it is significant given the fact that inmates are a relatively young population whose lifestyles and risky behavior have significantly reduced their morbidity.[3]

The treatment of patients with hypertension in correctional institutions is made more difficult because of the numbers involved and the lack of organizational capacity to manage it. For example, permission for inmates to keep their medications with their personal possessions is determined on a case-by-case basis and is often too restrictive. As a result, inmates lack timely access to medications to ensure continuity, they fail to receive timely follow-up assessment and treatment modification, and they lack opportunities to learn about self-management of their disease.

Correctional PAs can improve chronic hypertension care by ensuring that the patient's level of control and conditional status is properly categorized and that the patient is encouraged to gain self-management of his or her disease. Monitoring patient adherence through medication distribution systems and assessment of disease control are important strategies correctional PAs can use in managing their patients with hypertension.

MANAGING MENTAL HEALTH IN CORRECTIONAL INSTITUTIONS

When prisons were first developed in the United States, rehabilitation and social control dominated the debate as to what the main focus of imprisonment should be.[25] Little attention was given to mental health; however, since the 1980s, correctional institutions have evolved into repositories of mentally ill offenders. Today 20% of inmates have a serious persistent mental illness (SPMI).[26] Persons with SPMI deviate from social norms and acceptable behavior; as a result, they come to the attention of the criminal justice system. By default, correctional institutions warehouse individuals with SPMI. Ditton's[26] national study found that approximately 19% of all jail and prison inmates had severe mental illnesses. Although this study was performed before the introduction of mental health courts, the estimate of 20% of SPMI remains constant with other studies.[27]

Mental Health Screening

A little more than a quarter of federal inmates with mental health diagnoses have been incarcerated for three or more prior incarcerations. This is because mental health service efforts are often directed toward stabilization rather than treatment. The role of mental health is often seen as prompting individuals to adjust to the realities of incarceration. This short-term stabilization is a partial explanation why recidivism rates are so high because mentally ill inmates return to the community with little or no help, only to return to jail or prison.

The mental health capacities in U.S. jails are inadequate. In a study of correctional facilities,[3] it was found that 41.6% did not use a screening instrument to assess mental illness on newly arriving inmates. Rather, screening was generally performed by visual observation and inmate verbal report. Individuals who tested "positive" are referred to mental health for an in-depth and thorough mental health assessment, although some institutions did report that they use the Mental Health Screening Form III and the Beck Depression Inventory II (27.4% and 23%, respectively) to screen inmates for mental illness.

Suicide

Inmate suicides were the leading cause of death in 1983 (56% of all deaths), but because of improved standards and training, suicide rates have steadily declined. In 2002, the jail suicide rate was 47 per 100,000, compared with 129 per 100,000 inmates in 1983.[28] Prisons have steadily maintained their suicide rate of 16 per 100,000 since 1990 (from a high of 34 per 100,000 in 1980).[28] In comparison, jails have a suicide rate four times that of the national average, which in 2004 was 11.05 suicides per 100,000.[29]

Rates of inmate suicide are closely related to jail size. More than 40% of the nation's jails house fewer than 50 inmates, and in 2002, they had a suicide rate of 47 per 100,000 inmates.[28] These small jails had a suicide rate five times higher than the largest jail systems (an average daily population of at least 1500 inmates). Reasons for this phenomenon include lack of adequate staffing, insufficient training, inadequate housing, and failure to properly screen individuals into the jail.

Suicide prevention efforts begin with well-trained staff who aggressively conduct intake screening and provide ongoing assessment of all inmates entering the correctional facility. Five points in time are especially important in monitoring individuals for suicidal ideation during their confinement: initial admission into the facility, after adjudication when the inmate is returned to the facility from court, after receipt of bad news or after suffering any type of humiliation or rejection, confinement in isolation or segregation, and after a prolonged stay in the facility.[30]

Correctional PAs should take an active role in the screening and assessment process to identify inmate suicide risk. Being alert to behavioral cues that an inmate might be contemplating suicide is ultimately the strongest preventive measure that correctional staff can demonstrate. Correctional PAs can help to prevent inmate suicides by establishing trust with inmates, gathering pertinent information, and taking action through effective communication.

Gender Dysphoria

In the realm of transgender populations, PAs may find themselves on the forefront of evaluation, treatment, counseling, and medical management of individuals diagnosed with gender dysphoria. Gender dysphoria is defined in the *Diagnostic and Statistical Manual of Mental Disorder* (DSM-5) as "A strong and persistent cross-gender identification. It is manifested by a stated desire to be the opposite sex and persistent discomfort with his or her biologically assigned sex." Working with psychological services, PAs seeing transgender inmates are faced with ever-changing clinical practice guidelines as case laws are decided and further ethical responsibilities as more inmates identify themselves as lesbian, gay, bisexual, or transgender. This is an area of correctional medicine that requires culturally competent PAs for effective management.

Co-occurring Disorders

The relationship between drugs and crime is well established, with about half of state inmates and a third of federal prisoners reporting that they committed their current offense while under the influence of alcohol or drugs.[31] In 2002, 68% of jail inmates reported symptoms in the year before their admission to jail that met substance dependence or abuse criteria.[32] Studies consistently report that between 72% and 78% of inmates with mental illness have a co-occurring drug or alcohol abuse problem.[33] Yet despite this well-established relationship of mental illness, drugs, and crime, few jails and prisons use a formal validated screening instrument for drug abuse among their entering inmates.[34]

In a 2006 study, 81.9% of the jails and prisons surveyed reported that receiving screening (which constitutes observation and inquiring for alcohol or drug use) is the most often used method to assess for drug abuse.[34] About a third of the respondents indicated that they use the Addiction Severity Index (ASI) and the Alcohol Use Subscale (ASI-Alcohol) to screen for substance abuse disorders. Sadly, 16.4% of the respondents indicated that they use no instruments to screen for substance abuse. Correctional PAs should promote the use of accurate and timely screening instruments for substance abuse.

Correctional PAs should find additional guidance in treating inmates with drug abuse by reviewing *Principles of Drug Abuse Treatment for Criminal Justice Populations.* They will find support for comprehensive reentry services designed to minimize relapse and recidivism.[35]

SPECIAL ISSUES IN CORRECTIONS

Pain Management

One issue that challenges all corrections health professionals is how to differentiate between legitimate pain sufferers and those manifesting drug-seeking behavior. Nearly 70% of the incarcerated populations are charged with serious drug offenses and have some sort of drug-seeking behavior.[32] Distinguishing between a true chronic pain sufferer from an individual who is manipulating and seeking drugs is something that a correctional PA learns to do quickly.

The history is an important way to distinguish pain sufferers from manipulators. A true chronic pain sufferer is someone who has narrowed his or her selection of medications to actually find some, but not total, relief. The drug-seeking individual, on the other hand, will have a polypharmacy approach, often mixing classes of drugs "without finding any relief."

Associated pain with movement is another way to distinguish legitimate chronic pain sufferers from those exhibiting drug-seeking behavior. A legitimate chronic pain sufferer generally reports being pain free at rest, but an individual who expresses multifocal pain at rest may indeed have some drug manipulation issues.

Nonmalignant pain management in correctional institutions is complex. Because incarcerated populations have documented histories of trauma, mental illness, and substance abuse disorders, clinicians find it difficult to assess what and how much to prescribe to this population. Correctional PAs can find supplemental information by reviewing the NCCHC's *Position Statement on Chronic Pain Management*, which can be found at http://www.ncchc.org/position-statements.

End of Life

Several factors contribute to the incarcerated population's death rate. Data on prisoner deaths remain sketchy; however, limited studies have indicated that when compared with the same age groups of civilians (such as 55–65 years and 65 years and older), prisoners have significantly higher mortality rates from malignant neoplasms, chronic liver disease, pneumonia, septicemia, and HIV/AIDS.[36]

How are terminally ill inmates managed? In general, there are two options to managing terminally ill inmates in prison. The first is to compassionately release dying inmates to community settings. A compassionate or early medical release program permits terminally ill patients to return to the community and be housed in a home care setting, a hospice, or a long-term care skilled nursing facility. In this way, a terminally ill prisoner can return home to be near his or her family in the last stages of death. However, there are many barriers to the liberal use of compassionate release programming. A prisoner's criminal record, public safety concerns, statutory limitations, and public activism against release have prohibited the compassionate release of some prisoners. The lack of community resources to accept transferees from prisons or the lack of outside family support may in fact disqualify a prisoner for an early release. In addition, the approval process may be inordinately long. Approvals for early release may require an independent medical board, a judge, a prosecutor, and even public input before a decision is made to allow an individual to be released early and die outside the prison setting. It is common for prisons to release an inmate hours before he or she dies.

The second option is to create a correctional hospice program. There are a number of barriers to developing a hospice program, which include a lack of funding, a staff that is untrained in hospice care, and a prison culture that fosters suspicion and insensitivity. Approximately 85% of hospice patients receive Medicare coverage for services. Yet prisoners are not Medicare or Medicaid eligible, so any hospice-type service that is provided in correctional institutions is absorbed within the department budget or through pro bono activity by community hospice agencies. Most departments of corrections do not have formal hospice programs. Nearly 70% of terminally ill inmates are kept in infirmaries, about 10% are compassionately released, and 20% are cared for in a hospice program.[37] Thus, hospice training and experience among correctional health workers is limited. Finally, the prison culture hampers the implementation of hospice care. Many consider correctional institutions as places for harsh punishment, assuming an attitude that demonizes inmates, providing as few services as possible. This includes hospice care. Some staff members believe that palliative or hospice care would be "coddling prisoners"[37] and, as such, does not provide an appropriate tone for a prison. Another barrier to overcome is that inmates have a dim view of death and dying behind the "walls" and would rather be transferred to an outside hospital or have a compassionate release so they can be with family and friends during their last stages of life. State rules governing such releases are often not supportive for compassionate releases, so with an increase in the elderly inmate population and terminal illness, there will be more need for hospice services.

Correctional PAs are often involved in hospice and end-of-life care issues. Providing clinical support for a dying inmate is one aspect of that involvement, but correctional PAs can also be involved in providing support to staff and inmate volunteer workers who are involved in hospice care. Training of staff and providing psychological support are some of the ways that correctional PAs can be involved in hospice care.

One area of death that correctional PAs should not be involved in is executions. The mandate from professional organizations is clear on this point. The American Academy of Physician Assistants' policy prohibits PAs from participating in executions. The NCCHC standard and position statement for health care professionals prohibits the involvement of health staff in any aspect of the execution process.[38] The ethical conundrum of establishing a therapeutic relationship with a patient, only to participate in his or her termination of life, is one that few PAs face; nonetheless, many correctional PAs have had to face this and many other ethical dilemmas on a daily basis.

MANAGING ETHICAL CONFLICTS IN CORRECTIONAL INSTITUTIONS

Autonomy

Correctional health care is the nexus among criminal justice, public health, law, and ethics. And although the challenging ethical issues of the correctional health care field are similar to those in the community, the nature of prisons and jails limits autonomy and choice. Correctional medicine ethics is much more complex because there are no clear-cut guidelines for an ethical conduct of correctional health professionals.

The competing priorities between correctional interests and health interests continuously provide flashpoints of conflict and tension. For example, one cornerstone of medical ethics is patient freedom of choice. In a prison or jail setting, patients' choices of providers are limited. Their ability to choose or change health providers is limited and in many cases not an option. Likewise, if a PA is having difficulty communicating with a troublesome patient, there is little opportunity to change to a different health care professional. As a result, both the patient and PA are stuck with each other and must resolve their issues.

Issues such as informed consent and refusal of treatment are complex in correctional settings. Inmates have the right to be informed of the risks and benefits of proposed procedures and therapies and may refuse. However, can an inmate refuse treatment for a health condition that poses a risk to others? Correctional health staff are obligated to ensure the safety and public health of institutions. Medical isolation is usually the first step to contain an infectious inmate who refuses treatment. If the inmate remains recalcitrant, correctional health clinicians will obtain a court order to enact appropriate care. However, system disincentives, such as payment of a fee for health services or programming conflicts between sick call and court visits, might be causes for inmate refusals and should be analyzed. Other possible alternatives should be investigated.

The ethical conundrum is that when inmates are protesting their condition of confinement, refusal, such as hunger strikes or refusal to abide by custody rules, may be their only alternative. The dilemma that correctional health clinicians find themselves in is protecting the patient's health and life while honoring his or her efforts to effect system change. In these situations, correctional PAs need to educate and communicate with their patients and custody officials to alleviate conflict and improve clinical outcomes.

Justice

One ethical tenet is that patients are to be treated equally. Health care professionals are taught that they must remain neutral in their perspective about the patients they encounter and treat them accordingly. This ethical principle is put to the test every day in correctional medicine. How would you feel about treating a child molester who has diabetes?

Would a rapist with *Chlamydia* be treated any differently? This can be a major deterrent for many PAs who are new to correctional health care, and it can put their professional objectivity to the test every day. Regardless of their criminality, inmates should receive health care that is at community care standards.

Beneficence

The ethical principle of acting only for the benefit of the patient is *beneficence*. Correctional clinicians are challenged with regard to what constitutes beneficence for the patient or obligations to the state. For example, contraband in a correctional institution is a serious problem because it jeopardizes the safety and security of everyone. Body cavity searches are one method that correctional administrators use to ensure that contraband is not entering the facility. This presents a conflict for the correctional clinician who should conduct his or her actions with beneficence and resist efforts to have them conduct body cavity searches on their patients. Of course, if there is sufficient medical indication to conduct a body cavity search, then it should be performed.

Another issue that challenges the principle of beneficence is competency for execution. Establishing a therapeutic relationship is contingent on a goal to restore the individual to full function and thus improve his or her quality of life. It is antithesis to cases when the goal is restoring an individual's competency in order to carry out an execution sentence. The NCCHC position statement advises correctional clinicians that restoring an inmate to competency for the purposes of execution should be made by an independent expert and not by any health care professional regularly in the employment of or under contract to provide health care with the correctional institution or system holding the inmate.[38] This requirement does not diminish the responsibility of correctional health care personnel to treat any mental illness of death row inmates.

Confidentiality

In an environment where there are "no secrets," it is difficult to protect the confidentiality of inmates' health problems. Maintaining confidentiality and privacy of patient information is difficult under circumstances when control is not maintained by health staff. The use of per diem workers, visiting clinicians, and other temporary health care providers also complicates how confidentiality is maintained.

The principle of confidentiality ensures the patient that disclosure of specific information given to the provider during a course of treatment will remain confidential. Because this can be complicated in a jail or prison, correctional PAs have to work harder to gain patient trust in a therapeutic relationship. When an inmate tells a clinician that he broke his jaw "while slipping in the shower" or "tripping and hitting my bunk bed," the clinician needs to understand that pressing for more information could jeopardize the patient–clinician relationship. On the other hand, if an inmate tells the clinician, in the course of a clinical encounter, that his new tattoo was obtained in the cell block, the clinician has the responsibility of informing custody that there is a potential that contraband material (ink, needles) is present in the prison. Discerning the difference between patient-specific confidential information and information that must be shared with custody staff is a fine line that many correctional PAs must negotiate.

FUTURE DIRECTIONS

Correctional PAs serve to educate inmates about appropriate management of their acute and chronic health conditions, disease prevention, and healthy lifestyles in anticipation of release. The planning for release and continuity of care begins at intake.

The Patient Protection and Affordable Care Act (PPACA) will increase access to health insurance via Medicaid for many low-income individuals. What is not known is how returning inmates, with untreated mental health and substance abuse needs, will affect the changing public health landscape. As the PPACA regulation unfolds, its impact on correctional health care and the reentry population will need to be closely watched.

CONCLUSION

Unlike their noncorrectional colleagues, PAs who work in jails and prisons have unique challenges to their professional ethics and personal beliefs. Some are well suited for this work environment, but others do not fare well. This chapter has described the areas that are unique in correctional medicine, which are often not discussed in PA educational programs.

Why would a PA want to work in a jail or prison? After all, working conditions in U.S. prisons and jails are what you would expect in developing countries' health care systems, where patients often present to the clinic late in the course of their disease; they have self-medicated with legend drugs or traditional treatments; the health facilities are so poor that they may delay diagnosis; referrals (if needed) are not easily arranged; there are problems with shortages of trained staff; there is poor infection control and lack of follow-up

care; and the "patient may be unable (e.g., because of financial hardship) to fully adhere to treatment."[39]

Beyond the similarity between U.S. correctional institutions and those of developing countries, why would you want to provide health care to patients who are seeking to "game the system" or who have had little contact for health care services? The answer lies in the PA's role. Practicing correctional medicine creates an opportunity for PAs to advocate for individual and community health, two cornerstones of the profession.

As patient advocates, correctional PAs have the opportunity to make a difference in the lives of disadvantaged and disenfranchised populations who need specialists in public health, primary care, infectious disease, and chronic disease. PAs may see inmates in clinical, emergency, and consultation settings for their acute and chronic conditions. Jails and prisons are challenged in caring for inmates with physical disabilities, congenital issues, and sensory and cognitive deficits. Rising costs for care further challenge correctional administrators to review requests for compassionate release, transferring these costs to society.

Correctional PAs can advocate for improved conditions of confinement and improved health services, making improvements in clinical care and patient outcomes.

An average day in the life of a correctional PA is complete with clinical and administrative responsibilities (see Case Study 43.1). Seeing patients in a variety of settings such as segregation cells, sick call clinics, and inpatient settings while performing a number of administrative tasks is a dynamic that creates opportunities for correctional PAs to advocate for patient needs.

As advocates for public health, PAs working in corrections address issues that directly prevent the spread of disease into our communities and have an impact on eliminating health care disparity to disenfranchised populations.

CASE STUDY 43.1 A DAY IN THE LIFE OF A FEDERAL CORRECTIONAL PHYSICIAN ASSISTANT

7:00 AM Arrive at work. Exchange chit for keys, pepper spray, handcuffs, and radio. Enter the secure perimeter through sally ports (systematic gated entry). Check in box in the medical records area for inmate-related correspondence, including laboratory reports, consultation summaries, and new intake records, that require review and action before uploading into the electronic medical record.

7:20 AM Go to the segregation (SEG) unit, and conduct rounds to offer inmates an opportunity to address health issues. (The SEG unit is a seclusion unit that houses inmates restricted from the general population.)

8:00 AM Sign on to a computer to scan emails, perform required policy reviews, and complete required training activities.

8:15 AM Attend the morning report all-hands meeting to review patient health issues that occurred since the last meeting, overnight events, and the current day's schedule. Health services staff announcements are also made.

8:40 AM Address any urgent clinical issues deemed "same day" from the sick call triage clinic and follow up on issues addressed overnight by the covering clinical staff.

9:30 AM Scheduled sick call or chronic care clinic inmate appointments are seen, and all documentation is completed using the electronic medical record. This includes any visit records, orders, and consultation request. Emails are checked between visits.

11:00 AM Preview and confirm appointments scheduled for the next day; perform chart review for responding to inmate written inquires, complete transfer summary requests, and perform mortality record review and any required peer reviews.

12:00 noon Lunch

12:30 PM Afternoon scheduled appointments begin, including history and physical examinations for newly admitted inmates and preoperative clearances. At any time, an employee may present with a work-related injury for assessment. I may be assigned to act for the assistant health administrator who represents the Health Service Department in several institution meetings and be present during the midday inmate mealtime for "open house."

3:00 PM During the afternoon, inmates return from out-of-institution trips. They stop in for triage until cleared to return to the general population. As the afternoon winds down, there are numerous reports waiting to be completed, including prerelease paperwork; transfer paperwork; responses to the courts for medical study cases; required training; and any meetings called such as team meetings, staff meetings, and occasional continuing medical education sessions.
I meet with my clinical supervising physician to review chronic care and newly admitted inmate plans of care that encountered countersignatures throughout the day. The nonclinical duties are squeezed in as time permits. As the day winds down, I take another look at emails, check voicemail, and check my mailbox.

3:45 PM Shut down the computer. Return to the control area to exchange equipment for my personal chits, and exit the secure perimeter. Every day is full, and no two days are exactly alike.

CLINICAL APPLICATIONS

- Is the clinical management of infectious diseases such as HIV or hepatitis C any different in a prison or jail setting?
- Serious persistent mental illnesses are a great concern in prisons and jails. How can PAs be clinically prepared to manage patients with these conditions?
- Will it be safe to work or do a clinical rotation in corrections?

KEY POINTS

- Ensuring that inmates have access to health care services is a fundamental responsibility of correctional medical professionals. Inmates have a higher prevalence of health problems than the general population, both acute and chronic, that require well-trained health experts such as correctional PAs.
- Correctional health care is the nexus among criminal justice, public health, law, and ethics. Correctional medicine should not be quickly dismissed because it provides the opportunity to make a difference in the lives of disadvantaged and disenfranchised populations that need specialists in public health, primary care, infectious disease, and chronic disease.
- Correctional medicine is one of the cornerstones of public health in this country. As patient advocates, correctional PAs have an opportunity to make progress on eliminating health disparities.
- The safety of inmates, staff, and visitors takes priority in correctional institutions, and many decisions that would seem inconsequential in the free world take on great importance in corrections. PAs working in a correctional environment need to know that it is a constant balance between public safety and public health.
- The recruiting, training, and retaining of health professionals to work in correctional health care are difficult because prisons and jails do not have medical care as the primary mission.

AUTHOR DISCLOSURE STATEMENT

Robin N. Hunter Buskey, DHSc, PA-C, Senior Physician Assistant, U.S. Department of Justice, Federal Bureau of Prisons.

Opinions expressed are those of the author and do not necessarily represent the opinions of the Federal Bureau of Prisons or the U.S. Department of Justice.

ACKNOWLEDGMENTS

The author thanks R. Scott Chavez for his career commitment to excellence for correctional health care and for his creative wisdom for this chapter in the previous editions.

The author thanks Pieter VanHorn, PA-C, Senior Physician Assistant, Health Services Administrator, Federal Correctional Institution McKean, Lewis Run, Pennsylvania, for his review of the manuscript and valuable comments.

References

1. Harrison PM, Beck AJ. *Prison and jail inmates at midyear 2005* (Bureau of Justice Statistics Special Report, NCJ 213133). Washington, DC: National Criminal Justice Reference Service; 2006.
2. Hammett TM, Harmon MP, Rhodes W. The burden of infectious disease among inmates of and releases from U.S. correctional facilities. *Am J Public Health*. 2002;92:1789–1794.
3. National Commission on Correctional Health Care (2002). Health status of the soon to be released inmate (Vols. I and II). http://www.ncchc.org/health-status-of-soon-to-be-released-inmates. Accessed December 20, 2015.
4. Estelle v. Gamble, 429 U.S. 97 (1976).
5. Farmer v. Brennan, 511 U.S. 825 (1994).
6. Tillery v. Owens. 719 F. Supp 1256, 1286 (W.D.Pa. 1989) aff'd, 907 F.2d 418 (3rd Circ. 1990).
7. Johnson D. Legal issues related to managing the challenging mentally ill. Atlanta, GA: Presented at the National Commission on Correctional Health Care Conference; October 2006.
8. Thornton RL. *New Approaches to Staff Safety*. 2nd ed. Washington, DC: U.S. Department of Justice, National Institute of Corrections; 2002.
9. Human Rights Watch. *No Escape: Eale Rape in U.S. Prisons*. New York: Human Rights Watch; 2001.
10. Prison Rape Elimination Act of 2003. https://www.gpo.gov/fdsys/pkg/PLAW-108publ79/pdf/PLAW-108publ79.pdf. Accessed December 20, 2015.
11. Federal Bureau of Prisons. *Management of Methicillin-Resistant Staphylococcus aureus (MRSA) Infections*. Washington, DC: Federal Bureau of Prisons; 2012. http://www.bop.gov/resources/pdfs/mrsa.pdf. Accessed December 20, 2015.
12. MacNeil JR, Lobato MN, Moore M. An unanswered health disparity: tuberculosis among correctional inmates, 1993 through 2003. *Am J Public Health*. 2005;95:1800–1805.
13. Rao NA. Prevalence of pulmonary tuberculosis in Karachi central prison. *J Pakistan Med Assoc*. 2004;54(8):413–415.
14. Saunders DL, Olive DM, Wallace SB, et al. Tuberculosis screening in the federal prison system: an opportunity to treat and prevent tuberculosis in foreign-born populations. *Public Health Rep*. 2001;116(3):210–218.
15. Kraut JR, Haddix AC, Carande-Kulis V, Greifinger RB. *Cost-effectiveness of routine screening for sexually transmitted diseases among inmates in United States prisons and jails. In: Health Status of the Soon to Be Released Inmate. Vol. 2*. Chicago:

16. Spaulding AC, Jacob-Arriola K, Ramos KL, et al. Primary care in jail settings: report on a consultants' meeting. *J Correctional Health Care*. 2007;13(2):93–128.
17. Hunter Buskey RN, Mathieson K, Leafman JS, et al. The effect of blood glucose self-monitoring among inmates with diabetes. *J Correct Health Care*. 2015;21(4):343–354.
18. Beckwith CG, Poshkus M. HIV behind bars: meeting the need for HIV testing, education, and access to care. *Infect Dis Corrections Rep*. 2007;9(17):3–4.
19. Kavasery R, Altice FL. Routine HIV testing in jails: addressing the challenges. *Infect Dis Corrections Rep*. 2007;9(17):3.
20. Bernard K, Sueker JJ, Colton E, et al. Provider perspectives about the standard of HIV care in correctional settings and comparison to the community standard of care: how do we measure up? *Infect Dis Corrections Rep*. 2006;9(3):1–6.
21. U.S. Institute of Medicine. *The Hidden Epidemic: Confronting Sexually Transmitted Diseases* (a report prepared by the Committee on Prevention and Control of Sexually Transmitted Diseases). Washington, DC: National Academies Press; 1997.
22. Kahn RH, Joesoef R, Aynalem G, et al. Overview of sexually transmitted diseases. In: Puisis M, ed. *Clinical Practice in Correctional Medicine*. 2nd ed. Philadelphia: Mosby Elsevier; 2006:175–181.
23. Tedeschi SK, Bonney LE, Manalo R, et al. Vaccination in juvenile correctional facilities: state practices, hepatitis B, and the impact on anticipated sexually transmitted infection vaccines. *Public Health Rep*. 2007;122(1):44–48.
24. Cropsey KL, Kristeller JL. The effects of a prison smoking ban on smoking behavior and withdrawal symptoms. *Addict Behav*. 2005;30(3):589–594.
25. Rothman DJ. Perfecting the prison: United States, 1789–1865. In: Morris N, Rothman DJ, eds. *The Oxford History of the Prison: The Practice of Punishment in Western Society*. New York: Oxford University Press; 1998:102–116.
26. Ditton PM. *Mental Health and Treatment of Inmates and Probationers*. Washington, DC: Department of Justice; 1999.
27. Teplin LA. Psychiatric and substance abuse disorders among male urban jail detainees. *Am J Public Health*. 1994;84:290–293.
28. Mumola CJ. Suicide and homicide in state prisons and local jails. Bureau of Justice Statistics. August 2005. U.S. Department of Justice, Office of Justice Programs. NCJ 210036. http://www.bjs.gov/content/pub/pdf/shsplj.pdf. Accessed December 20, 2015.
29. Centers for Disease Control and Prevention. Suicide: facts at a glance, 2007. http://www.cdc.gov/ncipc/dvp/suicide/SuicideDataSheet.pdf. Accessed September 26, 2007.
30. Hayes L. *Guide to developing and revising suicide prevention protocols. NCCHC Standards for Health Services in Jails*. Chicago: National Commission on Correctional Health Care; 2003:159–164.
31. Mumola CJ, Substance abuse and treatment, state and federal prisoners. 1997; U.S. Department of Justice, Office of Justice Programs. NCJ 172871. http://www.bjs.gov/content/pub/pdf/satsfp97.pdf. Accessed December 20, 2015.
32. Karberg JC, James DJ. Substance dependence, abuse, and treatment of jail inmates, 2002. Bureau of Justice Statistics Special Report No. NCJ 209588. U.S. Department of Justice Office of Justice Programs. http://www.bjs.gov/content/pub/pdf/sdatji02.pdf. Accessed December 20, 2015.
33. McNiel DE, Binder RL, Robinson JC. Incarceration associated with homelessness, mental disorder, and co-occurring substance abuse. *Psychiatr Serv*. 2005;56(7):840–846.

National Commission on Correctional Health Care; 2002: 81–108. http://www.ncchc.org/filebin/Health_Status_vol_2.pdf. Accessed December 22, 2016.

34. Chavez RS. An assessment of U.S. jail and prison screening and treatment practices for drug abuse and co-occurring disorders. Atlanta: Poster presentation at the American Association for the Treatment of Opioid Dependence; 2006.

35. National Institute on Drug Abuse. Principles of drug abuse treatment for criminal justice populations (revised; NIH Publication No. 06–5316). https://d14rmgtrwzf5a.cloudfront.net/sites/default/files/txcriminaljustice_0.pdf. Accessed December 20, 2015.

36. Mumola CJ. Medical causes of death in state prisons; 2001-2004. Data Brief, U.S. Department of Justice, Office of Justice Programs. NCJ 216340. Bureau of Justice Statistics. http://www.bjs.gov/content/pub/pdf/mcdsp04.pdf. Accessed December 20, 2015.

37. Maull FW. Delivery of end-of-life care in prisons and jails. In: Puisis M, ed. *Clinical Practice in Correctional Medicine*. 2nd ed. Philadelphia: Mosby Elsevier; 2006:529–537.

38. National Commission on Correctional Health Care. Position statement on competency for executions, 1988, p. 195. standards for Health Services in Prisons. Chicago: National Commission on Correctional Health Care; reaffirmed 2012.

39. Chavez RS. The incarcerated male. In: Heidelbaugh J, ed. *Clinical Men's Health: Evidence in Practice*. Amsterdam: Elsevier; 2007:532–547.

The resources for this chapter can be found at www.expertconsult.com.

The faculty resources can be found online at www.expertconsult.com.

MILITARY MEDICINE

Ron W. Perry

The U.S. Military is us. There is no truer representation of a country than the people that it sends into the field to fight for it. The people who wear our uniform and carry our rifles into combat are our kids, and our job is to support them, because they're protecting us.
—Tom Clancy

It is appropriate that any physician assistant (PA) textbook include a chapter covering military medicine, as this profession began with four Vietnam Veterans (Navy Hospital Corpsmen) being selected to matriculate at the original Duke University PA Program in 1965. Since then, 200 accredited programs have come online here in the United States, with well over 100,000 PAs having faithfully and competently provided patient care over the past half century. The federal government continues to be the largest employer of PAs, with approximately 2800 active-duty PAs currently serving in the armed forces.

HISTORY OF MILITARY PHYSICIAN ASSISTANTS

Shortages in U.S. health care systems (civilian and military) during the 1960s resulted in needs not being fulfilled by physicians. Shortfalls in military physician recruiting were made more serious by the unpopular war in Vietnam. A decrease in the availability of health care providers to U.S. Department of Defense

(DoD) beneficiaries became a reality, and physician scholarship programs were initiated to bring more physicians into the military services. This shortage, however, was not relieved in the 4-year period of time it took for a physician to be educated. Even after a medical student had been selected to receive a scholarship that obligated him or her to military service, it took 5 years for a general medical officer (GMO) (who has no residency training) to be educated and up to 9 years for a board-eligible physician or surgeon to be trained. PAs and other physician extenders, such as nurse practitioners, were seen as the short-term answer to a potentially long-term problem.

By 1970, the DoD had initiated plans to start training PAs. In March 1971, the DoD answered a number of questions concerning the nature of the position, training, and degree of PA independence by issuing the following definition[1]:

The military Physician's Assistant is a skilled health professional who is not a physician but who by experience and formal training has become qualified to perform certain tasks formerly undertaken only by a physician. He works under the supervision of a medical officer, though he may at times serve some distance from the physician and receive instruction and guidance by telephone or other means of communication. He may perform selected tasks delegated to him by the physician supervisor who is responsible for his actions. His principal duties will involve direct contact with patients to obtain medical histories and to perform physical examinations, order appropriate laboratory and x-ray studies, interpret and record these data and prescribe limited therapy. He is considered to meet the criteria of the "Type-A" Physician's Assistant as defined by the Board of Medicine of the National Academy of Science, May 1970.

By 1971, the use of PAs in outpatient care was rapidly on the rise in military and civilian settings, but with approximately only 1800 PAs nationally, it was clear that the military would have to get into the business of training their own.[2] The Army and Air Force established their PA training programs in 1971. The school that Army PA students attended was the Medical Field Services School PA program at Fort Sam Houston, Texas. The Air Force started its training program at the School of Health Care Sciences, Sheppard Air Force Base. The Navy joined the Air Force program by 1972 but also later established its own training sites in Virginia and California before eventually sending students to train with the Army at Fort Sam Houston. The Coast Guard initially relied on recruiting civilian PAs or sending enlisted personnel to civilian PA programs but eventually joined the Air Force Sheppard program in 1990.

In all cases, those chosen for these programs were enlisted military members with broad military and medical backgrounds. The curriculum at each of these programs consisted of 1 year of didactic training at a military educational facility followed by a 1-year rotational clinical practicum in a military hospital. Upon successful completion of the 2-year programs, these new military PAs were credentialed by either the military hospital to which they were assigned or the military hospital that had medical supervision over their clinical practice. There was a lack of standardization and support in the military respective medical communities, leaving these initial PAs positioned within the enlisted and warrant officer ranks. By 1978, the Air Force began commissioning PAs as officers followed by the Navy in 1989, the Coast Guard in 1990, and the Army in 1992.

THE INTERSERVICE PHYSICIAN ASSISTANT PROGRAM

In 1996, the military services combined their various PA programs to form the Interservice Physician Assistant Program (IPAP), located at Fort Sam Houston, San Antonio, Texas (Fig. 44.1). The sponsoring institution was the Army Medical Department Center and School (AMEDDC&S), and IPAP was aligned under the Academy of Health Sciences. The AMEDDC&S

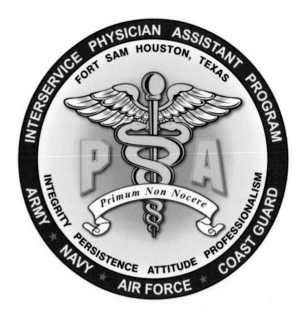

FIG. 44.1 ■ Logo of the Interservice Physician Assistant Program (IPAP). (Courtesy of the author, 2015.)

leadership reached an agreement with the University of Nebraska Medical Center (UNMC) that the latter would provide faculty and administrative support for the IPAP. This was followed by program accreditation through the Commission on Accreditation of Allied Health Education Programs (CAAHEP) in 1997. The Healthcare Interservice Training Advisory Board (HC-ITAB) formally consolidated and approved the new accredited program for the Army (including the Guard and Reserves), Navy (including the Marine Corps), Air Force (including the Air Guard), and Coast Guard. This new program convened its first class in April 1996.

The IPAP mission is to provide the uniformed services with highly competent, compassionate PAs who model integrity, strive for leadership excellence, and are committed to lifelong learning. Graduates are commissioned into the officer corps of their respective service and take their place beside other military health care professionals in providing medical services to active duty military personnel, their dependents, and retirees. It takes a dedicated and cohesive team of Army, Navy, Air Force, Coast Guard, and civilian faculty and staff to successfully lead military students with as few as 60 college semester hours through an extremely intense 29-month curriculum culminating in the Master of Physician Assistant Studies (MPAS) degree and commissioning as a military officer. The IPAP faculty and staff team at phase 1 are composed of PAs, physicians, science officers, and others. Phase 2 is primarily staffed with clinicians who precept and teach the PA students at 22 geographically diverse clinical military training sites.

From 1996 to 2001, the IPAP graduated PAs with a bachelor of science degree. Beginning in 2002, IPAP graduates earned a bachelor's degree at the end of phase 1 and an MPAS degree at the end of phase 2. In 2009, because of the wartime need for PAs in the DoD and Department of Homeland Security (DHS), the IPAP increased the throughput to up to 240 students per year (up to 80 entering in three classes). This led to a total yearly enrollment of up to 480 (240 in phase 1 and 240 in phase 2), solidifying the IPAP as the largest PA program in existence. Also in 2009, the IPAP was organizationally moved from the PA Branch to the newly created Graduate School located at the AMEDDC&S. The Graduate School is composed of graduate programs in physical therapy, nursing anesthesia, nutrition, social work, pastoral care, and health care administration. This change led to a dynamic graduate-level environment and culture of education, service, and research. When the *U.S. News and World Report* rankings were published in 2011 ("Best Graduate Schools in America"), all of the programs in the Graduate School were ranked among the best in the country. The IPAP was ranked 13th of PA programs nationally.

In 2010, the IPAP extended the length of the program from 24 to 29 months. This allowed the program to go from an extremely compact, three-trimester didactic format (in 12 months) to a more reasonable four-semester delivery over a 16-month period. The students must successfully complete 100 semester hours of competency-based curriculum in this period before advancing to phase 2. The clinical portion was also extended from 12 months to 13 months to facilitate the change in station move to a phase 2 training site for students and their families, as well as hospital orientation, Health Insurance Portability and Accountability Act, Advanced Cardiovascular Life Support (ACLS), and other necessary training courses. Upon successful completion of all phase 2 rotations and program requirements, the student is granted another 52 semester hours, for a 29-month program total of 152 semester hours.

IPAP graduates receive a certificate of completion (from the sponsoring institution, AMEDDC&S), which enables them to sit for the National Commission for Certification of Physician Assistants (NCCPA) certifying examination. They are also conferred an MPAS degree from the affiliate university. A competitive bid process determines the affiliate university, which is currently the University of Nebraska Medical Center. Military PAs take great pride in their PA program, and rightfully so. The IPAP moved higher in ranking in the March 2015

U.S. News and World Report rankings and is now ranked number 11 in the nation.[3] As of this writing, four of the past five graduating cohorts have scored a first-time pass rate of 100% on the NCCPA certification examination. The NCCPA PANCE 5-year first time pass rate average for the IPAP is 97%, which compares very favorably with notable academic programs such as Duke University (96%), which admits students with a minimum of a baccalaureate degree, over 1 year of direct patient care experience, and an annual throughput of 80 students.

RECRUITING CHALLENGES

The armed forces continue to rely heavily on the IPAP to meet their respective PA inventory shortfalls, and the IPAP works hard to meet that demand by producing an average of 169 new PAs every year. In addition, there are limited scholarship opportunities for civilian PA students who wish to serve as a military PA after graduation and NCCPA certification. However, PA attrition remains a significant challenge to force management and has led to the ongoing practice of recruiting fully qualified civilian PAs into military service. This recruitment into active duty or into the National Guard or Reserve components is problematic for several reasons. First, the United States just recently participated in two protracted, active wars going back to 2001, the longest time in our history. During this time, all PAs were guaranteed to be tapped for hazardous duty within 6 months of graduating or being commissioned into the military. This volunteering for harm's way is analogous to writing a check for "everything up to and including my life." In addition are the following reasons:

- Overall disparity in pay between the military services and the civilian sector:
  - The base pay of an O1 (second lieutenant/ ensign) with less than 2 years of creditable service is $35,211.[4]
  - The base pay of an O2 (first lieutenant/lieutenant junior grade) with less than 2 years of creditable service is $40,568.[4]
  - A PA accession may be brought into the military as an O2 if he or she has a master's degree as a PA along with NCCPA certification.
  - Since 2009, DOD PAs have been on more competitive footing. By signing a 4-year multiyear contract after completion of an initial service contract, PAs may receive up to $25,000 per year of Incentive Special Pay and Multiyear Specialty Pay. This bonus, however, is subject to change or be eliminated based on the needs

of the military. Also, all DoD PAs who have a medically related master's degree and NCCPA certification receive an additional $6000 per year of board certification pay. DoD PAs are also eligible for an additional $5000 per year of retention bonus pay. These bonuses have contributed favorably to PA retention and recruitment efforts.

- The median (50th percentile) salary of a civilian PA within the first year of practice in 2015 was $84,700.[5]
- Some civilian-trained PAs may be overwhelmed by military productivity standards, especially when coupled with the military's clinical support system and rules. The productivity expected (25+ patients per day) is not excessive; however, the support infrastructure (physical, fiscal, and personnel) is not as flexible and efficient as in some civilian health care systems.
- Adaptation to the role of a professional military officer first and to the role of medical provider second can be disconcerting and stressful.
- The scope and demands of military practice may be broader than some PA roles in civilian practice. Military PAs often practice fairly autonomously in remote and austere environments. It is expected that they will function by providing quality care with minimal support and consultation. It is common for a PA to rarely see the physician supervisor and to have only telephonic or radio contact on an as-needed basis.

SCOPE OF PRACTICE

Although military PAs principally work in primary care and family practice settings, they can also be found in acute care and emergency services. Specialization varies by branch of military, and many specialties are available. Military PAs may specialize in aviation medicine, bone marrow transplantation, cardiovascular perfusion, emergency medicine, occupational medicine, orthopedics, otolaryngology, oncology, public health, and general surgery. The credentials committee and military treatment facility commanders ensure the proper scope of practice for patient care and procedures. Hospital commanders define in writing the scope and limits of the clinical practice for each PA and designate the supervising physicians. Clinical privileges for PAs are determined on initial assignment, are reevaluated after any change of assignment, and are reviewed at least annually. While military PAs work in a wide variety of settings, the following core scope of privileges applies to all[6]:

The scope of privileges for the PA includes the evaluation, diagnosis, and treatment for patients of all ages with any symptom, illness, injury, or condition. PAs provide medical services within the scope of practice of the collaborating physician(s), including routine primary and preventive care of children and adults. PAs may refer patients to specialty clinics and assess, stabilize, and determine disposition of patients with emergent conditions.

Military PAs must keep abreast of innovations in primary patient care and combat medicine, continually ensuring deployment readiness. Eighty-percent of Army PAs are assigned to combat or field maneuver units; the remainder are assigned to outpatient care at installation hospitals or to administrative positions. Historically, most Navy and Air Force PAs were assigned to family practice or primary care clinics, but they are increasingly seen in combat operational roles at remote air bases, aboard ships, and with the Marines because of their participation and outstanding track record in Operations Desert Shield, Desert Storm, Iraqi Freedom, Enduring Freedom, and the global war on terrorism. Specialty-trained PAs must keep their skills current in their respective specialties and in family practice to maintain their interoperability and NCCPA certification.

ROLE OF PHYSICIAN ASSISTANTS IN THE MILITARY HEALTH SYSTEM

The Military Health System (MHS) is led by the Assistant Secretary of Defense for Health Affairs and includes several organizational areas such as TRICARE (health care program for over nine million beneficiaries worldwide), Force Health Protection and Readiness, military medical departments, and even civilian network facilities, providers, and partners. Within the MHS, military PAs and other health care professionals collaborate to ensure those in uniform are medically ready to deploy anywhere around the globe on a moment's notice. Not only do they ensure mission readiness, but they also deploy side by side with the warfighter. The MHS is more than just combat medicine; it is a complex system that incorporates health care delivery, medical education, public health, private sector partnerships, and cutting-edge medical research and development.[7]

Military medical centers, hospitals, and clinics are the core of the MHS, and PAs serve at every level. These facilities form an integrated network, although they are located on military bases and posts around the world. The MHS team at these facilities conducts

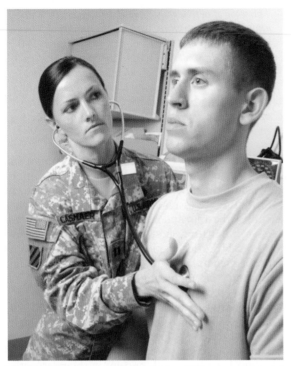

FIG. 44.2 ■ Army physician assistant (PA) at a troop medical clinic. Female PAs comprise approximately 25% of the active-duty PA community. (Photo courtesy of U.S. Army Recruiting Command, 2015.)

research and provides services for the treatment of exposures, injuries, and diseases related to military service and deployment. Warrior care also includes actively supporting wounded, ill, and injured service members in their recovery and reintegration or transition to civilian life.

In 2015, there were approximately 2800 PAs in all components of the armed forces. A majority of these PAs are working in primary care, family practice, emergency departments, troop medical clinics, or dispensaries (Fig. 44.2). PAs are considered by many to be the "gatekeepers" of the MHS. Having repeatedly been proven cost-effective, PAs are providing high-quality medical care while increasing accessibility to medical care for all DoD and DHS beneficiaries. Military PA roles are flexible and are not designed solely for peacetime or wartime. The majority of current military PAs have deployed at least once for 6 to 18 months (in a wartime role) and must remain in a deployment-ready status in between deployments.

Peacetime

Similar to their civilian counterparts, PAs in military service improve the productivity of a physician's practice, reduce patient wait time, manage emergencies effectively, reduce pressure on the physician, improve patient access to professional care, and lower the costs of that care. It must be noted that when PAs see patients, they are personally productive but also allow the physicians in their practice setting to see more complex patients. It has been hypothesized that PAs can see more than 80% of the patients in a given practice. This figure can be further defined by stating that PAs can effectively manage 80% of the disease or injury processes of their physician colleagues. Moreover, these 80% of disease processes may account for more than 90% of the patients seen.

The military PA community has achieved much in a relatively short time. It is common to find PAs serving as officers in charge of medical clinics or as department heads of large hospital units. PAs also serve as advisors to the services' Surgeons General and are actively engaged at the highest levels at the Defense Health Agency. Military PAs have opportunities to serve as executive and commanding officers at commands within the United States and abroad. Within the past few years, military PAs have also been selected to serve in senior leadership positions within the White House Medical Unit.

Wartime

Physician assistants have played extensive roles in all areas of responsibility (AORs) the United States is involved in. It is impossible to name all roles that PAs have filled, but here are just a few:

• Hospital commander
• Battalion commander
• Provincial reconstruction team medical chief (includes tribal and government official liaison duties)
• Clinic commander
• Medical representation for all echelons of care
• Joint chiefs of staff duty
• Consultants to major commanders
• Consultants to the surgeons general
• Clinicians on humanitarian missions
• Liaison or advisor to health education professionals in the AORs (medical schools, technician schools, and midlevel provider initiatives)

Wartime military PAs provide routine and resuscitative unit-level medical care and evacuation to sick, wounded, and injured personnel from forward combat locations. In the past, PAs were primarily assigned to second-echelon care positions. Currently, PAs can be found at every echelon of care, from the battlefield to tertiary care facilities in the United States. PAs contribute directly and significantly to mission and warfighter readiness. Specialty-trained PAs—those trained in orthopedics, general surgery, and emergency medicine—are used at every echelon of care. In wartime, PAs often perform the following functions:

- Conduct or supervise training of unit personnel in first aid, sanitation, personal hygiene, medical evacuation procedures, and the medical aspects of injury prevention.
- Arrange for a unit preventive psychiatry program that includes unit leader training in methods of preventing psychiatric disorders and combat stress casualties.
- Perform triage on and treat sick, wounded, or injured persons.
- Refer patients who require additional treatment to a facility capable of that care.

With the current battlefield being more fluid, PAs have adapted to the vertigo of change. It is remarkable that during recent combat operations, injuries that resulted in a 25% mortality rate in the 1960s now result in less than 10% mortality. The military PA has been an integral, engaged partner in battlefield care, research, and advancements in trauma management. Also of note is that more than 80% of all injuries are returned to duty by PAs.

SERVICE IMPACT

Although armed forces PAs have been largely used in primary care and for troop care in maneuver units, they are also educated and trained in the care of every type of DoD beneficiary. The additional use of specialty-trained PAs is cost beneficial and represents an optimal use of a health care resource to extend the capabilities not only of the primary care physician but also of the highly trained specialist physician. Although the military has been in the forefront of creating formalized residency and fellowship training programs for PAs, the DoD has been lagging in the use of PAs in specialty areas. The Army took the lead in enhancing its PA residency training by partnering with a civilian accredited university (currently Baylor University) to grant a doctorate degree for their residency graduates. New training opportunities became available as a result of the creation of the San Antonio Military Medical Center (SAMMC). It is composed of the Air Force's flagship hospital, Wilford Hall Medical Center, and the venerable Brooke Army Medical Center, which includes the Institute of Surgical Research, which encompasses the famous burn unit. Also included is the Center for the Intrepid (a world-class rehabilitation facility). The SAMMC also led to the creation of the San Antonio Uniformed Services Healthcare Education Consortium, which combined San Antonio–based military and civilian residency programs. This consortium brought Army and Air Force medical training together in 2010.

The daily working relationships of physician–PA partnerships foster unity of thought and medical logic that permit relative autonomy of practice by PAs when the military situation so dictates. PAs may be independently assigned to units that are deployed to remote areas of the world. In such instances, the medical decisions made by PAs follow accepted guidance and standards in that they are the senior medical officers on site.

Military PAs are justifiably proud to be members of this relatively new health care profession that provides an innovative level of medical care previously unavailable. Aside from a physician, no other health care provider can be substituted for a PA. PAs are the only midlevel providers who are educated according to the medical model to extend the capabilities of physician services in all treatment settings. Any discussion of the substitution of health care that PAs provide can be addressed only at the level of health care delivered—either increased, as with a physician, or decreased, as with a Hospital Corpsman or medic. Proper utilization of health care extenders such as PAs, along with nurses and medics, creates a health care team capable of delivering exceptional routine and emergency care under the direct or indirect supervision of a physician. The team works toward a common goal of improving the quality, accessibility, and cost-effectiveness of health care. PA utilization with Hospital Corpsmen and medics in such health care teams enhances the availability of care and provides an excellent role model for enlisted personnel who might be considering health care careers.

CASE STUDY 44.1 A DAY IN THE LIFE OF A MILITARY PHYSICIAN ASSISTANT

A day in the life of LTC Rick Villarreal, PA, Deputy Commander NATO Role IIE Hospital (ESP), Herat, Afghanistan. Hard to say what each day would bring, but suffice it to say, it was usually something related to the war in Afghanistan. We all tried to get into a routine, which many believed made the days, weeks, and months go faster. On this particular day, the morning had started off as per the usual. I did physical training at 0500 for an hour followed by personal hygiene, a light breakfast, and then morning report. It was otherwise a quiet morning; no sick call because it was Sunday, but being in a hospital, we were open 24/7. At around noon, I got a call on my medical cell phone, which was linked directly to the Medical Advisor (MEDAD) for the region where I was assigned. He stated that there had been an explosion of some type and that the two closest hospitals to the explosion had not been able to take the casualties, so we were up.

Information was sketchy as it usually was; we never really knew what we had until they were actually in our hospital. They estimated the casualty count at 15 to 20, all local nationals, and they would be coming in by coalition forces' medevac. Although we were fully staffed with four surgeons, an intensivist, a family physician, and a radiologist, I contacted a local forward operating base and asked their physician to come and assist if possible. I then contacted the Air Force fixed wing medical evacuation system and told them what I had coming in by helicopter and that I would need their assistance to further evacuate the casualties after I had them stabilized at our facility. In about 30 minutes, we had our facility fully ready to receive the casualties. The story now had more clarity; there had been an improvised explosive device on the back of flatbed truck. When the truck was driven onto an Afghan military installation, it was remotely detonated, injuring and killing multiple curious onlookers.

The Air Force medevac was in the air within 15 minutes of my call and arrived at my location just as the casualties were starting to arrive via helicopter. Of those who had survived the blast, we received 13, every casualty having eye injuries either to one or both eyes. I triaged and identified the four most serious casualties. We had four trauma beds in the hospital, all staffed by NATO military personnel, and they took the four immediately. Along with a senior medical noncommissioned officer, I continued to triage and treat the remaining casualties outside the hospital. With the help of the medevac crew, we stabilized the remaining 9 casualties and put all 13 on fixed wing medevac for evacuation to a larger medical facility. The total time from the initial call to the time all the casualties had been stabilized and evacuated was less than 4 hours.

I held an After Action Review immediately, and we reviewed all things that went well and identified those that could have been done better. I told the staff to get some rest and have a good dinner. On my way to my office, I received another call. An Afghan woman showed up at a NATO military installation, pregnant and not feeling well. Upon evaluation, there were no fetal heart tones, and the woman appeared septic. The clinic did not have the staff or facilities to take care of the patient. I identified a NATO physician and sent him by helicopter to the site. He further stabilized the patient and induced labor. The nonviable infant was delivered later that evening. Through an non-governmental organization (NGO), I facilitated the movement of the patient to an Afghan hospital. I was in contact with the helicopter as they were en route back to my location. They told me they had been instructed to land at a neighboring NATO installation because of an attack at my location. At that instant, my medical cell rang, and I was told that there was an explosion at one of the gates, and the tower guards were taking small arms fire. I got the staff together, and we prepared to take casualties; it was now midnight.

CONCLUSION

Military PAs serve in a diversity of settings with unique demands and are situated in the middle of the struggle among increases in demand for health services, quality of care, and cost containment. These demands are and will continue to be placed on all PAs, both military and civilian. Military PAs have committed to their challenges historically and will continue to meet or exceed the demands of patient care and operational readiness now and in the future. Military PAs are highly dedicated and honored members of the MHS. More important, military PAs are the trusted clinicians who serve with warfighters, 24/7, around the globe. Their job satisfaction and superb morale come with their commitment to doing the best job possible under any conditions.

John F. Kennedy's Inaugural Address in 1961 included: "My fellow Americans: ask not what your country can do for you; ask what you can do for your country." Service to the brave men and women of the U.S. military is surely an honorable and significant means by which to answer this call to service. Many thanks and much respect to all who have answered the call and lived a life of service to our country, the heroes who have and continue to protect this great country.

KEY POINTS

- Military PAs provide high-quality, cost-effective medical care.
- PAs are valued and respected members of the MHS.
- The number of PAs in the military fluctuates with the needs of the country.
- The working environment, mission, and focus of military PAs vary by the needs of the service employing them.
- PAs in the military have risen to new heights of leadership opportunities.

DISCLAIMER

The author is solely responsible for the contents of this chapter. It is not a position paper representing the Department of Defense, Department of Homeland Security, or any other governmental entity.

ACKNOWLEDGMENTS

The author extends a sincere, heartfelt appreciation to all current and prior military PAs who have dedicated themselves to answering the call of duty. You have made immeasurable, positive impacts on patients' lives around the world.

Thanks to Richard A. Villarreal, PhD, PA-C, and George R. Cunningham, MD, for their review, thoughtful feedback, and meaningful contributions to this chapter revision.

References

1. Department of the Army Historical Summary: FY 1971. http://www.history.army.mil/books/DAHSUM/1971/chV.htm. Accessed December 6, 2015.
2. Gray DP. Many Specialties One Corps: A Pictorial History of the U.S. Navy Medical Service Corps. *Virginia: Donning*; 1997.
3. *U.S. News & World Report.* Best physician assistant programs - 2015. http://grad-schools.usnews.rankingsandreviews.com/best-graduate-schools/top-health-schools/physician-assistant-rankings. Accessed December 6, 2015.
4. Defense Finance and Accounting Services. Military pay tables 2015. http://www.dfas.mil/militarymembers/payentitlements/military-pay-charts.html. Accessed December 6, 2015.
5. American Academy of Physician Assistants. AAPA 2015 Salary report. https://www.aapa.org/Store/detail.aspx?id=15NATSAL. Accessed December 6, 2015.
6. Centralized Credentials (CCQAS) for DoD PAs Version 2. https://ccqas.csd.disa.mil/Secured/Privileging/CLP-MTFPrivileges-Results.asp. Accessed January 7, 2013.
7. Military Health System. http://www.health.mil. Retrieved December 8, 2015.

The resources for this chapter can be found at www.expertconsult.com.

The faculty resources can be found online at www.expertconsult.com.

CHAPTER 45

INNER-CITY HEALTH CARE

Trenton Honda • Theresa Horvath

According to 2010 U.S. Census, 80.7% of the population lives in urban areas.[1] This large percentage is due, in part, to the inclusion of not only those who live within the city limits but also those who live in the increasingly dense "outer city," the suburbs surrounding urban areas. Although the population and physical geography of a city can contract and expand over time, cities are all characterized by dense, heterogeneous populations. Cities are also places where residents have more social contact and reliance on one another yet where the differences between poverty and wealth are starkly visible.

Neighborhood plays an important role in the individual experience as a city dweller. Wealthy urban neighborhoods give their inhabitants access to green spaces, physical safety, cultural opportunities, and wide options for food. Poorer neighborhoods can be isolated by these same factors. They tend to be located in areas that are less desirable geographically, such as near or on the edges of highways. They can be isolated from accessible transportation, sources of affordable housing, and access to fresh food. These neighborhoods disproportionately bear the burden of people with mental illnesses and addiction problems. Access to medical care is limited. Increasingly, these areas are inhabited by people of color. This is what is known as the "inner city."

There is no discipline of study known as "inner-city health," but "urban health" has become a well-recognized subdiscipline of public health. In 1998, the *Journal of Urban Health* was founded by the New York Academy of Medicine, which was a first attempt to join epidemiology with clinical medicine and health policy. In 2002, the International Society for Urban Health was founded to provide support to scholars engaged in research, interventions, and program evaluations of urban health issues.

An important focus of research in urban health has been to identify the multifaceted determinants of health and how they affect the poorest city dwellers. Depending on the determinant that is assessed, population density can be an attribute or a risk. This chapter delineates how health risks specific to cities affect those who are most vulnerable and describes measures created to address the underlying conditions that bring about illness and to sustain those in neighborhoods of greatest need.

HISTORY

Ring around the rosie
A pocketful of posies
Ashes, ashes
We all fall down.

The origins of this children's rhyme, first sung in the mid-14th century, reflects the horror of Bubonic Plague, which was responsible for killing as much as one third of the population of Europe.[2] Many centuries later, the Black Plague was found to be caused by *Yersinia pestis*, which is transmitted by the fleas harbored on household rats. Rats travel from home to home more easily in densely populated areas. Although there were no "cities" as such in Europe until centuries later, peasants lived clustered around feudal manors, and thus plague disproportionately affected these individuals. Not only did peasants live in closer proximity to one another, but there was also no place that they could go when their community became infected. Lords, on the other hand, often could escape into more rural areas and protect themselves and their families from contagion.

The social aspects of this pandemic were as terrible as the disease itself. Plague became seen as a curse from God. Religious cults emerged, and bizarre rituals developed whereby people would march through the streets flagellating themselves in an effort to purge their sins. More important, Jews became the scapegoat for this disease. Individual Jews were tortured into confessing that they contaminated wells and other public facilities. Eventually, this led to the mass burning of Jewish communities, often with their residents trapped inside. The use of scapegoats to vent frustration at the inability to stem devastating illness has been seen at other points in history as well, such as targeting all African immigrants for the recent Ebola outbreak in the United States. Scapegoats are an especially appealing explanation for mass illness in cities, where tainting shared resources such as the water supply, transportation, and food exchange become easy explanations when no other is apparent.

The disproportionate effects of contagious infections among urban poor, especially of members of racial or ethnic minorities, have occurred in the United States as well. The yellow fever outbreaks that occurred mostly in the mosquito-infested areas of southern cities such as Memphis, Savannah, and New Orleans throughout the 19th and early 20th centuries provide such an example. Yellow fever is caused by a virus spread by the *Aedes aegypti* mosquito. It can be highly contagious, leading to death in cases that progress to the toxic phase.[3] As with the plague, wealthier individuals fled these cities during the outbreaks. Those who were most vulnerable were recent immigrants to these cities. During the outbreak in New Orleans in 1858, public health measures were used only after wealthy citizens became infected.[4]

The first recorded outbreak of yellow fever occurred in Philadelphia in 1793. People became infected and died at such a rate that most of those able to care for the sick and dying, from health workers to grave diggers, refused to do so for fear of infection. Through an ironic series of events, African Americans became both the heroes and the victims of this outbreak. Once a thriving slave port, by 1793, Philadelphia had greatly curtailed its slave community. There was an active community of free blacks as well, whom some members of the white community excluded from their institutions and churches.

The African American community put aside these racial tensions, and under the leadership of Richard Allen, founder of the African Methodist Episcopal Church, volunteered to care for the ill. The response from the African American community was based on moral principles, yet a myth arose that African Americans carried immunity to the disease, which unfortunately was not the case. African Americans did die at a slower rate than whites, which was surprising given the level of their exposure, giving rise to a credible hypothesis that genotypic immunity existed among some African Americans. Nonetheless, after the epidemic subsided, a racial backlash ensued, and African Americans were blamed for financially profiting from their role.[4,5]

There are many examples that demonstrate that the poorest urban dwellers are the most affected by illness. Infectious disease outbreaks best show that when large numbers of people are affected, economic, cultural, ethnic, and racial factors predict that those with the fewest resources shoulder the greatest burdens. Therefore, treating this community during crises such as epidemics requires a holistic approach; social well-being and safety must be addressed along with medical treatment.

THE GROWTH OF THE URBAN ENVIRONMENT AND THE INNER CITY

Inner-city medical practice has become more important as the populations of both the United States and the world become increasingly urbanized. In the 1950s, 30% of the world's population lived in cities. The World Health Organization (WHO) estimates that as of 2014, 54% of the world's population lived in urban areas and projects that this will increase to 66% by 2050 (Fig. 45.1).[6]

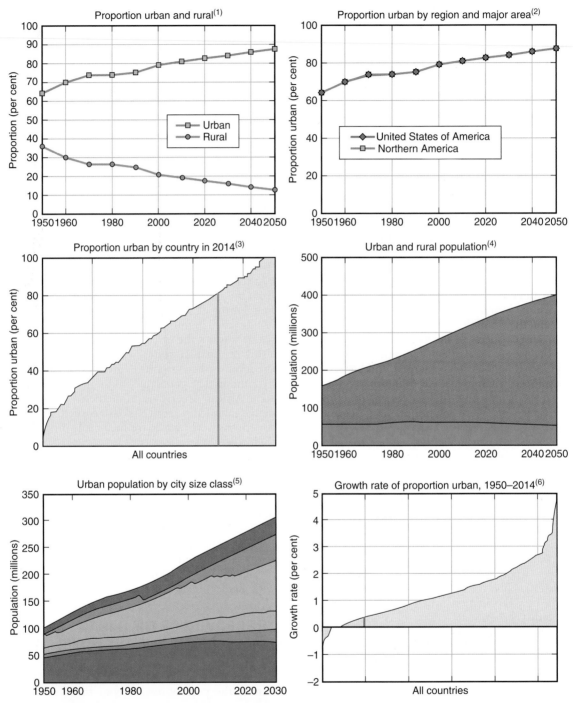

FIG. 45.1 ■ **Country profile: United States of America.** (Copyright 2014, United Nations, Population Divisions/DESA. United Nations. *World Urbanization Prospects, the 2014 Revision: Country Profiles.* http://esa.un.org/unpd/wup/Country-Profiles.)

Interestingly, recent demographic changes in cities have made the principles and eccentricities of inner-city health care germane to not only the inner city proper but also to more peripheral communities. Although traditionally the "inner city" refers to the historic center of a city, the increase in urban migration witnessed in the past half-century, coupled with the gentrification of many historic urban neighborhoods in large cities such as New York, has created the phenomenon of the "outer-inner city." This term refers to devalued suburban areas appropriating many of the traditional demographic, socioeconomic, and environmental qualities of the traditional inner-city environment.[7]

WHY INNER-CITY HEALTH CARE IS UNIQUE

Health care in the contemporary inner-city environment (including the outer-inner city) has been influenced greatly by these long-term, large-scale demographic changes. Those who live in inner-city environments tend to be of lower socioeconomic status, have less access to health care, have less education, and are more racially diverse than those who live in other urban environments. Additionally, the physical environments of the inner city tend to offer a dearth of infrastructure resources that would serve to support health while simultaneously increasing pollution.

DIVERSITY IN THE INNER CITY

The population of inner cities today is far more diverse than it was during the late 1960s when the term "inner city" began to be widely used. New waves of immigration from every corner of the globe have brought millions of new residents to the nation's ports of entry, and many of these immigrants have settled in the inner cities. The ethnic composition of these enclaves varies widely across America. Hispanics predominate in the southern tier of major cities, but the immigrant populations in northern cities are more diverse. They include large refugee populations from Southeast Asia, East Africa, and Central Europe, as well as Hispanic populations. The immigrant population of the United States has more than tripled since 1970.[8] Twenty-three percent of the U.S. population in 2010 was foreign born or first-generation American,[9] with the majority living in cities and their centers, up from 20% just 10 years earlier. This increase in diversity has created both challenges and opportunities

for America's cities and for health care providers. In addition to the barriers to health care that grow from economic disadvantage, they must confront barriers that grow from differences in language and culture as well.

In 2002, the Institute of Medicine (IOM) published a groundbreaking report titled *Unequal Treatment: Confronting Racial and Ethnic Disparities in Healthcare*.[10] This report documents racial and ethnic health care disparities described by more than 100 studies and offers recommendations. Disparities have been verified in health status, health care screening, testing, and treatment for many diseases and conditions. People of color generally have less favorable outcomes than whites.[10] Some examples of health disparities follow:

- African Americans die from asthma at rates three times higher than white Americans.[11]
- Asian Americans have hepatitis B at twice the rate of white Americans.[12]
- Both African Americans and American Indians are roughly twice as likely as white Americans to have diabetes.[13]
- Puerto Ricans have asthma at twice the rate of white Americans.[14]
- African American, Hispanic and Latino, and Asian patients with the same condition are less likely to be referred for or receive kidney transplantation than whites.[10]
- African Americans and Hispanics and Latinos with the same conditions are less likely to receive advanced cardiac procedures such as angioplasty.[10]
- African American patients with diabetes are less likely to have the appropriate glycosylated hemoglobin test, ophthalmologic visits, and influenza immunizations than whites.[10]

In 2012 the IOM published a follow-up report titled *How Far Have We Come in Reducing Health Disparities? Progress Since 2000: Workshop Summary*.[15] The report notes that, "although some progress has been made . . . no significant change in disparities had occurred for at least 70 percent of the leading health indicator objectives."[15] Although low socioeconomic status and decreased access to health care have both direct potential effects on health, the importance of the impact of racial and ethnic diversity on health cannot be overstated. Any examination of health and health behavior outcomes necessitates examination of sociocultural and environmental determinants of the outcome in the population. This theoretical approach, termed the "ecological model," is a contextual understanding of health and health behavior outcomes. Approaching problems from this orientation provides potential points of intervention that can be explored when a change in health outcomes is desired. Furthermore, when different populations are found to have unequal health outcomes, the ecological model is a sociobehavioral, rather than a purely biological, understanding of illness. Put more simply, the ecological environments in which "races" find themselves is what actually determines the difference in health outcome, not genetics.[16]

What then is responsible for the poorer health outcomes observed in multiple epidemiologic studies for people of color? One likely factor is institutional racism.[16] Institutional racism describes societal patterns or institutional behaviors that effectively impose negative conditions against identifiable groups on the basis of race or ethnicity. These negative conditions deleteriously affect the access to and quality of goods, services, and opportunities available to minorities.[16]

In fact, the state of being a minority in a population appears to itself convey some adverse health effects. Hue et al. (2008) investigated whether being a minority itself was related to health behaviors known to cause chronic disease.[17] They found that Asian Indians on a Caribbean island were significantly less physically active then the natives on the island. This was remarkable because data showed that Asian Indians in India were generally more active than the island natives. In this sense, race was important as a determinant of minority status only. As the demographics of the inner city continue to change, this finding is an important consideration.[17]

CASE STUDY 45.1

A 32-year-old African American mother presents to the community health clinic complaining about her youngest child wheezing for the past month. At night, she reports that she can often hear him coughing. Last night, it became so difficult for him to breathe that she called 911 because she doesn't have a car, and the subway was not running in the middle of the night. Her son spent the night in the county hospital emergency department receiving multiple nebulizer treatments while her two other children slept at a neighbor's house. The emergency department physician assistant (PA) referred her for an urgent follow-up. She reports that she is a single mother of three children. She and her children live in an "old factory" that was converted into studio apartments down in the center of town. She says she "hates" her apartment because it's always cold, nothing ever gets fixed, the water tastes terrible, and the paint is peeling off the walls. She reports a family history of asthma in both of the patient's siblings. She inquires, "Why do all of my children have asthma?"

Inner-city environments also tend to differ in the environmental exposures to which their denizens are exposed. The location of the inner city, whether at the historical center of a city or on the outskirts, often places living quarters in close proximity to traffic and industry and their attendant noise and pollution or, in the years since the decline of manufacturing, near the waste that those industries produced. These exposures have been associated with increased risks of malignancy, asthma, infectious disease, and cardiovascular disease.

Children are at increased risk from environmental toxicants for both biological and behavioral reasons. Children undergo rapid periods of growth and development. A toxic exposure during one of these phases can have much more dire physiologic consequences than exposures in fully developed individuals. Additionally, an exposure in childhood to a persistent chemical or to a mutagenic chemical has more time to cause its deleterious effects because of the longer remaining life of a child compared with an adult.[18]

Behaviorally, children tend to expose themselves to more environmental toxins than adults. This is because children tend to play outside in the dirt, often without protective clothing, and with not only integumentary but also alimentary exposure because of hand–mouth behaviors. Taken together, these behaviors increase their exposure to air pollution, pesticides, and lead in the soil and the household from degenerating paint and other environmental toxins.[18] When reading through Case Study 45.1, in addition to asthma treatment, what preventive health measures might be indicated for this patient?

CASE STUDY 45.2

A 43-year-old factory worker who emigrated from Central America with his family 6 years ago presents for evaluation of "peeing all night long." He states, through an interpreter, that for the past 3 months, he has been urinating four to five times per night. The voids are all large volume. Additionally, he reports that his clothes have been feeling "loose" recently. He and his mother, wife, and four children share a one-bedroom apartment. He states that he works 14 hours per day, so he is really not able to exercise at all. He used to play soccer back home, but he states the parks in his neighborhood aren't safe, so he stopped when he moved to the United States. When you query him about his diet, he states that his apartment has no kitchen, only a "hot plate," so he gets breakfast and lunch from the vending machine at work. On examination, you note a moderately obese Hispanic male in no acute discomfort. Urinalysis reveals 3+ glucose.

The inner city lacks many of the environmental characteristics that are supportive to a healthy lifestyle. Physical activity is negatively impacted by the lack of green space, built environments that are not conducive to outdoor exercise, and lack of public safety infrastructure. Because physical activity is an integral part of a healthy lifestyle, these deficits in the build environment directly and indirectly impact the incidence and prevalence of myriad chronic diseases, including hypertension, diabetes, cardiovascular disease, and cancer.[19]

The build environment of the inner city not only impacts physical activity but also access to food.[19] The WHO defines food security as "when all people at all times have access to sufficient, safe, nutritious food to maintain a healthy and active life." "Access" is further specified as referring to both physical and economic access, and a "healthy and active life" is defined as inclusive of both the nutritional needs of the population and the dietary preferences. The three pillars of food security identified by the WHO are as follows: food availability, food access, and food use.[19]

According to the U.S. Department of Agriculture (USDA), 14% of U.S. households in 2014 were food insecure, with 5.6% of these households having one or more members who decreased food consumption because of scarcity.[20] African Americans, households headed by a single woman with children, and those with high income-to-poverty ratios were the most likely to be insecure (Fig. 45.2). Geographically, the American South is disproportionately affected by food insecurity (Fig. 45.3).

Recently, inner-city environments have come under scrutiny for their lack of provision of access to healthy food to residents. The USDA has designated *low-income census tracts* where a substantial number of residents have *low access* to a supermarket or large grocery store as "food deserts."[21] Food deserts are ubiquitous in the United States (Fig. 45.4). Importantly, a food desert does not mean that there is no food and people are starving in these areas. On the contrary, obesity is often a major concomitant problem with food access in the United States. What is lacking in food deserts is unprocessed food that contributes to health and a healthy lifestyle, including fresh fruits and vegetables.[21] The lack of easy availability of healthy foods leaves residents with access to only highly processed, obesogenic, and diabetogenic foods that have been shown to contribute to a number of chronic diseases. A good example of a food desert is the city of Detroit. According to a 2012 report by the IOM, there is not one major chain grocery store within the city limits; residents must drive into the suburbs to purchase

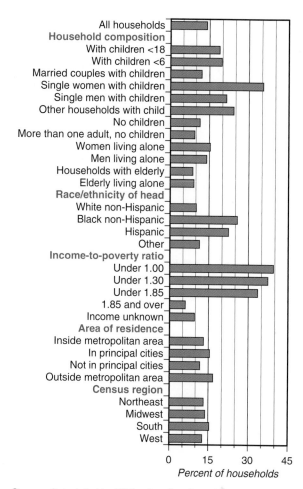

Source: Calculated by ERS using data from the December 2014 Current Population Survey Food Security Supplement.

FIG. 45.2 ■ Prevalence of food insecurity, 2014. (From U.S. Department of Agriculture. http://www.ers.usda.gov/topics/food-nutrition-assistance/food-security-in-the-us/keystatistics-graphics.aspx#.UiYOnD_8KSp.)

affordable fresh fruits and vegetables.[15] After reading Case Study 45.2, what nonpharmacologic interventions or recommendations would you make to this patient?

HEALTH CARE IN THE INNER CITY

Some of the differences in health care systems can be traced to the period of outmigration from the inner cities that occurred several decades ago. As the middle class left for the suburbs, many private practitioners went with them. Some hospitals closed or were defunded as well. Hospitals that remained faced a difficult prospect. With their base of paying patients moving away, they could either ally with teaching

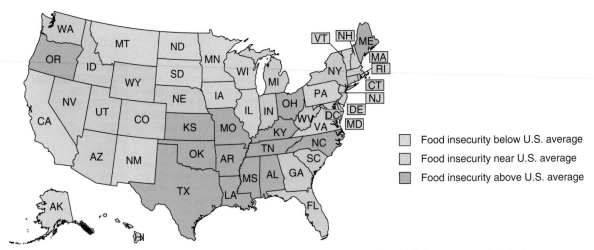

FIG. 45.3 ■ Prevalence of food insecurity, average 2012 to 2014. (From U.S. Department of Agriculture. http://map.feedingamerica.org/county/2014/overall.)

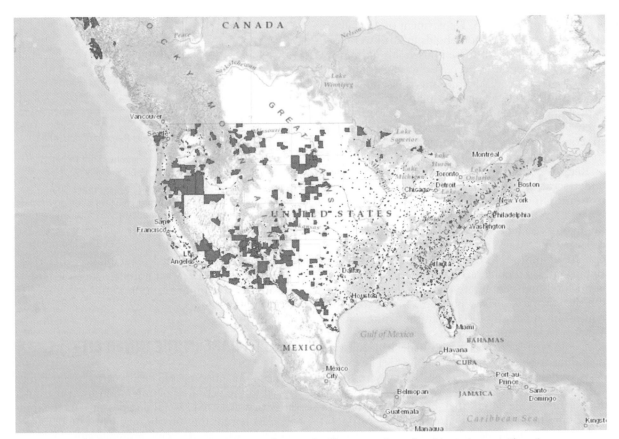

FIG. 45.4 ■ Low-income census tracts where a significant number of residents is more than 1 mile (urban) or 20 miles (rural) from the nearest supermarket. (From U.S. Department of Agriculture. *Food Access Research Atlas.* http://www.ers.usda.gov/data-products/food-access-research-atlas/go-to-the-atlas.aspx.)

hospitals and the training subsidies they received or attempt to become specialty centers capable of attracting patients from the suburbs.

Economics drove most private hospitals to become specialty centers, which dictated policies that had the effect of shutting out those who could not afford to pay the full cost of their care. Over time, inner-city populations became more and more dependent on public teaching hospitals for their care. The changing fee schedules of public health insurance programs such as Medicaid and Medicare mitigated this trend for a short time, but as the rates paid by these programs began to fall behind the costs of care, the trend accelerated.

As the population of the inner cities became more concentrated with poor people, private medical office practices faced increasing operational difficulties. More people were uninsured. The fees that Medicaid and Medicare paid the practices were too little to cover costs. The Patient Protection and Affordable Care Act of 2009 (PPACA) sought to expand the accessibility of insurance to individuals not otherwise covered by introducing subsidies and government-regulated health insurance marketplaces where individuals could purchase medical insurance. Exact estimates of how many people have been affected by the PPACA have been imprecise, but between the increase in Medicaid eligibility, coverage of young adults under their parents' plans, and those individuals not otherwise covered, millions of Americans have gained access to health care that they would not have otherwise been able to as a result of the PPACA. The effect that this coverage has had on the health of all Americans, and specifically on those of greatest need, has yet to be calculated.[22]

EFFECTS OF SOCIAL ISOLATION IN THE INNER CITY

Twenty-eight percent of the population in the United States lives alone, a trend that has been steadily rising since 1970 when single-person households constituted 17% of the total population.[23] Living alone does not predispose an individual to depression or early death. Many single householders prefer living alone. Living alone is, however, an important factor in social isolation that is a health risk, especially among older individuals and people with underlying illnesses. Social isolation is not feeling lonely; rather, it is having decreased contact with others. So although feeling lonely can exacerbate chronic health conditions, it is not a risk factor for morbidity or mortality per se.[24]

Social isolation can have magnified effects in the inner city. Natural occurrences such as extreme weather can have dire consequences in urban areas where residents do not have the aid of their family or neighbors. Eric Klinenberg performed a "social autopsy" of the 1995 heat wave disaster in Chicago in which 739 people died as a result of heat exposure. Their deaths were classified as heat-related "excessive death," meaning that despite their underlying health conditions, their deaths were directly attributable to heat exposure.[25] Klinenberg found that most of those who died were elderly, low income, African American, and living alone. He further found that the high degree of death in this population was caused by two things: The first was the lack of preparedness and response of emergency personnel to provide aid to low-income neighborhoods.[25] The second was that the social conditions, specifically social isolation, left many of those who perished without the social networks needed to leave their apartments.

Klinenberg contrasted two bordering low-income Chicago neighborhoods, North Lawndale and South Lawndale (called the Little Village). North Lawndale consists primarily of African American residents, and although it had been a thriving neighborhood decades prior, infrastructural necessities such as local businesses and places to shop had been abandoned, drug activity became rampant, and many older residents were frightened to leave their homes or even leave their windows open for fear of robbery or assault. Little Village consists primarily of Latino residents and has retained the support systems that North Lawndale lacks, both in terms of businesses and social cohesion. Although the degree of poverty among older adults was comparable between the two neighborhoods, North Lawndale had 19 heat-wave–related deaths (40 of 100,000), but South Lawndale had only 4 (4 of 100,000).[25]

There have been both quantitative and qualitative disputes with Klinenberg's findings. Browning and that although commercial decline did correlate with heat-related death, the lack of social networks and collective efficacy did not.[26] Duneier conducted a qualitative analysis of 16 of the victims through unstructured interviews with surviving family members and concluded that social isolation could not be proven among his informants but that drugs and alcohol were confounding factors.[27] Whether social isolation was the definitive factor or one of many factors, it is clear that poverty and living alone were risks for death in the 1995 disaster.

Since the attack on the World Trade Center in 2001, the focus of "urban disaster" preparedness has become terrorism rather than those caused by natural events. Although the health risks of those who were directly affected by the collapse of the Twin Towers were substantial, this type of event is uncommon. It is still more likely for an earthquake or hurricane to cause death and destruction in a city. One primary reason Hurricane Katrina, a combination of a natural event and inadequate preparedness, was so unprecedentedly devastating was because of the lack of rescue and recovery efforts on the part of local and federal governments. In this instance, the 2005 disaster of New Orleans had a lot in common with the 1995 disaster of Chicago. Although the natural event was inevitable, the degree to which the health, safety, and well-being of the victims were not adequately addressed increased the morbidity and mortality rates far beyond what they might have been. Both the health system and, perhaps more important, the municipal government were unable to play the role needed to prevent significant morbidity and mortality.

RECENT TRENDS IN THE INNER CITY

One important trend in the inner city has been the ongoing crisis in housing in the some of the nation's largest inner-city populations. Although "urban renewal" of the 1960s and 1970s was the most devastating factor on the physical integrity of poorer neighborhoods, the mortgage crisis and subsequent financial recession have had devastating effects on many cities, leaving vast numbers of properties uninhabited as individuals and families defaulted on loans.[28] This phenomenon has all but destroyed the city of Detroit, which had been on the brink of ruin before the housing crisis. Defaulting on loans has also left more families homeless. The urban infrastructure has not adequately provided for these individuals and families. School-age children have been especially hard hit, many of whom hide their homelessness from their peers and teachers if they are able to remain in school.

ROLE OF PUBLIC TEACHING HOSPITALS

Public teaching hospitals are key providers of care to inner-city, high-poverty populations. Teaching hospitals provide an important safety net to uninsured individuals, providing care to 37% of all those in need nationwide. In addition, teaching hospitals provide 24% of care to Medicaid patients.[29] In addition to the provision of care to those who could not otherwise afford it, these hospitals are major employers, often acting as the cornerstone of the inner city's economy.

Many patients hospitalized in these institutions have underlying illness that could be better managed by good primary care. More severe manifestations of disease states require longer hospital stays and more complex and costly care. Yet by virtue of caring for large numbers of both uninsured patients and patients for whom public insurance does not cover the full cost of care, these hospitals suffer chronic budget shortages. These shortages frequently manifest in overcrowding, outdated equipment, and rundown facilities.

There are also inherent contradictions in the multiple roles an urban public hospital must play. Teaching institutions must provide opportunities for students to learn. This role contributes to making specialty care and complicated medical procedures priorities over the more routine tasks involved in managing chronic illness. Therefore, although teaching hospitals afford poor communities tertiary care that might otherwise be absent, their role as community institutions responsible for providing their patients with continuity of care may be compromised as a result.

In response to community pressure and other factors, some teaching hospitals recognize their lack of attention to the treatment of chronic illness provision of preventive care. Some have made efforts to resolve this by establishing primary care departments and satellite clinics or by working with networks of community health centers (CHCs). However, these efforts can be curtailed by funding problems, leaving the populations of the inner cities overly dependent on the emergency department as their major source of care.[30]

ROLE OF PUBLIC HEALTH DEPARTMENTS

Urban public health departments have long played a vital role in the inner cities, especially in efforts to improve environmental health and sanitation and to control the spread of communicable disease. During the short-lived War on Poverty in the mid-1960s, some urban health departments used federal funds to provide additional services. Unfortunately, most of these services were funded through "categorical grants" targeted to a specific health care problem such as sickle cell anemia or family planning, and the service delivery was also organized according to these categories. This meant that health departments might be able to provide a number of screening services and immunizations for a child but might not be able to care for the child's ear infection or other needs for which no categorical funding was available.

At times, this pattern of service delivery resulted in extreme inefficiency. In the late 1970s, for example, it was common for women to be required to visit three different health department programs and undergo three different examinations to piece together basic gynecologic services that could easily have been provided in one primary care visit. This fragmentation occurred because services for sexually transmitted disease screening, birth control, and cervical cancer screening were organized categorically to more easily comply with federal reporting requirements.

In the recent past, many urban health departments have decategorized their services to more closely reflect the needs of their patients. A few have ventured into primary care either by offering services directly or through alliances with other providers. With the onset of the acquired immunodeficiency syndrome (AIDS) epidemic and the increased incidence of other communicable diseases in the inner cities, health departments have also worked hard to expand their capacity to fulfill their traditional mission of protecting the public health through education, prevention, and the control of communicable diseases.

ROLE OF COMMUNITY HEALTH CENTERS

Community health centers are federally funded organizations that provide primary medical and sometimes dental and behavioral services to residents of a defined geographic area that is medically underserved. More than 1300 health centers operate 9000 service delivery sites in every U.S. state; Washington, DC; Puerto Rico; the Virgin Islands; and the Pacific Basin care for nearly 23 million patients.[31] The CHCs are governed by a board, most of whose members are residents of the neighborhood and who receive their medical services from the CHC. They offer comprehensive preventive and primary care and provide services on a sliding-fee scale according to the patient's ability to pay.

Community health centers have reestablished the concept of primary care in many inner-city neighborhoods in which the family doctor had all but disappeared. They have created a model of care that is held to be more efficacious and cost-effective than other modes of care, and they have pioneered innovations in caring for disadvantaged populations. These clinics employ physicians, PAs, and nurse practitioners. They provide care in internal and family medicine, pediatrics, obstetrics and gynecology, mental health, and sometimes dental services.

Besides being an important safety net institution, CHCs are important to PAs in that they provide the venue to interact with the National Health Service Corps (NHSC). To pay back NHSC scholarships or to qualify for NHSC loan forgiveness programs, PAs and other clinicians must work at centers that meet federal definitions for medically underserved communities through Health Service Provider Area (HPSA) scores. CHCs are federally qualified health centers that universally meet this definition. Therefore, working at a CHC meets the employment requirements of all HRSA scholarships and loans.

INCREASING NEED FOR LANGUAGE LITERACY

Cities have always been places for new immigrants and homes to people who have not yet learned English. Ethnic enclaves of years ago, primarily from the countries of Europe, have given way to immigration from all corners of the globe. The number of languages and dialects that hospitals and CHCs now have to accommodate has grown exponentially as a result. Although traditionally, some providers have relied heavily on family members to translate medical encounters, confidentiality and power issues often prevented the clinician from gaining a full understanding of what the patient was attempting to communicate. Staff members who are fluent in another language may help, but many health faculties have been unable to meet the growing need for language fluency.

Because hiring individual interpreters may be prohibitively costly, especially in very diverse areas, some hospitals are beginning to use centralized language banks from which a provider can call and get translators in almost any language or dialect over the phone. This centralization of resources allows for a number of institutions to use the same translators. Because this service does not require the translator to be onsite, even a small number of individuals speaking a language rare for the community can be accommodated with translation services. With the obvious barriers to communication presented by speaking over the telephone notwithstanding, the quality of service provided to recent immigrants or older immigrants who have no interest in learning English may improve when their words are understood.

HOMELESS HEALTH CARE IN THE INNER CITY

The demographic change in America's inner cities is not the only change affecting the nature of health care delivery. The increase in homelessness also presents a challenge to the public health of a city. Health centers designed to serve relatively stable low-income families now find themselves caring for large numbers of homeless families, with little chance of providing continuity of care as patients move from one shelter to another or from one city to another. In response, Health Care for the Homeless Projects has been created in many inner cities, providing onsite health care in shelters and sometimes on the streets.

A study of homeless mothers and children in New York found increased depression in the mothers compared with nonhomeless mothers. Behavioral problems were also higher for the children, particularly for boys (up to three times higher) compared with their nonhomeless classmates.[32] Providers in the inner cities are also seeing increases in communicable diseases such as tuberculosis that seemed all but nonexistent in urban America just a few years ago. Together with the continuing crisis of human immunodeficiency virus (HIV) and AIDS, these infectious diseases, partly as a byproduct of immigration and homelessness, pose special challenges for the inner city.

In an effort to address this challenge, some health care providers have enlisted their professional organizations to provide enhanced understanding of these complex problems and to propose solutions. One example is that of the American College of Physicians, which commissioned senior research scientist Dennis Andrulis[33] to investigate inner-city health care. This resulted in a groundbreaking policy paper[34] that amplified the concept of the "urban health penalty." This is defined as "a condition that exists when healthier, more affluent persons leave the city and the remaining and new residents experience health problems that interact with the city's physical and economic deterioration."[35] He describes poverty zones where minorities are overrepresented, jobs are in short supply, and significant health problems result in premature death.[35] House and colleagues studied this effect further, finding a mortality hazard ratio of 2.25 for urban males compared with those in rural or small town settings.[36]

A 29-year epidemiologic study conducted by Lynch et al. from the University of Michigan School of Public Health stated in its conclusion, "sustained economic hardship leads to poorer physical, psychological, and cognitive functioning."[37] This may seem obvious to members of the communities and to health care providers working in inner cities. However, the Michigan study is able to draw a direct and clear connection between poverty and the increased incidence of illness.

Inner-city health care providers, practicing in large teaching hospitals, health departments, CHCs, or with private physicians, have had to struggle to continue providing care to people in the inner cities. They have demonstrated remarkable staying power and creativity in the face of the problems we have described. One example is that of Jeffrey Brenner, a primary care physician who works in Camden, New Jersey, considered to be the poorest, most dangerous city in the nation. Frustrated by the seemingly futile efforts to improve the health of his patients, he formed the Camden Coalition of Health Care providers who participate in his program of comprehensive preventive and primary care. He used a neighborhood mapping of recently discharged patients to identify the most vulnerable patients. He employed the help of other physicians around the city and formed interdisciplinary teams including a registered nurse, licensed practical nurse, and social worker. These teams visit individuals who have been recently discharged from hospitals and assess their medical and social needs, which are then referred to others in the coalition. This approach has not only avoided readmission for the sickest patients, but it has also been an enormous cost saver for the Camden safety net.[38] Winning a MacArthur Fellowship has allowed Dr. Brenner to replicate his sustainable and accountable care systems in 10 other cities, including Allentown, PA; Aurora, CO; Kansas City, MO; and San Diego, CA.

KEY POINTS

- The **ecological model** allows for a contextual understanding of health and health behavior outcomes. It permits a sociobehavioral, rather than a purely biological, understanding of illness.[16]
- **Social isolation** is not feeling lonely; rather, it is having decreased contact with others. It is a health risk particularly important for elderly city dwellers.[24]
- **Food deserts** are the USDA's designation of low-income census tracts where a substantial number of residents have low access to a supermarket or large grocery store.
- **Community health centers** are federally funded organizations that offer comprehensive preventive and primary care and provide services on a sliding-fee scale according to the patient's ability to pay.
- The **medical safety net** is the network of health care institutions that provide care to uninsured or underinsured individuals in a community.

References

1. United States Department of Commerce, United States Census Bureau. Frequently asked questions. https://ask.census.gov/faq.php?id=5000&faqId=5971

2. Cantor NF. *In the Wake of the Plague. The Black Death and the World It Made*. New York: The Free Press; 2001.

3. Patterson KD. Yellow fever epidemics and mortality in the United States, 1693-1905. *Soc Sci Med*. 1992 Apr;34(8): 855–865.

4. Reid-Pharr RF. *Conjugal Union, the Body, the House and the Black American*. New York: Oxford University Press; 1999.

5. Powell JH. *Bring Out Your Dead: The Great Plague of Yellow Fever in Philadelphia in 1793*. Philadelphia: University of Pennsylvania Press; 1993.

6. United Nations, Department of Economic and Social Affairs, Population Division, World Urbanization Prospects: The 2014 Revision, Highlights; 2014 (ST/ESA/SER.A/352).

7. Millington G. The outer-inner city: urbanization, migration and race in London and New York. Urban Research & Practice. 2012:5(1):6-25.

8. Gibson C, Jung K. Historical census statistics on the foreign-born population of the United States: 1850–2000. U.S. Census Bureau. http://www.census.gov/population/www/documentation/twps0081/twps0081.html. Accessed February 9, 2012.

9. Current population survey data on the foreign-born population. U.S. Census Bureau. http://www.census.gov/population/foreign/data/cps.html. Accessed February 9, 2012.

10. Smedley BD, Stith AY, Nelson AR. In: *Unequal Treatment: Confronting Racial and Ethnic Disparities in Healthcare*. Washington, DC: National Academies Press; 2002.

11. American Lung Association. State of lung disease in diverse communities 2010. http://www.lung.org/finding-cures/ourresearch/solddc-index.html. Accessed February 9, 2012.

12. Centers for Disease Control and Prevention. A comprehensive immunization strategy to eliminate transmission of hepatitis B virus infection in the United States. Recommendations of the advisory committee on immunization practices (ACIP) Part II: immunization of adults. *MMWR*. 2006;55(RR-16):1–33.

13. American Diabetes Association. Diabetes statistics. http://www.diabetes.org/diabetes-basics/diabetes-statistics/. Accessed February 9, 2012.

14. Centers for Disease Control and Prevention. 2007 National Health Interview Survey (NHIS) Data, Table 4–1. http://www.cdc.gov/asthma/nhis/07/table4-1.htm. Accessed February 9, 2012.

15. Anderson KM. *How Far Have We Come in Reducing Health Disparities?: Progress Since 2000: Workshop Summary*. Washington, DC: National Academies Press; 2012.

16. LaVeist TA, Isaac LA. *Race, Ethnicity, and Health: A Public Health Reader*. San Francisco: Jossey-Bass; 2012.

17. Hue O, Sinnapah S, Antoine-Jonville S, Donnet JP. Asian Indians of Guadeloupe are less physically active than their island counterparts. *Scand J Med Sci Sports*. 2008;19(2): 222–227.

18. Friis R. *Essentials of Environmental Health*. Sudbury, MA: Jones and Bartlett Learning; 2010.

19. World Health Organization. Food security. Retrieved from http://www.who.int/trade/glossary/story028/en/, 2016.

20. FAO Agricultural and Development Economics Division (June 2006). Food security. Retrieved from ftp://ftp.fao.org/es/ESA/policybriefs/pb_02.pdf.

21. United States Department of Agriculture. Food security in the U.S. 2016. Retrieved from http://www.ers.usda.gov/topics/food-nutrition-assistance/food-security-in-the-us/key-statistics-graphics.aspx.

22. Public Protection and Affordable Care Act, Title II, The Role of Public Programs. http://www.hhs.gov/healthcare/facts-and-features/key-features-of-aca/index.html.

23. Klinenberg Eric. *Going Solo. The Extraordinary Rise and Surprising Appeal of Living Alone*. New York: Penguin Publishing Group; 2012.

24. Steptoe A, Shankar A, Demakakos P, Wardle J. Social isolation, loneliness, and all-cause mortality in older men and women. Proceedings of the National Academy of Sciences of the United States of America. 2013;110(15):5797–5801.

25. Klinenberg Eric. *Heat Wave*. Chicago: Chicago University Press; 2002.

26. Browning CR, Wallace D, Feinberg SL, Cagney KA. Neighborhood social processes, physical conditions and disaster-related mortality: the case of the 1995 Chicago heat wave. *ASR*. 2006;71:661–678.

27. Duneier M. Ethnography, the ecological fallacy, and the 1995 Chicago heat wave. *ASR*. 2006;71:679–688.

28. Frey WH. The new metro minority map: regional shifts in Hispanics, Asians and Blacks from Census 2010. Washington, DC: The Brookings Institution; August 2011. http://www.brookings.edu/papers/2011/0831_census_race_frey.aspx. Accessed January 9, 2012.

29. American Association of Medical Colleges. Why teaching hospitals are important to all Americans. https://www.aamc.org/advocacy/campaigns_and_coalitions/gmefunding/factsheets/253374/teaching-hospitals.html. Accessed January 15, 2016.

30. Ruger JP, Richter CJ, Spitznagel EL, Lewis LM. Analysis of costs, length of stay, and utilization of emergency department services by frequent users: implications for health policy. *Acad Emerg Med*. 2004;11(12):1311–1317.

31. U.S. Department of Health and Human Services. HRSA Health Center Program. http://bphc.hrsa.gov/about/what-is-a-health-center/index.html. Accessed January 15, 2016.

32. San Agustin M, Cohen P, Rubin D, et al. The Montefiore community children's project: a controlled study of cognitive and emotional problems of homeless mothers and children. *J Urban Health*. 1999;76(1):39–50.

33. Andrulis DP. *The Urban Health Penalty: New Dimensions and Directions in Inner-City Health Care*. Philadelphia: American College of Physicians; 1997.

34. American College of Physicians. Inner city health care. *Ann Intern Med*. 1997;126:485–490.

35. Greenberg M. American cities: good and bad news about public health. *Bull NY Acad Med*. 1991;67:17–21.

36. House JS, Lepkowski JM, Williams DR, et al. Excess mortality among urban residents: how much, for whom, and why? *Am J Public Health*. 2000;90(12):1898–1904.

37. Lynch JW, Kaplan GA, Shema SJ. Cumulative impact of sustained economic hardship on physical, cognitive, psychological, and social functioning. *N Engl J Med*. 1997;337:1889–1895.

38. The MacArthur Foundation. MacArthur Fellows Program. Jeffrey Brenner. https://www.macfound.org/fellows/886/. Accessed January 16, 2016.

The resources for this chapter can be found at www.expertconsult.com.

The faculty resources can be found online at www.expertconsult.com.

RURAL HEALTH CARE

Steven Meltzer

WHY YOU SHOULD READ THIS CHAPTER

The physician assistant (PA) profession was envisioned and created in the 1960s to fulfill a growing gap in access to health care because of a shortage of primary care physicians. Using the field-tested skills of ex-military corpsmen as an "assistant to the primary care physician," it was believed that PAs could extend the practice reach of physicians to underserved communities and populations with less cost. Although changing demographics and trends have shifted PAs to more urban practices and less primary care focus, there remains tremendous potential for the profession to help shape the health of rural communities and individuals and continue to fulfill the vision of its originators.

WHAT IS RURAL, AND WHY DOES IT MATTER?

Our perspectives on the definition and culture of rural America today are very different from how we perceived rural in the mid-20th century or even in the current context of the 21st century. For many, the word *rural* often paints a vision of open farmlands; untouched forests; rolling hills; and a sparsely populated, rustic environment. Although many rural people do live in such surroundings, other rural residents live in areas just adjacent to urban areas, and their sense of being rural comes as much from their lifestyle as from the actual environment (Fig. 46.1).

The U.S. population shift since 1990, from rural to urban, occurred steadily as a result of changing

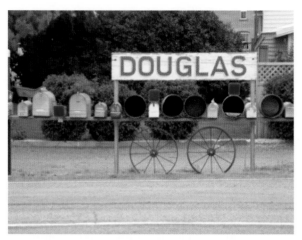

FIG. 46.1 ■ (Courtesy of Steven Meltzer, 2003.)

Population change by metro/nonmetro status, 1976–2012

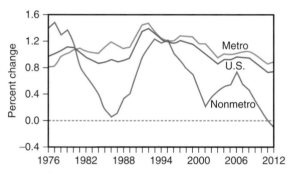

Note: Metro status changes for some counties in 1980, 1990, 2000, and 2010. Rates are imputed for 1989–1990, 1999–2000, and 2009–2010.

FIG. 46.2 ■ Rural-Urban Population Trends. (Source: U.S. Department of Agriculture, Economic Research Service, using data from the U.S. Census Bureau.)

lifestyles, economics, and postdepression and postwar transitions. In 1910, the rural population accounted for 71.6% of the total population but by 1940 had dropped to 52.2%; 1950 was the first time the U.S. population had become predominantly urban with only 43.9% rural. Over the past 60 years, rural communities continued to erode, and between 2010 and 2014, the rural population dropped from 19.3% to 15%, although some areas of high recreation and retirement options have seen increases.[1,2] The growth in urban populations was not primarily in the "core" inner cities; in fact, the majority of growth in urban areas from 1930 to the present was in the suburbs, increasing from 13.8% to 50% of the total urban population (80%)[2]; 65%

of all U.S. counties are classified an nonmetropolitan[2] (Fig. 46.2).

When considering rural America, caution should be used to not put everyone into the same basket; each rural community is distinct, and each U.S. region has distinct characteristics that help define its rurality. For example, small towns in rural New England are different in character from the open plains and communities of Montana or Wyoming; these characteristics reflect the economic, ethnic, and social differences unique to each area.

So why does defining "rural" matter? More than 40 federal programs use rural definitions to allocate facility and grant funding and support resources—for example, the National Health Service Corps, Rural Health Clinics (RHCs) and Federally Qualified Health Center (FQHC) designations, Critical Access Hospital (CAH) designation, and Universal Services Telecommunications Grants. In addition, the PA concept was envisioned at a time when there was a significant shortage of primary care physicians nationally, particularly in rural and suburban areas. Understanding the dynamics of rural health care, then, is important to understanding the evolution of the PA profession and future opportunities for PAs in rural practice settings.

CHARACTERISTICS OF RURAL POPULATIONS AND COMMUNITIES

Definitions of *Rural*

Federal and state policymakers are often required to define "rural" and "urban" in order to develop and apply policies appropriately. What seems like a simple task, however, can become complicated because agencies at both levels of government use differing methodologies to define these terms depending on the population targeted, geographic determinants, and the specific purpose of the program. There are at least three major federal agencies that define rural: the U.S. Census Bureau, the Office of Management and Budget, and the U.S. Department of Agriculture Economic Research Center. See complete definitions at http://ric.nal.usda.gov/what-rural. Because each agency defines *rural* differently, it can be a challenge for communities and health systems to know exactly which programs they quality for and how to access resources.

Frontier counties, another designation created for federal programs in 1990, were initially described as counties with very low population densities of no more than six people per square mile (compared with a national average of 73 years). The *frontier* designation was used inconsistently by the agencies that track rural populations and health, so a national consensus process was implemented by the Frontier Education Center and funded by the Federal Office of Rural Health Policy (FORHP) in 1997. The purpose of the process was to develop a new definition recognizing that "frontier" described not only physically isolated areas but also areas relatively isolated because of geography, weather, or other factors. The final report was published in April 1998 and provides a matrix, based on a maximum of 105 points, that can be used to determine the relative frontier status of any area. The determinants include population density per square mile, distance in miles to services and markets, and distance in time to services and markets.[3] The 2010 U.S. Census includes 445 "frontier" counties with populations of less than 6 people per square mile. See http://frontierus.org/frontier-definitions for complete definitions by application.

RURAL DEMOGRAPHICS

Several features set rural communities apart, such as employment, income, poverty, and age level as noted in Table 46.1.

In general, rural areas have higher rates of poverty, older adults, health disparities, low income, occupational injury, and unemployment. Rural populations are less likely to have health insurance, retirement plans, and other benefits because the majority of employers have fewer than 50 employees and often are not able to provide those benefits at reasonable cost, although the Patient Protection and Affordable Care Act (PPACA) of 2010 now provides some incentives for employers to do so. Workers are often seasonally employed and may work in high-injury occupations, such as mining, timber, fishing, and farming. Nonmetro populations typically have lower education levels than metro areas.

Although the prevailing impression of rural America is that it is primarily agricultural in nature, the percentage of population involved in traditional agricultural work (farming, forestry, mining, and fishing) reflects about 9.6% of industry[4]; still less than 6% of the U.S. population is directly involved in farming. Manufacturing (34.8%), tourism and recreation services (16.7%), and destination retirement living (16.5%) have accounted for the bulk of employment in nonmetro areas of the country for the past decade.[5-7] More recently, employment in the service sector has increased to 41%; government to 15.6%; and transportation, trade, and utilities to 17.3%.[4]

Farm productivity has continued to increase because of changes in technology, equipment, and techniques, and therefore the transformation of farmland to other uses has been much slower than the decline in employment. Farm households that do remain in agriculture are likely to also have nonfarm revenues from other sources to supplement income and maintain the farm. In addition to these changes, farmlands are under increasing pressure from urban fringe expansion to be sold and developed for large housing tracts, recreation areas, manufacturing plants, and retirement villages.[6,8]

Aging Populations

There are multiple challenges regarding the aging population in nonmetro areas stemming from factors such as outmigration of youth, aging in place of the existing population, increased migration of metro population to nonmetro areas, fewer health resources and access points, and declining number of rural health care services.[4]

The role of population aging on Medicare and access to health care will intensify, especially since the large baby boomer generation began to turn 65 years old in 2010. Key issues that will lead to changes include

- Nonmetro areas will continue to have an increasing percent of elderly population.
- Compared with metro areas, nonmetro older adults generally have lower incomes, lower educational attainment, and a higher dependence on Social Security income, creating demand for medical, social, and financial assistance.

TABLE 46.1 Selected Social and Economic Indicators, 2012 to 2015		
Indicator	Nonmetro	Metro
Unemployment (%),* 2015	5.8	5.4
Annual per capita earnings*	$31,415	$41,244
Median household income,* 2012	$41,198	$52,988
Poverty rate—overall (%),* 2014	18.1	15.1
By Age		
0–17 years of age, 2013	25.2	21.1
18–64 years of age	17.6	14.1
65 years of age and older	10.5	9.3

*Data from U.S. Department of Agriculture. *Rural Poverty & Well-being.* http://www.ers.usda.gov/topics/rural-economy-population/rural-poverty-well-being.aspx.

- There will be continuing difficulty in accessing health care because of a reduced number of primary care and specialty providers and services.
- One of the more recent trends that counteracts the previous information is the increasing number of metro aging populations that have moved and continue to move to nonmetro retirement communities typically adjacent to metro areas. This population group skews the data because they are often more affluent and mobile, have higher education levels, are more likely to be married than living alone, and typically have private insurance.[48]

Minority Population Trends

Compared with the 2000 U.S. Census, 2010 Census data show that racial and ethnic minorities increased from 18.3% of nonmetro residents to almost 20%, with Hispanics and Asians the fastest growing minority groups.[9] American Indian numbers increased also, but this is believed to be due to the increased number of people reporting American Indian heritage on the census questionnaires. The Hispanic rural population (9.3%) moved ahead of the African American population (8.2%) in the past decade and is now the fastest growing ethnic population in the rural counties, having a 46% increase since 2000. Less than 2% of the rural population is Native American, but that still comprises more than 50% of their total population. Asian, mixed race, and Pacific Islanders total less than 3% of the rural population.[9,10] It is important to note that Hispanic and African American minorities are tied historically and geographically to large areas of the country: African Americans are significantly overrepresented in the small and rural towns in the southeastern states, and Hispanics in the four states of Texas, California, New Mexico, and Arizona (slightly more than 50%).

Although immigration brings new and diverse populations to nonmetro areas, which can revitalize small towns economically and demographically, those same increases create pressures in the local economic structure and raise concerns about increased demands for social services, education, and barriers to assimilation. The Hispanic population had been primarily a rural-based group, with roughly 90% of all Hispanics living in nonmetro areas throughout the 1990s, but recent census data reflect a wider dispersion across the country and into more urbanized areas (suburban, 12.7%, and urban, 27.3%).[9,10] Although legal and illegal immigration generated the primary increase in the Hispanic population before 9/11, the subsequent decrease in illegal immigration from Mexico because of multiple major congressional acts significantly reduced the flow of Hispanics into the United States. The Hispanic population had the greatest increase in population by 46% in the past decade primarily because of increased birth rates.[9]

The influx of a broad mix of immigrants and the continuing shift among geographic areas creates significant challenges for rural communities that for generations have had populations based in European cultures, often from the same regions or cities. These changes require a paradigm shift for communities in regard to accommodating language differences in schools and businesses, religious beliefs and the availability of churches, clothing and food purchases, and social and health accessibility.

Rural America will continue to face many challenges with the continuing population shift to metropolitan areas and aging of the rural population, increasing presence of immigrant populations, changing economies, and lack of resources. Health policymakers will need to be creative in recognizing and meeting local, regional, and national health care needs.

ACCESS TO HEALTH CARE

The issue of access to health care is of great concern. The definition of access is informed by the context of people, place, provider, and payment. It can no longer be viewed as only being able to physically get to a source of care and the availability of services. As important is whether the type of facility and provider are appropriate for the care needed (individual or community) and what types of payment options are available. Lack of specialty physicians and advanced diagnostic and treatment modalities may still create access issues for rural populations with increased chronic disease and poverty.[11]

Geography plays an important role in limiting access because rural residents must often travel longer distances and may have natural boundaries, such as mountains, rivers, and federal parks and forests that have no through roads. Distance is often compounded by weather conditions, which can make travel hazardous or limit air evacuation efforts; twisty two-lane roads; and lack of public transportation in rural areas (Fig. 46.3).

The locations and availability of health and social services create access issues as well. Health care providers are often found in county seats or similar population centers and often are not able to provide adequate outreach to less populated areas for financial, staffing, or other reasons. Those with special needs—such as people with physical or mental disabilities—who may need personal assistance to access care are even more disadvantaged by these factors. In

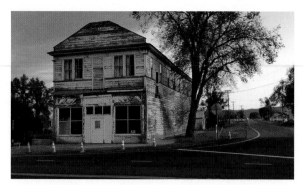

FIG. 46.3 ■ (Courtesy of Steven Meltzer, 2015.)

addition, federal and state programs set up to address these issues are often targeted toward children with special needs or older adults. Unfortunately, many rural communities do not have the population to qualify for the special funding or to support the services.

In looking at rural population data, it has been frequently noted in the past that many people did not have health care insurance, a significant barrier in accessing services. Rural populations tend on average to be older and poorer, have more chronic disease, and have lower levels of education, all of which can contribute to a lower health status and a higher need for health care. The 2010 Census showed there were 49.9 million people without health insurance in the United States—16.3% of the population; this was up from 46.6 million in 2006.

The PPACA attempted to meet several challenges of access to care by (1) increasing funding for health profession education and training programs, (2) increasing the availability of health clinics and centers to minimize distance factors, and (3) expanding insurance coverage through both the private and public sectors to cover more families and individuals. The debate rages as to its success, but research following the PPACA impacts show that the uninsured rate from 2008 to 2014 dropped 40% in states participating in the Medicaid expansion program and 29% in nonexpansion states.[12] Although the PPACA significantly expanded coverage that benefitted rural areas, legislation at the federal and state levels curtailed expansion in a number of states.

The 2010 Census shows that nationally, the metropolitan uninsured rate was 19% overall; the nonmetro rate (communities under 2500) was considerably higher at 23%. There are multiple reasons why there were fewer insured individuals: many small businesses could not afford to pay full benefits for their workers, and many rural jobs are seasonal or require only part-time work and therefore are not covered for benefits. Extended benefits to family members, dental coverage, and sick leave also have been less often available to workers.[13]

Another critical aspect of access to health care is the availability of qualified health professionals. Data from 2010 reflect that although slightly less than 20% of the population was rural, only 9% of physicians practice in those areas.[14,15] Looking at PAs in rural communities, Cawley et al. report that 12% of all PAs work in nonmetro areas, a decrease from 15% in 2010. For primary care PAs, the numbers increase to 22% working in rural versus 78% in urban settings.[14]

The 2013 American Academy of Physician Assistants (AAPA) Annual Survey notes that 17% of rural primary care PAs are employed in certified RHCs, FQHCs, and CAHs, reflecting the continued important role nonphysician providers play in ensuring access to health care services in underserved areas.[16] In addition to the general maldistribution of physicians, the imbalance of physicians by ethnicity as noted in the American Association of Medical Colleges (AAMC) 2014 report on Diversity in the Physician Workforce:

- Whites and Asians are overrepresented in the U.S. physician population. Whites comprise 72.4% of the 2010 U.S. population and 75% of the physician population. Asians and native Hawaiians and other Pacific Islanders comprise 5.2% of the U.S. population and 12.8% of the physician population.[17]
- Hispanics, blacks, and American Indians and Alaska Natives are underrepresented in the U.S. physician population, comprising 16%, 13%, and 0.9% of the U.S. population and 5.5%, 6.3%, and 0.5% of the physician population, respectively.[17]

This becomes an important note when considering the growth of Hispanic and other nonwhite populations in nonmetro areas, as well as the need for greater numbers of culturally and linguistically appropriate health care providers and facilities.

According to recent research, multiple media reports, and federal job sites, the growth of the PA profession continues to climb. Projections for the future indicate it will be one of the top jobs for the next decade or more, especially in rural and urban underserved areas. The challenge will be for the profession to capture potential applicants who increasingly match the new demographics of the nation and especially rural populations.

RURAL HEALTH CARE SYSTEMS: HOSPITALS, CLINICS, AND THE SAFETY NET

The health status of rural populations tends to be poorer than that of urban populations and is often compounded by higher levels of poverty, aging, and unemployment as noted earlier. Rural populations tend to have higher rates of chronic diseases, and health outcomes are dependent on factors such as adequate access to necessary and affordable health care services, distance and geography, and personal behaviors that contribute to poor health. Ethnic minorities, a growing population in rural communities as noted, have higher incidences of health disparities and lack of access to services, lack of health care insurance, and higher poverty rates. Census data from 2010 note that almost 10% (9.8%) of children younger than age 18 years were uninsured, as well as 20.8% of African Americans, 30.7% of Hispanics, and 11.7% of non-Hispanic whites.[9,13]

The health care delivery system in rural America is trying to respond to many and varied problems. Although some of these also exist in urban underserved areas, many are unique to rural America. The rural health care system is often more loosely organized than its urban counterpart and much more thinly spread. Its component parts are similar, but many of the more familiar ones are missing or are present in only skeletal form. What appears in any given system varies with the degree of remoteness and the resources of the community. Mounting evidence of the relative decline in rural health care includes the closure and deteriorating financial condition of local hospitals and, more important, the difficulty of recruiting and retaining physicians, midlevel providers (PAs and nurse practitioners [NPs]), nurses, and other health care personnel.

Over the past 4 decades, a wide range of health policies and programs have been developed and implemented to mitigate these issues and assist rural Americans in improving their personal and community health status. The overall effect has been to create a health care "safety net" that includes clinics, hospitals, free clinics, and public health services that improve access to care regardless of ability to pay.

HOSPITALS: TRANSITIONING MODELS OF SERVICE

Early Models

As the demographics and economic basis of rural communities changed over the past 4 decades, rural hospitals faced significant challenges in maintaining services, staff, and providers. Several federal initiatives were created to assist these hospitals in finding a new way to not only survive but also continue to meet community needs in a more effective and efficient way (Fig. 46.4).

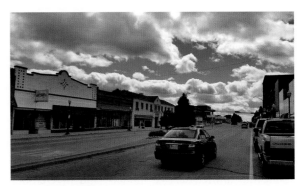

FIG. 46.4 ■ (Courtesy of Steven Meltzer, 2015.)

After World War II, as the nation's population was rapidly growing in suburban and rural areas, Congress passed the Hill-Burton Act in 1946 that gave hospitals, nursing homes, and other health facilities grants and loans for construction and modernization. State plans were to be developed to encourage expansion of health care facilities so that all people in the state would have access to care. By applying for and accepting the grants, the facilities agreed to provide free or reduced-cost emergency and other services to persons who were unable to pay, they had to serve all persons residing in the facility's area, and later they had to participate in the Medicare and Medicaid program. The Hill-Burton program stopped providing funds in 1997, but about 300 health care facilities nationwide are still obligated to provide free or reduced-cost care. Many of these facilities are still in their original buildings and struggle to find the capital resources to build new facilities or modernize.

During the 1970s and 1980s, the federal government experimented with a variety of alternative community hospital models to retain as much access to services while reducing costs and need for expansive facilities and staffing. The Medical Assistance Facility program authorized by Congress in 1990 set up a demonstration project in Montana to explore options around a limited services facility on a smaller scale than a fully accredited hospital. There were seven test sites and six control sites in Montana, and the model was deemed a relative success. It was also a significant opportunity for PAs and NPs because the model relied on use of midlevel practitioners to maintain access to care in these communities.

The Omnibus Budget and Reconciliation Act of 1989 established another alternative model: the Essential Access Community Hospital/Rural Primary Care Hospital (EACH/RPCH). This model was also based on a limited service facility staffed primarily by PAs and NPs, and there were test sites in seven states across the nation. The more rural RPCHs and larger EACHs were provided a higher cost-based Medicare reimbursement to improve financial stability, and the development of regional networks was encouraged.

Critical Access Hospitals

Congress later passed the Balanced Budget Act in 1997, which included provisions building on the successes of the MAF and EACH/RPCH models. The Medicare *Rural Hospital Flexibility Program* was established to continue to allow hospitals to refine the limited-service models, and in October 1999, all MAF and EACH/RPCH programs were grandfathered into the federally designated Critical Access Hospitals (CAH) program. Its purpose was to improve rural health by addressing access and quality of care issues for rural citizens through partnerships among the federal government, state government, rural CAHs, acute care urban hospitals, emergency medical services (EMS), and rural communities.[18]

The Flex Program consists of two separate but complementary components:
- A Medicare reimbursement program that provides reasonable cost reimbursement for Medicare-certified CAHs is administered by the Centers for Medicare & Medicaid Services (CMS).
- A state grant program that supports the development of community-based rural organized systems of care in participating states is administered by the Health Resources and Services Administration through the FORHP.

To receive funds under the grant program, states must apply for the funds and engage in rural health planning through the development and maintenance of a State Rural Health Plan that
- Designates and supports the conversion of CAHs
- Promotes EMS integration initiatives by linking local EMS with CAHs and their network partners
- Develops rural health networks to assist and support CAHs
- Develops and supports quality improvement initiatives
- Evaluates state programs within the framework of national program goals.

State entities, typically state offices of rural health, could apply for federal "Flex" grants to support the development of CAHs and networks to meet program objectives. As of March 2016, there are a total of 1331 active CAHs overseen by the FORHP.

Modifications to the program have resulted from the enactment of the Balanced Budget Refinement Act of 1999, the Benefits Improvement and Protection Act of 2000, and the Medicare Prescription Drug Improvement and Modernization Act (MMA) of 2003. These changes have been incorporated into the information presented below.

Criteria for Critical Access Hospital Certification

A rural hospital may be designated as a CAH if the following criteria are met:
- Owned by a public or nonprofit entity
- Located in a participating State Rural Hospital Flexibility state
- One or more of the following is true:
  - More than 35 miles from any other CAH or hospital
  - More than 15 miles from another hospital or CAH in mountainous terrain or in areas with only secondary roads
  - Designated a necessary provider under criteria published in the State CAH Plan
- Offers 24-hour emergency care
- Provides no more than 25 beds for acute care
- May operate distinct part units of up to 10 beds for psychiatric or rehabilitation services
- Keeps inpatients no more than an annual average of 96 hours except during inclement weather or other emergencies
- Meets staffing and other requirements established in General Acute Hospital or Primary Care Hospital licensing and the State Plan for CAHs
- Must have a formal agreement for participation as part of a rural health network. Rural health network defined as an organization of at least one CAH and one acute hospital[19]

Over the past decade, as hospitals faced further implementation costs for new federal policies and regulations, rural and small hospitals again faced financial challenges. To offset these requirements and costs, more recent policy developments include the FORHP's Small Rural Hospital Improvement (SHIP) Grant Program, which provides funding to small rural hospitals to help them do any or all of the following: (1) pay for costs related to the implementation of Prospective Payment Services (PPS), (2) comply with provisions of the Health Insurance Portability and Accountability Act (HIPAA), and (3) reduce medical errors and support quality improvement.

To be eligible for these grants, a hospital must be (1) *small*—49 or fewer available beds; (2) *rural*—located outside a metropolitan statistical area (MSA) or located in a rural census tract of an MSA as defined by the Goldsmith Modification or the Rural Urban Commuting Areas; and (3) *a hospital*, which is a non-federal, short-term, general acute care facility. All designated CAHs were included as eligible, as well as hospitals with 50 or fewer beds located in an area designated by any state law or regulation as a rural area or as a rural hospital. Unlike other programs, there is no requirement for matching funds with this program.[20]

More recently, the impacts of the PPACA, such as significantly increased numbers of patients seeking care and changes in reimbursement models, have pushed a number of CAH hospitals to the brink of closure. As of March 2016, there have been 71 hospital closures in the United States, mostly in the southern regions.[21] A variety of factors contribute to the closures, including changing demographics, declining services and inpatient and surgical care, increased Medicare and Medicaid patients (especially in states that did not participate in the Medicaid expansion program), long-standing marginal financial performance, and loss of providers. In addition, several congressional actions related to the PPACA have cut Medicare reimbursement, added more quality and value measures that increase costs, and reduced reimbursement for bad debts—all this in a postrecession environment in which rural areas are still trying to regain their economic footing.[22]

Some facilities have been able to "come back" as rehabilitation centers, nursing facilities, emergency outpatient facilities, or primary care clinics. The FORHP, National Rural Health Association, and North Carolina Rural Health Research Center at the University of North Carolina Chapel Hill are tracking closures and following how communities are responding.

Critical Access Hospitals—Physician Practice Mergers and Acquisitions

Over the past decade, the combination of recruitment and retention difficulties for rural practices, downward spiraling reimbursement payments from public and private payers, and added expense of new federal requirements such as electronic medical records encouraged the merging of rural physician practices with hospitals, many of which were CAH certified. As the overhead costs of owning and managing a practice continued to grow, physicians were more willing and interested in seeking relief through this mechanism. Additionally, such extended hospital linkages help capture market share by creating referral resources within the network. Under the PPACA health care reform requirements, creation of accountable care organizations (ACOs) and accountable community health (ACH) systems and implementation of meaningful use of electronic medical records have pushed more providers to seek collaborations that allow for flexibility and efficient use of resources to maintain adequate levels of local services.

Under the PPACA framework, health care networks (ACOs) would collaborate to lower costs, improve quality of care and services, and improve outcomes. By sharing resources and financial risk, the ACOs would receive better reimbursement, which would be shared proportionately among the partnering entities. In shifting toward a value-based reimbursement model, Medicare and other insurers anticipate overall health care costs will decrease over the next several years, with the difference used to help pay for the increased coverage of uninsured populations.

RURAL CLINICS: FRONTLINE ACCESS

Community and Migrant Health Centers

Access to health care for underserved populations such as migrant farm workers and their families was recognized as a problem as early as the 1960s. Congress passed the Migrant Health Act of 1962 (PL 87-692), which provided for the development of dedicated health clinics to serve the needs of these workers and families. President Lyndon Johnson's "War on Poverty" in the mid-1960s was responsible for passage of the Economic Opportunity Act of 1964, which increased access by creating Neighborhood Health Centers in urban areas with high poverty populations. All these centers were transferred to the Public Health Service in the early 1970s and later authorized in 1975 under Section 330 of the Public Health Service Act (PL 94-63). The new Community Health Centers (CHCs) were established to provide quality care to a wide range of underserved populations in both rural and urban areas and encouraged collaborative partnerships between public and private providers.

Over the next 2 decades, new programs were added to the CHC program to include the Migrant Health Center program, Healthcare for the Homeless Centers, and Public Housing Primary Care Program.[22] Later, the Omnibus Budget Reconciliation Acts of 1989, 1990, and 1993 created a new entity under Medicare and Medicaid known as FQHCs; the Social Security Act also expanded the definitions to add amendments describing FQHC look-alikes. These clinics received federal enhanced reimbursement but did not receive core federal grants under Section 330 for construction or operating costs.

Community health centers are characterized by five essential elements that differentiate them from other providers:

- They must be located in or serve a high-need community (i.e., Medically Underserved Areas [MUAs] or Medically Underserved Populations [MUPs]).

- They must provide comprehensive primary care services and supportive services, such as translation and transportation services that promote access to health care.
- Their services must be available to all residents of their service areas, with fees adjusted according to patients' ability to pay.
- They must be governed by a community board with a majority of members being health center patients.
- They must meet other performance and accountability requirements regarding their administrative, clinical, and financial operations.[23]

The Bush administration established the President's Health Centers Initiative in 2002, which was to increase the system by 1200 expanded or new access points, thereby pushing the number of patients served from approximately 15 million to 19.8 million. As of the end of 2014, there were more than 1278 CHCs with almost 9000 clinical service units serving 23 million people. Under current PPACA provisions, an additional $11 billion was allocated for the period 2010 to 2015 to expand the number of centers ($9.5 billion) to eventually serve 40 million people or about double current capacity. There is also $1.5 billion set aside to upgrade current facilities. Additional funds are also included under Title VII training to create Teaching Health Center collaboratives to increase the actual time medical students and residents spend in CHCs, RHCs, and other similar sites as part of their training.[24–26]

Community Health Centers often provide comprehensive health services, including medical, dental, mental health, pharmacy, and social services. Although there are no specific requirements, the CHCs use all types of health care providers, including PAs and NPs (15% of the CHC workforce). A 2004 study of CHC personnel shortages completed by Rosenblatt and colleagues[27] looked at the implications for the planned expansion under the President's Initiative and found that the CHCs were already understaffed and having difficulty recruiting and retaining providers. Rapid expansion under the PPACA has put even more pressure on the CHCs for recruitment and retention of health professionals at all levels.

The largest groups of physicians employed in CHCs are family physicians, internists, and pediatricians. Significantly, the study found that "in rural CHCs, 46% of the direct clinical providers of care are nonphysician clinicians (PAs, NPs, and certified nurse midwives [CNMs]) compared with 38.9% in urban CHCs." Obstetrician/gynecologists, psychiatrists, and dentists are the other main providers, although in much smaller numbers. Although there

has been a slight increase in the past couple years, given the significant declining trend in family medicine residency matches since 1997 (a loss of almost 52%) and the relatively small number of graduates of the other specialties noted, the recruitment and retention challenges facing CHCs with further expansion will increase proportionately.

Rural Health Clinics

The Rural Health Clinic Act of 1977 (PL 95-210) established CMS- and Medicare-recognized RHCs to help address the continuing shortages of health care access in rural areas. The purpose of the legislation was twofold: to increase access in rural, underserved communities and to encourage use of nonphysician providers such as PAs, NPs, and CNMs in collaborative models to expand the reach of physicians in those communities.

The RHC program was the first federal initiative to mandate the use of a team approach to health care delivery. Each federally certified RHC must have
- One or more physicians (does not have to be full time at the site)
- One or more PAs, NPs, or CNMs onsite and available to see patients 50% of the time the clinic is open for patients
- Written patient care policies developed by the physician; PA, NP, or CNM; and one practitioner not employed at the clinic
- The ability to provide emergency services to stabilize patients with life-threatening or acute illnesses
- An accurate and confidential and secure record-keeping system that is also in compliance with HIPAA regulations
- Diagnostic and treatment services commonly furnished in a physician's office, including the following laboratory services: chemical examinations of urine, hemoglobin or hematocrit, blood sugar, examination of stool specimens for occult blood, pregnancy test, and primary culturing for transmittal to reference laboratories

In addition, RHCs may have other services provided by arrangement to include
- Inpatient hospital care
- Specialized physician services
- Specialized diagnostic and laboratory services
- Interpreter for foreign language if indicated
- Interpreter for deaf and devices to assist communication with blind patients[28]

Initially, the RHC qualification process under PL 95-210 was onerous and excessively cumbersome. Congress had expected several thousand clinics to apply, but by 1990, there were only about 600. In the late 1980s and early 1990s, Congress reviewed the program to see why there were so many fewer clinics than expected. This resulted in a number of changes that improved the certification process, and by 1997, more than 3000 clinics were certified; in 2016, there were about 4000 clinics. The creation of the National Association of RHCs resulted in the availability of valuable technical assistance and networking support among clinics and clinicians. This association has also been effective in promoting RHCs at the state and community levels.

New Models for Frontier Communities

Discussions about how to serve more remote communities and populations began in 1997 with the establishment of the Rural Hospital Flexibility program. However, even the relaxed parameters of the CAH designation were not seen as reasonable for the outlying areas of Alaska, open spaces of Wyoming, or other remote areas of the country that did not have a hospital facility; there needed to be an expanded definition that would allow clinics to fill the gap in access to inpatient care. The Frontier Education Center (now the National Center for Frontier Communities), based in Arizona, helped spur the dialogue at state, regional, and national levels for more than a decade using the support of groups such as the National Rural Health Association.

As a result of these discussions, along with strong support from the congressional representatives from Alaska, the Medicare Prescription Drug Improvement and MMA of 2003 included provisions for testing a new model of clinics for more remote areas designated as the Frontier Extended Stay Clinic (FESC). There were two parts to the projected action: First, the MMA of 2003 gave authority to the CMS at the Department of Health and Human Services (DHHS) to conduct a demonstration program to reimburse extended-stay care received by Medicare beneficiaries. Second, the Consolidated Appropriations Acts of 2004, 2005, and 2006 included funding for the FORHP "to examine the effectiveness and appropriateness of a new type of provider, the FESC, in providing health care services in certain remote locations." This became the FESC Cooperative Agreement Program.[29] Applicants for this Cooperative Agreement competed nationally, and the Southeast Alaska Regional Health Consortium, an Alaska Native corporation, was awarded the funding. The Alaska FESC Consortium is a partnership of providers in Alaska and Washington state, as well as evaluators from the University of Alaska, Anchorage, and the Sheps Center at the University of North Carolina Chapel Hill.

A facility can be designated an FESC if it (1) is located in a community where the closest short-term acute care hospital or CAH is at least 75 miles away from the community or is inaccessible by public road and (2) is designed to address the needs of seriously or critically ill or injured patients who, because of adverse weather conditions or other reasons, cannot be transferred quickly to acute care referral centers or patients who need monitoring and observation for a limited period of time.

FUNDING AND REIMBURSEMENT FOR RURAL HEALTH SERVICES

Finances for rural facilities are complex and underscored by periodic changes at the state and federal levels. Important to recognize, however, are the various efforts to help stabilize rural hospitals and clinics, including the enhanced payments from Medicare for CAHs, RHCs, and CHCs (including FQHC look-alikes).

Rural populations have typically been described as older, poorer, having lower education achievement, including greater numbers of immigrants, and having more chronic disease; all of these elements contribute to a higher need for health care and more specialized care access. With 5 years of experience in implementation of the PPACA, we can see a change of trends and dynamics with greater numbers of insured individuals and families across the spectrum of race, ethnicity, age, and geographic location. The 2010 U.S. Census revealed that there were approximately 49.9 million people uninsured: 19% in urban areas and 23% in nonmetro areas of under 2500 population. The PPACA has allowed at least an additional 20 million so far to establish some level of health care insurance, with projections to 30 million by 2020.

Before the PPACA, many rural Americans struggled to find affordable health care, paying nearly half of all medical costs out of their own pockets. Many self-employed farmers, ranchers, and rural small business owners—some of the most critical contributors to strong rural economies—did not have access to the affordable insurance options that many people get through their employers. Under the Medicaid expansion program and the federal and state health marketplaces, many people have been able to purchase affordable insurance.

Unfortunately, because of a Supreme Court ruling in 2012, 24 states elected not to participate in the expansion program as of 2014; most of these states are in the southern section of the country where poverty and low-wage jobs are more common in rural areas, which creates a disproportionate burden on those people not able to access insurance. Reports indicate more than half of urban populations are able to access insurance through their workplaces, but rural areas have many smaller employers and part-time positions that may not offer any insurance options. Although some may be eligible for tax credits if their incomes are between 100% and 138% the federal poverty level, many will also fall in that "in-between" zone of making just too much to qualify for the available tax credits and therefore lower premiums.

Other significant barriers to access are absence of health plans willing to extend to rural areas or lack of providers, low population base, distance and time factors to get to primary care or hospital or specialty services, 24-hour coverage options, and fiscal protection of the safety-net providers via cost-based reimbursement.[30,31]

Rural Incentives for Providers

Recruitment and retention continue to be challenges for rural areas. Several programs implemented over the years to create incentives for providers to recruit and retain physicians in rural areas have been successful to some degree. These included a 10% Medicare bonus payment if the provider practiced in a Health Professional Shortage Area (HPSA) and, more recently as a part of the MMA 2003, an additional 5% bonus if the provider was also in a Physician Shortage Area. Such incentives can become meaningful financially if the practice is busy and has significant Medicare patients. Under the PPACA, physicians, hospitals, and CHCs will receive varying amounts of financial support to maintain and increase services. For example, the 10% bonus payment to physicians will be extended to all physicians in rural areas meeting specific criteria, such as 60% of services being "primary care services" as defined by the ACA.[30-33]

Other incentives programs include loan repayment and scholarship (state and federal—National Health Service Corps), state and local tax credits, malpractice premium reduction, a line of credit for home and clinic purchase, and various related support mechanisms.

RURAL HEALTH WORKFORCE ISSUES

Recruitment and retention of health care providers at every level and in every discipline for rural areas has remained a problem nationally even with the various programs and incentives described. Part of the problem is an absolute shortage of health professions available; the other factor is maldistribution toward specialty practices and location to urban and suburban communities.

Briefly, the shortages for medical practitioners for rural areas involve several factors:

- **Applicant pools:** Multiple studies have shown that medical school applicants increasingly come from urban, higher income areas and not from rural areas. Although the number of applicants waned for a short period several years ago, the medical school applicant pool rose from 39,000 in 2003 to 52,500 in 2015, and the number of matriculating students rose from 17,300 to 20,600 in the same period. Rural and racial/ethnic minority students are still very much in the minority, however. The AAMC, representing all the allopathic schools, challenged the existing 125 U.S. medical schools in 2002 to increase their student slots by 30% by 2019. Those schools are on target with increases and have been joined by a number of new medical schools now totaling 141. The American Association of Colleges of Osteopathic Medicine reports that, for the year ending 2015, there were 26,333 students enrolled in 31 osteopathic colleges in 46 locations nationally in 31 states.[32-34]

- **Lengthy timelines for completion of training:** The timeline for generalist physicians is a minimum of 11 years from start of an undergraduate program to the end of residency training; this increases with certain specialty programs, such as surgery, psychiatry, obstetrics and gynecology, and internal medicine subspecialties. As some disciplines moved to the master's or doctorate level, such as the Doctor of Physical Therapy (DPT), Doctor of Pharmacy (PharmD), and Doctor of Nursing Practice (DNP), additional time and cost are required to graduate and enter the workforce. Student debt is one the greatest challenges now facing medicine and other health profession students, with several new programs initiated under the PPACA to reduce those burdens.

- **Institutional capacity:** Classroom space and the availability of qualified faculty have been major barriers to meeting the significant shortages of nurses, as an example of this issue. State higher education budgets have not been a priority in many states, and resources are not available to support program expansion. The other factor is the inability of education programs to provide competitive salaries to attract personnel from the private sector. Nursing schools in particular have struggled to recruit and retain advanced nursing faculty because hospital and clinic salaries have increased significantly as a result of the nursing shortage nationally. For PA programs, the expansion of accredited programs in the past decade from 137 to 199 and the change to the master's degree as the entry level degree by 2020 have also created a gap of readily available academically prepared faculty for many of the same reasons as nursing.

- **Program availability:** Starting a new program or even expanding current programs is costly and has a long timeline because of approvals at the institutional and state levels. For example, 20 new allopathic medical schools have been started in the past 2 decades to try to meet the growing need. According to several recent studies published by the AAMC and Council on Graduate Medical Education on the physician workforce, major issues facing medicine include almost one third of currently practicing physicians aging to retirement in the next decade, with many of those older primary care physicians in rural areas; changing patterns of practice, with increased numbers of women physicians who take time off for child-rearing and may work fewer hours per week; and evidence that millennial physicians may take a more balanced perspective to work–home life and also work fewer hours than older physicians.[34] On the other hand, the number of PA programs increased dramatically from three programs in 1967 to 65 in the 1970s and 1980s to 154 in 2010 and 199 at the start of 2016, turning out about 7500 graduates each year.[35,36]

- **Changing discipline accreditation and graduation standards:** As noted earlier, some disciplines have moved to more advanced degrees over the past decade. This has lengthened training time, changed the demographics of the applicant pool, and potentially influenced practice site decisions. Increased costs of education and graduate debt load push providers toward higher paying jobs in urban areas rather than rural practices.

- **Recruitment costs and retention issues:** With physician recruitment costs averaging $30,000 or more just for the search company fees, frequent turnover of providers creates a financial drain on facilities. If start-up salaries, travel, and relocation costs are included, a typical recruitment cost could be closer to $100,000. Most sources indicate that good recruitment tactics result in better retention with satisfied providers and family. With the number of positions opening for PAs in specialty and generalist practices, there is a growing similarity in competition and recruiting costs for PAs

as well. These costs typically come from clinic and hospital budgets that are already marginal and take away from projected facility and staffing upgrades.

PHYSICIAN ASSISTANTS AND RURAL MEDICINE

Census data of the AAPA allow us to track PA involvement in rural health. The AAPA Annual Survey reported that in 2013, there were 93,098 individuals in practice.[16] The AAPA census notes that 32% are in primary care (compared with 38% in 2006, 48.5% in 2003, 52.7% in 1997, and 37% in 1986). The primary care field breakdown includes family and general medicine (44%), general internal medicine and specialties (14%), general pediatrics (5.7%), and obstetrics and gynecology (6.1%). Other prevalent specialties for PAs include general surgery and surgical subspecialties (26.6%), emergency medicine (10.3%), and the subspecialties of internal medicine (15%) and dermatology (3.3%).

Currently, 12% of PAs describe themselves as working in nonmetro settings, a drop from 22.7% in 2003 and 15% in 2010.[14] Almost 18.6% work in communities of fewer than 20,000. About 6.3% of primary care PAs were working in communities of fewer than 2500 in 2010.[37]

Recruitment and retention issues are similar to those of physicians, with multiple factors influencing rural practice. Factors such as the changing applicant pool with a significant increase in women applying and matriculating will have an increasing impact on practice profiles and lifestyles; women now account for 75% of matriculating students. A number of research studies have shown that women physicians and PAs tend to select urban practice settings to a greater extent than men. Another potential factor is the move by some institutions toward more advanced academic degrees, which may also affect rural deployment. A recent study of all PA graduates of the University of Washington MEDEX Physician Assistant program by Evans and colleagues[38] showed an almost inverse relationship between academic degrees awarded and rurality of employment, whereby graduates with higher degrees tend to practice to a greater extent in metro areas, a cause for concern for education programs targeting rural primary care.

Retention of rural PAs was examined by Larson and colleagues,[39] who found that a high percentage of PAs who started practice in rural areas (41%) were likely to leave for urban practice during the first 4 years and that female PAs were slightly more likely to leave than men. This was mitigated by urban PAs transitioning to rural settings (10%), however, thereby keeping the number of rural PAs between 15% and 20%. Issues related to leaving included difficulties around prescriptive authority, reimbursement, and availability of insurance. Factors influencing retention of rural PAs were published by Muus and colleagues[40] and included good relationships with the supervising physician and a relative degree of autonomy, reasonable practice hours and responsibilities, and satisfaction with living in the community.

FEDERAL AND STATE POLICY IMPLICATIONS FOR RURAL HEALTH CARE

Over the past several decades, there has always been a general lack of access to health care services in rural and frontier communities. Large-scale federal initiatives to deal with the problem consisted of provisions for medical research, construction of health centers, and money for medical education. Examples discussed earlier include the Hill-Burton Act of 1946, the Rural Health Clinic Act of 1977, implementation of Prospective Payment Systems and Diagnostic Related Group (PPS/DRG) payment in 1983, the Omnibus Budget Reconciliation Act of 1989, the Balanced Budget Act of 1997 and the Balanced Budget Revision Act of 1999, and more recently the MMA of 2003, all of which defined or redefined funding or facility opportunities for health care systems. The PPACA had significant implications for rural health.[12,30,31] Specific federal initiatives focused around the following areas:

- **Personnel:** Public Health Services Act Title VII (medicine and allied health) and VIII (nursing) funding for education, National Health Service Corps, 3R-Network
- **Reduction of inequities:** the creation of designations for HPSAs and medically underserved areas, enhanced Medicare and Medicaid reimbursement for rural clinics and hospitals
- **Support for the actual delivery system:** RHCs, Community and Migrant Health Centers, Rural Hospital Flex Program, FESC
- **Development of infrastructure to support the rural health care delivery system:** Area Health Education Centers (AHEC) Program, federal and state offices of rural health, and state primary care offices

The National Health Service Corps (NHSC), established in 1970, was designed to provide health personnel to the areas of greatest need. Initially, the NHSC was a program that linked scholarships with service obligations for "payback" in medically underserved communities. Although it was initially successful in placing new physicians—and later PAs, NPs, and CNMs—in needy clinics, the program was criticized when many providers moved on after their time was up. In response, the NHSC expanded its scope to include loan repayment and scholarship opportunities. This combination has given the NHSC more flexibility in responding to the needs of specific communities and individual providers. Over time, the NHSC has expanded the number of slots available to both PAs and NPs. The NHSC also supports the training of dentists and mental health providers. Although earlier studies showed a lack of retention, resulting disruption in continuity of care, a 2012 study revealed that 82% of placements stayed for at least 1 year after their initial obligation, and 55% stayed in place for 10 or more years.[41] New funding under the PPACA substantially increases the NHSC to expand both scholarship and loan repayment slots targeting FQHCs and RHCs and other underserved areas.

Parallel to the development of the NHSC, the federal government began investing directly in the training of primary care providers, including family medicine residencies and PA and NP educational training programs through Title VII/VIII of the Public Health Service Act. Funding formulas for these programs provided incentives for the development and support of rural training opportunities. Many PA programs specifically received support for the recruitment of individuals from rural communities to be trained for rural practice. Federal funding for these critical programs has increased significantly under the ACA, which is promoting enhanced recruitment to the health professions and expanded primary care training for physicians, PAs, allied health fields, and nursing. Specific funding to increase the number of PA programs and students has already been initiated, and new programs targeting the transition of military and veteran PAs have been developed and are expanding.

Federal designations—HPSAs, MUAs, and MUPs—are used to direct scarce public monies to areas of greatest need. As noted, these criteria are critically important to rural communities because eligibility for more than 40 programs—such as NHSC, Medicare bonus payments, RHCs and FQHC clinics, and CAHs—depend on these designations.

Although all three types of designations have been helpful in bringing more resources to rural America, they have also generated significant controversy. Some of the dissatisfaction has been with specific formulas—and cut-off points—in use at any given time. There has been a more general dissatisfaction with the cumbersome process involved in achieving these designations. The sad fact is that none of these designations gives a clear picture of the level of the "underservedness" that exists in this country. The granting of each of these designations involves a fairly high level of sophistication, the prior existence of an administrative infrastructure, and the availability of complex data sets. Thus, some of our most underserved areas have difficulty in meeting the administrative criteria for these designations even though they are clearly "eligible."

The creation of the Federal Office of Rural Health Policy (FORHP) was a significant juncture for rural communities. It was created by the federal government in 1987 and was tasked with promoting better health care service in rural America. The FORHP was also charged with keeping the DHHS advised on matters affecting rural hospitals and health care, coordinating activities within the department that relate to rural health care, and maintaining a national information clearinghouse. Working with government at federal, state, and local levels, as well as with associations, foundations, providers, and community leaders, it seeks solutions to rural health care problems. The FORHP does the following:

- Helps shape rural health policy
- Works with state offices of rural health
- Promotes rural health research
- Funds innovative rural health programs
- Provides support to the National Advisory Committee on Rural Health and Human Services
- Acts as a voice for the concerns of rural hospitals, clinics, and other rural health care providers
- Acts as a liaison with national, state, and local rural health organizations
- Works with minority populations in rural areas
- Sponsors a national clearinghouse of rural health information
- Evaluates programs[42]

A significant outcome of the FOHRP was the development of a matching grant program for state offices of rural health, which began in 1991, and has accomplished the creation of state offices in all 50 states. Each state office helps its local rural communities build health care delivery systems. Goals of the offices are to collect and disseminate information, provide technical assistance, help to coordinate rural health interests statewide, and support efforts to improve recruitment and retention of health professionals. Subsequently, the National Organization of State Offices of Rural Health was created as a representative body to provide states a voice in addressing legislative and policy issues at the national level.[42]

The AHEC has a mission "to enhance access to quality health care, particularly primary and preventive care, by improving the supply and distribution of health care professionals through community/ academic educational partnerships." The program was part of the Comprehensive Manpower Training Act of 1971, which Congress created to recruit, train, and retain a health profession workforce committed to underserved populations. The Health Education Training Centers (HETC) program was created in 1989 to provide programs for specific populations with persistent, severe unmet health needs, particularly along the southern border of the United States. Together the Area Health Education Center (AHEC) and HETC programs helped create a "town–gown" partnership between academic health centers and communities in addressing local community health needs. There are 53 academic health center AHEC programs with 231 regional centers operating in almost every state and the District of Columbia, connecting more than 120 medical schools and 600 nursing and allied health schools, all collaborating with AHECs to improve health for underserved and underrepresented populations.[43]

REQUISITES FOR RURAL PHYSICIAN ASSISTANTS

Depending on the type of practice setting—solo in a satellite clinic or in a multiphysician clinic—PAs benefit from having a broad range of skills beyond just their medical knowledge. Medical practice knowledge and skills can be helpful in not only managing clinic operations if necessary but also tracking their own contributions and value to the practice. This is helpful in negotiating salary or benefit increases, expanding scope of practice, or even supporting a need for more advanced education for skill enhancement.

A number of published papers indicate that confidence is one of the primary factors that contributes to the success and retention of PAs in rural areas.[44] Having confidence in your medical knowledge and skills provides the basis for a relatively high degree of autonomy, a significant factor in retention; this also enables PAs to engage the community through participation in outreach activities and social and community organizations. Factors that negatively affect retention include isolation (both from the precepting physicians and facilities and other professionals); frustration with lack of resources, such as equipment, no pharmacy in town, or inadequate transportation for patients to travel for referred care; or lack of support for vacations or continuing medical education time off.

Studies have also shown that PAs who grew up in rural or similar communities are more satisfied with rural practice; this is also true for spouses. Gender also plays a role in that women are less likely to seek or remain in rural settings for a variety of reasons. With more marriages including two professionals, adequate job opportunities for the non-PA spouse is an important factor in long-term family satisfaction.[43-45]

Rural PAs certainly need to have a level of confidence in their knowledge and skills to manage routine and emergency situations, and they should have all their advanced skill certifications updated as appropriate (e.g., Advanced Cardiac Life Support, Advanced Trauma Life Support, Pediatric Life Support). Familiarity with simple laboratory procedures, phlebotomy, taking routine radiographs, and enhanced computer skills can allow PAs to operate in a wider variety of settings comfortably, recognizing that often there are limited staff and ancillary services available locally.

Much of this may depend on the degree of remoteness and autonomy in the position, as well as the type of community population and practice. An important element of rural practice, which every PA needs to be mindful of, is the legal liability involved in autonomous decision making and recognizing their own knowledge level, as well as knowing the limits of the physician–PA relationship.

CHALLENGES AND REWARDS OF RURAL PRACTICE

Some liken the challenge or the attraction of rural practice to being "a little fish in a big pond." There are many opportunities in a smaller community to influence the health and well-being of individuals, as well as the community as a whole, whether it is assisting with sports team coverage, participating in teaching health subjects in the schools at all levels, establishing chronic disease management programs, teaching EMS classes, or being asked to serve on various boards and committees. As a health care professional, PAs are often seen as having advanced knowledge and skills that can serve the community in many ways.

Why consider rural practice? Many see the lifestyle as personally attractive, including a safer environment in which to raise a family, often a more relaxed lifestyle (except for on-call time), and accessibility to superb recreational facilities. Care should be taken, however, to ensure that each member of the family has input into the decision to move to a rural community. Access to social and recreational amenities may be lacking or far enough away to limit frequent trips. Salaries and benefits may be somewhat lower than in urban practices, but market forces determine ranges as much as size of the practice. It is not unusual to hear of starting salaries in the $85,000 to $100,000 range even in small communities as an incentive to practitioners to relocate; other initial benefits may include assistance with housing and moving expenses.

Professionally, there is often the opportunity to have a wider scope of practice. Some of the professional rewards that one finds in a rural setting include the ability to use most, if not all, of one's training. The most common exceptions to this are obstetric and surgical skills. Rural PAs usually have a much greater degree of independence (often regulatory as well as actual) than they would have in an urban setting, although this can be a two-edged sword because of the temptation to overstep limits. In rural practice, one can take pleasure in the fact that one can have a tremendous impact on the well-being of patients and can be involved in all aspects of their lives, from taking care of newborns and reinforcing parenting skills to helping ease the pain of an older patient who is dying. Rural PAs also find that they truly are meeting a need, one that might well go unmet if they were not present. Medical needs in underserved rural and inner-city areas are what PAs were originally created to meet. The PA profession has consistently shown that it can do an excellent job of meeting them.

> ### KEY POINTS
>
> Rural health involves a complex system that is determined in part by how we define "rural," the changing demographics of the population, state and federal programs that determine licensing, certification and funding, and meeting geographic challenges in accessing care. Rural communities and health care systems are always being challenged but have been resilient in meeting the health needs of their communities. Important issues include:
>
> - Health care reform implementation under the PPACA of 2010 has had significant impacts by increasing the number of people with insurance, increasing demand for access to services at all levels, and changing the way health care is organized and providers are reimbursed (e.g., PCMH, ACO, ACH, value versus quantity, Medicare and Medicaid changes). Challenges continue for rural health systems to remain viable.
> - Changing demographics of population dispersion across rural and urban counties, changes in population diversity, and lasting impacts of the recent recession on rural areas create the need for careful planning for health professions workforce and service delivery models.
> - Policy decisions, particularly at the federal level, often have unintended consequences for rural areas and health care. Issues such as health care reform, rigid immigration laws, decreased CMS reimbursement for physician services, and mandatory implementation of electronic medical records for Medicare reimbursement have all had significant effects on rural population access and health care system survival.
> - Health profession workforce projections suggest a significant shortfall in numbers of future physicians because of impending retirements in the next 2 decades of almost 30% of the MD and DO workforce, inadequate pipelines for replacements, and changing demographics within the profession. Studies suggest that alternative models using the growing numbers of PAs and NPs more effectively could significantly reduce that gap.
> - The PA profession was founded in part to meet the needs of rural and underserved communities and populations. As the profession has shifted to more advanced degrees and specialty practice, a majority female workforce, greater educational debt, and persistent state licensing challenges, what are the implications for PAs to continue to meet rural workforce needs? What are the potential incentives, skills, and other factors that would encourage rural practice?

References

1. Johnson K. Demographic trends in rural and small town America. Carsey Institute, Reports on Rural America Vol. 1, No.1, University of New Hampshire 2006, http://scholars.unh.edu/cgi/viewcontent.cgi?article=1004&context=carsey. Accessed June 2012.
2. Cromartie J. *Population & Migration*. Washington, DC: U.S. Department of Agriculture, Economic Research Service; May 26, 2012. http://www.ers.usda.gov/topics/rural-economy-population/population-migration.aspx. Accessed January 2016.
3. National Center for Frontier Communities. The Consensus Definition. http://www.frontierus.org/documents/consensus.htm. Accessed January 2012.
4. Rural Population and Migration. Trend 6—challenges from an aging population. Economic Research Service/U.S. Department of Agriculture. http://www.ers.usda.gov/Briefing/Population/Challenges.htm. Accessed February 1, 2007.
5. Jones CA, Parker TS, Ahern M, et al. Health status and health care access of farm and rural populations. Economic Research Service/U.S. Department of Agriculture, August 2009. http://www.ers.usda.gov/publications/eib57/. Accessed November 2015.
6. Ricketts TC. *Rural Health in the United States*. New York: Oxford University Press; 1999:3–19.
7. Rural Employment and Unemployment. Economic Research Service/U.S. Department of Agriculture. Updated January 2016. http://www.ers.usda.gov/topics/rural-economy-population/employment-education/rural-employment-and-unemployment.aspx. Accessed January 2016.
8. Reeder RJ, Brown DM. *Recreation, Tourism and Rural Well-being*. U.S. Department of Agriculture, Economic Research Report Number 7. August 2005.
9. 2010 Census Shows America's Diversity. U.S. Census news release, March 24, 2011. https://www.census.gov/newsroom/releases/archives/2010_census/cb11-cn125.html. Accessed November 2015.
10. Rural Population and Migration. Trend 5—diversity increases in nonmetro America. Economic Research Service/U.S. Department of Agriculture. http://www.ers.usda.gov/Briefing/Population/Diversity.htm. Accessed February 2007.
11. MacKinney AC. Access to rural health care: a literature review and new synthesis. RUPRI, August 2014. http://www.rupri.org/Forms/HealthPanel_Access_August2014.pdf. Accessed December 2015.
12. McBride T. The ACA's impact on rural areas. Powerpoint presentation at Washington University in St. Louis, MO, September 2015. http://cph.uiowa.edu/rupri/presentations/2015/The%20ACA%20Impact%20on%20Rural%20Areas.pdf. Accessed January 2016.

13. Overview of the uninsured in the United States. A Summary of the 2011 Current Population Survey Office of the Assistant Secretary for Planning and Evaluation. Department of Health and Human Services. http://aspe.hhs.gov/health/reports/2011/CPSHealthIns2011/ib.pdf. Accessed September 2012.

14. Cawley JF, Lane S, Smith N, Bush E. Physician assistants in rural communities. *JAAPA*. January 2016;29(1):42–45.

15. Physician Workforce Policy Guidelines for the United States 2004-2020 Council on Graduate Medical Education Sixteenth (COGME) Report. January 2005. http://www.hrsa.gov/advisorycommittees/bhpradvisory/cogme/reports/sixteenthreport.pdf. Accessed June 2012.

16. 2013 AAPA Annual Survey Report. https://www.aapa.org/WorkArea/DownloadAsset.aspx?id=2902. Accessed May 2014.

17. Diversity in the physician workforce. Facts and figures 2014. *AAMC*. http://aamcdiversityfactsandfigures.org. Accessed January 2016.

18. *HCFA Finalizes Rule to Improve Hospital, Emergency Treatment Access: Health Care Policy Report*. Washington, DC: Bureau of National Affairs; May 31, 1993.

19. Critical Access Hospitals. HRSA, Rural Health Information Hub. https://www.ruralhealthinfo.org/topics/critical-access-hospitals. Accessed December 2015.

20. Small Hospital Improvement Grant. Rural Assistance Center. U.S. Department of Health and Human Services. http://www.raconline.org/funding/details.php?funding_id=64.

21. 71 rural hospital closures: january 2010-present. Cecil G. Sheps Center for Rural Health Services Research. Chapel Hill: University of North Carolina; March 2016. http://www.shepscenter.unc.edu/programs-projects/rural-health/rural-hospital-closures/. Accessed March 2016.

22. Health Center History. Bureau of Primary Health Care/Health Resources Services Administration/DHHS. http://bphc.hrsa.gov/about/index.html. Accessed August 2012.

23. Federally Qualified Health Center Fact Sheet. DHHS/CMS/Medicare Learning Network. January 2013. https://www.cms.gov/Outreach-and-Education/Medicare-Learning-Network-MLN/MLNProducts/downloads/fqhcfactsheet.pdf. Accessed September 2015.

24. Creating health care jobs by addressing primary care workforce needs. http://www.hhs.gov/healthcare/facts-and-features/fact-sheets/creating-health-care-jobs-by-addressing-primary-care-workforce-needs/index.html. Accessed November 2015.

25. HRSA Health Center Expansion. DHHS/HRSA. http://bphc.hrsa.gov/about/healthcenterfactsheet.pdf. Accessed January 2016.

26. Teaching health center graduate medical education. DHHS/HRSA. http://bhpr.hrsa.gov/grants/teachinghealthcenters/index.html. Accessed January 2016.

27. Rosenblatt R, Andrilla CH, Curtin T, Hart LG. Shortages of medical personnel at community health centers. *JAMA*. March 1, 2006;293:1042–1049.

28. Rural Health Clinic Fact Sheet. DHHS/CMS/Medicare Learning Network. January 2016. https://www.cms.gov/Outreach-and-Education/Medicare-Learning-Network-MLN/MLNProducts/downloads/RuralHlthClinfctsht.pdf. Accessed January 2016.

29. Frontier Extended Stay Clinic (FESC) Cooperative Agreement Program. Office of Rural Health Policy/HRSA/DHHS. http://ruralhealth.hrsa.gov/funding/fesc.htmhttp://www.frontierus.org/index-current.htm. Accessed September 2012.

30. Coburn AF, Lundblad JP, MacKinney AC, et al. The Patient Protection and Affordable Care Act of 2010: impacts on rural people, places, and providers: a first look. RUPRI Health Panel. http://www.rupri.org/Forms/Health_PPACAImpacts_Sept2010.pdf. Accessed September 16, 2010.

31. Blumenthal D, Abrams M, Nuzum R. The Affordable Care Act at 5 years. *N Engl J Med*. June 18, 2015;372(25):2451–2458.

32. Medical school applicants, enrollees reach new highs. October 22, 2015. https://www.aamc.org/newsroom/newsreleases/446400/applicant-and-enrollment-data.html. Accessed January 2016.

33. Results of the 2014 Medical School Enrollment Survey. AAMC Center for Workforce Studies, April 2015. https://members.aamc.org/eweb/upload/Results%20of%20the%202014%20Medical%20School%20Enrollment%20Survey.pdf. Accessed January 2016.

34. Complexities of physician supply and demand: projections from 2013 to 2025. Report prepared by IHS, INC for the AAMC. March 2015. https://www.aamc.org/download/426242/data/ihsreportdownload.pdf. Accessed January 2016.

35. By the Numbers 2015. Physician Assistant Education Association (PAEA): 30th Annual Report on PA Education in the United States. http://paeaonline.org/research/annual-report-on-pa-educational-programs/. Accessed February 2016.

36. Accreditation Review Commission on Education of the Physician Assistant: Program data April 2015. http://www.arc-pa.com/acc_programs/program_data.html. Accessed January 2016.

37. Primary Care Workforce Facts and Stats. Agency for Wealthcare Research and Quality. https://www.ahrq.gov/research/findings/factsheets/primary/pcworkforceindex.html. December 28, 2016.

38. Evans T, Wick K, Brock D, Academic degrees and clinical practice characteristics, et al. The University of Washington Physician Assistant program: 1969-2000. *J Rural Health*. Summer 2006;22(3):212–219.

39. Larson EH, Hart LG, Goodwin MK, et al. Dimensions of retention: a national study of the locational histories of physician assistants. *J Rural Health*. 1999;15:391.

40. Muus KJ, Geller JM, Williams JD, et al. Job satisfaction among rural physician assistants. *J Rural Health*. 1998;14:100–108.

41. Federal Office of Rural Health Policy. http://hrsa.gov/ruralhealth/about/index.html. Accessed September 2012.

42. National AHEC Organization. http://www.nationalahec.org/about/AboutUs.html. Accessed November 2015.

43. Henry L, Hooker RS. Retention of physician assistants in rural health clinics. *J Rural Health*. Summer 2007;23(3):207–214.

44. Daniels ZM, VanLeit BJ, Skipper BJ, et al. Factors in recruiting and retaining professionals for rural practice: National Rural Health Association Workforce Issues Series. *J Rural Health*. 2007;23:62–71.

45. Henry LR, Hooker RS, Yates KL. The role of physician assistants in rural health care: a systematic review of the literature. *J Rural Health*. 2011;27:220–229.

The resources for this chapter can be found at www.expertconsult.com.

The faculty resources can be found online at www.expertconsult.com.

INTERNATIONAL HEALTH CARE

David H. Kuhns

The opportunity to work abroad in a clinical setting, whether updating the skills and knowledge of local providers for a couple of weeks or a longer term commitment of months providing essential health care to displaced populations suffering from the ravages of war, will likely have long-term effects for the physician assistant (PA) who rises to such a challenge. For many PAs, it is simply a heightened sense of adventure that makes such service appealing. For others, it is the heartfelt sense of moral obligation to help wherever in world the needs are great and the resources scarce. Regardless of the motive, such service as a PA will likely be a life-altering event.

Physician assistants have actively participated in the delivery of international health care since the inception of the PA profession. PAs work with many international organizations, both private and governmental. PAs have served, and continue to serve, with international relief organizations in Cambodia, Brazil, Tonga, Peru, Guatemala, Nicaragua, Syria, South Sudan, and Somalia, to name but a few. Other PAs are employed by private multinational corporations, supporting the oil-drilling and diamond mine crews above the Arctic Circle or providing primary care to expatriates and their families living in China and Saudi Arabia. Many more PAs serve with U.S.

Armed Forces throughout the world in a variety of environments where they are often tasked to provide medical care to the indigenous populations. Still other PAs work in other branches of the U.S. government. Some PAs serve as Peace Corps workers, although more experienced PAs serve as Peace Corps Medical Officers (PCMOs). As PCMOs, PAs provide the medical support for Peace Corps volunteers in a given country. PAs are employed by the U.S. Foreign Service and are also recruited for service with the Central Intelligence Agency. In addition, they will find opportunities through private corporations for deployment overseas in "hardship" environments such as Iraq and Afghanistan. In a much less volatile setting, American PAs have been working in the United Kingdom's National Health Service for the past 15 years. There they have served as both clinicians and role models for the recently qualified U.K.-trained PAs.

Physician assistants who want to practice internationally now have many more options than they did even just a few years ago. Nonetheless, the overall number of PAs who work internationally remains relatively small.

The actual clinical roles and responsibilities of international PAs are as varied and diverse as the many countries and cultures in which they work. Thus, for the same reasons that it is difficult to describe the role of a "typical" PA practicing anywhere in the United States, it is equally difficult to identify the "typical" PA role in foreign countries.

Physician assistants who choose to work in an international environment have many options. These options largely depend on the PAs themselves. First they must determine whether they will seek formal paid employment with financial compensation of salary and benefits or serve on a volunteer basis. PAs then need to identify the target population (expatriates or indigenous) they are interested in serving. After they have decided where, how, and with whom they want to work, PAs can begin an often lengthy application process. Passports, visa application forms, references, security clearances and background checks, screening health examinations, necessary vaccines, language skills and other pertinent training, and formal interviews are just some of the many steps that are likely to be required.

Working for the U.S. government, either in the capacity of the military PA or with other governmental organizations (e.g., Foreign Service), usually entails providing care to a generally young and otherwise healthy expatriate staff. The "standards of care" are expected to be similar to treatment for the same problem in a typical medical facility in the United States. Diagnostic equipment and supplies, although perhaps rudimentary, are likely to be familiar to even inexperienced providers. Advanced care may sometimes only be available by transporting the patient back to the continental United States by air ambulance.

At the other end of the health care spectrum is work in developing countries. Providing health care to indigenous populations through nongovernmental organizations (NGOs) can offer PAs a far greater challenge on many levels. Novice PAs (in terms of international experience) will likely face a rather unsettling experience when they come to realize that many of their preconceptions about what constitutes a "norm" in medical standards of care in the United States cannot, and for a variety of reasons *must not*, apply to the delivery of health care in a developing country. PAs may face medical conditions that they never imagined; disease states of which they know little or nothing; and an overwhelming lack of resources, such as hospitals without running water or an oxygen delivery system. Frequently, they will find that the medical and diagnostic equipment, if and when available, is rudimentary. Laboratory studies might be limited to determination of a hemoglobin value and microscopic examinations of urine and blood (for cell count and differential, as well as thick and thin prep slides for

---

BOX 47.1 PROFESSIONAL ORGANIZATIONS INVOLVED WITH INTERNATIONAL WORK FOR PHYSICIAN ASSISTANTS

- Physician Assistants for Global Health
  http://www.pasforglobalhealth.org
  pasforglobalhealth@gmail.com
- Fellowship of Christian Physician Assistants
  www.fcpa.net
  PO Box 7500
  Bristol, TN 37621
  FCPA@fcpa.net

---

malaria) and stool for ova and parasites. Unless they are fluent in the local language, common tasks such as diagnostic studies and hands-on physical evaluations frequently have to be done through local interpreters, thus increasing the time required for even a simple patient encounter. The organizations listed in Box 47.1 can provide additional information.

A PA who chooses to work with an indigenous population will have to decide if he or she wants shorter terms (e.g., 3–6 months doing emergency relief where conditions are likely to be stressful). The generally safer alternative is to work in developmental projects for longer terms (e.g., 9–12 months). These developmental projects typically have more infrastructure and are therefore likely to be in more stable countries.

A PA serving indigenous populations will likely confront many other hurdles beyond simple language differences. There may be significant cultural, societal, and religious issues to address. Despite these factors, and perhaps because of them, the rewards of investing oneself in such a venture are often immeasurable.

PRACTICAL CONSIDERATIONS

General Issues

The experience of many internationally experienced PAs demonstrates the need for a well-conceived plan. PAs who hope to practice internationally would be well advised to research all aspects of such a commitment. This section addresses a number of major hurdles that PAs have encountered. Although the following list of topics is comprehensive, it is by no means complete.

Box 47.2 presents a set of guidelines for PAs considering international work, which were adopted

1. Physician assistants (PAs) should establish and maintain the appropriate physician–PA team.
2. PAs should accurately represent their skills, training, professional credentials, identity, or service both directly and indirectly.
3. PAs should provide only services for which they are qualified via their education or experiences and in accordance with all pertinent legal and regulatory processes.
4. PAs should respect the culture, values, beliefs, and expectations of the patients, local health care providers, and the local health care systems.
5. PAs should be aware of the role of the traditional healer and support a patient's decision to use such care.
6. PAs should take responsibility for being familiar with and adhering to the customs, laws, and regulations of the country where they will be providing services.
7. When applicable, PAs should identify and train local personnel who can assume the role of providing care and continuing the education process.
8. PA students require the same supervision abroad as they do domestically.
9. PAs should provide the best standards of care and strive to maintain quality abroad.

From American Academy of Physician Assistants. *2016-2017 Policy Manual.* https://www.aapa.org/workarea/downloadasset.aspx?id=2147486552.

by the American Academy of Physician Assistants (AAPA) in 2015.

All PAs working internationally need to adhere to these guidelines, as well as to the AAPA's Guidelines for Ethical Conduct for the Physician Assistant Profession.

Licensure and Registration

There is no universal means by which PAs are permitted to work in a foreign country. In some cases whereby PAs are serving an expatriate patient population, official approval from foreign governments may be obtained through a series of clinical competency examinations. More often, PAs may be breaking new ground as they explore the ways by which they can perform the tasks and deliver the level of care for which they are trained. One such groundbreaker,

Donald Prater, worked in Nanjing, China, for a U.S.-based company, providing health care to hundreds of expatriates and their families who live in that region. Even though he was not providing medical services to the local residents, Chinese authorities required that he take the Chinese medical examination (in English) so that he could see his expatriate patients on a fee-for-service basis.

More commonly, governmental approval is awarded to the agency with which the PA is working (e.g., American Refugee Committee). Thus, the PA is allowed to work under the umbrella of that organization. Consequently, the agency typically requires that credentials and letters of recommendation be submitted as the first step in going "to the field." Experience indicates that PAs, as fully licensed, certified, and registered providers in the United States, can usually practice their clinical skills to the full scope of their training. However, the actual scope of practice for the international PA can, and often does, vary widely. It is important to remember that other international agencies such as Doctors Without Borders do not routinely recruit PAs because the majority of the countries where they work do not recognize the PA profession.

Physician–Physician Assistant Relationship

The physician–PA relationship in international settings can be informal or tightly structured. The supervising physician can be in immediate proximity, working alongside the PA in a refugee camp, or in the capital city of the country, accessible by radio or cell phone, while the PA is working remotely in the field. Another possibility is that the supervising physician may be based in the United States but available by satellite communications or another electronic format, a model that many private multinational companies follow. It is important to remember that because there are no distinct or universal rules that govern international PA practice (except those constraints of the state wherein the PA is duly licensed or registered), practice standards for PAs in international settings unfortunately remain vague and ill defined.

Malpractice

Although the myriad aspects of U.S.-based medical practice differ from those of international practice, and malpractice is not usually an issue in international practice, PAs must always provide the same high level of care for which they have trained, regardless of where in the world they find themselves. PAs should check with their malpractice insurance carriers before departing because insurance carriers rarely provide coverage outside the United States.

Physician assistants must never represent themselves as physicians, either at home or abroad. The problems that could occur as a result of such misrepresentation may be devastating for an individual PA and may even have long-reaching effects on the PA profession.

When a PA is working overseas, it remains his or her responsibility to account for absences from clinical practice at home. This may require that adequate documentation be provided for any extended absences, including formal verification from the international employer or the organization.

Continuing Education

Continuing medical education (CME), although not usually an issue for the other countries in which the PA may work, is nonetheless a requirement for maintaining licensure and certification. Maintaining certification by the National Commission on Certification of Physician Assistants (NCCPA) becomes an issue only if the PA is outside of the United States for 1 year or longer. From a practical perspective, Category 1 CME credits are best obtained either by "stockpiling" before leaving the United States or accessing web-based formats. Technologic developments can allow the globetrotting PA to access various Category 1 CME programs online from Internet cafes around the world.

Salaries

From PAs who work for a small NGO who may have to pay for all of their own travel and lodging expenses to the few lucky PAs who are fully employed by a multinational corporation that may compensate them generously, PAs working in the international arena will find that the range of salaries and benefits will be as varied as the types of positions that they may encounter.

QUALIFICATIONS

Medical Skills

The ability to work with limited or improvised resources is an essential skill. Of particular value is a reliance on a basic hands-on approach to medicine. To highlight this issue, Cameron McCauley, an experienced international PA, tells of a time during his PA training when he was learning to evaluate heart murmurs. Similar to many of his peers, he scoffed at the need for physical assessment skills when technology such as echocardiograms would confirm the diagnosis. Cameron was humbled many years later, when he found himself working in a remote village without any hope of accessing such technology. Instead, he used those basic physical diagnostic skills he had learned years before to determine that a young patient had a ventricular septal defect. The child was then referred to the distant capital city, where his diagnosis was confirmed and the defect was surgically corrected.

It is important to remember that there are usually few advanced resources available. The PA will seldom find advanced diagnostic options, such as ultrasonography or computed tomography, or even the basics of plain radiography. As an example of the paucity of resources that can be faced, when I worked in Kabul, Afghanistan, there was only one working electrocardiogram machine in the entire country. Often the nearest x-ray unit is hours away and can be reached only by driving over rough roads, with the patient bouncing along in the back of a beat-up Land Rover.

Tropical Medicine

Patients in developing countries typically do not have the same causes of morbidity and mortality as those in the United States. Instead of cancers and cardiovascular diseases, patients in developing countries typically succumb to the ravages of infectious diseases. Even such relatively straightforward illnesses as gastroenteritis, acute respiratory infections such as pneumonia, and measles are the leading causes of death. Treatment is usually simple if the patient can access the proper medication in time. Clinicians can spend years learning to specialize in infectious tropical disease; however, there are several short courses in American universities that can provide excellent training over a couple of weeks to a few months.

Public Health and Epidemiology

Because infectious diseases are so commonplace, especially in developing countries, a strong emphasis must be placed on prevention of these problems. Therefore, it is essential that PAs, especially those working in medical infrastructure development and public health capacity building, develop an understanding of the basic principles of public health. Many accredited schools of public health are available in the United States, but only a relative few offer specialty training in international health, and fewer still focus on refugee health and humanitarian emergencies.

Human Resource Management and Teaching Expertise

Frequently, PAs are sought not just as clinical providers but also as trainers or managers of local operations. In Jalalabad, Afghanistan, I served as the project medical coordinator for New Hadda, an emergency refugee camp of more than 80,000 people who, in the mid-1990s, had fled the fighting in Kabul, the capital, but were then unable to escape to neighboring Pakistan. Health care provided in the camp was the responsibility of the international humanitarian aid agency, Doctors Without Borders, which provided primary care through a series of clinics staffed by Afghan doctors and nurses. As the project medical coordinator, I was responsible for the overall delivery of medical care in the camp clinics, some limited clinical practice, and clinical teaching, as well as all aspects of public health in the camp. To accomplish this, I regularly collaborated with representatives from other local and international NGOs, the local Ministry of Health, the United Nations International Children's Emergency Fund (UNICEF), and the World Health Organization (WHO).

Language Skills

Speaking a second language (e.g., French, Spanish, Portuguese, Arabic) can open many doors and allow for an ease of communication with patients and professional counterparts. The alternative—total reliance on interpreters—can result in frustration for all parties involved. As a result, nuances in conversation during the medical history or examination process can be missed, and the interpreter can sometimes act as a screen, perhaps keeping details vague or even misleading the clinician.

OTHER CONSIDERATIONS

Stress

It is a well-known fact that living in harsh environments can be stressful. Accommodations are typically Spartan. Insects and vermin can plague your living space. The sound of gunfire can fill the air throughout the night. Adequate rest becomes a precious commodity. The days are often long and physically and sometimes emotionally demanding. In addition, working and living with the same group of people, day in and day out, provides additional challenges. It is common for expatriates working in the emergency setting of large refugee camp environments to work 7 days a week, 12 or more hours each day. Workers share a common feeling that there is so much work that needs to be done and so little time in which to do it. There must be some opportunity for rest and recuperation to avoid what many see as inevitable burnout. Therefore, many NGOs insist that workers take time away, to the extent that this can be done without affecting the operations of the project.

Medications and Standards of Treatment

Medications, if and when they are available, may not be familiar to the PA because they are sometimes antiquated by most Western standards. Usually, the latest multigenerational cephalosporins are unavailable, not just because of the cost but more often that resistance has not yet been a significant issue in the area. As a result, inexpensive but nonetheless effective drugs such as chloramphenicol or penicillin G are still used extensively.

Another common observation is that patients from the local population often expect that when they come to a clinic or a hospital, they will be treated and will always receive some sort of medication. A patient encounter in which the patient does not walk out with medications can be thought to be unsatisfactory from the patient's perspective, even though the PA may have otherwise given appropriate treatment and provided proper patient education. A visit without receiving medications can be viewed by the patient as substandard care.

Traditional Health Care

Maintaining an open mind is important when one is confronted with traditional and folk medicines. These methods, although usually unfamiliar to U.S.-born PAs, often play a significant role for patients. We must remember that after the PA and other international expatriate staff members leave, the responsibility for ongoing health care usually falls back onto the traditional health care worker.

In Afghanistan, I learned of the traditional "resuscitation" technique used by traditional birth attendants (TBAs) for stillborn infants. The TBA places the placenta on the face of the infant, with the thought that the placenta had provided life to the child in the womb, and it should do similarly after birth. To attempt to change this misconception would involve much work and more than a simple message that the TBA is "wrong." It is essential that changes be introduced according to a well-conceived approach. Undermining a community's confidence in a local provider would have long-term ramifications.

An awareness of how a community relies on traditional healers is important if one is to understand what that community expects of the PA. Expatriates must realize that their presence, however long, is still seen as transient by the indigenous populations. It is therefore important to remember that, especially in emergency relief settings, when the expatriate leaves, there will be little left but footprints in the sand.

Personal Health and Safety

Although working in war-ravaged and developing countries represents its own challenge, typically the greatest risk to expatriates occurs while they are traveling by car or truck. Injuries from motor vehicle accidents remain the primary reason for expatriates with Doctors Without Borders to return from the field for medical reasons. Other common maladies can range from the nuisance of common traveler's diarrhea to life-threatening cerebral malaria.

Land Mines and Unexploded Ordinance

More than 60 countries are still littered with millions of land mines, unexploded cluster bombs, and other munitions; these indiscriminate killers represent a significant threat not just to the local population but to expatriate relief workers as well. It is imperative that a mine-awareness training program be completed by expatriate PAs before they go to work in a land mine–infested country. PAs must always maintain a keen sense of safety when working in such an environment. Elizabeth Sheehan, a PA with vast international experience, tells of an incident when she was traveling through a heavily mined area of Cambodia. In front of her car, a cow was wandering down the dirt road. Suddenly, the cow exploded as it stepped onto a mine, showering Liz's car with cow parts.

Security

Expatriate PAs can sometimes find themselves in dangerous environments. Although they may be volunteers, the stipend of a few hundred dollars a month that they may receive is still significantly more than the average annual income for many locals. As a result, volunteer relief workers have been robbed, held hostage, and worse. There have been robberies, kidnappings, assaults, and even deaths among field workers of most major international relief organizations. Although the economic motivation for these acts seems clear, perhaps less obvious are the political overtones common in some developing countries. One such tragedy occurred on December 17, 1996, when six workers with the International Committee of the Red Cross in Chechnya were murdered as they slept. The reason for the attack was believed to be political. The murderers were never identified. In 2004, a team of five medical relief workers from Doctors Without Borders were ambushed and killed in Afghanistan.

Reentry

Returning home from an overseas experience often proves difficult, and returning PAs should not count on a smooth transition. Family members, other loved ones, and coworkers can seldom understand fully what the returned PA may have seen or experienced. Common experiences have been identified among returning relief workers. An example of such an experience is the "supermarket event." Kate Herlihy, who spent 2 years working for the American Refugee Committee in a Cambodian refugee camp, speaks of the disdain and shock that she felt when she entered a supermarket at home. She was overwhelmed by the variety of pet food after she had cared for starving people just a few days earlier.

More serious symptoms of posttraumatic stress disorder can also occur. Depression and even suicide have been reported in returned volunteers. It is therefore important to provide a mechanism for adequate debriefing on return and a means to follow up in a timely manner. Many international organizations offer psychological debriefings as part of ongoing support for their workers, paid and volunteer. It can be helpful to speak with a psychologist, psychiatrist, or other mental health expert if the PA has a difficult time with the reentry process.

Topics for Preparation

When a PA is considering taking the time to work overseas, it is important that he or she learn about all the possible aspects of such a commitment. The list below includes a selection of topics to be researched:

- What is the overall mission of the organization?
- What is the organizational approach to the problems—individual and curative, or more utilitarian public health focused, or perhaps a blend of both?
- What happens if you get to the field and you discover it is not what you had expected?
- What security parameters will be followed?
- Will the PA be self-sufficient, functioning outside the established health care system, or will he or she work alongside local counterparts in existing health support structures?
- Will there be a salary or a stipend for you as a volunteer?

- What will happen if you have a needlestick or some other HIV risk exposure?
- How will treatment be managed should there be an animal bite, where rabies cannot be ruled out?
- Who will pay the necessary expenses of your travel, room, and board?
- What provisions are made for your medical and psychological care both during and after a mission?
- Will you have time off while in the field? If so, what are the options for that time?
- What about repatriation to the United States in case of medical or family emergencies?
- What about life insurance?
- Will medical supplies and equipment be provided, or will you have to bring everything yourself?
- Is there a training or orientation program available, or will you be expected to go directly to the field?

- Is the situation stable enough for the PA to be accompanied by a spouse or other family member?
- How do you relax when you are under stress?
- How do you function in a team? How do you feel about living and working, day in and day out, in a cramped living space, often surrounded by smokers?
- What about the job that you will be leaving behind? Is there any chance that the job, as well as any promises regarding the security of that job, will not be maintained? If not, what is your fall-back plan?
- Case Study 47.1, written from my personal experience, illustrates the challenges and satisfactions of work in international health care.

CASE STUDY 47.1

For my first mission in 1994 with Doctors Without Borders, or *Médecins Sans Frontières (MSF)*, I had asked for a "stable" situation on which to cut my teeth. The reply from headquarters was that I had the opportunity to go to Somaliland (northwestern Somalia), where MSF had been working for almost a decade. The area was considered stable by MSF standards because it had been a couple of years since fighting had dominated the area. Somaliland was also hundreds of miles, and a separate and distinct country, from Somalia, where the situation around Mogadishu was much more volatile. Our project, based in the city of Burao, was to continue to strengthen the existing health structures, a 200-bed hospital and a series of 10 primary care clinics out in the "bush." This was to be accomplished through a collaborative effort with counterparts from the Somaliland Ministry of Public Health.

As the country medical coordinator, I was the leader of the small team of two other expatriates, a Dutch nurse and an English logistician, as well as about 40 local staff, consisting of doctors, nurses, and a variety of nonmedical support staff.

Because of improving health indicators, MSF was in the process of scaling back the team's overall operational involvement. As a result, my job was supposed to be primarily nonclinical. However, I was also told that I could probably integrate my clinical background into my daily work. Between regular meetings and negotiations with my counterpart, the hospital director, I would make ward rounds and discuss management of patients with the Somali doctors and nurses. Overall, it was proving a rather

interesting departure from my experience in emergency medicine. My focus was no longer centered on a single patient at a time as it was when I was working in the emergency department back home; instead, I now looked at improving the access to and the overall quality of medical care for a whole city and the regions beyond.

My first couple of weeks in Burao were overwhelming. I tried to establish some sense of order in my life. I had just left a busy emergency department in a tertiary care center in Portland, Maine, and I was now working in a hospital that lacked such amenities as running water or even continuous electricity for 24 hours a day. Goats and sheep wandered about the grounds of the hospital compound, leaving behind a different sort of "land mine" to discover. I could literally walk through a pile of sheep dung and then step into the operating theater. There, the patient could be found situated on a table with a large ceiling fan turning directly overhead. On the wards, patients lay on the bare springs of decrepit beds. If patients were fortunate enough to have a mattress or bed linens, the patient's family had provided them. Hospital windows had no intact glass or screens. The ceilings of the wards were stained from rain that had leaked through the countless bullet and shrapnel holes in the roof. During the rainy season, I saw the staff madly shuffling children in cribs around the room in a futile effort to avoid the many leaks that plagued the entire hospital. I developed an overwhelming sense of seeing that there was so much work that needed to be done and so little time or money to do what was really needed. Eventually, that sense of frustration grew less when, on several occasions, community elders would approach me and thank me for the "help that MSF was providing to this impoverished and forgotten country."

I eventually shifted my focus from trying to reproduce what I knew to be a standard of health care and turned to a more pragmatic approach. It would not matter if we could provide drugs, supplies, and diagnostic equipment such as x-ray machines, if they would then be lost to damage from the rains. We turned our focus to rehabilitating the infrastructure of the hospital—repairing the roof, replacing windows, and other simple efforts. Our efforts were starting to pay off. A sense of accomplishment was shared by the whole team. Unfortunately, our joy was short-lived. The political climate was changing acutely, and tensions were rising. The night air became quieter as people started to hoard their precious ammunition.

One particularly quiet night was suddenly disrupted by the sound of tanks rolling through the city streets. The next morning, the expatriate team was evacuated back to our base of operations in the adjacent country of Djibouti, a postage stamp–sized country located about 2 hours' flying time to the west. There we could relax over a beer and contemplate our next actions. Our downtime was limited to a short few hours. A freak storm had struck the area, resulting in a tremendous flash flood that hit the city of Djiboutiville. Walls of water spilled out of the rugged mountain areas and dumped into the flood plains from which the city arises. Shantytowns in the city's periphery suffered the most, with thousands of homes destroyed. More than 100 people were swept away by the rapidly rising waters, and hundreds of others escaped to safety when they were eventually plucked from roofs and treetops by helicopters sent by the local detachment of the French military. Although the fetid waters also struck the MSF office and forced my colleagues to flee to the roof, I was out of danger.

The flood was only the first blow. Another killer was stalking the population and awaiting the chance to pounce. With the flood came the opportunity for that culprit—cholera. Cholera is endemic in the area. These simple bacteria thrive in the milieu of a hot, humid environment and in the poor sanitation found in such a developing country. Untreated, cholera can result in a 50% mortality rate. Similar to so many other infectious diseases, the highest mortality rate is among the elderly, children, and those with significant medical problems. Within a few hours of exposure, the body responds to the infection with gastrointestinal symptoms. Abdominal cramps, nausea, vomiting, and profound diarrhea (often described as "rice water") in appearance, are the classic presentation.

The city was trying to recover from the flooding, dealing with the displacement from the floods, and planning for the inevitable cholera outbreak.

MSF responded by offering our assistance. Within the world of emergency medical relief, MSF is well known as an authority on managing cholera epidemics. With huge stores of prepackaged supplies available in European warehouses, MSF can respond to an emergency in a matter of days. The logistical support network is well organized and quite efficient, the product of many similar responses during the past decades. In just 3 days, two additional expatriate staff, an experienced nurse and a logistician, joined our team. The tents, intravenous (IV) fluids, chlorine for water treatment and disinfections, and the remainder of our cholera treatment center (CTC) supplies arrived the next day from Amsterdam. Our job was to establish a CTC near the hardest hit area of the city. The residents were already poor, with limited resources. Many were Somalis who had fled the fighting in their homeland and settled in Djibouti, awaiting peace in their homeland. In Djibouti, they lived in shanties—simple wood frame structures covered with corrugated sheets of metal and plastic sheeting. Drinking water supplies throughout the city had been contaminated. Children already suffered from malnutrition and were subject to malabsorption diarrheas.

As a novice to the ravages of cholera, I soon found myself in the uncomfortable role of being the senior medical person in charge of the CTC. The good news was that the treatment for cholera was simple: Replace fluids at a greater rate than they are being lost. If patients could tolerate oral fluids, they received oral rehydration salts (ORS). If unable to keep that down, patients received nasogastric (NG) feedings of ORS. If patients were profoundly dehydrated, as so many were, IV replacement of fluids was the only option left. The local staff that made up the backbone of our CTC were, as a rule, excellent in assessing and treating patients. My job was to ensure that we treated patients according to the protocols of the WHO. As the senior medical person on the scene, I was also the one to whom the staff turned if they were unable to place an NG tube or find an IV site.

I still recall treating a child about 2 years old, weighing only 6 or 7 kg (the result of chronic malnutrition). He was floppy and unresponsive, with poor skin turgor and sunken eyes, and in shock from the profound fluid loss of his vomiting and diarrhea. The child was held by one of the local nursing staff, suspended by his feet, while I waited for his neck veins to distend. I placed an external jugular line and started the process of rehydrating the child. Accustomed as I was to working in a level I trauma center, I was initially taken aback by the WHO protocol for the aggressive IV rate of 30 mL/kg/hr that is recommended in volume replacement for cholera. My skepticism ended when I saw the tremendous volume of liquid stools that just poured out of these children. To hold a child, floppy and lethargic, in shock from this dramatic gastroenteritis was eye-opening. Suddenly it became clear why cholera claims so many victims around the world each year. The days in the CTC were long and demanding, but my reward was seeing the child who had been at death's door a few hours earlier, now bright-eyed and alert in the arms of his grateful mother.

We soon handed over the day-to-day supervision of the CTC to the Djiboutian Ministry of Health. Meanwhile, our team made preparations to return to Somaliland. We learned that tens of thousands of civilians had fled the fighting in the cities and had returned to their traditional home in the Somali bush country. Because this displaced population had no provisions for medical care, MSF volunteered to help. My team was soon traveling back into Burao. There, we planned for a series of assessment missions to determine the extent of the problem we were facing.

It was on such a mission on December 23, 1994, that I found myself in the settlement of Hor Fadda, normally just a stopover in the desert for bands of nomadic shepherds. The "village" was little more than hundreds of simple huts surrounding a muddy watering hole the size of a tennis court. Countless goats, sheep, camels, and humans muddied the water as they all sought to quench their thirst. Surrounding the water hole were thousands of people who had fled the fighting in the capital city of Hargeisa. These refugees, mostly women, elderly men, and children (the young men were back in the city as fighters), were living in makeshift shelters constructed of branches and covered with plastic sheeting, while the men slept outside on the ground, wrapped from head to toe, shroudlike, with thin wool blankets. The only permanent structure in the village was a small, mud-walled hut that we converted to a temporary clinic where we initially treated patients. We then set up a large canvas tent that we had brought with us. That night, the tent would serve as our shelter. The following day, the tent served as the base for a clinic that provided health care to the 15,000 people in the camp.

Later that evening, we shared a meal of boiled mutton and rice. I sat back, enjoyed a cup of chai, relished the warmth from the fire, and took the time to relax a bit and to reflect on the events of the day. It had been a very long day that started at dawn with a 6-hour trip in an elderly Land Rover, bouncing over dirt roads, at times feeling like I was in the midst of a *National Geographic* special. The one thing that kept me from enjoying much of the journey was that the Somali countryside had been littered with land mines, the result of many years of civil war. We were now traveling roads that normally we would have avoided because of that threat from those hidden mines. However, now the stakes were different: Thousands of people were in need of assistance and, if we did not go, no one else was available. We traveled the well-worn roads and kept our fingers crossed.

After a very full day, we sat around the campfire, it was quiet—much quieter than I had yet experienced during my time on the horn of Africa. My thoughts turned to my loved ones, safe at home on the other side of the world. Christmas was less than a day away, and here I was, in the desert, half a world away, sitting around a campfire.

The silence was broken when Mohammed, one of the staff, asked me if I watched Western movies. I turned to see his toothy smile as he told me that the scene we were in was "just like in the movies." I chuckled and wondered what this man's image of America really was. I was surprised as he then described the typical cowboy scenario portrayed by John Wayne or Gary Cooper. He continued, "We could make a movie and call it *Night in Hor Fadda*," which caused us to laugh as we both continued to build the image upon the foundation that he had so accurately depicted.

It was during that evening that I realized how much I had experienced in a little over 2 weeks. I had been through the start of a civil war, a flash flood, a cholera outbreak, and a journey into the bush, where I had witnessed the devastating effects of war on civilians. Although physically and emotionally exhausted, I had survived. More important, at least to me, I felt good about what I had done. I started to lose some of my self-pity and instead started to feel that I was here for a purpose and that I had, in some small way, made a difference. Even today, many years later, on some clear nights as I look skyward, Mohammed's voice and handsome face echo in my mind. I smile when I see him.

CLINICAL APPLICATIONS

- If you were interested in a position in international health care, how would you research the opportunities for PAs? How would you match your skills to the health care needs and practice settings of international communities?
- If you secured an international position as a PA, how would you obtain information about the language, culture, politics, infrastructure, and health care system of the area? What else would you want to know before going to an international setting?

KEY POINTS

- Although sometimes dangerous, and usually clinically challenging, working as a PA in a developing country can also be demanding, both physically and emotionally. Nonetheless, it can be a rich and rewarding experience.
- Thoroughly researching the organization's mission statement and having a knowledge of the countries where they work will help you to better determine if you will be a fit in that organization.
- Personal preparation, including appropriate foreign language skills and supplemental training in tropical medicine, epidemiology, and disease control, will increase your marketability to international organizations.

The resources for this chapter can be found at www.expertconsult.com.

PATIENTS WITH DISABILITIES

Lisa K. Walker

In July 2005, the U.S. Surgeon General issued a Call to Action to Improve the Health and Wellness of Persons with Disabilities. According to this Call to Action, an estimated 54 million people of all ages, races, ethnicities, socioeconomic status, and education levels in the United States (20% of the population) are living with at least one disability. These disabilities range from spinal cord injuries causing paralysis to patients who are born with hearing loss or cognitive disabilities. More than 3 million people 15 years of age and older use a wheelchair. Another 10 million use a walking aid, such as a cane, crutches, or walker. Millions more live with hearing or visual losses that significantly impact activities of daily living (ADLs).[1] These numbers will increase significantly over the next 10 to 15 years with the aging of the baby boom generation. Despite these overwhelming statistics and the fact that July 26, 2015, marked the 20th anniversary of the signing of the Americans with Disabilities Act (ADA), the literature shows that significant disparities continue to exist when comparing the health of people with disabilities with that of the general population.[2-4] Access to acute and preventive health care services is lacking for these patients. Consequently, people with disabilities experience poorer health outcomes compared with the general population, according to the U.S. federal government's initiative Healthy People 2020.[5] Some of the barriers that prevent people with disabilities from receiving appropriate health care include physical barriers, inadequate communication, and attitudinal and social policy barriers. Adequate access to care is not only a legal obligation but also a necessity that could prevent catastrophic outcomes and prolong life. According to the Institute of Medicine's report "The Future of Disability in America," significant barriers still exist in hospitals and clinics that prevent patients with disabilities from accessing basic health care services.[6] These include physical access to facilities and equipment for patients with mobility impairments and access to information and communication for patients with visual, hearing, and cognitive disabilities. The report goes on to identify early education of health care professionals as a key in eliminating some of these barriers. Clearly, we can, and must, improve our knowledge, skills, and attitudes toward the care of patients with disabilities and do more to ensure equal access.

Disability can be defined many ways. The legal definition from the ADA is as follows:

A disabled person is someone with a physical or mental impairment that substantially limits one or more major life activities (as well as someone with a history of such an impairment or someone currently regarded as such).[7] This includes people with obvious, visible disabilities, as well as the majority of people with disabilities who have hidden conditions such as arthritis, diabetic neuropathy, or hearing loss.

Information in this chapter is designed to enable students to identify and eliminate many of the barriers faced by patients with disabilities, thereby improving health outcomes for this population. Each section addresses appropriate terms and definitions when working with patients with disabilities. This is followed by a discussion of the appropriate approach, common challenges, and methods to avoid errors in diagnosis and treatment when providing care to patients with specific disabilities, including patients who are deaf and hard of hearing, patients with mobility disabilities, patients with visual impairments (VIs), and patients with intellectual and developmental disabilities. Although evidence shows that patients with severe mental illness experience disparities in access to care, a comprehensive discussion of the primary health care needs of patients with mental illness is beyond the scope of this chapter.[2]

Many people with disabilities are accustomed to having others evaluate and circumscribe their lives and opportunities. Stereotypic and stigmatizing views of living with disabilities erect barriers to comprehensive care, such as limiting discussions of mental health or sexuality and overemphasizing isolated symptoms and diagnoses rather than overall health.

PROVIDING APPROPRIATE CARE FOR PATIENTS WHO ARE DEAF AND HARD OF HEARING

For the 28 million (1 in 10) Americans who are living with hearing loss, access to appropriate health care is limited primarily by the ability of the health care team to effectively communicate with the patient. A survey of people with varying degrees of hearing loss reveals that they often feel marginalized by their health care providers, that the "medical community holds a pathologic view of deaf people," and too often use inadequate modes of communication, such as lip reading, writing, or asking family members to interpret.[8]

Hearing loss can be defined in many ways. The severity of hearing loss is based on audiometric testing and measured in decibels.[9] In general, a person with severe hearing loss is unable to hear speech when a person is talking at a normal level, and those with profound hearing loss may only hear very loud sounds.[10] As with other types of physical disabilities, medical professionals view hearing loss as a condition that requires fixing, and people with intact hearing tend to think of deafness as a terrible loss. However, many people with hearing loss, particularly those who consider themselves part of the Deaf Community and communicate using American Sign Language (ASL), do not view themselves as ill or having suffered a tragic loss. Indeed, their deafness is as much a part of their identity as one's cultural or ethnic heritage. Conversely, not all persons with hearing loss identify with Deaf Culture and use ASL. These patients are more likely to view their deficit as a loss and seek remediation through medical intervention. This distinction is critical in your approach to and appropriate care of patients with hearing loss.

Terms and Definitions

Prelingual deafness: Deafness occurring before the acquisition of spoken language, either congenital or before the age of 2 or 3 years

Postlingual deafness: Deafness occurring after the acquisition of spoken language

Presbycusis: Loss of hearing as part of the aging process. Estimates are as high as 80% of those older than age of 65 years of age as having a hearing loss.

Deaf Culture or Deaf Community: A culture is defined by a group of people who share similar beliefs, customs, and language. If ASL is a deaf person's primary language, if he or she attended a school for the deaf, and if he or she seeks opportunities to socialize with other deaf people, then he or she most likely considers himself or herself part of the Deaf Culture. In this section of the text, you will see culturally deaf persons referred to as Deaf (capital "D") and persons who have a severe or profound hearing loss but do not affiliate with the Deaf Community as deaf (lowercase "d"). This is important in terms of identifying the most appropriate method of communication and therefore ensuring accessible, quality health care for individual patients with hearing loss.

American Sign Language (ASL): A visual-gestural language used by the Deaf Community in the United States. ASL is a true language, as different from English as any other language. It has a distinct word order and grammatical structure. It is not a visual representation of English nor is it rudimentary gestures. Signed languages are not universal. As a matter of fact, British Sign Language is practically incomprehensible to Deaf people raised in the United States. There is more similarity between ASL and French Sign Language because the development of ASL was heavily influenced by a Deaf teacher, Laurent Clerc, who came to the United States from France to teach deaf children in the late 1800s.

Interpreter: Someone who is fluent in two or more languages and renders messages from one spoken or signed language into another spoken or signed language.

It is important to note the use of the term *interpret* in contrast with the term *translate*, which means to render a message from one written language to another written language and is often incorrectly used when referring to interpreting. ASL interpreters have received special training. Some may have been raised in a Deaf family where ASL was their first language. They should have national or state certification to ensure competency in the language, knowledge of the interpreting process, and adherence to a professional code of ethics. In some states, sign language interpreting is a licensed profession.

Best Practices

Always ask patients what their preferred mode of communication is: lip reading and speaking, writing, or using an interpreter. Do not assume that all patients with hearing loss know sign language or are expert lip readers.

When working with a patient who prefers lip reading, speak in a normal tone of voice. Do not yell, exaggerate your lip movements, or speak excessively slowly. Maintain eye contact when speaking with your patient. Do not turn away or look down when speaking. Make sure the room is well lit and, if at all possible, avoid back lighting, such as standing in front of a bright window. Remember that facial hair may interfere with accurate lip reading. Be aware that a mask will interfere with effective communication if your patient is relying on lip reading.

A 2011 study of individuals with normal hearing revealed that mean-word recognition accuracy scores were barely greater than 10% correct when exposed to a video of a female talker with the sound removed.[3] For individuals relying on lip reading for communication, accuracy is significantly impacted, and much of the information must be gleaned from context and prior experiences. Therefore, it is important to have clear transitions from one topic to another. For example, if you are talking with a patient about his or her medication and then switch the topic suddenly

to his or her upcoming surgery, most lip readers will have difficulty following the conversation at that point. To ensure accuracy, always check for understanding. If something is not clear after one or two repetitions, try rephrasing the information or present it in writing. Do not say "Never mind" or "It's not important." This may be perceived as dismissive or condescending by the patient.

When working with a patient who prefers written communication, you will need to allow extra time for the encounter. Your communication with the patient should be written in short, simple phrases, but do not edit or eliminate information you would provide to any other patient. Avoid abbreviations and medical jargon. Do not assume a patient has fluency in written English. For many Deaf people who use ASL, English is their second language. Feel free to use brochures and patient education materials that are preprinted and readily available. Ask the patient to read any printed materials during the visit so that you can assess understanding. For lengthy visits requiring in-depth patient education (e.g., a patient newly diagnosed with diabetes), consider using Computer Assisted Real Time captioning (CART or C-Print). This service provides a transcriptionist who has special training and computer software that allows English text to be projected onto a screen as the speaker talks. Tablets and other handheld devices can also be used to facilitate written communication.

Health care facilities (public or private) are required to provide a sign language interpreter for Deaf patients who communicate in ASL. Interpreters can be scheduled through local medical centers or deaf service organizations, and some on-call availability is typical in major metropolitan areas. Interpreter requests should be made as soon as the need becomes known because there is a shortage of qualified interpreters in most communities. Video relay services are available at some locations, allowing immediate access to interpreters any time of the day or night. Not all Deaf people are comfortable with the video relay interpreters because trust plays a critical a role in potentially sensitive situations.

If you need to communicate with your deaf or hard-of-hearing patient by phone, you first need to assess his or her preferred mode of telecommunication. Many deaf people use text messaging or other computer-based communication such as email. Some rely on a telecommunication device for the deaf (TDD or TTY). Your clinic or hospital should be equipped with a TDD, but if it is not, you can use a telephone relay service similar to the video relay mentioned earlier by dialing 711 in most areas. There is no charge for this service. Some people with hearing loss have phone amplifiers and enough residual hearing to use the telephone directly. Never convey personal medical information through household members who can use the phone unless you have written permission from the patient.

Challenges

Many health care providers do not know how to access the services of an interpreter. Be proactive. Know the resources in your institution and your community so that you are able to locate qualified ASL interpreters. And be sure the office staff, those scheduling appointments or performing patient intake at your institution, are also familiar with these resources.

Patients do not always get sick on our schedule, and they may not be able to tell you their preferred mode of communication; therefore, it is critical to have an on-call list of interpreters for urgent or emergent visits. A sign language interpreter should have the skills to identify communication styles and recognize the communication needs of patients who are unable to do so. As always, if patients are able to communicate, ask first about their preferences before relying on a companion, family member, or interprete to determine the best approach to communication.

Methods to Ensure Access

If 80% of our diagnoses come from the history, then how important is clear and accurate communication with the patient in our ability to provide appropriate care? Working effectively with interpreters is key to providing good care to patients who do not or cannot use spoken English as a primary means of communication. An interpreter should be someone who has fluency in both languages (the language of the patient and that of the health care worker) and training in the role and ethics of interpreting. Guidance from the federal Department of Health and Human Services (DHHS) Office of Civil Rights makes it clear that a family member or friend should not be relied on to provide objective interpretation. And unless you are certain of a staff person's fluency and skill in functioning in the interpreter role, it is not advisable to use a staff member who happens to "know some signs" or "took some Spanish classes." Numerous examples (and lawsuits) exist regarding negative health outcomes as a result of using these well-intentioned but unqualified individuals to transmit medical information.

Interpreters have a distinct and limited role in medical settings. The ultimate goal is to facilitate communication, allowing all parties to function as autonomously and independently as anyone else in a similar situation. Interpreters are not advocates. They most likely do not know the medical or social history of the patient, nor would it be appropriate for them to share this information if they did know. Although they may periodically provide clarification, especially around cultural norms (this is called "cultural brokering"), it is not the role of an interpreter to explain things beyond what you have told the patient, check for understanding, or ensure appropriate follow-up. That is your job as the provider. The role of the interpreter is to afford individuals who do not share a common language the ability to effectively communicate with one another.[11]

Working with sign language interpreters differs in some subtle ways from working with a spoken language interpreter. Although spoken language interpreters usually prefer to position themselves so that they can see both you and the patient, sign language interpreters need to be beside and slightly behind the provider so that the patient can see the interpreter and provider at the same time. This positioning, particularly during history taking, enhances rapport and improves the clarity of communication.

Spoken language interpreters need to interpret consecutively (you speak and then pause and allow the interpreter to repeat what you have said in the patient's language) because they cannot interpret while you are speaking. Sign language interpreting can, for the most part, be done simultaneously. The interpreter will sign as you are speaking, usually a phrase or two behind you. You should address the patient directly. Do not say, "Tell him" or "Ask her." Expect pauses in the conversation as the interpreter completes a phrase and receives the patient's response. The patient will respond in his or her native language, and the interpreter will voice the patient's response in the first person. When you hear the interpreter say, "I have a pain in my side," he or she is simply repeating what was said or signed by the patient.

Interpreters may need to periodically ask for clarification of terms or concepts. If this is the case, a professional interpreter will make the request by stating, "The interpreter needs clarification." This allows for distinction in role and clarity for the participants as to who is speaking at any given time.

At times, a hearing sign language interpreter will work in tandem with a Certified Deaf Interpreter (CDI): someone who is Deaf, a native user of ASL, trained as an interpreter, and familiar with many communication modalities used by a wide range of deaf people. Deaf interpreters are typically needed to communicate with patients who do not use standard ASL such as those from other countries using that country's sign language or with Deaf people who have cognitive or physical barriers to using ASL and those who rely on idiosyncratic or "home" signs.

Interpreter errors do occur. One study revealed a mean of 31 errors per encounter made by interpreters in medical settings.[12] As you should for any patient with whom you do not share a common language, check with your deaf patient frequently for understanding. As a supplement to your onsite communication through the interpreter or with your lip-reading patients, provide a written copy of critical material (e.g., medication dosage changes or follow-up instructions) whenever possible. Give complete information regarding new or changed medication orders because there will likely be no interpreter available at the pharmacy.

CASE STUDY 48.1

A Deaf woman was in the emergency department (ED) for acute pharyngitis. She was accompanied by her mother, who is hearing. The patient, patient's mother, and physician assistant (PA) were all comfortable with having the mom interpret because she had developed fluency in ASL over the 20 years of raising her daughter. During the visit, as the provider was handing the patient her prescription, the provider asked if the patient was taking any medications. The patient said "No" even though she was taking oral contraceptive pills (OCPs). The appointment ended, and the patient went on her way, a prescription for antibiotics in hand. (Some medications can decrease the efficacy of OCPs and cause unintended pregnancy in some patients.)[4]

This is a classic example of why family or friends should never be substituted for professional interpreters. It is likely the patient may not have wanted her mother to know that she was taking birth control pills and she therefore didn't report it to the PA. The patient also has no reason to know that there might be an issue with taking OCPs and antibiotics together. The use of a professional interpreter allows for open communication between patient and provider without the interference or effects of a preexisting relationship interfering with accurate communication.

PROVIDING APPROPRIATE CARE FOR PATIENTS WITH MOBILITY DISABILITIES

As medical professionals, it is our duty to be aware of the challenges faced by millions of individuals with mobility disabilities in accessing proper medical care and to do everything we can to eliminate barriers. First and foremost, our role as PAs is to improve the health of all patients so that they can live full, productive, and independent lives. However, according to Healthy People 2020, patients with disabilities receive fewer screening and preventive services than their counterparts without disabilities.[2] Screenings such as mammography and Pap tests are often not done because of lack of equipment that is accessible to women with mobility disabilities, especially women who are wheelchair users. This lack of screening and prevention, compounded by inadequate accessibility to services, leads to unnecessary health disparities and poor outcomes (see Case Study 48.2).

Patients with mobility disabilities may rely on wheelchairs and other ambulatory aids as a primary means of mobilization; others may require no assistive devices at all. And although some individuals may only use a device temporarily, many need some form of ambulatory assistance on a permanent basis. Spinal cord injuries, stroke, cerebral palsy, amputations, and a variety of neuromuscular diseases (Huntington disease, muscular dystrophy, and multiple sclerosis, to name a few) are some of the more common reasons that individuals may rely on a wheelchair or ambulatory aid. As a health care provider, you should have a basic understanding of the special needs and complications associated with mobility disabilities.

Terms and Definitions

Spinal cord injury (SCI): Trauma causing damage to a segment of the spinal cord and nerve fibers. The location and degree of damage to the neurologic tissues determine the sensory, motor, and autonomic effect as a result of SCI.

Autonomic dysreflexia (AD): A potentially life-threatening increase in blood pressure, sweating, and other autonomic reflexes in reaction to some type of stimulus below the level of the lesion in a patient with a spinal cord injury. AD typically occurs in people with spinal cord injuries above T6.[13] The elevated blood pressure can lead to renal failure, cardiopulmonary failure, loss of consciousness, seizures, apnea, stroke, coma, and death.

Spina bifida: This neural tube defect results when the spinal cord, its surrounding nerves, or the spinal column develops abnormally during the first 28 days of gestation. It can affect the nervous, urinary, muscular, and skeletal systems, often causing bowel and bladder complications and paralysis below the spinal defect. In the United States, approximately 1500 infants are born with spina bifida each year.[14] The use of prenatal folic acid dietary supplementation has decreased the incidence of spina bifida and other neural tube defects.

Amputation: The surgical or traumatic loss of a limb or digits. There are approximately 1.9 million people living with limb loss in the United States. Each year, the majority of new amputations occur because of complications of the vascular system, especially from diabetes.

Phantom sensations and phantom pain: Sensations such as movement, touch, pressure, itching, posture, and heat and cold can still be felt, although the body part is no longer present. Patients with amputations often feel intense pain that comes from a missing limb, finger, or toe.

A comprehensive description of all conditions causing mobility disabilities, such as cerebral palsy, multiple sclerosis, muscular dystrophy, Huntington and Parkinson disease, and stroke, is beyond the scope of this chapter.

Best Practices

Patients with mobility disabilities should be treated with dignity in all aspects of the health care encounter. It is imperative that your interactions with the patient be respectful, appropriate, and reassuring. In addition to talking to your patient about his or her disability and inherent complications or conditions associated with it, you also need to address the same topics you address with every patient, such as immunizations, risk assessment, and sexual health. Studies show that patients with mobility disabilities suffer from increased morbidity and mortality when providers do not address *all* aspects of their health and well-being.[15]

When introduced to a person with a mobility disability, it is appropriate to offer to shake hands. People with limited hand use or those who wear an artificial limb can usually shake hands. Shaking hands with the left hand may be acceptable depending on the patient's cultural background. For those who cannot shake hands, touch them on the shoulder or arm to welcome them and acknowledge their presence.

It is important to respect the patient's personal space, including wheelchairs and other mobility aids. Avoid propelling the patient's wheelchair unless asked. Sit across from the patient in a chair for eye-to-eye contact. Do not squat down in front of the patient or stand over him or her as you converse. This may be perceived as offensive and demeaning by the patient.

If the patient arrives with an assistant or companion, address the patient directly. Do not assume that patients with spasticity, paralysis, or speech difficulties also have an intellectual disability. Most patients with mobility impairment have normal intelligence and can participate fully in their health care. Provide an opportunity for these patients to speak with you alone. Be aware that all patients with disabilities are at increased risk for abuse and neglect.

Your patient is your best resource when it comes to accommodations and assistance she or he may or may not need. If there are concerns about barriers to performing a comprehensive examination, such as undressing, accessing the examination table, and positioning, ask your patients with movement disabilities for their recommendations to remove these potential barriers. It is important to remember that not all mobility disabilities are the same. Each individual may use mobility devices of different types, transfer in different ways, and have varying levels of physical ability. Working with the patients is the best way to ensure safe, efficient, and accessible health care for all individuals with mobility disabilities.

To ensure that the patient with a mobility disability receives equal medical care to that received by a person without a disability, ask the patient to disrobe and perform the examination on the examination table if this is required to provide comprehensive, appropriate care. Ask if assistance is necessary with transfers and dressing and undressing, and be aware that offering assistance with these tasks may require additional time or the assistance of another individual. Never leave the patient unattended unless he or she asks to be left alone. You should be alert to the potential for fainting because of a gravitational pooling of blood when transferring the patient. Seek out rehabilitation specialists in your community for training and assistance. Ask the patient which positions are most comfortable during the examination, and ask if assistance is necessary before giving it. Examination tables with varying height capabilities, back supports, and whole-leg rests are available.[16] If your employer does not have an accessible examination table, you may want to discuss its value with the providers in your practice. An accessible table will benefit more than just your patients who use wheelchairs. Many patients, including older adults with arthritis and women in the last months of pregnancy, will appreciate a table that lowers, allows them to sit upright, and supports their legs.

Ensure that the patient is positioned comfortably if he or she is going to be sitting or lying still for an extended period of time. Pillows or pads may have to be adjusted between legs and wedged against the patient to decrease discomfort and reduce the risk of developing pressure sores. Patients with spasticity problems may need assistance holding still during procedures or examinations.

A complete examination should always include a sexual history. The sexual history is often neglected because of assumptions that people with limited mobility or paralysis cannot or do not have intimate relationships. These patients are still competent to maintain emotional and sexual relationships. The health care provider should perform the same inquiry for a patient with a mobility disability as he or she would for any other patient. It is also important to acknowledge the patient's needs, desires, anxieties, and questions pertaining to sexuality.

When examining a patient with a mobility disability, it is critical to perform a comprehensive visual inspection of the skin to assess for pressure sores and open wounds. Provide appropriate annual health promotion and disease prevention screenings, such as Pap smears, mammography, prostate and rectal examinations, and oral health examinations for all patients.

Challenges

Be cautious not to attribute all symptoms to an individual's primary disability. Patients with disabilities can present with heart disease, gastroenteritis, and migraines—all unrelated to their particular disabling condition. Do not let a patient's disability keep you from developing a comprehensive differential diagnosis list when assessing a patient's problem or symptoms. Careful medical management and skilled supportive care are necessary to prevent complications in the patient with a mobility disability. Functional goals are defined as realistic expectations of activities that individuals with mobility disabilities eventually should be able to perform. It is important to continue with long-term physical and occupational therapy treatments for patients to maintain function and maximize participation in the activities of work and life.

Certain health issues must be followed closely to prevent complications in patients with mobility disabilities. Difficulties such as urinary tract infections, pressure sores, and AD could become life threatening if not treated properly and promptly. Common serious challenges faced by these individuals include exaggerated reflexes, impaired cardiovascular function, loss of bladder and bowel control, loss of normal thermoregulation, lost or decreased breathing capacity; impaired cough reflexes, and muscle spasticity.

Autonomic dysreflexia is considered a medical emergency for the patient with a spinal cord injury. The patient may become *frightened* during an AD episode. You must remain calm and at the same time react quickly. It is critical to lower the patient's blood pressure as quickly as possible. This may be accomplished by raising the head of the examination table as high as possible. Sitting the patient straight up is best. Lower the legs and remove any abdominal binders and compression hose. You must remove or correct any potential stimulus, such as a vaginal speculum. Methods to prevent AD include performing a bowel program and catheterizations on a regular schedule, checking and emptying indwelling catheter leg bags often, changing catheters every 4 weeks to prevent any clogging, checking for pressure sores regularly, and maintaining good toenail hygiene to prevent ingrown toenails because any of these may trigger an episode of AD. It is important to educate the patient and caregivers about AD and the possible associated complications.

Methods to Ensure Access

Patients with mobility disabilities may find it difficult to access health care services primarily because of problems with physical accommodations. From parking to being able to get onto an examination table, people with mobility disabilities face many obstacles at medical facilities. Consequently, these patients are less likely to seek out and receive health services. As a health care provider, you can make a real difference in promoting the health of a population that is typically underserved.

When referring a patient for routine screening or specialty care, it is important to ensure there is accessible parking, including wheelchair van parking, which should include adequate space for a lift or ramp to deploy. Ensure that there is an accessible entrance to the facility and that it is clearly marked. Check to see if your local radiology service has an accessible mammogram machine that can accommodate patients in wheelchairs. When prescribing medication, ensure that the pharmacy can supply medication in easy-to-open containers that are accessible to individuals with hand disabilities. Office and medical staff should be educated to be respectful and to assume that a patient who is also a wheelchair user is likely to be fully employed, competent, and knowledgeable about self-care.

For more information about providing accessible care to patients with limited mobility, the DHHS in collaboration with the Department of Justice has produced an excellent guide for clinics and hospitals. This guide, titled *Access to Medical Care for Individuals with Mobility Disabilities*, can be viewed at http://www.ada.gov/medcare_ta.htm.

CASE STUDY 48.2

For 18 years, a patient with quadriplegia urged his primary care clinic to obtain an adjustable examination table, and for 18 years the clinic refused. He frequently underwent cursory examinations while seated in his wheelchair. It was not until he was hospitalized with an infected pressure ulcer and a successful ADA lawsuit was filed against the clinic that steps were taken to improve access for patients with mobility disabilities.[17] This story illustrates the need to look at our existing facilities and their accessibility *before* patients suffer from adverse outcomes.

PROVIDING APPROPRIATE CARE FOR PATIENTS WITH VISUAL IMPAIRMENTS

Approximately 10 million individuals who are blind or visually impaired live in the United States.[18] Approximately half of these individuals are older adults, and although the vast majority of people living with visual loss lead active and productive lives, unemployment statistics range from 50% to 75% for visually impaired adults. For people with visual loss, the biggest obstacle to improved quality of life, including access to appropriate health care, is overcoming assumptions and stereotypes regarding their abilities and challenges.

Terms and Definitions

Visual impairment (VI): Any vision problem that is severe enough to affect an individual's ability to carry out the ADLs. This may include people with low vision and those with no vision at all.

Legal blindness: A level of VI that has been defined by law to determine eligibility for benefits. It refers to central visual acuity of 20/200 or less in the better eye with the best possible correction, as measured on the Snellen vision chart, or a visual field of 20 degrees or less.

Total or profound blindness: Absence of vision or the ability to determine only the existence, not the source, of light (also called *light perception*)

Braille: A tactile code system of raised dots in specific patterns, representing printed letters and words, which is used by some visually impaired individuals. If you have materials available in Braille, ask your patient if Braille is preferred before offering them.

Dog guide: Assistance dogs trained to lead people with VIs around obstacles. Not all people with VIs use canes or dog guides. The use of dog guides and canes for mobility depends on personal preference and the individual's travel skills. The presence or absence of a cane or dog guide does not indicate the level of assistance a person might require to navigate a hallway or hospital room. The best way to find out if assistance is needed is to ask.

Sighted-guide technique: A specific technique for providing mobility assistance to a person with a VI. If a person with a VI accepts your offer of guidance, this technique should always be used. First, stand one step ahead of the person you are guiding. Tap the back of your hand against his or her hand. The person will grasp your arm directly above the elbow. Relax and walk at a comfortable, normal pace, always staying one step ahead of the person you are guiding. Pause when there is a change in terrain, such as a curb or set of stairs. Verbal cues are not necessary but may be helpful. Never walk away from the person you are guiding without warning or explanation. To guide the person to a seat, place the hand of your guiding arm on the back of the seat, and the person you are guiding will be able to find the seat.

Patients with VIs often receive less than optimal care because of assumptions made by health care providers.

> *I think it is really important that they know that most VI patients with diabetes can learn to measure insulin and monitor blood sugar and use a pump, so they don't just put them on the simplest routines and not the one that will give them the best management.*
> —A patient with diabetes and visual loss

Best Practices

Most people with VIs do not have hearing impairments or intellectual disabilities. Speak in a normal tone of voice, and communicate directly with the patient.

Relax. It is okay to say things such as "I see" or "It looks like . . .." Sighted references used in everyday conversation will not be offensive to your patients with VIs.

Introduce yourself by name and function, and state the reason you are there. Every time you enter the room of a person with a VI, state who you are even if you only left the room for a brief time. Be sure others do the same. Stay in one place when addressing the patient. It is difficult to face someone who is moving constantly. Let the patient know when you move from one place to another, and describe what you are doing (i.e., setting up for a procedure). It is disconcerting to hear drawers being opened and closed, instruments clanging, and wheels rolling across the floor when you do not know what is happening.

Most patients will not need assistance when changing, but do not forget to orient the patient to the room and the location of the gown. Be specific with directions, saying to your right, your left, or directly in front of you. Ask the patient if he or she needs assistance moving from the chair to the examination table. Guide patients using the sighted-guide technique described earlier, and make the patient aware if the step is pulled out before guiding him or her to the examination table. Always let the patient know when you are about to touch him or her for any reason but particularly for the different components of the physical examination.

Residual sight is critical to patients with any degree of VI. Routine eye examinations should be arranged. Changes in vision or new onset of eye symptoms may create tremendous anxiety and should be given your full concern and attention.

Challenges

There is a tremendous variety of residual sight in the visually impaired population. Some people can only see objects in the central field of vision (because of peripheral visual field deficits caused by glaucoma or retinitis pigmentosa), and others can only see at the periphery (as in macular degeneration). Some have only light perception, yet others can read a bold, 18-point font print with eyeglasses.

The patient's ability to use residual sight is greatly affected by lighting conditions and contrast. A patient may have difficulty navigating a dimly lit x-ray room or finding an examination table covered with white paper in a room painted white but has little or no trouble locating a dark blue chair on a white tile floor in the well-lit waiting room.

Methods to Ensure Access

Do not eliminate or abbreviate your history and physical examination. Include your usual patient education discussions even if the health maintenance you are recommending requires sight. For example, if you want your patient to collect stool samples for guaiac testing, describe the process for collecting a specimen, let the patient handle the materials used, and confirm that the patient will be able to follow through with the collection. Your patients with disabilities often have the best suggestions for modifications and accommodations that will allow them to participate in self-care.

Ask your patients how they prefer to receive their patient education materials. Some may request material in Braille, some may prefer a particular font style, and yet others may prefer to record your instructions on a handheld device. It is helpful to have a preprinted sheet of paper with a variety of font styles and sizes (Times New Roman and Arial are typically preferred) in bold and normal print. This will allow your patients to choose the style they are best able to read. Transferring your patient education materials to a Word document format will ensure accessibility for a majority of your patients with VIs.

CASE STUDY 48.3

An elderly woman with macular degeneration was brought to the ED after passing out in the grocery store. She was found to be severely anemic.

The patient had recently seen her primary care provider for symptoms of "diarrhea and fatigue." As a result of her syncopal episode and visit to the ED, a comprehensive history and thorough workup were pursued. Rectal bleeding was eventually revealed to be the source of her anemia.

It was not until this patient presented urgently to the ED that it became clear that what she had described as simple "diarrhea" was actually a much more serious symptom. It is important to be sensitive to these types of symptoms (those that rely on sight) in low-vision patients. Further investigation might be necessary in your visually impaired patients to avoid situations like the one described.

PROVIDING APPROPRIATE CARE FOR PATIENTS WITH INTELLECTUAL AND DEVELOPMENTAL DISABILITIES

In 2002, the U.S. Surgeon General issued the National Blueprint for Improving the Health of Persons with Mental Retardation (MR). Upon introduction of this Blueprint, the Surgeon General noted that "people with MR, their families, and their advocates report exceptional challenges in staying healthy and getting appropriate health services when they are sick."[19] The Blueprint outlines a broad set of goals for improving the health of persons with intellectual and developmental disabilities, which includes improved training of health care providers. The Blueprint states, "The number one issue is lack of training to support healthy lifestyles for individuals with MR across the lifespan" and notes that didactic and clinical training of all health care providers is critical in meeting the goals of improved health.[19] According to the Declaration on Health Parity for Persons with Intellectual and Developmental Disabilities, "Health services for persons with intellectual and developmental disabilities often continue to be discriminatory, inappropriate, inefficient, uninformed, and insufficient" (see Case Study 48.4).[20]

Terms and Definitions

Mental retardation: Although this term has been around for decades, its pejorative use and negative connotation has led to a change in its acceptance and use by those in the field of intellectual and developmental disabilities. The best example of this is the recent name change of the American Association on Mental Retardation (AAMR), a 130-year-old association representing developmental disability professionals, clients, and their families nationwide. In November 2006, the AAMR announced its new name, the American Association on Intellectual and Developmental Disabilities.[21] With this in mind, throughout the remainder of this section, this population will be referred to as patients with intellectual and developmental disabilities.

Intellectual and developmental disability: A developmental disability is not a mental disorder. It is a disability that originates before the age of 18 years and is characterized by limitations both in intellectual functioning and in adaptive behavior. Diagnosis is often based on an IQ test score of approximately 70 or below. An intellectual disability may be developmental or acquired. An acquired intellectual disability may be the result of a traumatic brain injury or stroke, for example. The functional abilities of the person with an intellectual or developmental disability can be positively affected by early intervention and individualized supports.

Autism spectrum disorders (ASDs): Previously called pervasive developmental disorders. A constellation of symptoms, which include a varying degree of impaired communication, difficulty with social interactions, and restricted, repetitive, and stereotyped patterns of behavior, are often seen. Although these disorders can be reliably detected by age 3 years and, in some cases, as early as 18 months, it is estimated that only 50% are diagnosed before kindergarten. This has a profound impact on functioning because at least 2 years of early (preschool) intervention has been shown to benefit long-term functional abilities in children with ASD. Many, but not all, people with ASD have some degree of intellectual disability, and one in four has a seizure disorder.[22]

Down syndrome: A chromosomal anomaly that occurs in 1 of every 733 live births, which causes developmental delay and is associated with a number of physical conditions. In addition to intellectual disabilities, children with Down syndrome may have congenital heart defects, thyroid disease, and blood and nervous system disorders. Until the past few decades, the average age of survival for a person with Down syndrome was only 19 or 20 years. With recent advancements in clinical treatment, up to 80% of adults with Down syndrome reach age 55 years, and many live even longer. People with Down syndrome are at much greater risk for developing Alzheimer disease than the general population.[23]

Traumatic brain injury (TBI): A blow or jolt to the head, or a penetrating head injury that disrupts the function of the brain. Severity ranges from "mild" (brief change in mental status) to "severe," resulting in long-term problems with independent function. Recent data show that approximately 1.7 million people sustain a traumatic brain injury annually.[24] Depending on the severity of the injury, functional limitations may include memory problems, difficulty with problem solving, managing emotions, and vocational skills.

Best Practices

Because of the great variety in functional ability, it is critical that you know your patients with intellectual and developmental disabilities. Taking the time to assess their communication, level of understanding, and ability to follow through in self-care will greatly increase your ability to provide appropriate care for these patients across the life span.

Even if the patient arrives with a caregiver (often staff or family member), engage the patient in the history taking, examination, and patient education process as much as possible. Begin with the assumption that the patient can participate in his or her care. As is the case with all patients with disabilities, if you are unsure, ask. When needed, check with caregivers or review available documentation to ensure accuracy, but do not assume that staff members are familiar with any given patient's medical history.[25]

Many people with intellectual and developmental disabilities are literal, concrete thinkers. Therefore, keep your communication simple and straightforward without being condescending or "talking down" to the patient. Avoid questions or instructions that require multitasking. If something requires several steps, ask the patient to complete one step before moving on to the next. Be thorough and inclusive. Discuss sexual health and assess for smoking, as well as drug and alcohol use, when appropriate.

Perform a comprehensive physical examination when appropriate. Take the time to explain what you will be doing, and answer any questions before you begin the examination. Visuals can be helpful. Make sure you schedule adequate time for the more sensitive examinations such as breast and genital examinations. Because people with intellectual and developmental disabilities are vulnerable to sexual abuse, these examinations should be approached with great sensitivity, and any reaction that makes you concerned about abuse should be thoroughly explored.

When discussing patient instructions or follow-up, give thorough explanations and always check for understanding. Simple written instructions should be provided. Ask the patient if he or she has any questions.

You should not hesitate to refer all patients for any recommended or required diagnostic screening. Routine health promotion and disease prevention should be provided to patients with intellectual and developmental disabilities, and as life expectancy continues to increase, more of these patients will be in need of screening examinations such as mammography and colonoscopy. Good communication with your patient, caregivers, and other health care providers will ensure that these patients will be able to successfully participate in any necessary testing. When obtaining consent for testing or procedures, you need to ask about guardianship. Many patients with intellectual and developmental disabilities are their own guardians and can consent independently.[26]

Challenges

Assessing your patient's ability to participate in his or her own health care takes time and patience. You will need to work with your facility, supervising physicians, and support staff to ensure quality and continuity of care for your patients with intellectual and developmental disabilities. As much as possible, these patients should be given the opportunity to make choices and experience self-determination in areas that affect their health.

Preventive health screening and education regarding lifestyle modification should be undertaken with all patients regardless of intellectual ability. You will need to get to know the auxiliary health services and providers in your area who are skilled in providing appropriate care for this population.

Methods to Ensure Access

A multidisciplinary approach and the enlistment of the assistance of experts in the field will ensure that your patients with intellectual and developmental disabilities get the best, most comprehensive care. The use of the patient-centered medical home model of care, which is defined by the Patient-centered Primary Care Collaborative as "a model or philosophy of primary care that is patient-centered, comprehensive, team-based, coordinated, accessible, and focused on quality and safety," can improve the provision of care for patients with intellectual and developmental disabilities, thereby improving access and outcomes.[27]

CASE STUDY 48.4

After several visits to his primary care provider for fever and rash, a 21-year-old man with a developmental disability was finally diagnosed with bacterial endocarditis. By the time he arrived at the hospital, he had developed bacteremia and shock. Before initiating any treatment, the providers responsible for his care in the hospital approached his parents and asked if "everything possible should be done." Horrified, they responded, "Of course!"

Before he fell ill, this young man was attending college classes, working part time, and participating in an active social life through a local service organization. To insinuate that a patient with a developmental disability deserves anything less than comprehensive, aggressive treatment of a life-threatening illness is inexcusable and constitutes illegal discrimination.

CLINICAL APPLICATIONS

- What experiences or encounters have you had with people with disabilities? How are people with disabilities portrayed in the media (movies, television)? How have these experiences and portrayals shaped your attitudes and opinions toward people with disabilities?
- Seek out opportunities to work with individuals with various disabilities during your clinical year. Ask them about their challenges and experiences in accessing the full range of health care services and how you can make accommodations to meet their needs.
- As a community service project with your classmates, offer to speak to local groups that provide support and services for people with disabilities about the PA profession and general health topics such as diet and exercise or cancer screening.

KEY POINTS

- Speak directly to the patient. If the patient has an assistant or companion in attendance, do not assume that the patient cannot answer his or her own questions. Listen attentively to your patients with disabilities to understand their background and individual functional needs. The patient is often your best source of information about his or her disability.
- Avoid stereotyping your patients. Do not make assumptions about anything (cognitive function, relationships, sexual activity).
- Become aware of the barriers to care that exist for your patients with disabilities, and work to eliminate these barriers. Advanced access planning in the clinic can save time and improve quality of care. Check accessibility when referring patients to diagnostic testing and specialty clinics.
- Treat every patient equally, providing the same services to patients with disabilities as you do to those without one. Do not take shortcuts. Do not eliminate information or services you would provide to any other patient.
- Focus on the patients' overall health and well-being, not just the disabling condition. Defining "health" as the absence of disability or chronic illness negatively affects people with disabilities. Most lead active, fulfilling lives that may include school, sports, work, community involvement, relationships, and parenting.

ACKNOWLEDGMENT

The author would like to acknowledge Mary Vacala, ATC, PA-C, the coauthor of this chapter in the previous edition.

References

1. Center of Assistive Technology. Cornucopia of disability information: disability statistics. Available from: http://codi.tamucc.edu/graph_based/.demographics/.awd/AWD.html. Accessed April 3, 2016.
2. Kennedy C, Salsberry P, Nickel J, et al. The burden of disease in those with serious mental and physical illness. *J Am Psychiatr Nurse Assoc.* 2005;11(1):45–51.
3. Altieri NA, Pisoni DB, Townsend JT. Some normative data on lip-reading skills. *J Acoust Soc Am.* 2011 Jul;130(1):1–4.
4. Bauer KL, Wolf D. Do antibiotics interfere with the efficacy of oral contraceptives? *J Fam Pract.* 2005;54(12):1079–1080.
5. Healthy People 2020. Disability and health. Available from: https://www.healthypeople.gov/2020/topics-objectives/topic/disability-and-health. Accessed April 3, 2016.
6. Field M, Jette A. The future of disability in America. Institute of Medicine Committee on Disability in America. Washington, DC: National Academies Press; 2007. http://www.nap.edu/catalog/11898/the-future-of-disability-in-america. Accessed April 3, 2016.
7. ADA National Network: Information, guidance, and training on the Americans with Disabilities Act. Available from: https://adata.org/faq/what-definition-disability-under-ada. Accessed April 3, 2016.
8. Iezzoni LI, O'Day BL, Killeen M, Harker H. Communicating about health care: observations from persons who are deaf or hard of hearing. *Ann Intern Med.* 2004;140(5):356–362.
9. American Speech-Language Hearing Association. Degree of hearing loss. Available from: http://www.asha.org/public/hearing/Degree-of-Hearing-Loss/. Accessed April 3, 2016.
10. Centers for Disease Control and Prevention. Hearing loss in children, types of hearing loss. Available from: http://www.cdc.gov/NCBDDD/hearingloss/types.html. Accessed April 3, 2016.
11. The National Council on Interpreting in Health Care. A National Code of Ethics for Interpreters in Health Care (July 2004) and National Standards of Practice for Interpreters in Health Care (September 2005). Available from: www.ncihc.org. Accessed April 3, 2016.
12. Flores G, Laws MD, Mayo SJ, et al. Errors in medical interpretation and their potential clinical consequences in pediatric encounters. *Pediatrics.* 2003;111(6 Pt 1):1495–1497.
13. Krassioukov A, et al. A systematic review of the management of autonomic dysreflexia following spinal cord injury. *Arch Phys Med Rehabil.* 2009;90(4):682–695.
14. Spina Bifida Homepage: Data and statistics. Available from: http://www.cdc.gov/ncbddd/spinabifida/data.html. Accessed April 3, 2016.
15. Reis JP, Breslin ML, Iezzoni LI, Kirschner KL. It takes more than ramps to solve the crisis of healthcare for people with disabilities. Available from: http://dredf.org/wp-content/uploads/2012/10/it-takes-more-than-ramps.pdf. Accessed April 3, 2016.
16. Center for Disability Issues in the Health Professions, Western University of Health Sciences. The importance of accessible examination tables, chairs and weight scales. Available from: http://webhost.westernu.edu/hfcdhp/wp-content/uploads/1-Brief-Tables-Scales.pdf. Accessed April 3, 2016.
17. Tamar Lewin. Disabled patients win sweeping changes from HMO. *New York Times;* April 2001. http://www.nytimes.com/2001/04/13/us/disabled-patients-win-sweeping-changes-from-hmo.html. Accessed April 3, 2016.
18. American Foundation for the Blind. Blindness statistics. Available from: http://www.afb.org/Section.asp?SectionID=15. Accessed April 3, 2016.
19. National Library of Medicine. Closing the gap: a National Blueprint for Improving the Health of Persons with Mental Retardation. Available from: http://www.ncbi.nlm.nih.gov/books/NBK44346/. Accessed April 3, 2016.

20. American Association on Mental Retardation. The Declaration on Health Parity for Persons with Intellectual and Developmental Disabilities. http://aaidd.org/news-policy/policy/position-statements/health-mental-health-vision-and-dental-care. Accessed December 28, 2016.

21. Newton Wellesley Committee for Community Living. The language of disability (pdf). http://www.nwwcommittee.org/pdf/the_language_of_disability_2012.pdf; Accessed April 3, 2016.

22. National Institute of Mental Health. Autism spectrum disorders. Available from: http://www.nimh.nih.gov/health/topics/autism-spectrum-disorders-pervasive-developmental-disorders/index.shtml. Accessed April 3, 2016.

23. National Down Syndrome Society. Down syndrome facts. Accessed from: http://www.ndss.org/Down-Syndrome/Down-Syndrome-Facts/. Accessed April 3, 2016.

24. Faul M, Xu L, Wald MM, Coronado VG. *Traumatic brain injury in the United States: emergency department visits, hospitalizations, and deaths*. Atlanta, GA: Centers for Disease Control and Prevention, National Center for Injury Prevention and Control; 2010.

25. The staff and students of STRIVE U. Focus group conducted by author. December 19, 2006.

26. Krauss MW, Gulley S, Sciegaj M, Wells N. Access to specialty medical care for children with mental retardation, autism, and other special health care needs. *Mental Retardation*. 2003;41(5):329–339.

27. Defining the Medical Home. Patient-centered Primary Care Collaborative. Available from: https://www.pcpcc.org/about/medical-home. Accessed April 3, 2016.

The resources for this chapter can be found at www.expertconsult.com.

CHAPTER 49

MASS CASUALTY NATURAL DISASTER

Nancy E. McLaughlin • Jeff W. Chambers • James C. Johnson III

Mass casualty incidents (MCIs) can result from both natural disasters, such as hurricanes, and human-made disasters, such as terrorist attacks. MCIs tax medical infrastructures and require urgent response from medical personnel from many different disciplines. Physician assistants (PAs) are being called on to respond to the urgent medical needs more frequently than in the past. Many times, PAs are first on the scene and take a leadership role in chaotic situations. In recent years, large-scale disasters such as 9/11 and Hurricane Katrina have raised concerns about our ability to respond in an effective and coordinated manner to the medical (and other) needs created by these disasters.[1]

The World Health Organization (WHO) defines *disaster* as "a serious disruption of the functioning of a community or a society causing widespread human, material, economic or environmental losses which exceed the ability of the affected community or society to cope using its own resources (ISDR)."[2] Natural disasters include such events as earthquakes, volcanoes, landslides, tsunamis, flooding (river or coastal), tornadoes, droughts, wildfires, sand or dust storms, blizzards, and infestations. Certain geographic locations are more prone to particular natural disasters. For example, whereas midwestern states are prone to tornadoes, western states might experience earthquakes and wildfires. Situational awareness is important to be prepared for natural disasters.

Vulnerability is the "degree to which a socio-economic system is either susceptible or resilient to the impact of natural hazards."[2] Vulnerability is determined by hazard awareness, infrastructure, public policy, and ability to implement disaster management procedures. Poverty remains one of the main causes of vulnerability.[2] There is no better illustration than the vulnerabilities present in Haiti on January 12, 2010, when a 7.0 earthquake struck the capital of Port-au-Prince, killing hundreds of thousands of people. Haiti remains one of the poorest countries in the Western Hemisphere. The Haitian government gave much attention to other natural disasters such as hurricanes and mudslides even though Haiti had a documented history of devastating earthquakes dating back to the 1770s. Haiti is located on the borders of the American and Caribbean tectonic plates, making it particularly vulnerable to earthquakes. In addition, because of deforestation of trees, lumber for buildings became expensive. Therefore, buildings shifted to concrete and stone structures that could not withstand the violent shaking during the earthquake. Building codes were either not enforced or were nonexistent. Buildings collapsed, trapping many beneath the ruble. Furthermore, first aid for emergency situations was not readily available, compounding the suffering and loss of life from this disaster. All of these vulnerabilities drastically increased the death toll from this natural disaster.

The WHO defines *mass casualty* as "an event which generates more patients at one time than locally available resources can manage using routine procedures. It requires exceptional emergency arrangements and additional or extraordinary assistance."[3] The phrase *mass casualty* conjures up images of 150 casualties waiting at several hospitals in a metropolitan area in such cases as the Boston Marathon bombings. By definition, mass casualty would also constitute a multivehicle accident with eight casualties being transported to a critical access hospital in a rural area. MCI events can be a result of a terrorist attack such as the events of 9/11. Another less publicized event is the train derailment in Graniteville, South Carolina, in 2005 that resulted in an immediate release of 46 tons of liquid chlorine near a textile mill where 183 people were working the night shift.[4] Each of these events has vastly different origins, but each resulted in an MCI.

The effects of an MCI or natural disaster can be mitigated with well-rehearsed emergency response teams and a prepared community. The community is deemed "recovered" when the health status of the community is restored to its pre-event state. In some instances, this can be a relatively short period of time, but other instances can take many years. The goals of emergency response are
1. Reverse the adverse health effects caused by the event.
2. Modify the hazard responsible for the event (reducing the risk of the occurrence of another event).
3. Decrease the vulnerability of the society to future events.
4. Improve disaster preparedness to respond to future events.[1]

Most MCIs and natural disasters come with little to no warning; therefore, it is essential that PAs have a solid foundation in disaster preparedness and emergency response. Understanding the cyclical pattern known as the disaster cycle is essential to understanding the four reactionary stages that occur after a catastrophic event. The four reactionary stages are
1. Preparedness
2. Response
3. Recovery
4. Mitigation and prevention[1]
Each stage varies in duration depending on the type of MCI or natural disaster experienced.

PRINCIPLES OF TRIAGE

Triage comes from the French verb "trier," which means "to sort." Triage of patients in a mass casualty or natural disaster situation often requires medical providers to alter their thought process about treating patients. Under normal circumstances, the sickest or worst injured get immediate medical attention, and often medical providers try to save the life of a patient at all costs. When medical personnel and medical supplies are limited, the critically injured and ill are passed over to help care for patients with a higher likelihood of surviving. Treatment is aimed at doing the most good for the most patients. By assigning priorities for treatment through triage principles, medical personnel make the most efficient use of available resources.[5]

There are three major reasons why triage is beneficial when responding to a natural disaster or MCIs. Triage categorizes patients who need rapid medical care to save life or limb. By separating out the minor injuries, triage reduces the urgent burden on medical facilities and organizations.[6] On average, only 10% to 15% of disaster casualties are serious enough to require overnight hospitalization.[6] By providing for the equitable and rational distribution of casualties among the available hospitals, triage reduces the burden on each to a manageable level, often even to "non-disaster" levels.[6] The disaster triage system in the United States is color coded: red, yellow, green, and black, as follows:
- **Red:** First priority, most urgent. Life-threatening shock or airway compromise present, but the patient is likely to survive if stabilized.
- **Yellow:** Second priority, urgent. Injuries have systemic implications but not yet life threatening. If given appropriate care, the patients should survive without immediate risk.
- **Green:** Third priority, nonurgent. Injuries localized, unlikely to deteriorate.
- **Black:** Dead. Any patient with no spontaneous circulation or ventilation is classified dead in a mass casualty situation. No cardiopulmonary

resuscitation (CPR) is given. You may consider placement of catastrophically injured patients in this category (dependent) on resources. These patients are classified as "expectant." Goals should be adequate pain management. Overzealous efforts toward these patients are likely to have deleterious effect on other casualties.[1]

Understanding principles of triage is essential for medical providers attending to casualties to save the most lives during an MCI or natural disaster.

CHEMICAL, BIOLOGICAL, RADIOLOGIC, NUCLEAR, EXPLOSIVES, AND ENVIRONMENTAL INCIDENTS

Mass casualty incidents and natural disaster events have been the scourge of humankind since antiquity. As we have moved into 21st century, the causes of disasters have expanded from the natural disasters and infectious disease pandemics of previous centuries to potential human-made events such as chemical, biological, radiologic, nuclear, and explosives (CBRNE) incidents that have the ability to produce widespread carnage very quickly. As the industrial age flourished, modern manufacturing processes began to use toxic chemicals in their daily operations. These chemicals are transported near urban areas via highways and railroads, which places the general public at great risk when accidental spills occur. Furthermore, these same modern manufacturing processes have allowed people to produce chemical, biological, and nuclear weapons capable of inflicting multitudes of casualties. Combined with the rise of rogue terrorist groups, the potential for one of these weapons of mass destruction being used against a civilian population is of grave concern. PAs, no matter the specialty they might practice in, need to have a basic understanding in the recognition and treatment of CBRNE injuries, as well as injuries that result from natural disasters.

Chemical Disasters

Ancient Greek myths spoke of the effectiveness of chemical warfare, and various agents have been used throughout the ages, culminating with the widespread use in World War I. Many of the chemical agent–related disasters in modern times are related to industrial accidents. One of the most famous chemical disasters was the December 3, 1984, Bhopal disaster in India that killed between 4000 and 20,000 people from exposure to methyl isocyanate.[7]

Disasters from chemical exposures create numerous casualties very quickly and place first responders in danger of also being contaminated. Proper decontamination of patients at the scene by trained civilian or military personnel takes priority before rendering medical care. Contamination of medical personnel and facilities risks not only the provider's health but may also place the ability of the hospital to receive casualties in jeopardy. First responders will usually be able to communicate the type of chemical agent involved to the receiving hospital, and treatment of patients should be focused on that contaminant. The injuries associated with chemical disasters depend on the class of agent involved. Some of the more common agents that may be encountered include

- **Choking agents** that target the pulmonary system such as chlorine and phosgene. These agents are lung irritants that cause injury to the lung–blood barrier, resulting in asphyxia.
- **Blood agents,** such as hydrogen cyanide, are rapidly lethal via halting cellular respiration. Treatment is the rapid removal of the victim from the environment, application of oxygen, and administration sodium nitrite.
- **Blister agents or vesicants,** such as mustard gas, are some of the most common chemical warfare agents. These oily substances act via inhalation and contact with skin. Blister agents affect the eyes, respiratory tract, and skin, first as an irritant and then by affecting cell metabolism. Blister agents cause large and often life-threatening skin blisters that resemble severe burns. The effects of mustard agents are typically delayed: Exposure to vapors becomes evident in 4 to 6 hours, and skin exposure is seen in 2 hours to 48 hours. Treatment is decontamination and supportive care targeted to address life-threatening respiratory compromise.
- **Nerve agents** are perhaps the most rapidly lethal chemical agents and result in respiratory paralysis and death in a matter of minutes. Nerve agents, such as sarin and VX, enter the body through inhalation or through the skin. The degree of symptom severity depends on the level of exposure. Classic symptoms of moderate to high doses of nerve agent result in pronounced secretion of mucus, bronchoconstriction, abdominal cramping, vomiting, involuntary urination and defecation, muscle weakness, convulsions, and death by suffocation. Treatment must be rapid to prevent death and include decontamination and administration of high doses of atropine and 2-PAM (2-pyridine aldoxime methyl) chloride. Supportive care must be aggressive because the physiological effects can continue long after nerve agent is reversed.
- **Riot control agents** (tear gas) are chemical compounds that temporarily make people unable to

function by causing irritation to the eyes, mouth, throat, lungs, and skin. The effects of exposure to a riot control agent last about 15 to 30 minutes after the patient has been decontaminated. Immediate signs and symptoms of exposure to a riot control agent include excessive tearing, eye burning, blurred vision, a runny nose, difficulty swallowing, chest tightness, coughing, and nausea and vomiting. Long-lasting exposure or exposure to a large dose of a riot control agent can result in blindness, glaucoma, and sometimes death from respiratory compromise. Treatment includes the removal of the patient from the environment, copious irrigation, and symptomatic treatment.

- **Toxins** are poisons produced by living organisms. One of the most well-known toxins is botulinum toxin. Botulinum toxin is produced by the bacteria *Clostridium botulinum* and is extremely lethal. The lethal dose has been estimated to be about 1 microgram if ingested and even less if inhaled. The incubation period is between 1 and 3 days at which time the patient presents with abdominal pain, diarrhea, visual changes, and muscular weakness. Paralysis ensues, compromising respiratory function, and asphyxia ensues. No specific treatment is available for botulinum toxin. Treatment is directed at supporting the cardiopulmonary system.

Biological Disasters

Biological disasters are diseases conveyed by biological vectors, including exposure to pathogenic microorganisms, toxins, and bioactive substances that can cause injury, illness, social, and economic disruption and death.[8] Biological disasters can be naturally occurring or can be human-made in the form of accidental release or bioterrorism. Naturally occurring biological disasters can be divided into epidemics and pandemics. An epidemic is a disease process affecting a disproportionately large number of individuals within a population, community, or region at the same time.[9] A pandemic is an epidemic that spreads across a continent or worldwide, such as the 1917 influenza pandemic.[9] Epidemics are common after tropical storms, floods, earthquakes, and wars when normal hygiene and sanitation services are disrupted. Examples of natural epidemics include the avian flu common in southeast Asia; the cholera outbreak in Haiti after the earthquake in 2010 as the result of improper sanitation protocols by Nepalese soldiers who were part of the United Nations forces; dengue fever and malaria outbreaks from mosquito-borne vectors; the Ebola outbreak in West Africa in 2015; and measles, which has a high mortality rate in developing countries.

Epidemics can also be the result of bioterrorism. Bioterrorism is a method that disseminates widespread panic in a population and produces a slow onset of mass casualties. Bioterrorism can be targeted to both a human population and an animal population, which can produce large-scale economic losses. Many of the common bioterror weapons such as smallpox, anthrax, and plague were weaponized by the United States and the Soviet Union after World War II. Although many of these bioweapon stocks were destroyed as the result of arms agreements, some stockpiles remain in the former Soviet Union. These stockpiles, as well as the scientific ability to produce these weapons, are sought after by terrorist groups. Recognizing bioterrorism is a critical first step in decreasing the number of casualties. Incidentally, frontline medical professionals may be the first to recognize health trends that indicate a bioterrorism attack.

Biological disasters present differently from chemical disasters. The vectors are different and can include agents dispersed into the air that may drift for miles; animals, including fleas, mice, mosquitoes, and livestock; food and water supplies; and from person to person such as smallpox. Unlike chemical agents, there is a lag time between exposure and the appearance of symptoms. This lag time gives the vector more time to expose a greater number of victims. Furthermore, it increases the time it takes before the disease is recognized, isolated, and treated. Three categories of biological agents can cause mass casualties:

- **Category A** (which pose the most risk to public health): These agents are easily disseminated from person to person and have a high mortality rate. These agents include smallpox, Ebola, Lassa fever, anthrax, plague, tularemia, and botulism. Special isolation precautions of contaminated patients are required. Consequently, multiple casualties can be devastating to the medical system as patients require an inordinate amount of resources.
- **Category B:** These agents are moderately easy to disseminate; have moderate morbidity and low mortality rates; and include alphaviruses, *Brucella* (brucellosis), *Burkholderia mallei* (glanders), *Coxiella burnetii* (Q fever), ricin, staphylococcus enterotoxin B, *Salmonella, Vibrio cholera,* and *Escherichia coli* O157:H7. Children, older adults, and immunocompromised individuals are more at risk for complications from these diseases. Early, aggressive treatment is critical in reducing the long-term morbidity of the diseases.
- **Category C:** These agents include many that have insect vectors, including Nipah, yellow fever, tick-borne hemorrhagic fever viruses, tick-borne encephalitis, and bacteria such as *Mycobacterium*

tuberculosis. Although these diseases have the potential for morbidity and mortality, they are less likely to be widespread public health threats.

Clinicians should be aware of the diseases that lend themselves to becoming bioweapons. Anthrax, smallpox, plague, tularemia, and brucellosis are diseases that are relatively easy to produce, inexpensive, readily spread from person to person, and can be "weaponized" for distribution over a wide area. Bioweapons are considered to be a "poor man's nuclear bomb" and can produce widespread casualties. For example, smallpox causes a one in five mortality rate. Furthermore, there are associated widespread panic and economic chaos. Unlike chemical weapons, where casualties would occur quickly after an attack, victims of bioterrorism would present days after the exposure with initial "flulike" symptoms. Be aware that with modern air travel, a bioterrorism victim on another continent may present to an emergency department (ED) or medical office in the United States with the early stages of the disease. It cannot be emphasized enough that a thorough travel history is obtained on every ill patient. Clinicians should inquire about friends and family members with similar symptoms and maintain a high index of suspicion if multiple patients present with similar symptoms. Clinicians should also become suspicious of an epidemic curve that rises and falls during a short period of time, an endemic disease rapidly emerging at an uncharacteristic time of the year, lower attack rates of people who have been indoors, clusters of patients arriving from a single location, and large numbers of rapidly fatal cases.[10] Isolation of the patient and those exposed to the patient should take first priority, including personal protective equipment (PPE) for all staff. Decontamination should only be considered in cases of gross contamination, and this determination needs to be made in conjunction with local and state health departments. Basic decontamination includes removal of clothing and bathing in soap and water. Clinicians should notify the hospital's infection control personnel, public health officials, law enforcement, emergency medical services (EMS), and the Centers for Disease Control and Prevention (CDC) promptly. Postexposure immunization and prophylaxis measures depend on the biologic agent involved. Furthermore, the determination on proceeding with an intervention should be made in conjunction with the local and state health departments. Treatment of patients should be directed at addressing presenting symptoms because exposure to many of the bioterror agents presents with respiratory or gastrointestinal complaints. Additionally, clinicians should be ready to address the potential for respiratory failure, hemorrhagic shock, or septic shock.

Nuclear and Radiologic Disasters

Nuclear and radiation disasters are, fortunately, uncommon in the United States. Although the prospect for a large-scale nuclear power disaster on the scale of the Fukushima, Japan, accident is remote, incidents involving radiologic dispersal devices (i.e., dirty bombs), occupational accidents, or even an explosion from an improvised nuclear device are possible events. Clinicians should be prepared for these events and be familiar with the types of nuclear and radiologic devices, decontamination methods, and recognition of radiation sickness and should have a basic knowledge of treatment for radiation injuries.

Improvised Nuclear Devices

Improvised nuclear devices are a type of nuclear weapon that generates four types of energy: a blast wave, intense light, heat, and radiation.[11] Depending on the size of the device, victims in the initial blast zone have an extremely high mortality rate from the blast wave. Furthermore, any survivors would sustain severe burns, blindness, and a rapid onset of acute radiation syndrome (ARS). ARS is caused by an irradiation of the entire body by a high dose of radiation over a few minutes.[9] The major cause of ARS is the depletion of immature parenchymal stem cells in certain tissues.[9] The radiation dose must be greater than 70 rads, from an external source of gamma rays. Symptoms include anorexia, fever, malaise, severe diarrhea, dehydration, and electrolyte imbalances. Death usually occurs in 3 days and is the result of infection, dehydration, and electrolyte imbalances. Mortality rates depend on the radiation dose received. As a general rule, nausea and vomiting that start within 4 hours of exposure are a poor prognosticator. Victims farther from the blast zone could expect radiation sickness and contend with contaminated food and water. Rapid decontamination and supportive care are critical to decreasing mortality and morbidity.

Radiologic Dispersal Devices (Dirty Bombs)

A "dirty bomb" is a device that is a more likely scenario in a radiologic terrorist attack. A dirty bomb or radiologic dispersal device (RDD) is a mix of radioactive material and a high explosive that does not create a nuclear blast but disperses the radioactive material over an area. Easy to produce, the potential radioactive material can include industrial waste or even the byproducts of common medical procedures. The danger from an RDD is from blast trauma. The radiation exposure is only a concern for people near the blast, and the potential for radiation exposure serves as a "fear weapon," possibly slowing first responders. Basic decontamination procedures need to be followed but should not impede rapid evaluation and treatment of trauma injuries.

Occupational Accidents and Radiologic Exposure Devices

Occupational accidents and use of radiologic exposure devices (REDs) are both situations when a person is exposed to radioactive material. In the case of occupational accidents, these are seen mostly in research facilities, hospitals, and some manufacturing operations. Exposure to an RED is a criminal attempt to expose victims to a radiation source, usually in a public place such as a food court or bus. In both situations, the physiologic response of the victim depends on the type and amount of exposure, the length of exposure, and what body part was exposed. High levels of exposure can result in ARS; however, the effects of low-dose exposure could take weeks to appear. Treatment is directed toward symptoms; however, the patient will require long-term monitoring specifically evaluating for leukopenia and bone marrow suppression with resultant infection.

Natural Disasters

By far, the most common type of mass casualty event seen worldwide is natural disasters. Depending on location, PAs should be prepared for natural disasters that are common to that location. The gulf coast and the eastern coast of the United States are prone to hurricanes, which can produce widespread devastation, resulting in not only mass casualties as the result of trauma (i.e., penetrating and crush injuries) but also infectious disease issues as the result of a loss of infrastructure and sanitation. The Midwest and the southern United States are prone to tornadoes. Tornadoes give very little warning and tend to cause injuries similar to those from hurricanes except in a smaller geographic area. The West Coast and Alaska are prone to earthquakes and tsunamis, which give little or no warning and generate widespread destruction. In the case of earthquakes, many of the injuries are crush injuries from collapsed structures or injuries related to resulting fires or explosions. Similar to hurricanes, earthquakes involve a wide area and can result in severe impairment of local fire departments and EMS to render care. Tsunamis result in widespread inland flooding and structure damage. Many of the deaths are the result of drowning; however, exposure to sewage, industrial chemicals, and waterborne pathogens can result in a widespread

public health emergency. By knowing what types of environmental events are common to an area, proper preparation can ensure a better outcome in the event of one of these disasters.

Hurricanes

Hurricanes have plagued the southeastern and the eastern United States, resulting in catastrophic loss of property and life. Hurricanes have become a bigger problem over the past 50 years because more people are living in coastal regions. Hurricanes damage by both wind and water. Wind damage, as the result of 150 plus–mph winds, result in the structural collapse of buildings, homes, and utilities as well as exposing people to wind-blown shrapnel, causing penetrating injuries. Water damage occurs as the wind pushes wave action inland, resulting in flooding and potential drowning deaths. Subsequent exposure to water-borne illnesses is a very real risk. People in poor health and older adults are susceptible to aggravation of preexisting health problems caused by a lack of medications, prolonged exposure to heat, and a lack of a clean water supply. The widespread devastation to health care facilities and transportation infrastructure makes treating and evacuating large numbers of patients problematic and usually requires a state or federal response. Hurricane Katrina highlighted the problematic nature of providing medical care in an environment where electricity, water, and transportation are absent. Clinicians should be ready to treat patients in poor conditions with limited supplies. Emphasis should be on the triage of patients with prompt evacuation to intact facilities. Many times such disasters require the assistance of ground and air military assets. Clinicians should be mindful to take care of themselves in this type environment with proper hydration, nutrition, and rest–work cycles to avoid fatigue and injuries.

Tornadoes

Tornadoes strike with little or no warning, usually in the spring and summer in the Midwest and the southeast United States. Although the destruction in usually confined to a narrow area, mortality and morbidity can be high. Winds exceeding 200 mph result in structure collapse and flying debris that produce crush injuries, penetrating injuries, and lacerations. Health care facilities should be prepared to receive ambulatory patients quickly after an event. Disaster protocols should be routinely rehearsed in tornado-prone areas and recall rosters updated to allow for a quick surge of staff to the ED. In some cases, the local hospital can be at "ground zero" from a tornado strike as happened in Joplin, Missouri. In these situations, the hospital is rendered inoperable, and the staff must deal with transferring inpatients to another facility as well as setting up a treatment area in whatever structure is available. Mutual aid compacts established beforehand between hospitals and states are critical to mitigating suffering and death. Routine disaster drills in conjunction with local emergency medicine services, hospitals, National Guard Medical Teams, and Federal Disaster Medical Assistance Teams (DMAT) can reduce confusion and provide for a quicker response in the event of a catastrophic tornado.

Earthquakes

Similar to tornadoes, earthquakes give little or no warning yet result in large areas of property destruction, injuries, and deaths. The West Coast and Alaska are known for catastrophic earthquakes, but large fault lines in the Midwest and Mississippi River Valley make this area prone to devastating earthquakes as well. Most of the injuries and deaths are the result of crush injuries, fires, and explosions. Earthquakes that strike areas with older structures not built to withstand earthquakes will result in a large-scale mass casualty event. Similar to a hurricane, local infrastructure (including medical facilities), may be inoperable, and roads may become impassable. Again, clinicians should be ready to follow their hospital's disaster plan and be prepared to see large numbers of patients with crush injuries, open fractures, head injuries, compartment syndrome, and lacerations. Clinicians should expect casualties to exceed their facilities' capabilities within a matter of hours. Patients standing the best chance of survival should be treated and evacuated first. Care must be taken not to exhaust material and manpower on patients with predictably poor outcomes. In addition, public health can become an issue. Rapid deployment of state and federal civilian and military assets is critical to provide nutrition, water, medical teams, supplies, heavy lift capability, and security. Hospital disaster plans should include yearly opportunities to interface with these state and federal assets.

Tsunamis

Tsunamis are enormous waves generated by an underwater earthquake, often thousands of miles away. Because of the Pacific Rim's earthquake activity, the West Coast of the continental United States, Alaska, and Hawaii are prone to tsunamis; however, any coastline is at risk. Tsunamis occur with little warning and are characterized by a sudden receding of the ocean and then the sudden development of waves that flood inland, sometimes for miles. The majority of deaths are from drowning. Injuries as the result of debris include crush injuries, lacerations, and fractures. Populations are affected by a lack of clean water, contaminated food, and exposure to the elements. Clinicians should be prepared not only to treat acute injuries but also to manage the aggravation of preexisting medical conditions and the procurement of lost medications in the at-risk populations.

Terrorism

Terrorism is the use of violence in the pursuit of political gains. Terrorism gained a foothold by various groups in the 1970s, culminating with the events of September 11, 2001. Terrorism can be from domestic sources, such as the Oklahoma City Federal Building bombing, or from foreign terrorist groups. PAs should be aware of potentially high-value terrorist targets in their communities and be prepared to respond to blast injuries, chemical exposures, biological exposures, radiation exposures, and penetrating injuries such as gunshot wounds. Potential targets include famous landmarks, transportation hubs, hotels, government offices, chemical factories, railcars and transfer trucks carrying sensitive materials, petroleum plants, nuclear facilities, and military installations, to name a few. Clinicians should practice situational awareness and know that in a mass casualty situation, there is the potential that an armed terrorist could present to a medical facility as a patient. Clinicians should be knowledgeable in regard to decontamination procedures and PPE in the event of a CBRNE attack. Protection of hospital staff and clinicians is of the utmost importance so as not to risk the ability of the facility to provide care.

Mass casualty incident and disaster preparedness is not a luxury in the 21st century. As threats grow from both natural and human-made sources, all PAs must be prepared to respond as frontline health care providers no matter their specialty. The threats can come from any place at any time. The best chance of mitigating suffering and death is proper training and preparation of the responding providers.

PREPARING BEFORE DISASTER STRIKES

Preparation for an MCI or disaster begins with education. PAs and the lay public should educate themselves on the types of disasters likely to occur in their respective regions. Situational awareness is a cornerstone of disaster preparedness. Situational awareness is the concept of observing one's environment to identify potential dangers. Determination of the likelihood of specific types of disasters requires an understanding of natural disaster patterns, surrounding industries and businesses that incorporate hazardous chemicals and processes, and potential terrorist targets (military bases, federal buildings, national landmarks, financial institutions, key infrastructure).

Evaluating natural disaster patterns allows individuals and disaster planners to direct the focus of their preparation as it relates to sheltering in place versus evacuation. For example, a person living in an area prone to tornadoes will need to plan for sheltering options that are accessible on short notice because evacuation time will be limited. Individuals should evaluate their homes and other locations they frequent for areas that offer maximum protection. The plan used to promote safety during a tornado is much different from the plan common in hurricane preparation. Whereas individuals caught in the path of a tornado have little time to escape, technology normally allows tracking of hurricanes for lengthy periods of time before landfall. This lead time allows the public to physically secure houses, commercial buildings, infrastructure, and so on. The lead time also allows for self-evacuation as well as assisted evacuation of special needs populations. Whether an individual is facing a quick-hitting tornado or a protracted threat from a hurricane, preplanning is key to protecting life and property.

Just as preplanning for natural disasters is required for increased survival, decreased injuries, and appropriate postdisaster medical response, preplanning is also required as it relates to human-made disasters and terrorism. Human-made MCI and disaster scenarios include but are not limited to industry-related accidents such as nuclear power plant malfunctions with large-scale radiation release, hazardous material (HAZMAT) release and contamination, structural collapse, and airline crashes. These types of incidents are unintentional, but terrorism is an intentional act causing, in this case, the disaster. Preplanning for human-made and terrorism-related disasters vary with the mechanism and location of the attack.

An appropriate and effective medical response to an MCI or disaster requires preplanning. Preplans are designed to provide a framework for responders to follow. MCI and disaster preplans are developed by governmental agencies at the local, state, and federal levels. Preplans are also common to private entities with special needs such as high-risk industrial processes, large numbers of employees, and special needs populations. Adherence to MCI and disaster preplans allows agencies from multiple jurisdictions, as well as agencies from different disciplines (medical,

fire, law enforcement, military), to work jointly rather than duplicating efforts or possibly inhibiting each other from performing required tasks. MCI and disaster preplans vary in complexity based on specific types of events, types and numbers of agencies involved, geographic areas covered, and so on. It is common for medical providers of varying levels to self-deploy to the scenes of MCIs or disasters to assist with medical care. Well-designed preplans take into account the tendency of individuals to respond independently and set up mechanisms to account for these responders, verify credentialing, and integrate them into the overall operational plan if needed. Although the impromptu response to the scene of an MCI or disaster may provide much-needed help for dispatched resources, medical providers interested in MCI or disaster response should explore opportunities to participate through defined roles within existing MCI and disaster response teams and preplans. Interested PAs will then be trained to function as members of the responding teams. Understanding how to practice medicine in an austere environment and how it differs in some aspects from conventional medicine will make a PA an asset on the scene rather than a liability. Trained MCI and disaster medical responders understand that medicine is a part of the operation but has to be planned and carried out in a manner that is governed by such concerns as scene safety, any ongoing law enforcement activity, and limitation of resources including personnel and supplies. As PAs, our tendency is to focus on the medical needs of the patient, providing the highest standard of care possible. Although focusing on the medical needs of our patients is completely appropriate in our conventional medical care settings, it could easily lead to dangerous tunnel vision at the scene of an MCI or disaster. Focusing on a patient's medical needs may cause us to miss the fact that he or she is lying in contact with a live high-voltage power line. The concept of triage medicine is important for the disaster medical responder. To make the decision to withhold CPR on a patient with no pulse in the setting of mass casualties who could benefit from immediate medical attention is not a decision that is easily made. Learning proper triage techniques and algorithms can assist medical responders in functioning in the MCI and disaster environment. PAs interested in local or regional response should contact their municipal or state Office of Emergency Management to discuss opportunities for service. Another option for PAs interested in MCI and disaster response is the National Disaster Medical System (NDMS).

The National Disaster Medical System (NDMS) is a federally coordinated system that augments the

Nation's medical response capability. The overall purpose of the NDMS is to supplement an integrated National medical response capability for assisting State and local authorities in dealing with the medical impacts of major peacetime disasters and to provide support to the military and the Department of Veterans Affairs medical systems in caring for casualties evacuated back to the U.S. from overseas armed conventional conflicts.[12]

The MCI and disaster response component of the NDMS includes NDMS Response Teams. The NDMS Response Teams include
• DMATs
• International Medical Surgical Response Team (IMSURT)

A DMAT is a team of medical providers of varying levels as well as support members including administrative and logistics personnel. The teams are based in various states across the nation and are designed to rapidly respond to MCI and disaster situations to augment local and regional medical response. PAs volunteering for assignment to a DMAT are considered intermittent federal employees when the DMAT is activated. The IMSURT is a specialized NDMS team capable of providing surgical and critical care services in the aftermath of an MCI or disaster. Similar to a DMAT, the IMSURT will augment local and regional resources.[12]

The NDMS falls under the Office of Emergency Management (OEM) within the U.S. Department of Health and Human Services Office of the Assistant Secretary for Preparedness and Response. The OEM also houses the Medical Reserve Corps (MRC).

The Medical Reserve Corps (MRC) is a national network of volunteers, organized locally to improve the health and safety of their communities. The MRC network comprises 998 community-based units and over 200,000 volunteers located throughout the United States and its territories.[13]

Physician assistants volunteering for the MRC are available to be used during MCI and disaster situations as well as disease outbreaks. The MRC also focuses on community health and health promotion.[12]

Physician assistants can learn more about volunteer options for NDMS at http://www.phe.gov and more about the MRC at http://www.medicalreservecorps.gov. The OEM also offers the Emergency System for Advance Registration of Volunteer Health Professionals. This is a state-based registry that health care volunteers can join to have their credentials and licensure validated. This registry allows PAs to be used on scene quicker in the case of an MCI or disaster because credentialing of responding providers can be a time-consuming process for administrative personnel on scene.[12] Further information about this registry can also be found at http://www.phe.gov.

Another recommended resource for PAs interested in MCI and disaster response is the website of the American Academy of Physician Assistants (AAPA), http://www.aapa.org, where PAs can access a document titled *The PA in Disaster Response: Core Guidelines.*[1]

Other websites with information related to MCI and disaster preparedness include
• Centers for Disease Control and Prevention. *Natural Disasters and Severe Weather.* http://emergency.cdc.gov/disasters/.
• American College of Surgeons. *Disaster Management and Emergency Preparedness.* http://www.facs.org/quality-programs/trauma/education/dmep.
• Federal Emergency Management Institute. *ICS Resource Center.* https://training.fema.gov/emiweb/is/icsresource.
• FEMA. *Community Emergency Response Teams.* https://www.fema.gov/community-emergency-response-teams.
• Centers for Disease Control and Prevention. *Guidelines for Field Triage of Injured Patients Recommendations of the National Expert Panel on Field Triage.* http://www.cdc.gov/mmwr/preview/mmwrhtml/rr5801a1.htm.

Physician assistants who are attached to disaster response teams or who hold positions requiring them to respond to MCI or disaster situations will likely have equipment provided to accomplish their assigned tasks. For individuals who will respond in a volunteer capacity, the following items should be considered when putting together a basic medical response load:
• PPE (gloves, eye protection, hand sanitizer)
• Tourniquets (commercial, improvised)
• Oral and nasal airways
• Advanced airways (if within scope of practice)
• Bag-valve mask
• Occlusive dressing for chest wounds (commercial, petroleum gauze, examination gloves)
• Large-bore needles for chest decompression (if within scope of practice)
• Bandages (various sizes)
• Hemostatic dressings
• Emergency or survival blankets (Mylar or other conductive material)

Just as preparation is a must for any disaster medical responder, it is equally vital for the public at large. News stories after disasters are filled with individuals lamenting a perceived lack of response to their basic needs. Individual preparedness is key to survival during and immediately after an event. The most effective mindset for individual disaster preparedness is the concept of all-hazard planning. All-hazard planning allows preparation across disaster types. The concept of all-hazard planning pushes disaster planners and individuals to focus on preparedness and response measures that would be generally effective regardless of the cause of the disaster. For instance, creating safe and effective evacuation routes from a facility would increase survival regardless of the cause of the evacuation (e.g., fire, chemical release, active assailant). The following suggestions can serve as a guide for individual disaster preparedness and are derived from information found on the CDC's website (http://emergency.cdc.gov/preparedness/kit/disasters/):

- Water (1 gallon per person per day)
- Food (nonperishable, prepackaged Meals Ready-to-Eat)
- Fire-starting material (commercially available, improvised)
- Candles (commercially available emergency candles)
- Knife including can opener
- Cell phone and charger (commercially available emergency charger)
- NOAA weather radio (battery powered, solar, hand crank)
- Flashlight
- Batteries
- Fishing line and hooks
- First aid kit
- Medications (prescription medications as well as desired over-the-counter medications)
- Emergency or survival blankets (Mylar or other conductive material)
- Cash
- Pet supplies (food, medications, leash)
- Maps
- Communication plans for family and friends during or immediately after event
- Preplanned meeting place for family and friends during or immediately after event[14]

As health care providers, PAs are regularly engaged in health promotion and disease prevention efforts. Educating our patients about MCI and disaster preparedness is an area of health promotion that is of vital importance and can impact not only our patients but public health efforts as well.

AFTER A CRISIS

Physician assistants play a vital role in caring for those who have lived through a mass casualty or natural disaster. Not only will they care for the victims of such tragedies, but they may also have to care for the first responders. Immediate medical needs are accessed to prevent loss of life and limb. Subsequently, other issues may arise well after the actual incident such as disease outbreaks caused by contaminated food and water. PAs need to maintain awareness of federal and state surveillance and reporting requirements regarding disease outbreaks to prevent full-blown epidemics. This information can be ascertained on individual state Department of Health websites or from the CDC's *Morbidity and Mortality Weekly Report (MMWR). MMWR* reports national and international incidents and gives up-to-date information on public health issues. It can be found at http://www.cdc.gov/mmwr.

Posttraumatic Stress Disorder

Posttraumatic stress disorder (PTSD) develops after a terrifying ordeal that involves physical harm or the threat of physical harm.[15] People who have PTSD continue to experience stress or are traumatized long after they are out of harm's way.[15] PTSD was once thought to be a mental disorder suffered by only war veterans, but it can be observed in any individual who has undergone a traumatic event such as a terrorist attack or a natural disaster. It should also be noted that PTSD can be observed in children.

Signs and symptoms of PTSD include the following three categories:

1. Reexperiencing symptoms
   - Flashbacks: reliving the trauma over and over, including physical symptoms such as a racing heart or sweating
   - Bad dreams
   - Frightening thoughts
2. Avoidance symptoms
   - Staying away from places, events, or objects that are reminders of the experience
   - Feeling emotionally numb
   - Feeling strong guilt, depression, or worry
   - Losing interest in activities that were enjoyable in the past
   - Having trouble remembering the dangerous event
3. Hyperarousal symptoms
   - Being easily startled
   - Feeling tense or "on edge"
   - Having difficulty sleeping or having angry outbursts[15]

Children with PTSD often present with bedwetting after having been previously toilet-trained, forgetting how or being unable to speak, acting out the scary event during play, or being unusually clingy.[15]

Recognizing the signs and symptoms of PTSD is imperative to diagnosing and ultimately treating those who have this debilitating condition.

Not everyone who experiences a traumatic event will go on to develop PTSD. Several risk factors and resilience factors have been identified to help determine who is at greatest risk of experiencing PTSD.[15]

Risk factors for PTSD include

- Living through dangerous events and traumas
- Having a history of mental illness
- Getting hurt
- Seeing people hurt or killed
- Feeling horror, helplessness, or extreme fear
- Having little or no social support after the event
- Dealing with extra stress after the event, such as loss of a loved one, pain and injury, or loss of a job or home

Resilience factors that may reduce the risk of PTSD include

- Seeking out support from other people, such as friends and family
- Finding a support group after a traumatic event
- Feeling good about one's own actions in the face of danger
- Having a coping strategy, or a way of getting through the bad event and learning from it
- Being able to act and respond effectively despite feeling fear[15]

The diagnostic criteria for PTSD as per the *Diagnostic and Statistical Manual of Mental Disorders*, 5th edition (DSM-5), identifies the trigger as exposure to actual or threatened death, serious injury, or sexual violation. The exposure must result in one or more of the following scenarios, in which the individual

- Directly experiences a traumatic event
- Witnesses the traumatic event in person
- Learns that the traumatic event occurred to a close family member or close friend
- Experiences first-hand repeated or extreme exposure to aversive details of the traumatic events[16]

The disturbance, regardless of its trigger, causes clinically significant distress or impairs the individual's social interactions and capacity to work or perform other important areas of functioning.[16] It is not the physiologic result of another medical condition, medication, drugs, or alcohol.[16]

Special Populations

Children, older adults, and people with mental impairments are all at higher risk for injury and illness after a disaster. Cognitive impairment and physical disability such as vision and hearing impairment make evacuating older adults and people with cognitive impairments more difficult. Older adults also have more chronic illnesses and are dependent on medication to maintain a stable state of health. Evacuation of these groups of people is often delayed to the point that it is too late, as seen during Hurricane Katrina. Furthermore, pediatric populations do not realize the gravity of a particular emergency situation and may not move to safety. In addition, they are dependent on adults to direct them, which may be difficult in places such as daycare centers where the adults are outnumbered by the children in need. Pediatric and geriatric populations are often more susceptible to infectious disease because of lowered immune responses.

CASE STUDY 49.1 ENVIRONMENTAL SCENARIO

On May 22, 2011, an EF5 tornado struck Joplin, Missouri, which created total devastation 1 mile wide and 14 miles long, killing 158 people, injuring 1150, and causing $2.8 billion of damage.[17] The local hospital, St. John's Regional Medical Center, was so severely damaged that it was deemed structurally compromised and had to be torn down. Six people died at St. John's; one was a visitor, but the other five were on ventilators that failed when the backup generator failed to start.[18] Because of the extreme damage to the hospital, it was unable to service the multiple casualties created by the tornado during the initial response.

IMPACT AND RESPONSE

The hospital sustained a direct hit from the tornado, causing windows and walls to be blown out; portions of the roof to fly off; and a loss of all power, communications, and water. Patients were evacuated to other facilities, and alternate care sites were established at a local high school. The incident command system was established, and additional personnel and supplies arrived, including the Missouri National Guard and the Department of Health and Human Services (DMAT, which provided an 8000-square-foot field hospital.[19]

DISCUSSION

The Joplin incident exemplifies the need for a hospital to have a thorough disaster plan and rehearse the plan routinely. Having contingency plans to establish patient care in another location in the event the hospital becomes a casualty is critical, especially in areas of the country with frequent tornadoes, earthquakes, and hurricanes. Clinicians must be prepared for an influx of casualties quickly that will include open fractures, lacerations, head injuries, crush injuries, and ocular injuries. Chronically ill patients will have lost access to medications; therefore, being able to provide medications, as well as basic nutrition, is critical to this now homeless population. Mitigating suffering until additional civilian and military assistance arrive can be extremely challenging with limited resources. PAs must be flexible and prepared to work in an austere environment with limited equipment and supplies for the first few days after the disaster. PAs must also remember self-care as well and use proper work–rest cycles so as to not become overwhelmed by the workload. Formal disaster and trauma training can provide invaluable skill sets for PAs who may be called on to respond in these situations.

CASE STUDY 49.2 DISASTERS

Incidents involving biological, chemical, terrorist, and natural disasters are a constant threat to public safety. The following incidents illustrate how these types of events impact the public and provide general concepts as to response and mitigation efforts of the health care team.

BIOLOGICAL EMERGENCIES

The 2001 anthrax attack was a bioterrorism event that occurred over the course of several weeks starting on September 18, 2001. Letters containing anthrax spores were mailed to several media outlets and to two U.S. senators, resulting in five deaths and 18 confirmed cases requiring treatment. Law enforcement was able to trace anthrax to the U.S. Army's biodefense lab at Fort Detrick, Maryland, and the attacks were believed to have originated from a civilian employee of the facility.

VICTIMS

Of the victims, 64% were male, ranging in age from 43 to 94 years, and all but two were known to have handled the mail.[9] Eleven cases were inhalational, and 12 were cutaneous, with all five deaths the result of inhalational anthrax, resulting in a 45% mortality rate.[9] The mean incubation period was 4 to 6 days.[9] Almost all the patients presented with fever, chills, fatigue, cough, nausea, vomiting, dyspnea, and sweats.[9]

IMPACT

The attacks followed on the heels of the September 11 attacks and caused a major disruption in government function by shutting down dozens of buildings, including the Senate office building for several days as well as mail-sorting facilities in Washington, DC. The Federal Bureau of Investigation estimated that total cost of the damage exceeded $1 billion.[20] The event sowed fear among the public in the wake of the attacks on Washington, DC, and New York, and it was initially suggested that the attacks were the work of a terrorist group or a foreign government in the run-up to the 2003 invasion of Iraq, which was later disproved.[21] As of 2014, several of the victims report lingering health problems, including shortness of breath and fatigue.

RESPONSE

The anthrax attack in 2001 required an unprecedented public health response.[22] The first patients presented to local EDs in New York and Florida seeking treatment for a skin condition.[9] Subsequent cultures of the wounds revealed cutaneous anthrax, and within 1 to 2 days, cases of inhalational anthrax were reported. Antibiotic prophylaxis was begun using oral ciprofloxacin, and isolation of patients and facilities was instituted. However, the epidemic overwhelmed the nation's laboratory workforce because more than 120,000 samples were tested in the ensuing days.[9] Public health workers were also overwhelmed with work, with one nine-state area generating 2817 bioterrorism calls in a 1-week period, almost all false alarms. An influx of patients with common viral symptoms concerned they had contracted anthrax swamped EDs, physician offices, and health departments for testing, which diverted medical and laboratory resources from needed areas.[9] Health care professionals also realized that many had no experience recognizing anthrax and were concerned about missing a case of a disease with such a high mortality rate.[9]

DISCUSSION

Surveillance and situational awareness are critical to the response of an infectious disease event. The PA should be alert and maintain an index of suspicion, especially if multiple patients present with the same symptoms. A tight cluster of casualties, dead animals in the area, and the presentation of an unusual disease are key indicators of a biological attack. Scene safety becomes urgent, and PAs and other personnel must don PPE. PAs should be familiar with the use of pre- and postexposure antibiotics as well as active and passive immunologic agents. Initial patient evaluation should focus on the airway, breathing, and circulation and supporting these systems. Base empiric treatment on physical findings until laboratory confirmation, but do not delay potential live-saving interventions. Initiate isolation precautions and notify the public health department as soon as possible. PAs play a critical role in outbreak identification and reducing the spread of the disease.

CASE STUDY 49.3 TERRORISM

On April 15, 2013, the Boston Marathon was well under way when two bombs built in pressure cookers and packed with shrapnel exploded about 200 yards and 12 seconds apart, killing three people and injuring 264.[23] Two self-radicalized brothers were implicated. One was killed in a shoot-out with police, and the second was captured. The explosion quickly produced a mass casualty situation that challenged the robust Boston emergency medical system.

IMPACT AND RESPONSE

Fortunately, medical help was immediately available because health care professionals were in attendance to support the runners. The availability of prompt first aid and the quick response of Boston Fire and EMS were critical in saving lives. Twenty-seven hospitals were used to treat 264 patients.[24] Lower extremity injuries were common because of the bombs' being placed on the ground. Seventeen amputations were performed, and many patients required multiple surgical debridements because of the vast amounts of nails and ball bearings loaded in the improvised explosive devices.

DISCUSSION

Terrorism resulting in a mass casualty event, whether it is from a high-yield explosive device, multiple improvised explosive devices, or a weapon of mass destruction, can quickly overwhelm a city's emergency medical response and hospital system. The need for local responders and hospitals to rehearse the Incident Management System and train together on a regular basis cannot be overemphasized. PAs who may be on the scene of such an event should practice scene safety and be aware of secondary explosive devices designed to injure first responders. Be prepared to establish a quick triage system and direct other first responders and bystanders to provide first aid care, including hemorrhage control, which many times is a preventable cause of mortality in blast events. As a hospital provider, being current in Advanced Cardiac Life Support (ACLS), Pediatric Advanced Life Support (PALS), and Advanced Trauma Life Support (ATLS) is very beneficial, and PAs should keep these skills current no matter the provider's subspecialty. Emergency medicine providers should routinely practice mass casualty drills and be prepared to work in teams as patients arrive. Preparation also allows for fluid integration of additional recalled providers as they arrive at the ED, thereby decreasing confusion. Providers should keep laboratory and radiographic studies to a minimum because ancillary hospital services can become saturated quickly. Incoming casualties should be retriaged frequently because a blast patient's condition can deteriorate quickly. The PA should keep in mind the concept of "salvage" and not definitive treatment at these initial stages. The fundamentals of shock resuscitation take priority, and early surgical intervention in crucial. Keep in mind the potential for psychological trauma as well in both patients and providers. PTSD is common after terrorist events, and early recognition and referral for counseling are important to help ameliorate long-term consequences.

CASE STUDY 49.4 CHEMICAL EMERGENCIES

On June 11, 2014, a 58-year-old woman presented via ambulance to a rural Jefferson County, Georgia, ED complaining of shortness of breath, nausea, vomiting, weakness, and an inability to move, which had begun earlier that day. In addition, her young grandson and two grandchildren had similar, but milder, symptoms. It was discovered that the patient's relative had used an agricultural insecticide inside her home called Fumitoxin, which when exposed to moisture emitted a phosphine gas. Phosphine, a colorless, odorless gas, is a lung-damaging agent that produces pulmonary edema and is fatal unless treated. The adult patient died; however, the children were treated and survived.

IMPACT AND RESPONSE

This scenario is an example of a chemical multicasualty versus mass casualty event. Although not the extent of chemical exposure one might see with a large industrial accident or in combat, this small, rural ED was saturated with critical patients quickly. By definition, a multicasualty event is an event with multiple patients, but the health care facility's resources are not exhausted. In a mass casualty event, the hospital's resources are exhausted, and additional resources must be used. Even though there were only four patients, this qualifies as a mass casualty event because of the severity of the injuries and the limited resources. In addition, multiple medical personnel were exposed, which required use of a HAZMAT team from another town for decontamination of personnel. The ED was closed until decontamination was completed.

DISCUSSION

Physician assistants must be familiar with potential chemical exposures and be able to recognize the signs and symptoms associated with common household and industrial agents. In addition, the potential for a terrorist attack with a chemical agent is a concern, especially in target-rich urban environments. Multiple patients presenting with a sudden onset of similar symptoms is a key sign of a chemical exposure. These exposures can quickly overwhelm a hospital because many patients will self-present, requiring emergent decontamination before entering the ED. As was demonstrated in the scenario, an ED can be quickly rendered inoperable by one patient who was not decontaminated.

Chemical agent exposure requires emergent decontamination and aggressive treatment to ameliorate suffering and death. PAs at the front lines of EDs, civilian and military disaster teams, and international nongovernmental organizations (NGOs) should have a working knowledge of potential agents and their treatment.

SUMMARY

Personal and community preparedness is the key to decreasing casualties in MCIs and natural disasters. A rapid coordinated response among EMS, law enforcement, military, and medical communities is imperative in times of emergencies. PAs are increasingly playing important roles in MCI and disaster management. Additional training in emergency and disaster management is becoming more important as PAs are finding themselves thrust into these situations. PAs also play an important role in providing their patient population with valuable information of emergency preparedness. As natural disasters and MCI become more prevalent, the role of PAs will continue to grow.

CLINICAL APPLICATIONS

- What are the most likely disasters in your area?
- Does your medical facility have an active shooter plan?
- How do you currently educate your patients on MCI and disaster preparedness?
- How would your medical practice or hospital cope with an MCI?

KEY POINTS

- PAs should have a basic knowledge of CBRNE threats.
- PAs should educate patients on emergency preparedness.
- PAs should be well versed on agencies and services that offer aftercare in the case of an MCI or natural disaster.
- PAs should consider getting advanced training in disaster response.

PERSONAL STORIES
Boston Marathon Bombings: The White Jacket

Dixie Patterson, PA-C

The white jacket. I have an immense amount of pride wearing it. As a cardiac surgery PA for the past 18 years, putting my white lab coat on over my scrubs each morning means we're about to start rounds on our postop patients. At the Boston Marathon, putting on that white Adidas medical volunteer jacket signifies I'm part of one of the best finish line medical teams out there.

I've always been passionate about cardiac surgery. I like to think it's an elegant precise work of art and fancy plumbing. Some describe it as hours of boredom interrupted by minutes of sheer terror. It's a challenge I readily accept and work hard to make sure my training prepares me for whatever happens. Most days are routine—critical care decisions, chest tubes, x-rays, and wound checks. But you always must be prepared for a code blue, a crashing patient, and potentially needing to open a postop patient's chest at the bedside. Controlled chaos. Operating on some of the largest blood vessels in the body, seeing blood is an everyday occurrence, but it's in an extremely controlled environment. Through a meticulous opening in a blue surgical drape, we fix broken valves and bypass blocked arteries. The surgeon and I are part of a skilled team, working alongside anesthesiologists, nurses, and perfusionists, all with the common goal of keeping that patient alive and getting him or her back home to loved ones.

I've also always been passionate about running. As a runner for 25 years, the Boston Marathon has always been the holy grail of marathons for me. I was honored to get to run it back in 2009. After moving to the Boston area a couple of years later, it only made sense for me to combine my love of medicine and running, so I proudly became a medical volunteer for the Boston Athletic Association (BAA), the group that organizes the Boston Marathon. The BAA prepares its volunteers to treat the problems most often seen after running 26.2 miles: dehydration; sodium imbalances; hyper- and hypothermia; orthopedic strains, sprains, fractures, and blisters; and the potential for fatal cardiac issues. The BAA medical team consists of doctors, PAs, nurses, physical therapists, psychologists, and massage therapists, all working together to help keep runners safe and get them back home to enjoy wearing that finisher's medal proudly.

The third Monday in April is a special day in Boston. It's not only an official holiday—Patriot's Day—but it's also the running of the Boston Marathon. The Red Sox always play an afternoon home game along the marathon course, and most people are off work to enjoy the day. Monday, April 13, 2013, was the kind of day runners dream of. The sky was sparkling blue with temperatures in the 50s and a slight tailwind. I was again volunteering in the finish line medical tent. It's located about 50 yards from the finish line. Our section of the tent was near the back opening, where Boston EMS had ambulances ready for transport if needed. Two other PAs and I were in charge of eight cots. Before the runners started, we had prepared our section with intravenous lines, space blankets, emesis basins, gauze, and other items we frequently use. We had some spare time and walked down Boylston Street to the finish line area to take some quick snapshots. Little did we know what would happen in that very area only 6 hours later. I remember remarking to my friends how it was a perfect day to run a marathon.

Because of the ideal weather, we weren't that busy in the med tent. The BAA sets up large-screen TVs in the tent so we can watch the race coverage while caring for runners. It was actually a fairly boring day—dehydration, blisters, nausea. We were never at full capacity. Hours of boredom interrupted by . . . BOOM! The tent shook. There was silence as we all looked around. Twelve seconds later . . . BOOM!

I've never heard a bomb before, but there was no doubt in my mind what those sounds had been. I looked at my friends and said they should text their husbands saying they were okay. Just then, the tent announcer stated that all physicians and PAs should go to the finish line for mass casualties. I remember turning back to my best friend (a medical administrator) and telling her to not look at what was about to come into the tent. Having nothing more than a roll of gauze in my hand, my other friend and I ran out of the tent onto Boylston Street. The smell of smoke was still in the air. Most of the spectators had already left the area. It was controlled chaos. The street, now void of runners, was full of white BAA jackets, wheelchairs, Boston EMS, policemen, and ambulances (Figs. 49.1 and 49.2). I ran across that hallowed finish line from the wrong direction and found a sea of people on the sidewalk. Blood, broken glass, the smell of smoke . . . it was eerily quiet.

Cardiac surgery has taught me to stay calm when things around me get crazy. You sort of develop a type of tunnel vision to concentrate on the one thing in front of you, allowing you to think as clearly as you can. A woman in her mid-50s had been lifted into a wheelchair but had open bilateral tibia and fibula fractures. I had a roll of gauze. This was far from the sterile blue drapes that I am so familiar with in the operating room. I focused on her left leg

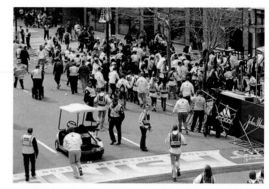

FIG. 49.1 ■ The finish line at the Boston Marathon (2013).

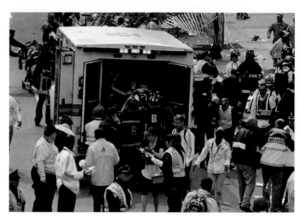

FIG. 49.2 ■ Scene at the Boston Marathon finish line (2013).

while someone else treated her right. Someone used a wooden fence slat to make a splint. Belts were used on her thighs for tourniquets. Stay calm . . . focus . . . hurry. I heard a policeman yelling, "Evacuate the area! We found another device!" That's all it took for my friend and me to run back to the med tent. Some patients were put into ambulances directly from the sidewalk, but most were whisked back to the tent for further triage and stabilization before transport.

There were more than 100 medical providers back in the tent. Everyone worked seamlessly together like we'd all been working together for years, to give these patients a fighting chance. Egos were left at the door. I have no doubt that many lives were saved that day because of the preparation, quick thinking, and selfless actions of everyone around the finish line. Still, three spectators were killed. If you'd have seen what I did, you'd have thought it had been many more. Despite my years in cardiac surgery, I'll never get used to pulling that sheet over a lifeless body. There in the tent, where hours earlier we had all eaten lunch on cots, I saw a twisted shoe sticking out from under a white sheet. I respectfully covered it.

After all patients were transported, we were ordered to evacuate the tent so they could sweep it for bombs. Somehow I had felt safe behind those canvas walls. It hit us all hard on the ride home what we had just witnessed. Luckily, we all had each other to lean on and still do. The BAA also had many debriefings and offered mental health services to those in need. And the world came to realize just what "Boston Strong" meant.

Our community came together in solidarity. And the following year, we showed the world that terrorism will not stop us from coming out on a beautiful Monday in April to run a historic race on Patriot's Day. I was lucky enough to get an invitational entry into the Boston Marathon the following year. I ran for all those who couldn't and in memory for those killed the year before. A year after the bombings, I ran those magical 26.2 miles, and in a healing moment for myself, I finally got to run across that hallowed finish line from the right direction (Fig. 49.3).

Haitian Earthquake, 2010: International Disaster Relief

Henry Curran, PA-C

My name is Henry Curran, and I have been a PA since 1976. During my career, I have worked in family practice, occupational medicine, sports medicine, urgent care, and emergency medicine fields. In 2001, I joined Georgia #3 DMAT, and as a member of this team, I have deployed to the G-8 Summit, hurricanes Ivan, Ophelia, Katrina, Ike, Isaac, and Sandy, and the Haiti earthquake. Although each of these deployments was unique in terms of environment, risk, physical requirements, mission, and skill set, for me, our deployment to Haiti was probably the most challenging.

Eventually, a Coast Guard C-130 arrived and first flew the Michigan team to Port-au-Prince and later returned to collect my team. After touching down in Haiti, we were loaded into mango trucks and taken to the U.S. Embassy to be given our field assignment. The detour to the Turks and Caicos separated us from our cache of equipment, so while our logistics people searched for our cache, we bedded down on the embassy grounds alongside a host of insects and malaria-carrying mosquitoes. Disaster work can be uncomfortable.

Outside the embassy walls, thousands of men, women, and children were in a line trying to get visas to leave the destruction and chaos. Many were

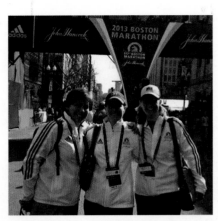

FIG. 49.3 ■ Dixie Patterson *(middle)* at the Boston Marathon finish line with her two best friends; on the right is Courtney Luck, PA-C. On the left is Heather McCormick, medical administrator (2013).

injured, and because they had been waiting for several days with only the food and water they were able to carry, most were dehydrated, especially the infants. Because they were so desperate to leave, they refused to give up their places in line to be cared for. Team members, using what resources could be scavenged, began offering what aid they could as they stood in line. Frustration is always a big part of disaster work.

Another consideration in disaster work is the personal toll it can take on responders. Haiti's January temperature and humidity are nearly the same and are in the high 90s. That along with daily aftershocks that rattled our nerves, lack of rest, and possibly a little PTSD associated with a recent in-flight near-death experience caused some team members problems, and two people were sent back to the United States.

At last, our cache was located between the runways at the airport, and we were given our mission to become a triage hospital for the U.S. Naval Hospital ship *USS Comfort*. We were assigned several dump trucks, and it was all hands on deck to hand load our equipment. With constant humanitarian aid being flown in on each side of us, we loaded our equipment and ourselves in the buckets of our trucks. We were driven for 2 hours to an abandoned landfill outside Port-au-Prince to set up our BOO (base of operation) (Fig. 49.4). Even though we all suffered some degree of heat injury and many had contusions from being jarred around with our equipment during transport, a small truck was waiting on us to repackage a woman with an open-book pelvic fracture, another with long bone fractures, and a young girl with amputations of several digits from her hands and feet. While the rest of the team began constructing our BOO, a

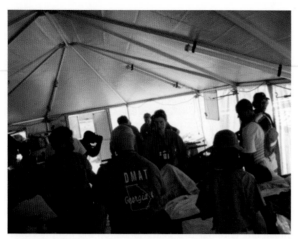

FIG. 49.4 ■ Haitian earthquake (2010), base of operation camp.

small squad was assembled to extract the patients form the back of a truck and hot load (rotors turning) them on to a helicopter for transport to the *Comfort*. The next several days became a blur, but essentially, it was a constant replay of this experience, as severely injured patients from French, German, Israeli, and NGO medical camps were sent to us and in turn were triaged by my team and loaded on, seemingly, unending flights to the advanced level care aboard ship. Most patients made it to the *Comfort* and to the expert care it offered, but unfortunately, some never made it and succumbed to their injuries. In one situation, the team sent a young victim home in a cab because she had a brain injury that was not salvageable. In a large-scale disaster, limited resources and definitive care must be reserved for those most likely to survive and withheld from those who are less likely to survive. Disaster medicine requires some really tough decisions.

Each morning and afternoon, a herd of goats calmly walked through our BOO. And no matter how chaotic the situation, someone would announce: "Here come the kids," which was followed shortly by "page a pediatrician." The goats heard this several times as they made their way through different sections of our BOO. During disaster work, we look for humor wherever we can find it. I don't know if the goats thought it was funny.

We certainly did not think it was funny when the prop wash from a helicopter destroyed our billeting tent (our home) and on another occasion our communications tent. We laugh about it now, so I guess time and distance make things funnier. At the time, it just became another test of our ability to adapt and get the job done.

Whether in the South Bronx after Hurricane Sandy or a landfill in Haiti, disaster medicine has inherent risk, and harsh environments challenge personnel. Frustration over limited resources should be expected.

Flexibility is a key attribute to a PA working in harsh environments. Medical resources available in the United States are not available in developing countries, especially in a disaster situation. PAs have to be aware that definitive care cannot be provided to every patient, and this can be a difficult concept for many clinicians. The concept of flexibility also extends to being able to handle unpredictable events. In one case, a Navy Seahawk helicopter knocked down the DMAT tents with its rotor wash, causing the team to improvise and rebuild the tent in the middle of seeing patients. After 2 weeks of seeing numerous patients, battling heat and austere conditions, and working long hours, the team returned to Atlanta. As the result of this deployment and other DMAT deployments to Hurricane Katrina, Hurricane Ike, and Hurricane Sandy, there are several key questions PAs need to ask themselves if they want to become involved in disaster medicine.

Disaster medicine is inherently dangerous, so is the PA willing to work in areas that can turn violent, where contracting an infectious disease is a certain risk, and where travel can be hazardous? The PA's physical ability and health are critical factors. Is the PA's ability to deliver care in an austere environment limited by obesity, orthopedic problems, or other health issues that require medications or can be affected by heat, dust, and basic living quarters (e.g., sleeping on the ground)? Can the PA adapt and not only perform his or her clinical job but also be willing to do other jobs (e.g., putting up tents, lifting heavy loads, cleaning floors)? Can the PA work as part of a team (in this case, a paramilitary structure) and subjugate one's own needs for the benefit of the team? If so, disaster medicine can be one of the most rewarding endeavors PAs can do in their professional careers. The need for engaged medical professionals will only grow, and PAs provide a perfect skill set for those in need.

References

1. The PA in disaster response: core guidelines. American Academy of Physician Assistants. https://www.aapa.org/WorkArea/DownloadAsset.aspx?id=3087. Accessed March 20, 2016.
2. Definitions. World Health Organization. http://www.who.int/hac/about/definitions/en/. Accessed March 20, 2016.
3. Mass Casualty Management System. World Health Organization. http://www.who.int/hac/techguidance/MCM_guidelines_inside_final.pdf. Accessed March 20, 2016.

4. Wenck M, Van Sickle D, et al. Rapid assessment of exposure to chlorine released from a train derailment and resulting health impact. *Public Health Rep.* 2007;122(6):784–792.

5. Ramesh A, Kumar S. Triage, monitoring, and treatment of mass casualty events involving chemical, biological, radiological, or nuclear agents. *J Pharm Bioallied Science.* 2010;2(3):239–247.

6. Hrdina CM, Coleman CN, et al. The "RTR" medical response system for nuclear and radiological mass-casualty incidents: a functional TRiage-TReatment-TRansport medical response model. *Prehospital Disaster Med.* 2009;24(3):167–178.

7. Bhopal trial: eight convicted over India gas disaster. BBC News. June 7, 2010. http://news.bbc.co.uk/2/hi/south_asia/8725140.stm. Accessed March 20, 2016.

8. National Disaster Management Authority Government of India. http://www.ndma.gov.in/en/. Updated December 11, 2015. Accessed March 20, 2016.

9. Medical management of chemical and biological casualties. U.S. Army Medical Research Institute of Chemical Defense, Aberdeen Proving Ground, MD.

10. Noah DL, Sovel AL, Ostroff SM, Kildew JA. Biological warfare training: infectious disease outbreak differentiation criteria. *Mil Med.* 1998;163:198–201.

11. Improvised nuclear device. Centers for Disease Control and Prevention. http://emergency.cdc.gov/radiation/pdf/infographic_improvised_nuclear_device.pdf. Accessed on March 20, 2016.

12. Public Health Emergency. U.S. Department of Health and Human Services. www.phe.gov. Updated December 10, 2015. Accessed March 20, 2016.

13. Medical Reserve Corps. U.S. Department of Health and Human Services. https://www.medicalreservecorps.gov/pageviewfldr/About. Updated November 20, 2015. Accessed March 20, 2016.

14. Emergency Response and Disaster Preparedness. Centers for Disease Control and Prevention. http://emergency.cdc.gov/preparedness/kit/disasters/. Accessed March 20, 2016.

15. Post-traumatic stress disorder. National Institute of Mental Health. http://www.nimh.nih.gov/health/topics/post-traumatic-stress-disorder-ptsd/index.shtml. Accessed March 20, 2016.

16. Post-traumatic stress disorder. American Psychiatric Association. http://www.dsm5.org/Documents/PTSD%20Fact%20Sheet.pdf. Accessed March 20, 2016.

17. National Weather Service central region service assessment, Joplin, Missouri, May 22, 2011. Department of Commerce. http://www.nws.noaa.gov/os/assessments/pdfs/Joplin_tornado.pdf. Accessed March 20, 2016.

18. Murphy K. Five patients who died in Joplin hospital suffocated. Reuters. May 24, 2011. http://www.reuters.com/article/us-usa-weather-tornadoes-hospital-idUSTRE74N7FB20110524#GdClWE5crClcjsYB.97. Accessed March 20, 2016.

19. Campbell C. Everything was wiped out as far as you can see. *Suburban Journals.* June 6, 2011. http://www.stltoday.com/suburban-journals/metro/news/everything-was-wiped-out-as-far-as-you-can-see/article_9366c593-0a0a-5f0f-aebc-314-fa55412f7.html. Accessed March 20, 2016.

20. Lengel A. Little progress in FBI probe of anthrax attacks. *The Washington Post.* April 8, 2008. http://www.washingtonpost.com/wp-dyn/content/article/2005/09/15/AR2005091502456.html. Accessed March 20, 2016.

21. Vargus E, Ross B, Osunsami S. Anthrax investigation/bentonite/cases [ABC Evening News video]. Nashville, TN: Vanderbilt Television News Archive, October 28, 2001. http://tvnews.vanderbilt.edu/program.pl?ID=716233. Accessed March 20, 2016.

22. Bioterrorism: Public health response to anthrax incidents of 2001. U.S. Government Accountability Office. http://www.gao.gov/products/GAO-04-152. October 15, 2013. Accessed March 20, 2016.

23. Straw J, Ford B, McShane L. Police narrow in on two suspects in Boston Marathon bombings. *New York Daily News.* April 17, 2013. http://www.nydailynews.com/news/national/injury-toll-rises-marathon-massacre-article-1.1319080. Accessed March 20, 2016.

24. Kotz D. Injury toll from Marathon bombs reduced to 264. *Boston Globe.* April 29, 2013. https://www.bostonglobe.com/lifestyle/health-wellness/2013/04/23/number-injured-marathon-bombing-revised-downward/NRpaz5mmvGquP7KMA6XsIK/story.html. Accessed March 20, 2016.

YOUR PHYSICIAN ASSISTANT CAREER

CHAPTER 50

LEADERSHIP SKILLS FOR PHYSICIAN ASSISTANTS

Ruth Ballweg

CHAPTER OUTLINE

SELECTING AND ADMITTING LEADERS

LEADERSHIP FOR CLINICIANS

PHYSICIAN ASSISTANTS IN LEADERSHIP

A LEADERSHIP SKILL SET FOR PHYSICIAN ASSISTANTS

ENTRY INTO LEADERSHIP

BENEFITS FROM LEADERSHIP ROLES

CONCLUSION

KEY POINTS

In the 50 years of the physician assistant (PA) profession, we have worked hard to be seen as flexible and caring clinicians who can increase health care access, cost effectively improve the efficiency of health care systems, and advance the health care quality movement. Our success in clinical roles has been well documented. Unfortunately, we've fallen behind in a major area: leadership! This chapter is intended to provide background, information, guidance, and examples for PAs and PA students beginning their leadership trajectory.

SELECTING AND ADMITTING LEADERS

The admissions process for PA programs selects for individuals whose priority is to provide clinical care. The acquisition of clinical knowledge, skills, and attitudes is emphasized. Unfortunately, the importance of PA leadership roles receives less attention.

LEADERSHIP FOR CLINICIANS

For clinicians, leadership is often defined too narrowly as encompassing only medical settings. In fact, it is important that PAs look at leadership in a larger context to include community organizations, educational institutions, sports, and even politics! It's important to see leadership skills as transferrable.

Skills and behaviors learned as a committee participant, board member, or officer in any organization can be transferred to other settings.

PHYSICIAN ASSISTANTS IN LEADERSHIP

California Congresswoman Karen Bass is an excellent example of PA leadership. In addition to being a PA and a former PA educator, she was a community leader in health care access issues. From there she ran for state legislature and then on to the U.S. Congress. It is increasingly common to see PAs as members of school boards; hospital leadership structures; and, of course, PA organizations.

Leadership is important for PAs at all levels. Leadership brings increased visibility and credibility to the profession. It also creates opportunities for PA input into policies and implementation. We have a lot to offer! Our goal should be to have a PA in every administrative structure where physicians are typically seen or represented.

Ideally, every PA program will place a value on a history of leadership in their admissions process, introduce PA students to faculty members with community leadership networks, and support student-led populations based projects with leadership opportunities. In addition, PA program faculty should encourage and support student career trajectories that include the consideration of future roles as clinical, academic, and health policy leaders.

Too often, clinicians deprecate administrative roles and leadership as tainted and thankless tasks. The attitude is "someone's got do it, but it isn't going to be me!" This view fails to take into account the potential to make things better—in both the short term and in the long term—for patients, clinicians, and the larger community.

In reflecting on their careers, many senior PAs say they are astounded at the opportunities that were made available to them. These PAs also recount stories of being drawn into leadership positions even though this was never their intention. They do, however recognize the contributions they have made, so they pride themselves as having "never said NO!" when faced with a leadership invitation. They didn't want to limit themselves or to limit the contribution that PAs can make in both clinical AND nonclinical settings.

A major advantage that PAs have in leadership roles is that we are already experienced in asking for help. PAs see this as a strength, not a weakness!

In a new administrative or leadership role, it's good practice to ask a lot of questions about everything from the history of the organization to unique terminology to the roles of everyone in the group. A first priority should be to schedule individual meetings to better understand the organization, its policies, and the cast of characters.

A LEADERSHIP SKILL SET FOR PHYSICIAN ASSISTANTS

The role of leaders is often mischaracterized as simply being the public and political face of an organization. This inaccurate view of leadership may also see some types of activities (e.g., officer or board member positions within an organization) as rewards or popularity contests rather than as work to be done. In fact, the skill set for an effective leader—at either the junior or senior level—includes processes to be understood and mastered rather than tasks to be checked off (Box 50.1).

In reviewing this list of skills and processes, most PAs are quick to notice the overlap with clinical work-ups, diagnosis, treatment, and follow-up. As PAs, we're used to gathering information, problem solving, and getting things done. That's what leaders do!

ENTRY INTO LEADERSHIP

A good leadership entry principle is to pick something that you care strongly about or that really needs doing. Many PA leaders describe their entry into leadership as involvement based on a commitment or passion

---

> ### BOX 50.1 SAMPLE LEADERSHIP SKILLS FOR PHYSICIAN ASSISTANTS
>
> Working with others
> Speaking up
> Asking questions
> Suggesting solutions
> Volunteering to be part of a group
> Volunteering to coordinate or lead a group
> Acknowledging the contributions of others
> Learning how meetings work
>   The importance of an agenda
>   The importance of minutes
>   Projected timeline or schedule
>   Making people feel welcome
>   Making people feel included
> Following up

that they have for a specific issue. It could be a health or patient care issue, it could be a hobby or personal sport, or it may be a personal issue for themselves or someone in their family. Of course, the leadership role may also be a part of an employment situation that is sought after by the PA or assigned by the employer.

BENEFITS FROM LEADERSHIP ROLES

Involvement in leadership roles often brings with it the opportunity for training—both in content and in context as well as in the specific leadership roles and responsibilities of the organization. This training can be a major benefit of investing time in a leadership position.

Leadership positions may require that you expand your perspective on an issue or that you even change the way you think about yourself. The issue may be more complex than you thought it was. Learning about the issue may also require that you meet people you wouldn't ordinarily have met, might not have had access to, or wouldn't have thought that you would ever agree with. These experiences can also be a major benefit of leadership roles and experiences.

Leadership roles also provide opportunities to be mentored or to mentor others. Sadly, the mentorship opportunities can be missed by an insufficient understanding of the potential for these relationships. Primarily, mentors are often thought to be senior people. In fact, peer mentors can be more accessible and offer more observations, feedback, and advice about current dilemmas and opportunities. Peer mentors—who are also contemporaries—are more likely to serve as long-term mentors, but senior mentors may be available only for specific situations and circumstances. Regardless of the type of mentor, it's wise to talk with mentors about values, goals, expectations, frequency of meetings and contacts, preferred communication methodology, and timelines. It's important to recognize that regardless of the type of relationship (e.g., mentor–mentee or peer mentors), both parties should be clear that each will gain something from the time spent.

CONCLUSION

For PAs and PA students, considering and accepting leadership positions can be a career-expanding opportunity. Based on our ability and experience in forming and developing relationships and our strong and effective communication skills, once involved in an organization, PAs are often promoted or move up into expanded leadership roles.

In speaking with senior PAs, most of them will say: "I had no idea where this career would take me . . . or my family." Leadership opportunities are clearly part of that growth. Advice from these senior PAs includes (1) don't limit yourself; (2) consider roles that you'll need to grow into; (3) keep an open mind; and probably most important, (4) use your imagination!

KEY POINTS

- Leadership is a key component of the PA role because PAs advocate for individual patients, for health care access, for optimum PA utilization, and for the health of the populations they serve.
- Leadership skills are transferrable from organization to organization and from issue to issue.
- PAs entering the career may not have considered the leadership roles that they will be called on to play throughout their careers.
- PA leadership extends beyond the career—and beyond medicine—into other leadership positions within their community and within a wide range of organizations.

The resources for this chapter can be found at www.expertconsult.com.

The faculty resources for this chapter can be found at www.expertconsult.com.

CHAPTER 51

BE A PHYSICIAN ASSISTANT EDUCATOR

Wallace Boeve • Karen Mulitalo • Elizabeth Rothschild • Joseph Zaweski

CHAPTER OUTLINE

ACADEMIC DIRECTOR	RESEARCH DIRECTOR AND DATA ANALYST
CLINICAL DIRECTOR	PROGRAM DIRECTOR
DIRECTOR OF ADMISSIONS	KEY POINTS

Physician assistant (PA) education is an exciting potential career for practicing PAs to consider. For PAs who enjoy teaching and mentoring students, becoming a PA educator offers many opportunities for career advancement, an enormous variety of tasks and experiences, a flexible lifestyle, and excellent benefits. This chapter provides an overview of PA education as a career and the specific roles held by PA educators within the program. Although educators perform different duties within the program based on their roles, all PA educators must have certain skills in common. Those who are considering PA education as a career should seek certain experiences to position themselves well to move into education.

All PA educators need experience in both clinical practice and teaching. Because most PA programs require at least 2 or 3 years of clinical practice experience for potential faculty, a PA who is interested in teaching should choose a generalist specialty as opposed to a narrow subspecialty. PAs who have only focused on total hip replacement surgeries, for example, may have difficulty explaining the intricacies of diabetes management to students. Laying a foundation for teaching with broad clinical experience, including general patient assessment, psychiatric assessment, and exposure to clinical procedures, sets up a PA well to move into education. A PA education position is not for people at the end of their PA clinical careers who are looking for semiretirement. Many years of clinical experience can prepare a PA for teaching; however, most new educators are surprised by the time-consuming nature of education, particularly during the first year. Whether creating lesson plans, developing curriculum, understanding PA program accreditation, maintaining clinical partnerships, or responding to students and administrators, the PA professoriate offers a wide variety of job tasks as well as a very flexible schedule in meeting those tasks. Clinical PAs should realize that they are likely to work more hours as PA educators than they did in clinical practice but that the tasks in education are less routine.

Before considering a full-time academic appointment, PAs who are interested in education should teach in both clinics and classrooms. Becoming a preceptor gives PAs experience in one-on-one mentorship of students and help PAs develop clinical teaching skills. Being a preceptor also gives PAs a window into the administrative aspects of the clinical year. PAs who are moving toward education should also seek opportunities to guest lecture or work as part-time PA faculty members. Part-time teaching gives exposure to academia without having to carry additional administration, service, or scholarship requirements like full-time faculty members. Taking the time to lecture or lead a small group allows PAs to improve their teaching techniques and to assess whether moving into full-time education is the best fit.

Physician assistants who are considering moving into full-time PA education should also seek opportunities to gain experience with PA professional organizations and in research. Professional organization involvement helps the clinical PA be more aware of current practice issues (e.g., reimbursement, legislative) that impact PA practice. PAs who participate in professional service also gain organizational skills and professional contacts, which will serve them well if they choose to enter PA education. Although PA programs have traditionally focused on the clinical education of PAs, more universities are requiring PA faculty to participate in the development of original research. Few PAs have research experience or expertise. PAs considering joining the faculty of a PA program should seek opportunities to be involved in research and bolster their expertise before moving into PA education. Potential opportunities include clinical research at your workplace or assisting the research conducted by PA professional organizations to which you belong.

As clinical PAs move into academia, they are often surprised at how different the culture of higher education is compared with the culture of health care institutions. A certain mystique exists among doctorally prepared professors. They often assume that everyone has taken the same path to the professoriate that they did: bachelor's degree, master's degree, and then doctorate. Particularly when the PA program is relatively new to the institution, other faculty often need some education to help them understand the differences in the structure of PA education and the qualifications of the PA faculty. PA programs are atypical within higher education. Many other graduate professional programs are offered part time or online. Administrators and other faculty may be shocked to learn that PA students are expected to be in class 32 to 40 hours per week. Few other graduate professional programs run year round. Unlike traditional academic master's degree programs, PA programs do not have an intensive research component, and PA education is not designed for a student to progress on to the doctorate. PA faculty need to understand the academic culture and assumptions to be able to effectively advocate for the PA program and its students. Every institution has policies and processes, but in higher education, these processes can be very entrenched. New faculty may feel frustrated by the bureaucracy, but maintaining a flexible attitude and taking the time to develop relationships on campus can mitigate the frustration and allow PA faculty to become happy members of the academic community.

ACADEMIC DIRECTOR

The primary role of the academic director of a PA program is to oversee, develop, and coordinate the didactic curriculum. Most students are familiar with a didactic curriculum as the traditional way of learning we experienced in undergraduate education. The content of each course comprises the essential pieces of the didactic phase. The academic director works with each member of the didactic faculty to ensure compliance with the program's published mission, goals, and educational objectives. These objectives must comply with the published standards of the Accreditation Review

Commission on Education for the Physician Assistant (ARC-PA), and it is the role of the academic director to ensure complete compliance. The academic director supervises and mentors faculty during the creation and implementation of course content. This process occurs at both an individual and team level, and hence it is important for the academic director to establish a robust process that incorporates the free flow of ideas and respectful debate during curriculum development.

Working with the program director and other members of the leadership team, the academic director establishes benchmarks for individual course and student performance. A scholastic benchmark is a measured criterion set by the faculty and program administrators for a course, an individual, or a program. An example of a course benchmark may be that 70% of students rate each course "above average" or better for organization. An individual student benchmark may be that each student maintains a 3.0 grade point average for each semester. These benchmarks help establish the goals for the program and, in this way, contribute to the overall quality of the program. Working with the assessment committee, the academic director participates in program self-analysis to identify areas where benchmarks have not been met in the didactic curriculum. An important role of the academic director is to identify performance improvement initiatives and to direct and manage implementation of these initiatives. The goal is to meet or exceed all established benchmarks. As the program changes and develops, benchmarks will need to be revised. New benchmarks may need to be set and old ones updated. Thus, the academic director needs to have a solid understanding of the various methods for course, student, and faculty evaluation. Student progress must also be tracked. The academic director identifies students at risk and develops remediation plans with the faculty. Seeing a student progress in knowledge and successfully complete a remediation plan is a very gratifying experience.

After the goals, objectives, and benchmarks are set for the program, the task turns to management of the didactic phase. Semester schedules must be created so that topics and modules are sequenced in the most effective manner to promote learning. For example, electrocardiography (ECG) instruction may ideally occur at the same time as cardiovascular disease and dysrhythmia management. However, the students' schedule may not accommodate instruction in all topics simultaneously, so the academic director and didactic faculty team must decide if ECG instruction can occur at another time. Course mapping is a technique used to visualize the timeline of all courses in a curriculum simultaneously.

This tool helps to ensure topics are distributed appropriately across the curriculum. In the previous example, while students are learning cardiovascular disease, they also need to be learn cardiac laboratory testing and interpretation, as well as procedures used for cardiac disease. Because these topics may be taught in separate courses, a curriculum map helps to determine the proper timeline.

Faculty development is another very important role for the academic director. Typically, individual didactic faculty are responsible for assigned courses within the curriculum. Some courses require expert guest lecturers to deliver specialized content. The academic director assists faculty with recruitment of guest lecturers and assists in the evaluation process of all lecturers. He or she reviews the evaluations of each instructor with the assigned faculty course director to provide guidance and quality control. Each faculty member needs to be familiar with different educational theories, learning domains, and styles of education. Test item writing is a critical skill for didactic faculty. Proficiency with spreadsheets, databases, and learning management systems is essential. The academic director must educate and mentor faculty in all these skills.

The role of the academic director requires competent leadership skills. He or she must be an effective communicator with personnel management and administrative proficiency. It is important for the academic director to create a productive environment and to model professional behavior for faculty. Directing the didactic curriculum is similar to conducting a band or chamber orchestra. There are many moving parts, and when organized appropriately, the outcome can be very rewarding for both the students and the professors. One of the most gratifying education experiences is to request a consult on a patient and to have one of your former students arrive on the scene, providing competent, effective medical care, and to realize the role you had in developing these PAs.

CLINICAL DIRECTOR

The clinical year of a PA program is a pivotal time for budding PAs. The hands-on knowledge gained during clinical training enables students to combine foundational medical knowledge with practical skills to competently care for patients. Faculty who work in this phase of the program, called clinical directors or clinical educators, have the unique opportunity to closely mentor, guide, and direct students through this advanced phase of PA education.

Physician assistant faculty who are involved in clinical education must be organized, energetic, adept at change, positive, and determined. No two days are alike for clinical educators, and those who enjoy flexible schedules and multifaceted work environments are well suited for this area of education. One day may involve driving to a rural clinic to observe and evaluate a student, another day may be spent writing and revising an examination, and another day may include meeting one on one with students or facilitating a small group.

A crucial aspect of clinical education is establishing and maintaining training sites. Clinical directors are involved in recruiting new preceptors, facilities, and hospitals. Recruitment may involve visiting clinics, meeting with hospital administrators, networking at regional and state meetings, or calling area providers to discuss new opportunities. After preceptors begin working with students, the faculty will continue to contact or visit them to maintain appropriate connections to the program as outlined by the institution policies and the ARC-PA's standards.

Clinical directors supervise the scheduling of student rotations. Unlike the academic phase of the program, during each class block, every student has an individual schedule that consists of an assigned course, location, and preceptor. For example, in the first block of the clinical schedule, the 50 students of the PA program will not be enrolled in a single common course but will be assigned various individual courses (e.g., pediatrics, women's health, surgery) that take place in up to 50 unique sites. Scheduling 50 students for 12 or more clinical placements is challenging and requires a large amount of legal and informational paperwork. Clinical directors may need to meet regularly with legal counsel and other administrators to develop clinical agreements called affiliations. These affiliation agreements are required to allow students to practice at clinical sites.

Fundamental to the educational process of these clinical courses is the development of a curriculum for each clerkship. Establishing a syllabus to guide the learner on clinical rotations is similar to the didactic phase of the program, but it must be adaptable to the various training sites where students are placed. Faculty may also use innovative techniques to assess the learning that takes place in the clinical year, including reflective writing pieces, projects, and portfolio assignments.

Evaluation of the clinical training phase of education is multifaceted and varies greatly by institution. Clinical faculty supervise, direct, and review this evaluation. Faculty may observe clinical skills, presentations, and patient examinations in the clinic as part of the evaluation process. Written or oral examinations usually are administered after the completion of required clinical experiences. These examinations may be written, scored, and revised by clinical faculty. Clinical faculty collect and review evaluations of students' clinical performance generated by preceptors to help determine their course grades.

There is no one specific path to becoming a clinical educator. The essential characteristics of a future clinical educator are to have a desire to mentor students accompanied by a willingness to work closely with preceptors in the most dynamic phase of PA education. There are, however, some strategic steps that may enhance one's future career as clinical faculty. An essential first step toward this faculty position is serving as a clinical preceptor. This clinical teaching allows a future faculty member to see the clinical year training requirements from a different viewpoint and go through the evaluation process as a preceptor. Serving as a preceptor or mentor to students from various institutions broadens the perspective of the clinical teacher. Involvement in local, regional, and state PA activities is also essential. The connections a PA can make while participating in professional service are essential for recruiting new preceptors to the program. By establishing this network of peers and colleagues, the faculty member will be at an advantage when engaging local and regional leaders. Many institutions ask alumni to visit and evaluate current students at distant sites. Contact your alma mater to offer your services to help in this assessment process and gain first-hand experience with student evaluations.

DIRECTOR OF ADMISSIONS

Many PA students have had experience with the admissions office at their PA program through various student activities such as giving tours, interviewing applicants, or hosting candidates. What is not always apparent to PA students is the depth of the admission process and the many months of work required to get an applicant to the interview day. Director of admissions is a complex and multifaceted faculty position. It is also one of the most rewarding positions in PA education. It is exciting to have the opportunity to meet and interact with an enthusiastic group of applicants who have worked years to get to the point of applying to PA school.

Physician assistant faculty who are involved in the admissions process must be good communicators, well organized, passionate about the PA profession, technologically savvy, and must possess a willingness to mentor pre-PA students. Admissions directors must also be willing to say "no" because not every applicant is a good fit at a specific program. Over the past few years, not only has there been a rapid growth of the PA profession, but there has also been a large increase in the number of applicants to PA school. Currently, approximately 20,000 individuals apply to PA school annually. Large increases in the numbers of applicants require PA programs to create streamlined processes to efficiently manage and review applications.

Before receiving applications, each PA program must establish its recruitment focus and outline its selection process. PA faculty may travel to area colleges or universities or other local and regional health care recruiting events. Many PA programs choose to manage admissions through the Central Application Service for Physician Assistants (CASPA). As of 2016, 212 PA programs participate in this online application service. As a part of CASPA, the admissions director is responsible for understanding the electronic application process, establishing secure access to the electronic applications, and training other faculty and staff members how to use the system. The Physician Assistant Education Association offers opportunities for faculty and staff who do admissions to receive training in both admissions processes and the use of CASPA.

The structure of the admissions process varies across programs, but each school must meet both the ARC-PA standards as well as institutional, state, and federal laws for a fair selection process. An important aspect of the admission director's leadership is to organize faculty participation and input for the process. Behind the scenes, each application is tracked for completion of all components (transcripts, references, and essays) and then evaluated by a member of the admissions committee. This committee may consist of other faculty, the program director, administrators, alumni, or community PAs. The admissions committee attempts to thoroughly evaluate each application to assess the "fit" of the potential student with the program, her or his readiness for the demanding coursework in PA school, and her or his potential success as a clinical PA. Although this is an enjoyable task, it is also quite time intensive because faculty are asked to read many applications over a short period of time. The goal of the committee's work is to narrow down the field and invite the most qualified applicants to campus for an interview. Other faculty, current or past students, and staff may take part in the interview process for the applicants who have made it to this phase of the process.

Participating in admission interviews, campus tours, and applicant hosting is an excellent way to get experience with admissions while still in PA school. As a practicing PA, becoming involved in the admissions process of area programs is also a great way to give back to the profession and to gain valuable experience. Even if the local program is not your alma mater, reach out and offer your services to assist with admissions or in mentoring pre-PA students. Gaining experience as an ambassador for the profession is a helpful practice that will demonstrate interest in a future faculty role in admissions. Some examples of this service include speaking to local school, college, or university groups (such as pre-PA interest groups, health career panels, science and math magnet programs); allowing pre-PA students to shadow you at work (let the local PA program or state PA organization know that you are available); and contacting the local area health education center office to let them know of your interest in working with students.

RESEARCH DIRECTOR AND DATA ANALYST

In addition to some of the more traditional academic positions within PA education, a few additional roles have been developed in recent years to meet the growing demands for quality graduate PA education. Depending on the nature of research requirements for students and faculty, as well as the institutional support for ongoing data analysis, PA programs may have one or more people who serve as research directors or data analysts. These roles vary by institution but offer great opportunities for collaboration and personal development.

Many programs require students to perform a research project or scholarly writing as part of their PA training. This project may require individual original research or development of a clinical literature review or may be a task for which students work on a social, medical, or professional research protocol together. Conducting original research requires students and faculty to abide by ethical and institutional requirements for proposal writing, human subjects protection, data collection, and thesis development. To ensure that students are properly guided through this process, many programs have developed the role of research director.

The research director assures compliance with program and institutional requirements for graduate-level research. Additionally, the research director may train other faculty members to serve as research mentors to students. The research director may also manage program databases, collaborate with other researchers, and communicate with institutional officials to assure quality and compliance in the collection, storage, and dissemination of data. In addition, many research directors design, execute, and publish their own original research studies. The research director can improve the reputation of the PA program by publishing regularly and representing the university and the program at scientific meetings. Faculty members who enjoy data analysis and writing, who relish mentoring students and other faculty, who are detail oriented, and who have a research background are ideal for this position.

The data analyst role may be held by a PA faculty member, a non-PA faculty member with a background in public health or statistics, or an administrative staff member. The data analyst is typically someone with expertise in statistics and data presentation. The data analyst works closely with the program director to develop and maintain data collection processes that support the program in several ways. First, the ARC-PA requires programs to routinely collect and analyze data on student performance, preceptor and employer perception of graduates, and alumni satisfaction to use to make improvements in the program. Second, programs often provide data to students on their own performance, particularly in the clinical year. Third, most universities require regular reporting of program data for university-wide accreditation and internal assessments.

A practicing PA or current PA faculty member who is considering becoming a research director or data analyst should seek to gain knowledge and experience in data collection, human subject protection, epidemiology, statistics, and clinical research. Many schools of public health offer introductory epidemiology and statistics courses in condensed formats or through online classes, both of which are more accessible to people who hold full-time positions. PAs who are practicing clinically will find that working on practice-related quality improvement research or clinical research can be great experience to bring to their faculty member position.

PROGRAM DIRECTOR

The role of the director of a PA program is one of the most crucial faculty roles. Program directors provide vision, direction, mentorship of faculty, administrative leadership, and oversight of the PA education program. The ARC-PA designates the program director as the administrative leader in the accreditation standards for PA education programs. He or she is responsible for several specific areas of program administration.

Program directors are responsible for effectively deploying faculty and staff within the program to implement the didactic and clinical portions of PA education. They are responsible for assuring that the programmatic structure allows for the most effective and efficient delivery of education to students. Program administration includes assuring that faculty and staff have the resources needed to carry out their responsibilities. Program directors also represent the program within the wider academic community and ensure that the faculty, staff, and students have access to campus resources and opportunities that increase the quality of educational experiences offered. The administrative duties of the PA program director are different from those of clinical work or teaching. Many times, these responsibilities are carried out through meetings with program faculty, staff, and other administrators within the academic community. Program directors must be familiar with various processes within the academic institution in which the program is located and be able to negotiate the politics of the institution on behalf of the program.

The program director is responsible for the fiscal management of the program and must have a full understanding of the costs of running a program. Program directors must be intimately acquainted with the process used by their institution to allocate and disburse funds to maximize the finances of the program. Some directors have direct responsibility for the budget and are solely responsible for funds spent for the program, but others may have a budget administrator housed within their academic department or school that allocates and manages funds for the program. Either way, the program director must have a very clear understanding of program expenses and how these expenses will be met through a program budget.

Programs must continually assess their programmatic processes and outcomes to assure they are providing quality education to PA students and adequate development of program faculty. The program director accomplishes this goal by gathering data and regularly analyzing it to assure the program is meeting or exceeding standards. The program director is responsible for ensuring these processes for program evaluation, data collection, and data analysis occur regularly throughout the academic year. Data collection for PA programs includes information on student performance such as tests or assessments, Physician Assistant National Certification Examination pass rates, and student evaluations and feedback. The data analyzed also include information about the effectiveness of program administration such as the rate of faculty turnover, faculty evaluation of program effectiveness, and whether there are enough faculty and staff to meet the program mission.

Physician assistant program curricula are in a continuous state of development and growth because of advances in medicine, new educational approaches, and the growth of the PA profession. The program director leads the faculty in planning and development of the curriculum and organizational structure to reflect these changes. Program development should also include the professional development of program faculty, planning for fiscal and physical space needs, facilitating an increased participation in national and professional organizations, and increasing the scholarly productivity of both faculty and students.

All PA programs must regularly undergo evaluation by the ARC-PA to continuing operating. This accreditation process involves meeting accreditation standards set forth by ARC-PA. The program director is responsible for working with the program faculty and staff to assure that all accreditation standards are met. The process includes regular reports on program progress in meeting standards, completion of an application for accreditation, a written self-study, and preparing the program for periodic site visits from ARC-PA representatives. Although the director is ultimately responsible for all parts of the accreditation process, program directors should be facilitatie faculty and staff to assist in the development of the report and the site visit itself.

Physician assistants and PA faculty who are considering becoming program directors should realize that the role is completely different from clinical practice and different still from the role of a PA faculty member. The role is far more administrative and requires skills in financial management and human resource management that are traditionally associated with clinical practice or general faculty roles. Aspiring program directors should have demonstrated leadership experiences throughout their career that show preparation for the role. Program directors should know how to manage people effectively, move faculty and staff toward a program mission or vision, and be able to collaborate with other members of the academic community. Effective communication skills are critical for program directors and are often included in the list of essential qualifications for program director positions. Because the program director is the leader of an academic program, those who are interested in becoming a program director should work toward obtaining an academic doctoral degree.

Because program directors lead a clinical training enterprise, they must have personal experience in clinical practice, either as a PA or as a doctor. This knowledge helps the program director provide effective oversight of program curriculum development and implementation. Experience as a member of the teaching faculty at a program can give program directors insight into the function and effective organizational structure of PA programs. A program director with previous experience in these areas will have a clearer understanding of curriculum development, program function, challenges of finding clinical sites, and developing effective teaching methods. A clinical and teaching background can also enhance the understanding of the challenges faculty, staff, and students may be experiencing and allow the program director to exercise good judgment in an executive capacity.

KEY POINTS

- PA education is a flexible and satisfying career to consider even as you enter clinical practice for the first time.
- Prospective educators should consider working in generalist medical and surgical specialties to acquire the expertise needed to effectively train primary care PAs.
- Serving as a clinical preceptor is an essential first step for aspiring PA educators.
- Those interested in working in PA education should also gain experience in classroom teaching, professional service, research, and quality improvement.
- Prospective program directors need strong clinical and educational experience. They also need to gain expertise in leading others, managing budgets and working within complex organizations.

The resources for this chapter can be found at www.expertconsult.com.

PROFESSIONAL SERVICE

Tamara S. Ritsema

The history of the physician assistant (PA) profession is the story of volunteers who made great strides for the profession and for patients against sometimes long odds. These pioneers worked tirelessly to secure recognition for the profession, obtain reimbursement for PA services, secure prescribing rights, and each of the other elements that allow American PAs to practice effectively. Other PAs have made incredible contributions through service to and advocacy for impoverished patients, patients with disabilities, abused women and children, and refugees. It would be easy to think that all the hard work is done and that newly graduated PAs are not needed in service to the profession or the community. This belief is sadly untrue. PAs still need to serve the profession for it to thrive.

WHAT IS PROFESSIONAL SERVICE?

Professional service is exactly what it sounds like: service by the PA to the profession itself or on behalf of the profession to others. Each PA can find a way to serve that matches her or his talents, availability, and interests. PAs have traditionally been involved in many types of service, including

1. **Volunteering with PA professional organizations:** PA professional organizations at the national, state, and institutional levels rely extensively on volunteer support to carry out their missions. Although our national organizations, such as the American Academy of Physician Assistants (AAPA), the PA Foundation (PAF), the National

Commission on Certification of Physician Assistants (NCCPA) Foundation, and the Physician Assistant Education Association (PAEA), each has a small number of full-time staff who work alongside volunteers, most other PA-related professional organizations rely almost exclusively on volunteers to complete the needed work. Without volunteers, the costs of providing services, lobbying legislators, organizing continuing medical education (CME) events, and so on would be prohibitive. In addition, having PAs direct these activities helps ensure that the profession is being effectively represented and that the services provided by the professional organizations are actually meeting the needs of PAs.

The minimum level at which each PA should serve the profession is by joining our national and state professional associations. Unfortunately, although the state and federal laws governing PA practice in most states are reasonably favorable, there are no guarantees that they will remain so. Many states have seen legislation proposed by other professions that would attempt to restrict PA practice in one way or another. Some of these legislative proposals have been so restrictive that they would have effectively made it impossible for PAs to practice at all in certain specialties. Other times, well-meaning politicians have proposed new legislation that inadvertently excludes PAs from performing an activity allowed for doctors and nurse practitioners. Sometimes regulatory bodies fail to include PAs as authorized providers in the regulations that govern medical practice nationally or on the state level. In 2013, for example, the author of the federal regulations on durable medical equipment (DME) excluded PAs from the list of providers who could authorize DME such as walkers and crutches for patients with TRICARE insurance, meaning PAs were unable to write prescriptions for these items for members of the armed services and their families![1] The only way to protect the legislative gains the profession has made is to have continuous monitoring of proposed legislation and regulations in each state and on the federal level. Monitoring legislation and regulations in real time requires money to hire either staff or a lobbying organization. Most clinical PAs have neither the time nor the expertise to monitor legislation and regulations on their own. Supporting your national and state professional organizations with your annual dues allows these organizations to have a stable funding stream with which they can develop services that benefit all PAs and allow you to continue your practice.

Beyond simply supporting your professional organizations with your membership funds, there are many opportunities to get involved with PA organizations on the state and national levels. State organizations need PAs to plan CME conferences, serve on the organization's board, represent the state in the AAPA House of Delegates, develop public relations strategies, monitor the finances of the organization, liaise with medical and nursing associations, run membership drives, advise student members, lobby on behalf of the profession, develop legislative strategies in conjunction with lawmakers, represent PAs to large employers across the state, and develop community service projects. The subcommittees that perform these duties are often looking for more people to assist them and are frequently very interested in having newly graduated PAs serve alongside more experienced PAs. Newly graduated PAs often have energy and exciting new ideas to share.

After you have a bit of experience in your specialty or have served at the state level, you may wish to begin serving at the national level. The AAPA and the PAF have a host of volunteer opportunities to serve on behalf of all PAs. The AAPA and the PAF need people to sit on scholarship committees; work to develop stronger relationships with the federal government; develop the annual AAPA conference; liaise to medical, specialty, and other health professions organizations; and raise money for philanthropic work. You might also consider working with a constituent organization of AAPA. Constituent organizations within AAPA are groups of PAs with unifying interests such as

particular specialties (e.g., psychiatry, nephrology), common characteristics (e.g., ethnicity, religion or sexual orientation), or specific interests (e.g., rural health, global health, administration, alternative medicine). Constituent organizations bring together PAs across the country to achieve common goals and to network. They may lobby for particular federal legislation or regulations. They often provide CME of specific interest to their members. They typically also provide support to their members facing particular challenges related to their specialty, cause, ethnicity, religion, or sexual orientation. Specialty constituent organizations often serve as the representatives of PAs to their medical specialty organizations. For example, the president of the Society for Physician Assistants in Pediatrics (SPAP) attends the annual American Academy of Pediatrics (AAP) meeting to speak on behalf of PAs and meet with AAP leadership regarding issues of mutual interest and concern to pediatricians and pediatric PAs. Volunteering on the national level provides exciting opportunities to meet new people and develop new leadership skills.

2. **Teaching and precepting students:** So many people invested in you to bring you into PA school and to get you through your PA training. Think of the people who patiently taught you to how to break bad news to a patient, how to suture, or how to deliver a baby. Although some of these people were paid to help you, many were volunteers. Most guest lecturers and clinical preceptors serve unpaid or are paid only a small stipend for their work. They teach students out of love of their profession, concern for patients, and passion for teaching medicine to others. Most PA programs like potential lecturers, laboratory instructors, and preceptors to have at least 1 year of clinical experience before they begin to teach. However, after you are settled into your practice, consider participating in the training of PAs. PA programs have many types of opportunities for involvement ranging from occasional involvement to regular commitment. Programs may simply need PAs with surgical experience to come 1 day each year to teach students how to scrub, gown, and glove. They often use PAs to lecture or lead small groups in their own area of clinical expertise. Many programs provide you with some guidance about best teaching practices as you get started with teaching, perhaps for the first time. Program faculty will always provide you with the instructional objectives for each session to guide you as you develop your material. As you gain experience and confidence in your teaching abilities, you will likely be

asked to develop and present more sessions as the years go by.

Precepting students is a way to make a huge contribution to both PA students and to your patients. Training future PAs to deliver high-quality care ensures the best care for our patients even after we move on. Precepting PA students is a significant investment of your time and energy, but it yields great returns as well. As you remember from your own PA training, PA students typically work full time with their preceptors, performing nearly all the tasks the preceptor performs. Becoming a preceptor means being willing to take students for a defined period (typically 4–6 weeks), allowing them to see patients themselves under your supervision, teaching the student through the lens of each patient visit, potentially assigning the student things to read and research, serving as a role model, and providing both daily and final feedback on their performance at your site. Some preceptors have students present nearly all year, but others choose to have students only at the times of the year when they believe they can provide the best educational experience for the students. Clinicians are often concerned that having a student present will slow them down as they see patients. Teaching does require taking time for the students, but savvy preceptors are often able to devise strategies to keep to the schedule while still allowing students time with patients. For example, sometimes students can perform time-consuming tasks such as patient education on behalf of the preceptor while the preceptor quickly sees several other patients. Working with students also encourages the preceptor to keep up with her or his specialty. Students often have questions to which preceptors do not know the answer, challenging the preceptors to do further research and expand their own knowledge base. Preceptors generally report that they love the personal interaction with the students. They enjoy getting to know them as people and seeing their skills and confidence develop over the course of the rotation. They also appreciate some of the perks that programs offer preceptors such as academic appointments to the university, access to the medical library through the university, and CME credit for teaching.[2]

If you are unable to precept students full time, you may still be able to do some precepting. Some PA programs send first-year students out to preceptors for a few afternoons a month to begin to learn to see patients, perform physical examinations, develop differential diagnoses, interpret laboratory studies and radiographs, and initiate treatment with an experienced PA or doctor.

Other programs even send students out only a few times per year just to practice patient interview or physical examination skills. Contact your local PA program to find out if they have a need for intermittent precepting that you might be able to fill.[3]

3. **Institutional or health system service:** Most hospitals and health systems have leadership by doctors and nurses in all areas of hospital management, including safety, operations, finance, human resources, and patient relations. Unfortunately, it is still relatively rare for PAs to be routinely included on these committees or in these leadership roles. These committees often wield tremendous power within a hospital or health system. PAs sometimes discover that policies have been made that substantially impact their ability to practice without any PA input whatsoever. PAs who wish to make an enormous and immediate impact on their own clinical environment should consider serving on committees within their medical center or health system. You should not wait to be invited to join these committees; instead, you should ask to be appointed to a committee in an area of your interest. Many PAs have had the experience of requesting to serve on a committee and receiving a response such as, "Well, we've never had a PA on that committee before, but now that you mention it, that's a good idea!" Consider working with a trusted physician or nursing colleague to advocate for you if the initial answer is no. Serving on a hospital or health system committee will give you enormous insights into your institution and the health system at large and will allow you to advocate for PAs and PA practice.

4. **Community service:** Another important means by which you can serve the profession is to serve your community. The PA profession was started, in part, to meet the needs of people who were not being properly served by the medical system at the time. Groups of PAs, individual PAs, and PA programs have always served their communities as part of their professional commitment to provide holistic care for patients. Knowing that our patients' health is affected as much by whether they have a safe place to live and food to eat as it is by medical care, many PAs are regularly involved in community service. The AAPA annually recognizes a PA for service with the PAragon Humanitarian Service award for outstanding achievement in serving marginalized people. PAs are working with victims of natural disasters, sexual assault and domestic violence survivors, linguistic and cultural minorities, homeless people, people with low levels of literacy, people with intellectual disabilities, and many others. They provide medical care, counseling, tutoring, food, mentoring,

preventive screening, and friendship. PAs partner with schools; hospitals; health systems; homeless shelters; and organizations such as Habitat for Humanity, the American Red Cross, and Boys and Girls Clubs of America. This service is the source of enormous satisfaction to the individual PAs, but their service also reflects well on the profession. PAs serving their communities demonstrate that our profession is committed to our patients beyond the reach of our clinical settings. Their service builds trust and confidence in PAs and the PA profession.

Physician assistants who decide to provide medical care on a volunteer basis need to be aware of some specific concerns. First, you must meet your state's requirements for physician supervision even if you are not being paid for your work. You will generally need to obtain a new delegation agreement or practice agreement with a supervising physician who also works at your volunteer site to cover your work there. It is essential for you to clearly understand and conform to the regulations your state has for supervision in PA practice. Failing to do so risks sanction by the state medical board. Second, you need to obtain malpractice coverage for your volunteer work if you are providing medical assessment and treatment services. Sometimes the organization has blanket coverage for all health professional volunteers, but it is not safe to assume this, and you should confirm any coverage before beginning to see patients. You may need to purchase a policy yourself to cover your work at the volunteer site. Third, your employment contract may have an exclusion clause preventing you from doing substantially the same work you do in your day job for another clinic in the same area. These exclusion clauses typically are meant to prevent you from moonlighting with a competitor, but you would not want to jeopardize your primary employment by inadvertently violating your contract. Most employers are happy to write an exception for a clinician who wishes to volunteer to care for medically underserved patients, but it is essential to clarify this issue with your primary employer before starting your volunteer work.

WHY SHOULD I GET INVOLVED IN PROFESSIONAL SERVICE?

Although serving others hopefully provides a benefit to those being served, people often overlook the potential benefits they receive by serving. Research shows that people who volunteer live longer, have lower levels of depression, and perform better in their primary employment.[4–6] Experienced PAs who engage in professional service often express that they believe they got more out of the experience than they put into it. Some of the specific benefits of professional service include

1. **To continue learning and develop new skills:** Most PAs have no experience with the process of getting a bill through a legislature. They are unlikely to have experience in planning a medical conference, raising money, or developing a public relations strategy. Volunteering as part of your state professional organization can enable you to develop all of these skills and more. Teaching PA students will force you to look for the answers to questions you have never previously considered. Volunteering at a homeless shelter may provide you with new insights on how to access the social services system to the benefit of your patients. These new skills may someday be the source of a second career or a new interest for you.

2. **To develop new relationships:** Working as a volunteer almost always involves meeting new people and forming new relationships. The shared commitment to the goal at hand, whether passing a piece of legislation or feeding hungry people, often accelerates the development of a personal connection among the volunteers. By definition, volunteers to the same cause share specific interests and values. Working with others to solve complex problems and achieve mutual goals bonds people together. Many PAs speak about how they have become close friends with someone through their volunteer commitments. These relationships can be the source of encouragement, the genesis of your next job, or a place where you gain a new perspective on an issue.

3. **To further your career:** Serving the profession may raise your personal profile among PAs and other health leaders. You may be profiled in a professional magazine or interviewed in the media for your work. You may have opportunities to speak or publish that arise from your professional service. Positive attention may bring you your next job or open other opportunities to you that you had not considered prior to your involvement.

4. **To positively influence the direction of the profession:** It is very easy to complain about what is happening to PAs and the PA profession in a time of substantial changes in the health system. It is far more difficult to engage and try to effect change. Those who sit at home and complain have no influence. Those who volunteer get to influence the strategies and approaches the profession will take to try to remedy the problems at hand. Volunteering with your health system, state organization, specialty organization, or the AAPA is a powerful way to have your voice heard.

5. **To help others in need:** American PAs are overwhelmingly drawn from the ranks of the middle and upper socioeconomic classes. Most PAs have been blessed with a good education and many opportunities for personal development. Few newly graduated PAs have dealt with serious health problems of their own. Other Americans have not been as fortunate. Serving those who have become ill, never had a quality education, or are victims of natural or economic forces beyond their control allows us to express appreciation for the advantages we have. Working closely with those in need changes our perspectives on life and society.

Volunteers enable charities to provide far more services to clients than they would be able to do if they had to rely on paid staff alone. The value of the medical care, literacy services, and food, however, goes beyond the financial. Providing services to those in need affirms their dignity and humanity. In addition, most people who regularly volunteer with those in significant physical need report that they learn much from the clients they serve and that the satisfaction they have in the relationships with those they serve is enormous.

6. **To give back to those who gave for you:** Over the past 50 years, many PAs and PA allies have given generously of their time and expertise to bring the profession to the point we are at today. The gains they made for the profession and for our patients are not set in stone, however. We must continue advocating for our profession and for our patients to maintain our scope of practice and to continue to advance the profession for future PAs and their patients. If every PAs serves the profession in one way or another, all the needs of the profession will be met.

HOW CAN I GET INVOLVED IN PROFESSIONAL SERVICE?

Just ask! Most organizations are eager for volunteers and have mechanisms to bring you on board and get you trained for your work. Research opportunities online. Speak to friends and colleagues. Phone your PA faculty to ask them about their experiences with professional involvement. Attend a state- or national-level CME conference and network there. Consider opportunities that may arise through your community, your house of worship, your workplace, or your specialty. There are limitless avenues for involvement. Pick one and get started!

KEY POINTS

- The continuation of the success of the PA profession is still dependent on the willingness of PAs to serve and represent their profession. The PA profession would not have made as many gains as it has without the sacrifices of many PAs in the past. PAs need to continue to serve the profession to ensure the success of the profession for the future.
- Many types of service exist for PAs. Every PA can find a way to serve that uses their interests and talents. Common types of service include service to PA professional organizations, teaching and precepting PA students, becoming members of institutional or health system committees, and community service.
- Professional service is a satisfying way to develop new skills, relationships, and interests. Volunteering not only helps PAs develop personally and professionally but may also result in new opportunities for them in the future.

References

1. Herman, L. TRICARE program; proposed clarification of benefit coverage of durable equipment and ordering or prescribing durable equipment. (2013). The American Academy of Physician Assistants. https://www.aapa.org/WorkArea/DownloadAsset.aspx?id=1284. Published September 11, 2013. Accessed December 8, 2015.
2. Latessa R, Colvin G, Beaty N, Steiner BD, Pathman DE. Satisfaction, motivation, and future of community preceptors: what are the current trends? *Acad. Med. J. Assoc. Am. Med. Coll.* 2013;88:1164–1170.
3. Accreditation Review Commission on Education for the Physician Assistant. Accredited US PA programs. http://www.arc-pa.org/acc_programs/. Published October 24, 2015. Accessed December 8, 2015.
4. Poulin MJ. Volunteering predicts health among those who value others: two national studies. *Health Psychol.* 2014;33:120–129.
5. Kim J, Pai M. Volunteering and trajectories of depression. *J. Aging Health.* 2010;22:84–105.
6. Rodell JB. Finding meaning through volunteering: why do employees volunteer and what does it mean for their jobs? *Acad Manage J.* 2013;56:1274–1294.

The resources for this chapter can be found at www.expertconsult.com.

The faculty resources can be found online at www.expertconsult.com.

CHAPTER 53

THE FUTURE OF THE PHYSICIAN ASSISTANT PROFESSION

Ruth Ballweg • Daniel T. Vetrosky

CHAPTER OUTLINE

KEY POINTS

As you have read the various sections and chapters in this book, the authors and editors hope you have learned about the history of the profession; how the profession developed throughout the years; what physician assistants (PAs) "really do" on a day to day basis; and the numerous roles, including direct and indirect medical positions, in which PAs are currently engaged. We also hope you have begun to think about the role you might be interested in or suited for, especially in these current times of innovative health care model development, access and delivery model changes, technological advances, and ever-changing reimbursement requirements. To paraphrase the author of Chapter 1, as many older and retired PAs continue to say, with great enthusiasm: "I had no idea where the PA career would take me or the many options and opportunities that would come along. Who knew?" That statement is as meaningful then as it is now!

We also hope that you will continue to use this book long after you have graduated and secured a job. Many of the chapters you used during your training can be very useful after you are in the workforce, especially if you want to change specialties. The chapters on other medical and surgical specialties can offer some insight as to what may be required, but keep in mind that every practice will vary with job description, protocol, and modes of practice. As you will see later in this chapter, the future of the profession is in your hands. The chapter on leadership will give you a means to become an effective and forward thinking leader. Continue to use this book as a resource and guide as you embark on the journey that is the PA profession.

So what will the future of the PA profession be? This question is best answered by revisiting why the PA profession was conceived and the developments that have occurred over the past 50 years of the profession: to facilitate access to health care for the United States by extending the physicians' medical practice through the use of passionate people trained in the medical model by physicians. This has been admirably accomplished, and as you have experienced through your education, new and innovative teaching models have been developed that broaden the topics being taught while continuing to adhere to the medical model of health care education. You will also note that although physicians still lecture to classes, the majority of PA program faculty are now PAs. Program chairs used to be physicians, and now the majority are PAs. More exciting is the appointment of PAs to associate dean and dean's positions in universities and colleges. There are many more examples of the expanding roles and opportunities for PAs such as congressmen and-women; military leaders in all branches, including the White House, Federal Bureau of Investigations, and Central Intelligence Agency; hospital administrators; National Institutes of Health and Centers for Disease Control and Prevention researchers; and most exciting, PA consultants, teachers, and clinicians for developing PA programs in Canada and overseas! By way of these examples, the answer to the initial question depends on the willingness of you and other graduates to be innovative, involved, and adventuresome!

How can you affect the future of the profession? First and foremost, be the best health care provider and patient advocate you can. Be ethical, sympathetic, understanding, and nonjudgmental in your dealings with patients, staff, community, and the profession. Be an active member of the interprofessional community, and above all, be a lifelong learner. Stay up-to-date with medical treatment and diagnostic innovations that will evolve during your professional tenure. Stay appraised of your state's requirements, the state's PA and medical professional societies, national PA organizations, medical specialty organizations, and the national health care changes that are inevitable. Our profession has exemplified the aforementioned traits and has moved us forward along the path of growth and professional recognition. You can help influence the future of the profession by saying "yes" to committee membership and many other leadership opportunities as mentioned in Chapter 1.

What is the future of the PA profession? The first word that comes from the "crystal ball" and current news reports is *growth*—demand in the usual medical and surgical disciplines as well as growth in new areas of medicine such as interventional radiology, oncology, pathology, genetics, and forensics, to name a few. Other growth areas are in contract services with the government, both overt and covert. An exciting area of growth is that of international clinical and educational positions. The second and third words that come from both the future and the past are *innovation* and *willingness*—innovation to see the possibilities for the profession and willingness to pursue the avenues to accomplish those potentials. With these words, *innovation* and *willingness*, as operative stimuli for the current and new PAs come the technological advances that are inevitable in the practice of medicine. In the beginning of the profession, there were no computed tomography or magnetic resonance imaging scanning technologies. Now we have the ability to expand these scanning technologies with three-dimensional (3D) image compilation, arteriography, and the use of positron emission computed tomography scanning to view disease processes, including tumor identification and spread. We are now able to view these scanning reports and images online or via a disk. 3D printing technologies are allowing medicine to literally print anatomic structures and eventually working organs. The electronic medical record is now a requirement that has helped practices, hospital and diagnostic laboratories, and radiologic services to be in touch with each other, albeit with some glitches. As this modality continues to develop, it will benefit continuity of care. The PA profession is in a position to not only use the technology to its fullest but also to be innovators in developing better and more user-friendly interfaces. With that being said, technology is marvelous, timely, informative, and helpful. It is also mystical, borders on sorcery, and is clearly impersonal. Do not let bauds, bytes, check boxes, computers, programs, or apps supplant the touch of humanity. Communicate with your eyes, your hands, and your hearts. Communicate with your personality and not with a computer or tablet!

There will be many more future changes in the medical field, including new diagnostic modalities, novel physical examination instrumentation, and innovative therapeutic medications and interventions. Embrace them and become responsible practitioners, keeping in mind that not every advance in medicine can or should be used or will fit every patient. Be lifelong learners for your patients' sake.

The future of the profession is in your hands! Be steadfast (no pun intended) advocates of the profession, and be responsible medical practitioners by remembering the following Key Points, many of which echo this book's first chapter.

KEY POINTS

- The principle and culture of medical and clinical roles is about lifelong learning. Embrace new innovations, but be responsible users of new and old technology. One size does not fit all.
- Develop a support system of peers, senior mentors, supervising doctors, and others to serve as a foundation for the long-term decisions that you make about the future of your career.
- Effective leaders are needed to promote the changing access to health care and ensure continued quality in health care provision. The PA profession has moved ahead because PAs have been willing to say "yes" to leadership opportunities. Please consider leadership as a building block and part of your PA career.
- Be innovative, willing, and responsible providers of health care. You are the future of the PA profession and its continued growth and position in the practice of medicine.

We suggest you refer to the ARC-PA website to review the ARC-PA standards and other valuable resources: www.arc-pa.org

INDEX

Note: Pages followed by *b*, *t*, or *f* refer to boxes, tables, or figures, respectively.